D1400924

EVALUATION of Orthopedic and Athletic Injuries

SECOND EDITION

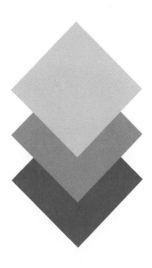

CHAD STARKEY, PHD, ATC

Associate Professor
Northeastern University
Bouvé College Health Sciences
Boston, Massachusetts

JEFFREY L. RYAN, PT, ATC

Clinical Director
Hahnemann Sports Medicine Center
Hahnemann University Hospital
Philadelphia, Pennsylvania

EVALUATION of
Orthopedic and Athletic Injuries

SECOND EDITION

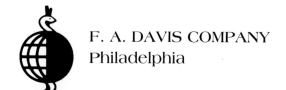

F. A. DAVIS COMPANY
Philadelphia

F. A. Davis Company
1915 Arch Street
Philadelphia, PA 19103
www.fadavis.com

Printed in the United States of America

Last digit indicates print number: 10 9 8 7 6

Acquisitions Editor: Jean-François Vilain
Developmental Editor: Maryann Foley
Cover Designer: Louis J. Forgione

As new scientific information becomes available through basic and clinical research, recommended treatments and drug therapies undergo changes. The author(s) and publisher have done everything possible to make this book accurate, up to date, and in accord with accepted standards at the time of publication. The authors, editors, and publisher are not responsible for errors or omissions or for consequences from application of the book, and make no warranty, expressed or implied, in regard to the contents of the book. Any practice described in this book should be applied by the reader in accordance with professional standards of care used in regard to the unique circumstances that may apply in each situation. The reader is advised always to check product information (package inserts) for changes and new information regarding dose and contraindications before administering any drug. Caution is especially urged when using new or infrequently ordered drugs.

Library of Congress Cataloging-in-Publication Data

Starkey, Chad, 1959-
   Evaluation of orthopedic and athletic injuries / Chad Starkey,
Jeffrey L. Ryan.—2nd ed.
      p. cm.
   Includes bibliographical references and index.
   ISBN 10: 0-8036-0791-1 (alk. paper) ISBN 13: 978-0-8036-0791-0
   1. Sports injuries. I. Ryan, Jeffrey L., 1962-   .II. Title.
RD97 .S83 2001
617.1'027—dc21
                                        2001028774

I wish that I were writing this dedication for you, instead of to you
I cannot hear the violins, but I know that they're out there
All the meanwhile I'm trying to figure out if I'm still just about glad
Or just about sad

—cas

To Nancy, Lisa, and Kaley, for your love, support, and making me laugh.
To our angels, Jack and Caitlyn, you are with us always.

—jlr

Preface

We had to set two primary goals for the second edition of *Evaluation of Orthopedic and Athletic Injuries*. First, we wanted to include the most comprehensive and current information. Secondly, we have worked closely with the developmental editors and production staff to assure that the information presented in this text is as user-friendly as possible.

Several features are new to this edition. We have added "Boxes" to present observational findings, goniometric measurements, resisted range of motion/manual muscle tests, ligamentous tests, and special tests to each chapter. Likewise, tables and other recurring items are presented in the same format from chapter to chapter.

We have added two new chapters to this addition. The Assessment of Posture and General Medical Conditions expands upon the content of the first edition. We have also presented the spinal column in two separate chapters, one describing the thoracic and lumbar spine and the other dealing only with the cervical spine. Two new appendices, Assessment of Muscle Length and Functional Testing have also been added.

To maintain consistency from chapter to chapter, we relied on the muscle origins, insertions, actions, and innervations described in Kendall, FP, and McCreary, EK: Muscles: Testing and Function, ed 4. Williams & Wilkins, Baltimore, 1993 and Hislop, HJ, Montgomery, J, and Connelly, B. in Daniels, L, and Worthingham, C: Muscle Testing: Techniques of Manual Examination, ed 6. WB Saunders, Philadelphia, 1995. The procedures used for goniometric evaluation were based on Norkin, CC and White, J: Measurement of Joint Motion: A Guide to Goniometry (ed 2). FA Davis, Philadelphia, 1995.

We would like to take this opportunity to extend our thanks to specific individuals at the FA Davis Publishing Company. First, a heartfelt "merci beaucoup" to our publisher, Jean-François Vilain. Jean-François had the faith and vision for the first edition of this text that helped us see it to fruition. Without his support, none of this would have been possible. We have made it a tradition to poke a little fun at him in the preface, but this time we'll be nice. Have a long, healthy, relaxing retirement. And good luck with those English classes!

We also would like to thank our Developmental Editors, Sharon Lee and Maryann Foley, who have kept this project on track and on schedule. The improved presentation of this text is a tribute to their diligence to detail. Additionally, many thanks to the students and faculty at Northeastern University who volunteered their time for the photo shoots (and numerous reshoots!).

The following individuals have added their expertise through the careful review of the second edition:

Sara Brown, MS, ATC
Athletic Training Program Director
Boston University
Boston, MA

Scott Doberstein, MS, LATC, CSCS
Head Athletic Trainer/Lecturer
University of Wisconsin – La Crosse
La Crosse, WI

Kevin Curley, MD
Non-Operative Sports Medicine Fellow
Pennsylvania Hospital
Philadelphia, PA

Thomas V. Gocke, III, MS, ATC/L, PA-C
Athletic Trainer/Physician Assistant
Raleigh Orthopaedic Clinic
Raleigh, NC

Marsha L. Grant-Ford, PhD, ATC
Glassboro, NJ

Kevin Guskiewicz, PhD, ATC
Athletic Training Program Director
University of North Carolina – Chapel
  Hill
Chapel Hill, NC

**William R. Holcomb, PhD, ATC/L,
  CSCS**
Program Director/Athletic Training
  and Sports Medicine
University of Northern Florida
Jacksonville, FL

Glen Johnson, MD
Parkcrest Surgical Associates, Inc.
Assoc. Prof. of Orthopedics
Washington University School of
  Medicine
St. Louis, MO

Pete Koehneke, MS, ATC
Chair/Associate Professor of Sports
  Medicine and Exercise Science
Canisius College
Buffalo, NY

Sheri Martin, MPT, ATC
Assistant Clinical Specialist
Northeastern University
Boston, MA

Mark A. Merrick, PhD, ATC
The Ohio State University
Indiana State University
Columbus, OH

James B. Sullivan, DPM, ATC
North Smithfield Podiatry
North Smithfield, RI

Paula S. Turocy, EdD, ATC
Athletic Training Department
  Chair/Assoc. Prof.
Duquesne University
Pittsburgh, PA

Bruce M. Zagelbaum, MD, FACS
Clinical Instructor of Ophthalmology
Manhasset, NY

The authors encourage feedback (including questions) about this text. Please feel free to contact us: Chad Starkey (chadstarkey@aol.com) and Jeff Ryan (jeffryan1@home.com).

Chad Starkey
Jeff Ryan

Contributors

Chapter 1
Cultural Considerations in the Evaluation Process
  (BOX 1–1)
RENÉ REVIS SHINGLES, MS, ATC

Assistant Professor
Athletic Training Education Program
Department of Physical Education and Sport
Central Michigan University
Mt. Pleasant, Michigan

Chapter 3
SHERI MARTIN, MPT, ATC

Athletic Training Program
Northeastern University
Boston, Massachusetts

Chapter 9
G. MONIQUE BUTCHER, PHD, ATC/L

Assistant Professor, Athletic Training
Coordinator, Graduate Biomechanics
Department of Sport and Exercise Sciences
Barry University
Miami Shores, Florida

PETER S. ZULIA, PT, ATC

Director
Oxford Physical Therapy and Rehabilitation, Inc.

Instructor
Athletic Training Program
Department of Physical Education, Health and Sports Studies
Miami University
Oxford, Ohio

Contents

CHAPTER 5

The Ankle and Lower Leg

CHAPTER 6

The Knee

CHAPTER 7

The Patellofemoral Articulation

CHAPTER 8

The Pelvis and Thigh

CHAPTER 9

Evaluation of Gait

CHAPTER 10

The Thoracic and Lumbar Spine

CHAPTER 11

The Cervical Spine

CHAPTER 12

The Thorax and Abdomen

CHAPTER 13

The Shoulder and Upper Arm

CHAPTER 14

The Elbow and Forearm

CHAPTER 15

The Wrist, Hand, and Fingers

The Eye

The Face and Related Structures

CHAPTER 18

Head and Neck Injuries

CHAPTER 21

General Medical Conditions

APPENDICES

The Injury Evaluation Process

Structure governs function. In the human body, anatomy is the structure and physiology and *biomechanics* are the functions. An understanding of the structure and function of the human body is required for a competent evaluation of injuries and illnesses. The evaluation process is the search for dysfunctional anatomy, physiology, or biomechanics. Because the body is an integrated machine, knowledge of the specific structure and function of individual body parts must be expanded to include the relationship between these parts in producing normal movement (biomechanics); when injured, in producing abnormal movement *(pathomechanics);* and, when ill, in producing abnormal physiology *(pathology).*

The successful management and rehabilitation of injuries depends on an accurate initial assessment of the condition. Accuracy depends on the precision and thoroughness of the evaluation technique. Although the evaluation process is often thought of as the initial assessment of an injury, it is actually an ongoing process throughout all phases of recovery. The effectiveness of the treatment and rehabilitation protocol, and their subsequent modification, is based on the ongoing reevaluation of the patient's functional status. Skill in evaluating injuries is based on the accuracy of the conclusion reached and the efficiency with which it was performed.

Regardless of whether the evaluation is an initial *triage* of the injury or a reevaluation of an existing condition, a *systematic* and methodical evaluation model leads to efficiency and consistency in the evaluation process and assists in developing proficiency in the special skills needed to achieve an accurate assessment.

 ## SYSTEMATIC EVALUATION TECHNIQUE

This chapter describes the evaluation model used throughout this text and introduces the members of the health care team. This model is only one of many systems that could be used (Fig. 1–1). Any model may be used, as long as it meets two important criteria: (1) each step of the model is justified and (2) the model is followed throughout the evaluation, with any changes made to meet the specific task at hand.

To better organize, interpret, and monitor a patient's progress and develop treatment priorities, obtaining *objective data* is important whenever possible. *Baseline measurements* obtained during the initial evaluation are recorded and referenced during subsequent reevaluations to document the patient's progress and identify the need for changes in the patient's treatment and rehabilitation protocol.

DESCRIPTION OF THE EVALUATIVE MODEL

The evaluation model used in this text is a seven-step process. Each step is designed to obtain specific information. The individual steps, as well as the components of each step, are presented sequentially, with one task completed before another is begun. After the examiner is familiar with the evaluation process, tasks can be combined and the sequence altered, such as in-

---

Biomechanics   The effect of muscular forces, joint axes, and resistance on the quality and quantity of human movement.

Pathomechanics   Abnormal motion and forces produced by the body, most often occurring secondary to trauma.

Pathology   A condition produced by an injury or disease.

Triage   The process of determining the priority of treatment.

Systematic   Orderly; based on a specific sequence of events.

Objective data   Finite measures that are readily reproducible regardless of the individual collecting the information.

Baseline measurements   The initial physical findings, either from the pre-season physical examination in the athlete or upon the initial evaluation during an injury or illness.

History

Determine the mechanism of injury and onset of the symptoms, and question the patient about any associated sounds or sensations at the time of injury. Ascertain any relevant history of prior injury to the involved and uninvolved sides. The history continues throughout the evaluation based on subsequent findings.

Inspection

Compare the involved and uninvolved sides for signs of swelling, deformity, differences in skin color and texture, muscle tone, and other bilateral differences. The inspection process begins during, or prior to, history taking and continues throughout the evaluation.

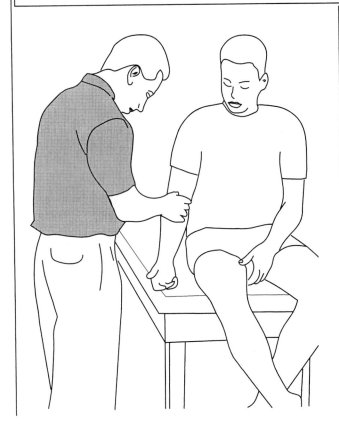

Palpation

Identify areas of point tenderness, crepitus, swelling, malalignment of a joint or bone, or other types of deformity.

Range of Motion Tests

Determine a joint's ability to move actively and passively through a range of motion and the joint's muscles' ability to generate tension through resisted range of motion or manual muscle tests.

Ligamentous Tests

Apply a stress in one of the cardinal planes to a joint's ligaments and/or capsule.

Special Tests

Apply a stress (often in multiple planes) to isolate a specific anatomical structure or function.

Neurological Tests

Assess motor and sensory nerve function. Identify normal reflex loops. Not required for all evaluations.

FIGURE 1–1. Injury evaluation model used in this text. History and inspection are performed throughout the examination process. Note that several evaluation models may be used.

specting the injured area while conducting the history or concurrently using inspection and palpation during the assessment of posture.

The Role of the Noninjured Paired Structure

Neglecting the opposite, or noninjured, body part is a common flaw when learning to evaluate injuries. The noninjured body part provides an immediate reference point to help determine the relative dysfunction of the injured body part. In the case of an injury to one of the extremities, the individual may use the noninjured limb to demonstrate the mechanism of injury or the move-

ments that produce pain (Table 1–1). Because of the importance of the uninvolved body part, it is necessary to dedicate a portion of the history process to identifying a prior or existing injury that may influence the bilateral comparison.

Although the role and importance of the noninjured body part is clear, it is not as clear where it fits into the evaluation process. One school of thought is to perform each task on the noninjured body part first before involving the injured side. The underlying rationale is that the patient's apprehension will be decreased if the evaluation is first performed on the noninjured structure. The other school of thought suggests that testing

Table 1–1
ROLE OF THE NONINJURED LIMB IN THE EVALUATION PROCESS

Segment	Relevance
History	Serves as a reference point when normal (i.e., no history of injury or preexisting condition) for the patient to compare what is being experienced in the injured body part; the patient may demonstrate the mechanism of injury using the noninjured limb
Inspection	Provides a reference for symmetry and color of the superficial tissues
Palpation	Provides a reference for the comparison of bilateral symmetry of bones, alignment, tissue temperature, or other deformity as well as the presence of increased tenderness
Range of motion testing	Provides a reference for range of motion, strength, and painful arcs
Ligamentous and capsular tests	Provides a reference for end-feel, relative laxity, and pain
Special tests	Provides a reference for pathology of individual ligaments, joint capsules, and musculotendinous units, and the body's organs
Neurologic tests	Provides a reference for bilateral sensory, reflex, and motor function

the uninvolved limb first may actually increase the patient's apprehension and cause *muscle guarding.* This text assumes that the noninjured body part will be evaluated first, although the urgency of some acute injuries, *dislocations,* for example, may cause the evaluation of the noninjured limb to be omitted.

 CLINICAL EVALUATIONS

Clinical evaluations, whether in an athletic training room, physical therapy facility, or physician's office, are performed in a relatively controlled environment compared with on-field evaluations. In the clinic, the evaluator has luxuries that are not available on the field, including evaluation tools (e.g., tape measures, *goniometers*), references, medical records, and, perhaps most importantly, time.

HISTORY

The most important portion of an examination is the patient's medical history. The rest of the examination and any special studies being used help confirm the information derived from the history. The history provides information about the structures involved and the extent of the tissue damage. Perhaps the single most important piece of information obtained during the history-taking process for an acute injury is the injury mechanism, and for chronic conditions, any change in training routines, equipment, or postures. This information helps identify the forces that were placed on the body and, potentially, the injured tissues.

Taking a medical history relies on the ability to communicate with the patient. The quality of information gained from the patient's response will be equal to your ability to communicate. An often-unrecognized barrier to performing an evaluation is sociocultural differences between the patient and clinician that can hinder communication between the involved parties and influence the manner in which the rest of the evaluation is performed. An awareness of these differences can facilitate communication and improve patient care (Box 1–1).

Open-ended questions are useful during the history-taking process because they allow the patient to describe the nature of the complaint in detail. For instance, rather than asking a closed-ended question that can be answered with "yes" or "no," such as, "Does it hurt when you raise your arm?," use an open-ended question such as, "What causes your pain?"

The medical file is a valuable resource for referencing baseline information, establishing the previous history of injury, providing documentation regarding the rehabilitation program, and identifying any factors that may predispose further injury. Professional standards of practice and state licensure laws usually require accurate documentation of pertinent findings of the subjective (e.g., pain) and objective (e.g., girth measure-

Muscle guarding Voluntarily or involuntarily assuming a posture to protect an injured body area, often through muscular spasm.

Dislocation The complete displacement of the articular surfaces of two joints.

Goniometer A device used to measure the motion, in degrees, that a joint is capable of producing around its axis.

Box 1–1
CULTURAL CONSIDERATIONS IN THE EVALUATION PROCESS

When performing an evaluation, the information gained must be pertinent and accurate to arrive at the proper assessment. Miscommunication often can occur because of differing cultural conventions between the examiner and the patient, possibly leading to an incorrect impression, inappropriate care, or patient noncompliance.[1,2] Therefore, to minimize this risk, practitioners should learn to:

- Involve patients in their own health care.
- Understand cultural groups' attitudes, beliefs, and values as related to issues of health and illness.
- Use cultural resources and knowledge to address health care problems.
- Develop care plans that are holistic and include patients' cultural needs.

Just as developing good evaluations skills takes time, energy, and commitment, so does providing culturally competent care. "Culture" is the values, beliefs, and practices shared by a group and influences an individual's health beliefs, practices, and behaviors. Evaluating patients within a cultural context helps the examiner gain accurate information. It also conveys that you care about the patient as a person, not as a body part or injury (e.g., "my ACL patient").

Some religions specifically prohibit or limit the amount of medical intervention that can occur. A portion of the pre-participation medical examination should identify any of these limitations. In an acute injury situation, this problem is compounded if the patient is unconscious.

Remember that culture is always present, operating and influencing the interchange in every evaluation (whether the interaction is between different cultures or within the same culture). Here are a few cultural aspects to consider during the evaluation process.

HISTORY

- Convey respect: Patients, particularly adult patients, are addressed formally (Miss, Mr., Mrs., Ms.) unless otherwise directed to do so by the patient.
- Language: Barriers can exist when English is spoken as a second language or if the patient does not speak English. Likewise, barriers can exist even when speaking the same language or dialect. Some communication interventions include:
  - Determine the level of English fluency.
  - Obtain the use of an interpreter, if needed.
  - Recognize that dialects are acceptable.
  - Avoid stereotyping because of language and speech patterns.
  - Clarify slang terms.
  - Use jargon-free language.
  - Use pictures, models, or materials written in the patient's language.
  - Speak more slowly, not more loudly.
  - Ask about one symptom at a time.

To ensure understanding, have the patient paraphrase your instructions. If you are working in a setting where other languages are spoken, consider learning the languages of the clientele or obtain the services of an interpreter. If an interpreter is used, speak to the client, not the interpreter.

- Verbal versus nonverbal communication: The actions of the examiner can be just as important as what is said (or not said). If a person has difficulty understanding what you are saying, he or she will increase his or her reliance on secondary forms of communication such as body language and facial expressions.
- Narrative sequence: Examiners often ask history questions and expect answers in a chronological order. However, not all patients describe the history chronologically. Some relay what happened episodically, indicating those "episodes" deemed important to the injury. Allow the patient to respond to the question in the sequence he or she feels comfortable. Taking notes will help in gaining the pertinent information.
- Family considerations: Including immediate and extended family in the decision-making process is often important. Family members can assist with therapeutic regimens, thereby ensuring compliance.

INSPECTION

- Skin assessment (coloration and discoloration): When inspecting dark-pigmented skin for pallor, cyanosis, and jaundice, check the mucous membranes, lips, nail beds, palms of hands, and soles of feet to determine the problem.
- Skin conditions: be aware that keloids, scars that form at the site of a wound and grow beyond its boundaries, are most common in black or African-American patients (see Figure 1–4). Ascertain if the patient is prone to keloids, particularly if surgery is indicated.

(continued)

Box 1–1
CULTURAL CONSIDERATIONS IN THE EVALUATION PROCESS (continued)

ISSUES REGARDING PHYSICAL CONTACT

- Religious considerations: Permission must be granted before touching any patient. In some cultures and religions, the act of physically being touched or exposing body areas may carry with it certain moral and ethical issues.
- Gender considerations: The standard for the "appropriateness" of touching can be influenced by the gender of the patient and the clinician. Some patients may not feel comfortable being examined by an individual of the opposite gender. If a clinician is of the opposite gender of the patient, the process should be observed by a third party (e.g., another clinician, coach, teammate, parent, or guardian).

Not all individuals in a given ethnic or racial group behave the same way. The levels of acculturation and social economic status are just two factors that influence health-care beliefs and practices. Therefore, use this information as a guide during the evaluation process. Further information may be obtained from the following sources:

Office of Minority Health, U.S. Department of Health and Human Services: 800-444-6472
Center for Cross-Cultural Health (A clearing house of information, training, and research): 612-624-4668
Resources for Cross-Cultural Health Care: 401-588-6051

ments) evaluation, goals for the patient, a treatment plan, and daily treatment logs with periodic reevaluations. The National Collegiate Athletic Association (NCAA) has recommended the inclusion of specific components of the collegiate athlete's medical record (Box 1–2).[3]

For athletic injuries, practice and game videos can be used to help identify the mechanism of injury. These films may allow the medical team to actually view the mechanism and circumstances surrounding the injury.

The following information should be obtained during the history-taking process:

- **Mechanism of the injury:** How did the injury occur? The description of the mechanism of injury (e.g., "I rolled my ankle in") helps to visualize the involved structures and the forces placed on them. Was the trauma caused by a single traumatic force *(macrotrauma)*, or was it the accumulation of repeated forces, resulting in an *insidious* onset of the *symptoms (microtrauma)*?
- **Relevant sounds or sensations at the time of injury:** What sensations were experienced? Did the patient or bystanders hear any sounds, such as a "pop" that could be associated with a tearing ligament or a bone fracturing? Determining the relationship between true physical dysfunction and the reported sensations is useful. For example, true "giving way" or *instability* would involve the *subluxation* of a joint. The physical sensation of a joint's giving way, but without true joint subluxation, indicates pain inhibition or weakness of the surrounding muscles.
- **Location of the symptoms:** Where does the individual perceive the pain? In many cases, the location of the pain correlates with the damaged tissue. However, pain may also be referred from another source, so the evaluator must be familiar with *referred pain* patterns, which are discussed in the appropriate chapters of this text. Ask the patient to point to the area of pain. Using one finger to isolate the area of pain is more likely to isolate the involved structure or structures, as opposed

to describing the painful area by waving the hand over a general area, indicating *diffuse* pain.

- **Onset and duration of symptoms:** When did this problem begin? With acute macrotrauma, the *signs* and symptoms tend to present themselves immediately. The signs and symptoms associated with chronic or insidious microtrauma, such as *overuse syndromes*, tend to progressively worsen with time and continued stresses. The severity of overuse conditions may be graded based on the duration of time since the onset of symptoms and the amount of associated dysfunction to the body part (Table 1–2).

Macrotrauma A single force resulting in trauma to the body's tissues.

Insidious Of gradual onset; with respect to symptoms of an injury or disease having no apparent cause.

Symptom A condition not visually apparent to the examiner, indicating the existence of a disease or injury. Symptoms are usually obtained during the history-taking process.

Microtrauma Accumulation of subtraumatic forces at the cellular level that eventually causes injury to the tissue.

Instability Giving way or subluxation of a joint during functional activity that causes pain and inability to complete the activity.

Subluxation The partial or incomplete dislocation of a joint, usually transient in nature; the joint surfaces relocate as the forces causing the joint displacement are relieved.

Referred pain Pain at a site other than the actual location of trauma. Referred pain tends to be projected outward from the torso and distally along the extremities.

Diffuse Scattered or widespread.

Sign An observable condition that indicates the existence of a disease or injury.

Overuse syndrome Injury caused by accumulated microtraumatic stress placed on a structure or body area.

Box 1–2
NCAA GUIDELINE 1B: MEDICAL EVALUATIONS, IMMUNIZATIONS, AND RECORDS

- History of injury, illness, pregnancy, and surgery of both athletic and nonathletic origin
- Physician referrals and subsequent feedback regarding treatment, rehabilitation, and disposition
- Preparticipation and preseason medical questionnaire detailing the following items:
  - Illnesses suffered (acute and chronic)
  - Surgery and hospitalization
  - Allergies
  - Medications taken on a regular basis
  - Conditioning status
  - Injuries suffered (acute and chronic; athletic and nonathletic)
    - Cerebral concussions sustained
    - Episodes involving the loss of consciousness
    - *Syncope*
    - Exercised-induced asthma or bronchospasm
    - Loss of paired organs
    - Heat-related injury
    - Cardiac conditions, including those involving the immediate family
    - *Sudden death* in a family member younger than age 50 years
    - Family history of *Marfan syndrome*
- Immunization records:
  - Measles
  - Mumps
  - Rubella
  - Hepatitis B
  - Diphtheria
  - Tetanus
- Other documentation, signed by the athlete and parent if the athlete is under age 18 years
  - Release of medical records
  - Consent to treatment

Table 1–2
CLASSIFICATION SYSTEM FOR OVERUSE INJURIES

Stage	Presentation of Symptoms	Functional Ability
I	Pain after activity	Little dysfunction initially; pain with movement increasing as the patient nears stage II
II	Pain during and after activity	Pain with movement of the body part, with associated decreased performance; in the latter stages, dysfunction of the body part may make the patient unable to perform activity
III	Constant pain	Great loss of function during all activities

- **Description of symptoms:** How is the pain described? Is it sharp, dull, or achy? Is it intermittent or constant? Does the patient describe other symptoms, such as weakness or *paresthesia?* Does he or she describe dysfunction of the body part or the inability to perform an activity?

Syncope Fainting caused by a transient loss of oxygen supply to the brain.

Sudden death Unexpected and instantaneous death occurring within 1 hour of the onset of symptoms; most often used to describe death caused secondary to cardiac failure.

Marfan syndrome A hereditary condition of the connective tissue, bones, muscles, and ligaments. Over time, this condition results in degeneration of brain function, cardiac failure, and other visceral problems.

Paresthesia The sensation of numbness or tingling, often described as a "pins and needles" sensation, caused by compression of or a lesion to a peripheral nerve.

- **Changes in the symptoms:** Are there any factors that change the intensity of the symptoms, including specific postures, motions, treatments and modalities, and medication?
- **Previous history:** Is there a history of previous injury to the body area? Are there any possible sources of weakness from a previous injury? If there is a history of injury to this body part, ask the patient to describe and compare this injury with the previous injury. Was the onset similar? Do the present symptoms duplicate the previous symptoms?

A history of injury to the body area, prior medical conditions, and *congenital* conditions can predispose the person to further injury or influence the evaluation findings. If the injury appears to be a chronic condition or if previous injury to this body part has occurred, prior medical referral and subsequent treatment and rehabilitation protocol must be determined:

- When did this episode occur? Has it reoccurred since the initial onset?
- Who evaluated and treated this injury previously?
- What diagnosis was made?
- What was the course of treatment and rehabilitation?
- Was surgery performed or medication administered?
- Did the previous treatment plan decrease the symptoms?

Apparent musculoskeletal injuries that fail to resolve over time warrant special attention. The signs and symptoms of certain tumors and other systemic pathologies may masquerade as overuse injuries, strains, *sprains,* and other inflammatory conditions.[4]

- **Related history to the opposite body part:** How does the injured body part compare with the uninjured side? Much of what is deduced during the examination of an injury is based on the findings of the injured body part and comparison with those of the uninjured side. Any previous injury to the uninvolved side that may affect the findings of any bilateral comparison must be determined.
- **General medical health:** What is the athlete's general health status? Athletes are often assumed to be in prime physical health. Unfortunately, this is not always correct. Evaluate anyone undergoing a preparticipation physical examination and subsequent update for any congenital abnormality or disease that may affect the evaluation and treatment of the injury. Current advances in medical treatment, including the use of medications, have allowed people to participate in athletics who previously would have been medically disqualified. These problems must be taken into consideration in the evaluative and treatment process.

At the conclusion of the history-taking process, a clear picture is formed of the events causing the injury; predisposing conditions that may have led to its occurrence; and the activities, motions, and postures that increase the symptoms. This portion of the evaluation is a dialogue between the examiner and the patient. Do not hesitate to "follow leads" to fully ascertain all the facts regarding the person's condition. The history may be expanded upon during the remainder of the evaluation, backtracking or asking further questions relevant to the patient's condition.

Although the physical aspect of the evaluation holds the immediate priority, the patient's psychological and emotional state must also be considered. People react differently to injury, with varying levels of pain tolerance, apprehension, fear, and desire to return to activity. The evaluation process may be adjusted based on the patient's psychological status. For instance, a patient who is apprehensive or fearful during the evaluation may relax if the examiner takes extra time to explain each of the steps in the evaluation process. Creating a comfortable setting for the patient will facilitate the evaluative process.

The information gained and the impression formed during the history-taking process is confirmed or refuted during the rest of the examination.

INSPECTION

During a clinical evaluation, the inspection process begins as soon as the patient enters the facility. At this time, *gait,* posture, and functional movement patterns are observed. Inspection continues throughout the history-taking process. Candid observation of the patient may provide information concerning his or her "natural" postures and movement patterns. Any guarding or "carrying" postures in which the patient splints the body part in a protective position can be noted.

Visually inspect the area for signs of **gross deformity** or other obvious injury, including serious bleeding, signs of fracture, and swelling. Signs of joint displacement or bony fracture warrant the termination of the evaluation and the immediate referral to a physician. Careful bilateral inspection may reveal subtle differences in otherwise healthy-looking body parts (Fig. 1–2).

Congenital   A condition existing at or before birth.

Sprain   The stretching or tearing of ligamentous or capsular tissue.

Gait   The sequential movements of the spine, pelvis, knee, ankle, foot , and upper extremity when walking or running.

Gross deformity   An abnormality that is visible to the unaided eye.

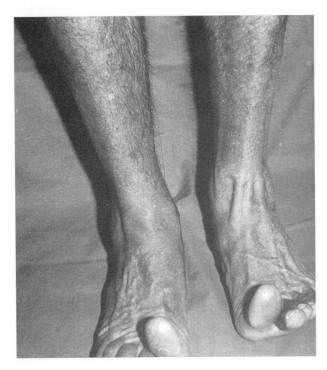

FIGURE 1–2. What's wrong with this picture? (The answer is given in the legend of Figure 1–3.) The patient has few functional complaints other than decreased strength during dorsiflexion of the right ankle. There is no history of trauma to the body area. Carefully examine both ankles to determine the cause of these complaints.

Inspect the injured body part and compare the results with the opposite structure for:

- **Gross deformity:** Are there signs of fracture or joint dislocation? These may be revealed through disrupted contour of long bones, significant differences in bilateral symmetry, or malalignment of joints. If a dislocation or fracture is suspected, the presence of any other significant trauma must be ruled out. The evaluation is terminated, emergency management procedures are implemented (e.g., splinting, checking for a *distal* pulse and *sensation*), and the person transported to a medical facility.
- **Swelling:** Does the involved body part show signs of swelling? Is the swelling localized or diffuse? The amount of time since the onset of the injury should be determined. The amount of swelling should be measured in a quantifiable manner using girth measurements (Box 1–3) or volumetric measurements (Fig. 1–3).
- **Bilateral symmetry:** Are bilateral body parts the normal mirror images of each other? Inspect the problematic area and compare it with its counterpart, noting any discrepancies between the two.
- **Skin:** Does the area show redness that may be associated with inflammation? Is a contusion present, indicating direct impact? Has *ecchymosis* settled in around or distal to an injured structure? Are there

signs of previous trauma, *keloids,* or surgical scars (Fig. 1–4)?
- **Infection:** Does the body area show signs of infection (e.g., redness, swelling, pus, red streaks, swollen *lymph nodes*)? Infections can strike both open and closed wounds.

The inspection process continues throughout the remainder of the examination. Over time, the patient may become less apprehensive and begin to move the limb more freely.

PALPATION

Palpation, the process of touching and feeling the tissues, allows the examiner to detect tissue damage that cannot be visually observed by comparing the findings of one body part with those of the opposite one. It also helps to identify areas of point tenderness. Palpation is performed in a specific sequence, beginning with structures away from the site of pain and progressively moving toward the damaged tissues. Thus, different potential sources of pain can be ruled out and possible involved secondary structures can be identified.

One method of sequencing is to palpate the bones and ligaments first and then palpate the muscles and tendons, and then, finally, locate any other areas such as pulses. The second form of sequencing is to palpate all structures (e.g., bones, muscles, ligaments) farthest from the suspected injury and then palpating progressing toward the injured site. Regardless of the palpation strategy that is used, all pertinent structures must be palpated. During the palpation, make note of the following potential findings:

- **Point tenderness:** Palpate toward the injured area, visualizing the structures that lie beneath the fingers. Accurately identifying the painful structure being palpated greatly assists in identifying the traumatized tissues. Compare any structure demonstrating increased tenderness with the *contralateral* structure. Certain

---

Distal Away from the midline of the body, moving toward the periphery; the opposite of proximal.

Sensation The ability of the athlete to perceive sensory stimuli such as touch discrimination or temperature.

Ecchymosis A blue or purple area of skin caused by the movement of blood into the skin.

Keloid Hypertrophic scar formation secondary to excessive collagen.

Lymph nodes Nodules located in the cervical, axillary, and inguinal regions, producing white blood cells and filtering bacteria from the bloodstream. Lymph nodes become enlarged secondary to an infection.

Contralateral Pertaining to the opposite side of the body or the opposite extremity.

Box 1–3
GIRTH MEASUREMENT

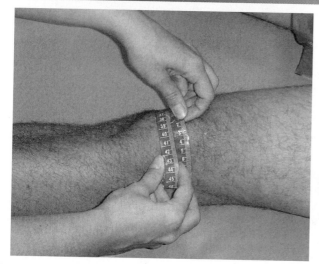 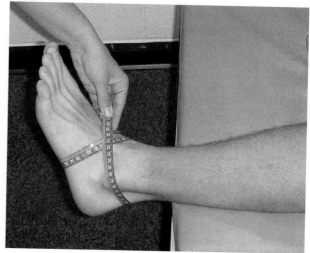

POSITION OF THE PATIENT	Supine
EVALUATIVE PROCEDURE	**1.** To determine capsular swelling, identify the joint line using prominent bony landmarks. To determine muscular atrophy, make incremental marks (e.g., 2, 4, and 6 in) from the joint line.
	2. Do not use a measuring tape made of cloth (cloth tapes tend to stretch and cause the markings to fade).
	3. Lay the measuring tape symmetrically around the body part, being careful not to fold or twist the tape. Use a figure-8 technique to measure ankle girth. Position the tape across the malleoli proximally and around the navicular and the base of the fifth metatarsal distally.
	3. Pull the tape snugly and read the circumference in centimeters or inches.
	4. Take three measurements and record the average.
	5. Repeat these steps for the uninjured limb.
	6. Record the findings in the medical file.
POSITIVE RESULTS	A significant difference in the girth between the two limbs, based on factors such as lower or upper extremity, side dominance, and so on.
IMPLICATIONS	Increased girth across the joint line: swelling Increased girth of muscle mass: hypertrophy Decreased girth of muscle mass: atrophy

areas of the body (e.g., the anatomical snuff box, orbital rim, costochondral joints) are normally tender. Palpation must elicit increased tenderness of the structure relative to the surrounding structures and the same structure on the opposite side of the body.

- **Trigger points:** Note any trigger points that may be found in muscle and, when palpated, refer pain to another body area. Attempt to determine the cause-and-effect relationship between the symptoms and the patient's pathology.
- **Change in tissue density:** Palpate for differences in the density or "feel" of the tissues that possibly indicate muscle spasm, hemorrhage, edema, scarring, myositis ossificans, or other conditions.

- **Crepitus:** Note a crunching or crackling sensed with the rubbing of tissues. Termed *crepitus,* this may indicate a fracture when felt over bone or inflammation when felt over tendon, *bursa,* or joint capsule. Crepitus can also occur when air enters the tissues such as after an orbital fracture or pneumothorax.

Crepitus   Repeated crackling sensations or sound emanating from a joint or tissue.

Bursa (plural, bursae)   A fluid-filled sac that decreases friction between adjoining soft tissues or between soft tissue and bones.

FIGURE 1–3. Volumetric measurement. **(A)** The tank is filled with water up to the specified level and the limb is gently immersed. **(B)** The overflow water is collected and poured into a calibrated beaker to determine the mass (volume) of the limb. Answer to Figure 1–2: The right tibialis anterior tendon is ruptured. Note the absence of its tendon as it crosses the joint line.

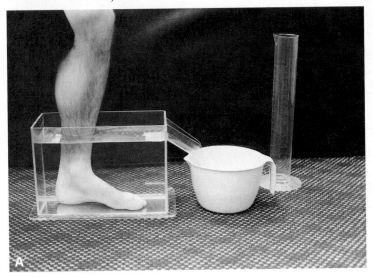
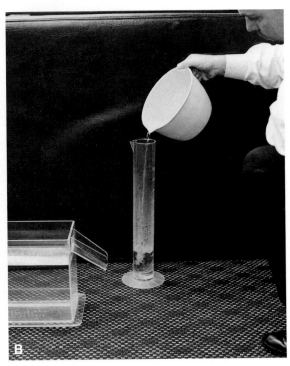

- **Symmetry:** Compare muscle tone, joint surfaces, and bony prominences bilaterally.
- **Increased tissue temperature:** Feel for increased temperature of the injured area relative to the surrounding sites, which usually indicates an active inflammatory process.

Some clinicians prefer to delay the palpation process until the end of the evaluation because this is often the most painful aspect of the evaluation. Excess pain with palpation can produce apprehension, causing the patient to guard the area and alter the remainder of the evaluation.

RANGE OF MOTION

Assessment of the patient's ability to move the limb through the range of motion actively, passively, and against resistance helps to quantify the person's current functional status. As with all evaluation tools, make comparisons bilaterally and, when possible, against established *normative data.* Complete tests for a particular body part must include all the motions allowed by the joint. Additionally, the joints *proximal* and distal to the affected joint may also need to be evaluated. Although a motion may be common to many joints (e.g., *flexion*), some motions, such as ankle *inversion,* are found in only

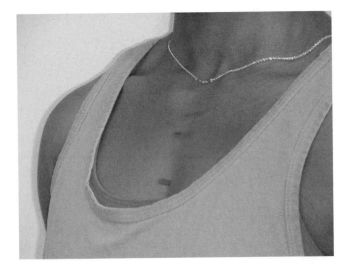

FIGURE 1–4. Keloid formation. These firm, nodular masses represent the overdevelopment of collagen-rich scar tissue. Keloid formation is most prevalent among African Americans.

Normative data Normal ranges of data collected for comparison during the evaluation of an athlete. On many measures, athletes have norms different from the general population.

Proximal Toward the midline of the body; the opposite of distal.

Flexion The act of bending a joint and decreasing its angle.

Inversion The movement of the plantar aspect of the calcaneus toward the midline of the body.

Box 1–4
GONIOMETRIC EVALUATION

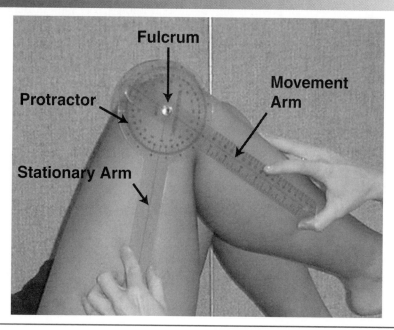

Fulcrum

Protractor

Movement Arm

Stationary Arm

GONIOMETER SEGMENTS	PROTRACTOR:	Measures the arc of motion in degrees. Full-circle goniometers have a 360° protractor; half-circle goniometers have a 180° protractor.
	FULCRUM:	The center of the goniometer's axis of rotation
	STATIONARY ARM:	The portion of the goniometer that extends from, and is part of, the protractor
	MOVEMENT ARM:	The portion of the goniometer that moves independently from the protractor around an arc formed by the fulcrum
PROCEDURE		1. Select a goniometer of the appropriate size and shape for the joint being tested.
		2. Position the joint in its starting position.
		3. Identify the center of the joint's axis of motion.
		4. Locate the proximal and distal landmarks running parallel to the joint's axis of motion.
		5. Align the goniometer's fulcrum over the joint axis.
		6. Align the stationary arm along the proximal body segment and the movement arm along the distal segment.
		7. Read and record the starting values from the goniometer.
		8. Move the distal joint segment through its range of motion.
		9. Reapply the goniometer as described in Steps 5 and 6.
		10. Read and record the ending values from the goniometer.

one joint. Those motions found in only one joint are most often overlooked during an assessment.

The evaluation of active and passive range of motion may be made grossly by observation of the evaluator or, more precisely, objectively measured with the use of a goniometer (Box 1–4). The patient's age and gender influence range of motion. In the high school and college-aged population, women have a greater range of motion in all planes than men do. Range of motion decreases after age 20 years for both genders, but this decrease occurs to a greater extent in women.[5,6]

Active Range of Motion

Active range of motion (AROM) is evaluated first, unless it is *contraindicated* by immature fracture sites or recently repaired *soft tissues*. Evaluating the AROM

Contraindication   Procedure that may prove harmful given the athlete's current condition.

Soft tissues   Structures other than bone, including muscle, tendon, ligament, capsule, bursa, and skin.

first allows you to determine the patient's willingness and ability to move the body part through the range of motion. An unwillingness to move the extremity could signify extreme pain, neurologic deficit, or possible *malingering*.

While the joint is actively moved through all the possible motions in the *cardinal planes*, the ease with which the movement is made and the total range of motion produced is observed (Fig. 1–5). Any compensation or abnormal movement in the surrounding structures also are noted. The patient may verbally or nonverbally describe a *painful arc* within the range of motion.

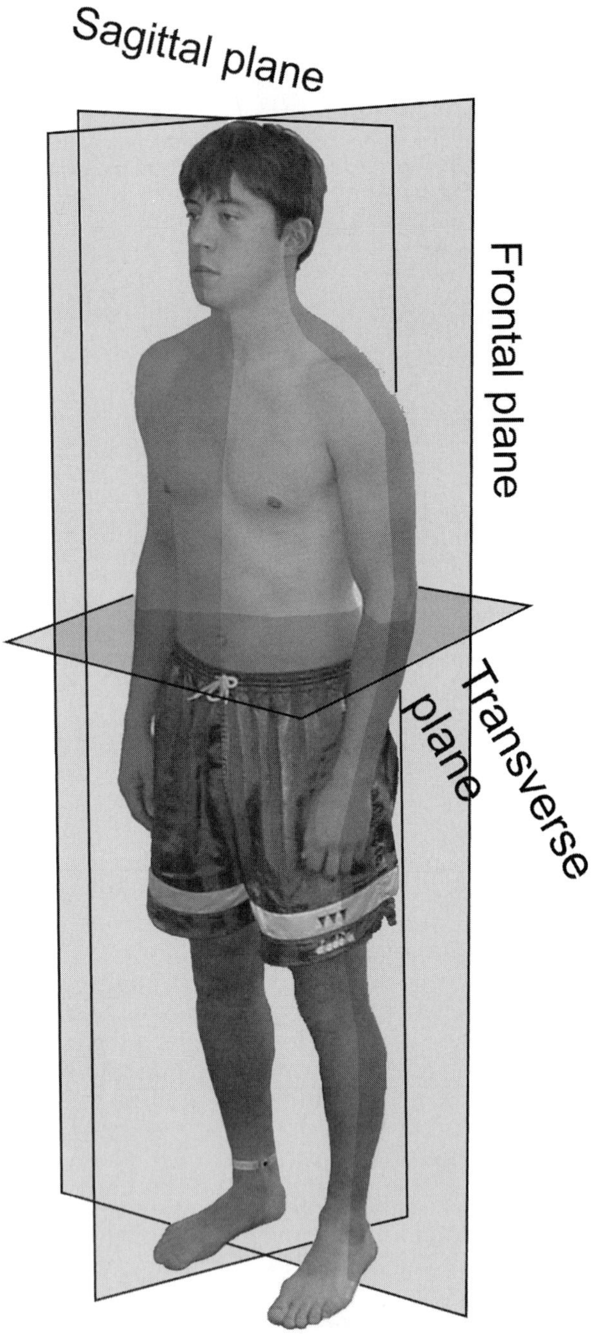

Passive Range of Motion

After AROM is checked, passive range of motion (PROM) is evaluated for the quantity of available movement and the *end-feel* of the tissues as they reach the limit of the available range of motion. The different end-feels as established by Cyriax are listed in Table 1–3.[7] Certain movements have particular normal end-feels (e.g., elbow *extension* should have a hard or bony end-feel). It is necessary to be familiar with these end-feels so pathological limits to range of motion can be identified (Table 1–4).

Useful information can be obtained by comparing the range of movement obtained for AROM with that obtained for PROM. Typically, PROM is greater than AROM. When AROM and PROM are equal and both fall short of the expected range of motion, capsular adhesions or joint tightness may be restricting the motion. AROM that is less than PROM signifies a muscular weakness or a lesion within the active *contractile tissue* that is causing pain and inhibiting motion.

Resisted Range of Motion

Resisted range of motion (RROM) testing can be performed through the joint's entire range of motion or, more commonly, tested isometrically through the use of a *break test*. In a break test, the amount of strength available within a muscle or muscle group is determined by trying to overcome the force of the contrac-

FIGURE 1–5. The cardinal planes of the body. The sagittal plane divides the body into left and right sides. The transverse plane bisects the body into superior and inferior or proximal segments. The frontal (coronal) plane divides the body into anterior and posterior segments.

Malingering   Faking or exaggerating the symptoms of an injury or illness.

Cardinal planes   Imaginary lines dividing the body into upper and lower (transverse planes), anterior and posterior (frontal plane), and left and right (sagittal plane) relative to the anatomic position.

Painful arc   An area within a joint's range of motion that causes pain, representing compression, impingement, or abrasion of the underlying tissues.

End-feel   The specific quality of movement felt by an examiner moving a joint to the end of its range of motion.

Extension   The act of straightening a joint and increasing its angle.

Contractile tissue   Tissue that is capable of shortening and subsequently elongating; muscular tissue.

Break test   An isometric contraction against manual resistance provided by the examiner; used to determine the athlete's ability to generate a static force within a muscle or muscle group.

Table 1–3
PHYSIOLOGICAL (NORMAL) END-FEELS

End-Feel	Structure	Example
Soft	Soft tissue approximation	Knee flexion (contact between soft tissue of the posterior leg and posterior thigh)
Firm	Muscular stretch	Hip flexion with the knee extended (passive elastic tension of hamstring muscles)
	Capsular stretch	Extension of the metacarpophalangeal joints of the fingers (tension in the palmar capsule)
	Ligamentous stretch	Forearm supination (tension in the palmar radioulnar ligament of the inferior radioulnar joint, interosseous membrane, oblique cord)
Hard	Bone contacting bone	Elbow extension (contact between the olecranon process of the ulna and the olecranon *fossa* of the humerus)

Table 1–4
PATHOLOGICAL (ABNORMAL) END-FEELS

End-Feel	Description	Example
Soft	Occurs sooner or later in the ROM than is usual or occurs in a joint that normally has a firm or hard end-feel; feels boggy	Soft tissue edema Synovitis
Firm	Occurs sooner or later in the ROM than is usual or occurs in a joint that normally has a soft or hard end-feel	Increased muscular tonus Capsular, muscular, ligamentous shortening
Hard	Occurs sooner or later in the ROM than is usual or occurs in a joint that normally has a soft or firm end-feel; feels like a bony block	Osteoarthritis Loose bodies in joint Myositis ossificans Fracture
Empty	Has no real end-feel because end of ROM is never reached owing to pain; no resistance felt except for patient's protective muscle splinting or muscle spasm	Acute joint inflammation Bursitis Abscess Fracture Psychogenic origin

tion. Although RROM tends to assess the strength of muscle groups throughout the full range of motion within the cardinal planes, **manual muscle tests** are used to isolate individual muscles within their functional planes of motion. RROM tests should not be performed when the patient is unable to voluntarily contract the injured muscle or is unable to perform AROM tests or if an underlying fracture site is not healed or the involved soft tissues are not yet healed.

Resisted testing of contractile tissues can be assessed with various grading scales, but the results are negated if the contraction causes pain (Table 1–5). With the exception of neurologic involvement, the use of these grading scales to quantify strength in athletes and others involved in strenuous physical activity is rarely beneficial (Fig. 1–6). RROM testing in a younger active population is particularly useful in determining any lesion that may be causing pain in a contractile tissue (Table 1–6).

During manual resistance, the limb is stabilized proximally to prevent other motions from compensating for weakness of the involved muscle. Resistance is provided distally on the bone to which the muscle or muscle group attaches, not distal to a second joint (Fig. 1–7). **Compensation** occurs when postural changes are used to substitute for a loss of motion or weakness, such as using shoulder girdle elevation to compensate for a loss of glenohumeral *abduction.* Compensation

Fossa   A depression on a bone.

Abduction   Lateral movement of a body part away from the midline of the body. In the feet, the movement is in reference to the midline of the foot.

Table 1–5
GRADING SYSTEMS FOR MANUAL MUSCLE TESTS

Verbal	Numerical	Clinical Finding
Normal	5/5	The patient can resist against maximal pressure; The examiner is unable to break the patient's resistance.
Good	4/5	The patient can resist against moderate pressure.
Fair	3/5	The patient can move the body part against gravity through the full range of motion.
Poor	2/5	The patient can move the body part in a gravity-eliminated position through the full range of motion.
Trace	1/5	The patient cannot produce movement, but a muscle contraction is palpable.
Gone	0/5	No contraction is felt.

may also occur through muscular **substitution,** especially by more proximal muscle groups, as the patient attempts to overcome weaknesses of the muscle being tested by recruiting other muscles (e.g., upper trapezius recruitment during shoulder abduction to compensate for a torn supraspinatus tendon). When the patient uses compensatory motions, the amount of resistance used against the contraction should be reduced.

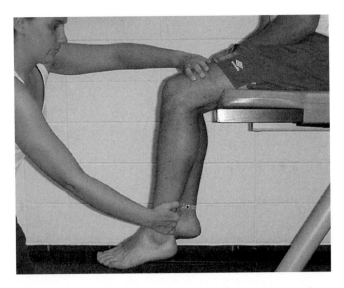

FIGURE 1–6. Manual muscle test in the gravity-eliminated position. With the knee flexed to 90°, the hamstrings are neither assisted by or work against the force of gravity during a break test. During resisted range of motion between 0° and 90°, the hamstrings are assisted by gravity. From 90 to the terminal ranges of flexion, the hamstrings must also overcome the effects of gravity in addition to the manual resistance provided.

Table 1–6
FINDINGS IN RESISTED RANGE OF MOTION TESTS

Strength	Pain	Clinical Indication
Good	None	Normal
Good	Present	Minor contractile soft tissue injury
Weak	Present	Significant contractile soft tissue injury
Weak	None	Neurologic deficit or chronic contractile soft tissue injury

LIGAMENTOUS AND CAPSULAR TESTS

Ligamentous and capsular tests evaluate the structural integrity of the *noncontractile tissues* surrounding a joint. Sprains of ligamentous tissue are generally graded on a three-degree scale (Table 1–7). Ligamentous and capsular tests can also help to confirm an injury history that predisposes the joint to subluxation, dislocation, or both.

Testing involves the application of a specific stress to a tissue to assess its laxity. However, a distinction must be made between laxity and instability. Laxity is a clinical sign and instability is the symptom.[8] Laxity describes the amount of "give" within a joint's supportive tissue. A person may have congenital laxity throughout all of his or her joints, which may be determined by

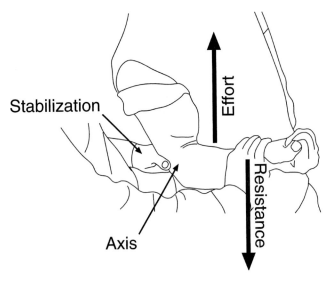

FIGURE 1–7. Performing manual resistance tests. The extremity is stabilized proximal to the joint being tested while resistance is provided distal to the joint.

Noncontractile tissues Ligamentous and capsular tissue surrounding a joint.

Table 1–7
GRADING SYSTEM FOR LIGAMENTOUS LAXITY

Grade	Ligamentous End-Feel	Damage
I	Firm (normal)	Slight stretching of the ligament with little, if any, tearing of the fibers. Pain is present, but the degree of laxity roughly compares with that of the opposite extremity.
II	Soft	Partial tearing of the fibers. There is increased glide of the joint surfaces upon one another or the joint line "opens up" significantly when compared with the opposite side.
III	Empty	Complete tearing of the ligament. the motion is excessive and becomes restricted by other joint structures, such as secondary restraints or tendons.

generalized measures, such as having the patient attempt to pull the thumb to the forearm (Fig. 1–8). Instability is a joint's inability to function under the stresses encountered during functional activities. The amount of joint laxity does not always correlate with the degree of joint instability.[9]

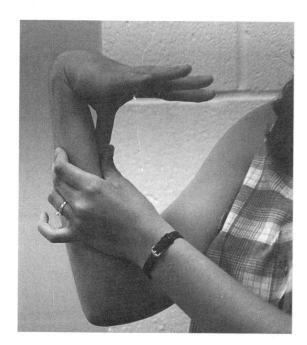

FIGURE 1–8. Determining systemic laxity. Some patients may be naturally lax in all of their joints. A simple test to determine laxity is to have the patient try to pull his or her thumb to the forearm. If this can be accomplished, it may be assumed that all of the patient's joints are lax.

All ligamentous tests are evaluated bilaterally and, whenever possible, compared with baseline measures. The proper joint angle must be obtained to isolate specific tissues within the joint. Performing ligamentous tests with the joint in the incorrect position can yield false results.

SPECIAL TESTS

Special tests involve specific procedures applied to a joint to determine the presence of pathomechanics. Therefore, these tests are unique to each structure, joint, or body part. Take special care to perform the test precisely as described to properly stress the involved tissue. As with all tests, a bilateral comparison must be performed. Examples of special tests include the impingement test in the shoulder or the McMurray's test for a meniscal tear.

NEUROLOGIC TESTS

Neurologic tests involve an ***upper and lower quarter screen*** of sensation, motor function, and ***deep tendon reflexes.*** Neurologic tests are used to identify nerve root impingement, peripheral nerve damage, central nervous system (CNS) trauma, or disease. Any neurologic signs must be determined so that proper management techniques may be performed. Lower quarter screens are presented in Box 1–5, and upper quarter screens are presented in Box 1–6.

Neurologic testing is not required for all injuries. During the clinical evaluation of orthopedic injuries, neurologic examination is indicated when the patient complains of numbness, paresthesia, unexplained muscular weakness, or pain of unexplained origin, or has sustained a cervical or lumbar spine injury.

Sensory Testing

Sensory testing involves a bilateral comparison of light touch discrimination, using a light stroke within the central portion of the ***dermatome*** to avoid overlap of

---

Upper and lower quarter screen Assessments of the neurologic status of the peripheral nervous system of the upper and lower extremities, through the evaluation of sensation, motor function, and deep tendon reflexes, respectively.

Deep tendon reflex An involuntary muscle contraction caused by a reflex arc in the spinal cord, initiated by the stretching of receptors within a tendon.

Dermatome An area of skin innervated by a single nerve root.

Box 1–5
LOWER QUARTER NEUROLOGICAL SCREEN

Nerve Root Level	Sensory Testing	Motor Testing	Reflex Testing
L1		Lumbar plexus	None
L2		Lumbar plexus	Partial
L3		Femoral n.	Partial
L4		Deep peroneal n.	Patellar t.
L5		Deep peroneal n.	Patellar t.
S1		Tibial n.	Achilles t.
S2	P. femoral cutaneous n.	Intrinsic foot/toe muscles Lateral plantar n.	Achilles t.

Box 1–6
UPPER QUARTER NEUROLOGICAL SCREEN

Nerve Root Level	Sensory Testing	Motor Testing	Reflex Testing
C5	Axillary n.	Axillary n.	Biceps brachii
C6	Musculocutaneous n.	Musculocutaneous n. (C5 & C6)	Brachioradialis
C7	Radial n.	Radial n.	Triceps brachii
C8	Ulnar n. (mixed)	Median & palm. interosseous n.	None
T1	Med. brachial cutaneous n.	None	None

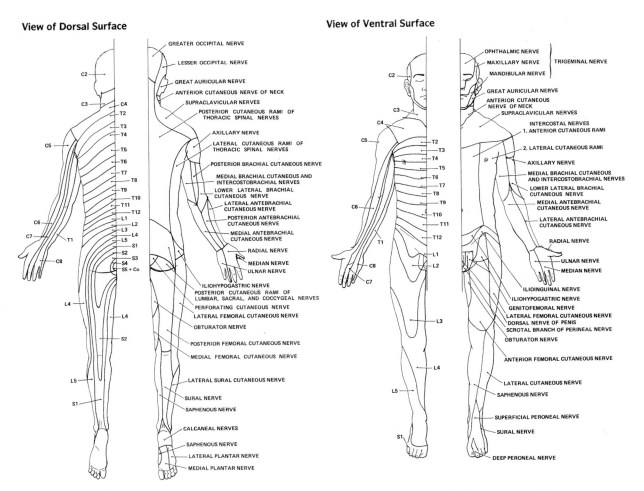

View of Dorsal Surface

View of Ventral Surface

Cutaneous innervation of the back of the body. Dermatomes are on the left, and peripheral nerves are on the right.

Cutaneous innervation of the front of the body. Dermatomes are on the left, and peripheral nerves are on the right.

FIGURE 1–9. The body's dermatomes. These charts describe the area of skin receiving sensory input from each of the nerve roots. Note that there are many different dermatome references, thus explaining the inconsistencies from text to text.

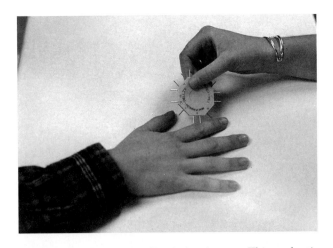

FIGURE 1–10. Two-point discrimination test. This evaluative procedure is used to determine the degree of sensory loss. A negative test result, results in the patient's feeling both points touching the skin; a positive test result occurs if the patient is unable to discriminate the two points.

multiple nerve roots (Fig. 1–9). The stroke should be felt to an equal extent on each side. Sensory tests using sharp and dull discrimination, hot and cold discrimination, and two-point discrimination may be used to perform a peripheral nerve injury assessment (Fig. 1–10).

Motor Testing

Manual muscle tests are used to test the *motor neurons* that are innervating the upper and lower extremities (see Box 1–5 and Box 1–6). Although innervation of all muscles tends to overlap, some muscles are more commonly tested for each nerve root. Whichever muscles are chosen, the clinician must be consistent in testing these muscles with a standard pattern of assessment.

Motor neurons Neurons that send signals from the central nervous system to the muscular system.

Table 1–8
DEEP TENDON REFLEX GRADING

Grade	Response
0	No reflex elicited
1	Hyporeflexoria: Reflex elicited with reinforcement (pre-contracting the muscle)
2	Normal response
3	Hyperreflexoria: Hyperresponsive reflex

Reflex Testing

Deep tendon reflexes (DTRs) provide further information about the integrity of the cervical and lumbar nerve roots. However, reflex testing is limited because not all nerve roots have a DTR. In an active population, DTRs may be graded using a four-point scale (Table 1–8).

Appendix A describes the reflex tests commonly used in the evaluation of orthopedic and peripheral nerve injuries. Increased response to a reflex test indicates an *upper motor neuron lesion,* while decreased responses could signify a *lower motor neuron lesion.*

ACTIVITY-SPECIFIC FUNCTIONAL TESTING

Although tools such as *isokinetic dynamometers* are valuable, a working knowledge of the patient's functional demands is still required (Fig. 1–11). Functional testing should indicate a person's ability to perform the tasks required for sports, work, or the basic activities of daily living (ADLs). Functional tests are typically designed to assess how multiple components of the body

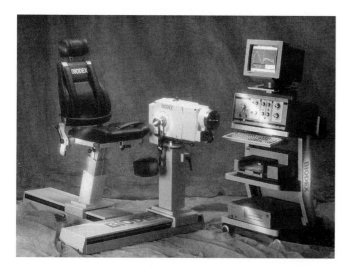

FIGURE 1–11. Isokinetic dynamometer used in determining muscular strength, power, and endurance.

work together to produce functional activity (e.g., one leg hop for distance, range of motion, strength, and balance). These assessments are then expanded to replicate the activity to be performed by the patient under the precise demands faced during real-life situations (e.g., running, jumping, stair climbing, stacking boxes on a pallet). Specific functional tests are described in Appendix B.

 ON-FIELD EVALUATION OF ATHLETIC INJURIES

On-field injuries are divided into ambulatory and athlete-down types. Because ambulatory conditions are marked by the athlete's coming to the clinician to be evaluated, little difference is evident between ambulatory evaluation and clinical evaluation. However, the amount of time available to perform the evaluation may be decreased during game competition.

Athlete-down conditions are signified by the athletic trainer's responding to the athlete and the situation. In order of their importance, the on-field evaluation must rule out:

- Inhibition of the cardiovascular and respiratory systems
- Life-threatening trauma to the head or spinal column
- Profuse bleeding
- Fractures
- Joint dislocation
- Peripheral nerve injury
- Other soft tissue trauma

Based on the findings of this triage, the immediate *disposition* of the condition must be determined. This includes the on-field management of the injury, the safest method of removing the athlete from the field, and the urgency of referring the athlete for further medical care.

On-field evaluations are best performed with two responders. In cases of head or spine trauma, one responder is responsible for stabilizing the spine, and the other performs the needed evaluations. For non-catastrophic conditions, one responder conducts the

Upper motor neuron lesion A lesion proximal to the anterior horn of the spinal cord that results in paralysis and loss of voluntary movement, spasticity, sensory loss, and pathological reflexes.

Lower motor neuron lesion A lesion of the anterior horn of the spinal cord, nerve roots, or peripheral nerves resulting in decreased reflexes, flaccid paralysis, and atrophy.

Isokinetic dynamometer A device that quantitatively measures muscular function through a preset speed of movement.

Disposition The immediate and long-term management of an injury or illness.

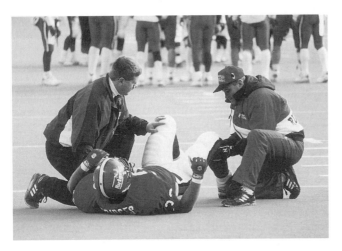

FIGURE 1–12. On-field evaluation performed by two responders. One responder calms and communicates with the athlete while the second performs the tests. This method is considered to be the optimal method for handling on-field injuries, especially in emergency situations.

on-field evaluation. The other responder calms and communicates with the athlete and controls the surrounding scene (Fig. 1–12).

When one athletic trainer is responsible for the on-field evaluation of an injury, a clear communication and evaluation protocol must be established (Fig. 1–13). In all instances, the coaching staff and other personnel should receive regular training in cardiopulmonary resuscitation (CPR) and be prepared to lend assistance in the event of a *catastrophic* injury.

A communication plan must be established for game-day on-field injuries. The use of pre-established

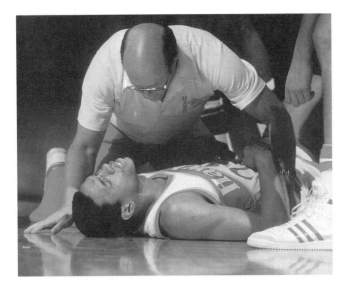

FIGURE 1–13. One examiner responding to an on-field injury. This method requires that the individual perform the evaluation, communicate with the athlete, and, if necessary, summon emergency personnel.

hand signals or walkie-talkies allows the individuals conducting the on-field evaluation to communicate with the sidelines. In this manner, the need for emergency equipment, special response equipment, the team physician, other emergency personnel, and transport squad can be relayed quickly.

Each sport at each level of competition has rules governing the on-field evaluation of injuries during sanctioned competition. In most cases, the official must summon assistance onto the field or court and in some cases, such as wrestling, the evaluation must be completed and the disposition of the athlete determined in a limited period of time. Otherwise, the athlete is disqualified from competition. The medical staff is responsible for becoming familiar with the pertinent rules governing the administration of medical assistance. Before each contest, the athletic trainer should meet with the officials and clarify these points. It is also important to discuss procedures with on-site emergency personnel to facilitate communication in case a need arises for their assistance.

ON-FIELD HISTORY

The injury history can be obtained from the athlete as well as from bystanders who witnessed the injury. However, if the athlete is unconscious or disoriented, as much information as possible is obtained from those who witnessed the episode. The history portion of the on-field evaluation is relatively brief compared with that associated with the clinical evaluation. The primary information to be gained includes:

- **Location of the pain:** Identify the site of pain as closely as possible. Although the athlete may be holding an area of his or her body, do not assume that this is the only site of trauma because multiple injuries may have occurred.
- **Peripheral symptoms:** Question the patient about the presence of pain or numbness that radiates into the distal extremities, suggesting spinal cord, nerve root, or peripheral nerve trauma.
- **Mechanism of the injury:** Identify the force that caused the injury (e.g., contact vs. non-contact injuries).
- **Associated sounds and symptoms:** Note any reports of a "snap" or "pop" at the time of injury that may indicate a tearing of ligaments or tendons or may be related to the fracture of a bone.
- **History of injury:** Identify any relevant history of injury that may have been exacerbated by the current trauma or may influence the physical findings during the current evaluation.

Catastrophic   An injury that causes permanent disability or death.

In cases in which the injury is apparent, such as an obvious fracture or dislocation, the history of the injury often becomes irrelevant. In these cases, rule out head and spinal trauma, attempt to calm the athlete, rule out injury to other body areas while initiating appropriate management of the condition, and, when appropriate, treat the athlete for shock.

ON-FIELD INSPECTION

In an athlete-down situation, the observation process begins as soon as the individual is in the responder's sight. Therefore, much of this process occurs before the history-taking process. During this time, observe for the following:

- **Is the athlete moving?** An athlete who is moving his or her body normally, holding an injured body part, or writhing in pain indicates consciousness, an intact CNS, and cardiovascular function. Far more critical are athletes who show no signs of movement or who are seizing, indicating possible CNS trauma. Do not move an unconscious athlete unless CPR is to be started, the athlete is to be transported to the hospital via an emergency squad, or the athlete regains consciousness and a safe extraction method has been determined. All unconscious athletes should be managed as if they are suffering from cervical spine trauma (see Chapter 18).
- **What is the position of the athlete?** Is the athlete prone, supine, or side-lying? Is a body part in an awkward position? Is any gross deformity evident? These factors take on added importance if the athlete is unconscious and must be moved to begin CPR.
- **Is the athlete conscious?** If the athlete is not moving when the responder arrives at the scene, determine the level of consciousness. This is most easily accomplished by speaking to the athlete and attempting to gain some type of verbal feedback or gesture.
- **Primary survey:** If the athlete is unconscious, the inspection process takes the form of a primary survey. This uses the ABC technique of assessing the **A**irway, checking for **B**reathing, and checking for **C**irculation.
- **Inspection of the injured area:** This process is an abbreviated version of the steps presented during the clinical evaluation section, specifically observing for signs of a fracture, joint dislocation, or swelling.
- **Secondary survey:** Observe and palpate the other body areas, noting for the presence of any bleeding, gross deformity, or other signs of trauma to other parts of the body.

ON-FIELD PALPATION

Two major areas to palpate include the bony structures and soft tissues. Findings of possible fractures, joint dislocations, or *neurovascular* inhibition warrant terminating the evaluation and transporting the athlete to a hospital.

Palpation of the Bony Structures

- **Bony alignment:** Palpate the length of the injured bone to identify any discontinuity. Although fractures of long bones (e.g., femur, humerus) are often accompanied by gross deformity, those of smaller bones may present no outward signs.
- **Crepitus:** Note any *crepitus,* associated with fractures, swelling, inflammation, or air entering the subcutaneous tissues.
- **Joint alignment:** If the injury involves a joint, palpate along the joint line to determine whether the joint is assuming its normal alignment.

Palpation of the Soft Tissues

- **Swelling:** Swelling immediately after the injury is often associated with a major disruption of the tissues. The exception to this is trauma to bursae, which tend to swell disproportionately to the severity of the injury.
- **Painful areas:** Areas that result in pain when palpated can indicate trauma to underlying tissue.
- **Deficit in the muscles or tendons:** Severe tearing of a muscle or tendon can result in a palpable defect.

ON-FIELD RANGE OF MOTION TESTING

While evaluating acute injuries on the field, range of motion and functional testing provide information about the athlete's ability and willingness to move the involved extremity. AROM is the most important test to be performed while the athlete is still on the field. PROM and RROM can be reserved for the sideline or clinical evaluation. If the athlete's injury involves the lower extremity, functional testing is expanded to include the body part's ability to bear weight.

On-field functional testing should not be performed in the presence of a suspected fracture, dislocation, or muscle or tendon rupture. An approach to assessing the athlete's function in a progressive manner includes:

- **Active range of motion:** The athlete is asked to move the limb through the range of motion, while the quality and quantity of movement are noted.
- **Passive range of motion:** The degree of muscular damage is assessed by placing the muscle on stretch.
- **Resisted range of motion:** If the active and passive range of motion test results are normal, break pressure is used to determine the involved muscles' ability to sustain a forceful contraction.

Neurovascular   Pertaining to a bundle formed by nerves, arteries, and veins.

• **Weight-bearing status** (lower extremity injuries): If the athlete is able to complete the AROM, PROM, and RROM tests, he or she can be permitted to walk off the field, with assistance if necessary. If the athlete is unable to perform these tests or signs and symptoms of a potential fracture or dislocation exist, the athlete is removed from the field in a non-weight-bearing manner.

ON-FIELD LIGAMENTOUS TESTING

The purpose of on-field ligamentous testing is to gain an immediate impression of the integrity of the ligaments involved in the injury before muscle guarding or swelling masks the degree of instability. Often, on-field ligamentous testing involve only the single-plane tests, which are then compared with the opposite side. Because these evaluations are being performed on the playing surface, ligamentous testing is often performed in less than ideal conditions.

ON-FIELD NEUROLOGIC TESTING

Neurologic testing becomes particularly important in the on-field evaluation of the athlete with a suspected head or spine injury. A thorough evaluation can ensure the proper management of these potentially catastrophic injuries. When responding to acute on-field neurologic injuries, knowledge of tests for cranial nerve and cervical nerve root involvement are needed. These tests are described in Chapters 11 and 18.

After the dislocation of a major joint or the fracture of a large bone, the integrity of the distal neurovascular structures must be determined. Bony displacement may impinge on or lacerate the nerves, arteries, and veins supplying the distal portion of the extremity. The specific processes for identifying these deficits are described in the appropriate chapters of this text.

REMOVAL OF THE ATHLETE FROM THE FIELD

A decision must be made regarding how and when to remove the athlete from the playing area, including the safest manner possible. If a fracture, dislocation, gross joint instability, or other significant musculoskeletal trauma is suspected, the involved body part must be splinted so the injured area and the joints proximal and distal to it are immobilized (Fig. 1–14).

Several methods may be used to assist in removing the athlete from the field (Fig. 1–15). The type of extraction method used is based on the severity and type of injury being managed. With most upper extremity injuries, the body part may be immobilized and the athlete then is walked off the field. With cases of lower extremity injuries, in which the athlete is unable to bear weight or upright posturing is contraindicated, several types of stretchers may be used. Injury to the spine requires the use of a spine board and rigid cervical collar.

 TERMINATION OF THE EVALUATION

During an evaluation, a finding may be so profound that no other information need be collected; management procedures are implemented and the patient is immediately referred to an appropriate medical facility. Such findings include (but are not limited to) obvious fractures or dislocations, gross joint instability, and neurovascular deficits (Table 1–9). The clinician's discretion must be used on a case-by-case basis to determine when further medical evaluation and care is indicated. When the severity of the condition is uncertain, always err on the side of caution.

 STANDARD PRECAUTIONS AGAINST BLOODBORNE PATHOGENS

Blood, synovial fluid, saliva, and other bodily fluids can potentially transmit bloodborne pathogens such as the *hepatitis B virus (HBV)* and the *human immunodeficiency virus (HIV)*.[10] All bodily fluids must be treated as though they contain these viruses.[11] The treatment of acute injuries that involve bleeding, the handling of mouthpieces, postsurgical wounds, and the handling of soiled dressings and instruments in the clinical setting must all be managed with caution (Fig. 1–16).

The use of *standard (universal) precautions* against bloodborne pathogens serves to reduce the possibility of accidental exposure to these pathogens (Table 1–10). These methods of protecting against accidental exposure include using gloves, *biohazard* disposal containers, and washing soiled towels, uniforms, and other

---

Hepatitis B virus (HBV)   A virus resulting in inflammation of the liver. After a 2- to 6-week incubation period, symptoms develop, including gastrointestinal and respiratory disturbances, jaundice, enlarged liver, muscle pain, and weight loss.

Human immunodeficiency virus (HIV)   The virus that causes acquired immune deficiency syndrome (AIDS).

Standard (universal) precautions   Universally accepted guidelines concerning bloodborne pathogens in patient-clinician interactions.

Biohazard   A substance that is toxic to humans, animals, or the environment.

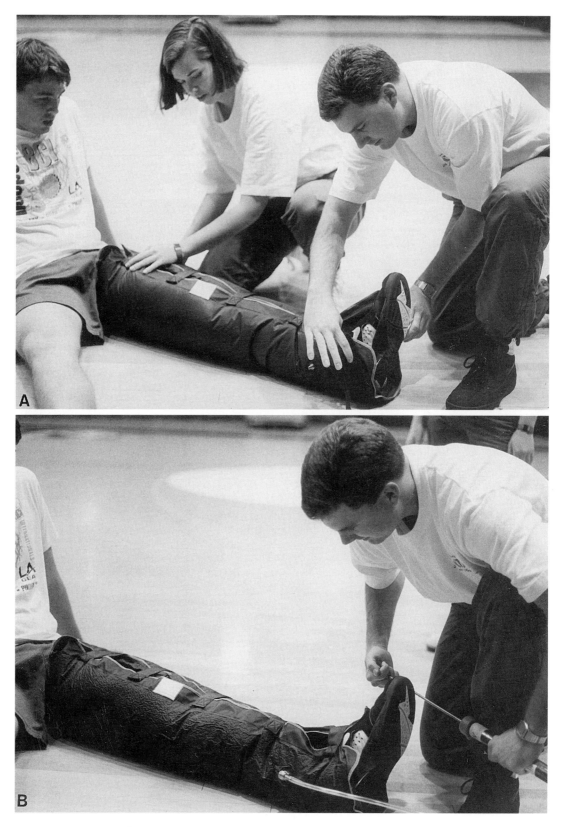

FIGURE 1–14. Use of a vacuum splint to immobilize the injured area. The splint should be of sufficient size to immobilize the joints proximal and distal to the injured area.

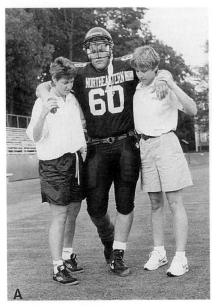

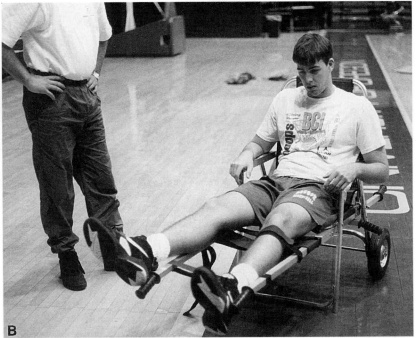

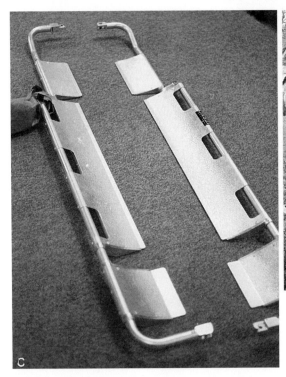

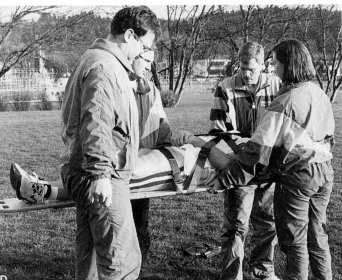

FIGURE 1–15. Various athlete extraction techniques: **(A)** assisted walking; **(B)** pull cart; **(C)** scoop stretcher; and **(D)** full spine board.

Table 1-9

CONDITIONS WARRANTING TERMINATION OF THE EVALUATION

Segment	Findings to Warrant Immediate Physician Referral
History	Reports of the inability to feel or move one or more limbs (confirm with neurologic screen) Reports of significant chest pain Description of a general medical condition that could affect the outcome of the evaluation Reports of difficulty breathing (e.g., anaphylaxsis)
Inspection	Obvious fracture Obvious joint dislocation
Palpation	Disruption in the contour of bone, indicating a fracture or joint dislocation Gross joint instability Malalignment of joint structures
Range of motion testing	Third-degree muscle tears
Ligamentous testing	Gross joint instability
Special tests	Gross joint instability
Neurologic tests	Neurologic dysfunction Sensory dysfunction Motor dysfunction Absent or diminished reflexes

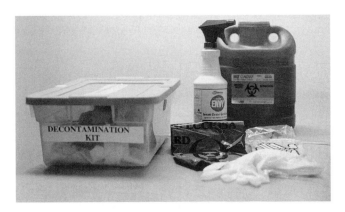

FIGURE 1–16. Use of standard precautions in the management of open wounds. Appropriate personal safeguards include the use of rubber gloves to protect the hands from blood, a disinfectant to clean up blood, and proper methods of disposing of soiled dressings and instruments.

material separately, according to the accepted guidelines. Your institution should have established policies and procedures and conduct an annual in-service defining the steps used in protecting employees from exposure to bloodborne pathogens while preventing possible transmission of disease from the clinician to the patient.

 THE ROLES OF DIFFERENT HEALTH CARE PROFESSIONALS

A patient may become involved with health care providers who assume various roles in the evaluation, treatment, and rehabilitation of patient injuries. The roles and duties are established before the start of the athletic season. Members of the health care team must

Table 1–10
STANDARD PRECAUTIONS AGAINST BLOODBORNE PATHOGENS

Protect skin and mucous membranes against exposure to blood and other fluids through the use of a barrier membrane, such as rubber gloves.

Immediately wash skin coming into contact with a potential carrying agent with soap and water.

Clean contaminated surfaces, such as tables and countertops, with a 1:10 mixture of household bleach and water.

Dispose of all used needles, scalpels, and so on in a proper manner using a biohazard container.

Refrain from having staff members with open, draining sores or skin lesions from providing direct patient care until the condition clears.

Bag soiled linen or uniforms and wash them separately from other items in hot water and detergent.

be aware of their position and be willing to relinquish control, referring the patient whenever necessary. Five key players on the health care team that may become involved in the evaluation of injured athletes include the athletic trainer, physical therapist, school nurse, emergency medical technician, and physician. The following is a description of the possible roles that the team members may play. For care to be successful, each team must develop its own specific roles within the legal guidelines of its state and work cooperatively. In addition, a patient may need the services of other health care practitioners, such as nutritionists, exercise physiologists, and sports psychologists.

ATHLETIC TRAINER

The athletic trainer has the knowledge base to take the athlete from the time of initial injury through evaluation, treatment, rehabilitation, and on to full return to activity. The athletic trainer is also the coordinator of the health care team when the injured athlete is a member of an organized team. The athletic trainer is usually the only health care team member to be a full-time employee of the institution, placing the athletic trainer in a medical, legal, ethical, and fiscal position of responsibility for team members' health care. The hiring of an athletic trainer as a full-time staff member is perceived as a benefit over contracting such services from a *sports medicine* clinic or hospital. Both the athlete and the organization benefit from the athletic trainer's being a full-time staff member whose duties and responsibilities are solely those of meeting the needs of injured athletes and of the institution.

PHYSICAL THERAPIST

The physical therapist can be a vital member of the evaluation and rehabilitation team of injured athletes. The physical therapist has a broad base of evaluation skills for orthopedic and nonorthopedic injuries and illnesses. Certain physical therapists have refined their evaluation and rehabilitation skills specifically for athletic injuries through either continuing education or specialization and competence in sports physical therapy as established by the Sports Physical Therapy Section of the American Physical Therapy Association.

It is more common to find the physical therapist as a member of the athlete's health care team when the athlete is a recreational athlete or a member of an institution that does not employ a full-time athletic trainer. In

Sports medicine *The application of medical and scientific knowledge to the prevention (including training methods and practices), care, and rehabilitation of injuries suffered by individuals participating in athletics.*

these cases, the physical therapist is vital to the overall rehabilitation process. Unless obtaining further education or training in the emergency management of athletic injuries, the physical therapist should refrain from situations in which such duties are performed. In these situations, it is prudent to defer to the athletic trainer or emergency medical technician.

SCHOOL NURSE

The school nurse in high school settings is a valuable addition to the health care team of athletes. Working with the athletic trainer, the school nurse aids in maintaining records, caring for non-athletic injuries and illnesses, educating, and counseling. The athletic trainer and school nurse need to maintain open lines of communication concerning the care of athletes.

EMERGENCY MEDICAL TECHNICIAN

The emergency medical technician (EMT) possesses valuable skills to be offered as a member of the athletic health care team. The EMT is competent in the emergency management of injury and illness, but the type of care provided depends on the qualifications of the individual EMT (Table 1–11). The roles and responsibilities of the emergency medical squad (EMS) must be determined and communicated before the start of each season. This planning process eliminates many questions that may arise during the most inopportune moments in the management of an acute injury.

One of the primary concerns in the transportation of injured athletes is that of equipment. Procedures of management of athletes who wear equipment that may interfere with normal practices of emergency care must be established before the time of an injury. Many pieces of equipment, such as football helmets and face masks, are designed to allow access to the athlete's face. Guidelines, such as the management of face masks and helmets as well as any piece of equipment, should be jointly established by the athletic trainer, EMTs, and team physicians before the start of the season rather than having them debate about it during a crisis situation.

Table 1–11
CLASSIFICATION OF EMERGENCY MEDICAL TECHNICIANS

Level	Skills
EMT-A	Trained in basic ambulance services
EMT-D	Trained in defibrillator use
EMT-I	Trained in defibrillator use, intravenous infusion administration, and endotracheal intubation
EMT-P	Paramedic; provides the highest level of prehospital care

PHYSICIAN

The patient must have access to a licensed physician (medical doctor or doctor of osteopathy).[12] Because it is not fiscally or physically practical for a physician to be present at all practices and games, athletic trainers assume the primary role for the evaluation and emergency management of athletic injuries when the physician is absent.

One physician directs the athlete's health care team and is responsible for the overall medical care provided to athletes. Historically, an orthopedic surgeon or general practitioner is aided by specialists in internal medicine, dentistry, cardiology, psychology, and so on (Table 1–12).

Table 1–12
MEDICAL SPECIALTIES

Specialty	Description
Cardiology	Specialist in ailments of the heart
Dentistry	Specialist in the prevention, diagnosis, and treatment of diseases of the teeth and gums
Endodontics	A branch of dentistry that specializes in the care of the pulp of the tooth
Family (primary care)	A physician who provides comprehensive, continuing care that is not limited by the patient's age, gender, or particular body area
Gynecology	Specialist in the care and treatment of the female reproductive system
Internal medicine	A physician who treats diseases and injuries of the internal organs by means other than surgery
Ophthalmology	Specialist in the treatment of eye injuries and disorders
Oral surgery	Physician who performs surgery on the teeth, jaw, and associated structures
Orthopedics	Specialist in the treatment of the skeletal, articular, and muscular systems
Osteopathy	A field of medicine that views the body in a systemic manner and uses physical techniques, medicines, and surgery to restore normal function; osteopathic physicians use the designation "DO" (Doctor of Osteopathy)
Pediatrics	Specialist in the medical care of children
Physiatrist	A physician who specializes in physical medicine
Radiology	Specialist in diagnosis of radiographs and other imaging techniques
Resident	Member of the hospital staff who is gaining clinical training after an internship

Other health care team members must recognize when to refer an athlete to the physician. The physician also needs to understand the proper role of the other health care team members.

◆ DOCUMENTATION

An injury evaluation normally includes physical contact between the patient and the clinician. At times, the physical contact may involve areas of the patient's body, such as the pelvic region or the chest in female patients, that call for the utmost in discretion. Regardless of the area of physical contact or the gender of the patient and clinician, the patient must always give **informed consent** for the clinician to perform the evaluation.

Informed consent should include a statement that the patient understands that physical contact will occur and gives the clinician permission to proceed with the evaluation process. Furthermore, the patient understands that if he or she becomes uncomfortable with the physical contact during the evaluation, he or she can ask the examiner to stop. Informed consent may be established in the form of a signed written statement or, in the case of an on-field injury during athletics, it may be verbal in nature if a signed form is not already on file. A patient suffering a medical emergency may not be able to give consent for treatment. In this case, a clinician's duty to provide emergency medical care overrides obtaining consent. Certain religions may limit the type of care rendered to the patient (see Box 1–1).

The findings of the initial and follow-up evaluations and any subsequent referrals must be documented in the patient's medical record. Besides serving a legal purpose, medical records have an important practical purpose. Through the use of clear, concise terminology and objective findings, the medical record serves as a method of communicating the patient's current medical disposition to all who read it.

The initial injury report serves as the baseline when planning the treatment and rehabilitation program. Through reevaluating the patient's condition and comparing it with the initial findings, the patient's progress may be monitored and subsequent adjustments made in the rehabilitation plan.

◆ REFERENCES

1. Murray, SO: Ethnic differences in interpretive conventions and the reproduction of inequality in everyday life. *Symbolic Interaction,* 14:187, 1991.
2. Spector, RE: *Cultural Diversity in Health and Illness* (ed 4). Stamford, CT, Appleton & Lange, 1996.
3. Halpin, T, and Dick, RW: *NCAA Sports Medicine Handbook,* 1999–2000 (ed 12). Indianapolis, National Collegiate Athletic Association, 1999, pp. 8–9.
4. Wnorowski, DC: When tumors pose as sports injuries. *Physician and Sportsmedicine,* 26:98, 1998.
5. Grimston, SK, et al: Differences in ankle joint complex range of motion as a function of age. *Foot and Ankle* 14:215, 1993.
6. Kendall, FP, and McCreary, EK: The lower extremity. In Kendall, FP, and McCreary, EK: *Muscles: Testing and Function* (ed 3). Baltimore, Williams & Wilkins, 1983, p 145.
7. Norkin, CC, and White, DJ: *Measurement of Joint Motion: A Guide to Goniometry* (ed 2). Philadelphia, FA Davis, 1995, p 9.
8. Snyder-Mackler, L, et al: The relationship between passive joint laxity and functional outcome after anterior cruciate ligament surgery. *Am J Sports Med,* 25:191, 1997.
9. Harter, RA, et al: A comparison of instrumented and manual Lachman test results in anterior cruciate ligament-reconstructed knees. *Athletic Training: Journal of the National Athletic Trainers Association* 25:330, 1990.
10. Occupational Health and Safety Administration: Bloodborne pathogens. *http://www.osha-slc.gov/SLTC/bloodbornepathogens/index.html*
11. American Academy of Pediatrics Committee on Sports Medicine and Fitness: Human immunodeficiency virus and other bloodborne viral pathogens in the athletic setting. *Pediatrics,* 104:1400, 1999.
12. Rich, BSE: "All physicians are not created equal." Understanding the education background of the sports medicine professional. *Journal of Athletic Training* 28:177, 1993.

2 Injury Nomenclature

Effective communication between members of the medical team relies on the use of standardized, consistent terminology. Each member of the team must be able to accurately describe the condition to physicians, other allied health personnel, the patient, the patient's family and, in the case of work with athletes, the coach.

During an evaluation, the signs and symptoms of an injury allow the clinician to differentiate between conditions that seem similar. In some cases, this distinction may be the deciding factor between a successful treatment and rehabilitation outcome or causing harm. For instance, treatment for a patient with lower leg pain would be much different if the pain was caused by a stress fracture than if it was caused by a muscle strain.

 ## SOFT TISSUE INJURIES

Soft tissue injuries, the most common form of orthopedic trauma, include trauma to the muscles and their tendons, skin, joint capsules, ligaments, and bursae. These injuries affect performance by hindering the motion at one or more joints, decreasing the ability of the muscle to produce force, creating joint instability, or mechanically limiting the amount of motion available to the joint.

MUSCULOTENDINOUS INJURIES

Injuries to a muscle belly or tendon adversely affect the muscle's ability to contract fully, forcibly, or both because of mechanical insufficiency or pain. If the *musculotendinous unit* has been mechanically altered through partial or complete tears, the muscle can no longer produce the forces required to perform simple movements or meet the demands required by athletic or work activity. Partial muscle or tendon tears cause decreased force production secondary to pain elicited during the contraction. Complete tears of the unit result in the muscle's inability to produce any force.

Strains

Strains are noncontact injuries to muscles and tendons caused by excessive tension within the muscle fibers.[1] **Tensile forces** are produced when the muscle is stretched beyond its normal range of motion, causing the fibers to tear. Muscle fibers can also be traumatized by **dynamic overload,** occurring when the muscle generates more force than its fibers can withstand. The amount of tension produced during dynamic overload, such as during an *eccentric muscle contraction,* is an elongating force exerted on the body distal to a muscle's attachment.

The grading of the severity of the strain is based on the number and extent of the fibers that have been traumatized. A three-degree scale is used[2]:

- **First-degree strains** involve stretching of the fibers. Pain increases as the muscle contracts, especially against resistance, and the site of injury is point tender. Swelling may also be present.
- **Second-degree strains** involve the actual tearing of some of the muscle fibers and may cause ecchymosis. These injuries present with the same findings as first-degree strains but are more severe.
- **Third-degree strains** involve the complete rupture of the muscle, resulting in a total loss of function and a palpable defect in the muscle. Pain, swelling, and ecchymosis are also present.

Muscle strains tend to occur at the junction between the muscle's belly and its tendon, most frequently

Musculotendinous unit   The group formed by a muscle and its tendons.

Eccentric muscle contraction   A contraction in which the elongation of the muscle is voluntarily controlled. Lowering a weight is an example of an eccentric contraction.

involving the distal junction.[3–6] With first- and second-degree strains, local tenderness is present over the site of the injury (i.e., pain is elicited at the injury site when the muscle is either actively shortened or passively elongated). Resisted range of motion results in decreased strength secondary to pain or the muscle's mechanical inability to produce force. In third-degree strains, the muscle is incapable of producing force. The patient may attempt to compensate through the use of other muscles and through body position. No tension within the muscle is felt with passive elongation and, after the initial pain has subsided, pain may be minimal to nonexistent.

Depending on the depth of the muscle relative to the skin, swelling and ecchymosis may be visible. The force of gravity can cause these fluids to accumulate distal to the actual site of the injury (Fig. 2–1). The muscular defect, often palpable in second-degree strains, may be visible as well as palpable in third-degree strains (Table 2–1).

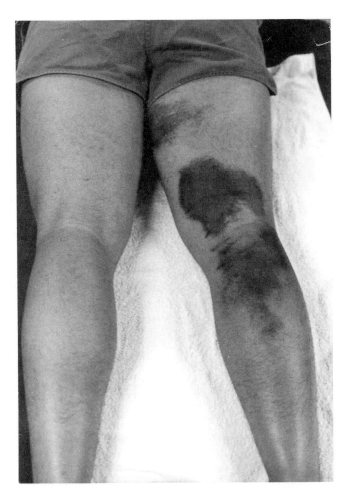

FIGURE 2–1. Ecchymosis associated with a muscular strain. Gravity causes blood that has seeped into the tissues to drift inferiorly.

Tendinitis

As indicated by the "-itis" suffix, tendinitis is inflammation of the muscle tendon. Although tendinitis may result from a single traumatic force, it most commonly arises from repetitive microtrauma being placed on the structure. This insult to the tendon activates an inflammatory process (Table 2–2). With chronic inflammation, the tendon thickens.

Tendinitis is the inflammation of the structures encased within the tendon's outer layering.[8] **Tenosynovitis,** an inflammation of the synovial sheath surrounding a tendon, is more common in the hands and feet because of the relatively small size of the tendons located there. Over time, adhesions can develop, causing restricted movement of the tendon within its sheath. Not all tendons are encased by a synovial sheath. Some are encased by a peritendinous layering of thick tissue. Such inflammation is termed **peritendinitis.**[9] The signs and symptoms of tenosynovitis are similar to those of tendinitis, except that the pain tends to be more localized and crepitus is more pronounced.

The clinical grading of tendinitis is based on when symptoms occur:

- **First-degree tendinitis** is marked by pain and slight dysfunction during activity.
- **Second-degree tendinitis** results in decreased function and pain after activity.
- **Third-degree tendinitis** is characterized by constant pain that prohibits activity.

Prolonged tendinitis or a single traumatic force can result in a partial (part of the tendon is disrupted) or full (the tendon is completely disrupted) tearing of a tendon. An exception to this is in the rotator cuff tendons of the glenohumeral joint. These tears are termed partial-thickness or full-thickness tears, referring to the depth of the tear rather than to how much of the tendon is torn. Therefore, a full-thickness tear, although it penetrates through the depth of the tissue, may have part of the tendon still intact.

Calcium formation within the tendon, **calcific tendinitis,** may also develop with long-term tendinitis. The calcium build-up within the substance of the tendon causes pain with active contraction. Over time, it may lead to decreased range of motion and decreased strength.

Active range of motion may produce pain at the end of the range of motion, especially if the tendon meets a bony structure. Passive motion in the muscle's *antagonistic* direction results in pain as the tendon is stretched. The dynamic tension produced during resisted range of motion testing results in pain, decreasing the amount of force produced (Table 2–3).

Antagonistic   In the opposite direction of movement (e.g., the antagonistic motion of extension is flexion).

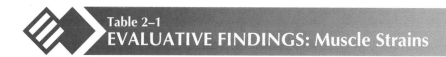

Table 2–1
EVALUATIVE FINDINGS: Muscle Strains

Examination Segment	Clinical Findings	
History	*Onset:*	Acute. Pain is located at the site of the injury, which tends to be at or near the junction between the muscle belly and tendon. The distal musculotendinous junction is most often involved.
	Pain characteristics:	Pain is located at the site of the injury, which tends to be at or near the junction between the muscle belly and tendon.
	Mechanism:	Strains usually result from a single episode of overstretching or overloading of the muscle but are more likely to result from eccentric loading.[7]
	Predisposing conditions:	Muscle tightness and improper warm-up before activity may predispose individuals to strain.
Inspection	Ecchymosis is evident in cases of severe muscle strains. Gravity causes the blood to pool distal to the site of trauma. Swelling may be present over the involved area. In severe cases, a defect may be visible in the muscle or tendon. If the strain involves a muscle of the lower extremity, the patient may walk with a limp.	
Palpation	Point tenderness exists over the site of the injury, with the degree of pain increasing with the severity of the injury. A defect or spasm may be palpable at the injury site.	
Range of motion	*AROM:*	Pain is elicited at the injury site. In the case of second- or third-degree strains, the patient may be unable to complete the movement.
	PROM:	Pain is elicited at the injury site during passive motion in the direction opposite that of the muscle, placing it on stretch.
	RROM:	Muscle strength is reduced. Pain increases as the amount of resistance is increased. Third-degree strains result in total a loss of function.

AROM = active range of motion; PROM = passive range of motion; RROM = resisted range of motion.

Table 2–2
MECHANISMS LEADING TO TENDINITIS

Mechanism	Implications
Microtrauma	Repetitive tensile loading, compression, and abrasion of the working tendons. Insufficient rest periods allow for the accumulation of the microtrauma, possible leading to tendon failure.
Macrotrauma	A single force placed on the muscle, causing discrete tearing within the tendon or at the musculotendinous junction. This area becomes the weak link when the forces of otherwise normal activity are sufficient to cause further inflammation.
Biomechanical alteration	The alteration of otherwise normal motion with redistribution of the forces around a joint, resulting in new tensile loads, compressive forces, or wearing of the tendons. Examples of this include running on uneven terrain or using poor technique with sporting equipment such as a tennis racquet.

Myositis Ossificans

Myositis ossificans is the formation of bone within a muscle belly's *fascia* and its intramuscular extensions close to the bone (Fig. 2–2).[10] The *etiology* of myositis ossificans can be traced to the genetic formation of abnormal tissue (myositis ossificans progressiva), neurologic disease, bloodborne disease (myositis ossificans circumscripta), or trauma (myositis ossificans traumatica). This text addresses only myositis ossificans traumatica.

Myositis ossificans occurs secondary to a traumatic injury such as a deep contusion or, less frequently, a muscle strain. Most commonly, the quadriceps femoris, hip adductor group, or biceps brachii muscles are affected.[10] The formation of the ossified area can be traced to an

Fascia A fibrous membrane that supports and separates muscles and unites the skin with the underlying tissues.

Etiology The cause of a disease (also the study of the causes of disease).

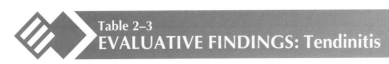

Table 2–3
EVALUATIVE FINDINGS: Tendinitis

Examination Segment	Clinical Findings	
History	***Onset:***	Occurs gradually or is chronic
	Pain characteristics:	Pain exists throughout the tendon.
	Mechanism:	Results from microtraumatic forces applied to the tendon
	Predisposing conditions:	History of muscle tightness, poor conditioning, increase in the frequency, duration, and/or intensity of training, changes in footwear or surfaces
Inspection	Swelling may be noted.	
	If the inflammation involves a tendon of the lower extremity, the patient may walk with a limp or demonstrate some other compensatory gait.	
	Inflammation involving the upper extremity results in abnormal movement patterns.	
	Many tendons are not directly visible or palpable.	
Palpation	The tendon is tender to the touch.	
	Crepitus or thickening of the tendon may be noted.	
Range of motion	***AROM:***	Pain in the tendon is possible throughout the range of motion as force is generated within the tendon.
	PROM:	Pain is elicited during the extremes of the range of motion as the tendon is stretched. Pain can be elicited earlier in the ROM in more severe cases.
	RROM:	Strength is decreased by pain. Pain is increased when the joint is isometrically stressed in its non–weight-bearing position.[8]

error in the body's healing process and a delay in the proper treatment of the initial trauma.[10,11] After the injury, fibroblasts begin to transform into *osteoblasts* and *chondroblasts*, giving rise to the formation of immature bone.

Calcification appears on radiographic examination approximately 3 weeks after the injury. As the size of the mass continues to expand, it becomes palpable. The joint's range of motion is affected as the bony mass impedes the muscle's ability to function (Table 2–4). For this reason, it

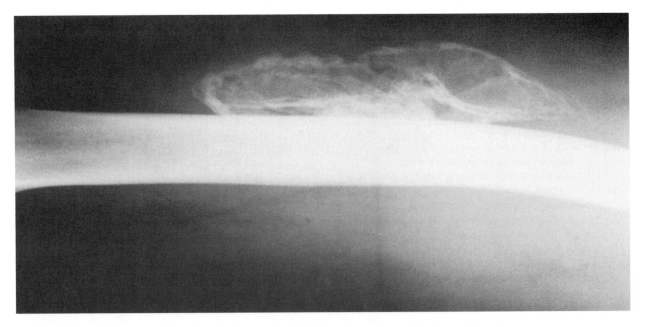

FIGURE 2–2. Radiograph of myositis ossificans. This calcification has occurred in the biceps brachii of a football lineman who sustained multiple blows to the muscle during the act of blocking.

Osteoblasts Cells concerned with the formation of new bone. **Chondroblasts** A cell that forms cartilage.

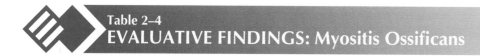

Table 2–4
EVALUATIVE FINDINGS: Myositis Ossificans

Examination Segment	Clinical Findings	
History	**Onset:**	The initial trauma is a **hematoma** caused by a single acute or repeated blows to the muscle. The ossification occurs gradually.
	Pain characteristics:	Pain occurs at the site of ossification, usually the site of a large muscle mass that is exposed to blows (e.g. the quadriceps femoris or biceps brachii muscles).
	Mechanism:	Calcium within the muscle fascia secondary to an abnormality in the healing process.
	Predisposing conditions:	History of myositis ossificans
Inspection	A superficial bruise may be noted. Edema of the distal joint closest to the site injury occurs. Ecchymosis may be present.	
Palpation	Acutely, the muscle is tender. As the ossification develops, it may become palpable within the muscle mass. Swelling and warmth may be felt at the site of injury. A fever may develop.[10]	
Range of motion	**AROM:**	As the ossification grows, the number of contractile units available to the muscle decreases. Antagonist motion is painful secondary to decreased flexibility within the affected muscle mass.
	PROM:	Decreased secondary to pain and adhesions within the muscle
	RROM:	Decreased secondary to pain; the ossification does not allow the muscle to contract normally
Special tests	Radiographic examination shows the ossification as it matures. A bone scan may be positive in the earlier stages.	

AROM = active range of motion; PROM = passive range of motion; RROM = resisted range of motion.

is very important to differentiate between muscle strains and contusions versus the formation of ossification.

Bursitis

Bursae are fluid-filled sacs that serve to buffer muscles, tendons, and ligaments from other friction-causing structures and facilitate smooth motion. Although common sites of bursa formation do exist, such as over the patella and olecranon process, bursae develop over areas where they are needed to reduce friction. Normally, bursae cannot be specifically palpated unless they are inflamed. The triggering event causing bursitis is irritation of the bursal sac secondary to a disease state, increased stress, friction, or a single traumatic force that activates the inflammatory process.

The clinical findings of bursitis depend on the location of the involved structure. Bursae that are immediately subcutaneous can enlarge greatly. However, the swelling remains localized within the sac. Often the underlying joint can be moved without causing pain. Bursae separating tendinous, bony, or ligamentous tissues often cause exquisite pain during all forms of joint movements, possibly limiting the degree of motion available to the joint.

Bursal inflammation can also be the result of local or systemic infection. Lacerations, abrasions, or puncture wounds entering a bursa can introduce an infectious agent, resulting in the subsequent enlargement of the bursa. A *staphylococcal infection* can localize within a bursa, producing symptoms resembling an overuse syndrome. Bursal infections may be accompanied by red streaks along the extremity and enlarged proximal lymph nodes. An analysis of the bursal fluid is required to determine the cause of the bursitis (Table 2–5).[12]

JOINT STRUCTURE INJURIES

The most prevalent soft tissue injuries involving the joint structures are those involving the capsular and ligamentous tissues.[13,14] Ligamentous injury to the knee, elbow, and shoulder are also quite prevalent. These injuries directly affect the **joint's stability** manner during movement.

Hematoma   A collection of clotted blood within a confined space (hemat = blood; oma = tumor).

Staphylococcal infection   An infection caused by the *Staphylococcus* bacteria.

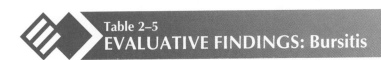

Table 2–5
EVALUATIVE FINDINGS: Bursitis

Examination Segment	Clinical Findings	
History	*Onset:*	Acute in the case of direct trauma to the bursa; insidious in the case of overuse or infection.
	Pain characteristics:	Pain occurring at the site of the bursal sac.
	Mechanism:	**Chemical:** Calcium or other chemical deposits within the bursa activating the inflammatory response.
		Mechanical: Repetitive rubbing of the soft tissue over a bony prominence or a direct blow, possibly related to improper biomechanics.
		Septic: Viral or bacterial invasion of the bursa.
	Predisposing conditions:	Improper biomechanics, poor padding of at-risk bursae (e.g., suprapatellar bursa, olecranon bursa).
Inspection	Local swelling of bursae can be very pronounced, especially those located over the olecranon process and patella.	
	Chronic or septic bursitis may appear red.	
Palpation	Point tenderness is noted over the site of the bursa.	
	Localized heat and swelling may be noted.	
Range of motion	*AROM:*	Pain may be noted.
	PROM:	Pain is produced if the motion causes the tendon or other structure to rub across the inflamed bursa.
	RROM:	Pain limits RROM. As the muscle contracts, it compresses the bursal sac.

Sprains

Sprains occur when a joint is forced beyond its normal anatomical limits, resulting in the stretching or tearing of the ligaments, joint capsule, or both. Although ligaments are commonly thought of and presented as discrete structures, they are often thickened areas within the joint capsule. When torn, the ligaments that are within the joint capsule or part of the joint capsule produce more swelling than the ligaments that are *extracapsular* because of the associated disruption of the capsule (Table 2–6).

The three degrees of sprains, based on the amount of laxity produced by the injury relative to the opposite limb are as follows (see also Table 1–7):

- **First-degree sprain:** The ligament is stretched with little or no tearing of its fibers. No abnormal motion is produced when the joint is stressed, and a firm *end-point* is felt. Local pain, mild point tenderness, and slight swelling of the joint are present.
- **Second-degree sprain:** Partial tearing of the ligament's fibers has occurred, resulting in joint laxity when the ligament is stressed. A soft but definite end-point is present. Moderate pain and swelling occur and a loss of the joint's function is noted.
- **Third-degree sprain:** The ligament has been completely ruptured, causing gross joint laxity, possible instability, and an empty or absent end-point. Swelling is marked, but pain may be limited secondary to tearing of the local nerves. A complete loss of function of the joint is usually noted.

Joint Subluxation

A subluxation involves the partial or complete disassociation of the joint's articulating surfaces that may spontaneously return to their normal alignments. The amount of force required to displace the bones is often sufficient to cause soft tissue or bony injury. Stretching and tearing of the joint capsule and ligaments and bony fractures must be suspected after a subluxation.

Subluxating joints are a progressive condition in which each subluxation predisposes the joint to subsequent episodes resulting from stretching of the supporting structures. All first-time subluxations must be evaluated by a physician, who should indicate how to manage subsequent subluxations of the joint.

Clinically, joint subluxations are often identified by a reported history of the "joint's going out and then popping back in." The joint's range of motion is limited by pain and instability. Chronically, the joint displays instability during ligamentous and capsular testing. These tests may produce an **apprehension response,** meaning that the patient displays anxiety that a specific test will cause the joint to again subluxate (Table 2–7).

Extracapsular Outside of the joint capsule.

End-point The quality and quantity at the end of motion for any stress applied to a tissue.

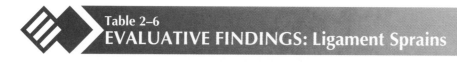

Table 2–6
EVALUATIVE FINDINGS: Ligament Sprains

Examination Segment	Clinical Findings	
History	*Onset:*	Acute
	Pain characteristics:	Pain is localized to the site of injury with first-degree sprains. As the severity of the sprain increases, the pain is radiated throughout the joint. A "popping" sensation or sound may be reported by the patient.
	Mechanism:	Sprains result from tensile forces caused by the stretching of the ligament.
	Predisposing conditions:	A history of a sprain can predispose the ligament to further injury. Shoe wear that increases the friction between the shoe–surface interface may increase the chance of lower extremity sprains. Women have a greater risk of some knee ligament sprains, but the exact cause has not been determined.
Inspection	Swelling of the joint is evident. Ecchymosis may form at and distal to the site of injury.	
Palpation	Point tenderness is noted over the ligament. The entire joint may be tender.	
Functional tests	*AROM:*	Limited by pain in the direction that stresses the involved ligament (or ligaments)
	PROM:	Limited by pain, especially in the direction that stresses the involved ligament (or ligaments)
	RROM:	Manual resistance throughout the ROM is painful. Isometric contractions may not produce as intense pain.
Ligamentous tests	The ligament can be stressed by producing a force through the joint that causes the ligament to stretch. The examiner should note the amount of increased laxity compared with the opposite side, as well as the quality of the end-point. The end-point should be distinct and crisp. A soft, "mushy," or absent end-point is a sign of ligamentous rupture.	
Special tests	These are determined by the particular joint being examined.	

AROM = active range of motion; PROM = passive range of motion; ROM = range of motion; RROM = resisted range of motion.

Table 2–7
EVALUATIVE FINDINGS: Joint Subluxations

Examination Segment	Clinical Findings	
History	*Onset:*	Acute or chronic. Chronic subluxation can occur as the joint's supportive structures are progressively stretched.
	Pain characteristics:	Pain occurs throughout the involved joint. Associated muscle spasm may involve the muscles proximal and distal to the joint.
	Mechanism:	Joint subluxation results from a stress that takes the joint beyond its normal anatomical limits.
	Predisposing conditions:	History of joint subluxation; congenital hyperlaxity
Inspection	Swelling may be present. No gross bony deformity is noted because the joint relocates.	
Palpation	Pain elicited along the tissues that have been stretched or compressed.	
Functional tests	*AROM:*	Possibly limited owing to pain and possible instability.
	PROM:	Possibly limited owing to pain and possible instability.
	RROM:	Muscular strength is decreased secondary to pain and joint instability.
Ligamentous tests	Pain is elicited during stress testing of the involved ligament (or ligaments). Laxity of the tissues is present, particularly post-acutely. The patient may note instability and react to guard against this by contracting the surrounding musculature or pulling away, an apprehension response.	
Special tests	These vary according to the body part being tested.	

AROM = active range of motion; PROM = passive range of motion; RROM = resisted range of motion.

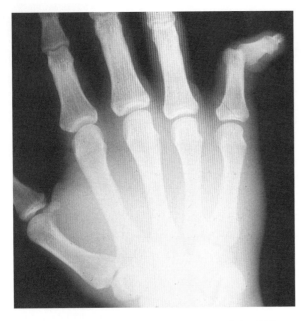

FIGURE 2–3. Radiograph of a dislocation of the fifth proximal interphalangeal joint (PIP joint).

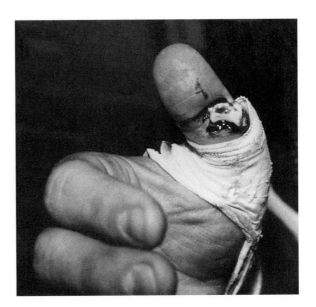

FIGURE 2–4. Open dislocation of the thumb's interphalangeal joint. Note the glossy appearance of the proximal articular surface. There appears to be a defect of the hyaline cartilage on the ulnar side of the bone.

Joint Dislocation

Dislocations involve the disassociation of the joint's articulating surfaces caused by forces that rupture many of the joint's soft tissue restraints. Joint dislocations result in obvious deformity and therefore normally do not require any evaluative tests (Fig. 2–3). In some instances, the dislocation may cause the joint surfaces to protrude through the skin (Fig. 2–4).

Because of the inherent risk of injury to bony, vascular, neurologic, or other soft tissue structures, reduction of the dislocation should not be attempted before radiographic examination. The reduction procedure should be performed by a physician. When a major joint (e.g., the shoulder, knee, ankle) is dislocated, the presence of the distal pulse and the normal sensory distribution of the involved extremity must be established (Table 2–8). Dislocations of major joints are medical emergencies. The possible involvement of the neurovascular structures increases the urgency for prompt medical treatment.

Table 2–8
EVALUATIVE FINDINGS: Joint Dislocations

Examination Segment	Clinical Findings	
History	*Onset:*	Acute or chronic. Chronic dislocation as the joint's supportive structures are progressively stretched
	Pain characteristics:	At the involved joint
	Mechanism:	Dislocation caused by a stress that forces the joint beyond its normal anatomical limits
Inspection	Gross joint deformity may be present and swelling is observed.	
Palpation	Pain is elicited throughout the joint. Malalignment of the joint surfaces may be felt.	
Functional tests	ROM is not possible because of the disruption of the joint's alignment.	
Ligamentous tests	These are contraindicated when the joint is dislocated.	
Special tests	Except for checking neurovascular injury, these are contraindicated when the joint is dislocated.	
Neurologic tests	Sensory distribution distal to the dislocated joint must be established.	
Comments	Dislocations of the major joints represent medical emergencies. The presence of the distal pulse must be established. A lack of circulation to the distal extremity threatens the viability of the body part.	

ROM = range of motion.

Table 2–9
EVALUATIVE FINDINGS: Capsular Synovitis

Examination Segment	Clinical Findings	
History	***Onset:***	Insidious; often subsequent to a previous injury to the joint
	Pain characteristics:	Pain occurring throughout the entire joint, causing aching at rest and increased pain with activity
	Mechanism:	Synovitis often begins folllowing an injury to a joint. The resulting inflammatory reaction triggers inflammation within the synovium.
	Predisposing conditions:	Underlying pathology within the joint
Inspection	The joint may appear swollen.	
	The patient may move the joint in a guarded manner.	
	Joints affected by synovitis do not appear red.	
	Presistent synovitis can result in muscle ***atrophy*** secondary to pain and decreased joint ROM.	
Palpation	Warmth may be felt.	
	A "boggy" swelling is present.	
	No distinct area of point tenderness is usually present.	
Functional tests	***AROM:***	Limitations exist within the ***capsular pattern*** of the joint.
	PROM:	Normally, this is greater than AROM but is still limited by pain.
	RROM:	Weakness secondary to muscle guarding
Ligamentous tests	In the absence of underlying pathology to the ligaments, the ligamentous test result is negative. Pain may be elicited by stretching the inflamed tissues.	
Special tests	Same findings are produced as for ligamentous testing	
Comments	The signs and symptoms of synovitis may mimic those of an infected joint.	

AROM = active range of motion; PROM = passive range of motion; ROM = range of motion; RROM = resisted range of motion.

Synovitis

The inflammation of a joint's capsule often occurs secondary to the presence of existing inflammation in or around the joint that spreads to the *synovial membrane* (Fig. 2–5). The patient complains of "bogginess" within the joint and tends to hold it in a position that applies the least amount of stress on the capsule's fibers (usually a position between the extremes of the joint's range of motion). The remaining signs and symptoms of synovitis are similar to those of bursitis, but the swelling is more diffuse (Table 2–9).

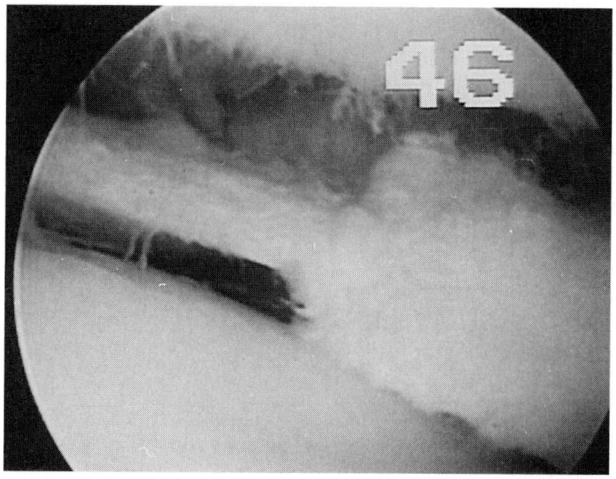

ARTICULAR SURFACE INJURIES

The articular or *hyaline cartilage* lining a bone's joint surface may be acutely injured or damaged as the result of degenerative changes caused by aging. Most of these injuries are irreversible and result in chronic joint pain, dysfunction, or both.

FIGURE 2–5. Illustration of synovitis of the knee joint capsule. The hairlike strands emerging from the top border of the joint represent inflammation of the synovial capsule.

Atrophy   A wasting or decrease in the size of a muscle or organ.

Capsular pattern   A pattern of decreased motion associated with injury of a joint's capsular tissue. Capsular patterns are specific to each joint.

Synovial membrane   The membrane lining a fluid-filled joint.

Hyaline cartilage   Cartilage found on the articular surface of bones, especially suited to withstand compressive and shearing forces.

Table 2–10
EVALUATIVE FINDINGS: Osteochondral Defects

Examination Segment	Clinical Findings	
History	**Onset:**	Acute or insidious
	Pain characteristics:	Complaints of pain in the joint during weight-bearing activities, depending on the site of the defect, the entire joint may be painful secondary to a synovial reaction (see Synovitis)
	Mechanism:	Acute: A rotational or **axial load** placed on two opposing joint surfaces. The resulting friction results in a tearing away of the cartilage. Chronic: A progressive degeneration of the articular cartilage.
	Predisposing conditions:	None
Inspection	Effusion is present.	
Palpation	The joint line may be tender from the defect, but the defect itself is usually not palpable. Tenderness may also be caused by synovitis.	
Functional tests	**AROM:**	Limited owing to pain and swelling
	PROM:	Increased relative to the AROM but still limited by pain and swelling
	RROM:	Decreased strength occurs, secondary to pain.
Special tests	The defect may be present on standard radiographic examination. Better imaging is obtained through the use of MRI.	

AROM = active range of motion; MRI = magnetic resonance imaging; PROM = passive range of motion; ROM = range of motion; RROM = resisted range of motion.

Osteochondral Defects

Fractures of a bone's articular cartilage and the progressive softening of this cartilage are collectively referred to as osteochondral defects (OCDs). The severity of an OCD is based on the depth of the defect. Partial-thickness OCDs involve the outer layering of the articular cartilage. Full-thickness OCDs expose the underlying bone (Fig. 2–6). As the depth of the defect increases, the stresses applied to the underlying bone are increased, resulting in pain during activity. The amount of disability found after an OCD also depends on the location of the defect on the articular surface. If the defect is located in an area of high joint forces, the disability secondary to pain is increased (Table 2–10).

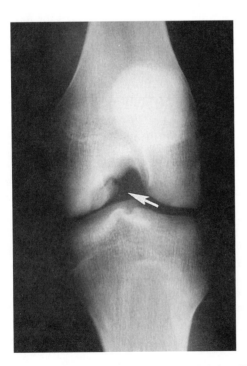

FIGURE 2–6. Radiograph of an osteochondral defect. Note the small fracture line on the medial portion of the trochanteric groove.

OSTEOCHONDRITIS DISSECANS

Characterized by dislodged fragments of bone within the joint space, osteochondritis dissecans is a lesion of the bone and articular cartilage resulting in the delamination of the subchondral bone. Osteochondritis dissecans is categorized into two groups based on the age of onset. **Juvenile osteochondritis dissecans** affects patients younger than age 15 years, and **adult osteochondritis dissecans** affects patients age 15 years or older.[15] Osteochondritis dissecans can affect most joints, but the talus, femur, patella, capitellum, and humeral head are most frequently affected.

The bony fragment may be stable within the joint or free floating within the joint space, where it can cause

Axial load A force applied through the long axis of a bone or series of bones.

Table 2–11
EVALUATIVE FINDINGS: Osteochondritis Dissecans

Examination Segment	Clinical Findings	
History	**Onset:**	Insidious or acute
	Pain characteristics:	Pain occurring within the joint, increasing with motion and possibly absent when the joint is at rest
	Mechanism:	Insidious: Progressive degeneration of the joint structures. Acute: Trauma causing a piece of bone or cartilage to break free and enter the joint space.
Inspection	Swelling around the joint may be noted. The patient tends to hold the joint in a pain-free position.	
Palpation	The affected joint may feel warm secondary to inflammation. Pain may become specific on palpation along the joint line.	
Functional tests	AROM, PROM and RROM may be reduced secondary to the loose body's lodging between the joint surfaces, creating a mechanical block against movement.	
	AROM:	May be limited by pain, **contracture**, or locking secondary to a loose body
	PROM:	May be limited by pain, contracture, or locking secondary to a loose body
	RROM:	May be limited by pain or contracture
Comments	Osteochondritis dissecans is categorized by the age of onset, juvenile (under age 15 years) and adult (age 15 years or older).	

AROM = active range of motion; PROM = passive range of motion; RROM = resisted range of motion.

greater problems of pain, loss of range of motion, and decreased joint function (Fig. 2–7). The underlying cause resulting in the destruction of bone has been proposed to be *ischemia,* trauma, and degenerative changes.[16–18]

The chief complaints include increasing pain, episodes of the joint "locking," and an inability to function. The onset is usually not related to any specific trauma. The complaints of pain are usually specific to the area of the affected joint. As the condition progresses, the joint's range of motion decreases and the patient's ability to produce forceful contractions of the surrounding muscles declines (Table 2–11).

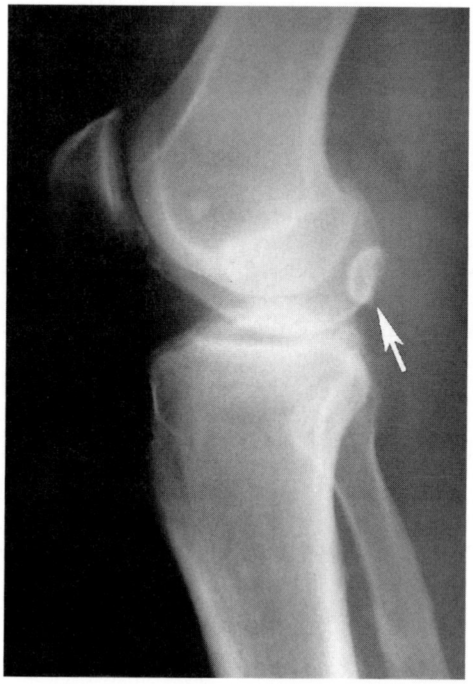

Arthritis

Although there are several causes for arthritis, the degeneration of a joint's articular surface, the most common type found in athletes, is **osteoarthritis.** This chronic condition most often affects the body's weight-bearing joints, especially the knees. With time, the articular surfaces begin to degenerate, and the regenerative process causes bony outgrowths on what should be an otherwise smooth surface (Fig. 2–8). This degeneration of the articular cartilage can eventually lead to the complete destruction of the cartilage and the exposure of the subchondral bone. Flaking pieces of bone can result in loose bodies and chronic synovitis.

The outward signs and symptoms of osteoarthritis depend on the duration of the condition. Acute cases present with minimal swelling and redness. Typically, the chief complaint is pain during joint motion while the joint surfaces are compressed. When the problem

FIGURE 2–7. Radiograph of a free-floating body in the joint space.

Contracture A pathological shortening of tissues causing a decrease in available motion.

Ischemia Local and temporary deficiency of blood supply caused by the obstruction of blood flow to a body area.

Table 2–12
EVALUATIVE FINDINGS: Arthritis

Examination Segment	Clinical Findings	
History	***Onset:***	Insidious
	Pain characteristics:	Pain occurs throughout the involved joint.
	Mechanism:	Osteoarthritis develops secondary to trauma and irregular biomechanical stresses' being placed across the joint.
		Rheumatoid arthritis is caused by a systemic disorder that activates an inflammatory response in the body's joints.
	Predisposing conditions:	For osteoarthritis, previous trauma to the joint has occurred. Rheumatoid arthritis is associated with a family history of the disorder. Certain occupations and obesity may overload the joints, causing increased forces over time.
Inspection	In chronic cases, gross deformity of the joint is noticed. Individuals with cases of shorter duration present with swelling.	
	When arthritis affects the joints of the lower extremity, an ***antalgic*** gait is produced.	
Palpation	Warmth and swelling are identified in the affected joint.	
	The articular surfaces, when and where palpable, are tender to the touch.	
Functional tests	***AROM:***	May be limited by pain, often becoming contractured as the condition progresses
	PROM:	These findings are equal to those of AROM testing.
	RROM:	This is decreased secondary to pain.
Ligamentous tests	Test results may be positive if a deformity has developed, causing the stressed capsule and ligaments to elongate over time.	
Special tests	Radiographic examination and other imaging techniques show degenerative changes within the joint.	

AROM = active range of motion; PROM = passive range of motion; RROM = resisted range of motion.

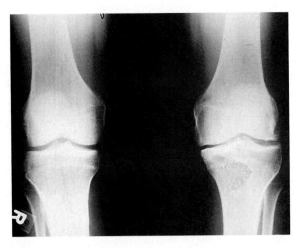

FIGURE 2–8. Radiograph of an arthritic joint. Note the loss of definition in the joint space of the left knee (on the right above).

becomes chronic, the patient suffers from unremitting pain and the inability to function. The affected area may be marked by obvious deformity (Table 2–12).

Rheumatoid arthritis is a systemic condition that affects the articular cartilages of multiple joints. As this condition worsens, the joints appear to be hard and nodular, with even simple movement resulting in pro-

found pain. The patient often has a family history of rheumatoid arthritis and his or her hand and multiple other joints are affected. Additionally, the patient may experience associated medical complications from the disease.

◆ BONY INJURIES

Bony injuries tend to be more traumatic than soft tissue injuries because of the large forces causing the fracture. In cases of acute fractures to the *long bones*, the ribs, and the spine, proper initial management of the injury must be used to minimize the chance of a permanent, possibly fatal, disability.

Injuries to bones of the pediatric and adolescent populations bring a unique set of challenges to the evaluation. The presence of *growth plates* as a weak link in

Antalgic   Having a pain-relieving quality; analgesic.

Long bones   A bone possessing a base, shaft, and head.

Growth plates   The area of bone growth in skeletally immature individuals; the epiphyseal plate.

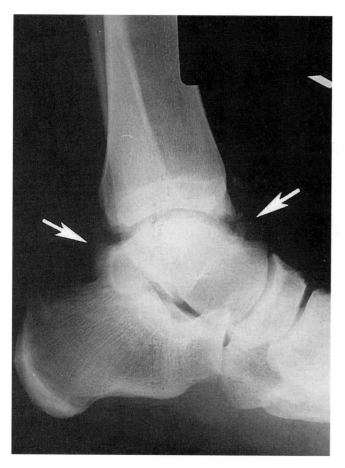

FIGURE 2–9. Radiograph of exostosis of the subtalar joint.

the skeleton presents problems in traumatic fractures and overuse injuries. Always be cognizant of the potential for growth plate injury in these populations.

EXOSTOSIS

Wolff's law states that a bone remodels itself in response to forces placed on it, a naturally occurring phenomenon that allows bones to adapt and become stronger.[19] Growth of extraneous bone, exostosis, can occur as a stress reaction from injury or from irregular forces being placed on the bone (Fig. 2–9). The bone develops an exostosis at the site of the stress that may become painful and, in some cases, forms a mechanical block against movement (Table 2–13).

APOPHYSITIS

Sometimes termed "growing pains," apophysitis is an inflammatory condition involving a bone's growth plate. In adolescents, the growth plate represents the weak link along the bone. Some of these growth areas serve as, or are close to, the attachment sites for the larger, stronger muscle groups in the body. Tightness of these muscles or repetitive forces applied to the bone by these muscles can result in inflammation and the eventual separation of these areas away from the rest of the bone (Fig. 2–10).

Apophysitis often includes a history of a recent rapid growth spurt. As the skeleton rapidly matures, the muscular tissues do not fully adapt to the new bone

Table 2–13
EVALUATIVE FINDINGS: Exostosis

Examination Segment	Clinical Findings	
History	**Onset:**	Insidious
	Pain characteristics:	Exostosis involving the extremities most often results in the localization of pain and other symptoms.
		Spinal exostosis can result in pain being referred along the distribution of affected nerve roots.
	Mechanism:	Exostosis is the result of repeated strain placed on a bone or the bony insertion of a tendon.
	Predisposing conditions:	Previous trauma to the area
Inspection	Deformity may be noted over the site of pain.	
Palpation	Point tenderness is present. A defect, in the form of a bony outgrowth, may be palpable.	
Functional tests	**AROM:** Limited secondary to pain and/or bony block	
	PROM: Equal to AROM	
	RROM: Reduced secondary to pain and/or bony block	

AROM = active range of motion; PROM = passive range of motion; RROM = resisted range of motion.

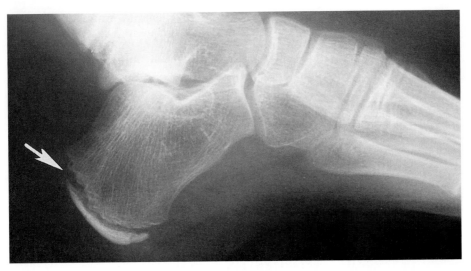

FIGURE 2–10. Radiograph of calcaneal apophysitis.

length and apply increased stress to the growth plate. Lack of flexibility may be a contributing cause, but after apophysitis has occurred, the flexibility of the muscle group attaching to the site further decreases. Resistance exercises (e.g., weight lifting) result in pain as the forces generated are transmitted to the affected area.

FRACTURES

Classification schemes of bony fractures are based on the location of the fracture relative to the rest of the bone (Box 2–1); the magnitude of the fracture line or lines (Box 2–2); the shape and direction of the fracture (Box 2–3); and the fracture's duration of onset. Although it is common practice, the use of relatively nondescriptive terms (e.g., boxer's fracture: fracture of the fourth or fifth metacarpal) or the identification of a fracture type by an individual's name (e.g., Colles' fracture: fracture of the distal radius that is displaced dorsally) tends to become corrupted over time and may be less accurate.

Avulsion Fractures

Avulsion fractures involve the tearing away of a ligament's or tendon's bony attachment (Fig. 2–11). Except for the case of large tendons (e.g., the patellar tendon), this injury may easily be missed because of the relatively small fracture site and the similarity to sprains or strains and their mechanisms. Tendon avulsions can also occur if a muscle is forcefully contracted and the attachment site is pulled away from the rest of the bone. When large tendons are involved, obvious deformity results as the tendon recoils from the fracture site. With smaller tendons or ligaments, pain is described at the fracture site and point tenderness is elicited. The stress testing of the joint may display the signs and symptoms of a third-degree sprain or strain.

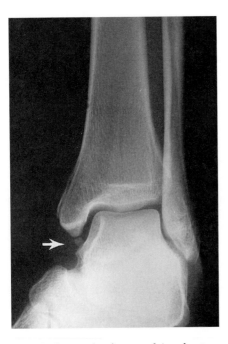

FIGURE 2–11. Radiograph of an avulsion fracture of the attachment of the deltoid ligament.

Diaphysis   The shaft of a long bone.

Prognosis   The course that a disease or injury is expected to take.

Epiphyseal line   The area of growth found between the diaphysis and epiphysis in immature long bones.

Box 2–1

TERMINOLOGY USED TO DESCRIBE THE FRACTURE LOCATION

Diaphyseal fractures involve only the bone's *diaphysis* and are associated with a good *prognosis* for recovery, barring any extenuating circumstances.

Epiphyseal fractures involve the fracture line crossing the bone's unsealed *epiphyseal line* and can have long-term consequences by disrupting the bone's normal growth. Epiphyseal fractures may mimic soft tissue injuries by resembling joint laxity during stress testing.

Articular fractures disrupt the joint's articular cartilage, which, if improperly healed, results in pain and decreased range of motion and can lead to arthritis of the joint.

Box 2–2

TERMINOLOGY USED TO DESCRIBE THE RELATIVE SEVERITY OF THE FRACTURE LINE

Fracture lines not completely disassociating the proximal end of the bone from its distal end are described as **incomplete fractures.**

Fracture lines with complete disassociation between the two ends of the bone are termed **undisplaced fractures** if the two ends of the bone maintain their relative alignment to each other.

The loss of alignment between the two segments is termed a **displaced fracture** and may jeopardize the surrounding tissues.

When a displaced fracture exits the skin, and **open fracture** (compound fracture) occurs.

Box 2–3
TERMINOLOGY USED TO DESCRIBE THE SHAPE OF THE FRACTURE LINE

Depressed fractures occur from direct trauma to flat bones, causing the bone to fracture and depress.

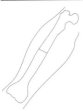

Transverse fractures are caused by a direct blow, **shear force,** or tensile force being applied to the shaft of a long bone and result in a fracture line that crosses the bone's long axis.

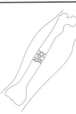

A **comminuted fracture** can result from extremely high-velocity impact forces leading to the shattering of bone into multiple pieces. This type of fracture often requires surgical correction.

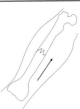

A **compacted fracture** results from **compressive forces** placed through the long axis of the bone. One end of a fractured segment is driven into the opposite piece of the fracture, often leading to a shortening of the involved limb.

A **spiral fracture** results from a rotational force placed on the shaft of a long bone, such as twisting the tibia while the foot remains fixated. The fracture line assumes an S-shape along the length of the bone.

Longitudinal fractures, which most commonly occur as the result of a fall, have a fracture line that runs parallel to the bone's long axis.

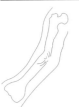

Greenstick fractures, generally specific to the pediatric and adolescent population, involve a displaced fracture on one side of the bone and a compacted fracture on the opposite side. The name is derived from an analogy to an immature tree branch that has been snapped.

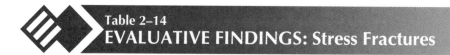

Table 2-14
EVALUATIVE FINDINGS: Stress Fractures

Examination Segment	Clinical Findings	
History	*Onset:*	Insidious; the patient cannot report a single traumatic event causing the pain
	Pain characteristics:	Pain tends to radiate from the involved bone but may become diffuse.
	Mechansim:	Cumulative microtrauma causes stress fractures.
	Predisposing conditions:	Overtraining, poor conditioning, and improper training techniques may be noted.
Inspection	Usually no bony abnormality is noted. Soft tissue swelling and redness may be present.	
Palpation	Point tenderness exists over the fracture site.	
Functional tests	All motions are generally within normal limits.	
Special tests	Long bone compression test Percussion along the length of the bone Bone scans or other imaging techniques	

Stress Fractures

Although stress fractures most commonly occur in the lower extremities, this condition can be found in any bone that absorbs repetitive stress. [20,21] Stress fractures present as a complex injury because of their nondescript initial findings and their tendency to mimic the signs and symptoms of soft tissue injuries. Stress fractures occur when the bone's osteoclastic activity outweighs osteoblastic activity, causing a weakened area along the line of stress. If the external stress is not reduced (e.g., the patient continues running), the bone eventually fails.

The history reveals a chronic condition caused by repetitive stresses to the involved area. There may have been a recent change in the patient's workout routine, including changes in equipment, playing surfaces, frequency, duration, or intensity. Because of the related reduction in levels of estrogen and progesterone, *amenorrheic* women may be predisposed to developing stress fractures.[22] With specific palpation, an area of exact tenderness can be discerned along any bony surface. Compression of long bones may result in increased pain (Table 2–14).

 ### NEUROVASCULAR PATHOLOGIES

Trauma to the neurovascular structures (i.e., nerves, arteries, and veins) is often a consequence of joint dislocation, bony displacement, or concussive forces. If untreated, vascular disruption can lead to the loss of the affected body part. Neurologic inhibition can lead to the loss of function in the involved part.

PERIPHERAL NERVE INJURY

Entrapment injuries to the peripheral nerves are common at the ankle, elbow, wrist, and cervical spine. Peripheral nerves located more distally from the spinal column have a greater probability of regeneration than a lesion that occurs more proximal to the CNS.

In some cases, nonneurologic tissue or swelling entraps the nerve, causing dysfunction in the form of paresthesia and muscular weakness. This condition is most commonly seen at the ulnar tunnel, pronator teres muscle, carpal tunnel, and tarsal tunnel. In each case, the complaints are of specific pain patterns and paresthesia. With careful manual muscle testing, muscle weakness may be elicited. Although these syndromes may be suspected on evaluation, they are confirmed through electrodiagnostic testing.

Stretch injuries to peripheral nerves may be divided into three categories based on the pathology and the prognosis for recovery. *Neurapraxia* is the mildest form of peripheral nerve stretch injury. The nerve, *epineurium,* and *myelin sheath* are stretched but remain intact. Symptoms are usually transient and include

---

Shear forces Forces from opposing directions that are applied perpendicular to a structure's long axis.

Compressive forces A force applied along the length of a structure, causing the tissues to more closely approximate one another.

Amenorrheic (amenorrhea) The absence of menstruation.

Neurapraxia A stretch injury to a nerve resulting in transient symptoms of paraesthesia and weakness.

Epineurium Connective tissue containing blood vessels surrounding the trunk of a nerve, binding it together.

Myelin sheath A fatty-based lining of the axon of myelinated nerve fibers.

burning, pain, numbness, and temporary weakness on clinical evaluation.

Axonotmesis involves a disruption of the axon and the myelin sheath, but the epineurium remains intact. The signs and symptoms are the same as for neurapraxia, but axonotmesis has a longer duration. Because the axon undergoes *wallerian degeneration,* the return of normal innervation is unpredictable and sustained weakness may be experienced.

Neurotmesis, a complete disruption of the nerve, is the most severe form of peripheral nerve injury. The prognosis for the return of normal innervation is poor. This injury occurs under extremely high forces and usually entails *concurrent* injury to bones, ligaments, and tendons. Many times a nerve *graft* or tendon transfer is required to return function to the extremity. These procedures meet with limited success and are not conducive to the return to competitive athletics.

COMPLEX REGIONAL PAIN SYNDROME (REFLEX SYMPATHETIC DYSTROPHY)

Complex regional pain syndrome (CRPS), also known as reflex sympathetic *dystrophy* (RSD), is an exaggerated, generalized pain response after injury, involving intense or unduly prolonged pain that is out of proportion to the severity of the injury, *vasomotor* disturbances, delayed functional recovery, and various associated *trophic* changes.[23] Although CRPS is definitively diagnosed by a physician, the clinician must be aware of the common early findings so a timely referral can be made. These findings may include:

- Pain that is disproportionately increased relative to the severity of the injury
- Superficial hypersensitive areas (e.g., pain when clothing touches the skin)
- Edema
- Decreased motor function, leading to dystrophy
- Muscle spasm
- Dermatologic alterations, including the integrity of the skin, skin temperature changes, hair loss, and changes in the nailbed
- Vasomotor instability: *Raynaud's phenomenon, vasoconstriction, vasodilation, hyperhydrosis*
- Skeletal changes, including *osteoporosis*

The prognosis for patients with CRPS is extremely variable, but early intervention appears to improve the probability of a favorable outcome, making early recognition and referral a priority. Intervention includes rehabilitation with modalities and therapeutic exercise.[24] Symptomatic relief can be obtained through the use of various medications, including narcotics, central nervous system depressants, epidural injections, and muscle relaxants to reduce sympathetic activity.[23,25] In unyielding cases, surgical dissection of the nerve may be required to prevent the pain causing nerve transmission.[25]

◆ IMAGING TECHNIQUES

Various forms of imaging techniques used to view the body's subcutaneous structures are referenced throughout this text. Although the physician orders and subsequently interprets these results, a knowledge of the application of these techniques is valuable to the clinician. Table 2–15 presents these imaging techniques and their most advantageous uses.

RADIOGRAPHS

The most common imaging technique used in the evaluation of orthopedic injuries is radiography, or x-ray examinations (Fig. 2–12). Discovered in 1895, the use of x-rays marked the first time in the history of medicine that the internal structures could be viewed without invasive techniques.[26] Before this, the only method of viewing the internal structures was to actually cut the individual open.

Radiographic examination uses *ionizing radiation* to penetrate the body. Depending on the density of the

---

Wallerian degeneration Degeneration of a nerve's axon that has been severed from the body of the nerve.

Neurotmesis Complete loss of nerve function with little apparent anatomic damage to the nerve itself.

Concurrent Occurring at the same time.

Graft An organ or tissue used for transplantation. An allograft is a donor tissue transplanted from the same species. An autograft tissue is transplanted from within the same individual.

Dystrophy The progressive deterioration of tissue.

Vasomotor Pertaining to nerves controlling the muscles within the walls of blood vessels.

Trophic Pertaining to efferent nerves controlling the nourishment of the area they innervate.

Raynaud's phenomenon A reaction to cold consisting of bouts of pallor and cyanosis, causing exaggerated vasomotor responses.

Vasoconstriction A decrease in a vessel's diameter.

Vasodilation An increase in a vessel's diameter.

Hyperhydrosis Excessive or profuse sweating.

Osteoporosis Decreased bone density common in postmenopausal women.

Ionizing radiation Electromagnetic energy that causes the release of an atom's protons, electrons, or neutrons. Ionizing radiation is potentially hazardous to human tissue.

Table 2–15
SELECTED IMAGING TECHNIQUES AND THEIR USE IN DIAGNOSING ORTHOPEDIC AND ATHLETIC INJURIES

Technique	Best Use
Radiography	Standard: Bone lesions, joint surfaces, and joint spaces Arthrogram: Capsular tissue tears and articular cartilage lesions Myelogram: Pathologies within the spinal canal
CT	Bony or articular cartilage lesions and some soft tissue lesions, especially when quantifying detailed lesions (e.g., size and location; useful in identifying tendinous and ligamentous injuries in varying joint positions)
MRI	Soft tissue structures, especially ligamentous and meniscal injuries
Bone scan	Acute bony change determination but may produce false-positive findings, especially in endurance athletes
Ultrasonic imaging	Tendon and other soft tissue imaging

CT = computed tomography; MRI = magnetic resonance imaging.

The interpretation of radiographic images can be simplistically based on the ABCs method:[27]

- **A–Alignment:** The clinician observes for the normal continuity of the bones and joint surfaces and the alignment of one bone to another.
- **B–Bones:** Bones should have normal density patterns, presenting with uniform color throughout the bone as compared bilaterally. Areas of decreased density appear as darkened areas within the bone. Fractures and abnormal bony outgrowths such as exostosis can also be visualized.
- **C–Cartilage:** Although cartilage itself does not produce a radiographic image, the cartilage and ligamentous structures are inspected for what does not appear. The joint spaces should be smooth and uniform.
- **S–Soft tissue:** Although soft tissue cannot be imaged, swelling within the confines of the soft tissue or between the soft tissue and the bones can be determined. Additionally, the outline of soft tissues and even pockets of edema within soft tissue can be identified with adjusted exposure techniques.

Assessment of a joint's ligamentous integrity often requires the use of imaging techniques, during which stress is applied to a joint to measure the amount of laxity, a stress radiograph (Fig. 2–13). This requires application of a force that stretches the ligament during the x-ray exposure, allowing for the measurement of excessive motion, determining a third-degree ligament injury, or ascertaining the amount of overall joint laxity.

Other forms of radiographic screening involve the use of radio-opaque dyes that are absorbed by the tissues, allowing visualization by radiographic examination. Collectively known as **contrast imaging,** arthrograms, myelograms, and angiograms have various applications to specific body systems. With the availability of magnetic

underlying tissues, the radiation is absorbed or dispersed in varying degrees. High-density tissues such as bone absorb more radiation and are therefore more difficult to penetrate than less-dense tissue. The exposure to radiation leaves an imprint on special x-ray film, producing the familiar radiographic image. Overexposure to ionizing radiation is hazardous, and care must be taken to protect the reproductive organs through the use of a lead apron.

FIGURE 2–12. Stress radiograph for inversion of the ankle.

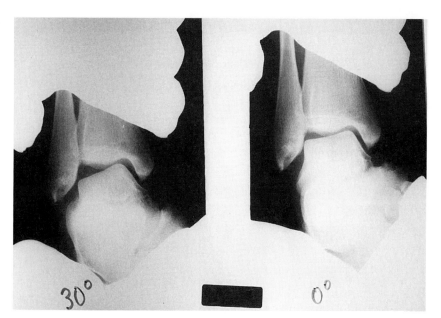

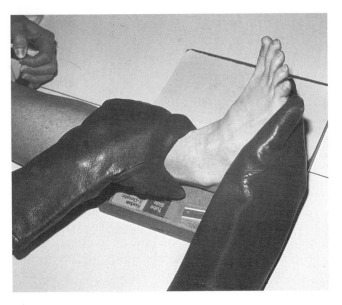

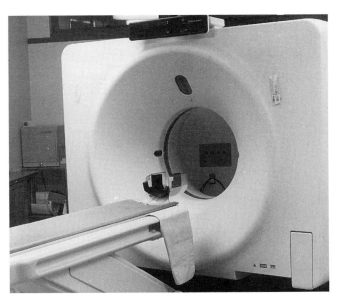

FIGURE 2–13. Setup of the stress radiograph shown in FIGURE 2–12.

FIGURE 2–14. Setup of a CT scan.

resonance imaging (MRI) techniques, these types of studies are less frequently used in the diagnosis of orthopedic injuries.

COMPUTED TOMOGRAPHY (CT) SCAN

Computed tomography (CT) scan uses many of the same principles and technology as radiography but is used to determine and quantify the presence of a specific pathology rather than as a general screening tool.

In the case of CT scans, the x-ray source and x-ray detectors rotate around the body (Fig. 2–14). Instead of the image's being produced on film, a computer determines the density of the underlying tissues based on the absorption of x-rays by the body, allowing for more precision in viewing soft tissue. This information is then used to create a two-dimensional image, or slice, of the body.[26] These slices can be obtained at varying positions and thicknesses, allowing physicians to study the area and its surrounding anatomical relationships (Fig. 2–15).

FIGURE 2–15. CT scan of a cranium.

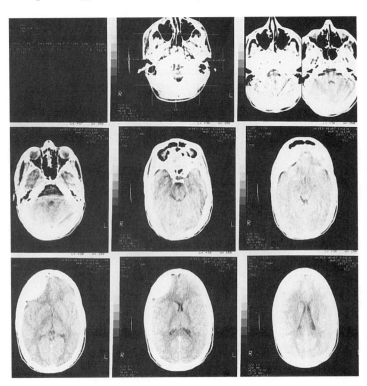

FIGURE 2–16. MRI image showing the knee in cross section.

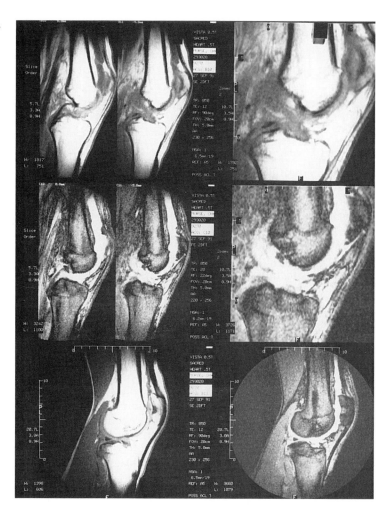

MAGNETIC RESONANCE IMAGING (MRI)

Perhaps the greatest innovation in the noninvasive diagnosis of subcutaneous pathology, MRI acquires a detailed picture of the body's soft tissues (Fig. 2–16). Similar to a CT scan, MRI is generally used to identify specific pathology or visualize a soft tissue structure (e.g., an anterior cruciate ligament sprain) rather than being used as a general screening tool. Compared with other imaging techniques, MRI offers superior visualization of the body's soft tissues, including swollen and inflamed tissues.

These images are obtained by placing the patient in an MRI tube that produces a magnetic field, causing the body's hydrogen nuclei to align with the magnetic axis (Fig. 2–17). The tissues are then bombarded by radio waves, causing the nuclei to resonate as they absorb the energy. When the energy to the tissues ceases, the nuclei return to their state of equilibrium by releasing energy, which is then detected by the MRI unit and transformed by a computer into images.[26]

Unlike the ionizing radiation associated with radiographs and CT scans, the energy used during the MRI process produces no known harmful effects. The only known limitations to the administration of this procedure lie with individuals who suffer from claustrophobia (who are fearful of entering the imaging tube) or those who have some types of implanted metal plates

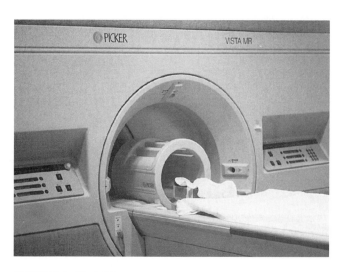

FIGURE 2–17. MRI generator.

or screws. Further technological advances will soon eliminate these contraindications by minimizing the effects of the imaging tube and reducing the level of magnetism to the point that metal implants can be safely exposed.

BONE SCAN

Bone scans are a form of nuclear medicine used to detect bony abnormalities that are not normally visible on a standard radiograph. The patient receives an injection of a *radionuclide* Tc-99m, a *tracer element* that is absorbed by areas of bone undergoing remodeling. These areas appear as darkened spots on the image and must be correlated with clinical signs and symptoms (Fig. 2–18). Bone scans can identify common pathologies, including degenerative disease, bone tumors, and stress fractures of the long bones and the vertebrae.[28]

ULTRASONIC IMAGING

Many internal organs and certain soft tissue structures, such as tendons, can be imaged using ultrasonic energy. The energy produced by ultrasonic imaging devices is similar to that used during therapeutic ultrasound treatments. However, imaging energy has a frequency of less than 0.8 MHz. Through a technique similar to sonar on a submarine, a computer detects the amount of sound that is reflected away from the tissues and creates a two-dimensional image of the subcutaneous structures (Fig. 2–19).

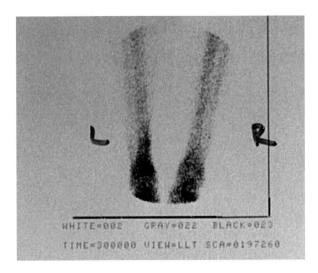

FIGURE 2–18. Bone scan of the lower extremity. The darkened areas indicate "hot spots" of high uptake of the tracer element.

◆ **REFERENCES**

1. Garrett, WE, Duncan, PW, and Malone, TR: *Muscle Injury and Rehabilitation.* Baltimore, Williams and Wilkins, 1988, p 9.
2. Rachun, A (ed): *Standard Nomenclature of Athletic Injuries.* Monroe, WI, American Medical Association, 1976.
3. Almekinders, LC, Garrett, WE, and Seaber, AV: Pathophysiologic response to muscle tears in stretching injuries. *Transactions of the Orthopedic Research Society* 9:307, 1984.
4. Almekinders, LC, Garrett, WE, and Seaber, AV: Histopathology of muscle tears in stretching injuries. *Transactions of the Orthopedic Research Society* 9:306, 1984.
5. Garrett, WE, et al: Biomechanics of muscle tears in stretching injuries. *Transactions of the Orthopedic Research Society* 9:384, 1984.

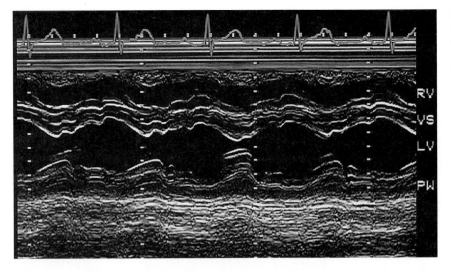

FIGURE 2–19. Ultrasonic image (mode echocardiogram) of the heart, showing normal left ventricular size and wall thickness. (RV 5 right ventricle; LV 5 left ventricle; VS 5 ventricular septum; PW 5 posterior wall.)

Radionuclide   An atom undergoing disintegration, emitting electromagnetic radiation.

Tracer element   A substance that is introduced into the tissues to follow or trace an otherwise unidentifiable substance or event.

6. Garrett, WE, et al: The effect of muscle architecture on the biomechanical failure properties of skeletal muscle under passive extension. *Am J Sports Med* 16:7, 1988.
7. Davies, GL, Wallace, LA, and Malone, TR: Mechanisms of selected knee injuries. *Phys Ther* 60:1590, 1980.
8. Gross, MT: Chronic tendinitis: Pathomechanics of injury, factors affecting the healing response, and treatment. *Journal of Orthopedic and Sports Physical Therapy* 16:248, 1992.
9. Frey, CC, and Shereff, MJ: Tendon injuries about the ankle in athletes. *Clin Sports Med* 7:103–118, 1988.
10. Kaeding, CC; Sanko, WA and Fischer, RA: Myositis ossificans. Minimizing downtime. *Physician and Sportsmedicine,* 23:77, 1995.
11. Estwanik, JJ: Contusions and the formation of myositis ossificans. *Physician and Sportsmedicine* 18:53, 1990.
12. It's bursitis, but which type? *Emerg Med* 21:71, 1989.
13. Starkey, C: Injuries and illnesses in the National Basketball Association: A 10-year perspective. *Journal of Athletic Training,* 35:161, 2000.
14. Garrick, JG, and Requa, RK: Role of external support in the prevention of ankle sprains. *Med Sci Sports Exerc* 5:200, 1973.
15. Sailors, ME: Recognition and treatment of osteochondritis dissecans of the femoral condyle. *Journal of Athletic Training,* 29:302, 1994.
16. Gardiner, JB: Osteochondritis dissecans in three members of a family. *J Bone Joint Surg Br* 37:139, 1955.
17. Woodward, AH, and Bianco, AJ: Osteochondritis dissecans of the elbow. *Clin Orthop* 110:35, 1975.
18. Lindholm, TS, Osterman, K, and VanKkae, E: Osteochondritis dissecans of the elbow, ankle, and hip. *Clin Orthop* 148:245, 1980.
19. Starkey, C: The injury response process. In Starkey, C: *Therapeutic Modalities* (ed 2). Philadelphia, FA Davis, 1999.
20. Ward, WG, Bergfeld, JA, and Carson, WG: Stress fracture of the base of the acromial process. *Am J Sports Med* 22:146:1994.
21. Yasuda, T, et al: Stress fracture of the right distal femur following bilateral fractures of the proximal fibulas. A case report. *Am J Sports Med* 20:771, 1992.
22. Roberts, WO: Primary amenorrhea and persistent stress fracture. A practical clinical approach. *Physician and Sportsmedicine,* 23:33, 1995.
23. Muizelaar, JP, et al: Complex regional pain syndrome (reflex sympathetic dystrophy and causalgia): Management with the calcium channel blocker nifedipine and/or the alpha-sympathetic blocker phenoxybenzamine in 59 patients. *Clin Neurol Neurosurg,* 99:26, 1997.
24. Sherry, DD: Short- and long-term outcomes of children with complex regional pain syndrome type I treated with exercise therapy. *Clin J Pain,* 15:218, 1999.
25. Kurvers, HA: Reflex sympathetic dystrophy: Facts and hypotheses. *Vasc Med,* 3:207, 1998.
26. D'Orsi, CJ: Radiology and magnetic resonance imaging. In Greene, HL, Glassock, RJ, and Kelley, MA: *Introduction to Clinical Medicine.* Philadelphia, BC Decker, 1991, p 91.
27. Schuerger, SR: Introduction to critical review of roentgengrams. *Phys Ther* 68:1114, 1988.
28. Patton, DO, and Doherty, PN: Nuclear medicine studies. In Greene, HL, Glassock, RJ, and Kelley, MA: *Introduction to Clinical Medicine.* Philadelphia, BC Decker, 1991, p 81.

3

Assessment Of Posture

SHERI L. MARTIN, MPT, ATC

Posture is the position of the body at a given point in time. Ideal posture is characterized by specific landmarks being aligned with the force of gravity, keeping the body as close to physiological equilibrium as possible.[1] Proper posture requires the least amount of muscular effort, resulting in reduced stress on the joints and surrounding structures. Correct postures can improve performance, decrease abnormal stresses, and reduce the development of pathological conditions.

Faulty posture is a position that deviates from ideal posture, requires an increased amount of muscular activity, and places an increased amount of stress on the joints and surrounding soft tissues.[2] Clinically, it is difficult to determine if the faulty posture is the result of muscle imbalances, caused by overuse of certain muscles during the *activities of daily living* (ADLs), or if the imbalances are the result of faulty posture. Restrictions in normal movement patterns may cause the body to acquire compensatory postures that still allow a functional motion to occur. Over time, these postures can result in muscle imbalances and soft tissue dysfunction that is presented in the form of *connective*, muscular, *myofascial*, nervous, or *inert tissue* pathology.[3]

The average person does not consider the effects of posture until pain or discomfort is experienced. People do not seek medical attention simply because they feel their posture is poor. They may seek medical attention because they are experiencing some type of pain or are experiencing an inability to function in a previously normal manner. Pain related to postural deviations is a common clinical occurrence.

Postural assessment is used to determine if certain postural deviations may be contributing factors in the patient's pain or dysfunction. The patient is in a static, nonfunctional position during clinical postural assessment that does not represent the natural postures assumed during ADLs. The different postures that the patient is exposed to during athletic, school, home, and work activities also must be identified and evaluated during the examination.

This chapter presents the relationship between correct posture, common postural deviations, and associated pain and dysfunction. The cause-and-effect relationship between faulty posture, common compensatory motions, and associated musculoskeletal dysfunctions is also discussed.

◆ CLINICAL ANATOMY

Before understanding how deviations in one region of the body affect another region, a review of some anatomical concepts is needed. The musculoskeletal system is designed to function in a mechanically and physiologically efficient manner to use the least possible amount of energy. The change in position of one joint results in the predictable change in position of the other interrelated joints.[4] When a postural deviation or skeletal malalignment occurs, other joints in the kinetic chain undergo compensatory motions or postures to allow the body to continue to move as efficiently as possible.

THE KINETIC CHAIN

The body is a series of kinetic chains in which different joints are either directly or indirectly linked together. In the kinetic chain concept, movement occurring at one joint causes movement to occur in an adjacent joint. This original movement causes a "chain reaction" of movements up or down the associated kinetic chain.

Activities of daily living (ADLs) The skills and motions required for in the day-to-day activities of life.

Connective tissue Tissue that supports and binds other tissue types.

Myofascial tissues A muscle and its associated fascia.

Inert tissues Noncontractile soft tissue, including the joint capsule and ligaments supporting the joint capsule.

Kinetic chains are classified as being **open chain** (non–weight-bearing) or **closed chain** (weight-bearing). Because the definition of open- and closed kinetic chain motions become blurred, the terms "weight-bearing" and "non–weight-bearing" are often used instead. The lower extremity-pelvis-lumbar complex functions primarily in a closed kinetic chain; the upper extremity, scapulothoracic, and cervical spine function primarily in an open kinetic chain.[4]

A closed kinetic chain movement is any movement in which the distal segment meets sufficient resistance or is fixated, such as the weight-bearing limb during walking or the upper extremity during push-ups or weight lifting. Because of the interdependency of each

joint within a closed chain, the joints involved in the chain undergo predictable changes in position in response to a change in position of another joint along the chain. A step up is an example of closed kinetic chain movement. The distal segment, the foot, is fixed as the body moves in relation to the base of support (Fig. 3–1A). As the knees flex to begin the squat, the ankles must dorsiflex and the hips must flex to allow the motion to occur.

An open kinetic chain is characterized by the distal portion of the chain moving freely in space, such as raising the leg off the ground (Fig. 3–1B). As the hip flexes in this open chain movement, the knee and ankle are not required to change positions. Some open chain movements

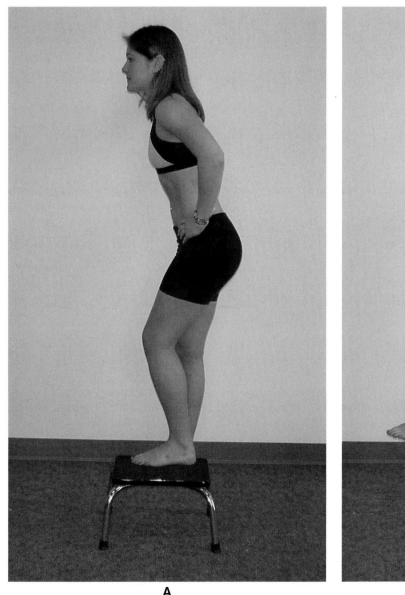 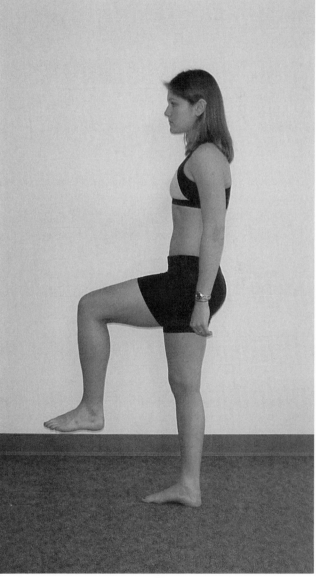

A   B

FIGURE 3–1. (A) Closed and **(B)** Open Kinetic Chains (left leg). Closed kinetic chains are formed when the extremity is weight-bearing; open kinetic chains occur during non–weight-bearing activities.

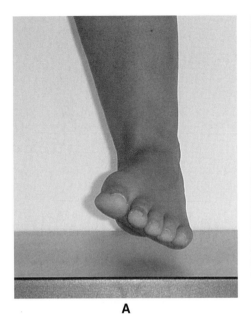

A

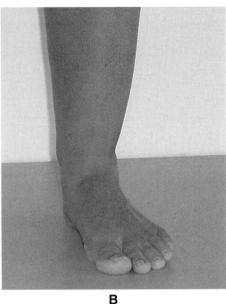

B

FIGURE 3–2. (A) Uncompensated (STJ Neutral) and **(B)** Compensated forefoot varus.

can be isolated to a specific joint. For example, as the wrist is flexed in an open chain environment, the elbow and shoulder do not undergo any changes in position.

The idea that different regions of the body function in a kinetic chain is an important concept to understand when assessing posture and attempting to determine the cause of a specific postural deviation. A soft tissue dysfunction or bony anomaly occurring in one region of the kinetic chain can affect the proximal or distal associated joints and soft tissue structures, causing a specific postural deviation. The body attempts to compensate for these deviations to maintain as much efficiency in movement and function as possible. An example of this compensatory strategy involves a structural condition of the foot called *forefoot varus.* If the body were unable to compensate for the abnormal position of the forefoot, a person would walk on the outside of the foot, not a very functional or efficient motion. To maxi-

mize propulsion and reduce the effect on gait, the foot compensates by excessively pronating at the subtalar joint (STJ) to reach a foot-flat position (Fig. 3–2). Because the lower extremity functions as a kinetic chain, excessive pronation at the subtalar joint causes excessive internal rotation of the tibia, leading to internal rotation of the femur, possibly changing the position of the hip joint and lumbar spine and altering patellar tracking (Table 3–1).[5]

The compensatory postures assumed by the body cause symptoms when the joint range of motion is excessive and produces joint stress; is excessive in its duration; or occurs at, or within, an inappropriate time.[4,6] If one motion is restricted, other joints in the area may compensate to allow for greater efficiency of movement.[7]

Another example of a kinetic chain in which a pathological soft tissue condition creates compensatory motion is termed *adhesive capsulitis.* In adhesive capsuli-

Table 3–1
EXAMPLES OF COMPENSATORY STRATEGIES OF THE BODY

Skeletal Malalignment	Compensatory Strategies					
	Subtalar Joint	Tibia	Tibiofemoral Joint	Femur	Hip Joint	Pelvis and Lumbar spine
Forefoot or rearfoot varus	Excessive pronation	Excessive internal rotation	Flexion	Excessive internal rotation	Flexion	Anterior rotation and excessive lumbar extension
Forefoot or rearfoot valgus	Excessive supination	Excessive external rotation	Extension	Excessive external rotation	Extension	Posterior rotation and excessive flexion

Forefoot varus Inversion of the forefoot relative to the rearfoot.

Adhesive capsulitis Inflammation of a joint capsule that restricts its range of motion.

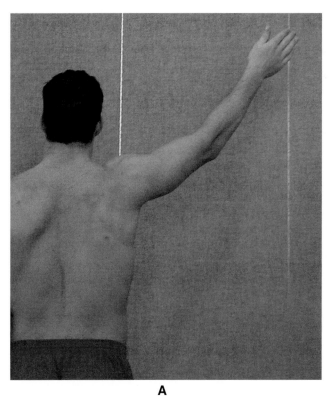
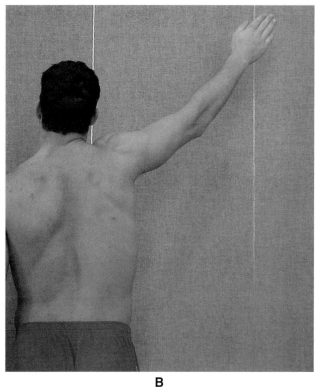

A   B

FIGURE 3–3. (A) Normal scapulohumeral elevation. **(B)** Scapulohumeral elevation compensated with increased upper trapezius activity.

tis, the **arthrokinematic** motions of the glenohumeral (GH) joint are decreased, prohibiting normal elevation of the humerus. Because the scapulothoracic articulation is part of the upper extremity kinetic chain, it compensates for the hypomobility of the GH joint by allowing excessive upward scapular rotation, to permit functional humeral elevation (Fig. 3–3). When compensatory movement patterns or postures occur over a prolonged period of time, they become "learned" and the body interprets them as being correct.[7]

Not all compensatory postures are detrimental. Some compensatory postures allow the body to function more efficiently, with less discomfort, or both. Such is the case for someone with *spinal stenosis* in the lumbar spine. The individual assumes a flexed posture in the lumbar spine (decreased lumbar lordosis) to increase the space in the vertebral canal caused by the narrowing that occurs with spinal stenosis. All findings of a postural evaluation must be interpreted before attempting to correct a postural deviation that has developed to compensate for a specific pathology.

MUSCULAR FUNCTION

Muscles produce joint motion and provide dynamic *joint stability.* To properly perform these roles, the muscles must be of an adequate length and must function in a proper manner. Muscles that are functionally too short or too long during activity can produce adverse stress on the joints, work inefficiently, or create the need for compensatory motions. An indication of whether a muscle's length is normal, shortened, or elongated begins during a thorough postural inspection. Further objective assessment of individual muscle length must occur later in the initial evaluation to reinforce what has been identified in the postural assessment (Table 3–2).

Table 3–2
MUSCLE LENGTH AND THE ABILITY TO PERFORM FUNCTION

Muscle Length	Ability to Provide Stability	Ability to Provide Mobility
Normal	Efficient	Efficient
Shortened	Efficient	Inefficient
Elongated	Inefficient	Efficient

Arthrokinematic Action and reaction of articular surfaces as a joint travels through its range of motion.

Spinal stenosis A narrowing of the vertebral foramen through which the spinal cord or spinal nerve root pass.

Joint stability The integrity of a joint when it is placed under a functional load.

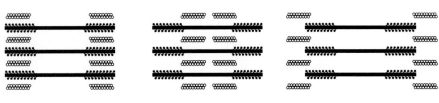

Resting State   Active Insufficiency   Passive Insufficiency

FIGURE 3–4. Relationship of actin and myosin cross bridges. When the muscle is in its resting state, there is full communication between the actin and myosin, allowing for a strong contraction. During active insufficiency, the muscle has contracted to its fullest point and the filaments can no longer slide. When the muscle is fully elongated, passive insufficiency, there is decreased communication between the actin and myosin, decreasing the strength the muscle can generate.

MUSCULAR LENGTH-TENSION RELATIONSHIPS

The **muscular length-tension relationship** describes how a muscle is capable of producing different amounts of tension (force), depending on its length. The tension-developing capacity of a muscle occurs within the *sarcomere* unit at the crossbridges formed between *actin* and *myosin* myofilaments. The optimal relationship between length and tension is the joint position where the muscle can generate the greatest amount of tension (force). At this length, the interaction of crossbridges between actin and myosin filaments within the sarcomere is at their most efficient position.

If a muscle is in a shortened or lengthened position, the interaction of crossbridges between actin and myosin filaments is reduced because there is either too much or too little overlap (Fig. 3–4). **Active insufficiency** occurs when a muscle is shortened and the actin and myosin myofilaments are overlapped to the point where maximum tension cannot be produced. **Passive insufficiency** occurs when the muscle is lengthened and the actin and myosin myofilaments lack sufficient overlap to generate force. In passive insufficiency, the muscle cannot generate sufficient tension to be effective in providing proper movement or stability.[7]

AGONIST AND ANTAGONIST RELATIONSHIPS

A muscle that contracts to perform the primary movement of a joint is termed the **agonist muscle.** The **antagonist muscle** performs the opposite movement of the agonist muscle and must reflexively relax to allow the agonist's motion to occur. This reflexive response is termed reciprocal inhibition. The biceps brachii and triceps brachii muscles are an example of an agonist and antagonist. During elbow flexion, the biceps brachii is the agonist performing the action of elbow flexion. The antagonist is the triceps brachii because it performs elbow extension. The triceps brachii must reflexively relax and elongate while the biceps brachii contracts to allow normal, smooth elbow flexion. If an antagonist muscle did not receive an inhibitory impulse to relax, but instead received an excitatory stimulus of the same magnitude as the agonist, the joint would not move because both sets of muscles would be contracting.

The concurrent contraction of the agonist and antagonist muscles, **co-contraction,** is a technique often used when working on dynamic stability of a joint. The smooth, deliberate movements of the body during normal ADLs are allowed to occur because of this excitatory/inhibitory reflex loop between the agonist and antagonist muscle groups. Proper balance between the lengths of the agonist and antagonist muscle groups is also necessary to maintain correct posture and avoid undue stress on the involved joints.

MUSCLE IMBALANCES

Understanding the concepts of optimal length-tension relationships and agonist versus antagonist muscles allows better comprehension of the implications of muscle imbalance. Muscle imbalances are characterized by an impaired relationship between a muscle that is over-activated, subsequently shortened and tightened and another that is inhibited and weakened.[8] Table 3–3 presents some of the common causes of muscle imbalances.

Different muscle types exhibit different patterns of activity in response to pain, postural deviations, or soft tissue dysfunction.[7,8] Skeletal muscles are classified as being either postural (also referred to as tonic) or phasic (Table 3–4). Postural muscles primarily function to support the body against the forces of gravity. They are composed of a higher percentage of slow twitch muscle

Sarcomere   A portion of striated muscle fiber lying between two membranes.

Actin   A contractile muscle protein.

Myosin   A contractile muscle protein.

Table 3–3
CAUSES OF MUSCLE IMBALANCES

Cause	Result
Nerve injury	Paralysis, muscle weakness, or muscle spindle inhibition
Pain	Inhibition or overactivation of muscle activity
Joint effusion	Reflexive inhibition of muscle activity
Poor posture	Alteration in muscle length–tension relationship
Repetitive activity of one muscle group	Adaptive shortening and increased recruitment

Table 3–4
POSTURAL AND PHASIC MUSCLES

Common Postural Muscles	Common Phasic Muscles
Sternocleidomastoid	Scalenes
Pectoralis major	Subscapularis
Upper trapezius	Lower trapezius
Levator scapula	Rhomboids
Quadratus lumborum	Serratus anterior
Iliopsoas	Rectus abdominis
Tensor fascia latae	Internal obliques
Rectus femoris	External obliques
Piriformis	Gluteus minimus
Hamstring group	Gluteus maximus
Short hip adductors	Gluteus medius
Gastrocnemius	Vastus medialis
Soleus	Vastus lateralis
Erector spinae	Tibialis anterior
Longissimus thoracic	Peroneals
Multifides or rotatores	
Tibialis posterior	

fibers, are slower to fatigue, and do not respond as quickly when activated.[8] Postural muscles have a greater tendency to become overactivated and shortened in response to stresses or pain (Table 3–5). *Trigger points* are soft tissue manifestations commonly seen in postural muscles undergoing stresses.[8]

Phasic muscles are primarily responsible for movement of the body. Having a higher proportion of fast twitch muscle fibers than postural muscles, phasic muscles contract more quickly and with a greater amount of force. Phasic muscles tend to rapidly fatigue because of the higher percentage of fast twitch fibers and have a greater tendency to become weak and inhibited in response to pain.[8] Muscle strains and tendinitis are common soft tissue dysfunctions seen in phasic muscles when under stress.

After a muscle becomes overactivated and shortened and its antagonist is weakened, the muscular balance around the joint it crosses becomes altered, changing the forces exerted on the joint. The overactivated muscle influences the way in which the underlying joint (or joints) moves and the amount of compression or distraction that occurs at that joint.[7] Muscle imbalances ex-

pend more energy and create inefficient and stressful movement patterns and postures for the body.[8,9]

When designing a rehabilitation program to correct a muscle imbalance, the initial focus is on elongating the shortened, overactivated muscle group before strengthening the inhibited and weakened group.[8] An inhibited, weakened muscle cannot sufficiently gain strength until the antagonist muscle is closely restored to its normal muscle length.[8]

SOFT TISSUE IMBALANCES

Muscle imbalances can also lead to abnormal compressive or shear forces being produced within the joint (or joints) crossed by those muscles. A joint's capsule and surrounding ligaments undergo adaptive changes (i.e., remodeling) from prolonged overstressing or understressing of the structure. Faulty posture and associated muscle imbalances can alter the position of joints, causing an increase in stress on different portions of the joint capsule and surrounding ligaments. While areas of a joint capsule that are continually stressed may elongate, areas (usually opposite areas) that are slack and not stressed may undergo adaptive shortening. The shoulder provides an example of a common inert soft tissue imbalance. A person who has pronounced rounded, forward shoulders for an extended time can experience adaptive shortening of the posterior portion and elongation of the anterior portion of the GH capsule. To compensate for rounded, forward shoulder

Table 3–5
POSTURAL VERSUS PHASIC MUSCLES

Characteristic	Postural Muscles	Phasic Muscles
Function	Support body against forces of gravity	Movement of the body
Muscle fiber type	Higher percentage of slow-twitch fibers	Higher percentage of fast-twitch fibers
Response to dysfunction	Become overactivated and tightened or shortened	Become inhibited and weakened
Common soft tissue dysfunction	Prone to trigger points	Prone to strains and tendinitis

Trigger point A pathological condition characterized by a small, hypersensitive area located within muscles and fasciae.

posture, the humeral head externally rotates so that the hands assume a somewhat normal posture. This reduces normal functional stresses on the posterior capsule, which, in turn, adaptively shortens. This position is further exaggerated as the anterior chest muscles adaptively shorten to maintain the posture while the middle and lower trapezius elongate.

◆ CLINICAL EVALUATION OF POSTURE

Posture plays both direct and indirect roles in the onset of overuse injuries. Overuse injuries are characterized by pain with an insidious onset, usually brought upon by repetitive tasks performed in specific postures.[10] When evaluating any type of musculoskeletal injury, a general observation of posture must occur early in the assessment process.

The clinical evaluation of posture is not an exact science.[11] The tools and techniques used are often not valid or reliable.[12,13] Although the use of radiographs, photographs, and computer analyses are the most objective and accurate methods for determining skeletal postural deviations,[14,15] clinical tools such as **plumb lines,** goniometers, flexible rulers, and inclinometers can increase the validity and reliability of the evaluation (Fig. 3–5).[15]

Clinically, posture may be described by the terms normal, mild (25% deviation from normal), moderate (50% deviation), and severe (75% deviation).[15] This is a subjective method for quantifying postural deviations demonstrating fair to poor inter-tester reliability.[15] Whenever possible, use measurements to further quantify skeletal malalignments causing postural deviations. Objective, quantifiable measurements can also assist in determining whether the current treatment plan is effective and if the patient's posture is improving.

The use of inspection and palpation in the assessment of posture varies from that during the evaluation of specific body areas. Although inspection and palpation are described as separate entities in this chapter, in practice these two segments take place simultaneously, each validating or refuting the findings of the other. As posture is being observed, the clinician simultaneously palpates to determine specific positions of joints and structures. The use of palpation to identify areas of point tenderness is not emphasized during the assessment of posture.

Posture is commonly assessed in two positions: standing and sitting. Additionally, assessing posture in any other static or dynamic positions that produce the patient's symptoms is important.. This would include any posture assumed by the patient for a prolonged period during the day or during normal ADLs. Certain movements can be performed before assessing a person's posture to assist in reinforcing that a natural, habitual posture is being assumed. The patient can be instructed to perform a sequence of movements referred to as the **orthoposition** and self-balancing position to obtain a relatively natural posture.[16,17] To ensure that the patient is standing in a relaxed, natural posture when beginning a postural assessment, have the patient perform the following sequence of movements:[16,17]

1. Have the patient march in place 10 times.
2. Roll the patient's shoulders forward and backward three times.
3. Have the patient nod his or her head and neck forward and backward five times.
4. Have the patient inhale and exhale deeply.

HISTORY

A concise and thorough history, at the beginning of the initial evaluation, assists in determining whether postural dysfunction is contributing to the patient's pathology and symptoms (Table 3–6). Repetitive tasks while maintaining a certain posture can lead to overuse injuries as well, so the history needs to identify any repetitive motions that are routinely performed.

If the mechanism of injury (MOI) for a particular injury has an insidious onset and symptoms have gradually increased over time, then the history needs to further explore the person's day-to-day tasks and postures. If the MOI can be traced to a specific force at a particular time, the history determines the factors that might have predisposed the patient to the injury. How-

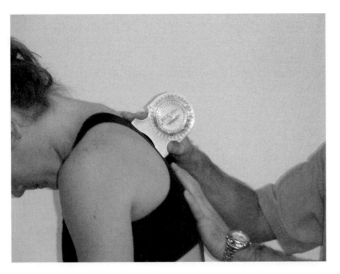

FIGURE 3–5. An inclinometer can be used to the measure range of motion for body parts where a goniometer would not be practical.

Plumb line   A string and pendulum that hangs perpendicular to surface.

Orthoposition   Normal or properly aligned posture.

Table 3–6
FACTORS INFLUENCING POSTURE

Factor	Example
Neurologic problems	Winging of the scapula secondary to inhibition of the long thoracic nerve
Muscle weakness	Increased pelvic angles secondary to weak abdominal muscles
Hypermobile joints	Genu recurvatum
Hypomobile joints	Flexion contracture
Decreased soft tissue flexibility	Decreased pelvic angles secondary to tightness of the hamstring muscles
Muscle imbalances	Forward shoulder posture caused by tightness of the pectoralis minor and elongation of the middle and lower trapezius
Bony abnormalities	Toe in or toe out posture secondary to internal or external tibial torsion
Leg length discrepancies	Functional scoliosis
Pain	Antalgic posture (e.g. side bending cervical spine to decrease compression on a nerve root)
Lack of postural awareness	Behavioral in nature (e.g., slouching in chair)

ever, in this case, improper posture may have contributed to the present symptoms.

The following information should be obtained to determine whether posture is contributing to the current pathology:

- **Mechanism of injury:** What is the mechanism of injury? Many overuse injuries associated with postural faults have an insidious onset with no specific cause of the pain. A nonspecific mechanism or time of injury may indicate that the injury is possibly caused by poor posture. Common responses pointing toward possible postural involvement in an injury may include:

  ○ Lack of awareness of one instance that caused the pain (insidious onset)
  ○ Pain worsening as the day progresses
  ○ Description of posture-specific pain
  ○ Complaints of intermittent pain
  ○ Vague or generalized pain descriptions
  ○ Initially starting as an ache that has progressively worsened over time.

- **Type, location, and severity of symptoms:** Are the symptoms constant or intermittent? Are they worse during a certain time of the day (e.g., morning, afternoon, evening)? Many postural dysfunctions are worse, or produce more symptoms, in the evening after the individual has maintained the posture all

day. Which positions or postures increase or decrease the symptoms? If the symptom is primarily pain, then what type of pain is it, burning, sharp, aching, pulsating? Is the patient experiencing paresthesia? If so, is it constant or intermittent? Where does it radiate?

- **Side of dominance:** Is the right or left side dominant? If one side is used for most, if not all tasks, then imbalances are likely to occur, exposing the patient to overuse injuries.

- **Activities of daily living:** What is the patient's usual day like? Many people have repetitive daily schedules. Which types of activities does the patient perform and for what duration or frequency? To better understand the motions associated with specific pain-producing tasks, it is helpful to have the patient demonstrate specific motions as they are being described. (Table 3–7).

- **Driving, sitting, and sleeping postures:** Has anything been changed in the person's daily routine over the past few months? (Table 3–8). Do any postures decrease the patient's discomfort?

- **Specific postures causing discomfort:** Do specific postures repeatedly cause the same type of symptoms?

- **Level and intensity of exercise:** Is exercise performed on a regular or sporadic basis or not at all? Has the exercise routine changed in any way? Does the patient warm up and cool down properly?

- **Medical history:** Has this problem occurred before? If so, was medical attention sought and what treatments were rendered? Are there any medical problems that should be identified? A general health questionnaire may be helpful to use before the evaluation to uncover any medical conditions.

INSPECTION

Ensure that the area used for postural assessment is private to protect the modesty of the patient and is a comfortable temperature. When possible, have males wear only shorts that are relatively short in length to expose the majority of their legs. Have females also wear shorts that expose most of their legs and a halter-type top that exposes the whole back. Shoes should be removed to allow observation of foot positions and the orthoposition is to be reinforced to ensure a natural, habitual posture. Do not inform the patient that his or her posture is being assessed at this time. A patient who is aware of this will become conscious about his or her posture and may stand more erect than usual.

A systematic approach should be taken when assessing posture so as not to overlook a specific region. The evaluation process may start at the foot and work superiorly or vice versa. This chapter describes posture starting at the feet and working superiorly. Whenever comparing bilaterally for symmetry, place your eyes at the same level as the region you are observing.

Table 3–7
EXAMPLES OF DAILY STRESSES AND THEIR POSSIBLE RESULTING PATHOLOGIES

Activity	Associated Tasks	Possible Postural Deviations	Possible Soft Tissue Dysfunctions	Corrections
Desk job	Computer use: Is the station ergonomically correct? Is it a multi-use station?	FHP, FSP, general postural faults caused by muscle fatigue or poor postural sense throughout trunk and upper quadrant	Soft tissue syndromes of the cervical, thoracic, and shoulder regions, including, myofascial syndromes, muscle imbalances, muscle strains, thoracic outlet syndrome, carpal tunnel syndrome, or other nerve entrapment syndromes throughout the upper extremity	1. Proper ergonomic design of work station 2. Frequent breaks with performance of postural exercises and stretches 3. Maintenance of proper sitting posture at work
	Telephone use: How is the phone held? Is the phone cradled between the ear and shoulder? Is the same side used?	Prolonged cervical lateral flexion, shoulder elevation	Adaptive shortening of cervical lateral flexors, lengthening of contralateral muscles, myofascial syndromes in all the above areas mentioned, joint or nerve root related problems in the cervical spine caused by compression of one side (narrowing of intervertebral foramen and compression of the ipsilateral facet joints)	Use a telephone headset to maintain the head in the neutral position and leave the hands free to perform other tasks with minimal strain
	What type of chair is used? Is it ergonomically correct?	Inadequate lumbar support: Leads to "slouched" posture and flexed lumbar, thoracic spine, forward shoulder posture, and FHP Inadequate arm rests: Leads to increased upper extremity work causing fatigue of shoulder girdle muscles	Muscle imbalances throughout trunk, shoulder girdle region, upper extremities; myofascial syndromes; TOS at any of three entrapment sites (anterior or mid scalenes, first rib and clavicle, pec minor and rib cage); other nerve entrapment syndromes	1. Ergonomically correct chair with adequate lumbar support and arm rests at correct height 2. The chair placed correctly in front of the computer and not angled to perform computer work and other tasks at the same time. 3. Frequent breaks from computer work to perform postural exercises or stretches 4. Maintenance of proper sitting posture at work.
	Are bifocals worn? Are regular glasses worn? Is there glare on the computer screen?	Forward head posture, forward shoulder posture from straining to read the screen	TMJ dysfunctions; myofascial syndromes; joint and nerve dysfunctions; muscle imbalances	1. Change of computer screen angle or height 2. Change of glasses as needed 3. Use of anti-glare screens and shields; decrease in glare from overhead fluorescent lighting

Category	Questions	Assessment	Possible Pathology	Recommendations
Manual labor	Frequency of bending, lifting, repetitive motions? (If possible, the patient should demonstrate the actual positions assumed and motions performed.)	Improper bending encompassing flexed lumbar spine; decrease use of leg muscles or increase use of back muscles; flexed thoracic and cervical spine with increase stress of soft tissue structures of back; combined motions of lumbar spine flexion and rotation; position also increasing the pressure within the lumbar discs	Muscle imbalance; myofascial syndrome; muscle strains or ligamentous sprains; joint or disc pathology	1. Teaching of proper lifting technique: maintenance of lumbar lordosis; flexing at hips; use of legs rather than back muscles; maintenance of cervical lordosis or thoracic kyphosis; use of pivoting with feet versus rotation of spine when turning 2. Perform extension exercises throughout day to counteract flexion 3. Use assistive devices to lift heavy objects; use more trips with less weight per trip; and use partner to lift heavy and bulky objects
	Repetitive overhead tasks?	Cervical spine in prolonged extension; upper extremities overhead requiring increased rotator cuff and scapular stabilizer muscle strength or endurance	Muscle imbalances; cervical spine facet joint or nerve compression; myofascial syndromes; with the presence of a FSP, patients are more prone to shoulder impingement syndromes	1. Frequent breaks from overhead activities 2. Use of stool or device to attempt to keep work at eye level
Student	Is any specific equipment used repetitively?	Repetitive motions with use of specific tool increasing stress on certain tissues	Muscle imbalances; tendinitis; strains; nerve entrapment syndromes	1. Stretching of muscles used during operation of tools 2. Ergonomically correct tools
	Is a backpack used? How heavy is the backpack?	FHP; FSP; flexed trunk and lumbar spine	Myofascial syndromes; TOS; facet or disc pathology; ligamentous sprains; muscle strains; muscle imbalances	1. Use of both shoulder straps while carry backpack to avoid carrying the weight over one shoulder 2. Limiting the weight of the backpack
Athletics	Sport and position? Frequency, duration and intensity of involvement?	Possible overuse injuries or overtraining techniques based on the sport and position played; identification of relationship between changes in the pattern of participation and the onset of symptoms (e.g., surfaces, direction)	Myofascial syndrome; muscle strains or ligamentous sprains; muscle imbalances	1. Conditioning to ready specific tissues to the rigors of the sport and position. Proper stretching before and after participation 2. Change in training regimen as necessary 3. Change of position 4. Increased awareness of stresses
	Specific positions during participation that cause pain?	Changes of postural alignments or positions that place increased or imbalanced stresses on tissues	Overuse injuries; muscle imbalances; microtrauma to soft tissues	1. Proper balancing of workout or practice to adequately alter stresses on tissues (frequent change of surface, direction, or position) 2. Conditioning specific to the rigors of the sport and position

FHP = forward head posture; FSP = forward shoulder posture; TMJ = temporomandibular joint; TOS = thoracic outlet syndrome.

Table 3–8
DRIVING, SITTING AND SLEEPING POSTURES

ADL	Posture	Possible Postural Deviations	Postural Correction
Driving	Inadequate lumbar support?	Flexion of lumbar spine and thoracic spine, FSP, and FHP	Use lumbar support cushion
	Reclined seat angle—hips flexed less than 90°?	Flexion of lumbar and thoracic spine; increased scapula protraction; excessive arm elevation to reach steering wheel; FSP; FHP	Adjust seat angle so hips are at 90° of flexion
	Seat distance too far from steering wheel and pedals?	Flexion of lumbar and thoracic spine; protraction of scapula; FSP; FHP; increased pelvis and leg activity to reach for pedals	Adjust seat distance so elbows and knees are flexed approximately 30° to 45°; the hands should reach the steering wheel and the thoracic spine and scapula should maintain contact with the seatback
	Frequency, length of time spent driving?	Increased fatigue, muscle imbalances, and overuse syndromes when incorrectly postured with prolonged sitting position	1. Use correct posture while driving 2. Take frequent rest stops and perform stretching exercises (e.g., spinal extension, hamstring stretches)
Sitting	Although some sitting postures are covered in Table 3–7, it is important to identify all different types of sitting postures assumed throughout the day	See Table 3–7 for description of postural deviations while sitting.	Use proper sitting posture that incorporates the following: body weight slightly anterior to ischial tuberosities; maintenance of normal lumbar lordosis; hips slightly higher than knees; feet flat on floor; shoulder maintained in a "back and down" position (retracted and depressed); arms supported at the proper height to maintain good shoulder position; head retracted and in a neutral position Keep in mind that everyone's posture may vary from the above description; the key is to understand what correct posture entails for that individual and to work from that position, changing various amounts of each movement to find a more "correct or functional" position for each individual
Sleeping	Mattress support (firm or soft)? Recent change in mattress?	A soft mattress may not provide adequate support; firm mattresses may be too rigid to conform to the natural curves of the body	Change mattress according to desired support
	Number of pillows used? Type of pillow used?	Using too many pillows places the head and neck in excessive lateral flexion toward the opposite side during sleeping; may cause prolonged compression and distraction at the neck on the weight-bearing side Too few or soft pillows will not maintain normal spinal curvature	Use an adequate number (and size) of pillows to maintain the head in the neutral position while sleeping
	Sleep posture?	Different positions place abnormal stresses on the soft tissues or may perpetuate postural changes	Use positions that are not at the extremes of motion (i.e., too much flexion or extension); use pillows to maintain positions such as between the legs when sidelying

FHP = forward head posture; FSP = forward shoulder posture.

62

OVERALL IMPRESSION

The first aspect of a postural assessment is the determination of the patient's general body type. There are three basic categories of body types: ectomorph, mesomorph, and endomorph. A person's body type is largely inherited and can assist in indicating a person's natural abilities and disabilities. However, body type does not necessarily dictate how that person may function (Box 3–1).[18]

VIEWS OF POSTURAL INSPECTION

Posture is inspected from all views or planes with the body in orthoposition: lateral (sagittal plane), anterior (frontal plane), and posterior (frontal plane). A **plumb line** may be used to assist the clinician in detecting postural deviations. When using a plumb line, align the patient using the feet as the permanent landmark. Position the plumb line slightly anterior to the lateral malleolus from the lateral view and equidistant from both feet from the anterior and posterior views. Box 3–2 presents ideal posture in each of the three planes.

Lateral View

Observation of posture from the lateral view involves making determinations of the anterior and posterior alignment of the body relative to the frontal plane. A person standing in ideal posture from the lateral view has landmarks at different regions of the body bisecting or relative to the plumb line (see Box 3–2). Table 3–9 lists common postural deviations noted from the lateral view.

Table 3–9
DEVIATIONS NOTED FROM THE LATERAL VIEW

Body Region	Deviation from Ideal Posture	Structural Relationships
Talocrural joint	Dorsiflexion	Knee flexion, hip flexion
	Plantarflexion	Genu recurvatum, knee extension, hip extension
Knee joint	Lateral epicondyle posterior to plumb line	Knee hyperextension (genu recurvatum), ankle plantarflexion
	Lateral epicondyle anterior to plumb line	Knee flexion and ankle dorsiflexion
Hip joint	Greater trochanter posterior to plumb line	Hip flexion, anterior pelvic tilt, increased lumbar lordosis
	Greater trochanter anterior to plumb line	Hip extension, posterior pelvic tilt, decreased lumbar lordosis
Pelvic position	Angle between ASIS and ipsilateral PSIS Greater than 10°: Anterior pelvic tilt	Increased lumbar lordosis, hip flexion
	Angle between ASIS and ipsilateral PSIS less than 8°: Posterior pelvic tilt	Decreased lumbar lordosis, hip extension
Lumbar spine	Lumbar vertebral bodies anterior to plumb line: Increased lumbar lordosis	Anterior pelvic tilt, hip flexion
	Lumbar vertebral bodies posterior to plumb line: Decreased lumbar lordosis	Posterior pelvic tilt, hip extension
Thoracic spine	Mid-thorax posterior to plumb line: Increased thoracic kyphosis	Forward head posture, forward shoulder posture, shortened anterior chest musculature
	Midthorax anterior to plumb line: Decreased thoracic kyphosis	Inability to flex through thoracic spine, possible shortened thoracic paraspinal muscles
Shoulder joint	Acromion process posterior to plumb line: Retracted shoulders or scapulae	Decreased thoracic kyphosis
	Acromion process anterior to plumb line: Rounded shoulder or protracted scapulae	Forward head posture, increased thoracic kyphosis, shortened anterior chest musculature, poor postural control of the scapula
Cervical spine	Lower cervical vertebral bodies posterior to plumb line: Decreased cervical lordosis	Straightened cervical spine, muscle imbalances
	Lower cervical vertebral bodies anterior to plumb line: Increased cervical lordosis	Forward head posture, forward shoulder posture, muscle imbalances
Head position	External auditory meatus posterior to plumb line: Head retraction	Straightened cervical spine, muscle imbalances
	External auditory meatus anterior to plumb line: Forward head posture	Forward shoulder posture, muscle imbalances, suboccipital restrictions

ASIS = anterior superior iliac spine; PSIS = posterior superior iliac spine.

Box 3-1
CLASSIFICATIONS OF BODY TYPES

	Ectomorph	Mesomorph	Endomorph
Description	Slender, thin build; relatively low body weight	Medium, athletic build, relatively average body weight	Short, stocky build; relatively high body weight
Joint shape	Small, flat joint surfaces	Medium joint surfaces	Large, concave-convex joint surfaces
Muscle mass	Minimal muscle bulk, thin muscles	Medium muscle build	Thick muscle mass
Joint mobility	Increased	Within normal limits	Decreased
Joint stability	Decreased	Within normal limits	Increased

Box 3–2

ASSESSMENT OF IDEAL POSTURE

Lateral	Anterior	Posterior
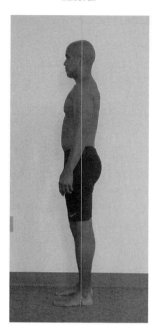	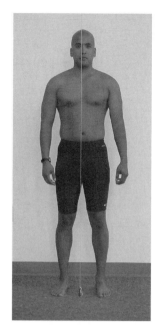	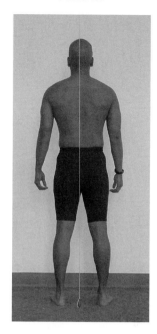

Alignment relative to plumb line: | **Alignment relative to plumb line:** | **Alignment relative to plumb line:**

Lateral

Alignment relative to plumb line:

Lower Extremity
- Lateral malleolus: Slightly posterior
- The tibia should be parallel to the plumb line and the foot should be at a 90° angle to the tibia
- Lateral femoral condyle: Slightly anterior
- Greater trochanter: Plumb line bisects

Torso
- Mid thoracic region: Plumb line bisects

Shoulder
- Acromion process: Plumb line bisects

Head and Neck
- Cervical bodies: Plumb line bisects
- Auditory meatus: Plumb line bisects

Anterior

Alignment relative to plumb line:

Lower Extremity
- Feet: Evenly spaced from plumb line
- Tibial crests: Slight external rotation
- Knees: Evenly spaced from plumb line
- Patella: Facing anteriorly
- Consistent angulation from joint-to-joint
- The lateral malleoli, fibular head, and iliac crests should be bilaterally equal

Torso
- Umbilicus: Plumb line bisects
- Sternum: Plumb line bisects
- Jugular notch: Plumb line bisects

Shoulder
- Acromion processes: Evenly spaced from plumb line
- Shoulder heights equal or dominant side slightly lower
- Deltoid, anterior chest musculature bilaterally symmetrical and defined

Head and Neck
- Head is bisected by plumb line
- Nasal bridge: Plumb line bisects
- Frontal bone: Plumb line bisects

Posterior

Alignment relative to plumb line:

Lower Extremity
- Feet evenly spaced from plumb line
- Feet in slight lateral rotation: Lateral 2 toes are visible
- Knees evenly spaced from plumb line
- Consistent angulation from joint-to-joint

Torso
- Median sacral crests: Plumb line bisects
- Spinous processes: Plumb line bisects
- Paraspinals bilaterally symmetrical

Shoulder
- Scapular borders: Evenly spaced from plumb line
- Acromion processes: Evenly spaced from plumb line
- Deltoid, posterior musculature bilaterally symmetrical
- Shoulder heights equal or dominant side slightly lower

Head and Neck
- Cervical spinous processes: Plumb line bisects
- Occipittal protuberance: Plumb line bisects

Anterior View

For the anterior view, the plumb line bisects the midline of the body in the sagittal plane. The major regions of the body are observed from this view and bilateral symmetry is compared (see Box 3–2). Table 3–10 presents common postural deviations that may be observed from the anterior view.

Posterior View

Many observations found in the posterior view help to confirm the findings from the anterior view (see Box 3–2). The plumb line should be of equal distance from both feet, bisecting the spinal column or trunk and head. From the posterior view, observe for bilateral symmetry of the major regions of the body. Table 3–11 presents postural deviations that may be observed from the posterior view.

INSPECTION OF LEG LENGTH DISCREPANCY

A leg length discrepancy can be a contributing factor to lower limb and back pathology.[19] The three categories of leg length discrepancies include; structural (true), functional (apparent), and compensatory (Table 3–12).[19–21] Although the most accurate method for determining unequal leg lengths is by radiograph evaluation, several methods can be used clinically.[22,23]

The most clinically reliable way of determining a leg length discrepancy is the pre-measured block method (Box 3–3). The most common, yet least reliable, method of determining a leg length discrepancy is measuring the distance between the **anterior superior iliac spine** (ASIS) and medial malleolus to determine a structural leg length difference and from the navel to the medial malleolus to identify a functional leg length difference (Fig. 3–6). Functional leg length discrepancies can be caused by pelvic obliquity.

Table 3–10
POSTURAL DEVIATIONS OBSERVED FROM THE ANTERIOR VIEW

Body Region	Deviation from Ideal Posture	Structural Relationships
Feet	Internally rotated feet (pigeon toed)	Internal rotation of tibia, femoral anteversion, or STJ pronation
	Externally rotated feet (duck feet)	External rotation of tibia, femoral retroversion, or STJ supination
STJ	Flattened medial arch	Excessive STJ pronation, internal tibial rotation
	High medial arch	Excessive STJ supination, external tibial rotation
Tibial position	External tibial rotation: Tibial crests positioned lateral to midline	Femoral retroversion, STJ supination, lateral positioning of patella
	Internal tibial rotation: Tibial crests positioned medial to midline	Femoral anteversion, STJ pronation, medial positioning of patella
Patellar position	Squinting patellae	Internal tibial rotation, femoral anteversion, STJ pronation
	Frog-eyed patellae	External tibial rotation, femoral retroversion, STJ supination
Leg positions	Genu varum	Increased angle of inclination of femur, femoral retroversion, STJ supination
	Genu valgum	Decreased angle of inclination of femur, femoral anteversion, STJ pronation
	Tibial varum	Structural deformity of the tibias causing excessive STJ pronation
Pelvic position	The iliac crests asymmetrical	Leg length discrepancy, scoliosis
	The ASIS asymmetrical	One ilium is rotated either anteriorly or posteriorly, leg length discrepancy, or congenital anomaly
Chest region	Pectus carinatum: Outward protrusion of the chest and sternum	Structural anomaly
	Pectus excavatum: Inward position of the chest and sternum	Structural anomaly
Shoulder region	The shoulder heights asymmetrical	Scoliosis
Head and cervical spine	The head side bent or rotated; asymmetrical muscle mass of neck	Poor postural sense, overuse of one side, torticollis (congenital deformation or acute spasm of the sternocleidomastoid muscle)

ASIS = anterior superior iliac spine; STJ = subtalar joint.

Table 3–11
POSTURAL DEVIATIONS OBSERVED FROM THE POSTERIOR VIEW

Body Region	Deviation from Ideal Posture	Structural Relationships
Calcaneal position	Calcaneal varum Calcaneal valgum	STJ in a supinated position STJ in a pronated position
Posterior leg musculature	Asymmetry in girth or definition of musculature	Leg side dominance Atrophy caused by injury or immobilization of one side
Iliac crest heights	Asymmetry of iliac crest heights	Possible leg length discrepancy Scoliosis
Back musculature	Asymmetry between mass or definition of erector spinae musculature	Side dominance or overuse of one side of the musculature (e.g., crew) Scoliosis
Spinal alignment	The spinous processes not in vertical alignment	A structural or functional scoliosis Asymmetry of scapula Asymmetry of spinal musculature Asymmetry of rib cage
Scapular position	Unequal height	Side dominance Scoliosis Muscle imbalance caused by paralysis or weakness of musculature
	Excessively protracted or asymmetrically protracted	Muscle imbalance Poor posture Scoliosis Forward shoulder posture Forward head posture
	Asymmetrically rotated	Muscle imbalance Side dominance Forward shoulder posture Forward head posture
	Winging scapula	Poor posture Muscle imbalance Muscular weakness
Shoulder heights	Shoulder heights unequal	Scoliosis Dominant side Scapula positioning
Neck musculature	The upper trapezius hyertrophied in relation to other periscapula muscles	Overused in normal upper extremity activities or overemphasized in weight lifting Side dominance
Head position	The head not sitting in a vertical position in relation to the neck	Caused by muscle imbalance Poor postural, proprioceptive sense
	Side bend, rotated	Compensation for scoliosis Torticollis (acquired or congenital)

STJ = subtalar joint.

Table 3–12
LEG LENGTH DIFFERENCES

Category Type	Description	Possible Causes
Functional or apparent leg length	Secondary to pelvic obliquity The asymmetry of the pelvis' altering the functional standing position and giving the appearance that one leg is longer or shorter than the other	Muscle weaknesses or imbalances around the pelvic region, unilateral hyperpronation of the foot, or any altered mechanics of the lower extremity
Structural or true leg length	Secondary to an actual difference in the length of the femur or the tibia of one leg compared with the other	Possibly from disruption in the growth plate of one of the long bones or a congenital anomaly
Compensatory leg length	A change in the joint angle of the foot, ankle, knee, or hip to compensate for other factors giving the appearance that one leg is longer than the other, yet they are equal	Factors such as pain, scoliosis, biomechanical changes

An actual difference in lengths of the femurs or tibias can be assessed in the supine position with the feet placed flat and in equal positions on the examining table with the knees flexed to 90 degrees. Observing the height of the knees from the anterior view will determine whether one tibia is longer than the other. Observing the length of the knees from the lateral view determines whether one femur is longer than the other (Fig. 3–7).[24] During weight bearing, the attitude of the feet can also provide evidence of a leg length discrepancy. The foot on the shorter leg supinates and the foot on the longer leg pronates in an attempt to compensate for the discrepancy in length (Fig. 3–8).

PALPATION

When assessing posture, accurate palpation of key landmarks assists in identifying various postural deviations.

Lateral Aspect

- **Pelvic position:** Palpate the ASIS and **posterior superior iliac spine** (PSIS) on the same side, placing marks on these landmarks to improve consistency. The relationship between the ASIS and PSIS, normally 9° to 10°, indicates if the pelvis is properly positioned or is rotated anteriorly or posteriorly (Box 3–4).

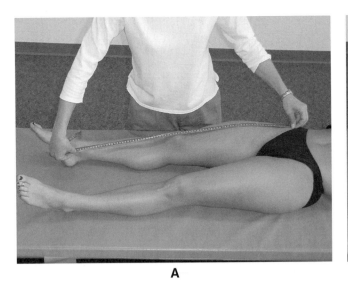
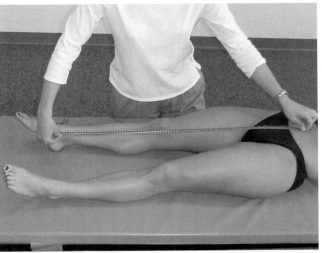

A

B

FIGURE 3–6. (A) Test for the presence of a structural (true) leg length discrepancy. Measurements are taken from the anterior superior iliac spine to the medial malleolus. Bilateral discrepancies of greater than 1/4 inch are considered significant. **(B) Test for the presence of an functional (apparent) leg length discrepancy.** Measurements are taken from each medical malleolus to the umbilicus. This test is meaningful only if the test for a true leg length difference is negative.

Box 3–3
MEASURED BLOCK METHOD OF DETERMINING LEG-LENGTH DISCREPANCIES

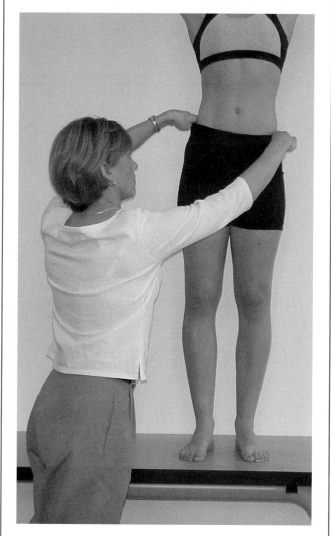 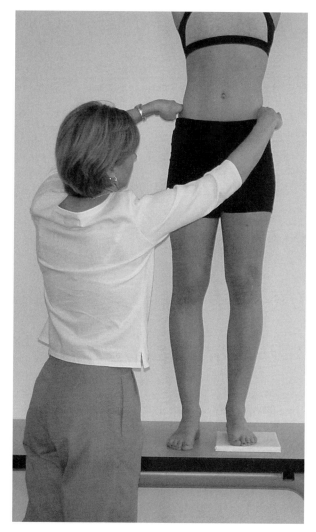

PATIENT POSITION	Standing with the feet shoulder-width apart and the weight evenly distributed
POSITION OF EXAMINER	Standing in front of the patient
EVALUATIVE PROCEDURE	The starting levels of the iliac crests are noted. Blocks of known thickness (measured in millimeters) are placed under the shorter leg until the iliac crests are of equal height. The leg length difference is calculated by totaling the sum of the heights of the individual blocks.
POSITIVE TEST	A leg length difference of greater than 0.7 cm (¼ in) is considered significant.
COMMENT	When the iliac crests are level, observe the heights of the ASIS. If the ASIS are not an equal height, then the patient has an asymmetrical pelvis.

ASIS = anterior superior iliac spine.

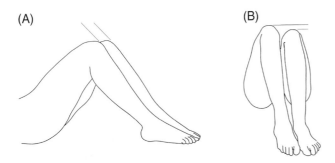

FIGURE 3–7. Clinical discrimination between femoral and tibial leg length differences. (A) When viewing the patient from the lateral side, an increased anterior position of one knee indicates a discrepancy in the lengths of the femurs. (B) When viewing the knees from the front, a difference in height indicates a discrepancy in the lengths of the tibias.

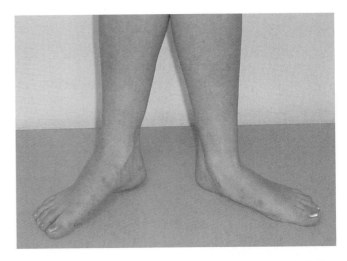

FIGURE 3–8. Foot posture associated with leg length difference. The foot on the long-leg side (the patient's left foot) is pronated while the foot on the short-leg side is supinated.

Anterior Aspect

- **Patellar position:** Before palpating for patellar position, ensure that the patient is standing comfortably with the feet symmetrically rotated and in an equal stance. Patellar position is observed while the patient is standing, laying supine, long sitting, and during dynamic positions. To assist in determining patellar position, place the thumbs on the medial borders of the patellae and the index fingers on the lateral borders. Further information regarding patellar position can be found in Chapter 7.
- **Iliac crest heights:** Palpate the lateral portions of bilateral ilia moving superiorly until reaching the most superior aspect of the iliac crests. Place the palmar aspects of the index and middle fingers on top of the iliac crests as if forming two "table tops." When you have located the landmarks, determine if your hands

are level and that the iliac crest heights are equal (Fig. 3–9). If one hand is higher than the other, then the iliac crests are unequal.
- **Anterior superior iliac spine (ASIS) heights:** Trace your thumbs down the anterior portion of both iliac crests until coming to the ASIS protuberance. Hook the thumbs on the most inferior ridges of the ASIS to ensure that the same aspect of the ASIS is being palpated on both sides. Determine whether your thumbs are level and the ASIS are of equal height (Fig. 3–10).
- **Lateral malleolus and fibula head heights:** Bilaterally palpate the most prominent projections of the lateral malleolus to determine if each is of equal height. Repeat this process for the fibular heads.

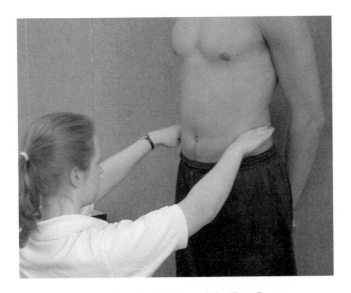

FIGURE 3–9. Finding the Heights of the Iliac Crests.

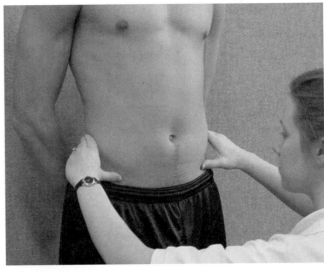

FIGURE 3–10. Identifying the Anterior Superior Iliac Spine.

Box 3–4

INSPECTION OF PELVIC POSITION

Neutral	Anterior Pelvic Tilt	Posterior Pelvic Tilt
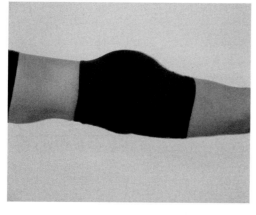	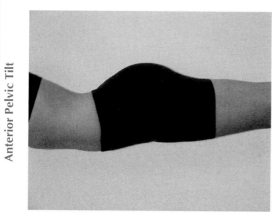	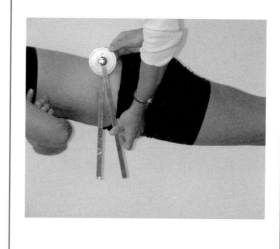
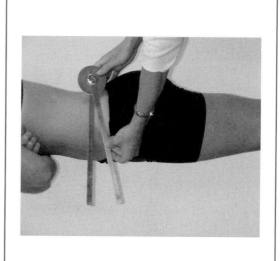	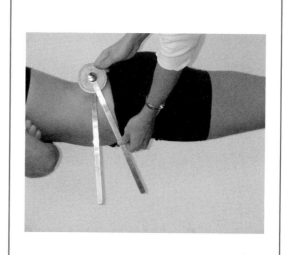	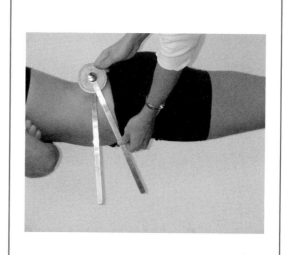
8 to 10° angle between the ASIS and PSIS	More than a 10° angle between the ASIS and PSIS	Less than an 8° angle between the ASIS and PSIS

ASIS: anterior superior iliac spine; PSIS: posterior superior iliac spine.

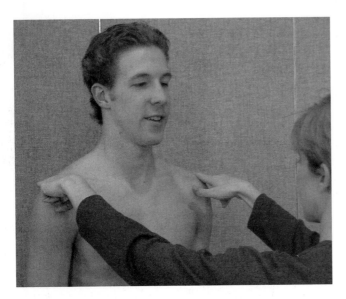

FIGURE 3–11. Identifying the Level of the Shoulders

- **Shoulder heights:** Place the palmar aspect of the index and middle fingers on the superior surface of the acromion processes. The fingers should sit flatly on both acromion processes and be parallel to the ground (Fig. 3–11).

Posterior Aspect

Many of the same landmarks used for the anterior view are also used in the posterior view. This section only discusses landmarks that are specific from the posterior view.

- **PSIS positions:** Keeping the index and middle fingers in the position for measuring iliac crest heights, angle the thumbs 45° downward and medially. Palpate for the PSIS, a relatively large, round protuberance, and hook your thumbs under the inferior edges of the PSIS. Determine if your thumbs are at equal heights (Fig. 3–12).
- **Spinal alignment:** Starting from the cervical vertebrae, trace your finger down each spinous process to the sacrum. A lateral deviation where more than one spinous process is not aligned vertically may reflect scoliosis. Refer to the section of this chapter on the spine for definitions of functional versus structural scoliosis.
- **Scapular position:** Evaluate the scapula for bilateral elevation or depression, *protraction* or *retraction*, rotation, and *winging* (Box 3–5).

FUNCTIONAL TESTS

Muscle length assessment can be performed after completing the postural assessment to objectively measure if specific muscles may be shortened or elongated, causing or contributing to any postural deviation that

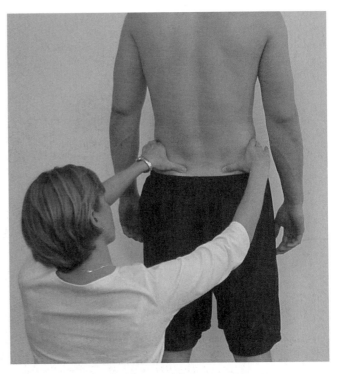

FIGURE 3–12. Palpating the Posterior Superior Iliac Spines

was observed. You cannot assume that a muscle is shortened just because a certain type of posture was observed. For example, a patient demonstrates an increase in anterior pelvic tilt. It might be assumed that the patient has tight rectus femoris or iliopsoas muscles that are causing the deviation. However, objective, measurable testing must occur to confirm this assumption. As with all aspects of an evaluation, assessing muscle length must have standard measures and be as objective as possible. However, for some muscle groups it is difficult to objectively measure the length. In these cases, a general estimate and comparison to the contralateral side or normative values is sufficient.

Before assessing the length of a muscle, rule out any bony or soft tissue restrictions that could be involved in the joint or joints that the muscle crosses.[8] Specific, measurable tests are available for many of the *two-joint muscles* that commonly create postural problems

---

Protraction (scapular)   Movement of the vertebral borders of the scapula away from the spinal column.

Retraction (scapular)   Movement of the scapular vertebral borders toward the spinal column.

Winging (scapular)   The inferior angle of the scapula lifting away from the thorax.

Two-joint muscles   A muscle that exerts its force across two different joints and whose strength depends on the position of those joints.

Box 3–5
INSPECTION OF SCAPULAR POSTURE

Scapular Elevation/Depression

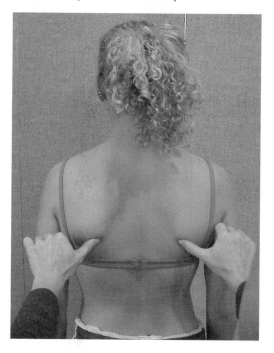

The height of the scapula are compared using the inferior angle as a landmark.

Scapular Protraction/Retraction

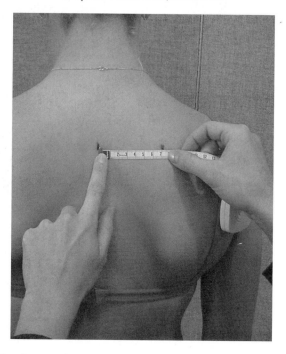

The distance from the T3 spinous process to the medial border of the scapula is measured. The normal value is 5 to 7 cm. An increased distance represents a protracted scapular position, a decreased distance, a retracted scapula.

Scapular Rotation

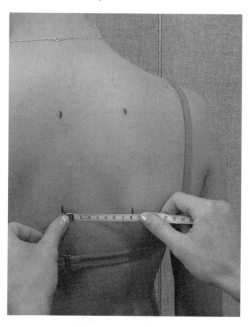

The distance from the T7 vertebrae to the inferior angle of each scapula is measured. An increased distance indicates an upwardly rotated scapula.

Scapular winging

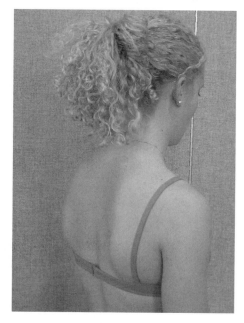

Elevation of the inferior angle of the scapula. Scapular tipping is characterized by the vertebral border lifting away from the thorax.

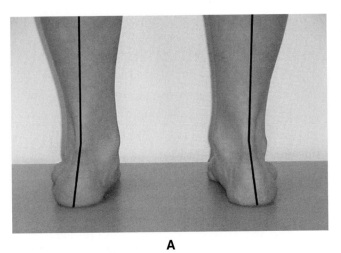
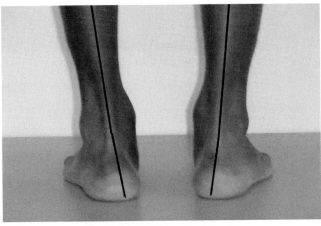

FIGURE 3–13. Alignment of the calcaneus and tibia. **(A)** Calcaneal eversion (Calcaneovalgus). **(B)** Calcaneal inversion (Calcaneovarus).

as they become shortened in length. When assessing muscle length for most of the *one-joint muscles,* the normal ranges (measurements) for passive joint range of motion are normally used. A goniometer used to measure joint angles assists in the objectivity of muscle length assessment. Appendix C presents techniques for assessing muscle length.

◆ COMMON POSTURAL DEVIATIONS

Many people in today's society have less than ideal posture. However, not all postural deviations cause pathology. Clinicians must be able to identify normal posture, *asymptomatic* deviations, and postural deviations possibly causing soft tissue dysfunction and pain. When evaluating postural deviations, keep in mind that any potential muscle imbalances can either cause the poor posture or be a result of the poor posture. Postural deviations also can be a result of skeletal malalignment, anomalies, or a combination thereof. The next section discusses some common postural deviations observed for each joint.

FOOT AND ANKLE

Hyperpronation

Excessive pronation is characterized by *adduction* and *plantarflexion* of the talus and *eversion* of the calcaneus while the foot is weight bearing (refer to Table 4–1 for a description of foot pronation and supination while weight bearing and non–weight bearing). The medial longitudinal arch also tends to be flattened with excessive pronation.

Two weight-bearing methods used to measure hyperpronation are the Feiss line and navicular drop tests

(see Chapter 4, Boxes 4–1 and 4–11). The subtalar neutral position is another common method to determine non–weight-bearing foot hyperpronation. In this position, the clinician is observing for forefoot or rearfoot varus, structural causes of hyperpronation, which is the cause of a number of postural deviations in the lower extremity (Fig. 3–13).

Supination

Excessive weight-bearing supination is characterized by abduction and *dorsiflexion* of the talus and inversion of the calcaneus. A heightened medial longitudinal arch is also commonly observed. Observation of forefoot or rearfoot valgus positions in the subtalar neutral position during non–weight bearing can be structural causes for excessive supination. Excessive supination can lead to a number of different postural deviations in the lower extremity.

One-joint muscles   A muscle that only exerts force across one joint.

Asymptomatic   Without symptoms.

Adduction   Medial movement of a body part toward the midline of the body.

Plantarflexion   Extension of the ankle; pointing the foot and toes.

Eversion   The movement of the plantar aspect of the calcaneus away from the midline of the body.

Dorsiflexion   Flexion of the ankle; pulling the foot and toes toward the tibia.

THE KNEE

Genu Recurvatum

This postural deviation is noted when the knee axis of motion is significantly posterior in relation to the plumb line, the person has greater than 5 degrees of knee hyperextension as measured with a goniometer, or the hyperextension is asymmetrical. A person with genu recurvatum often stands with his or her knees "locked" in an extreme extended position (Box 3–6). Genu recurvatum may be congenital or may be caused by pathology such as an anterior cruciate ligament sprain.

Genu Valgum

Genu valgum is a medial angulation of the femur and tibia occurring at the knee. Normally, a slight medial angulation at the knee is present. However, with exces-

sive genu valgum ("knock-kneed"), the knees are visibly closer together than the ankles during stance. Objectively measuring a person's Q angle determines if excessive genu valgum is present (see Chapter 7).

Genu valgum occurs because of structural anomalies at the hip, contributing muscular weaknesses occurring at the hip, or secondary to hyperpronation of the feet. Genu valgum can lead to a number of different postural deviations in the lower extremity, such as increased foot pronation, internal tibial rotation, medial patellar positioning, and internal femoral rotation.

Genu Varum

Genu varum ("bow-legged") is a lateral angulation of the femur and tibia occurring at the knee. The knees are further apart than the ankles while a person with genu varum is standing. Measuring the Q angle also objectively determines the presence of genu varum.

Box 3–6
GENU RECURVATUM

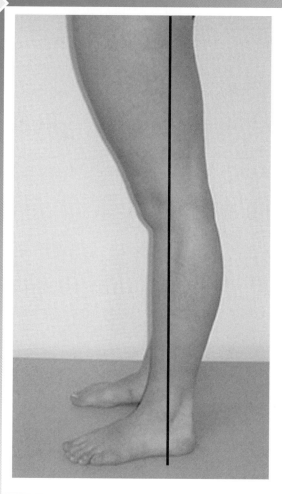

Possible causes	Hypermoility of joints/lax ligaments (commonly seen in ectomorph body type) Poor postural sense
Possible adverse effects	Increased stress on the ACL Increased tension on the posterior and posterolateral soft tissue structures Compressive forces on the anterior and medial compartments of the tibiofemoral joint

ACL = anteriocruciate ligament.

Genu varum occurs because of structural anomalies at the hip or from excessive supination of the feet. A number of different postural deviations in the lower extremity can occur because of genu varum; these include foot supination, external tibial rotation, lateral patellar positioning, and external femoral rotation. See Figure 6–16 for photographs of genu varum and genu valgum.

SPINAL COLUMN

Hyperlordotic Posture

This postural deviation entails an increase in the lumbar lordosis without compensation in the thoracic or cervical spines (Box 3–7). A person who demonstrates an increased lower lumbar lordosis (anterior convexity)

Box 3–7
HYPERLORDOTIC POSTURE

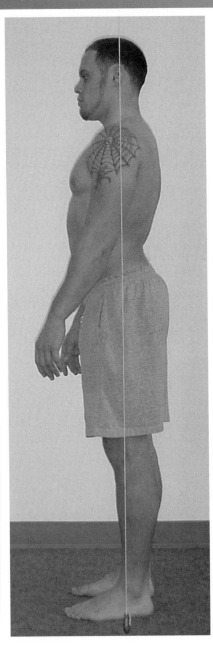

Joints involved	Lumbar spine, pelvis, hip
Possible cause	Tightened or shortened hip flexor muscles or back extensors Weakened or elongated hip extensors or abdominals Poor postural sense
Possible adverse effects	Increased lumbar lordosis Anterior pelvic tilt Hip assuming a flexed position
Possible associated compressive or distractive forces and pathological conditions	Increased shear forces placed on lumbar vetebral bodies secondary to psoas tightness Increased compressive forces on lumbar facet joints Adaptive shortening of the posterior lumbar spine ligaments and the anterior hip ligaments Elongation of the anterior lumbar spine ligaments and the posterior hip ligaments Narrowing of the lumbar intervertebral foramen

may have acquired this posture secondary to adaptive shortening of the hip flexors, rotating the ilia anteriorly and pulling the lumbar spine anteriorly. A large anterior abdominal mass, including during pregnancy, poor postural awareness, ligamentous laxity, and muscle weakness may also increase lumbar lordosis.

Kypholordotic Posture

Kypholordotic posture is similar to the hyperlordotic posture in that the patient has an increase in total lumbar lordosis; however, there is also a compensatory increase in thoracic kyphosis as an attempt to maintain the spine in a position of equilibrium (Box 3–8). In the kypholordotic posture, increases in the normal curvature are seen in both the lumbar and thoracic spines. The cervical spine also increases in lordosis and assumes a forward head posture (FHP) in an attempt to compensate for the other regions of the spinal column. With this posture, adaptive changes in the lengths of the muscles can be observed throughout the entire trunk.

Box 3–8
KYPHOLORDOTIC POSTURE

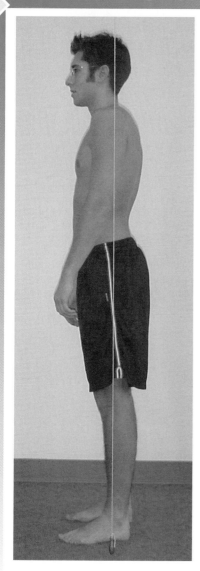

Joints involved	Pelvis, hip joint, lumbar spine, thoracic spine, cervical spine

Possible cause	Poor postural sense
	Muscle imbalance:
	    Tightened or shortened hip flexors or back extensors
	    Weakened or elongated hip extensors or trunk flexors

Possible adverse effects	Anterior pelvic tilt Hip joint flexion Increased lumbar lordosis (extension) Increased thoracic kyphosis (flexion)
Possible associated compressive or distractive forces and pathological conditions	Adaptive shortening of anterior chest musculature Elongation of thoracic paraspinal musculature Increased compressive forces on anterior structures of thoracic vertebrae and posterior structures of lumbar vertebrae Increased tensile forces on ligamentous structures in posterior aspect of thoracic spine and anterior aspect of lumbar spine Increased compression of lumbar facet joints Increased compression of thoracic anterior vertebral bodies Forward head posture Forward shoulder posture

Swayback Posture

Swayback posture is often referred to as a position of instability. With this deviation, the person relies on postural stability primarily from their ligaments rather than that of muscular support (Box 3–9). Individuals demonstrating a swayback posture commonly exhibit an ectomorph or a lax ligamentous mesomorph body type. The joints of these individuals' bodies are usually at the ends of their ranges, placing excessive strain on the surrounding ligamentous structures. In ideal posture, stability occurs because of a balance of static support from the ligamentous structures as well as a dynamic support from surrounding muscles.

Box 3–9
SWAYBACK POSTURE

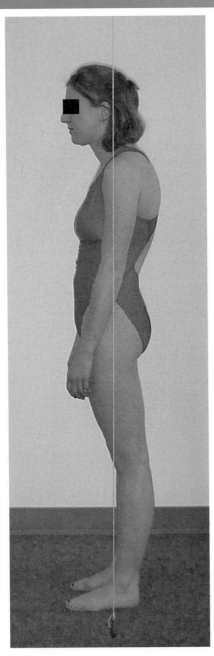

Joints involved	Knee joint, hip joint, lumbar spine, lower thoracic spine, cervical spine
Possible cause	Ectomorph body type: hypermobility of joints Poor postural sense Tightened or shortened hip extensors Weakened or elongated hip flexors or lower abdominals Decreased general muscular strength
Possible adverse effects	Genu recurvatum Hip joint extension Posterior pelvic tilt Anterior shift of the lumbosacral region Lumbar spine in neutral or minimal flexed position Increase in lower thoracic, thoracolumbar curvature (increase in lower thoracic kyphosis to cause posterior shift of trunk to compensate for anterior shift of L5/S1)
Possible associated compressive or distractive forces and pathological conditions	Elongation or increased tensile forces on the ligamentous structures at the anterior hip joint and posterior aspect of the lower thoracic spine Adaptively shortened or increased compressive forces on the posterior ligamentous structures at the hip joint and anterior aspect of the lower thoracic spine Increased tensile forces on the soft tissue structures of the posterior knee; compressive forces on anterior knee Result in increased stresses on joints; increased shearing forces L5/S1 Forward head posture Forward shoulder posture

Flat Back Posture

An individual displaying a flat back posture has lost the normal "S" shaped curvature of the spine in the sagittal plane (Box 3–10). The thoracic and lumbar curvatures are decreased and the spine is relatively straight. Often an associated FHP occurs to counteract the posterior displacement of the thoracic and lumbar spines. A decreased lumbar lordosis is associated with a posterior pelvic tilt.

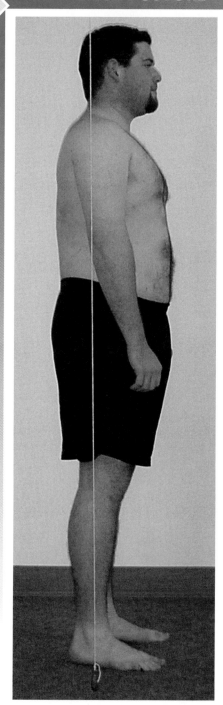

Box 3–10
FLAT BACK POSTURE

Joints involved	Hip joint, lumbar spine, thoracic spine, cervical spine
Possible causes	Shortened or tightened hip extensors, abdominal musculature Weakened/elongated hip flexors, back extensors Poor postural sense
Possible adverse effects	Extended hip joint Posterior pelvic tilt Flexed lumbar spine (decrease lumbar lordosis) Extended thoracic spine (decreased thoracic kyphosis) Flexed middle and lower cervical spine, extended upper cervical spine (FSP)
Possible associated compressive or distractive forces and pathological conditions	Adaptive shortening of soft tissue, compressive forces in posterior hip joint, anterior lumbar and mid-low cervical spines, posterior thoracic and upper cervical spines Elongation of soft tissue, tensile forces on the anterior hip joint, posterior lumbar and middle and lower cervical spines, anterior thoracic and upper cervical spines FHP resulting as compensation for the posterior displacement of the spine Knee flexion possibly occurring for the same reason

FHP = forward head posture; FSP = forward shoulder posture.

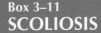

Box 3–11
SCOLIOSIS

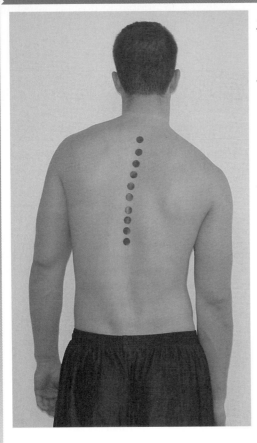

Joints involved	Thoracic and lumbar vertebrae
Possible causes	Structural scoliosis: Anomaly of vertebrae Functional scoliosis: Muscle imbalance, leg length discrepancy
Possible adverse effects	Rotation of one or more vertebrae Compresson of one facet joint; distraction of the opposite facet joint Shortened or tightened trunk muscles on concave side of the curvature Weakened or elongated trunk muscles on convex side of the curvature
Possible associated compressive or distractive forces and pathological conditions	Disc pathology Soft tissue pathology as the body attempts to compensate and maintain head posture Sacroiliac joint dysfunction Decreased mobility of spine and chest cage Asymmetry in chest expansion with deep breathing Decreased pulmonary function (if excessive in thoracic region) If caused by limb length inequality: 　Degenerative changes in lumbar spine, hip, knee joints in longer limb 　Muscle overuse on longer limb caused by increased muscle activity 　S-I joint dysfunction 　Excessive pronation of longer limb with dysfunctions associated with pronation 　Alteration of pattern of mechanical stresses on joint involved—structural

Scoliosis

Scoliosis involves the presence of lateral curvature of the spinal column (Box 3–11). Scoliosis is named for the side of convexity and the region of the spine in which it is observed. There are two types of scoliosis: functional and structural. Functional scoliosis occurs as the spine attempts to compensate to maintain the head in a neutral position and keep the eyes level. It is usually caused by a muscular imbalance, muscular guarding, a pelvic obliquity, or a limb length discrepancy. A structural scoliosis is caused by a defect or congenital bony anomaly of the vertebrae. A subcategory of structural scoliosis is *idiopathic* scoliosis. Idiopathic scoliosis makes up 2 to 4 percent of the population, affecting females more often than males.[25] Idiopathic scoliosis is structural in nature but does not involve bony abnormalities of the vertebral body. The exact cause of idiopathic scoliosis is not clear. However it seems to be multifactorial, based on heredity and involving musculoskeletal and neurologic factors.[25] To assist in determining whether a scoliosis is structural or functional, observe the patient's spine during erect posture and then during a forward flexed (trunk) posture. A structural scoliosis is present in both positions. In contrast, functional scoliosis is demonstrated only while the individual stands erect and disappears during spinal flexion.

SHOULDER AND SCAPULA

Forward Shoulder Posture

Forward shoulder posture (FSP) is characterized by protraction and elevation of the scapulae and a forward, rounded position of the shoulders that may also involve scapula winging and internal humeral rotation (Box 3–12).[1,3,26] FSP often occurs concurrently with forward head posture.

Idiopathic　Of unknown origin.

Box 3–12
FORWARD SHOULDER POSTURE

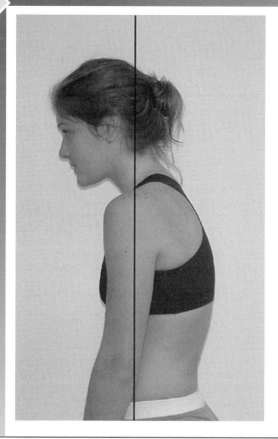

Joints involved	Scapulothoracic articulation Glenohumeral joint Thoracic spine Cervical spine
Possible causes	Tightened, shortened, or overdeveloped anterior shoulder girdle muscles (pectoralis major, pectoralis minor) Weakened or elongated interscapula muscles (mid trap, rhomboid, low trap) Poor postural awareness Abnormal cervical and thoracic spine sagittal plane arrangements[27] Postural muscle fatigue Large breast development Repetitive occupational and sporting positions[18]
Possible adverse effects	Humeral head is displaced anteriorly Forward head posture
Possible associated compressive or distractive forces and pathological conditions	Thoracic outlet syndrome Abnormal scapulohumeral rhythm and scapula stability Acromioclavicular degeneration Bicipital tendonitis Impingement syndrome Trigger points, myofascial pain in periscapular muscles Abnormal biomechanics of GH joint

Forward shoulder posture, observed from the lateral view, is associated with an anterior displacement of the acromion process in relation to the plumb line. Some common causes of FSP include poor postural sense (i.e., a person assuming a "slouched" posture); adaptively shortened anterior chest muscles (pectoralis major or minor); associated elongation of the posterior interscapula muscles (lower and middle trapezius, rhomboids); and abnormal cervical and thoracic spine sagittal plane curvatures, altering the resting position of the scapula.[1,27]

Several consequences result from the presence of prolonged FSP. Biomechanical changes in the shoulder girdle can cause any number of the following soft tissue dysfunctions: degeneration of the acromioclavicular joint; bicipital or rotator cuff tendinitis or impingement; muscular weakness; myofascial pain and trigger points; posterior capsular tightness; abnormal scapulohumeral rhythm; and can be attributed to the presence of excessive and habitual flexion of the back.[28–32] Adaptive shortening of the pectoralis minor or the anterior and middle scalene muscles can compress the subclavian artery, vein, and medial cord of the brachial plexus, resulting in **thoracic outlet syndrome**.[31,33,34] An FSP can also be associated with traction placed on the brachial plexus at the origin of the suprascapular and dorsal scapular nerves, causing associated pain and muscle weakness of the supraspinatus, infraspinatus, and rhomboids in which they innervate.[34]

Scapula Winging

Scapula winging can occur because of weakness of the periscapula muscles, especially the serratus anterior and middle and lower trapezius, and often occurs secondary to trauma to the long thoracic nerve. Scapula stabilization is essential for allowing normal arm mobility and biomechanics of the shoulder joint.

HEAD AND CERVICAL SPINE

Forward Head Posture

Forward head posture (FHP), the anterior displacement of the head relative to the thorax, is a common postural deviation.[35] Observed from the lateral view, FHP is characterized by the external auditory meatus aligning

Box 3–13
FORWARD HEAD POSTURE

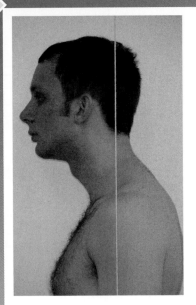

Joints involved	Cervical spine GH joint Thoracic spine
Possible causes	Wearing of bifocals Poor eyesight and need for glasses Muscle fatigue and weakness Poor postural sense Compensatory mechanism for other postural deviations (occupational activities and ADLs)
Possible adverse effects	Flexion of lower cervical spine Flattening or flexion of mid-cervical spine Extension of upper cervical spine Effects the normal GH joint motion
Possible associated compressive/distractive forces and pathological conditions	Adaptively shortened suboccipital muscles (capital extensors), scalenes, upper trapezius, and levator scapula Elongated and weakened anterior cervical flexors and scapular depressors Hypomobile upper cervical region with compensatory hypermobility of the mid-cervical spine Abnormal shoulder (GH joint) biomechanics; decrease in shoulder elevation Tempomandibular joint dysfunction[12,18] Thoracic outlet syndrome involving the anterior and mid-scalene region Myofascial pain periscapula muscles and posterior cervical muscles[36] Muscle overuse of posterior cervical and upper shoulder girdle muscles to maintain head in forward posture[36] Forward shoulder posture

ADL = activity of daily living; GH = glenohumeral.

anterior to the plumb line and anterior to the acromion process (Box 3–13). This posture results in flexion of the lower cervical spine, flattening or flexion of the mid-cervical spine, and extension of the upper cervical spine (suboccipital region).

Causes of FHP include poor postural sense, use of bifocal lenses, muscle fatigue, FSP, and the need for glasses.[18,36] Several possible dysfunctions of the cervical spine, shoulder, temporomandibular joint, and general upper quadrant can occur as a result of FHP.[12,18,36] The head weighs approximately 13 lbs. Displacing this weight anteriorly on the cervical spine increases the amount of muscular activity in the posterior neck muscles and upper shoulder girdle muscles.[31]

Forward head posture can also affect normal shoulder elevation. Elevation of the upper extremity requires cervical spine extension. If the mid and lower cervical spine remains in a flexed position, then full shoulder elevation cannot occur.[37] Certain muscle imbalances also result when FHP occurs concurrently with FSP (Table 3–13). Normally, the external auditory meatus aligns with the acromion process of the shoulder. If these landmarks do not align, note whether the patient is assuming an FSP. The patient then has both FSP and FHP even though the two landmarks are in alignment.

Table 3–13
COMBINATION OF FORWARD HEAD POSTURE AND FORWARD SHOULDER POSTURE

Muscles that Become Overactivated and Tightened	Muscles that Become Inhibited and Weakened
Pectoralis major Pectoralis minor Upper trapezius Upper rhomboids Levator scapulae	Lower trapezius Middle trapezius Serratus anterior

Table 3–14
INTERRELATIONSHIP BETWEEN JOINTS

Structure or Interconnecting Joints	Position of One Joint or Structure	Effect of Position of Other Joint or Structure
STJ and tibia	STJ pronated	Internal tibial rotation
	STJ supinated	External tibial rotation
Tibia and femur	Internal tibial rotation	Internal femoral rotation
	External tibial rotation	External femoral rotation
Tibiofemoral joint and the talocrural joint	Knee joint flexed, decreasing the angle between tibia and foot	Dorsiflexion of the talocrural joint
	Knee joint hyperextended, increasing the angle between tibia and foot	Plantarflexion of the talocrural joint
Femur and tibia	Femoral anteversion	Internal tibial rotation*
	Femoral retroversion	External tibial rotation*
Femur and patella	Internal femoral rotation	Squinting patellae
	External femoral rotation	Frog-eye patellae
Pelvic position and the hip joint	Pelvis in an anterior pelvic tilt, decreasing the angle between the pelvis and femur	Flexion of the hip joint
	Pelvis in a posterior pelvic tilt, increasing the angle between the pelvis and femur	Extension of the hip joint
Position of the pelvis and the lumbar spine	Pelvis in an anterior pelvic tilt, flexing the sacrum (nutation) and extending the lumbar spine	Increased lumbar lordosis
	Pelvis in a posterior pelvic tilt, extending the sacrum (counter nutation) and flexing the lumbar spine	Decreased lumbar lordosis

*The patient may attempt to compensate for femoral anteversion by excessively externally rotating the tibia in order to maintain the feet positioned straight ahead, the opposite is also true for the patient with femoral retroversion.
STJ = subtalar joint.

 INTERRELATIONSHIP BETWEEN REGIONS

Because each body part is closely linked to corresponding body parts, it is difficult to determine whether poor postural habits cause muscle imbalances, soft tissue dysfunctions, or pain or whether these conditions were the cause and poor posture was the result (Table 3–14). It is more important to understand the relationship and importance of correcting these factors because it is impossible to determine which was the cause or the effect after the fact.

Postural assessment is an important part of the evaluation process. Recognizing postural faults and establishing a plan to work toward correcting or minimizing these faults is an essential role for a clinician. Most soft tissue dysfunctions that have a gradual, insidious onset have, at least, a minimal postural component. This postural component may result in or cause imbalances between agonist and antagonist muscle groups or inert soft tissue structures. Clinicians must learn to investigate and observe the entire body and the interrelationships between regions when evaluating a specific body part. Learning to look at the "whole picture" makes someone a more effective clinician and more successful in treating patients.

DOCUMENTATION OF POSTURAL ASSESSMENT

Documentation of posture needs to be concise, yet as detailed as possible for the clinician to correlate possible postural involvement while interpreting other pertinent findings from the overall initial evaluation. Table 3–15 presents a sample postural assessment that would be recorded in the objective portion of an initial evaluation using the SOAP note documentation style. A sample of a standard postural assessment form can be found in Figure 3–14.

The following are guidelines for documenting posture:

- Document the view that is being observed (i.e., anterior, posterior, right lateral, left lateral).
- Quantify each postural deficit using minimum (min), moderate (mod), or severe (sev) and, whenever possible, objectively measure the deficits. When measuring the deficit, note the specific landmarks

Standard Postural Assessment Form

Name: _____

Clinician: _____

Painful area: _____

Date: _____

Duration of symptoms (months): _____

ANTERIOR VIEW

POSTERIOR VIEW

Alignment of plumb line with trunk: _____

Alignment of plumb line with head: _____

Calluses, bunions, blisters on feet: _____

Note calluses, blisters on heels: _____

Lower Extremity

Arch Position:	□ pes planus	□ pes cavus	□ neutral
Subtalar Joint:	□ pronated	□ supinated	□ neutral
Tibia Position:	□ medial rotation	□ lateral rotation	□ neutral
Patella Position	□ squinting	□ frog-eyed	□ neutral
Leg Position:	□ genu valgum	□ genu varum	□ neutral

Q-angle: □ left: _____ □ right: _____

Muscle mass/girth comments: _____

Other comments: _____

Lower Extremity (Posterior)

Calcaneal Position:	□ genu valgum	□ genu varum	□ neutral
Leg Position:	□ genu valgum	□ genu varum	□ neutral

Muscle mass calves: _____

Muscle mass posterior thighs: _____

Pelvis/Trunk

Iliac crest symmetry: _____

ASIS symmetry: _____

Abdominal muscle mass: _____

Chest Shape: □ pectus excavatum □ pectus recurvatum □ normal

Spinal Alignment: □ scoliosis □ neutral

Iliac crest symmetry: _____

PSIS symmetry: _____

Gluteal muscle mass: _____

Shoulder Girdle, Cervical Spine, and Head

Shoulder Position: □ internally rotated □ externally rotated □ neutral
Shoulder Heights: □ right elevated right □ depressed □ neutral
Head Position: □ side bent □ rotated □ neutral

Pectoral muscle mass: _____

Upper trapezius muscle mass: _____

Shoulder Girdle, Cervical Spine, and Head

Scapula Positions: _____

Elevation/depression: _____

Protraction/retraction: _____

Upward/downward Rotation: _____

Winging: _____

Periscapula muscle mass: _____

Upper trapezius muscle mass: _____

Shoulder height: _____

Head Position: □ side bent □ rotated □ neutral

LATERAL VIEW: RIGHT or LEFT (circle which):

Note Alignment of following structures relative to plumb line:

Lat. Malleolus:	□ anterior	□ posterior	□ bisecting
Talocrural Joint:	□ plantarflexed	□ dorsiflexed	□ neutral
Lat. Femoral Epicondyle:	□ anterior	□ posterior	□ bisecting
Knee Position:	□ flexed	□ extended	□ neutral
Greater Trochanter:	□ anterior	□ posterior	□ bisecting
Mid-Thorax:	□ anterior	□ posterior	□ bisecting
Acromion Process:	□ anterior	□ posterior	□ bisecting
Cervical Vertebral Bodies:	□ anterior	□ posterior	□ bisecting
External Auditory Meatus:	□ anterior	□ posterior	□ bisecting
Pelvic Position:	□ ant. rotation	□ post. rotation	□ neutral
Shoulder Position:	□ forward	□ neutral	
Head Position:	□ forward	□ neutral	

Lumbar Spine Position: _____

Thoracic Spine Position: _____

Cervical Spine Position: _____

Shoulder/Head: _____

LATERAL VIEW: RIGHT or LEFT (circle which):

Note Alignment of following structures relative to plumb line:

Lat. Malleolus:	□ anterior	□ posterior	□ bisecting
Talocrural Joint:	□ plantarflexed	□ dorsiflexed	□ neutral
Lat. Femoral Epicondyle:	□ anterior	□ posterior	□ bisecting
Knee Position:	□ flexed	□ extended	□ neutral
Greater Trochanter:	□ anterior	□ posterior	□ bisecting
Mid-Thorax:	□ anterior	□ posterior	□ bisecting
Acromion Process:	□ anterior	□ posterior	□ bisecting
Cervical Vertebral Bodies:	□ anterior	□ posterior	□ bisecting
External Auditory Meatus:	□ anterior	□ posterior	□ bisecting
Pelvic Position:	□ ant. rotation	□ post. rotation	□ neutral
Shoulder Position:	□ forward	□ neutral	
Head Position:	□ forward	□ neutral	

Lumbar Spine Position: _____

Thoracic Spine Position: _____

Cervical Spine Position: _____

Shoulder/Head: _____

FIGURE 3–14. Sample postural assessment form.

84

Table 3–15
DOCUMENTATION OF A FULL POSTURAL ASSESSMENT IN THE OBJECTIVE PORTION OF AN INITIAL EVALUATION USING SOAP FORMAT

View	Characteristics
Anterior	Min pes planus B feet
	Mod B squinting patellae
	Mod B genu valgum
	Min ↑ R ASIS
	Min B IR shld, R>L
Posterior	Min B calcaneal valgum
	Mod B genu valgum
	Min ↓ R PSIS
	Min B protraction scapulae, R>L
Left lateral	Min genu recurvatum
	Mod ant pelvis tilt, 20°
	Min ↑ lumbar lordosis
	Min FHP
Right lateral	Mod genu recurvatum
	Mod ant pelvis tilt, 20°
	Min ↑ lumbar lordosis
	Min FHP

ASIS = anterior superior iliac spine.
PSIS = superior posterior iliac spine.

used, specific positions measured, or any specific techniques used to measure them. This will assist in reproducibility of the measurement.

- Document the side of the body where the deficit occurs. If it involves unequal heights, choose whether to document the higher or lower side and then be consistent with your documentation.
- Use arrow symbols (↑↓) to represent increases or decreases regarding asymmetries in height.
- Use greater than (>) and less than (<) symbols to represent regions of muscle mass that are larger or smaller than the contralateral side.
- Document in an outline form (rather than paragraph form) to make the assessment easier to read and identify specific regions quickly.
- Document only postural deficits in the assessment. If a region of the body is normal, it does not require documentation.
- Use standard medical abbreviations to make documentation more concise.
- Use an asterisk (*) to emphasize a significant finding by placing the * beside the deficit.
- When evaluating an upper quarter injury, include the pelvis, lumbar spine, and all joints proximal to the injury in the postural assessment.
- When evaluating a lower quarter injury, include the lumbar spine, pelvis, and all joints distal to the painful site in the postural assessment.
- Include the entire body in the postural assessment of a patient with a spinal injury.

◆ **REFERENCES**

1. Kendall, FP, and McCreary, EK: *Muscles: Testing and Function* (ed 3). Baltimore, Williams & Wilkins, 1983.
2. Kisner, C and Kolby, LA: *Therapeutic Exercise: Foundations and Techniques* (ed 3). Philadelphia, FA Davis, 1996.
3. Kendall, HO, Kendall, FP, and Boynton, DA: *Posture and Pain.* Huntington N.Y, Robert E. Krieger Publishing Co., Inc, 1970, p. 15,153.
4. Riegger-Krugh, C, and Keysor, JJ: Skeletal malalignments of the lower quarter: Correlated and compensatory motions and postures. *J Orthop Sports Phys Ther*, 23:164, 1996.
5. Massie, DL, and Haddox, A: Influence of lower extremity biomechanics and muscle imbalances on the lumbar spine. *Athletic Therapy Today*, 4:46, 1999.
6. Tibierio D: Pathomechanics of structural foot deformities. *Phys Ther*, 68:1840, 1988.
7. Whilt SG, Sahrmann SA. Ch 16 A Movement system approach to management of musculoskeletal pain. In Grant, R: *Clinics in Physical Therapy: Physical Therapy of the Cervical and Thoracic Spine.* New York, Churchill Livingstone, 1994.
8. Jull, GA, and Janda, V: Muscles and motor control in low back pain: assessment and management. In Twomey, LT and Taylor, JR (eds): *Physical Therapy of the Low Back* (ed 2). New York, Churchill Livingstone, Inc., 1994, pp. 253–277.
9. Mannheimer, JS, and Rosenthal, RM: Acute and chronic postural abnormalities as related to craniofacial pain and temporomandibular disorders. *Dent Clin North Am* 35:185, 1991.
10. Krivickas, LS: Anatomical factors associated with overuse sports injuries. *Sports Med*, 24:132, 1997.
11. Novack, C, and Mackinnon, S: Repetitive use and static postures: A source of nerve compression and pain. *J Hand Ther*, 10:151, 1997.
12. Harrison, AL, Barry-Greb, T, and Wojtowicz, G: Clinical measurement of head and shoulder posture variables. *J Orthop Sports Phys Ther*, 23:353, 1996.
13. Garrett, TR, Youdas, JW, and Madson, TJ: Reliability of measuring forward head posture in a clinical setting. *J Orthop Sports Phys Ther*, 17:155, 1993.
14. Raine, S, and Twomey, LT: Head and shoulder posture variations in 160 asymptomatic women and men. *Arch Phys Med Rehabil*, 78:1215, 1997.
15. Peterson, DE, et al. Investigation of the validity and reliability of four objective techniques for measuring forward shoulder posture. *J Orthop Sports Phys Ther*, 25:34, 1997.
16. Greenfield, BH, et al: The influence of cephalostatic ear rods on the positions of the head and neck during positional recordings. *Am J Dentofacial Orthop*, 95:312, 1989.
17. Molhave, A: *A Biostatic Investigation of the Human Erect Posture.* Munkgard, Copenhagen, 1958.
18. Paris, SV and Loubert, PV: *Foundations of Clinical Orthopaedics.* Institute Press, Division of Patris Inc., 1990.
19. Ferguson, BRL: Limb length discrepancies. *J Am Podiatr Med Assoc*, 82:33, 1992.
20. Beal, MC: A review of the short leg problem. *J Am Osteopath Assoc*, 50:109, 1950.
21. Botte, RR: An interpretation of the pronator syndrome and foot types of patients with LBP. *J Am Podiatr Med Assoc*, 71:243, 1981.
22. Friberg O, Nurminen M, Korhumen K, et al: Accuracy and precision of clinical estimation of leg length inequality and lumbar scoliosis: comparison of clinical and radiographical measurements. *Int Disability Studies*, 10:45–53, 1988.
23. Hoyle DA, Latour M, and Bohannon, RW. Intraexaminer, interexaminer, and interdevice comparability of leg length measurements obtained with measuring tape and metrecom. *J Orthop Sports Phys Ther*, 14: 263–68, 1991.
24. Hoppenfeld, S: Physical examination of the hip and pelvis. In Hoppenfeld, S (ed): *Physical Examination of the Spine and Extremities.* New York, Appleton-Century-Crofts, 1976, p 165.
25. Byl, NN, et al: Postural imbalance and vibratory sensitivity in patients with idiopathic scoliosis: implications for treatment. *J Orthop Sports Phys Ther*, 26:60, 1997.

26. DiVeta, J, Walker, ML, and Skibinski, B: Relationship between performance of selected scapula muscles and scapula abduction in standing subjects. *Phys Ther*, 70:470, 1990.

27. Culham E, and Peat M. Spinal and shoulder complex posture: measurement using the 3S pace isotrak. *Clin Rehabil*, 7:309, 1993.

28. Ayub, E: Posture and the upper quarter. In Donatelli, RA (ed), *Physical Therapy of the Shoulder*. (2nd ed) New York, Churchill Livingstone, 1991.

29. Greenfield, B, et al: Posture in patients with shoulder overuse injuries and healthy individuals. *J Orthop Sports Phys Ther*, 21:287, 1995.

30. Knudsen, HO: *Posture: Sitting, Standing, Chair Design and Exercise.* Springfield, IL, Charles C. Thomas Publishers, 1988, p. 125, 314–315.

31. Langford, ML: Poor posture subjects a worker's body to muscle imbalance, nerve compression. *Occup Health Saf*, 63:38, 1994.

32. Travell JG, and Simons DG: *Myofascial Pain and Dysfunction. The Trigger Point Manual.* Baltimore, Williams & Wilkens, 1984.

33. Kopel, HP, and Thompson, WAL: *Peripheral entrapment neuropathies* (ed 2). New York, Robert E Krieger, 1976.

34. Howell, JW: Evaluation and management of thoracic outlet syndrome. In Donatelli RA (ed), *Physical Therapy of the Shoulder* (ed 2). New York, Churchill Livingston, 1991.

35. Willford, CH, et al: The interaction of wearing multifocal lenses with head posture and pain. *J Orthop Sports Phys Ther*, 23:194, 1996.

36. Garrett, TR, Youdas, JW, and Madison, TJ: Reliability of measuring forward head posture in a clinical setting. *J Orthop Sports Phys Ther*, 17:155, 1993.

37. Lee, DG: "Tennis elbow": A manual therapist's perspective. *J Orthop Sports Phys Ther*, 8:134, 1986.

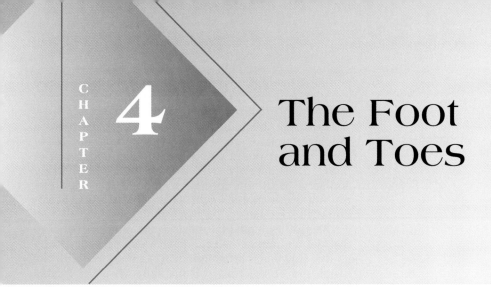

The Foot and Toes

The foot and toes perform a diverse range of tasks in combination with the ankle and lower leg. When standing, the foot provides a stable platform to balance and support the body. The foot acts as a rigid lever during the toe-off phase of gait and as a shock absorber during the initial contact phase (Fig. 4–1). When running, the foot is required to absorb and dissipate weight that is equal to three to eight times that of body weight.[1] In conjunction with the ankle, the foot and toes must be able to adapt to uneven terrain.

The foot, toes, and ankle are highly interrelated. Therefore, so is the evaluation of these areas. The evaluation of the foot and toes is described in this chapter, and the evaluation of the ankle and lower leg is discussed in Chapter 5. Despite this artificial delineation between the two areas, an evaluation of the foot and toes should also encompass an ankle evaluation and vice versa. In addition, some conditions may necessitate examining the entire lower extremity and lumbar spine along with a gait analysis.

◆ CLINICAL ANATOMY

The foot relies on intimate and precise relationships among the various surrounding structures. True one-on-one articulation between its bones is rare. This type of articulation tends to be limited to the joints of the toes. The majority of the remaining bones have multiple articulations with their contiguous structures. Muscular action and support are provided by the foot's *intrinsic* muscles and *extrinsic* muscles originating from the lower leg.

Formed by 26 bones and sesamoids, the foot is divided into three sections: the **rearfoot**, the **midfoot**, and the **forefoot** (Fig. 4–2). The **tarsals** consist of the calcaneus, talus, navicular, cuboid, and three cuneiforms. Originating from the distal tarsals, each of the five **metatarsals (MTs)** leads to the proximal **phalanges.** Each toe consists of three phalanges (proximal, middle, and distal), with the exception of the great toe, which has only two bones (proximal and distal).

FIGURE 4–1. Phases of gait for the right foot as defined by the Los Ranchos Medical Center system of gait analysis. This system, described in Chapter 9, divides the gait into weight-bearing and non–weight-bearing portions.

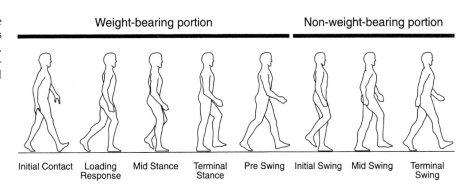

Weight-bearing portion | Non-weight-bearing portion

Initial Contact   Loading Response   Mid Stance   Terminal Stance   Pre Swing   Initial Swing   Mid Swing   Terminal Swing

---

Intrinsic   Arising from within the body.

Extrinsic   Arising from outside of the body.

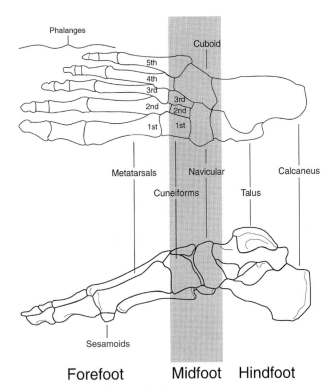

FIGURE 4–2. Anatomical zones of the foot. The talus and calcaneus form the rearfoot (rearfoot); the 3 cuneiform, the navicular, and the cuboid form the midfoot; and the 5 metatarsals, 14 phalanges, and 2 sesamoid bones form the forefoot.

REARFOOT

The **rearfoot**, formed by the calcaneus and talus, provides stability and shock absorption during the initial stance phase of gait and serves as a lever arm for the Achilles tendon during **plantarflexion** of the foot and ankle. The calcaneus is the largest of the tarsal bones. Its most prominent feature is the posteriorly projecting **calcaneal tubercle.** The large size of this tubercle provides a mechanically powerful lever for increasing the muscular force produced by the triceps surae muscle group (gastrocnemius, soleus, and plantaris). The large calcaneal body is the origin or insertion for many of the ligaments and muscles acting on the foot and ankle.

Arising off the anterior superior medial surface of the calcaneal body, the **sustentaculum tali** assists in supporting the talus (Fig. 4–3). On the inferior surface of the sustentaculum tali is a groove through which the tendon of the flexor hallucis longus passes. The lateral portion of the anterior calcaneus articulates with the cuboid. Projecting off the lateral side of the calcaneus, the **peroneal tubercle** assists in maintaining the stability and alignment of the peroneal tendons. Here, the

peroneal tendons diverge, with the peroneus brevis running superior to the tubercle and the peroneus longus traveling inferior to it.

The distal tibia and fibula form an articular mortise in which the talus sits (Fig 4–4). The inferior surface of the **talus** is marked by anterior, middle, and posterior *facets.* These facets provide a base for weight bearing and serve as the site for ligaments to attach. The superior surface is marked with facets that allow articulation with the tibia.

The saddle-shaped talus acts as the interface between the foot and ankle. Its unique shape is necessitated by its five functional articulations: (1) superiorly with the distal end of the tibia, (2) medially with the medial malleolus, (3) laterally with the lateral malleolus, (4) inferiorly with the calcaneus, and (5) anteriorly with the navicular. There are no muscular attachments on the talus.

MIDFOOT

Serving as the shock-absorbing segment of the foot, the **midfoot** is composed of the navicular, three cuneiforms, and the cuboid bones. The *keystone* of the medial longitudinal arch, the **navicular,** articulates anteriorly with the three cuneiforms, the cuboid laterally, and the talus posteriorly. The medial aspect of the navicular gives rise to the navicular *tuberosity,* the primary insertion for the tibialis posterior muscle.

The **cuboid** articulates with the third cuneiform and navicular medially, the fourth and fifth MTs anteriorly, and the calcaneus posteriorly. A palpable *sulcus* is formed anterior to the cuboid tuberosity and posterior to the base of the fifth MT, where the peroneus longus begins its course along the foot's *plantar* surface.

Adding to the flexibility of the midfoot and forefoot, the three **cuneiforms** are identified by their relative position on the foot: medial (first), intermediate (second), and lateral (third). Each cuneiform articulates with the navicular posteriorly, the corresponding MT anteriorly, and its contiguous cuneiform medially and laterally. The lateral border of the third cuneiform also articulates with the medial aspect of the cuboid.

Facet   A small, smooth, articular surface on a bone.

Keystone   The crown of an arch that supports the structures on either side of it.

Tuberosity   A nodulelike projection off a bone, serving as an attachment site for muscles and ligaments; referred to as a tubercle in the upper extremity.

Sulcus   A groove or depression within a bone.

Plantar   The weight-bearing surface of the foot.

FIGURE 4–3. Anatomy of the foot showing prominent bony landmarks and sites of ligamentous and muscular attachments.

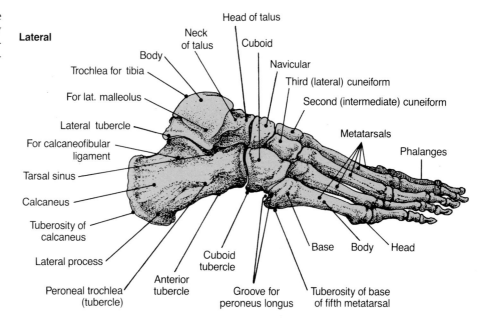

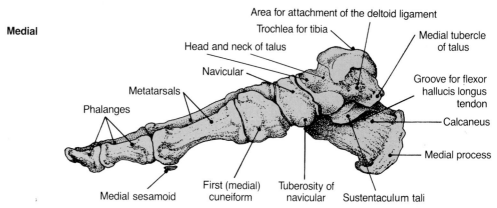

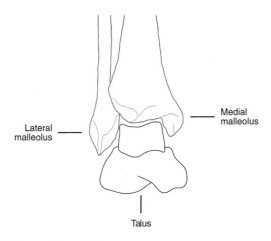

FIGURE 4–4. The ankle mortise. The articulation formed by the talus, tibia, and fibula. The subtalar joint is formed by the articulation between the inferior talus and the superior portion of the calcaneus.

FOREFOOT AND TOES

The **forefoot and toes,** formed by the five MTs and 14 phalanges, act as a lever during the preswing phase of gait. The five MTs may be conceptualized as miniature long bones, each having a proximal base, body, and distal head. The MTs are referenced numerically from medial (first) to lateral (fifth). Proximally, the bases of the first three MTs articulate with the corresponding cuneiform, although the second MT also has an articulation with the first and second cuneiform. The fourth and fifth MTs articulate with the cuboid. Although not true articular joints, each of the MT heads articulates with the proximal phalanx of the corresponding toe and loosely with the neighboring MT heads.[2] Like the MT heads, the bases articulate with the contiguous MTs, but with a tighter fit.

Table 4–1
SUMMARY OF NON–WEIGHT-BEARING AND WEIGHT-BEARING SUBTALAR MOTIONS

	Component Movements of Subtalar Supination/Pronation	
Motion	**Non–Weight Bearing**	**Weight Bearing**
Supination	Calcaneal inversion (or varus) Calcaneal adduction Calcaneal plantarflexion	Calcaneal inversion (or varus) Talar abduction (or lateral rotation) Talar dorsiflexion Tibiofibular lateral rotation
Pronation	Calcaneal eversion (or valgus) Calcaneal abduction Calcaneal dorsiflexion	Calcaneal eversion (or valgus) Talar adduction (or medial rotation) Talar plantarflexion Tibiofibular medial rotation

Like the MTs, each **phalanx** also has a base, shaft, and head, but these are on a much smaller scale. The toes also are numerically referenced as one through five from medial to lateral.

ARTICULATIONS AND LIGAMENTOUS SUPPORT

The ligaments joining the tarsal bones of the foot may be collectively grouped into three sets: (1) the thin *dorsal* tarsal ligaments, (2) the relatively thick plantar tarsal ligaments, and (3) the *interosseous* tarsal ligaments that stretch between contiguous bones and interrupt the synovial cavities. The specific names given to these ligaments typically reflect the bones to which they are connected.

Subtalar Joint

Located at the junction between the inferior surface of the talus and the superior surface of the calcaneus, the subtalar (talocalcaneal) joint has three articular facets. The **posterior articulation** is a concave facet on the talus. The **anterior** and **middle articulations** are convex facets. Obliquely crossing the talus and calcaneus is the tarsal canal, a sulcus that allows for the attachment of an intra-articular ligament.

It is often incorrectly stated that the motions occurring at the subtalar joint are inversion and eversion. The subtalar joint is a uniaxial joint with 1 degree of *freedom of movement*: supination and pronation.[3] The triplanar motion of the talus occurs around a single joint axis, allowing the component elements of pronation and supination to occur:

> **Supination**: inversion + adduction + plantarflexion
>
> **Pronation**: eversion + abduction + dorsiflexion

Although these motions may be discussed as individual elements, they do not occur independently of each other.[3] The relationship between these motions is influenced by the weight-bearing and non–weight-bearing status of the foot (Table 4–1). The difference between weight-bearing and non–weight-bearing function occurs because the talus becomes a moving structure during weight bearing, producing motion at the forefoot and midtarsal, subtalar, and talocrural joints.[4] When non–weight bearing, the calcaneus moves on the talus.

Because no muscles attach to the talus, the stability of the subtalar joint is derived from ligamentous and bony restraints. The **interosseous talocalcaneal ligament** lies in the tarsal canal. In addition to assisting in maintaining the alignment between the talus and calcaneus, this ligament serves as an axis for talar tilt and divides the subtalar joint into two articular cavities. A second intra-articular ligament, the **ligamentum cervicis**, lies laterally in the tarsal canal. Collateral support is gained from the lateral and medial (deltoid) ankle ligaments. One *slip* of the deltoid ligament, the **medial talocalcaneal ligament**, provides medial intrinsic support to the subtalar joint, and the **lateral talocalcaneal ligament** provides lateral support. Anterior glide of the talus on the calcaneus is partially restrained by the **posterior talocalcaneal ligament.**

Midfoot

The **talocalcaneonavicular (TCN) joint** and the **calcaneocuboid (CC) joint** represent the junction between the rearfoot and midfoot. The TCN joint is formed by the articulation between the talar head, the posterior aspect of the navicular, and the anterior border of the cal-

---

Dorsal (foot)   Referring to the superior portion of the foot and toes.

Interosseous   Between two bones.

Freedom of movement   The number of cardinal planes in which a joint allows motion.

Slip   A distinct band of tissue arising from the main portion of a structure.

caneus and its sustentaculum tali. The most important soft tissue support of this joint is provided by the **plantar calcaneonavicular ("spring") ligament.** Spanning the range from the sustentaculum tali to the inferior surface of the posterior navicular and blending in with the deltoid ligament of the ankle, this ligament forms a "socket" for the talar head, providing support for the medial longitudinal arch.

Formed by the anterior border of the calcaneus and the posterior aspect of the cuboid, the CC joint is reinforced by the plantar and dorsal **calcaneocuboid ligaments.** Further support is gained from the **long plantar ligament** and **plantar fascia** originating from the plantar surface of the calcaneus and inserting on the cuboid and the second, third, and fourth MTs.

The **midtarsal joint** is formed by the articulations of the tarsal bones located perpendicular to the long axis of the foot, the talonavicular and calcaneocuboid joints. Together, the midtarsal joint increases the range of motion (ROM) during inversion and eversion and allows the forefoot to compensate for uneven terrain.

Forefoot

The junction between the midfoot and forefoot is demarcated by the **tarsometatarsal joints** (Lisfrancs joint). Here the five MTs articulate with the bones of the midfoot in a gliding manner. Proximal and distal **intermetatarsal joints** are formed between the bases and heads of contiguous MTs. Permitting a slight amount of dorsal/plantar glide, the proximal joints are bound together by the **plantar, dorsal,** and **interosseous ligaments.** The distal joints are secured by the **deep transverse ligament** and the interosseous ligament.

A condyloid articulation between the MTs and the toes, the **metatarsophalangeal (MTP) joints** allows flexion and extension, and limited degrees of abduction, adduction, and rotation of the toes. Articular and fibrous joint capsules surround each joint. The plantar portion of the capsule is reinforced by the **plantar fascia** and thickened portions of the capsule, the **plantar ligament.** The medial and lateral joint capsule is reinforced by **collateral ligaments.**

With the exception of the first toe (hallux), each toe has two **interphalangeal (IP) joints:** a proximal interphalangeal (PIP) joint and a distal interphalangeal (DIP) joint. The hallux only has one IP joint. These hinge joints allow only flexion and extension to occur. Similar to the MTP joints, each joint is reinforced by the plantar and dorsal joint capsule and collateral ligaments.

MUSCLES ACTING ON THE FOOT AND TOES

The intrinsic foot muscles are those originating on one of the bones of the foot and directly influence the motion of the foot and toes. The extrinsic foot muscles originate on the lower leg or the distal aspect of the femur. The extrinsic foot muscles influence motion at the talocrural and knee joints, in addition to movement at the foot and toes (Tables 4–2 and 4–3).

Intrinsic Muscles of the Foot

The foot's intrinsic muscles are grouped into four layers (Table 4–4). The **superficial layer** contains the primary abductor of the first toe, the abductor hallucis; the primary abductor of the fifth toe, the abductor digiti minimi; and the secondary flexor of the second through fifth toes, the flexor digitorum brevis (Fig. 4–5). The **middle layer** is formed by the quadratus plantae, a muscle that, when contracted, changes the angle of pull for the flexor digitorum brevis and the lumbricals that flex the MTP joints and extend the IP joints. The tendons of the flexor hallucis longus and flexor digitorum longus also pass through this layer. The **deep layer** consists of the secondary flexors of the first and fifth toes, the flexor hallucis brevis and the adductor hallucis and the flexor digiti minimi brevis. The **interosseous layer,** found beneath the deep layer, contains the plantar and dorsal interossei. The three plantar interossei adduct the lateral three toes and the four dorsal interossei abduct the middle three toes (in relation to the second MT).

Extrinsic Muscles Acting on the Foot

The muscles that cross the talocrural or subtalar joints affect the position of the foot. The long toe extensors, extensor hallucis longus (EHL), and extensor digitorum longus assist in ankle dorsiflexion. The EHL also inverts the foot. The extensor digitorum longus everts the foot, but this action is weak. The flexor hallucis longus assists in plantarflexion and adduction and inversion of the foot and ankle. The flexor digitorum longus also plantarflexes the ankle while inverting the foot. The remaining muscles are described in detail in Chapter 5. Table 5–1 contains further information about the action of the extrinsic muscles on the foot.

ARCHES OF THE FOOT

Serving primarily as shock absorbers to buffer and dissipate the *ground reaction forces*, the three arches of the foot also serve to increase the foot's flexibility. The normal arches are more prominent in the non–weight-bearing position than in the weight-bearing position. When non–weight bearing, the medial longitudinal arch is the most noticeable; the lateral longitudinal arch and the transverse arch are less distinct. With weight bearing, the arches flatten as the foot contacts the ground at multiple points: the head of the first MT, the head of the fifth MT, and the calcaneus.

Ground reaction forces Forces applied to the feet when there is contact with the floor or ground; these are equal, but in the opposite direction of the forces applied by the feet to the floor or ground.

Table 4–2
POSTERIOR AND PLANTAR MUSCLES ACTING ON THE ANKLE, FOOT, TOES

Muscle	Action	Origin	Insertion	Innervation	Root
Abductor digiti minimi	Flexion of the 5th MTP joint Abduction of the 5th MTP joint	• Lateral portion of the tuber calcanei • Proximal lateral portion of calcaneus	• Lateral portion of the proximal 5th phalanx	Lateral plantar	S1, S2
Abductor hallucis	Abduction of the 1st MTP joint Assists flexion of the 1st MTP joint Assists in forefoot adduction	• Medial calcaneal tuberosity • Flexor retinaculum • Plantar aponeurosis	• Plantar surface of the medial base of the 1st toe's proximal phalanx	Medial plantar	L4, L5, S1
Adductor hallucis	Adduction of the 1st MTP joint Assists in flexion of the 1st MTP joint	Oblique head • Bases of 2nd through 4th metatarsals • Tendon sheath of peroneus longus Transverse head • Plantar surface of 3rd, 4th, and 5th metatarsal heads	• Lateral surface of the base of the 1st toe's proximal phalanx	Lateral plantar	S1, S2
Flexor digiti minimi brevis	Flexion of the 5th MTP joint	• Plantar surface of the cuboid • Base of the 5th metatarsal	• Plantar aspect of the base of the 5th metatarsal	Lateral plantar	S1, S2
Flexor digitorum brevis	Flexion of the 2nd through 5th PIP joints Assists in flexion of the 2nd through 5th MTP joints	• Medial calcaneal tuberosity • Plantar fascia	• Via four tendons, each having two slips, into the medial and lateral sides of the proximal 2nd through 5th phalanges	Medial plantar	L4, L5, S1
Flexor digitorum longus	Flexion of 2nd through 5th PIP and DIP joints Flexion of 2nd through 5th MTP joints Assists in ankle plantarflexion Assists in foot inversion	• Posterior medial portion of the distal two thirds of the tibia • From fascia arising from the tibialis posterior	• Plantar base of distal phalanges of the 2nd through 5th toes	Tibial	L5, S1

Muscle	Action	Attachment	Insertion	Nerve	Root
Flexor hallucis brevis	Flexion of 1st MTP joint	• Medial side of the cuboid bone's plantar surface • Slip from the tibialis posterior tendon	• Via two tendons into the medial and lateral sides of the proximal phalanx of the first toe	Medial plantar	L4, L5, S1
Flexor hallucis longus	Flexion of 1st IP joint Assists in flexion of 1st MTP joint Assists in foot inversion Assists in plantarflexion of the ankle	• Posterior distal two thirds of the fibula • Associated interosseous membrane and muscular fascia	• Plantar surface of the proximal phalanx of the 1st toe	Tibial	L4, L5, S1
Gastrocnemius	Ankle plantarflexion Assists in knee flexion	Medial head • Posterior surface of the medial femoral condyle • Adjacent portion of the femur and knee capsule Lateral head • Posterior surface of the lateral femoral condyle • Adjacent portion of the femur and knee capsule	• To the calcaneus via the Achilles tendon	Tibial	S1, S2
Interossei, dorsal	Abduction of the 3rd and 4th digits Assists in flexion of the MTP joints Assists in extension of the 3rd, 4th, and 5th IP joints	• Via two heads to the contiguous sides of the metatarsal bones	• Lateral portion of the bases of the 2nd, 3rd, and 4th proximal phalanges • The medial border of the second phalanx also receives the interossei arising between the 2nd and 3rd metatarsal	Lateral plantar	S1, S2
Interossei, plantar	Adduction of the 3rd, 4th and 5th digits Assists in flexion of the MTP joint Assists in extension of the 3rd, 4th, and 5th, IP joints	• Base and medial aspect of the 3rd, 4th, and 5th metatarsals	• Medial portion of the bases of the 3rd, 4th, and 5th proximal phalanges	Lateral plantar	S1, S2
Lumbricals	Flexion of the 2nd through 5th MTP joints Assists in extension of the 2nd through 5th IP joints	• Tendons of flexor digitorum longus	• Posterior surfaces of the 2nd through 5th toes via the tensor digitorum longus tendons	1st: Medial plantar 2nd to 5th Lateral plantar	1st: L4, L5, S1 2nd to 5th: S1, S2

Table 4–2 (continued)
POSTERIOR AND PLANTAR MUSCLES ACTING ON THE ANKLE, FOOT, TOES

Muscle	Action	Origin	Insertion	Innervation	Root
Peroneus brevis	Eversion of foot Assists in ankle plantarflexion	• Distal two thirds of the lateral fibula	• Styloid process at the base of the 5th metatarsal	Superficial peroneal	L4, L5, S1
Peroneus longus	Eversion of the foot Assists in ankle plantarflexion	• Lateral tibial condyle • Fibular head • Upper two thirds of the lateral fibula	• Lateral aspect of the base of the 1st metatarsal • Lateral and dorsal aspect of the 1st cuneiform	Superficial peroneal	L4, L5, S1
Plantaris	Ankle plantarflexion Assists in knee flexion	• Distal portion of the supracondylar line of the lateral femoral condyle • Adjacent portion of the femoral popliteal surface • Oblique popliteal ligament	• To the calcaneus via the Achilles tendon	Tibial	L4, L5, S1
Quadratus plantae	Modifies the flexor digitorum's angle of pull Assists in flexion of the 2nd through 5th MTP joints	Medial head • Medial calcaneus Lateral head • Lateral calcaneus	• Dorsal and plantar surfaces of the flexor digitorum longus	Lateral plantar	S1, S2
Soleus	Ankle plantarflexion	• Posterior fibular head • Upper one third of the fibula's posterior surface • Soleal line located on the posterior tibial shaft • Middle one third of the medial tibial border	• To the calcaneus via the Achilles tendon	Tibial	S1, S2
Tibialis posterior	Inversion of the foot Assists in ankle plantarflexion	• Length of the interosseous membrane • Posterior, lateral tibia • Upper two thirds of the medial fibula	• Navicular tuberosity • Via fibrous slips to the sustentaculum tail; cuneiforms; cuboid; and bases of the 2nd, 3rd, and 4th metatarsals	Tibial	L4, S1

DIP = distal interphalangeal; IP = interphalangeal; MTP = metatarsophalangeal; PIP = proximal interphalangeal.

Table 4-3

ANTERIOR AND DORSAL MUSCLES ACTING ON THE ANKLE, FOOT, TOES

Muscle	Action	Origin	Insertion	Innervation	Root
Extensor digitorum longus	Extension of the 2nd through 5th MTP joints Assists in extending 2nd through 5th PIP and DIP joints Assists in foot eversion Assists in ankle dorsiflexion	• Lateral tibial condyle • Proximal three fourths of anterior fibula • Proximal portion of the interosseous membrane	• Via four tendons to the distal phalanges of the 2nd through 5th toes	Deep peroneal	L4, L5, S1
Extensor digitorum brevis	Extension of the 1st though 4th MTP joints Assists in extension of the 2nd, 3rd, and 4th PIP and DIP joints	• Distal portion of the superior and lateral portion of the calcaneus • Lateral talocalcaneal ligament • Lateral portion of the inferior extensor retinaculum	• To the dorsal surface of the base of the first phalanx (syn: extensor hallucis brevis) • Proximal phalanges of the 2nd, 3rd, and 4th toes and to the distal phalanges via an attachment to the extensor digitorum longus tendon	Deep peroneal	L5, S1
Peroneus tertius	Eversion of the foot Dorsiflexion of the ankle	• Distal one third of the anterior surface of the fibula • Adjacent portion of the interosseous membrane	• Dorsal surface of the base of the 5th metatarsal	Deep peroneal	L4, L5, S1
Extensor hallucis longus	Extension of the 1st MTP joint Extension of the 1st IP joint	• Middle two thirds of the anterior surface of the fibula • Adjacent portion of the interosseous membrane	• Base of the distal phalanx of the 1st toe	Deep peroneal	L4, L5, S1
Tibialis anterior	Dorsiflextion of the ankle Inversion of the foot	• Lateral tibial condyle • Upper one half of the tibia's lateral surface • Adjacent portion of the interosseous membrane	• Medial and plantar surface of the 1st cuneiform • Medial and plantar surfaces of the 1st metatarsal	Deep peroneal	L4, L5, S1

DIP = distal interphalangeal; IP = interphalangeal; MTP = metatarsophalangeal; PIP = proximal interphalangeal.

Table 4–4
LAYERS OF THE FOOT'S INTRINSIC MUSCLES

Layer	Muscles
1st superficial layer	Abductor hallucis Flexor digitorum brevis Abductor digiti minimi
2nd middle layer	Tendon of flexor hallucis longus Tendons of flexor digitorum longus Quadratus plantae Lumbricals
3rd deep layer	Flexor hallucis brevis Adductor hallucis Flexor digiti minimi brevis
4th interosseous layer	Plantar interossei Dorsal interossei

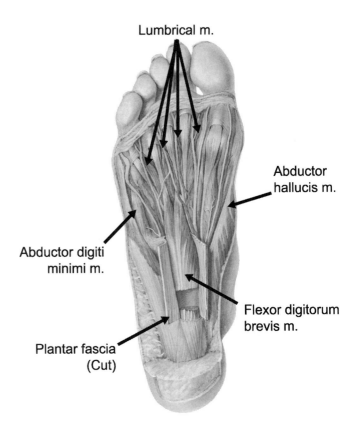

FIGURE 4–5. The superficial layer of the foot's intrinsic muscles is formed by the abductor digiti minimi, the abductor hallucis, and the flexor digitorum brevis muscles. The lumbrical muscles are a component of the middle muscle layer.

Medial Longitudinal Arch

Five bones form the prominent medial longitudinal arch: the calcaneus, talus, navicular, first cuneiform, and first MT (Fig. 4–6). The bony, ligamentous, and muscular arrangement of the medial arch allow a greater amount of motion than that allowed by the other arches of the foot. Serving as the keystone, the navicular bone is the stabilizing element between the anterior and posterior sides of the arch. Because the navicular bone plays an important role in supporting the medial longitudinal arch, dysfunction of this bone or the structures that support and reinforce the bone leads to dysfunction of the arch as a whole.

Ligamentous support of the medial arch is obtained from the plantar calcaneonavicular ("spring") ligament, the long plantar ligament, the deltoid ligament, and the plantar fascia. A slip from the spring ligament to the

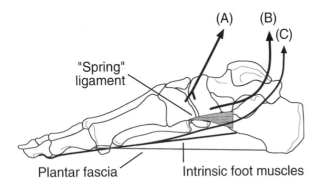

FIGURE 4–6. Soft tissue support of the medial longitudinal arch. Dynamic support is obtained through the **(A)** tibialis anterior, **(B)** tibialis posterior, **(C)** flexor hallucis longus muscles. The spring ligament is assisted by the plantar fascia and intrinsic foot muscle in bowing the arch.

ankle's **deltoid ligament** also assists in providing superior support of the navicular. A second slip supports the talus.

Primary support of the medial longitudinal arch is obtained from the three slips of the **plantar fascia.**[1] The central slip, originating off the medial calcaneal tubercle and inserting into the distal plantar aspects of each of the five digits, is the longest and thickest (Fig. 4–7). As the central slip progresses down the length of the foot, it gives rise to two other slips, one deviating medially and the other deviating laterally. The function of the plantar fascia is complimented by many of the foot's intrinsic muscles and ligaments. The plantar fascia is attached to the overlying plantar skin.[5]

The plantar fascia supports the medial and lateral longitudinal arches in a manner similar to the way a bow string functions to give the bow a curve. By longitudinally supporting the proximity of the calcaneus to the MT heads, the plantar fascia bows the foot's long arches. Because of the fascia's attachment on the phalanges, extending the toes draws the calcaneus toward

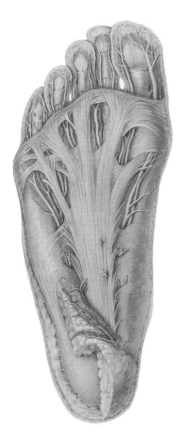

FIGURE 4–7. Plantar fascia. The central slip attaches to each of the five toes. Extending the toes tightens the fascia, increasing the curvature of the medial longitudinal arch.

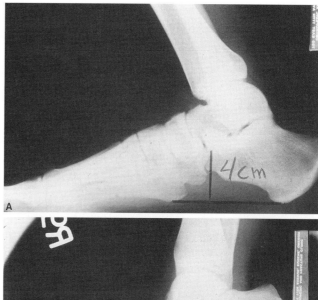

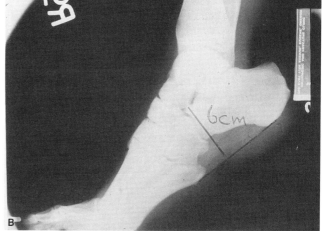

FIGURE 4–8. Windlass effect of the plantar fascia on the medial longitudinal arch. **(A)** The height of the medial arch when the foot is fully weight bearing **(B)** Extending the toes causes the plantar fascia to tighten, resulting in an increase in the height of the arch.

the MT heads. As a result, the arches become further extenuated, owing to a windlass effect (Fig. 4–8).

During static weight bearing, muscles provide little support to the medial arch. However, during walking, a force couple is formed between the tibialis anterior and the tibialis posterior, drawing the arch proximally and superiorly to supinate the foot. Dysfunction of this force couple can place additional stress on the foot's bony and soft tissue structures, possibly leading to lower leg pathologies such as medial tibial stress syndrome or tibialis posterior tendinitis.

Lateral Longitudinal Arch

Lower and more rigid than the medial longitudinal arch, the lateral arch is composed of the calcaneus, the cuboid, and the fifth MT. Although the lateral longitudinal arch is often considered a unique structure, it is actually a continuation of the medial arch. The arch itself is rarely the site of injury.

Transverse Metatarsal Arch

The transverse MT arch is formed by the lengths of the MTs and tarsals and is shaped by the concave features along the inferior surface of the MTs. The arch originates at the MT heads and remains present to the point where it fades on the calcaneus (Fig 4–9). The first and fifth MT heads are the weight-bearing structures. The second MT forms the apex of the arch. Structural support of this arch is derived from the intermetatarsal ligaments and transverse head of the adductor hallucis muscle.

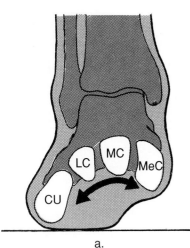 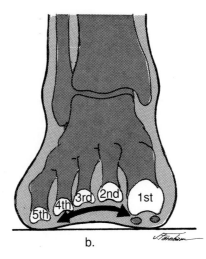

FIGURE 4–9. Transverse metatarsal arch. **(A)** At the midtarsal joints; CU = cuboid, LC = lateral cuneiform, MC = middle cuneiform, MeC = Medial cuneiform. **(B)** At the distal metatarsals.

◆ CLINICAL EVALUATION OF FOOT AND TOE INJURIES

When evaluating foot injuries, an evaluation of the ankle complex is often included. Additionally, evaluation of the lower extremity, lumbar spine, and gait also may be necessary. Having the patient dressed in shorts during the examination helps to expedite the evaluation of these structures.

HISTORY

A detailed and accurate history of recent and prior incidence of foot pain is needed to accurately evaluate this body area. An acute onset of symptoms should lead the examiner to suspect bony trauma. Insidious pain may arise from inflammation of a ligamentous or muscular structure or from the development of a stress fracture.

- **Location of the pain:** Pain in the foot may arise from trauma to its intrinsic structures or secondary to compensation for improper lower leg biomechanics. Pain may be referred from the lumbar or sacral nerve roots, the sciatic nerve, or the femoral nerve or one of their branches (Table 4–5).

  - **Retrocalcaneal pain:** Pain along the posterior aspect of the calcaneus may result from inflammation of the retrocalcaneal bursa, inflammation of the Achilles tendon, or os trigonum pathology (see Chapter 5). Retrocalcaneal bursa pain is more isolated to the area between the Achilles and the calcaneus; the pain associated with tendonitis may be more diffuse.

  - **Heel pain:** Pain in the heel may be the result of plantar fasciitis or a heel spur, especially if the pain is located on the medial plantar aspect. In the absence of a mechanism of injury to this area, pain may be referred from the lumbar nerve roots or their peripheral nerves.

  - **Medial arch pain:** The medial arch can be the site of pain for **tarsal tunnel syndrome,** a midfoot sprain, plantar fasciitis, navicular fracture, or tibialis posterior tendonitis. Compression of the posterior tibial nerve, tarsal tunnel syndrome, radiates a sharp, burning pain and paresthesia to the medial arch.

  - **Metatarsal pain:** Pain specifically located on a MT that worsens over time can indicate a stress fracture. This pain should be differentiated from pain arising from between the MTs, possibly the result of impingement of the intermetatarsal nerves. The pain caused by both conditions carries the common trait of worsening with activity. **Metatarsalgia** is nondescript pain arising from the MTs.

  - **Great toe pain:** Pain and dysfunction in the great toe can be disabling and alter the gait cycle. Pathology within the MTP joint, such as **hallux rigidus** or **hallux abducto valgus,** is characterized by diffuse pain throughout the joint during hyperextension and flexion. Pain localized to the plantar surface of the joint may be caused by a sesamoid fracture or inflammation of the sesamoids **(sesamoiditis).** The first MTP joint is often the first part of the body to demonstrate the signs and symptoms of *gout,* characterized by swelling, redness, and severe pain. Dorsal pain can originate from an ingrown toenail.

Gout   A form of arthritis marked by inflammation and pain in the distal joints.

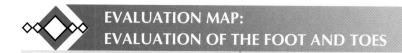

1. HISTORY

Location of the Pain
Heel
Medial arch
Metatarsal
Toes
Lateral arch

Onset of Injury
Acute onset
Insidious onset
Mechanism of injury
Playing surface
Running distance
Running duration
Shoes

2. INSPECTION

General Inspection
Callus and blisters
Foot type

Toes
Morton's alignment
Claw toes
Hammer toe
Hallux valgus
Bunion
Corns
Ingrown toenail
Subungual hematoma

Medial Structures
Medial arch

Lateral Structures
Fifth metatarsal

Dorsal Structures

Plantar Surface
Plantar warts
Callus

Posterior Structures
Achilles tendon

Foot Alignment
Forefoot varus
Forefoot valgus
Rearfoot varus
Rearfoot valgus

Non–Weight Bearing
Inspection of foot alignment
Assessment of talar position

3. PALPATION

Medial Structures
First MTP joint
First metatarsal
First cuneiform
Navicular
Talar head
Sustentaculum tali
Spring ligament
Medial talar tubercle
Calcaneal dome
Flexor hallucis longus
Flexor digitorum longus
Tibialis posterior
Posterior tibial artery

Lateral structures
Fifth MTP joint
Fifth metatarsal
Styloid process
Cuboid
Lateral border of the calcaneus
Peroneal tendons

Dorsal structures
Sinus tarsi
Dome of the talus
Cuneiforms
Rays
Tibialis anterior
Extensor hallucis longus
Extensor digitorum longus
Extensor digitorum brevis
Inferior extensor retinaculum
Dorsalis pedal artery
Intermetatarsal neuromas

Plantar structures
Medial calcaneal tubercle
Plantar fascia
Sesamoid bones of the great toe

Metatarsal heads

4. RANGE OF MOTION TESTS

Toes Active ROM
Flexion
Extension

Toes Passive ROM
Flexion
Extension

Toes Resisted ROM
Flexion
Extension

Related Motions
Subtalar joint
Inversion
Eversion
Talocrural joint
Dorsiflexion
Plantarflexion

5. LIGAMENTOUS CAPSULAR TESTS

MTP and IP Joints
Valgus stress testing
Varus stress testing

Metatarsal and Tarsal Joints
Intermetatarsal glide
Tarsometatarsal joint glide
Midtarsal joint glide
Mobility of the first ray

6. NEUROLOGIC TESTS

Tarsal tunnel
Peroneal nerve
Sciatic nerve
Lumbar or sacral nerve root
impingement

7. SPECIAL TESTS

Arch Pathologies
Test for supple pes planus
Feiss' line
Navicular drop test

Tarsal Tunnel Syndrome
Tinel's sign

Metatarsal/Phalanx Fracture
Long bone compression test

Intermetatarsal Neuroma
Pencil Test

Table 4–5
POSSIBLE PATHOLOGY BASED ON THE LOCATION OF PAIN

			Location of Pain			
	Proximal (Calcaneus)	Distal (Toes)	Plantar	Dorsal	Medial	Lateral
Soft tissue injury	Calcaneal bursitis Retrocalcaneal bursitis Achilles tendon inflammation*	Corns Hallux rigidus IP sprain MTP sprain	Callus Plantar fasciitis Plantar fascia rupture Plantar warts Intermetatarsal neuroma Tarsal tunnel syndrome	MTP sprain Forefoot sprain	Medial arch pathology Plantar fasciitis Tarsal tunnel syndrome Tibialis posterior* Turf toe syndrome	Peroneal tendinitis*
Bony injury	Calcaneal fracture Calcaneal spur Calcaneal cyst	Phalanx fracture Arthritis or inflammation	Sesamoiditis Sesamoid fracture Heel spur	Metatarsal stress fracture Talus fracture Tarsal coalition	Navicular stress fracture Bunion Hallux rigidis	Cuboid fracture Fifth metatarsal fracture (especially at the base)

*Discussed in Chapter 5.
IP = interphalangleal; MTP = metatarsophalangeal.

○ **Lateral arch pain:** Compression of the posterior tibial nerve as it passes through the tarsal tunnel can cause pain radiating along the lateral arch. Acutely, pain may be isolated to the lateral arch after fractures of the fifth MT. Pain arising from peroneal tendinitis may radiate into the lateral foot (see Chapter 5).

• **Onset and mechanism of injury:** The duration of the symptoms and pain that worsens or diminishes with specific activities provide insight about the nature of the injury and the tissues involved.

• **Acute onset**

○ The acute onset of foot injuries can occur from a rotational force being applied along the longitudinal axis as the foot lands on an uneven surface. These irregular positions place an increased force across the bones and ligamentous structures as they are stressed beyond their end ROM. A direct blow to the phalanges or MTs may result in their fracture. Ligaments can be avulsed from their attachment site if the joint is forced beyond its normal ROM. Avulsion of muscle attachments may result from forceful contractions as the patient attempts to maintain balance during activity.

• **Insidious onset**

○ **Playing surface:** In athletic activities, changing from a playing surface of one density to a surface with a different density may precipitate injury. For example, a change from running on an indoor rubberized track to running outdoors on pavement alters the ground reaction forces and stability that are distributed through the foot, ankle, and lower leg. Moving to a harder surface may result in an increased load being placed through these structures. Moving to a softer or rubberized surface increases eccentric loading of the muscles because of the surface's rebounding effect.

○ **Distance and duration:** Altering the components of the training regimen may increase or change the forces placed on the body and hinder the foot's ability to accommodate, resulting in overuse injuries. Ask the patient if he or she has significantly increased the distance, duration, or intensity of training. With increased stresses, the muscles providing dynamic support to the foot become fatigued, resulting in altered biomechanics.

○ **Shoes:** Training shoes that no longer provide adequate support may produce injury-causing forces at the foot. Changing either competitive or casual footwear (such as high heels) may alter the biomechanics of the lower extremity and redistribute forces in the foot. Ask the patient if he or she has been wearing shoes that are excessively worn or of an inappropriate type. Also find out if the patient has a new pair of shoes for competition or

daily wear. Also ask if the patient wears orthotics. If so, ascertain the reason for their use, for what activities they are worn, and the last time they were fitted.

INSPECTION

Even before the formal evaluation takes place, the inspection process begins by observing the patient entering the facility. At this time, note whether the individual was assisted into the facility, is currently using crutches or a cane, or has any gross dysfunction in gait. During the history-taking process, note any bilateral gross deformity, swelling, or redness in the foot, toes, and ankle (Fig. 4–10). Inspect the patient's daily casual and participation footwear for irregular wear patterns and for the appropriateness relative to the activity.

First, inspect the feet while they are in the non–weight-bearing position and then compare these findings with those obtained while the feet are weight bearing and during gait. In the non–weight-bearing position, the foot normally assumes its natural alignment. While weight bearing, the foot reveals the way it compensates for structural abnormalities of the foot, the lower extremity, and the body as a whole. Refer to Chapter 9 for more information about the evaluation of gait.

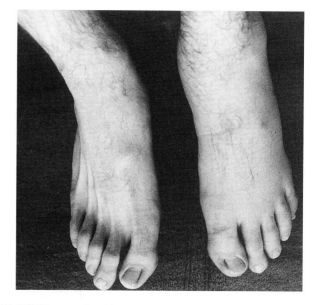

FIGURE 4–10. Swelling of the foot. Without first gathering a history of the injury, it cannot be determined whether this swelling is caused by trauma to the foot or ankle or from a lower leg or knee injury. If the leg is kept in a *gravity-dependent position*, edema will migrate distally.

Gravity-dependent position The extremity or body part is placed at a level that is lower than the heart, increasing intravascular pressure and hindering venous return.

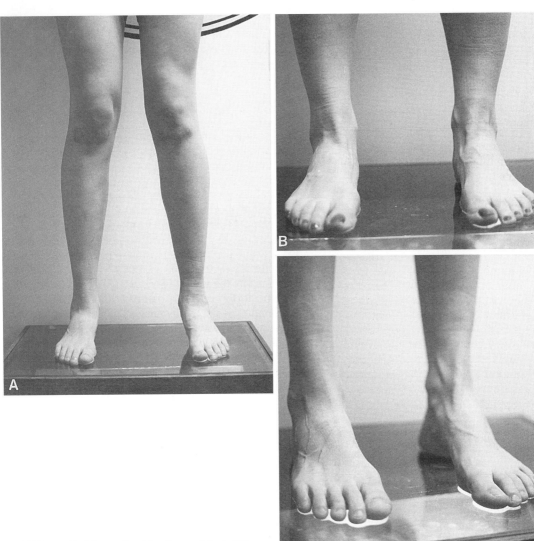

FIGURE 4–11. Three classifications of feet: **(A)** pronated, **(B)** normal, **(C)** supinated.

General Inspection of the Foot

- **Foot type:** Observe the foot from the anterior and posterior views to determine its general type: pronated, neutral, or supinated (Fig. 4–11). Feet that deviate from the neutral position represent either a structural abnormality within the foot or the foot's adaptation to a structural deficit in the leg, pelvis, or spine. Abnormal foot posture may also be the result of neurologic or disease states. To be classified as pronated or supinated, the observations must meet the extremes of each of the three categories presented in Table 4–6. Otherwise, the foot should be classified as neutral (Box 4–1).
- **Calluses and blisters:** Inspect the foot and toes for blisters and calluses, possibly indicating improperly fitting shoes, poor biomechanics, or underlying bony or soft tissue dysfunction. Blisters may be the result of dermatologic conditions such as *tinea pedis* or indicate areas of increased pressure caused by friction or irritation from the foot rubbing against the shoe. Calluses develop as the result of long-term pressures. Their presence under the MT heads may indicate a biomechanical abnormality. Those under the calcaneus are usually the result of an improper gait pattern.[6]

Tinea pedis A fungal infection of the foot and toes.

Table 4–6
CLASSIFICATION SCHEME FOR THE CLINICAL DEFINITION OF FOOT TYPE (WEIGHT BEARING)*

Pronated Foot	Supinated Foot
• The calcaneus must be everted greater than 3° from perpendicular relative to the position of the ground.	• The calcaneus must be inverted greater than 3° from perpendicular relative to the position of the ground.
• A medial bulge must be present at the talonavicular joint, indicating excessive talar adduction.	• A medial bulge must not be present at the talonavicular joint, indicating excessive talar adduction.
• The medial arch must be low. This is determined by Feiss' line, formed by connecting the points formed by the head of the first MT, the navicular tubercle, and the medial malleolus (see Box 4–1).	• Using Feiss' line, the arch must be high.

*Each of the three criteria under each of the column headings must be met for the foot to be classified as such; otherwise, the foot should be categorized as neutral.

Inspection of the Toes

- **General toe alignment:** The common toe malalignments are presented in Box 4–2.
- **Morton's alignment:** This condition, also referred to as Morton's toe, results in a greater amount of force transmitted along the second *ray* during push off, causing *hypertrophy* of the second MT. This may be a predisposing condition for MT stress fractures.[7] A callus may be present under the second MT head. Morton's toe has been associated with increased callus formation, pain, and hallux rigidus.[8]
- **Claw toes:** Claw toes are commonly associated with pes cavus. A callus may be found over the dorsal portion of the PIP joint and on the plantar surface of the MTP joint and, in some cases, on the tips of the toes.
- **Hammer toe:** Hammer toes often develop as either the long toe extensors or long toe flexors substitute for weakness of the primary dorsiflexors or plantarflexors. They often occur after injury, such as a rupture of the plantar fascia, or with neuromuscular disease states. A callus may be located on the dorsal surface of the PIP joint, resulting from friction against the shoe. In most cases, this deformity affects

only one ray and may be caused by improperly fitting shoes (especially during the growth years), hereditary factors, elongation of the plantar fascia, or hallux valgus.[9]

- **Hallux abducto valgus:** Hallux abducto valgus (also referred to as simply "hallux valgus") is also characterized by increased ROM during extension and flattening of the medial longitudinal arch.[10] Hallux valgus may be congenital; result from improperly fitting footwear such as pointed-toed shoes; or be traced to disease states such as *cerebral palsy,* rheumatoid arthritis, or osteoarthritis.[11] Pain and dysfunction may also result from a bunion over the first MTP joint that forms secondary to the valgus deformity or secondary to the dislocation of the first MTP joint's *sesamoid bones.*

  ○ **Bunion:** Formed by the development and subsequent inflammation of a bursa, bunions are characterized by redness, inflammation, and tenderness on the medial aspect of the first MTP joint. Causes of bunions include hallux valgus and poorly fitting shoes. A smaller **bunionette** may form on the lateral aspect of the fifth MTP joint.

- **Corns:** Also referred to as clavus, corns are a thickening of the stratum corneum and tend to occur in non–weight-bearing areas. Corns may be sensitive to the touch.

  ○ **Hard corns** (heloma dura), located in areas that receive excessive pressure, appear as hard, granular nodules on the skin. Hard corns tend to form on the toes and PIP joints. Because of the resultant biomechanical changes in foot function, hard corns progress distally.[12]

  ○ **Soft corns** (heloma molle) form between the toes. The web space between the fourth and fifth toes is the most common site. Dampness in the web space serves to moisten the corn, thus keeping it soft. The moisture together with the dark, warm environment predispose the lesion to infection and *ulceration.*

Ray The series of bones formed by the metatarsal and phalanges.

Hypertrophy The increase in the cross-sectional size of a muscle, bone, or organ.

Cerebral palsy A birth-related neurologic defect that results in motor dysfunction.

Sesamoid bone A bone that lies within a tendon.

Ulceration An open sore or lesion of the skin or mucous membrane that is accompanied by inflamed and necrotic tissue.

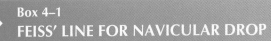

Box 4–1
FEISS' LINE FOR NAVICULAR DROP

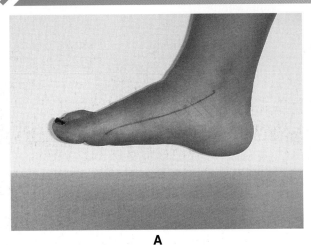 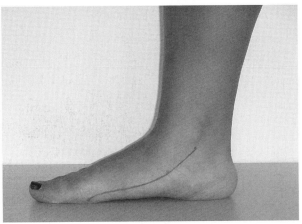

A	**B**

With the patient in a non–weight-bearing position, a line is drawn from the apex of the medial malleolus and the plantar aspect of the 1st MTP joint. The displacement of the navicular tubercle is marked when the patient bears weight.

PATIENT POSITION	Sitting with the feet off the end of the table
POSITION OF EXAMINER	Positioned at the patient's feet
EVALUATIVE PROCEDURE	With the patient non–weight bearing, the examiner identifies and marks the apex of the medial malleolus and the plantar aspect of the 1st MTP joint. A line is drawn connecting the marks over the first MTP joint and the medial malleolus **(A)**. Mark the position of the navicular tubercle. The patient stands with the feet approximately 1 ft apart and the weight evenly distributed. The examiner should check that the line drawn previously still connects the apex of the medial malleolus and the plantar aspect of the first MTP joint. The new position of the navicular tubercle is marked **(B)**.
POSITIVE TEST RESULT	A navicular that drops two thirds or greater the distance to the floor.
IMPLICATIONS	Hyperpronated foot.

MTP = Metatarsophalangeal.

- **Ingrown toenail:** These most often involve the great toe. The corners of the nail should be inspected for intrusion into the skin (Fig. 4–12). The areas of ingrowth cause disruption and subsequent infection of the skin surrounding and beneath the nailbed, causing it to appear red and swollen.
- **Subungual hematoma:** Localized trauma to the toenail can result in the formation of a hematoma beneath the nail, called a subungual hematoma (Fig. 4–13). Commonly found in the great toe, the resulting collection of blood turns the nail a dark purple and causes pain from pressure being placed on the involved nerve endings. A subungual hematoma may form secondary to a fracture of the distal phalanx or may be caused by a falling object or other compressive forces.

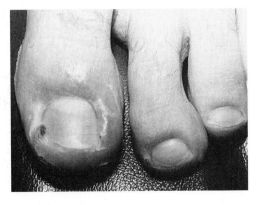

FIGURE 4–12. Ingrown toenail. This painful condition results from abnormal growth patterns of the nail, causing it to imbed within the skin.

Box 4–2
PATHOLOGICAL TOE POSTURES

	Claw Toes	Hammer Toes	Morton's Toes	Hallux Abducto Valgus
Observation				
Illustration				
Deviation	Contracture of the interosseous or lumbrical muscles (or both)	Contractures of the associated toe extensors and flexors; inability of the interosseous muscles to hold the proximal phalanx in the neutral position	Although it appears that the 2nd toe is longer than the 1st, Morton's toe is formed by the 1st metatarsal being shorter than the 2nd.	Over time, there is a gradual and progressive subluxation of the 1st MTP joint. A bunion will develop on the medial border of the 1st MTP joint.
Posture	Hyperextension of the MTP joint and flexion of the PIP and DIP joints. Claw toes affect the lateral four toes.	Hyperextension of the MTP and DIP joints and flexion of the PIP joints of the lateral four toes.	The attitude of the foot is normal, but the 2nd toe extends beyond the great toe.	The 1st MTP joint exceeds an angle of 20° in the frontal plane and the 1st and 2nd toes overlap.

DIP = distal interphalangeal; PIP = proximal interphalangeal; MTP = metatarsophalangeal.

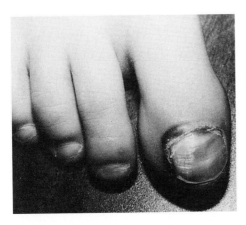

FIGURE 4–13. Trauma to the toe can result in bleeding under the nail, a subungual hematoma. Often, the blood must be drained from beneath the nail.

Inspection of the Medial Structures

- **Medial longitudinal arch:** Spanning from the calcaneus to the first MTP joint, the medial longitudinal arch is more prominent when the foot is non–weight bearing. In the non–weight-bearing position, observe if the arch is abnormally flattened (pes planus) or heightened (pes cavus). A detailed evaluation of the arch is presented in the Pathologies and Related Special Tests Section of this chapter.

Inspection of the Lateral Structures

- **Fifth metatarsal:** Normally, the foot's lateral border is relatively straight, especially along the shaft of the fifth MT. Inspect the length of the bone for deviation of its contour, which indicates a fracture.

Inspection of the Dorsal Structures

The tendons of the long toe extensors and the small mass of the extensor digitorum brevis thinly cover the dorsal surface of the foot laterally. Observe the dorsal aspect of the foot for swelling, discoloration, or abnormal bony alignment.

Inspection of the Plantar Surface

When inspecting the length of the plantar surface of the foot, pay particular attention to the condition of the skin and the presence of callus formation or blisters, as noted previously.

- **Plantar warts:** Plantar warts are a common dermatologic abnormality afflicting the foot's plantar aspect (Fig. 4–14). Caused by the virus *Verruca vulgaris*, plantar warts are usually localized in calloused skin in areas of excessive weight-bearing stresses. However, they may develop anywhere on the plantar aspect of the foot. Plantar warts, typically more focal than an ordinary callus, can be point tender. The patient often complains of the sensation of "stepping on a pebble."

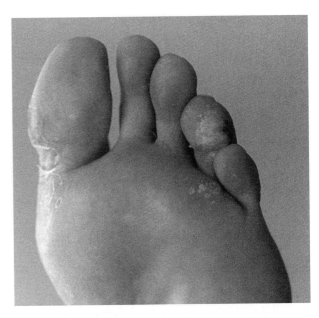

FIGURE 4–14. Plantar warts. This condition results in point tenderness and masks the normal skin markings, thus distinguishing it from callus.

Plantar warts mask the normal *whorls* and skin markings, thus differentiating them from callus build-up.

Inspection of the Posterior Structures

- **Achilles tendon:** With the patient in the weight-bearing position, observe the relationship of the Achilles tendon to the tibia. Normally these two structures are in alignment. Bowing of the tendon may be an indication of pes planus (Fig. 4–15). Refer to Chapter 5 for more information regarding Achilles tendon pathology.
- **Calcaneus:** Retrocalcaneal exostosis (also referred to as Haglaund's deformity or "pump bumps") can be associated with rearfoot varus (Fig. 4–16).

Non–Weight-Bearing Inspection of Foot and Calcaneal Alignment

An assessment of foot alignment requires comparative measures taken when the foot is weight bearing and again when the foot is non–weight bearing. To assess the position of the foot while it is non–weight bearing, position the patient in a prone position so that the feet and ankles are lying over the edge of the examination table.

- **Assessment of talar position:** Assess for the subtalar neutral position with the patient weight bearing, prone, or in the seated position. With the right foot as an example, place the left thumb and index fin-

---

Whorls Swirl markings in the skin. Fingerprints are images formed by the whorls on the fingertips.

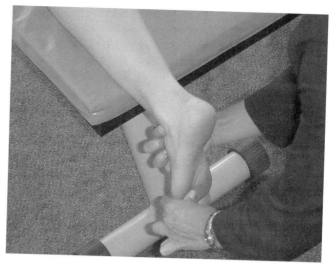

FIGURE 4–17. Finding the neutral position of the talus. Subtalar neutral is found when the talus fits symmetrically within the mortise.

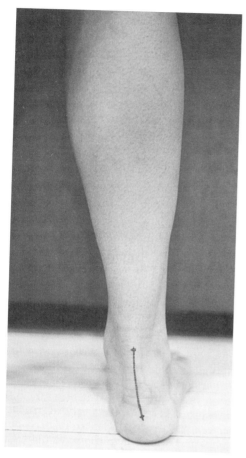

FIGURE 4–15. Achilles tendon alignment in an individual with pes planus. Note the valgus alignment of the calcaneus as noted by the inward bowing of the Achilles tendon.

gers on the anterior aspect of the foot over the sides of the talar dome. Using the right hand, grasp the foot from the lateral side and invert and evert the foot and ankle until the neutral position of the foot is determined (Fig. 4–17). The talus is in its neutral position when it is aligned symmetrically between the thumb and index finger. After talar neutral is found, note the alignment of the forefoot and rearfoot. The reliability of this technique depends on the skill and experience of the clinician.[4]

Mobility of the first ray: Assess the tarsometatarsal joint and the first MTP joint for normal mobility. Pes planus is often marked by hypermobility of the first ray; pes cavus may result in a rigid ray.

Inspection of Foot Alignment

Inspection of the alignment of the forefoot relative to the rearfoot can be performed with the patient in the weight-bearing position, the non–weight-bearing position, or both. (Fig. 4–18). The inferior displacement

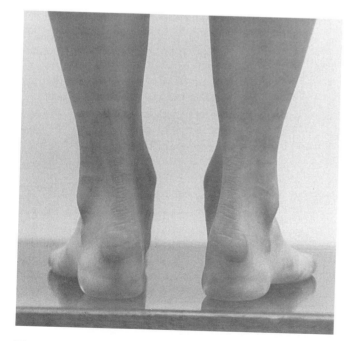

FIGURE 4–16. Retrocalcaneal exostosis, "pump bumps."

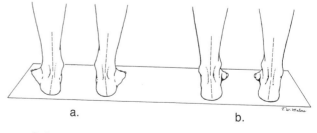

Calcaneovalgus   Calcaneovarus

FIGURE 4–18. (A) Rearfoot valgus (calcaneovalgus), pronation of the subtalar joint caused by eversion of the calcaneus. **(B)** Rearfoot varus (calcaneovarus), supination of the subtalar joint associated with calcaneal inversion.

of the navicular in the weight-bearing position relative to the non–weight-bearing position significantly influences the weight-bearing attitudes of the forefoot and rearfoot.[13] Refer to Chapter 9 for a description of the pathomechanics arising from these foot postures.

- **Foot posture:** With the subtalar joint it its neutral position, identify the forefoot and rearfoot postures (Box 4–3).
- **Plantarflexed first ray:** Observe the first ray. A first ray that is plantarflexed at the tarsometatarsal joint causes the ray to be located inferior to the remaining four rays. Plantarflexed first rays are associated with a cavus foot or can be acquired in the presence of genu varum and may be confused with forefoot valgus.

PALPATION

To make palpation easier, position the patient so the foot and ankle extend off the end of the examination table. Include the related ankle structures during the palpation phase of a foot evaluation.

Palpation of the Medial Structures

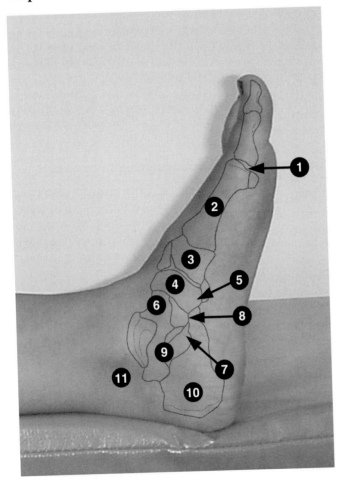

1. **First MTP joint:** Begin by locating the articulation between the proximal phalanx of the first toe and the first MT. Palpate the area for tenderness or increased skin temperature that may indicate acute injury to the ligamentous structures, chronic inflammatory conditions of the tendons or articular structures, or disease states such as **gout.**
2. **First metatarsal:** From the first MTP joint, palpate the length of the first MT, noting any crepitus, bony deformity, or pain elicited along the shaft. Because the dorsal and medial surfaces and part of the plantar surface of this bone are easily palpated, gross fractures can be identified with relative ease.
3. **First cuneiform:** Identify the base of the first MT as it articulates with the first cuneiform by the attachment of the tibialis anterior. To make this bone more palpable, ask the patient to actively plantarflex the ankle. This motion causes the base of the first MT to be depressed on the cuneiform, making this junction more palpable.
4. **Navicular:** Palpate proximally from the first cuneiform to locate its articulation with the medial border of the navicular.
5. Move posteriorly from the articulation to find the prominent medial **navicular tuberosity (5).** The navicular serves as the keystone of the medial longitudinal arch. As such, any dysfunction of this bone results in dysfunction of the arch as a whole.
6. **Talar head:** Palpate the talar head, immediately proximal and superior to the navicular. This structure is more easily located by inverting and everting the forefoot. When the forefoot is in eversion, the talar head is more prominent medially.
7. **Sustentaculum tali:** Palpate the sustentaculum tali, located distal to the medial malleolus, a protrusion off the calcaneus. Serving as an attachment site for the spring ligament and providing inferior support to the talus, this structure is not always easily identifiable.
8. **Spring ligament:** Palpate the plantar calcaneonavicular ligament from its origin off the sustentaculum tali to its insertion on the navicular. In cases of pes planus or forefoot sprains, this ligament may become very tender to the touch or feel thickened.
9. **Medial talar tubercle:** Palpate proximally and superiorly from the spring ligament to locate the small projection off the proximal-medial border of the talus, immediately adjacent to the anterior margin of the medial malleolus. The medial talar tubercle serves as a site of attachment for part of the deltoid ligament.
10. **Calcaneus:** From the medial talar tubercle, palpate inferiorly to locate the posterior flare of the calcaneus; continue to palpate to the site of the Achilles tendon attachment.

Hypermobile Possessing excessive mobility.

Box 4-3
PATHOLOGICAL FOOT POSTURES

	Forefoot Varus	Forefoot Valgus	Rearfoot Varus	Rearfoot Valgus
Observation				
Illustration				
Deviation	With the rearfoot (calcaneus and talus) in the neutral position, the 1st MT is elevated relative to the 5th MT.	With the rearfoot in the neutral position, the 5th MT is elevated relative to the 1st MT.	The calcaneus is inverted relative to the long axis of the tibia and may be related to a varus alignment of the tibia or a calcaneus that does not completely derotate during fetal development.	The calcaneus is everted relative to the long axis of the tibia and can be associated with a valgus tibial alignment. Rearfoot valgus is rarely observed.
Compensated	During static weight bearing, the forefoot compensates by inverting and overpronating. During gait, there is an increased period of pronation as the 1st MT has farther to travel before contacting the ground.	During gait, the 1st MT strikes the ground prematurely, resulting in eversion of the forefoot and supination.	The rearfoot is rigid, increasing supination during non-weight bearing, but increases the amount of time that the calcaneus is relatively inverted and pronated during gait.	The rearfoot becomes *hypermobile*, resulting in increased pronation.

MT = metatarsal.

11. **Medial tendons:**

○ **Flexor hallucis longus:** The bulk of this muscle, hidden beneath the gastrocnemius and soleus muscles, is not palpable until its tendon begins its path posterior to, and around, the medial malleolus. It is difficult to distinguish this tendon from the other structures in the area. As the tendon begins its course along the plantar aspect of the foot, it again is no longer palpable until it inserts on the distal phalanx of the great toe. Resisting flexion of the great toe makes this tendon more prominent as it passes across the plantar aspect of the first MTP joint and courses to its attachment site.

○ **Flexor digitorum longus:** Similar to the flexor hallucis longus, the mass of the flexor digitorum longus is not identifiable as it lies beneath the bulk of the gastrocnemius and soleus muscles. Its tendon is palpable, although not uniquely identifiable, as it passes posterior to, and around, the medial malleolus. As it passes along the plantar aspect of the foot, it is no longer palpable until it inserts on the plantar aspect of the second through fifth toes.

○ **Tibialis posterior:** The tibialis posterior can be palpated from its attachment on the medial aspect of the navicular and is more prominent if the patient actively inverts the foot. In the presence of pathology, the tendon and its attachment become sensitive to the touch.

Palpation of the Lateral Structures

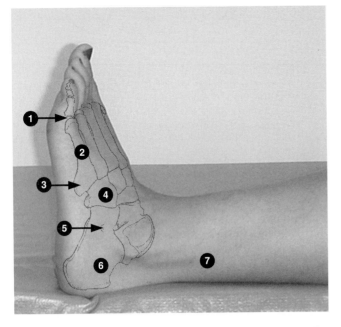

1. **Fifth MTP joint:** Locate the articulation between the fifth toe and fifth MT. Palpate the joint for tenderness arising from ligament or articular damage.

2. **Fifth metatarsal:** From the fifth MTP joint, palpate the length of the fifth MT and note any pain or discontinuity in the bone's shaft. This structure, especially at its proximal end, is the site of acute injuries and stress fractures.

3. **Styloid tuberosity:** The base of the fifth MT is marked by a laterally projecting styloid tuberosity (process), the site where the peroneus brevis tendon attaches. Covered by a bursa, this structure is commonly avulsed as the peroneus brevis tendon is pulled from its attachment.

4. **Cuboid:** Locate the cuboid by palpating immediately proximal to the styloid process. The groove through which the peroneus longus passes beneath the foot is at the middle portion of the lateral aspect of the cuboid.

5. **Peroneal tubercle:** The peroneal tubercle is the most prominent bony landmark on the calcaneus, located inferior and anterior to the most distal portion of the lateral malleolus. The peroneal tubercle marks the point at which the peroneus longus and brevis tendons diverge after jointly passing posterior to the lateral malleolus.

6. **Lateral border of the calcaneus:** From the cuboid, continue to palpate toward the rearfoot. The junction between the cuboid and the calcaneus is often indistinct.

7. **Peroneal tendons:** Locate the bony lateral portion of the distal one third of the fibula. The tendons of peroneus longus and brevis may be palpated as a single structure as they course posterior to the distal third of the fibula and pass beneath the lateral malleolus. The tendon's paths split at the peroneal tubercle. From this point, the peroneus brevis tendon can be palpated to its insertion on the styloid process of the fifth MT. The peroneus longus tendon can be palpated to the point where it passes through the peroneal groove between the fifth MT's styloid process and the anterior margin of the cuboid. Here it disappears on the plantar aspect of the foot. The peroneus longus' insertion can be palpated on the medial and inferior surface of the first cuneiform and lateral base of the first MT. Injury to these structures may result in pain at the base of the fifth MT and cuboid.

Palpation of the Dorsal Structures

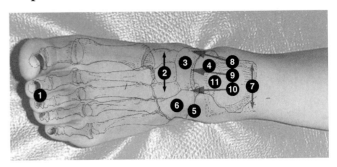

1. **Rays:** Starting with the distal phalanx, palpate the toes through the length of their associated MTs,

noting any deformity, crepitus, or pain elicited during the process.

2. **Cuneiforms:** Although the cuneiforms are indistinguishable from each other to the touch, approximate their locations relative to the first three MTs. The three cuneiforms each articulate with the first three MTs; by palpating the length of the MTs to their bases, the individual cuneiforms can be identified (see Fig. 4–2).

3. **Navicular:** Palpate posteriorly from the cuneiforms to locate the navicular.

4. **Dome of the talus:** Palpate posteriorly and somewhat laterally from the navicular to find the dome of the talus. This structure is more easily located if the foot and ankle are placed in inversion and plantarflexion, allowing the dome's lateral border to become palpable from under the ankle mortise.

5. **Sinus tarsi:** Locate the sinus tarsi located anterior to the lateral malleolus. Normally, this landmark appears as a depression in the forefoot, marking the site of the extensor digitorum brevis muscle. With chronic conditions such as arthritis or after acute trauma, including ankle sprains, tarsal fractures, or dislocations, the sinus may fill with fluid and become sensitive to the touch (Fig. 4–19).

6. **Extensor digitorum brevis:** Palpate the origin and proximal muscle belly of the extensor digitorum brevis in the sinus tarsi when the toes are actively extended. The tendinous slips to each of the toes become indistinguishable as they pass under the long toe tendons. The most medial portion of the extensor digitorum brevis muscle and its tendon attaching on the first toe is often referred to as a separate muscle, the **extensor hallucis brevis.**

7. **Inferior extensor retinaculum:** Palpate the inferior extensor retinaculum along its entire length as it traverses the entire upper portion of the foot. As the tendons of tibialis anterior, EHL, and extensor digitorum longus pass over the talus and tarsals, their proximity to the bones during dorsiflexion is maintained by the inferior extensor *retinaculum.*

8. **Tibialis anterior:** Invert the subtalar joint and dorsiflex the ankle to make the tibialis anterior tendon more palpable at the point where it inserts on the first cuneiform. As the tendon crosses the talocrural joint, it is easily palpable but quickly loses its identity as it flares into its musculotendinous junction.

9. **Extensor hallucis longus:** Locate the EHL tendon by palpating laterally from the tibialis anterior tendon. When the great toe is extended, palpate the tendon's length from the tibialis anterior to its flare into the distal phalanx. Continue to palpate the length of the EHL to its origin on the middle half of the anterior fibula and adjacent interosseous membrane.

10. **Extensor digitorum longus:** Palpate lateral to the EHL for the tendon of the extensor digitorum longus. Although the central portion of the tendon is difficult to palpate, palpate its individual slips to the lateral four toes, prominent on the dorsal aspect of the foot when the toes are extended.

11. **Dorsalis pedis pulse:** Locate the dorsalis pedis artery lying between the tendons of EHL and extensor digitorum longus. With the ankle in the neutral position, palpate the dorsalis pedis pulse and compare it with the opposite extremity. A unilateral absence or decreased pulse may indicate a vascular obstruction such as **anterior compartment syndrome** (see Chapter 5).

Palpation of the Plantar Structures

The plantar surfaces of the calcaneus and the MT heads are padded by fatty deposits and overlying thick skin, making it difficult to identify specific bony structures and muscles. The examiner must rely on approximations and functional tests in identifying and determining many painful tissues.

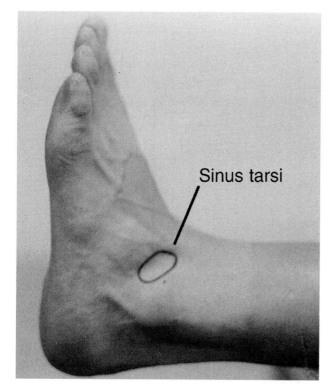

FIGURE 4–19. The sinus tarsi. This area becomes swollen and tender following a wide range of trauma to the foot and ankle.

Retinaculum A ligamentous tissue serving as a restraining band to hold other tissues in place.

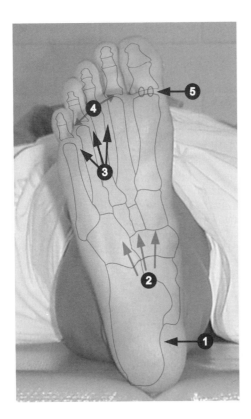

ing the toe to make the plantar fascia more prominent. Then trace the fascia back to its origin on the medial calcaneal tubercle. The anterior ridge of the medial calcaneal tubercle is the attachment site of the plantar fascia and the flexor digitorum brevis muscle. The medial border of this structure is the site of origin of the abductor hallucis. Pain elicited during palpation of this area may indicate a **plantar fasciitis** or a **heel spur** (Fig. 4–20).

2. **Plantar fascia:** Palpate the plantar fascia from its origin on the calcaneus through its length and breadth to its attachment on each of the MT heads, noting any painful areas within this structure. Individuals suffering from plantar fasciitis may demonstrate tenderness along the length of the fascia.

3. **Intermetatarsal neuroma:** Apply gentle pressure to the area between the MTs. Nerves located in this area can become inflamed and cause dysfunction of the foot and lower extremity.

4. **Metatarsal heads:** Beginning with the first MTP joint, palpate each of the MT heads, noting for the presence and integrity of the transverse arch. The pads under the first and fifth MT heads should be the thickest because they are the primary weight-bearing areas of the forefoot.

5. **Sesamoid bones of the great toe:** Palpate along the plantar surface of the first MT to reach the first MTP joint. At this point, two small sesamoid bones can be felt in the flexor hallucis brevis tendon. Inflammatory conditions of these bones, **sesamoiditis,** or fractures elicit pain to the touch or while weight bearing, especially during the toe-off phase of gait, when pressure is applied to the ball of the foot and the joint is extended. The onset of sesamoiditis has

1. **Medial calcaneal tubercle:** Locate the medial calcaneal tubercle by identifying the point where the heel pad begins to thin and merge into the medial longitudinal arch. From this point, move to the medial ridge and apply pressure upward and toward the calcaneus. The medial calcaneal tubercle may also be located by dorsiflexing the ankle and extend-

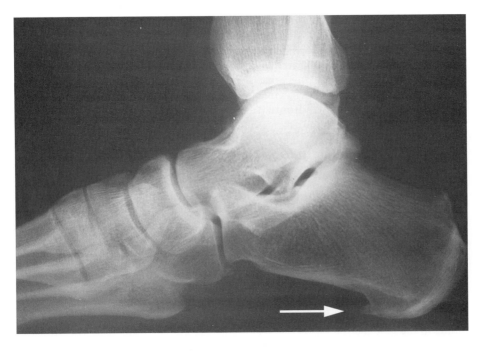

FIGURE 4–20. X ray of a heel spur. A form of exostosis, heel spurs are an abnormal bony outgrowth of the calcaneus. Note the hooklike projection arising from the anterior border of the calcaneal tuberosity.

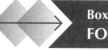

Box 4–4
FOOT GONIOMETRY

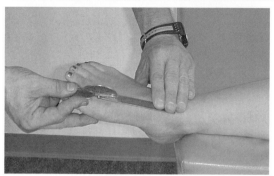
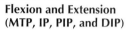
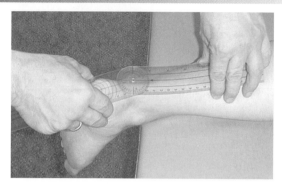

	Flexion and Extension (MTP, IP, PIP, and DIP)	Rearfoot (Subtalar) Inversion and Eversion
PATIENT POSITION	Supine	Prone
GONIOMETER PLACEMENT		
FULCRUM	Positioned over the dorsal aspect of the joint being tested	Centered over the Achilles tendon with the axis bisecting the malleoli
STATIONARY ARM	Centered on the midline of the bone proximal to the joint being tested	Centered on the midline of the lower leg
MOVEMENT ARM	Centered on the midline of the bone distal to the joint being tested	Centered over the midline of the calcaneus

DIP = distal interphalangeal; IP = interphalangeal; PIP = proximal interphalangeal; MTP = metatarsophalangeal.

been linked to *rigidity* of the first ray (cavus foot structure).

RANGE OF MOTION TESTING

The relatively limited amount of motion available to the IP joints makes it difficult to accurately measure ROM for these joints. This section describes the ROM tests for the MTP joints only. The results of these tests should be compared bilaterally to determine any pathological conditions at these joints. Goniometric measurement of foot and toe motion is presented in Box 4–4. Plantarflexion, dorsiflexion, inversion, and eversion tests for the ankle are described in Chapter 5.

Active Range of Motion

The greatest ROM occurs at the first MTP joint, allowing 75 to 85 degrees of extension and 35 to 45 degrees of flexion (Fig. 4–21). To prevent compensatory motion, the first MTP joint must permit 60 to 65 degrees of extension; otherwise, excessive pronation occurs during gait. The ROM available to the MTP joints decreases at each subsequent lateral joint. Active motion at the fifth MTP joint is negligible.

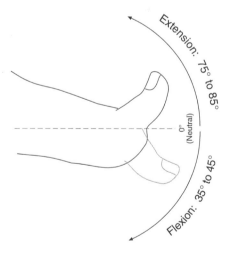

FIGURE 4–21. Active range of motion for flexion and extension of the great toe's metatarsophalangeal joint. The range of motion decreases with each subsequent joint from the first MTP joint to the fifth.

Rigidity A pathological loss of a joint's motion or a soft tissue's elasticity.

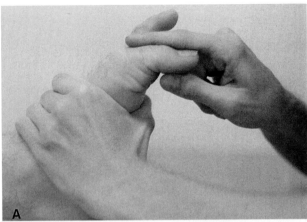

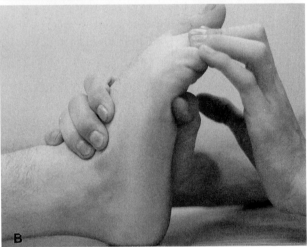

FIGURE 4–22. Passive flexion of the **(A)** great toe and **(B)** lateral four toes.

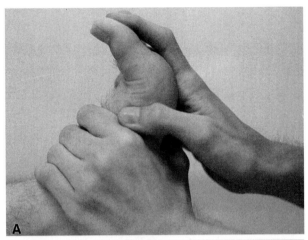

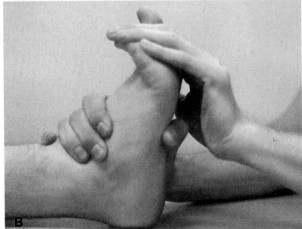

FIGURE 4–23. Passive extension of the **(A)** great toe and **(B)** lateral four toes.

Passive Range of Motion

Because the muscles acting on the lateral four toes are different from those acting on the hallux, determine passive motion for the first toe alone and the motion at the lateral four toes as a unit.

- **Flexion:** Stabilize the forefoot proximal to the MT heads. To prevent contribution from the IP joints, apply pressure on the dorsal portion of the proximal phalanx (Fig. 4–22). The normal end-feel for flexion is firm owing to tension of the dorsal fibers of the joint capsule and the collateral ligaments.
- **Extension:** Maintain stabilization as described for measurement of passive flexion, but apply pressure to the proximal phalanx's plantar aspect (Fig. 4–23). A firm end-feel arises from the capsule's plantar fibers and the short flexor muscles.

Resisted Range of Motion

Resisted ROM testing of the great toe is conducted separately from that of the lateral four toes (Box 4–5).

LIGAMENTOUS AND CAPSULAR TESTING

With the exception of the MTP and IP joints, identifying trauma to specific ligaments and joint capsules of the foot is difficult. This section describes how to isolate stresses to the ligaments stabilizing the toes and the general integrity of the midfoot's soft tissues.

Metatarsophalangeal and Interphalangeal Joints

The MTP and IP joints are supported by the medial and lateral collateral ligaments (MCL and LCL). The dorsal

Box 4–5

RESISTED RANGE OF MOTION FOR THE TOES

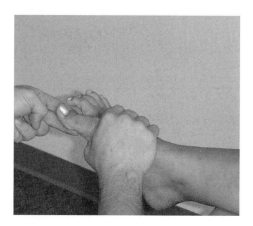
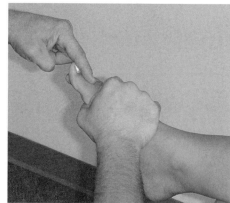

Flexion	Extension

STARTING POSITION	The joint being tested is placed in the neutral position	
STABILIZATION	The forefoot is stabilized by grasping the metatarsals proximal to their heads.	
RESISTANCE	**Great toe:** along the entire length of the toe's plantar aspect **Lateral four toes:** on their plantar aspect	**Great toe:** along the entire length of the toe's dorsal aspect **Lateral four toes:** on their dorsal aspect
MUSCLES TESTED	**Great toe:** Flexor hallucis longus, flexor hallucis brevis **Lateral four toes:** Flexor digitorum longus, flexor digitorum brevis, flexor digiti minimi brevis, dorsal interossei (MTP joint flexion), plantar interossei (MTP joint flexion), lumbricals (MTP flexion)	**Great toe:** Extensor hallucis longus, extensor hallucis brevis **Lateral four toes:** Extensor digitorum longus, extensor digitorum brevis, dorsal interossei (IP joint extension), plantar interossei (IP joint extension), lumbricals (IP joint extension)

IP = interphalangeal; MTP = metatarsophalangeal.

and plantar surfaces of these articulations are reinforced by the joint capsule. Passive *overpressure* in flexion, as described in the Passive Range of Motion section of this chapter, is used to determine the integrity of the dorsal joint capsule; passive overpressure in extension evaluates the integrity of the plantar capsule.

The application of a *valgus force* stresses the MCL of the joint. A *varus force* stresses the LCLs (Box 4–6). Compare the results of this examination with those obtained when the test is repeated on the same joint on the opposite extremity.

Intermetatarsal Joints

The deep transverse MT ligaments and the interosseous ligaments secure the MT heads in a relatively stable alignment. Forces causing an abnormal amount of glide between any two MT heads can result in trauma to these ligaments. Testing intermetatarsal glide, thus du-

plicating the mechanism of injury, can be used to evaluate the integrity of these ligaments (Box 4–7). Compare the amount of glide bilaterally.

Tarsometatarsal Joints

The integrity of the tarsometatarsal joint ligaments are assessed through joint play and glide tests. The tarsometatarsal joints are evaluated by assessing the

---

Overpressure   A force that attempts to move a joint beyond its normal range of motion.

Valgus force   A lateral force applied toward the body's midline (medially).

Varus force   A medial force applied from the body's midline outward (laterally).

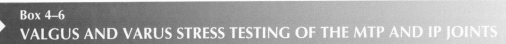

Box 4–6
VALGUS AND VARUS STRESS TESTING OF THE MTP AND IP JOINTS

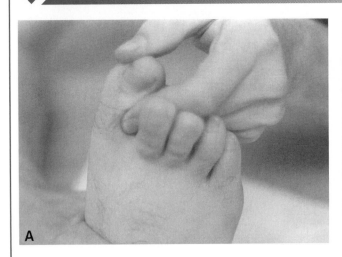
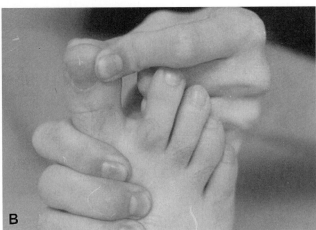

Stress testing of the toe's capsular ligaments: **(A),** Valgus stress applied to the interphalangeal joint; **(B),** varus stress applied to the metatarsophalangeal joint.

PATIENT POSITION	Supine or sitting
POSITION OF EXAMINER	Standing The proximal bone stabilized close to the joint to be tested The bone distal to the joint being tested grasped near the middle of its shaft Care is necessary to isolate the joint being tested.
EVALUATIVE PROCEDURE	**Valgus testing (A):** The distal bone is moved laterally, attempting to open up the joint on the medial side. **Varus testing (B):** The distal bone is moved medially, attempting to open up the joint on the lateral side.
POSITIVE TEST	Pain or increased laxity when compared with the same joint on the opposite extremity
IMPLICATIONS	**Valgus test (A):** MCL sprain of the involved joint **Varus test (B):** LCL sprain of the involved joint

IP = interphalangeal; LCL = lateral collateral ligament; MCL = medial collateral ligament; MTP = metatarsophalangeal.

amount of motion during dorsal and plantar glide (Box 4–8).

Midtarsal Joints

The ligaments of the midtarsal joints are evaluated by dorsal and plantar glide of the cuneiforms (Box 4–9).

NEUROLOGIC EXAMINATION

The foot and toes are supplied by the L4 to S2 nerve roots. Neurologic dysfunction of the nerve roots or in-dividual nerves can radiate symptoms to the foot. When neurologic symptoms (e.g., numbness, muscle weakness, reflex deficits) are present, the source of the dysfunction, such as whether a nerve root or a periph-eral nerve lesion is involved, must be determined.

To identify nerve root pathology refer to the Lower Quarter Neurologic Screen in Chapter 1 (Box 1–5). Pathologies that can result in local neurologic dysfunc-tion include entrapment of the posterior tibial nerve (tarsal tunnel syndrome) and interdigital neuroma. Per-oneal nerve trauma and anterior compartment syn-drome (discussed in Chapter 5) can also radiate symp-toms into the foot (Fig 4–24).

Box 4–7
INTERMETATARSAL GLIDE TEST

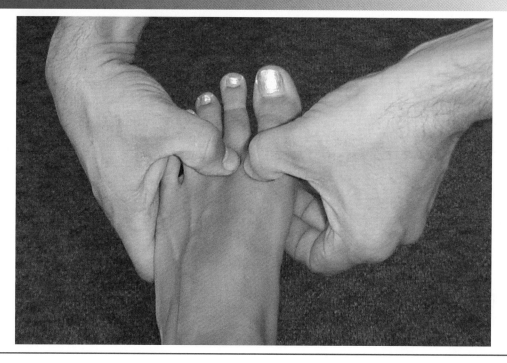

Assessment of the amount of intermetatarsal glide between the 1st and 2nd metatarsal heads.
Perform this test for each of the four articulations formed between the five metatarsals.

PATIENT POSITION	Supine or sitting on the table with the knees extended
POSITION OF EXAMINER	Standing in front of the patient's feet One hand grasping the first MT head; the other grasping the second MT head
EVALUATIVE PROCEDURE	The two MT heads are moved in opposite directions (plantarly and dorsally and then dorsally and plantarly). This procedure is repeated by moving to the lateral MT heads until all four intermetarsal joints have been evaluated.
POSITIVE TEST	Pain or increased glide compared with the opposite extremity
IMPLICATIONS	Trauma to the deep transverse metatarsal ligament, interosseous ligament, or both Pain without the presence of laxity may indicate the presence of a neuroma

MT = metatarsal.

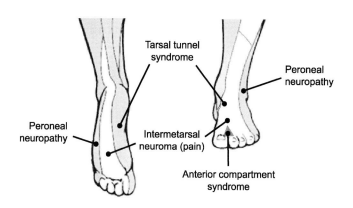

FIGURE 4–24. Peripheral neurological symptoms in the foot.

Box 4–8
TARSOMETATARSAL JOINT GLIDES

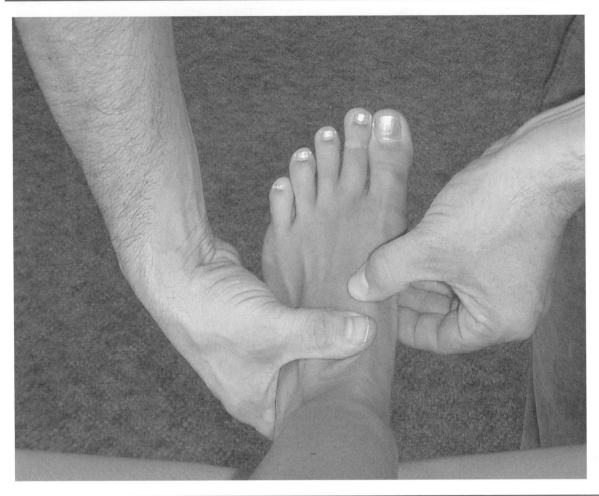

Assessment of the amount of glide between the tarsals and the base of the metatarsals. Perform this test on each of the five tarsometatarsal joints.

PATIENT POSITION	Supine Knee flexed and the heel stabilized by the edge of the table
POSITION OF EXAMINER	Standing or sitting in front of the patient's foot One hand gasping the distal tarsal row The opposite hand gasping the metatarsal being glided
EVALUATIVE PROCEDURE	The metatarsal is glided dorsally on the tarsal and then glided plantarly on the tarsal. Repeat for each joint
POSITIVE TEST	Pain associated with movement Increased or decreased glide relative to the opposite foot
IMPLICATIONS	Increased glide: ligamentous laxity Decreased glide: joint adhesions, articular changed causing coalition of the joint

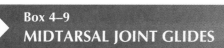

Box 4–9
MIDTARSAL JOINT GLIDES

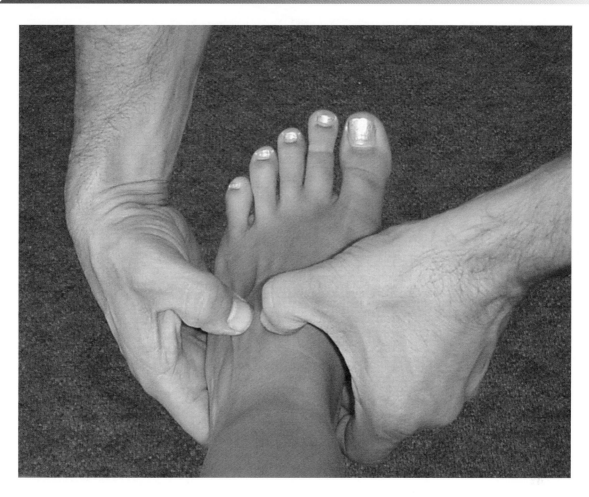

Assessment of the amount of joint glide between the tarsals.

PATIENT POSITION	Supine Knee flexed and the heel stabilized by the edge of the table
POSITION OF EXAMINER	Standing or sitting in front of the patient's foot Grasp the plantar and dorsal aspect of one tarsal with the stabilizing hand. The opposite hand grasps the adjacent tarsal in a similar manner
EVALUATIVE PROCEDURE	One tarsal is glided dorsally and then plantarly on the stabilized tarsal Repeat for each tarsal joint
POSITIVE TEST	Pain associated with movement Increased or decreased glide relative to the opposite foot
IMPLICATIONS	Increased glide: ligamentous laxity Decreased glide: joint adhesions, articular changes causing coalition of the joint

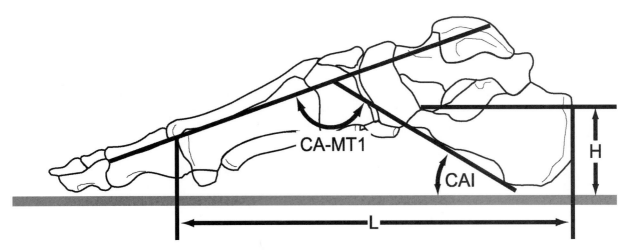

FIGURE 4–25. Calculation of arch height and length taken from a weight-bearing radiograph. H = Height; L = Length; CA-MT1 = Calcaneal 1st metatarsal angle; CAI = Calcaneal inclination.

◆ PATHOLOGIES AND RELATED SPECIAL TESTS

Many of the conditions affecting the normal function of the foot may be traced to improper biomechanics of the foot itself or the result of compensation by the foot for biomechanical deficits elsewhere in the lower extremity.

ARCH PATHOLOGIES

Although abnormalities of the arch may be caused by acute trauma or disease states, they more commonly occur congenitally. Many athletes successfully compete throughout long careers with pes planus or pes cavus. Increasing or decreasing the height of the arch alters the biomechanical function of the subtalar and mid-tarsal joints. These conditions become a concern when they become painful or result in pathologic biomechanical dysfunction elsewhere in the lower extremity. Possible ramifications of altered arch structure include plantar fasciitis, heel spurs, and patellofemoral pain for pes planus and claw toes; MT stress fractures; or a plantar fascia rupture for pes cavus. Poor foot posture also increases the risk of the patient's acquiring overuse injuries.[6]

Arch height can be computed by several different methods. The most accurate is a lateral weight-bearing radiograph of the foot from which the following measures are determined: (1) the height of the medial longitudinal arch, (2) the height-to-length ratio, and (3) the calcaneal-first MT angle (Fig. 4–25).[14] The height of the arch itself is a less significant finding than the actual change in height that occurs when the foot goes from a non–weight-bearing to a weight-bearing position as measured by navicular drop.

Pes Planus

Pes planus is characterized by the lowering of the medial longitudinal arch, giving this condition its colloquial name, **"flat feet"** (Fig. 4–26). The onset of pes planus can be traced to a congenital origin, biomechanical changes, or acute trauma. Pes planus itself results in biomechanical changes in all three planes of the foot and ankle, especially affecting the function of the subtalar and calcaneocuboid joints.[15] The lowered arch causes the talus to tilt medially and the navicular to displace inferiorly, making the talus more prominent (talar beaking).

Acute pes planus can occur after trauma to the structures supporting the medial longitudinal ligament, in-

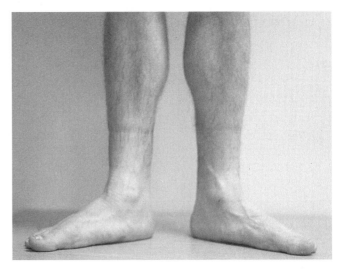

FIGURE 4–26. Pes planus. Note the absence of the medial longitudinal arch.

cluding rupture of the plantar fascia, tears of the plantar ligaments, calcaneonavicular (spring) ligament sprains, or the rupture of the tibialis posterior or tibialis anterior tendon.[1,16-18] Traumatic, symptomatic pes planus can also be related to a fracture of an **accessory navicular** (Fig. 4–27). The accessory navicular is an abnormal osseous outgrowth on the navicular that, when present, serves as a partial attachment site for the tibialis posterior. Loss of the union between the accessory navicular and the navicular itself results in a decrease in the effectiveness of the tibialis posterior in supporting the medial arch.

Mechanical factors leading to pes planus include weakness of the tibialis posterior, tibialis anterior, and the toe flexors. Stretching or weakness of the supporting ligaments, especially the spring ligament, results from the plantar-medial displacement of the talus, further increasing the amount of weight-bearing pronation. These events may be triggered or exaggerated by postural abnormalities of the spine and lower extremity to which the foot must adapt during weight bearing. Also, they may progress over time after a strain or rupture of the posterior tibialis tendon.

Pes planus is classified as being either rigid (structural) or flexible (supple). Rigid pes planus, possibly associated with **tarsal coalition,** is marked by the absence of the medial longitudinal arch when the foot is both weight bearing and non–weight bearing. With supple pes planus, the arch appears normal during non-weight bearing but disappears when the foot is weight bearing (Box 4–10).

Two tests can be used to determine the severity of navicular displacement when the foot transitions from non–weight-bearing to weight-bearing status. The Feiss' line provides an estimation of the proportion of navicular drop relative to a line spanning the distance of the plantar aspect of the first MTP joint and the medial malleolus (See Box 4–1). A quantitative measure of pronation can be calculated using the **navicular drop test** (Box 4–11).[13,19] Navicular drop is the distance between the original height of the navicular (in subtalar joint neutral position) to the final weight-bearing position of the navicular in a relaxed stance.[20]

Supple pes planus may be corrected with the use of firm or soft orthotic material (depending on the specific foot characteristics) to reduce the amount and velocity of navicular drop.[13] Semirigid orthotics or motion-control shoes may be used for pes planus to decrease certain biomechanical deficiencies such as excessive pronation.

Left untreated, pes planus can result in MT stress fractures, low back pain, and other musculoskeletal problems in the lower extremity and spine.[14] Evidence has also established a relationship between pes planus and a predisposition to anterior cruciate ligament (ACL) tears. The tibia internally rotates as the navicular drops during pronation, causing the ACL to tighten as it wraps around the posterior cruciate ligament (see Chapter 6).[21]

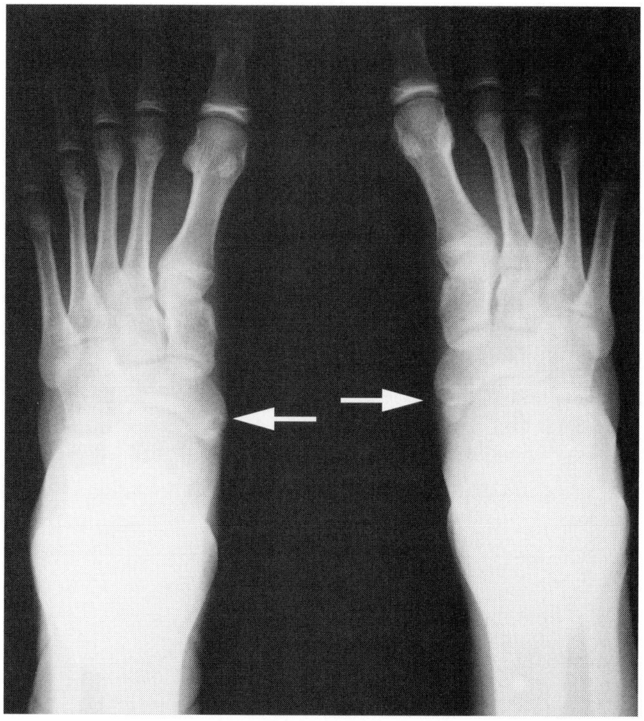

Pes Cavus

Appearing as a high medial longitudinal arch, pes cavus is often a congenital foot deformity. However, certain neurologic or disease states such as upper motor neuron lesions or cerebral palsy may result in its presence.[22] Hypertrophy of the peroneus longus muscle relative to the tibialis anterior has also been traced to cavus deformities.[23] This foot type is associated with a generalized stiffness and impaired ability to absorb ground contact forces. During running, pes cavus results in increased pressure loads on the forefoot and rearfoot.[6]

A spreading and apparent drop of the forefoot relative to the rearfoot caused by the depression of the MT heads is noted during inspection of the area (Fig. 4–28). The dorsal pads under the calcaneus and the MT heads appear smaller than in a "normal" foot. The lateral four toes may be clawed. Over time, calluses may be found over the PIP joints.

In the case of congenital pes cavus, treatment approaches are often symptomatic, and soft orthotics or shoes with soft midsoles may be used to decrease or counter pathomechanical motion and to dissipate forces. Advanced conditions may be corrected through a plantar facial release, a surgical technique in which the plantar fascia is sectioned, allowing the medial longitudinal arch to drop.[5]

FIGURE 4–27. Accessory navicular. The arrows identify the bony outgrowths associated with an accessory navicular.

Box 4–10
TEST FOR SUPPLE PES PLANUS

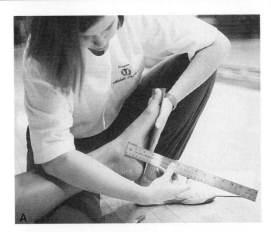

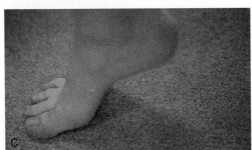

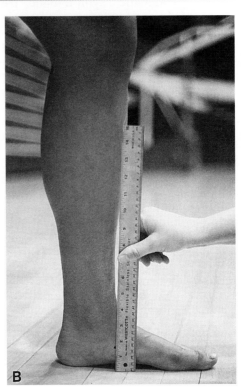

Supple pes planus. The patient displays a normal arch in the non–weight-bearing position **(A).** In weight bearing, the arch disappears (ruler added for demonstrative purposes) **(B).** When the patient performs a toe raise, the arch returns by means of the windlass effect **(C).**

PATIENT POSITION	Sitting on the edge of the examination table
POSITION OF EXAMINER	Positioned at the patient's foot
EVALUATIVE PROCEDURE	With the patient in a non–weight-bearing position the examiner notes the presence of a medial longitudinal arch **(A).** The examiner instructs the patient to stand so that the body weight is evenly distributed **(B).**
POSITIVE TEST	The presence of a medial longitudinal arch when non–weight bearing disappears when weight bearing To confirm the presence of supple pes planus, note if the arch reappears as the patient performs a toe raise **(C).**
IMPLICATIONS	If the medial longitudinal arch disappears when weight bearing, a supple pes planus is present. If no arch is present while in a non–weight-bearing position, a rigid pes planus is present.
COMMENT	This test is only meaningful when the medial longitudinal arch is present with the patient in a non–weight-bearing position.

Box 4–11
NAVICULAR DROP TEST

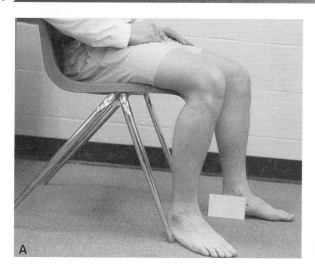

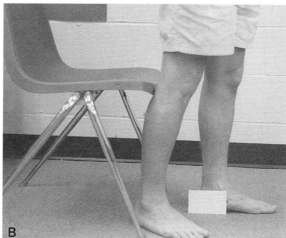

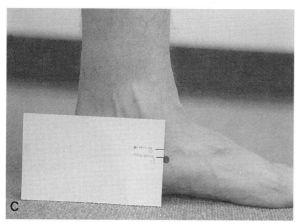

The navicular drop test is used to assess hyperpronation of the foot by measuring the height of the navicular tuberosity while the foot is non–weight-bearing **(A)** to weight-bearing **(B)** and measuring the distance of the inferior displacement **(C)**.

PATIENT POSITION	Sitting with both feet on the floor. A noncarpeted surface is recommended.
POSITION OF EXAMINER	Kneeling in front of the patient.
EVALUATIVE PROCEDURE	The subtalar joint is placed in the neutral position with the patient's foot flat against the ground, but non–weight-bearing. With the patient non–weight-bearing, a dot is placed over the navicular tuberosity. A 3 × 5 index card is positioned next to the medial longitudinal arch. A mark is made on the card corresponding to the level of the navicular tuberosity **(A)**. The patient stands with the body weight evenly distributed between the two feet, and the foot is allowed to relax into pronation. The new level of the navicular is marked on the index card **(B)**. The relative displacement (drop) of the navicular is determined by measuring the distance between the two marks in millimeters **(C)**.
POSITIVE TEST	The navicular drops greater than 10 mm.[13]
IMPLICATIONS	Hyperpronated foot.

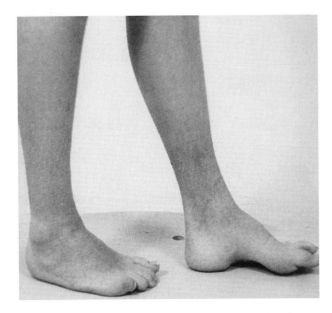

FIGURE 4–28. Pes cavus, abnormally high medial arches.

Increased height of the medial longitudinal arch may be a predisposing condition to MT, tibial, and femoral stress fractures.[14] Pes cavus may also be associated with spinal scoliosis, although the cause-and-effect relationship has not been established.[23]

Transverse Metatarsal Arch Pathology

Architecturally, the transverse MT arch is supported through a buttress formed by the medial and lateral longitudinal arches, with dynamic support provided by the peroneus longus muscle.[24] Normally, the transverse MT arch is only slightly visible during non-weight bearing, possibly being obscured by the fat pad covering the plantar aspect of the MT heads. During static weight bearing, the arch flattens, with the first MT head and sesamoids bearing 33 percent of the body weight while the remaining four toes equally assume the rest of the load.

A deficiency in the transverse MT arch can produce pain under the heads of the second through fifth MTs. The development of an intermetatarsal neuroma is possible as the nerves become compressed between the MT heads. Inspect and palpate the plantar aspect of the involved foot and compare it with the uninvolved side.

PLANTAR FASCIITIS

Inflammation of the plantar fascia or the interface between the fascia and the first layer of intrinsic muscles can be traced to a single traumatic episode, repeated stress, biomechanical deficits, the presence of a heel spur, or nerve entrapment.[25] Abnormal foot types such as pes planus or pes cavus may be predisposing factors for this condition. Biomechanical dysfunction can also be the result of medial heel pain caused by the entrapment of the medial calcaneal nerve or the nerve innervating the abductor digiti quinti muscle.[25] The onset of plantar fasciitis can occur after significant changes in activity intensity and duration, prolonged standing, training errors, or weight gain.[9] Bilateral fasciitis may be caused by underlying disease states of nervous, vascular, muscular, or connective tissue.[26]

Plantar fasciitis and heel spurs were once thought to be closely related. It was believed that shortening of the plantar fascia caused an outgrowth (i.e, a heel spur) to appear on the medial calcaneal tubercle. Although heel spurs and plantar fasciitis may occur concurrently, their presence may be coincidence (see the Heel Spurs section of this chapter). Regardless of the relationship between these two conditions, a heel spur has the potential for negatively impacting the foot's biomechanics, leading to plantar fasciitis.

Trauma to the plantar fascia may lead to inflammation, a pulling away of its origin from the calcaneus, a strain of its tissues, or its complete rupture. Inflammation of this structure may also result in tearing-type injuries secondary to the functional shortening of its tissues. Over time, tightness of the triceps surae muscle group occurs, resulting in a valgus heel position at heel strike. During push off, dorsiflexion and supination are restricted, further increasing the amount of tension placed on the plantar fascia. As a result, muscle strength during gait is weakened.[27]

Typically, pain is centralized around the plantar fascia's origin on the medial calcaneal tubercle. However, the fascia may be tender along its entire length. A common symptom of plantar fasciitis is pain when stepping out of bed in the morning or stepping on the foot after a period of non–weight bearing. Initially, the patient's chief complaint is pain in the heel when resting after activity. Weakness may be demonstrated during resisted plantarflexion; dorsiflexion also is decreased.[27] As this injury progresses, pain is experienced with the onset of activity, subsiding secondary to stretching of the tissues and increased blood flow to the area. In the chronic stage, the pain is almost always constant (Table 4–7).

When accompanied by pes planus or pes cavus, plantar fasciitis may be considered a symptom of changes in the foot's biomechanics.[28] In this event, the arch's biomechanics must be corrected to alleviate the plantar fasciitis. The presence of a heel spur or hallux abducto rigidus may cause a significant decrease in the amount of strength and ROM available to the foot. Decreased strength and ROM in the plantarflexors and dorsiflexors can lead to plantar fasciitis.[27]

Conservative treatment of patients with plantar fasciitis includes the use of orthotics and heel cups and stretching of the plantar fascia and the muscles of the lower extremity. Dorsiflexion splints may be used when the patient is at rest. These devices place the ankle in dorsiflexion to passively maintain the length of the triceps surae and the plantar fascia. Physicians may

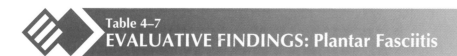

Table 4–7
EVALUATIVE FINDINGS: Plantar Fasciitis

Examination Segment	Clinical Findings	
History	***Onset:***	Either acute or insidious
	Pain characteristics:	Pain centralized near the medial calcaneal tubercle and can be spread throughout the fascia. Pain may be described when weight bearing and is worsened after being in a non–weight-bearing position. Pain is especially noticeable when the patient rises from bed in the morning.
	Mechanism:	Acute; forced dorsiflexion of the ankle combined with toe extension
		Insidious: Increased activity, additional distance when running, changing surface, or using a new or different shoe type or brand.
	Predisposing factors:	Subtalar valgus, foot pronation, pes cavus, pes planus, Achilles tendon or triceps surae tightness, leg length discrepancy, or weight gain
Inspection	In some cases, swelling may be noted on the plantar aspect near the calcaneus.	
	Pes planus or pes cavus may be noted.	
Palpation	Pain is at or near the origin of the plantar fascia that, on occasion, runs the length of the plantar fascia.	
Functional tests	Pain may be experienced during both active and passive ankle dorsiflexion and toe extension because of the stretch placed on the plantar fascia.	
	AROM: Decreased dorsiflexion ROM	
	PROM: Decreased dorsiflexion ROM	
	RROM: Decreased strength during plantar flexion, especially when weight bearing (e.g., doing single-leg toe raises)	
Ligamentous tests	Not applicable	
Neurologic tests	Tinel's sign to rule out posterior tibial nerve entrapment (tarsal tunnel syndrome)	
Special tests	None	
Comments	Plantar faciitis may result secondary to pes planus or pes cavus.	

AROM = active range of motion; PROM = passive range of motion; ROM = range of motion; RROM = resisted range of motion.

elect to use ***corticosteroid*** injections for problem cases, but this technique has been associated with ruptures of the plantar fascia. Most patients respond well to conservative care, but those suffering from bilateral inflammation respond less favorably.[9,26]

Chronic plantar fasciitis can lead to tightness of the triceps surae muscle group. As the calf muscles tighten, they move the foot into plantarflexion, increasing and prolonging the tension on the plantar fascia as it attaches at the calcaneal tubercle.

Heel Spur

A heel spur is a hook-shaped bony outgrowth (exostosis) found on the medial calcaneal tubercle (see Fig. 4–20). This condition was once thought to be a consequence of a shortened plantar fascia's leading to exostosis of its attachment on the calcaneus. However, surgical and radiographic investigations have determined that heel spurs are commonly located at the origin of the short toe flexor muscles rather than on the fascia's attachment site.[26]

Although plantar fasciitis and a heel spur can occur simultaneously, the cause-and-effect relationship between the two conditions is unclear.[26] Calcaneal pitch angle may be a predictor of heel spurs and plantar fasciitis,[29,30] and the prevalence of heel spurs increases with age.[31]

The signs, symptoms, and treatment of a heel spur are similar to those of plantar fasciitis (see Table 4–7). However, heel spurs tend to have a gradual onset and the chief complaint is pain during the heel-strike phase of gait. However, 15 percent of asymptomatic adults have been found to have spurs.[32] Evaluate the triceps surae muscle group for tightness that is associated with plantar fasciitis and heel spurs.

Conservative treatment is similar to that used for those with plantar fasciitis. Surgical intervention may be required for spurs that do not respond to conservative treatment, are unusually large, or impair neurovascular function.

Plantar Fascia Rupture

Dorsiflexion of the foot combined with extension of the toes exerts a tensile force to the plantar fascia. If the force of this stretch is sufficient, the fascia can avulse from its bony attachment on the calcaneus or rupture its central slip. A low (shallow) calcaneal pitch angle

---

Corticosteroid A substance that permits many biochemical reactions to proceed at their optimal rates (e.g., tissue healing).

may place individuals at increased risk of suffering a plantar fascia rupture (see Figure 4–25).[29,30] The risk of rupture is increased after corticosteroid injections.[5,9]

The patient has immediate difficulty bearing weight secondary to pain. The terminal stance, midstance, and pre-swing phases of gait are painful. The area may be swollen and discolored because of soft tissue swelling and bleeding. Soon after the rupture, the patient may demonstrate an acute hammer toe deformity on the involved foot (see Box 4–2).[9]

TARSAL COALITION

Tarsal coalition is a bony, fibrous, or cartilaginous union between two or more tarsal bones. A hereditary condition, tarsal coalition most often affects the calcaneonavicular, talonavicular, or talocalcaneal joints[15,33] The resulting signs, symptoms, and dysfunction depend on the joints involved in the coalition. Tarsal coalition clinically resembles rigid pes planus and may be related to *peroneal spastic flatfoot.* The patient displays limited subtalar motions leading to further stress at the midtarsal area with eventual collapse of the longitudinal arches.

Rigidity of the foot reduces the amount of external rotation at the ankle. Thus, compensatory forces are concentrated distal to the subtalar joint. The calcaneus assumes a valgus position relative to the tibia, and the forefoot abducts, the arch flattens, and the navicular overrides the talus to cause talar beaking (Fig. 4–29).[15,34] As the peroneals contract, especially the peroneus longus, spasm and pain result.[15]

Tarsal coalition most often affects or becomes symptomatic in preteens. The initial finding often follows an inversion ankle sprain, an injury that is predisposed by subtalar joint coalition.[15,35] Age appears to have a relationship with the joints most commonly involved in tarsal coalition: the talonavicular joint for children age 3

to 5 years; the calcaneonavicular joint for those age 8 to 12 years; and the talocalcaneal joint for those age 12 to 16 years.[15]

Clinically, tarsal coalition is exhibited as a rigid flatfoot with calcaneal valgus and abduction of the forefoot that is unchanged when the patient is in a weight-bearing position (rigid pes planus).[15] Palpation over the involved joint may cause pain.

Tarsal coalition is differentiated from other foot problems by the limitations in subtalar motion. It also can be identified by radiographic examination. A definitive diagnosis of tarsal coalition is made through the use of radiographs for bony fusion, computed tomography (CT) scans, or magnetic resonance imaging (MRI) for cartilaginous or fibrous coalition.[15] Any rigidity in the rearfoot may indicate tarsal coalition, warranting referral to a physician for further evaluation.

If detected in its early stages, tarsal coalition usually responds well to immobilization, the use of orthotics, or both.[15,36] When surgery is performed to release the coalition before any secondary degenerative changes occur, the prognosis is excellent.[37]

TARSAL TUNNEL SYNDROME

Tarsal tunnel syndrome (TTS) is caused by the entrapment of the posterior tibial nerve or one of its medial or lateral branches as it passes through the tarsal tunnel. The definition of TTS has been expanded to include compressive lesions of the posterior tibial nerve proximal to the retinaculum, under the deep fascia of the leg, and distally under the abductor hallicus muscle.[38]

Anatomically, the tarsal tunnel is bordered anteriorly by the tibia and the talus and laterally by the calcaneus. The flexor retinaculum forms a fibrous roof that is attached to the sheaths of the tibialis posterior, flexor hallicus longus, and flexor digitorum longus tendons (Fig 4–30).[39] The tunnel itself is compartmentalized by fascial membranes, or septa, which tightly bind the posterior tibial nerve, predisposing it to compressive forces.[38]

The onset of TTS has been traced to several different factors. Acute TTS may be caused by acute trauma, including tarsal fracture or dislocation, hyperplantarflexion, or eversion. It can also be the result of overuse injuries. Predisposing conditions include ganglion formation, fibrosis, arthritis, or other disease states such as diabetes.[38,40–42] Anatomical factors that may lead to the onset of TTS include *nonunion fractures* of the sustentaculum tali, muscle anomalies, or anterior entrapment of the nerve by the extensor hallicus brevis mus-

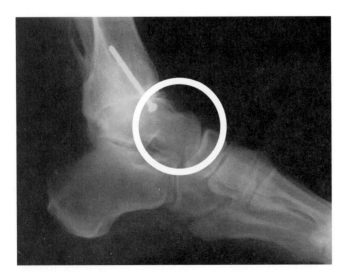

FIGURE 4–29. Talar beaking associated with tarsal coalition. The screw implanted in the tibia is for an unrelated condition.

Peroneal spastic flatfoot A lowering of the medial foot caused by spasm of the peroneus longus muscle.

Nonunion fracture The incomplete healing of a bone that has not demonstrated signs of healing over the prior three-month period.

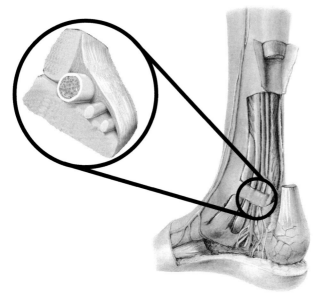

FIGURE 4–30. The tarsal tunnel. The bony surface of the tarsal tunnel is formed by the tibia, talus, and calcaneus, with the roof being formed by the flexor retinaculum.

cle.[43–45] Biomechanically, rearfoot varus, pronated feet, an unstable medial longitudinal arch, and internal tibial rotation place an increased stress load on the posterior tibial nerve, predisposing it to TTS.[46]

The primary patient complaints are diffuse pain, burning, or numbness along the plantar and medial aspect of the foot that increases with activity and decreases with rest. Approximately one third of patients report pain arising from the medial malleolus and radiating into the medial lower leg, midcalf, and, occasionally, the medial heel (Table 4–8).[39] Cold intolerance and increased pain when wearing low-cut or high heel shoes may also be described.[29] Muscular function is often normal. A positive Tinel's sign is often elicited along the path of the nerve inferior and distal to the medial malleolus (Fig. 4–31).

Tarsal tunnel syndrome may easily be confused with the symptoms produced by plantar fasciitis. However, close examination of the symptoms assists in differentiating between the two conditions.[40] Pain produced by TTS is commonly located along the medial portion of the heel and arch; with plantar fasciitis, pain is localized near the fascia's insertion on the calcaneus.

Table 4–8
EVALUATIVE FINDINGS: Tarsal Tunnel Syndrome

Examination Segment	Clinical Findings	
History	**Onset:**	Acute or insidious
	Pain characteristics:	Pain, numbness, and paresthesia occur along the plantar or medial aspects of the foot. Cold intolerance of the involved foot may be described.
	Mechanism:	Compression of the posterior tibial nerve (or its branches) within the tarsal tunnel. This pressure may also involve the vascular structures within the tunnel. A history of a plantarflexion–eversion mechanism injury to the ankle may be described. TTS also possibly associated with fracture, dislocation, or inflammation of the tarsals or local ganglion formation.
	Predisposing factors:	Prior tarsal fracture or dislocation; history of eversion ankle injury; pronated feet; arthritis; nonunion fracture of the sustentaculum tali; inflammation of the extensor retinaculum.
Inspection		Inspection of the foot is normally unremarkable. However, in chronic cases, trophic changes of the foot and nails may be noted. Inspection of the medial longitudinal arch reveals signs of pes planus, a condition often associated with TTS.
Palpation		Palpation over the tibial nerve and its branches results in tenderness, especially in the area of the tarsal tunnel and with nerve passage beneath the flexor retinaculum.
Functional tests	**AROM:**	Motor function of the intrinsic and extrinsic muscles is often normal.
	PROM:	Forced plantarflexion and eversion may increase symptoms secondary to pressure from the flexor retinaculum.
	RROM:	Normal
Ligamentous tests		Not applicable
Neurologic tests		The Tinel sign may be positive inferior and distal to the medial malleolus. Sharp or dull and two-point discrimination may be decreased along the medial and plantar aspects of the foot.
Special tests		Not applicable
Comments		Symptoms of TTS may closely resemble those of other foot maladies, especially plantar fasciitis. Presence of TTS is confirmed through electrical diagnostic studies or MRI.

AROM = active range of motion; PROM = passive range of motion; RROM = resisted range of motion; TTS = tarsal tunnel syndrome.

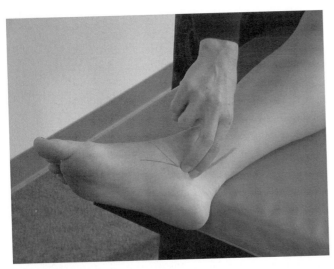

FIGURE 4–31. Location of Tinel's sign for tarsal tunnel syndrome. Tapping over the path of the posterior tibial nerve refers pain into the foot and toes.

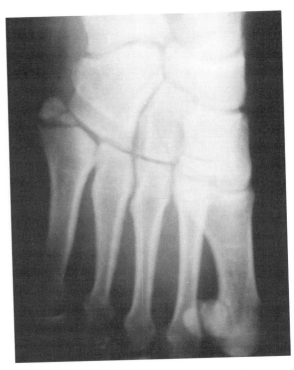

FIGURE 4–32. Fracture of styloid process of the fifth metatarsal.

Whereas stretching and exercise often decrease the pain produced by plantar fasciitis, activity increases the pain caused by TTS. A definitive diagnosis of TTS is made through electrodiagnostic studies, MRI, or ultrasonic imaging.[29,38,47]

A complete evaluation of the lower extremity is required to identify the cause of TTS. A common finding is pes planus in which hyperpronation increases the traction stress placed on the nerve, prolonging its recovery. The use of an orthotic to control the amount of pronation is recommended when treating patients with this condition.[48] Surgical intervention may be needed to release the compressive forces placed on the posterior tibial nerve. Results are most successful when the compression occurs within the tarsal tunnel itself.[29]

METATARSAL FRACTURES

Fracture of the MTs can result from direct trauma or overuse. Acute fractures occur secondary to compressive, tensile, rotational, or crushing forces. Stress fractures have a more insidious and complex onset. The toe flexors assist the foot in dissipating the forces placed on the MTs. Fatigue or general weakness of the toe flexors increases the amount of strain placed on the MTs, increasing the risk of fractures.[49] The presence of diabetes mellitus also increases the risk of MT fracture.[50]

The base of the fifth MT is particularly prone to avulsion fractures (Fig. 4–32). The body counters against inadvertent inversion of the foot and ankle by contracting the peroneals, everting the foot and bringing it back to its proper orientation. If the force of the contraction is too great, the peroneal brevis tendon can be avulsed from its attachment on the styloid process of the fifth MT. This mechanism, when associated with pain, crepitus, and swelling over the insertion site, strongly sug-

gests a fracture. The signs and symptoms of an avulsion fracture of the fifth MT's styloid process are clinically similar to that of a **Jones' fracture,** a fracture of the fifth MT 1 cm distal to the proximal diaphysis (Fig. 4–33).[51]

Stress fractures of the MTs, the most common site, are related to biomechanical abnormalities of the foot.[52] Predisposing conditions include dysfunction of the first MTP joint, neuropathy, metabolic disorders (including diabetes and osteoporosis), and rearfoot malalignment.[53] Because of the prevalence of osteoporosis, postmenopausal women are at increased risk of stress fractures.[54]

During weight bearing, hypomobility increases the amount of stress placed on the midfoot and hypermobility increases the amount of stress placed on the forefoot. Over time, the individual begins to experience local pain associated with activity. Stress fractures of the MTs have been termed **march fractures** because of their prevalence in new military recruits. If unrecognized and untreated, a stress fracture can progress to the stage of a gross fracture.

The signs and symptoms of an acute fracture may include obvious deformity and the presence of a *false joint* over the fracture site. The suspicion of acute frac-

False joint Abnormal movement along the length of a bone caused by a fracture or incomplete fusion.

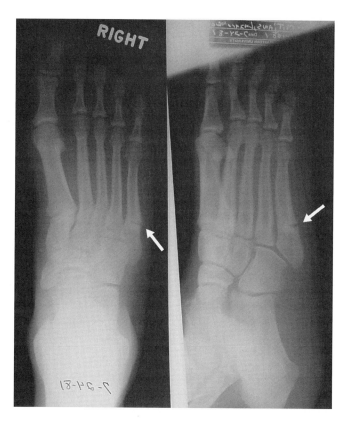

FIGURE 4–33. Radiograph of a Jones' fracture, a fracture of the fifth MT 1 cm distal to the styloid process.

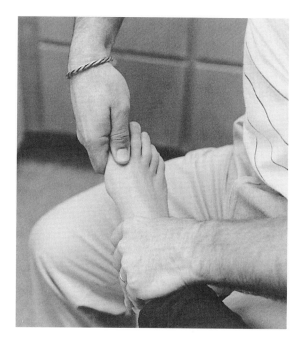

FIGURE 4–34. Long bone compression test for suspected fractures of the metatarsals. A longitudinal force is placed along the shaft of the bone. In the presence of a fracture, compression of the two fragments results in pain and possibly the presence of a "false joint."

tures may be further substantiated by the use of the long bone compression test (Fig. 4–34). ROM of the joints above and below the fracture site may be limited because of pain.

Stress fractures are characterized by a dull pain over the fracture site that increases with activity and decreases with rest. This condition must be differentiated from other foot conditions. Pain may be referred to the MTs secondary to TTS or an intermetatarsal neuroma. Additionally, pain may arise from irritation of the interosseous muscles, be caused by an inflammatory condition such as periosteitis, or have a vascular origin. Any suspected fracture to the MTs requires immediate immobilization and non–weight bearing while the patient is referred to a physician (Table 4–9).

Management of patients with these conditions depends on the type and location of the fracture. Avulsion fractures may be managed with soft casting requiring 4 weeks for recovery.[55,56] Fractures of the MT shaft or neck typically require immobilization and weight bearing to tolerance for 4 to 6 weeks. Because of their propensity for a non-union, Jones' fractures require 8 weeks of immobilization followed by weight bearing in a cast as tolerated.[56] Jones' fractures often require surgical fixation.

Phalangeal Fractures

Phalangeal fractures occur when a longitudinal force is applied to the bone, such as kicking an immovable ob-

ject, or secondary to a crushing force, such as a weight falling on the toes (Fig. 4–35). Signs and symptoms of a fractured phalanx include deformity, pain, and crepitus. While running or walking, pain is experienced during toe-off. Although this condition results in pain and an *antalgic gait*, few treatment options exist. After a fracture has been confirmed through radiographic examination, the treatment consists of rest, the use of a hard-soled shoe to prevent flexion of the toes, taping the affected toe to the one next to it ("buddy taping"), and possibly the use of crutches. Surgical intervention may be required if the fracture disrupts the articular surface.

INTERMETATARSAL NEUROMA

Intermetatarsal neuromas (interdigital neuroma) are caused by the entrapment of a nerve between two MT heads.[57] This condition is also referred to as **plantar neuroma**. When the nerve entrapment occurs between the third and fourth MTs, the condition is termed **Morton's neuroma**. The third common digital (plantar)

Antalgic gait A limp or unnatural walking pattern caused by pain, trauma, or dysfunction of the lower extremity.

Table 4–9
EVALUATIVE FINDINGS: Metatarsal Fractures

Examination Segment	Clinical Findings	
History	**Onset:**	Acute, or in the case of stress fractures, insidious
	Pain characteristics:	Pain occuring along the shaft of the metatarsal, radiating into the intermetatarsal space
	Mechanism:	Acute: Direct trauma to the metatarsal (e.g., being stepped on), dynamic overload (e.g., avulsion of the peroneus brevis tendon), or rotational (e.g. inversion of the foot). Insidious: Repetitive stresses placed along the shaft of the metatarsal or compression arising from the contiguous metatarsals (e.g., "march fracture"). The symptoms typically increase with activity and decrease with rest.
	Predisposing factors:	Patients with a history of long-term diabetes mellitus are at an increased risk of pedal fractures. Pes planus, pes cavus, Morton's toe, or subtalar varus or valgus may predispose the individual to metatarsal stress fractures. Stress fractures may also be induced by change in footwear, increased intensity or duration of training, and changing running surfaces. Postmenopausal women are at an increased risk of stress fractures.
Inspection	In acute injures, gross deformity or swelling may be visible along the shaft of the bone. Stress fractures may reveal no significant outward signs, but inflammation around the painful area may be present.	
Palpation	Tenderness and crepitus may be present over the site of acute fractures of maturing stress fractures. A *false joint* may be present with acutely fractured metatarsals.	
Functional tests	**AROM and PROM:**	Movements that compress the bone, mainly dorsiflexion of the ankle or rotation of the foot, typically result in pain.
	RROM:	In all planes, RROM normally results in pain. These symptoms are replicated when weight bearing.
Ligamentous tests	Not applicable	
Neurologic tests	Not applicable	
Special tests	Long bone compression test	
Comments	The presence of acute fractures must be confirmed through radiographic examination. Bone scans or MRIs are required to definitively diagnose stress fractures in their early stages.	

AROM = active range of motion; PROM = passive range of motion; RROM = resisted range of motion.

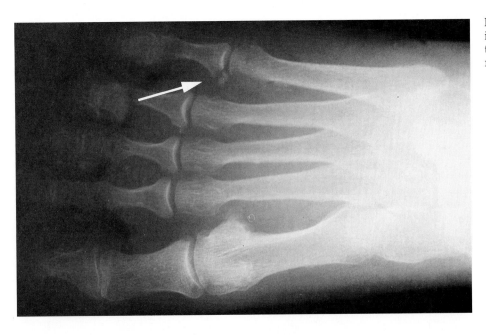

FIGURE 4–35. Fracture of the proximal phalanx of the fifth toe. Note the fracture line crossing the proximal medial process.

FIGURE 4–36. Determination of the presence of an intermetatarsal neuroma. The eraser end of a pencil is used to apply pressure to the intermetatarsal space, compressing the nerve ending.

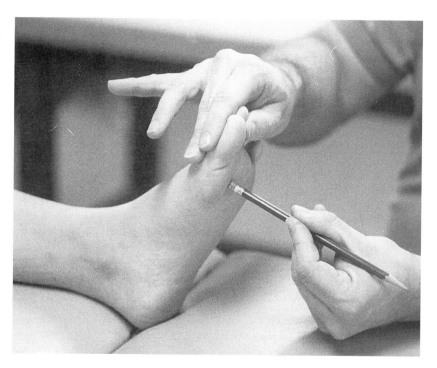

nerve is most commonly affected.[58,59] The communicating branch of the lateral plantar nerve has also been implicated with Morton's neuroma.[58]

Prolonged pressure on the involved nerve results in a degenerative neuropathy and formation of fibrotic nodules and edema around the nerve. The exact relationship of this buildup and the diagnosis of a neuroma is unclear.[59,60] Over time, *demyelination* of the nerve occurs.[60]

Excessive motion, a thickened and shortened transverse intermetatarsal ligament, and hyperpronation predispose individuals to intermetatarsal neuromas. Activities that increase weight-bearing pressure on the forefoot, such as wearing pointed-toed and high heels shoes, can trigger the signs and symptoms.[59] Women are more likely to be affected with this condition than men. Also, a high likelihood exists for reoccurrence in the same foot.[59,61]

The chief complaints, closely resembling those of a MT stress fracture, include pain in the anterior transverse arch radiating to the toes, the plantar aspect of the foot, and, occasionally, projecting up the ankle and lower leg. Numbness and paresthesia in the digits may also be described. An increase in intermetatarsal pressure during weight bearing on the forefoot increases pain.[62] The symptoms increase when the patient is wearing shoes, especially if the shoes are tight fitting. Patients report relief of the symptoms when the footwear is removed. A nodule may be felt between the involved MT heads. Tenderness may be increased by extending the digits and dorsiflexing the foot during palpation. Squeezing the transverse arch, thus compressing the MT heads, replicates the symptoms. The eraser end of a pencil may be used to apply pressure directly to the neuroma, resulting in an increase in the symptoms (Fig. 4–36).

Patients suspected of suffering from an intermetatarsal neuroma need to be referred to a physician for further evaluation and definitive diagnosis. Ultrasonography is a highly reliable method of identifying the location and size of intermetatarsal neuromas.[61,63]

Initial treatment includes modification of footwear (i.e., the patient should avoid wearing shoes that increase symptoms), the use of orthotics to decrease intermetatarsal pressure, and the use of oral antiinflammatory medication.[64,65] Corticosteroid or local anesthetic injections may be used for symptomatic relief. However, this form of treatment seldom resolves a neuroma.[64,66] In advanced cases, surgical excision of the neuroma provides dramatic relief of the symptoms.[59,64]

HALLUX RIGIDUS

Progressive degeneration of the first MTP joint's articular surfaces can result in limited motion (hallux limitus) or complete *ankylosis* (hallux rigidus).[67] The joint degeneration is caused by osteoarthritis; rheumatoid arthritis; gout; and advanced hallux valgus, synovial effusion, or other chondral erosions affecting the articular surfaces.[68–71] The etiology of hallux limitus and hallux rigidus may be related to an irregularly flattened MT head, hypermobility of the first ray, or a long first MT leading to degeneration-causing forces on the joint.[67]

Demyelination   Loss of a nerve's fatty lining.

Ankylosis   Immobility of a joint.

Morton's toe has been associated with hallux rigidus, especially in female dancers.[8]

As the condition progresses, the MT head erodes (chondritis dessicans) or a fracture occurs through the articular surface (osteochondritis dessicans).[69] The axis of joint motion shifts from the center of the MTP to its plantar aspect. If untreated, spastic contractures and fusion of the joint (ankylosis) occur.[69,71] In some cases, the sesamoids located under the first MTP joint may hypertrophy, further decreasing ROM.[69] Irregularity of the joint surfaces results in pain. The subsequent loss in ROM affects the terminal stance and pre-swing phases of gait (see Fig 4–1).

Feet affected by hallux rigidus may develop a palpable exostosis on the dorsal aspect of the joint. Extension of the first MTP joint is limited by the phalanx's striking the exostosis. Similar to what happens with arthritis, the joint is prone to pain and swelling, especially after activity. Radiographic examination is used to definitively diagnose this condition (Fig. 4–37).

Conservative treatment includes the use of passive ROM exercises to maintain extension in the joint and the use of orthotics to decrease hyperextension forces on the first MTP joint. Corticosteroid injections assist in decreasing inflammation. If the condition progresses, thereby limiting extension and affecting gait so that regular ambulation becomes antalgic, surgical intervention may be required. The most common surgical procedure, a cheilectomy, involves the removal of the distal dorsal aspect of the first MT and the superior half of the joint surface and other areas of exostosis.[72,73] Removal of the bone decreases pain and restores extension to the joint, allowing a more normal gait pattern.

FIRST METATARSOPHALANGEAL JOINT SPRAINS

Sprains of the first MTP joint are one of the most common sports injuries to the foot. The injury usually occurs as the foot is planted and the foot and the ankle is subsequently dorsiflexed. As the shoe grasps the playing surface, body weight and forward momentum force the first MTP joint into hyperextension. Sprains of the plantar MTP joint capsule have been termed **"turf toe"** because of the reportedly high instance of this injury during competition on artificial turf.[74]

Pain in the joint during the push-off phase of gait, active joint motion, or manual resistance, or when attempting quick stops are common complaints of patients with first MTP joint sprains. The joint is painful to the touch and ROM is limited. A radiograph is needed to rule out fracture to the MT or phalanx.

Athletes, especially those who compete barefooted, are also susceptible to varus and valgus sprains of the MTP joints. A varus force is applied to the joint capsule and collateral ligaments when the toes are bent toward the body's midline. An outward bending results in a valgus force being placed on the capsule. On rare occasions, the MTP joint may dislocate.

Management of sprains of the first MTP involves removing aggravating stresses through the use of crutches, a firm shoe insole, or other immobilization device. The physician may prescribe the use of oral or injectable antiinflammatory medications.

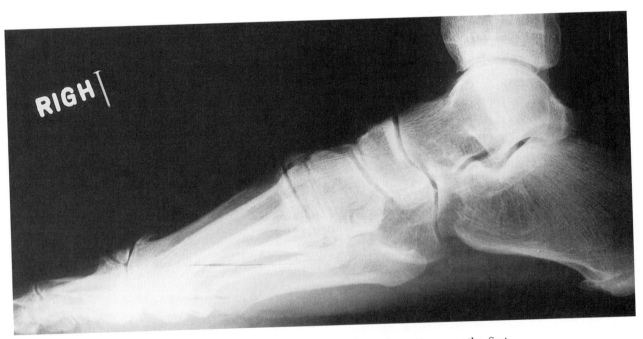

FIGURE 4–37. X-ray view of hallux rigidus. The wedge-shaped bony formation over the first metatarsophalangeal joint serves as a mechanical block in limiting extension.

ON-FIELD EVALUATION OF FOOT INJURIES

Although it is possible for an athlete to walk off the playing area with a fracture, especially if it involves the toes, significant trauma to the foot and toes usually results in the athlete's inability to bear weight without pain. The location of the pain and mechanism of injury act as a guide for on-field injury evaluation. Not all of the steps described in this section apply to all injuries.

With any sign or symptom indicating a bony fracture or joint dislocation, terminate the evaluation, splint the foot and ankle, and refer the athlete to a physician. The inability to bear weight without pain as well as the inability to push off or hop on the involved foot also indicates the need to keep the athlete from further competition. After the athlete is moved to the sideline or the sports medicine facility, the remaining evaluation proceeds, as described earlier in this chapter.

EQUIPMENT CONSIDERATIONS

Only the most severe cases, based on the degree of pain, reports of a "crack" or "pop," or obvious trauma such as bleeding through the shoe, warrant removal of the shoe or sock while the patient is on the playing surface. (Chapter 5 provides a description of removing footwear and ankle braces.)

ON-FIELD HISTORY

Question the athlete about his or her history relating to the mechanism of injury, the location of the pain, any sounds associated with its onset, and the athlete's willingness and ability to bear weight on the injured limb. Pain may also radiate to the foot from the lumbar or sacral plexus or after trauma to the peroneal nerve or anterior compartment syndrome.

ON-FIELD INSPECTION

Observe the posture of the athlete. Is the individual remaining down on the field or court or is the athlete hopping off or being assisted off the playing surface? The shoe itself will prohibit a direct inspection of the foot. If the footwear is removed while the athlete is still on the field, note the integrity of the joints, any gross deformity of the long bones, or the presence of gross swelling or discoloration.

If a significant injury such as a fracture or dislocation is evident during the initial inspection, perform a secondary survey to rule out the presence of unrecognized trauma. Then immobilize the body part and refer the athlete for medical evaluation.

ON-FIELD PALPATION

With the exceptions of the plantar and superior aspects of the calcaneus and the talus, the bones of the foot are relatively subcutaneous, assisting in the identification of crepitus or other deformities through palpation.

- **Bony palpation:** The presence of a fracture or dislocation must be ruled out.

  ○ Palpate the lengths of the five rays to rule out discontinuity in the bony shafts or joints.
  ○ Palpate the tarsals, calcaneus, talus, and the medial and lateral malleoli for point tenderness or crepitus that may indicate a gross or avulsion fracture or dislocation.

- **Soft tissue palpation:** The forces placed on the foot can be sufficient to significantly strain or rupture its tendons, fascia, or ligaments.

  ○ **Plantar fascia:** Palpate the length of the plantar fascia to identify areas of point tenderness. Pain arising from the medial calcaneal tubercle may signify a rupture of the plantar fascia.
  ○ **Anterior musculature:** Palpate the anterior musculature. Hyperplantarflexion of the ankle or an eccentric contraction of the tibialis anterior can result in a strain, rupture, or avulsion of its tendon, leading to tenderness of these structures. This mechanism may also result in a fracture of an **accessory navicular.**
  ○ **Medial musculature:** Palpate the tibialis posterior, flexor hallicus longus, and flexor digitorum longus, which pass posterior to the medial malleolus. These tendons may be impinged by eversion of the subtalar joint. The tibialis posterior may be strained in response to an inversion mechanism.
  ○ **Posterior musculature:** Palpate the posterior musculature. Achilles tendon ruptures are common in athletics. (Refer to Chapter 5 for more information on this condition.)
  ○ **Lateral musculature:** Palpate the peroneal muscles as they pass posterior to the lateral malleolus. An inversion and plantarflexion mechanism followed by contraction of the peroneals can result in an avulsion of the peroneus brevis attachment from the styloid process of the fifth MT.

ON-FIELD RANGE OF MOTION TESTS

Range of motion testing during this phase of the evaluation is most likely limited to flexion and extension of the toes, inversion and eversion of the foot, and plantarflexion and dorsiflexion of the ankle. If these can be performed without pain or signs of a fracture or dislocation, the athlete can attempt to bear weight, as described in Chapter 1.

ON-FIELD MANAGEMENT OF FOOT INJURIES

Except in rare circumstances, most foot injuries do not require the athlete to be transported directly from the playing field to the hospital. Acute trauma such as Achilles tendon ruptures, ankle fractures, and ankle dislocations are discussed in Chapter 5.

PLANTAR FASCIA RUPTURES

Splint suspected plantar fascia ruptures with the foot and ankle in a slightly plantarflexed position or instruct the athlete not to bear weight. Fit the athlete with crutches and refer the individual to a physician or doctor of podiatric medicine.

FRACTURES AND DISLOCATIONS

Remove athletes from the field in a non–weight-bearing manner if a fracture or dislocation is suspected. After further evaluating the athlete on the sideline, immobilize his or her foot, fit the athlete for crutches, render appropriate immediate treatment, and refer the patient to a physician.

 ## REFERENCES

1. Huang, CK, et al: Biomechanical evaluation of longitudinal arch stability. *Foot Ankle*, 14:353, 1993.
2. Draves, D: *Anatomy of the Lower Extremity*. Baltimore, Williams & Wilkins, 1986, p. 126.
3. Norkin, CC, and Levangie, PK: The foot-ankle complex. In Norkin, CC, and Levangie, PK (eds): *Joint Structure and Function: A Comprehensive Analysis*, ed 2. Philadelphia, FA Davis, 1992, pp. 388–393.
4. Picciano, AM, Rowlands, MS, and Worrell, T: Reliability of open and closed kinetic chain subtalar joint neutral positions and navicular drop test. *J Orthop Sport Phys Ther*, 18:553; 1993.
5. Kitaoka, HB, Luo, ZP, and An, K: Effect of plantar fasciotomy on stability of arch of foot. *Clin Orthop*, November:344, 1997.
6. Sneyers, CJL, et al: Influence of malalignment of feet on the plantar pressure patterns in running. *Foot Ankle Int*, 16:624:1995.
7. Krivickas, LS: Anatomical factors associated with overuse sports injuries. *Sports Med*, 24:132, 1997.
8. Ogilvie-Harris, DJ, Carr, MM, and Fleming, PJ: The foot in ballet dancers: The importance of second toe length. *Foot Ankle Int*, 16:144, 1995.
9. Acevedo, JI, and Beskin, JL: Complications of plantar fascia rupture associated with corticosteroid injection. *Foot Ankle Int*, 19:91, 1998.
10. Klaue, K, Hansen, ST, and Masquelet, AC: Clinical, quantitative assessment of first tarsometatarsal mobility in the sagittal plane and its relation to hallux valgus deformity. *Foot Ankle*, 15:9, 1994.
11. Marchinko, DE: The complex deformity known as hallux abducto valgus. In Marchinko, DE (ed): *Comprehensive Textbook of Hallus Abducto Valgus Reconstruction*. Chicago, Mosby, 1993, pp. 1–5.
12. Brainard, BJ: Managing corns and plantar calluses. *Physician and Sportsmedicine* 19:61, 1991.
13. Mueller, MJ, Host, JV, and Norton, BJ: Navicular drop as a composite measure of excessive pronation. *J Am Podiatr Med Assoc*, 83:198, 1993.
14. Saltzman, CL, Nawoczenski, DA, and Talbot, KD: Measurement of the medial longitudinal arch. *Arch Phys Med Rehabil*, 76:45, 1995.
15. Kulik, SA, and Clanton, TO: Tarsal coalition. *Foot Ankle Int*, 18:286, 1996.
16. Borton, DC, and Saxby, TS: Tear of the plantar calcaneonavicular (spring) ligament causing flatfoot. A case report. *J Bone Joint Surg Br*, 79:641, 1997.
17. Rule, J, Yao, L, and Seeger, LL: Spring ligament of the ankle: normal MR anatomy. *AJR Am J Roentgenol*, 161:1241, 1993.
18. Kitaoka, HB, Luo, Z, and An, K: Three-dimensional analysis of flatfoot deformity: Cadaver study. *Foot Ankle Int*, 19:447, 1998.
19. Beckett, ME, et al: Incidence of hyperpronation in the ACL injured knee: A clinical perspective. *Journal of Athletic Training*, 27:58, 1992.
20. Brody, D: Techniques in the evaluation and treatment of the injured runner. *Orthop Clin North Am*, 13:542, 1982.
21. Loudon, JK, Jenkins, W, and Loudon, KL: The relationship between static posture and ACL injury in female athletes. *J Orthop Sport Phys Ther*, 24:91; 1996.
22. Ramcharitar, SI, Koslow, P, and Simpson, DM: Lower extremity manifestations of neuromuscular diseases. *Clin Podiatr Med Surg*, 15:705, 1998.
23. Carpintero, P, et al: The relationship between pes cavus and idiopathic scoliosis. *Spine*, 19:1260, 1994.
24. Thordarson, DB, et al: Dynamic support of the human longitudinal arch. A biomechanical evaluation. *Clin Orthop*, July:165, 1995.
25. Sammarco, GJ, and Helfrey, RB: Surgical treatment of recalcitrant plantar fasciitis. *Foot Ankle Int*, 17:520, 1996.
26. Powell, M, et al: Effective treatment of plantar fasciitis with dorsiflexion night splints: A crossover prospective randomized outcomes study. *Foot Ankle Int*, 19:10, 1998.
27. Kibler, WB, Goldberg, C, and Chandler, TJ: Functional biomechanical deficits in running athletes with plantar fasciitis. *Am J Sports Med* 19:66, 1991.
28. Middleton, JA, and Kolodin, EL: Plantar fasciitis: Heel pain in athletes. *Journal of Athletic Training* 27:70, 1992.
29. Bailie, DS, and Kelikian, AS: Tarsal tunnel syndrome: Diagnosis, surgical technique, and functional outcome. *Foot Ankle Int*, 19:65, 1998.
30. Prichasuk, S, and Subhadrabandhu, T: The relationship of pes planus and calcaneal spur to plantar heel pain. *Clin Orthop*, Sept:192, 1994.
31. Riepert, T, et al: Estimation of sex on the basis of radiographs of the calcaneus. *Forensic Sci Int*, 77:133, 1996.
32. Leach, RE, Seavey, MS, and Salter, DK: Results of surgery in athletes with plantar fasciitis. *Foot and Ankle* 7:156, 1986.
33. Stormont, DM, and Peterson, HA: The relative incidence of tarsal coalition. *Clin Orthop* 181:24, 1983.
34. Clarke, DM: Multiple tarsal coalitions in the same foot. *J Pediatr Orthop*, 17:777, 1997.
35. Kelo, MJ, and Riddle, DL: Examination and management of a patient with tarsal coalition. *Phys Ther*, 78:518, 1998.
36. Vincent, KA: Tarsal coalition and painful flatfoot. *J Am Acad Orthop Surg*, 6:274, 1998.
37. O'Neill, DB, and Micheli, LJ: Tarsal coalition: A followup of adolescent athletes. *Am J Sports Med*, 17:544, 1989.
38. Frey, C: Magnetic resonance imaging and the evaluation of tarsal tunnel syndrome. *Foot and Ankle*, 14:159, 1993.
39. Mann, RA: Tarsal tunnel syndrome. In Mann, RA, and Coughlin, MJ (eds): *Surgery of the Foot and Ankle*. St. Louis, Mosby-Year Book, Inc, 1993, p. 554.
40. Jackson, DL, and Haglund, B: Tarsal tunnel syndrome in athletes. Case reports and literature review. *Am J Sports Med*, 19:61, 1991.
41. Stefko, RM, Lauerman, WC, and Heckman, JD: Tarsal tunnel syndrome caused by an unrecognized fracture of the posterior process of the talus (Cedell fracture). *J Bone Joint Surg Am*, 76:116, 1994.
42. Sammarco, GJ, Chalk, DE, and Feibel, JH: Tarsal tunnel syndrome and additional nerve lesions in the same limb. *Foot and Ankle*, 14:71, 1993.
43. Myerson, MS, and Berger, BI: Nonunion of a fracture of the sustentaculum tali causing a tarsal tunnel syndrome: A case report. *Foot Ankle Int*, 16:740, 1995.

44. Sammarco, GJ, and Conti, SF: Tarsal tunnel syndrome caused by an anomalous muscle. *J Bone Joint Surg Am*, 76:1308, 1994.

45. Kanbe, K, et al: Entrapment neuropathy of the deep peroneal nerve associated with the extensor hallicus brevis. *J Foot Ankle Surg*, 34:560, 1995.

46. Daniels, TR, Lau, JT, and Hearn, TC: The effects of foot position and load on tibial nerve tension. *Foot Ankle Int*, 19:73, 1998.

47. Masciocchi, C, Catalucci, A and Barile, A: Ankle impingement syndromes. *Eur J Radiol*, 27(S1):S70, 1998.

48. Mann, RA, and Baxter, DE: Diseases of the nerves. In Mann, RA, and Coughlin, MJ (eds): *Surgery of the Foot and Ankle*, ed 6. St Louis, CV Mosby, 1992, p. 543.

49. Sharkey, NA, et al: Strain and loading of the second metatarsal during heel-lift. *J Bone Joint Surg Am*, 77:1050, 1995.

50. Wolf, SK: Diabetes mellitus and predisposition to athletic pedal fracture. *J Foot Ankle Surg*, 37:16, 1998.

51. Kavanaugh, JH, et al: The Jones' fracture revisited. *J Bone Joint Surg*, 60A:776, 1978.

52. Brukner, P, et al: Stress fractures: A review of 180 cases. *Clin J Sport Med*, 6:85, 1996.

53. Weinfeld, SB, Haddad, SL, and Myerson, MS: Metatarsal stress fractures. *Clin Sports Med*, 16:319, 1997.

54. Kaye, RA: Insufficiency stress fractures of the foot and ankle in postmenopausal women. *Foot Ankle Int*, 19:221, 1998.

55. Weiner, BD, Linder, JF, and Giattini, JF: Treatment of fractures of the fifth metatarsal: A prospective study. *Foot Ankle Int*, 18:267, 1997.

56. Clapper, MF, O'Brien, TJ, and Lyons, PM: Fractures of the fifth metatarsal: Analysis of a fracture registry. *Clin Orthop*, June:238, 1995.

57. Thompson, FM, and Deland, JT: Occurrence of two interdigital neuromas in one foot. *Foot and Ankle*, 14:15, 1993.

58. Frank, PW, Bakkum, BW, and Darby, SA: The communicating branch of the lateral plantar nerve: a descriptive anatomic study. *Clin Anat*, 9:237, 1996.

59. Wu, KK: Morton's interdigital neuroma: A clinical review of its etiology, treatment, and results. *J Foot Ankle Surg*, 35:112, 1996.

60. Bourke, G, Owen, J, and Machet, D: Histological comparison of the third interdigital nerve in patients with Morton's metatarsalgia and control patients. *Aust N Z J Surg*, 64:421, 1994.

61. Levine, SE, et al: Ultrasonographic diagnosis of recurrence after excision of an interdigital neuroma. *Foot Ankle Int*, 19:79, 1998.

62. Holmes, GB: Quantitative determination of intermetatarsal pressure. *Foot Ankle*, 13:532, 1992.

63. Sobiesk, GA, et al: Sonographic evaluation of interdigital neuromas. *J Foot Ankle Surg*, 36:364, 1997.

64. Bennett, GL, Graham, CE, and Mauldin, DM: Morton's interdigital neuroma: A comprehensive treatment protocol. *Foot Ankle Int*, 16:760, 1995.

65. Nunan, PJ, and Giesy, BD: Management of Morton's neuroma in athletes. *Clin Podiatr Med Surg*, 14:489, 1997.

66. Rasmussen, MR, Kitaoka, HB, and Patzer, GL: Nonoperative treatment of plantar interdigital neuroma with a single corticosteroid injection. *Clin Orthop*, May:188, 1996.

67. Vanore, JV, and Corey, SV: Hallux limitus, rigidus, and metartarso-phalangeal joint arthrosis. In Marchinko, DE (ed): *Comprehensive Textbook of Hallus Abducto Valgus Reconstruction*. Chicago, Mosby, 1993, pp. 209–221.

68. Ahn, TK, et al: Kinematics and contact characteristics of the first metatarsophalangeal joint. *Foot Ankle Int*, 18:170, 1997.

69. Camasta, CA: Hallux limitus and hallux rigidus: Clinical examination, radiographic findings, and natural history. *Clin Podiatr Med Surg*, 13:432, 1996.

70. Weinfeld, SB, and Schon, LC: Hallux metatarsophalangeal arthritis. *Clin Orthop*, Apr:9, 1998.

71. Lichniak, JE: Hallux limitus in the athlete. *Clin Podiatr Med Surg*, 14:407, 1997.

72. Mackay, DC, Blyth, M, and Rymaszewski, LA: The role of cheilectomy in the treatment of hallux rigidus. *J Foot Ankle Surg*, 36:337, 1997.

73. Iqbal, MJ, and Chana, GS: Arthroscopic cheilectomy for hallux rigidus. *Arthroscopy*, 14:307, 1998.

74. Tewes, DP, et al: MRI findings of acute turf toe. A case report and review of anatomy. *Clin Orthop*, July:200, 1994.

C H A P T E R

5

The Ankle
and Lower Leg

Ankle injuries are common in athletes, accounting for 20 to 25 percent of all athletic time-lost injuries.[1-3] During athletic competition, the ankle's muscular, capsular, and bony structures must absorb and dissipate normal and abnormal forces. Ankle sprains have a relatively high reinjury rate because of the residual instability and the subsequent loss of the joint's sense of position caused by injury to its joint proprioceptors.

The lower leg offers a significant challenge to the clinician's evaluation and management skills. Seemingly minor injuries, such as contusions, can have severe consequences resulting from compression of the neurovascular structures of the ankle, foot, and toes. Trauma or dysfunction of the ankle and lower leg muscles can lead to biomechanical changes, potentially causing injurious gait deviations. Conversely, different foot types can cause gait pattern deviations that stress the muscles and bones of the lower extremity.

◆ CLINICAL ANATOMY

The lower leg is formed by the tibia and fibula (Fig. 5–1). The junction of the distal tibia, fibula, and talus is referred to as the **ankle mortise** (Fig. 5–2). Discussion of the ankle must also include the rearfoot, midfoot, and fifth metatarsal (MT) because of the ligamentous and muscular attachments to these structures.

A normal anatomic relationship between the tibia and fibula is required for proper biomechanics of the knee proximally and the ankle and foot distally. These bones function to distribute the weight-bearing forces along the limb, allowing the ankle mortise to produce the range of motion (ROM) needed for walking and running.

The **tibia** is the primary weight-bearing bone of the lower leg. Its distal articular surface forms the roof of the ankle mortise; the medial malleolus forms the shallow medial border of the mortise and provides a broad site for the attachment of the **deltoid ligaments.**

Many of the muscles acting on the ankle, foot, and toes originate off the anterolateral and posterior bor-

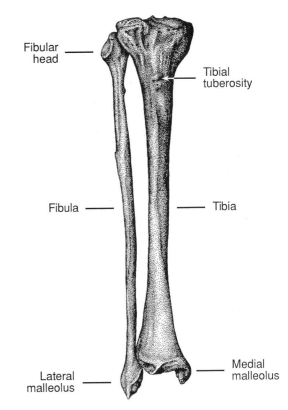

FIGURE 5–1. Long bones of the lower leg and their primary bony landmarks.

ders of the tibial shaft. The relatively flat anteromedial border is covered by a thin layer of soft tissue, predisposing the *periosteum* to contusions in this area. The periosteum of the tibial shaft may become inflamed at the site of muscular attachment secondary to overuse syndromes. The **interosseous membrane** arises off the

---

Periosteum A fibrous membrane containing blood vessels covering the shafts of long bones.

136

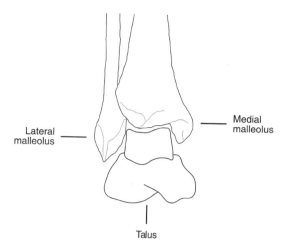

Lateral malleolus

Medial malleolus

Talus

FIGURE 5–2. Ankle mortise—the articulation formed by the distal articular surface of the tibia and its medial malleolus, the fibula's lateral malleolus, and the talus.

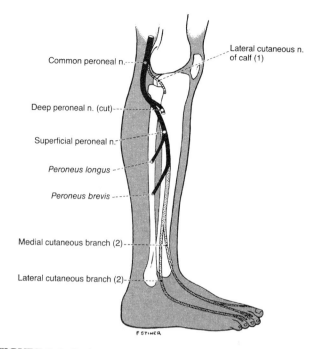

Common peroneal n.

Lateral cutaneous n. of calf (1)

Deep peroneal n. (cut)

Superficial peroneal n.

Peroneus longus

Peroneus brevis

Medial cutaneous branch (2)

Lateral cutaneous branch (2)

F STINER

FIGURE 5–3. Path of the peroneal nerve. The common peroneal nerve courses behind the fibular head, exposing it to potential injury. Trauma at this site causes a weakness in plantarflexion, eversion, and dorsiflexion.

length of the lateral tibial border and attaches to the length of the medial fibula, binding the bones together.

Lateral to the tibia is the **fibula.** A long, thin bone, the fibula (1) serves as a site of muscular origin and attachment, (2) serves as a site of ligamentous attachment, (3) provides lateral stability to the ankle mortise, and (4) serves as a pulley to increase the efficiency of the muscles that run posteriorly to it.

The fibula's function as a weight-bearing bone is not fully understood. The amount of force transmitted through the fibula has been reported to range from 0 to 12 percent of the total body weight.[1,2,4] Clinically, the percentage of body weight carried along this bone is inconsequential. However, trauma to the fibula decreases its ability to serve in its previously described roles.

The upper two thirds of the fibular shaft, with the exception of the fibular head, is protected by overlying muscle. A close relationship is found between the fibula and the peroneal nerve, which innervates the lower leg's anterior and lateral compartment (Fig. 5–3). The nerve courses subcutaneously just posterior to the fibular head, making it vulnerable to injury. The distal one third of the fibula, a common fracture site, becomes more superficial and begins to thin immediately proximal to the lateral malleolus.

The lateral malleolus provides a site of attachment for the lateral ankle ligaments. The lateral malleolus extends farther distally than the medial malleolus does, forming the lateral wall of the ankle mortise. The lateral malleolus is mechanically superior at limiting eversion than the medial malleolus is at limiting inversion. The lateral ankle is a common site for sprains possibly resulting in avulsion of the ligaments from the lateral malleolus, especially when the ankle is inverted.

The superior articulating portion of the **talus,** the **trochlea,** is quadrilateral in shape and almost entirely covered with articular cartilage. Its anterior surface is broader than its posterior surface (Fig. 5–4). The medial

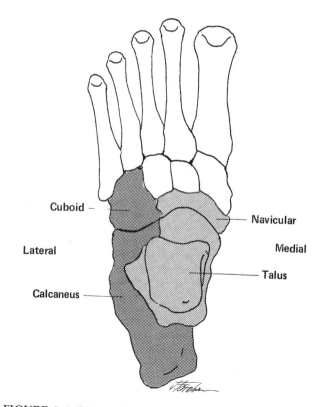

Cuboid

Navicular

Lateral

Medial

Talus

Calcaneus

FIGURE 5–4. View of the superior articular surface of the talus. Its wide anterior edge fits tightly in the mortise when the ankle is dorsiflexed.

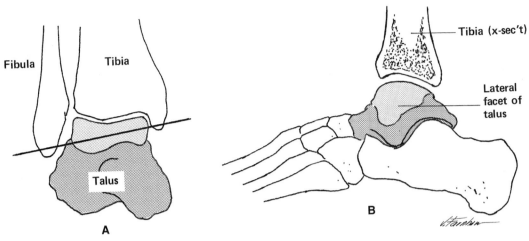

FIGURE 5–5. The talocrural joint in the **(A)** transverse and **(B)** frontal planes. The axis of motion in the transverse plane is indicated.

border of the talus articulates with the medial malleolus; its lateral border articulates with the lateral malleolus; and its superior surface articulates with the tibia. Its inferior surface articulates with the calcaneus, forming the subtalar joint.

RELATED BONY STRUCTURES

The insertion of the Achilles tendon on the **calcaneal tubercle** provides the foot with a mechanical advantage. Forming a long lever arm, the calcaneus provides increased power during gait (see Fig. 4–3). The large body of the calcaneus also provides a site of attachment for some of the ankle's ligaments.

The **navicular** bone is located anterior to the talus along the foot's medial arch. This bone serves as one of the sites of insertion for the tibialis posterior muscle. It also supports the medial longitudinal arch via the plantar calcaneonavicular "spring" ligament. Positioned along the lateral longitudinal arch, the **cuboid** is anterior to the calcaneus. The base of the **fifth metatarsal** articulates distally with the anterolateral portion of the cuboid. The fifth MTs serve as the site of attachment for the peroneus brevis and, along with the cuboid, provides a passageway for the route of the peroneus longus along the foot's plantar aspect.

ARTICULATIONS AND LIGAMENTOUS SUPPORT

Isolated movements of a single joint in a single plane do not occur during functional movements of the ankle complex. Pure *uniplanar* injuries are almost nonexistent because of the ankle's intimate anatomic relationship with the structures of the foot. The majority of injuries to the ankle involve the lateral structures, resulting from an inversion stress accompanied by plantarflexion of the foot.

Talocrural Joint

Formed by the articulation between the talus, tibia, and fibula, the talocrural joint is a close-fitting articulation, especially as it nears its *closed-packed position* of dorsiflexion. A modified *synovial hinge joint*, the talocrural articulation has one degree of freedom of movement: dorsiflexion and plantarflexion. The axis of rotation runs obliquely, connecting the points just distal to the inferior tips of the lateral and medial malleolus (Fig. 5–5). The talocrural joint is surrounded by a joint capsule. Most of the ligaments described in this section are actually areas of increased density in the capsule (the exception to this is the calcaneofibular ligament, which is extracapsular). Tearing the ankle ligaments usually results in damage to the joint capsule and irritation of the synovial lining.

Three ligaments provide lateral support to the talocrural joint so that at least one is taut regardless of the relative position of the talocalcaneal unit (Fig. 5–6). The **anterior talofibular (ATF) ligament** originates off the anterolateral surface of the lateral malleolus, following a path to insert on the talus near the sinus tarsi. This ligament is tight during plantarflexion, resists the motion of inversion of the talocalcaneal unit in the plantarflexed position, and limits anterior translation of the talus on the tibia.

The **calcaneofibular (CF) ligament** is an extracapsular structure with an attachment on the outermost por-

Uniplanar Occurring in only one of the cardinal planes of motion.

Closed-packed position The point in a joint's range of motion at which its bones are maximally congruent; the most stable position of a joint.

Synovial hinge joint A joint separated by a space filled with synovial fluid.

FIGURE 5–6. Lateral ankle ligaments. The calcaneofibular ligament is an extracapsular structure; the anterior and posterior talofibular ligaments are thickenings in the joint capsule.

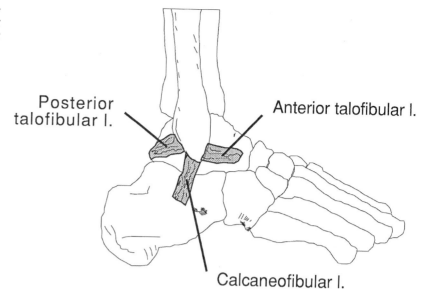

tion of the lateral malleolus. It courses inferiorly and posteriorly to its insertion on the calcaneus.[5] The CF ligament is the primary restraint of talar inversion within the midrange of talocrural motion.

Arising from the posterior portion of the lateral malleolus, the **posterior talofibular (PTF) ligament** takes an inferior and posterior course to attach on the talus and calcaneus. This is the strongest of the three lateral ligaments and is responsible for limiting posterior displacement of the talus on the tibia.

Four ligaments that, as a group, comprise the **deltoid ligament** provide medial ligamentous support (Fig. 5–7). The **anterior tibiotalar (ATT) ligament** originates off the anteromedial portion of the tibia's malleolus and inserts on the superior portion of the medial talus. The **tibiocalcaneal (TC) ligament** arises from the apex of the medial malleolus with attachment on the calcaneus directly below the medial malleolus. The **posterior tibiotalar (PTT) ligament** spans the posterior aspect of the medial malleolus, attaching on the posterior portion of the talus. As a group, these three ligaments prevent eversion of the talus. The **tibionavicular (TN) ligament** runs beneath and slightly posterior to the ATT ligament, inserting on the medial surface of the navicular bone to limit lateral translation and lateral rotation of the tibia on the foot. The ATT and TN ligaments are taut when the subtalar joint is plantarflexed. The TC and PTT ligaments tighten during dorsiflexion.

FIGURE 5–7. Medial "deltoid" ankle ligament showing the four individual ligaments.

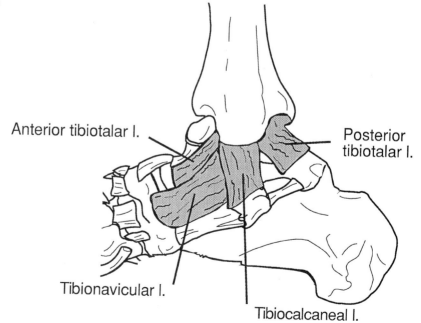

Interosseous Membrane

The interosseous membrane, a strong fibrous tissue acting to fixate the fibula to the tibia, also serves as part of the origin for many of the muscles acting on the foot and ankle. A small proximal opening allows passage of the tibia's anterior neurovascular structures. Distally, the membrane blends into the anterior and posterior tibiofibular ligaments to support the distal tibiofibular *syndesmosis joint.*

Distal Tibiofibular Syndesmosis

The integrity of the ankle mortise relies on the functional relationship between the tibia and fibula. This union is a syndesmosis joint where a convex facet on the fibula is buffered from a concave tibial facet by dense, fatty tissue. The syndesmosis is maintained by the **anterior and posterior tibiofibular (tib-fib) ligaments** and an extension of the interosseous membrane, the **crural interosseous (CI) ligament** (Fig. 5–8). This structural arrangement allows for rotation and slight spreading of the mortise while still maintaining joint stability. The CI ligament functions as a fulcrum to motion at the lateral malleolus, so a small

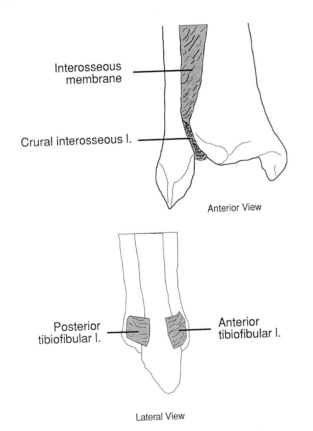

FIGURE 5–8. Distal tibiofibular syndesmosis with the talus removed for clarity. The anterior view shows the role of the interosseous membrane and the crural interosseous ligament in maintaining lateral restraint of the fibula. The lateral view shows the role of the tibiofibular ligaments in preventing anterior and posterior displacement of the fibula on the tibia.

amount of malleolar movement results in a large amount of movement at the tibiofibular joint.[6] During dorsiflexion, the distal fibula moves laterally away from the tibia and glides superiorly, bringing the interosseous membrane and tibiofibular ligaments into a more horizontal alignment. When the ankle is plantarflexed, the fibula is pulled inferiorly and medially toward the tibia and the ligamentous structures take a vertical alignment.[7] Excessive eversion or dorsiflexion can result in a widening of the ankle mortise, with possible injury to the ligaments supporting the syndesmosis.

The Subtalar Joint

The subtalar joint provides 1 degree of freedom of movement, inversion and eversion. The motions of the subtalar joint, the talocrural joint, and the midtarsal joints combine together to produce the functional motions of pronation and supination. (Chapter 4 provides more information about the subtalar joint.)

MUSCLES OF THE LOWER LEG AND ANKLE

The lower leg is divided into four compartments: the anterior, lateral, superficial posterior, and deep posterior (Fig. 5–9). Each compartment contains muscles and neurovascular structures that are tightly bound by fascial linings. Intracompartmental injury can result in the accumulation of fluids that increase the pressure within the compartment, obstructing the flow of blood to and from the area and placing pressure on the nerves. The action, origin, insertion, and innervation of each muscle are described in Table 5–1.

Anterior Compartment Structures

The muscles of the anterior compartment, the tibialis anterior, the extensor hallucis longus (EHL), the extensor digitorum longus (EDL), and the peroneus tertius all act as dorsiflexors at the ankle (Fig. 5–10). The most superficial of these muscles, the **tibialis anterior,** is the prime mover for ankle dorsiflexion and subtalar joint inversion. In addition to their functions at the toes, the **extensor hallucis longus** assists during foot inversion; the **extensor digitorum longus** contributes to eversion. The **peroneus tertius** runs parallel with the fifth tendon of the EDL, but its attachment on the dorsal surface of the fifth MT causes this muscle to make a stronger contribution to eversion than dorsiflexion.

Crossing the anterior portion of the ankle mortise is the extensor retinaculum, whose superior and inferior bands give it a Z shape (Fig. 5–11). The retinaculum

Syndesmosis joint A relatively immobile joint in which two bones are bound together by ligaments.

FIGURE 5–9. Cross section of the lower leg, indicating the muscles and neurovascular structures located in each of the four compartments. "Vessels" refer to the associated artery, vein, and lymphatic vessel.

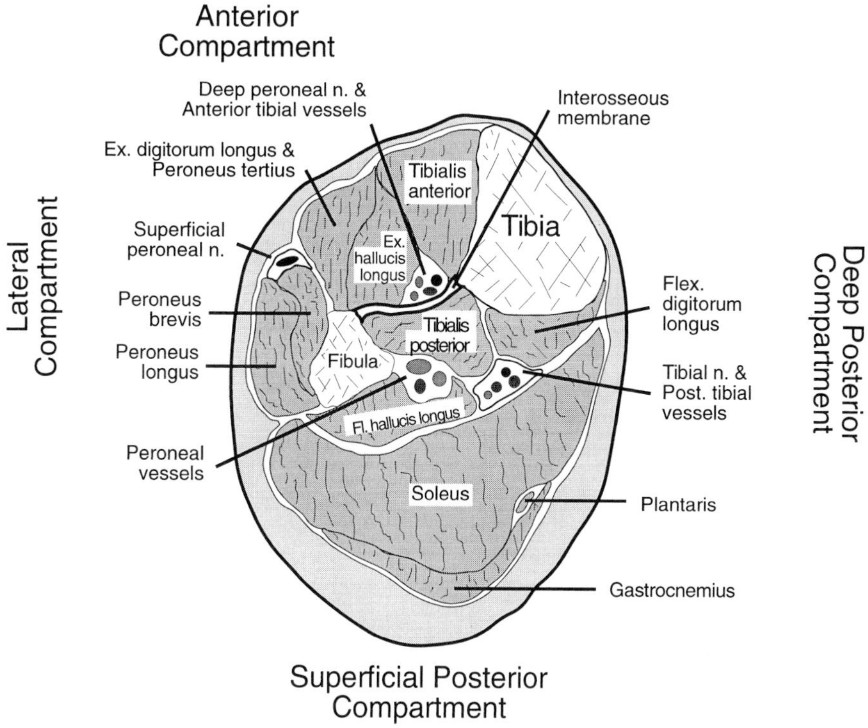

Anterior Compartment

Deep peroneal n. & Anterior tibial vessels

Ex. digitorum longus & Peroneus tertius

Superficial peroneal n.

Peroneus brevis

Peroneus longus

Peroneal vessels

Lateral Compartment

Interosseous membrane

Tibialis anterior

Ex. hallucis longus

Tibia

Tibialis posterior

Fibula

Fl. hallucis longus

Soleus

Flex. digitorum longus

Tibial n. & Post. tibial vessels

Deep Posterior Compartment

Plantaris

Gastrocnemius

Superficial Posterior Compartment

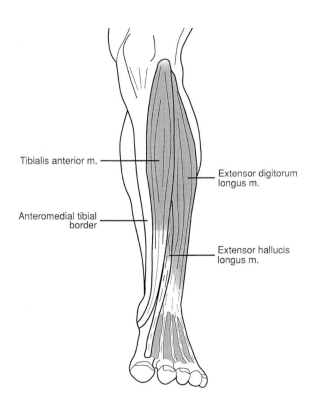

FIGURE 5–10. Muscles of the anterior compartment: the tibialis anterior, extensor hallucis longus, and extensor digitorum longus. The peroneus tertius is not shown.

Tibialis anterior m.

Anteromedial tibial border

Extensor digitorum longus m.

Extensor hallucis longus m.

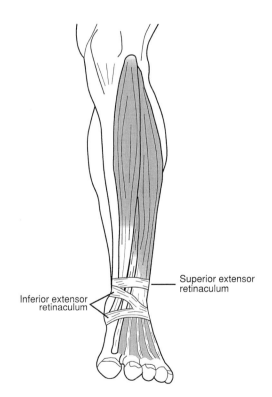

FIGURE 5–11. Extensor retinaculum formed by the inferior and superior bands. These structures prevent the muscles of the anterior compartment from bowing during dorsiflexion.

Superior extensor retinaculum

Inferior extensor retinaculum

Table 5–1
MUSCLES ACTING ON THE FOOT AND ANKLE

Muscle	Action	Origin	Insertion	Nerve	Root
Extensor digitorum longus	Extension of the 2nd through 5th MTP joints Assists in extending the 2nd through 5th PIP and DIP joints Assists in foot eversion Assists in ankle dorsiflexion	• Lateral tibial condyle • Proximal three-fourths of anterior fibula • Proximal portion of the interosseous membrane	• Via four tendons to the distal phalanges of the 2nd through 5th toes	Deep peroneal	L4, L5, S1
Extensor hallucis longus	Extension of the 1st MTP joint Extension of the 1st IP joint	• Middle two-thirds of the anterior surface of the fibula • Adjacent portion of the interosseous membrane	• Base of the distal phalanx of the 1st toe	Deep peroneal	L4, L5, S1
Flexor digitorum longus	Flexion of the 2nd through 5th PIP and DIP joints Flexion of the 2nd through 5th MTP joints Assists in ankle plantarflexion Assists in foot inversion	• Posterior medial portion of the distal two-thirds of the tibia • From fascia arising from the tibialis posterior	• Plantar base of distal phalanges of the 2nd through 5th toes	Tibial	L5, S1
Flexor hallucis longus	Flexion of the 1st IP joint Assists in flexion of the 1st MTP joint Assists in foot inversion Assists in plantarflexion of the ankle	• Posterior distal two-thirds of the fibula • Associated interosseous membrane and muscular fascia	• Plantar surface of the proximal phalanx of the 1st toe	Tibial	L4, L5, S1
Gastrocnemius	Ankle plantarflexion Assists in knee flexion	Medial head • Posterior surface of the medial femoral condyle • Adjacent portion of the femur and knee capsule Lateral head • Posterior surface of the lateral femoral condyle • Adjacent portion of the femur and knee capsule	To the calcaneus via the Achilles tendon	Tibial	S1, S2
Peroneus brevis	Evasion of foot Assists in ankle plantarflexion	• Distal two-thirds of the lateral fibula	• Styloid process at the base of the 5th metatarsal	Superficial peroneal	L4, L5, S1

Muscle	Action	Proximal Attachment	Distal Attachment	Innervation	Nerve Root
Peroneus longus	Eversion of the foot Assists in ankle plantarflexion	• Lateral tibial condyle • Fibular head • Upper two-thirds of the lateral fibula	• Lateral aspect of the base of the 1st metatarsal • Lateral and dorsal aspect of the 1st cuneiform	Superficial peroneal	L4, L5, S1
Peroneus tertius	Eversion of the foot Dorsiflexion of the ankle	• Distal one-third of the anterior surface of the fibula • Adjacent portion of the interosseous membrane	• Dorsal surface of the base of the 5th metatarsal	Deep peroneal	L4, L5, S1
Plantaris	Ankle plantarflexion Assists in knee flexion	• Distal portion of the supracondylar line of the lateral femoral condyle • Adjacent portion of the femoral popliteal surface • Oblique popliteal ligament	• To the calcaneus via the Achilles tendon	Tibial	L4, L5, S1
Soleus	Ankle plantarflexion	• Posterior fibular head • Upper one-third of the fibula's posterior surface • Soleal line located on the posterior tibial shaft • Middle one-third of the medial tibial border	• To the calcaneus via the Achilles tendon	Tibial	S1, S2
Tibialis anterior	Dorsiflexion of the ankle Inversion of the foot	• Lateral tibial condyle • Upper one-half of the tibia's lateral surface • Adjacent portion of the interosseous membrane	• Medial and plantar surfaces of the 1st cuneiform • Medial and plantar surfaces of the 1st metatarsal	Deep peroneal	L4, L5, S1
Tibialis posterior	Inversion of the foot Assists in ankle plantarflexion	• Length of the interosseous membrane • Posterior, lateral tibia • Upper two-thirds of the medial fibula	• Navicular tuberosity • Via fibrous slips to the sustentaculum tali, cuneiforms, cuboid, and bases of the 2nd, 3rd, and 4th metatarsals	Tibial	L4, S1

DIP = distal interphalangeal; IP = interphalangeal; MTP = metatarsophalangeal; PIP = posterior interphalangeal.

143

serves to secure the distal tendons of the muscles of the anterior compartment as they cross the talocrural joint, preventing a bowstring effect during dorsiflexion or toe extension. The medial portion of the inferior band holds the tibialis anterior and extensor hallucis longus close to the dorsum of the foot. A loop on the lateral border of the retinaculum wraps around the four tendinous slips of the extensor digitorum longus, holding them laterally and against the dorsum of the foot.

Branching off the common peroneal nerve near the fibular head, the **deep peroneal nerve** runs from the upper portion of the fibula along the interosseous membrane behind the tibialis anterior. This nerve and its subsequent branches innervate most of the muscles located within the anterior compartment and on the dorsum of the foot. Supplying the anterior compartment with blood, the **anterior tibial artery** passes through the superior portion of the interosseous membrane to follow the path taken by the deep peroneal nerve. A branch of the anterior tibial artery, the **dorsalis pedis artery,** supplies blood to the dorsum of the foot.

Lateral Compartment Structures

The **peroneus longus** and **peroneus brevis** form the bulk of the lateral compartment. The peroneus longus is the most superficial of these muscles, with its belly covering all but the most inferior portion of the peroneus brevis and its tendon. The peroneus brevis lies beneath the peroneus longus as the tendons pass behind the lateral malleolus where they share a common synovial sheath. The peroneal tendons are held in position behind the malleolus by the **superior and inferior peroneal retinacula.** Their paths diverge as they clear the retinaculum and approach the peroneal tubercle. The peroneus brevis tendon courses to the styloid process on the base of the fifth MT, while the peroneus longus tendon runs a path along the plantar aspect of the foot to attach to the base of the first MT and first cuneiform. As a group, these muscles are strong evertors of the foot and contribute to plantarflexion (Fig. 5–12)

The lateral compartment contains the **superficial peroneal nerve,** which is responsible for innervating the peroneus brevis and peroneus tertius. Together with the common peroneal nerve, it also innervates the peroneus longus. Arising off the posterior tibial artery, the **peroneal artery** runs lateral to the interosseous membrane, supplying blood to the lateral compartment and lateral ankle.

Superficial Posterior Compartment Structures

The gastrocnemius, soleus, and plantaris collectively form the triceps surae muscle group (Fig. 5–13). The **gastrocnemius** and **plantaris** are two-joint muscles, each having origins on the posterior aspects of the femoral

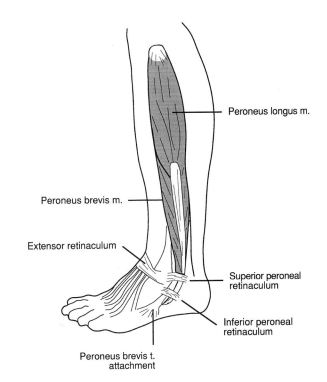

FIGURE 5–12. Muscles of the lateral compartment: the peroneus longus and brevis. The superior and inferior peroneal retinacula maintain the alignment of the peroneal tendons so that their angle of pull plantarflexes and everts the foot.

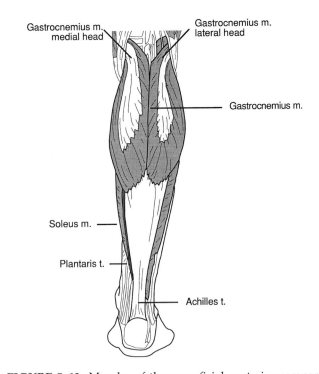

FIGURE 5–13. Muscles of the superficial posterior compartment: the gastrocnemius, soleus, and plantaris. This group of muscles is collectively referred to as the "triceps surae."

condyles. The **soleus,** originating off the posterior tibia, is the only member of the triceps surae group to cross only one joint. The gastrocnemius and soleus have a common insertion on the calcaneus via the Achilles tendon. Some anatomy texts also include the plantaris as a part of the anteromedial portion of the Achilles tendon complex and insertion. Whereas the gastrocnemius and soleus are prime movers during plantarflexion, the gastrocnemius is most involved when the knee is extended.

Traveling between the medial and lateral heads of the gastrocnemius and running deep to lie between the soleus and the tibialis posterior (located in the deep posterior compartment) is the longest branch of the sciatic nerve, the **tibial nerve.** Supplying the innervation for all of the muscles in the superficial and deep posterior compartment, branches of the tibial nerve continue to the plantar aspect of the foot after coursing around the medial malleolus. The **posterior tibial artery** follows the same course as the tibial nerve.

Deep Posterior Compartment Structures

The **tibialis posterior** is the only muscle of the deep posterior compartment acting exclusively on the foot and ankle (Fig. 5–14). Because of its angle of pull, this

muscle is a primary adductor of the forefoot while also assisting in plantarflexion and inversion. The remaining two muscles of the deep posterior compartment, the **flexor digitorum longus** and the **flexor hallucis longus,** primarily act to flex the toes and secondarily act to plantar flex and invert the ankle.

BURSAE

Two major bursae are associated with the lower leg and ankle. The **subtendinous calcaneal** (retrocalcaneal) **bursa** is found between the Achilles tendon and the calcaneus, decreasing friction between these two structures. Lying between the posterior aspect of the Achilles tendon and the skin is the **subcutaneous calcaneal bursa,** which protects the Achilles tendon from direct trauma and decreases friction from the skin and footwear.

 CLINICAL EVALUATION OF THE ANKLE AND LOWER LEG

The following describes a model evaluation of the ankle and lower leg. Both the ankles and lower legs must be exposed during this examination to facilitate inspection and palpation of the foot and ankle. A complete examination of an ankle injury may require a concurrent evaluation of the foot and knee.

HISTORY

During the history-taking process for a patient with an ankle or lower leg injury, the onset and mechanism of injury, the duration of the symptoms, and any previous history of injury to the involved or uninvolved limb must be established. The patient's responses to the following list guide the remainder of the history-taking process and form the framework on which the rest of the examination is based.

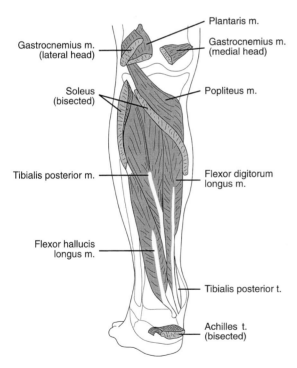

Gastrocnemius m.
(lateral head)

Soleus
(bisected)

Tibialis posterior m.

Flexor hallucis
longus m.

Plantaris m.

Gastrocnemius m.
(medial head)

Popliteus m.

Flexor digitorum
longus m.

Tibialis posterior t.

Achilles t.
(bisected)

FIGURE 5–14. Muscles of the deep posterior compartment: the tibialis posterior, flexor hallucis longus, and flexor digitorum longus. The superficial muscles have been removed to show the deep compartment. A common mnemonic, "**T**om, **D**ick, **A**nd **N**ervous **H**arry," is used to describe the structures that pass behind the medial malleolus: **t**ibialis posterior, flexor **d**igitorum longus, tibial **a**rtery, tibial **n**erve, and the flexor **h**allucis longus.

- **Location of the pain:** Identify the painful area as specifically as possible so that the subsequent portions of the evaluation emphasize the suspected structures involved (Table 5–2). The lower leg and ankle may also be areas of referred pain arising from anterior compartment syndrome, tarsal tunnel syndrome, the peroneal nerve, and sciatic nerve or lumbar nerve root impingement.
- **Nature or type of pain:** Pose specific questions to determine how the symptoms are aggravated by certain activities and how these symptoms are affecting athletic participation or normal daily activities.
- **Onset:** Identify the onset of symptoms to determine if there has been acute trauma such as a sprain, strain, fracture, or if there has been a gradual onset of symptoms as with overuse syndromes.

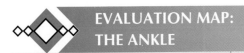

EVALUATION MAP: THE ANKLE

1. HISTORY

Location of the Pain
Nature or type of pain
Onset
Injury mechanisms
Level of activity and conditioning
    regimen
History of injury

2. INSPECTION

General Inspection
    Weight-bearing status
    General bilateral comparison
    Swelling

Lateral Structures
    Peroneal muscle group
    Distal one-third of the fibula
    Lateral malleolus

Anterior Structures
    Appearance of the lower leg
    Contour of the malleoli
    Talus
    Sinus tarsi

Medial Structures
    Medial malleolus
    Medial longitudinal arch

Posterior Structures
    Gastrocnemius–soleus complex
    Achilles tendon
    Bursae
    Calcaneus

3. PALPATION

Lateral Structures
    Fibular shaft
    Interosseous membrane
    Anterior and posterior tibiofibular
        ligament

Calcaneofibular ligament
Anterior talofibular ligament
Posterior talofibular ligament
Peroneal tubercle
Cuboid
Base of the 5th metatarsal
Peroneus longus and brevis
Peroneal retinaculum

Anterior Structures
    Anterior tibial shaft
    Dome of the talus
    Extensor retinacula
    Sinus tarsi
    Tibialis anterior
    Long toe extensors
    Peroneus tertius

Medial Structures
    Medial malleolus
    Deltoid ligament
    Sustentaculum tali
    Spring ligament
    Navicular and navicular tubercle
    Talar head
    Tibialis posterior
    Long toe flexors

Posterior Structures
    Gastrocnemius–soleus complex
    Achilles tendon
    Subtendinous calcaneal bursa
    Subcutaneous calcaneal bursa
    Dome of the calcaneus

Palpation of pulses
    Posterior tibial artery
    Dorsalis pedis artery

4. RANGE OF MOTION TESTS

AROM
    Plantarflexion and dorsiflexion
    Inversion and eversion

PROM
    Plantarflexion and dorsiflexion
    Inversion and eversion

RROM
    Dorsiflexion
    Plantarflexion
        Gastrocnemius
        Soleus
    Inversion
    Eversion

5. LIGAMENTOUS TESTS

Anterior Talofibular Ligament Instability
    Anterior drawer test

Calcaneofibular Ligament Instability
    Inversion stress test (talar tilt)

Ankle Syndesmosis Instability
    Kleiger's test
    Squeeze test

Deltoid Ligament Instability
    Eversion stress test (talar tilt)
    External rotation test

6. NEUROLOGIC TESTS

Anterior compartment syndrome
Peroneal nerve involvement
Sciatic nerve involvement
Lumbar nerve root involvement

7. SPECIAL TESTS

Lower Leg Fractures
    Squeeze test

Stress Fracture
    Bump test

Achilles Tendon Pathology
    Thompson test

Neurovascular Pathology
    Homan's sign

AROM = active range of motion; PROM = passive range of motion; ROM = range of motion; RROM = resisted range of motion.

Table 5–2
POSSIBLE TRAUMA BASED ON THE LOCATION OF PAIN (EXCLUDING GROSS INJURY)

	Location of Pain			
	Lateral	**Anterior**	**Medial**	**Posterior**
Soft tissue	Inversion ankle sprain Syndesmosis sprain Capsular impingement Subluxating peroneal tendons Peroneal muscle strain Peroneal tendinitis Interosseous membrane trauma Peroneal nerve trauma	Extensor retinaculum sprain Syndesmosis sprain Tibialis anterior or long toe extensor strain Tibialis anterior or long toe extensor tendinitis Anterior compartment syndrome Interosseous membrane trauma Anterior tibiofibular ligament sprain	Evasion ankle sprain Capsular impingement Tibialis posterior strain Tibialis posterior tendinitis	Triceps surae strain Achilles tendinitis Achilles tendon rupture Subtendinous calcaneal bursitis Subcutaneous calcaneal bursitis Deep vein thrombophlebitis Posterior tibiofibular ligament sprain
Bony	Lateral ligament avulsion Lateral malleolus fracture Fibular stress fracture Fifth MT fracture Peroneal tendon avulsion Arthritis	Tibial stress fracture Talar fracture Talar osteochondritis Arthritis Periosteitis	Medial ligament avulsion Medial malleolus avulsion Medial malleolus fracture Arthritis	Calcaneal fracture Arthritis Os trigonum trauma

MT = metatarsal.

- **Injury mechanism:** In the case of macrotrauma, determine the mechanism of injury to identify the general area of the structures affected and the type of injury involved (Table 5–3). Chronic or insidious disorders require more in-depth questioning to determine the factors surrounding the cause of pain.
- **Changes in activity and conditioning regimen:** Attempt to develop a "picture" of recent activities to evaluate chronic or insidious conditions. For overuse injuries, establish whether the patient has:

  ○ Significantly increased the duration, intensity, frequency, or type (i.e., added hills) of exercise. When available, the athlete's personal training log is useful in determining excessive increases in exercise intensity.
  ○ Changed shoe brands or styles or is competing in old, worn-out shoes.
  ○ Switched from participating on a surface of one texture and density to one of a different type.
  ○ Recently begun wearing orthotics, changed the type of orthotic worn, or recently discontinued the use of orthotics.

- **Prior history of injury:** Question the patient and, if available, review the patient's medical file regarding the history of injury to both the involved and uninvolved extremities and the lumbar spine. Patients with a history of previous ankle sprains may demonstrate excess laxity and decreased *proprioception*. Other injuries to the lower extremity or lumbar spine may present with biomechanical changes in gait.

INSPECTION

Much of the observation phase occurs while the patient is not weight bearing. Then these results are compared with the weight-bearing findings.

Proprioception   The athlete's ability to sense the position of one or more joints.

Table 5–3
MECHANISM OF ANKLE INJURY AND THE RESULTANT TISSUE DAMAGE

Uniplanar Motion	Tensile Forces	Compressive Forces
Inversion	Lateral structures: Anterior talofibular ligament, calcaneofibular ligament, posterior talofibular ligament, lateral capsule, and peroneal tendons; lateral malleolus fracture	Medial structures: Medial malleolus, deltoid ligament, and medial neurovascular bundle
Eversion	Medial structures: deltoid ligament, tibialis posterior, and long toe flexors	Lateral structures: Lateral malleolus and lateral capsule
Plantarflexion	Anterior structures: Anterior capsule, long toe extensors, and extensor retinaculum Lateral structures: Anterior talofibular ligament	Posterior structures: Posterior capsule, subtendinous calcaneal bursa, subcutaneous calcaneal bursa, os trigonum, and talus fracture
Dorsiflexion	Posterior structures: Triceps surae, Achilles tendon Lateral structures: Posterior talofibular ligament	Anterior structures: Anterior capsule, syndesmosis, and extensor retinaculum

General Inspection

- **Weight-bearing status:** Begin the inspection process as the patient enters the facility or walks off the field. At this point, the weight-bearing capacity of the involved limb should be noted, including:

  o Did the patient enter the facility with ease or was an antalgic gait present?

  o Was the limb externally rotated, suggesting a possible lack of ankle dorsiflexion caused by pain or restriction?

- **General bilateral comparison:** Observe both lower extremities, noting redness, pallor, or other obvious deformity.
- **Swelling:** Determine the amount of swelling using girth or volumetric measurements (see Box 1–3).

Inspection of the Lateral Structures

- **Peroneal muscle group:** Inspect the length of the peroneal muscle group. The tendons may be seen as they course posteriorly and inferiorly around the lateral malleolus, being held in position by the superior and inferior peroneal retinacula (see Fig. 5–12). The tendons will become more visible if the patient is able to actively invert and evert the foot.
- **Distal one third of the fibula:** Note the contour and symmetry of the distal one third of the fibula as it becomes superficial proximal to the lateral malleolus. Any discontinuity in the bone's shaft or the formation of edema over this portion of the shaft may indicate a possible fibular fracture.
- **Lateral malleolus:** Keep in mind that very little soft tissue covers the lateral malleolus, making its shape easily identifiable. Even mild ankle sprains can result in swelling that obscures the malleolus and peroneal tendons (Fig. 5–15). Any formation of ecchymosis around and distal to the lateral malleolus may signify acute trauma such as a sprain or fracture.

Inspection of the Anterior Structures

- **Appearance of the anterior lower leg:** Inspect the anterior lower leg for skin color and edema. Anterior compartment syndrome may present with reddened or shiny skin or pitting edema. If these signs coincide with paresthesia in the web space between the first and second toes, decreased dorsiflexion strength, and/or absence of the dorsalis pedis pulse, immediately refer the patient to a physician or emergency room.
- **Contour of the malleoli:** Observe the malleoli, which should be prominent as they project from the tibia and fibula. Swelling can obscure these structures. Edema between the tibia and fibula above the distal tibiofibular joint and the distal one third of the interosseous membrane may indicate a syndesmotic sprain.
- **Talus:** If the patient is capable of bearing weight, observe the bilateral symmetry of positions of the tali. In the case of leg length discrepancies, one foot has a

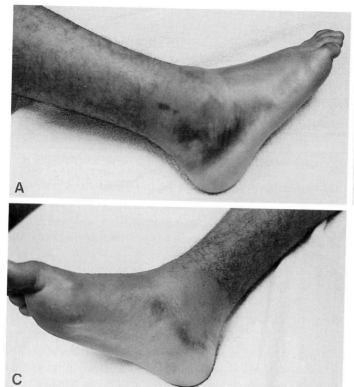

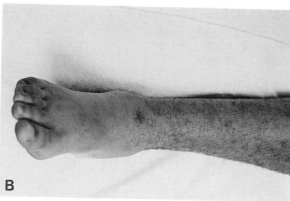

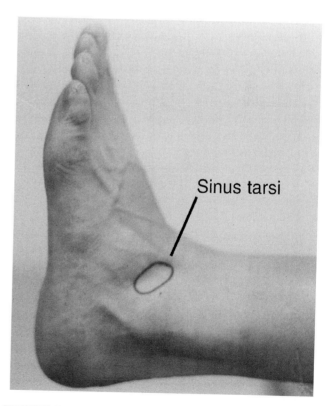

FIGURE 5–15. Damage to the lateral ankle capsule can result in the collection of edema around and distal to the malleolus. Note the distortion of the normal ankle contours and medial formation of ecchymosis.

prominent medial talus caused by pronation of the longer leg; the shorter leg maintains a somewhat neutral or supinated position (see Fig. 3–8).

With the patient still standing, note the presence of the medial longitudinal arch. If this arch is not adequately supported, the medial aspect of the talus rotates inward and the navicular drops inferiorly. Excessive protrusion of the talus can be seen from the anterior as well as the posterior view. Lower leg pain, such as periosteitis or tendinitis of the tibialis anterior or tibialis posterior muscles, is often associated with this deformity. The medial movement of the talus and subsequent flattening of the medial longitudinal arch fatigue the musculature and place strain on their periosteal attachments on the tibia.

- **Sinus tarsi:** Observe the sinus tarsi, an indentation formed over the lateral aspect of the talus, noting for its normally concave shape. After injury to the anterior talofibular ligament or fractures about the ankle, the area fills with fluid, resulting in loss of its normal indentation in the proximal foot (Fig. 5–16).[8]

Inspection of the Medial Structures

- **Medial malleolus:** Similar to the lateral malleolus, the medial malleolus is superficial, with little soft tissue covering it. Its appearance should be distinct without obvious deformity or the presence of edema.

FIGURE 5–16. Location of the sinus tarsi. This depression may become swollen and painful secondary to trauma to the foot or ankle.

- **Medial longitudinal arch:** Observe for the normal concave appearance of the medial longitudinal arch, which should be maintained with the patient both bearing weight and non–weight bearing. Pes planus (flatfoot) results in the superior portion of the talus' tilting medially, causing increased stress on its ligamentous and muscular structures and altering gait biomechanics. Pes cavus, a high medial arch, results in a supinated foot, and a potential predisposition to inversion ankle sprains or stress fractures caused by limited shock-absorbing capacity.

Inspection of the Posterior Structures

- **Gastrocnemius-soleus complex:** Bilateral comparison should indicate calf musculature of approximately equal size, shape, and mass. *Atrophy* may be present if the leg has been immobilized or the S1 or S2 nerve root or the tibial or sciatic nerves are impaired. Tearing of the muscle may result in depressions in the skin, especially at the musculotendinous junction with the Achilles tendon. Unexplained redness and swelling of the posterior calf could indicate deep vein *thrombophlebitis.*
- **Achilles tendon:** The prominent Achilles tendon is seen as it tapers from the musculotendinous junction to its insertion on the calcaneus. Achilles tendon ruptures may present with a visible defect if the tear occurs in its middle or distal portion. Proximal tendon tears may present with no visible defects.
- **Bursae:** Inspect the calcaneal bursae for swelling, redness, or other signs of inflammation.

- **Calcaneus:** The calcaneus is normally very distinct, with little soft tissue covering its medial and lateral borders. The presence of a thickened area at the insertion of the Achilles tendon is sometimes associated with retrocalcaneal pain. This thickening, an exostosis, may be caused by the footwear's rubbing on this area, possibly associated with subcutaneous calcaneal bursitis (see Chapter 4).

PALPATION

Palpation of the Fibular Structures

1. **Common peroneal nerve:** Palpate the common peroneal nerve as it passes behind the lateral portion of the fibular head and then branches into its deep and superficial branches.
2. **Peroneus longus and brevis:** Locate the peroneus longus muscle from its origin on the fibular head and palpate the muscle belly along the upper two thirds of the lateral fibula. The tendons of both the peroneus longus and brevis are palpable along the distal one third of the fibula and as they course posterior to the lateral malleolus. As these tendons approach the peroneal tubercle, they diverge so that the peroneus longus tendon passes through the groove in the cuboid to follow a course along the plantar aspect of the foot, at which point it is no longer palpable. The location where the peroneus longus begins to pass beneath the cuboid is a common site of tendon ruptures.[9] The peroneus brevis tendon travels a shorter distance to its attachment on the base of the fifth MT.

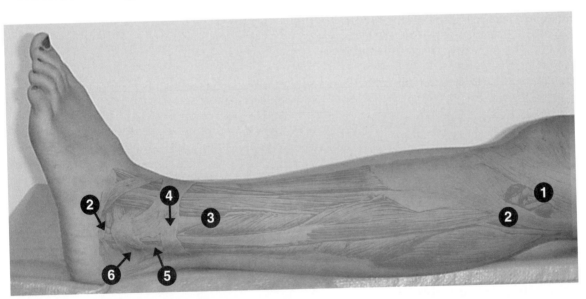

Atrophy A wasting or decrease in the size of a muscle or tissue.

Thrombophlebitis Inflammation of a vein and the subsequent formation of blood clots.

3. **Fibular shaft:** Begin by locating the fibular head and palpate along the length of the shaft over the bulk of the peroneals until the bone reemerges along its distal third. Apply gentle pressure over the distal one third of the fibular shaft, noting any pain and discontinuity in the bone, which may indicate the presence of a fracture.

4. **Anterior and posterior tibiofibular ligaments:** Locate the attachment of the anterior and posterior tibiofibular ligaments on the fibula just superior to the lateral malleolus. Palpate anteriorly along the length of the anterior tib-fib ligament to its attachment on the anterolateral portion of the tibia. Direct palpation of the posterior tib-fib ligament is difficult because of the peroneal tendons. Tenderness along these structures or the interosseous membrane may indicate a syndesmotic ankle sprain.

5. **Interosseous membrane:** An area of the interosseous membrane may be palpated in the ankle syndesmosis between the distal fibula and tibia. Begin palpating the posterior tibiofibular joint line, just superior to the lateral malleolus and progress superiorly until the fibula becomes covered by the mass of the peroneal muscles.

6. **Superior peroneal retinaculum:** Palpate the superior peroneal retinaculum as it projects off of the superior portion of the lateral malleolus. This structure may be painful after an acute tear or stretching.

Palpation of the Lateral Ankle

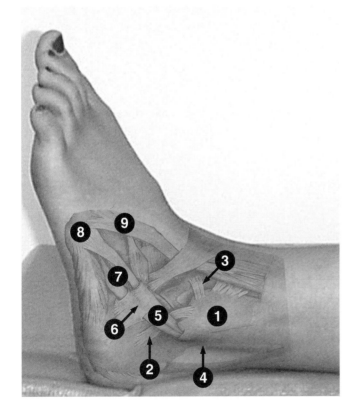

1. **Lateral malleolus:** Keep in mind that the lateral ligamentous structures may be avulsed from their origin on the malleolus or their insertion on the talus or calcaneus through the tensile forces associated with inversion. This pathology causes point tenderness, swelling, and crepitus. The distal portion of the lateral malleolus may be "knocked off" by the calcaneus during excessive eversion of the calcaneus. Long bone fractures may be ruled out using the **squeeze** or **bump test**.

2. **Calcaneofibular ligament:** Locate the origin of the CF ligament on the distal tip of the malleolus. The ligament becomes palpable as it leaves the malleolus and crosses the joint space, taking an oblique course to insert posterior to the peroneal tubercle. The CF ligament is usually the second structure damaged during inversion ankle sprains because it absorbs the greatest amount of stress when the talocrural joint is in the neutral position.

3. **Anterior talofibular ligament:** Locate the origin of the CF ligament and move anteriorly on the malleolus to find the origin of the ATF ligament on the inferior portion of the anterolateral malleolus. Running a course somewhat parallel to the plantar surface of the foot when the foot is in neutral position, the ATF ligament attaches on the anterolateral aspect of the talus near the sinus tarsi. The ATF ligament is not normally palpable.

4. **Posterior talofibular ligament:** From the origin of the calcaneofibular ligament, move upward and posteriorly around the malleolus to locate the PTF ligament. This ligament is not directly palpable, but pressure should be applied over the point of its insertion on the posterior portion of the talus. In most cases, the PTF ligament is damaged only in severe ankle sprains or dislocations.

5. **Peroneal retinaculum:** Palpate the space between the posterior portion of the lateral malleolus and the calcaneus for pain elicited over the superior peroneal retinaculum where the peroneal tendons pass beneath it. Follow the length of the tendons to locate the inferior peroneal retinaculum immediately below the lateral malleolus, along the lateral aspect of the calcaneus. Tears in these structures, especially the superior retinaculum, result in **dislocating** or **subluxating peroneal tendons**.

6. **Peroneal tubercle:** Feel for a small nodule located anterior to the attachment of the CF ligament and inferior to the distal tip of the lateral malleolus. The peroneal tubercle marks the point on the calcaneus where the peroneus longus and brevis tendons diverge. In cases of peroneal tendinitis or rupture of the distal peroneal retinaculum, this area is tender to the touch.

7. **Cuboid:** Palpate anteriorly from the peroneal tubercle to locate the cuboid bone as it lies proximal to the base of the fifth MT. This bone is rarely injured but may become tender secondary to ligamentous injury or inflammation of the peroneal tendons.

8. **Base of the fifth metatarsal:** Palpate anteriorly from the cuboid to find the base of the fifth MT and its laterally projecting flare, the styloid process. This structure may be avulsed from the shaft after the forceful contraction of the peroneus brevis muscle as the muscle attempts to counteract inversion of the ankle.

9. **Peroneus tertius:** Locate the peroneus tertius where it rises from the distal half of the anterior surface of the fibula. Palpate distally along the length of the muscle belly and tendon to the insertion point on the dorsal aspect of the base of the fifth MT. The tendon is most palpable as it crosses the joint anterior to the lateral malleolus. It is identifiable by being the most lateral of the muscles on the anterior aspect of the lower leg. The peroneus tertius is not present in the entire population.

Palpation of the Anterior Structures

1. **Anterior tibial shaft:** Locate the patellar tendon's attachment on the tibial tuberosity. The anteromedial portion of the tibia is subcutaneous and therefore palpable along its length to its medial malleolus. Pay special attention to the anterior ridge of the tibia where the tibialis anterior and long toe flexors attach, as well as to the periosteum and posterior border of the shaft along the origin of the tibialis posterior. These areas may become inflamed secondary to overuse and improperly described as "shin splints" (Box 5–1).

2. **Tibialis anterior:** Locate the origin of the tibialis anterior on the anterolateral portion of the proximal tibia and palpate distally along the length of the muscle belly. Near the distal one third of the medial tibia, the belly begins to merge into a thick, round tendon. Palpate the tendon to its insertion on the cuneiform and first MT.

3. **Extensor hallucis longus:** Have the patient actively extend the great toe to make the EHL tendon palpable at its insertion. Continue to palpate the length of the EHL as it passes lateral to the tibialis anterior to its origin on the middle half of the anterior fibula and adjacent interosseous membrane. The tendon eventually becomes obscured by the tibialis anterior muscle.

4. **Extensor digitorum longus:** Locate the tendon of the extensor digitorum longus lateral to the extensor hallucis longus. Active extension of the toes causes the EDL tendons to standout on the dorsal aspect of the toes and foot. Palpate the individual slips on the lateral four toes up though its common tendon.

5. **Dome of the talus:** Have the patient plantarflex the ankle to allow the anterior dome of the talus to be exposed from under the ankle mortise. Pain along this area is common with ankle synovitis and impact injuries to the ankle joint.

6. **Extensor retinacula:** Palpate the extensor retinacula for signs of tenderness as the tendons pass under them (see Fig. 5–12). The superior extensor retinaculum is palpated along the anterior aspect of the distal leg, just proximal to the tibiofibular joint. The inferior extensor retinaculum is palpated laterally beginning at the area of the inferior peroneal retinaculum and proceeds across the dorsum of the foot to the medial aspect of the midfoot. The retinacula may become traumatically injured during forceful, sud-

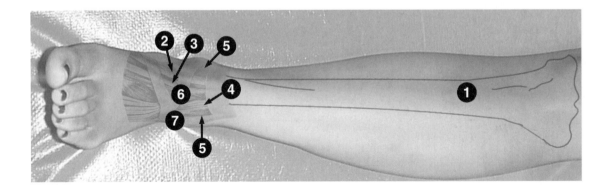

den dorsiflexion, or the tendons passing under it may become inflamed secondary to friction.

7. **Sinus tarsi:** Locate the sinus tarsi between the lateral malleolus and the neck of the talus. This area may become swollen and painful to the touch following ATF ligament injury, arthritic changes in the ankle, or fracture of the talus (see Fig. 5–16).

Palpation of the Medial Structures

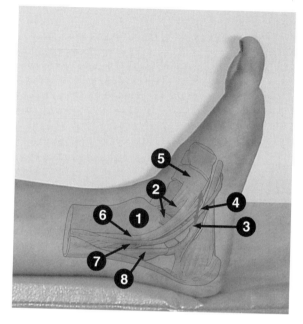

1. **Medial malleolus:** Palpate the entire border of the medial malleolus, noting any pain that may be elicited at the attachment sites of the medial ligaments or crepitus possibly indicating a fracture. Continue to palpate up the posteromedial tibial border, noting any pain that arises along the periosteal lining.

2. **Deltoid ligament:** Palpate the mass of the deltoid ligament as it encircles the lower portion of the medial malleolus. For all practical purposes, the individual ligaments forming this complex cannot be distinguished from each other.

3. **Sustentaculum tali:** Palpate approximately one finger's width inferior from the medial malleolus to locate the calcaneal sustentaculum tali. This structure supports the talus and is an attachment site for the spring ligament.

4. **Spring ligament:** Locate the spring ligament's origin on the sustentaculum tali and palpate along its route distally to its insertion on the navicular bone. The spring ligament becomes stretched in cases of chronic pes planus or torn in acute pronation or rotation of the forefoot.

5. **Navicular and navicular tuberosity:** Identify the navicular tuberosity (tubercle) by the attachment of the tibialis posterior. Palpate the navicular bone for signs of tenderness that possibly indicate tibialis posterior tendinitis, a sprain of the spring ligament, or a stress fracture. Pain elicited during palpation of this structure can also indicate an inflamed **accessory navicular.**

6. **Tibialis posterior:** Keep in mind that the belly of the tibialis posterior is not distinctly palpable as it lies under the gastrocnemius and soleus muscles. Its tendon passes behind and around the medial malleolus and becomes most palpable at its insertion on the navicular tubercle.

7. **Flexor hallucis longus:** Palpate the FHL tendon as it begins its path behind and around the medial malleolus. Note that it is difficult to distinguish this tendon from the other structures in the area. As the tendon begins its course along the plantar aspect of the foot, it is no longer palpable until it inserts on the distal phalanx of the great toe.

8. **Flexor digitorum longus:** Similar to the flexor hallucis longus, palpate the FDL tendon, although not uniquely identifiable, as it passes behind and around the medial malleolus. As it passes along the plantar aspect of the foot, it is no longer palpable until it inserts on the plantar aspect of the second through fifth toes.

Palpation of the Posterior Structures

1. **Gastrocnemius-soleus complex:** Palpate the gastrocnemius from its dual origin on the lateral and medial femoral condyles. Giving rise to a large muscle mass, the belly of the gastrocnemius is palpated

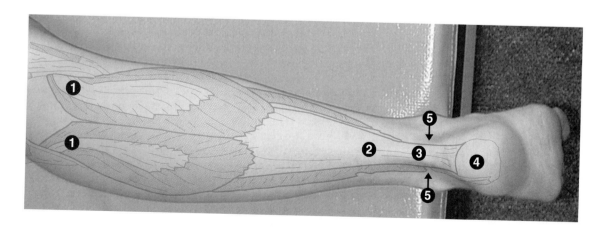

in its entirety as it forms the bulk of the posterior calf musculature. The soleus, which is covered by the gastrocnemius muscle, is not always directly palpable.

2. **Achilles tendon:** From its attachment on the calcaneus, palpate the length of the Achilles tendon proximally to where it blends with the triceps surae muscle group. This tendon should feel firm and ropelike, with a gradual, symmetrical increase in its width as you progress proximally. Palpate the Achilles tendon and its musculotendinous junction for symptoms of tendinitis or an **Achilles tendon rupture,** in which a gap in the tendon may be felt.

3. **Subcutaneous calcaneal bursa:** Isolate the subcutaneous calcaneal bursa, located between the posterior aspect of the Achilles tendon and the skin, by pinching the skin that overlies the tendon. In chronic inflammatory conditions, this bursa may be enlarged and thickened, forming "pump bumps" (see Fig. 4–9).

4. **Calcaneus:** Locate the posterior flare of the calcaneus and continue to palpate to the site of the Achilles tendon attachment. The calcaneal dome is located just anterior to the subtendinous calcaneal bursa. Pain elicited from adolescent patients during palpation of this area may indicate calcaneal apophysitis near the Achilles tendon's insertion on the calcaneus (see Chapter 4).

5. **Subtendinous calcaneal bursa:** Isolate this structure between the posterior aspect of the calcaneus and the anterior portion of the Achilles tendon by squeezing the soft tissue on either side of the Achilles tendon.

Palpation of Pulses

- **Posterior tibial artery:** Palpate the posterior tibial artery, located between the flexor digitorum longus and flexor hallucis longus tendons as they pass behind the medial malleolus. Supplying blood to the foot, the presence of this pulse must be established after any significant lower extremity bone fracture or joint dislocation. Note that swelling along the medial joint line may mask the presence of this pulse and make its detection difficult.

- **Dorsalis pedis artery:** A branch of the anterior tibial artery, the dorsalis pedis pulse may be palpated between the extensor digitorum longus and extensor hallucis longus tendons as they pass over the cuneiforms. The presence of this pulse after lower extremity fracture or dislocation and in those individuals suspected of having an anterior compartment syndrome must be established. This pulse is not readily detectable in all people. In the absence of a pulse on the involved side, make sure that the pulse is identifiable on the uninvolved extremity.

RANGE OF MOTION TESTING

The ROM available to the talocrural joint can be affected by muscular tightness, bony abnormalities, or soft tissue constraints. To allow for proper gait, the talocrural joint must provide 10 degrees of dorsiflexion

Table 5–4 **MUSCLES CONTRIBUTING TO FOOT AND ANKLE MOVEMENTS**	
Dorsiflexion	**Inversion**
Extensor digitorum longus	Extensor hallucis longus
Extensor hallucis longus	Flexor digitorum longus
Peroneus tertius	Flexor hallucis longus
Tibialis anterior	Tibialis anterior
	Tibialis posterior
Plantarflexion	**Eversion**
Flexor digitorum longus	Extensor digitorum longus
Flexor hallucis longus	Peroneus brevis
Gastrocnemius	Peroneus longus
Peroneus brevis	Peroneus tertius
Peroneus longus	
Plantaris	
Soleus	
Tibialis posterior	

during walking and 15 degrees during running. When dorsiflexion is limited, the foot compensates by increasing pronation during the weight-bearing phases of gait. This compensation results in biomechanical changes in the lower extremity that predisposes the individual to overuse injuries.

For the purposes here, plantarflexion and dorsiflexion are defined as the movement taking place at the talocrural joint, and inversion and eversion describe the motion occurring at the subtalar joint (Table 5–4; see Table 5–1 for nerve innervations). The use of goniometric measurements of plantarflexion and dorsiflexion and inversion and eversion is described in Box 5–2.

Active Range of Motion

- **Plantarflexion and dorsiflexion:** Spanning a range of 70 degrees, normal active ROM occurs as 20 degrees of dorsiflexion and 50 degrees of plantarflexion from the neutral position (Fig. 5–17).

- **Inversion and eversion:** Accounting for a total of 25 degrees, the predominant movement occurs as 20 degrees of inversion from the neutral position and 5 degrees of eversion from neutral (Fig. 5–18).

Passive Range of Motion

- **Plantarflexion and dorsiflexion:** Dorsiflexion is measured once with the knee extended to determine the overall influence of the triceps surae group and then again with the knee flexed to determine the influence of the soleus. The normal end-feel for both plantarflexion and dorsiflexion is firm, owing to soft tissue stretch of the anterior joint capsule, deltoid ligament, and ATF ligament during plantarflexion and of the Achilles tendon during dorsiflexion. After injury, the amount of ROM lost is greater during plantarflexion than in dorsiflexion. However, loss of dor-

Box 5–2
GONIOMETRY: ANKLE

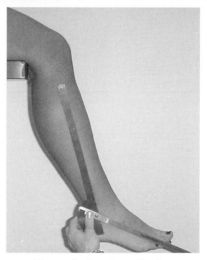

Plantarflexion–Dorsiflexion

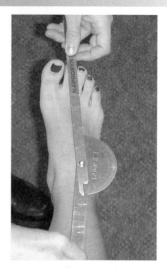

Inversion–Eversion

PATIENT POSITION	Sitting or lying supine with the knee flexed to at least 30° to release the triceps surae muscle group; dorsiflexion is then re-evaluated with the knee extended	
GONIOMETER ALIGNMENT		
FULCRUM	Centered over the lateral malleoulus	Over the talocrural joint line, centered between the malleoli
STATIONARY ARM	Aligned with the long axis of the fibula	Centered over the long axis of the tibia
MOVEMENT ARM	Parallel with the long axis of the 5th metatarsal	Over the 2nd metatarsal

siflexion is more debilitating in the long term because of the resultant changes in gait mechanics.

- **Inversion and eversion:** The patient should lie supine during the measurement of subtalar inversion and eversion, although less reliable measurements may be made with the patient sitting. The tibia and fibula are stabilized to prevent hip or lower leg rotation. The normal end-feel during neutral inversion is firm secondary to soft tissue stretch from the lateral

ankle ligaments (especially the CF ligament) and the peroneus longus and brevis muscles. A hard end-feel may be presented during eversion because of the fibula's striking the calcaneus. The end-feel may be firm because of stretching of the medial joint capsule and musculature. After injury, the capsular pattern loss is greater for inversion than for eversion.

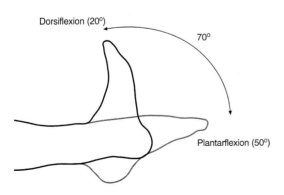

FIGURE 5–17. Range of motion for plantarflexion and dorsiflexion. Tightness of the Achilles tendon limits dorsiflexion.

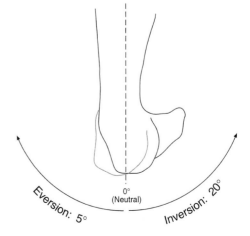

FIGURE 5–18. Range of motion for inversion and eversion.

Box 5-3
RESISTED ANKLE RANGE OF MOTION

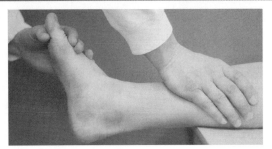
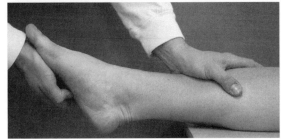

	Dorsiflexion	**Plantarflexion**
STARTING POSITION	Plantarflexion or neutral	Dorsiflexion or neutral; extend the knee to check the triceps surae as a group; flex the knee to at least 30° to isolate the soleus
STABILIZATION	Anterior aspect of the distal lower leg	Anterior aspect of the distal lower leg
RESISTANCE	Dorsum of the foot	Plantar aspect of the foot
SUBSTITUTION	Extension of the toes indicates that the extensor digitorum longus or extensor hallucis longus is contributing to the motion	Inversion of the foot indicates that the tibialis posterior, flexor digitorum longus, and/or flexor hallucis longus is contributing to the motion.
MUSCLES TESTED	Tibialis anterior, extensor digitorum longus, extensor hallucis longus, peroneus tertius	Gastrocnemius, soleus, tibialis posterior, peroneus longus, peroneus brevis, peroneus brevis, plantaris, flexor hallucis longus

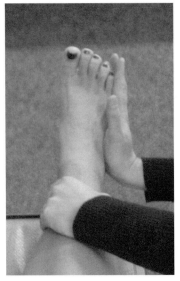

	Eversion	**Inversion**
STARTING POSITION	Inversion or neutral	Eversion or neutral
STABILIZATION	Distal lower leg	Distal lower leg
RESISTANCE	Lateral aspect of the foot	Medial aspect of the foot
SUBSTITUTION		Flexion of the toes could indicate substitution of the flexor hallucis longus or flexor digitorum longus muscles for the tibialis posterior
MUSCLES TESTED	Peroneus longus, peroneus brevis, extensor digitorum longus, peroneus tertius	Tibialis anterior, tibialis posterior, flexor hallucis longus, flexor digitorum longus

FIGURE 5–19. Toe-raise test for plantarflexion. **(A)** With the knee extended to include the gastrocnemius. **(B)** With the knee flexed to isolate the soleus muscle.

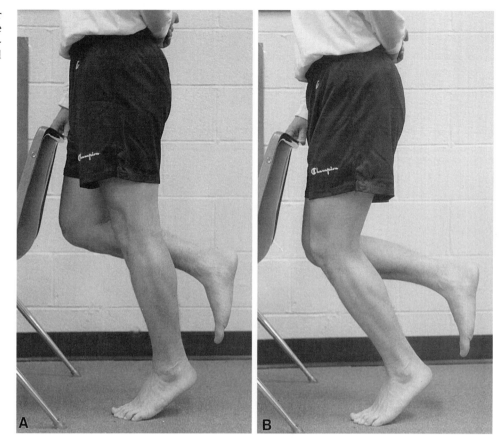

Resistive Range of Motion

Resisted ROM testing is presented in Box 5–3. Because the plantarflexor group is so powerful, it is often necessary to test these muscles using a unilateral heel-raise. The patient is asked to perform a set of 10 toe raises holding onto a sturdy object for balance (Fig. 5–19). Weakness in the plantarflexor group is evidenced by the inability to complete the test, inclining forward, or bending the knee when the gastrocnemius is being isolated.

TESTS FOR LIGAMENTOUS STABILITY

Range of motion tests stress the ligaments of the ankle complex, especially during passive ROM testing (see Table 5–3). Tests for ligamentous stability are still performed as a unique section of the clinical examination with emphasis placed on joint play and ligament-specific tenderness and pain.

Test for Anterior Talofibular Ligament Instability

The combined motions of ankle plantarflexion and subtalar inversion and supination place a strain on the ATF ligament, which serves to prevent anterior translation of the talus relative to the ankle mortise. The anterior drawer test is used to determine the integrity of the ATF (Box 5–4).

Test for Calcaneofibular Ligament Instability

The inversion stress test (talar tilt test) is used to determine whether the calcaneofibular ligament has been injured (Box 5–5). This test also stresses the anterior and posterior talofibular ligaments.

Test for Deltoid Ligament Instability

The distal projection of the lateral malleolus limits the amount of ankle eversion. Many of the injuries to the deltoid ligament are caused by rotational forces. The **eversion stress test** (Box 5–6) is used to evaluate injury resulting from a pure eversion mechanism. The **external rotation test** (Kleiger's test) is used to determine injury to the deltoid ligament caused by a rotatory stress or injury to the syndesmosis, with the results differentiated by the location of pain (Box 5–7).

Box 5–4
ANTERIOR DRAWER TEST

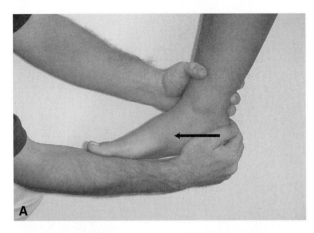

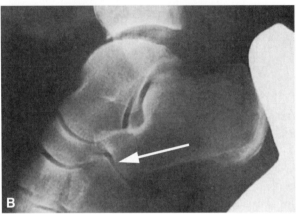

(A) Anterior drawer test to check the integrity of the anterior talofibular ligament.
(B) Radiographic view of a positive anterior drawer test. Note the anterior displacement of the talus relative to the tibia.

PATIENT POSITION	Sitting over the edge of the table with the knee flexed to prevent gastrocnemius tightness from influencing the outcome of the test.
POSITION OF EXAMINER	Sitting in front of the patient One hand stabilizes the lower leg, taking care not to occlude the mortise. The other hand cups the calcaneus while the forearm supports the foot in a position of slight plantarflexion.
EVALUATIVE PROCEDURE	The calcaneus and talus are drawn forward while providing a stabilizing force to the tibia
POSITIVE TEST	The talus slides anteriorly from under the ankle mortise compared with the opposite side (assuming it is normal). There may be an appreciable "clunk" as the talus subluxates and relocates, or the patient may describe pain.
IMPLICATIONS	Tear of the anterior talofibular ligament and the associated capsule
MODIFICATION	The test may be performed with the patient supine, but the knee must be kept in a minimum of 30° flexion to eliminate the influence of the gastrocnemius muscle.

Box 5–5
INVERSION STRESS TEST (TALAR TILT)

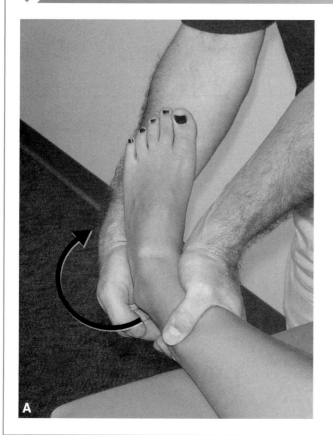

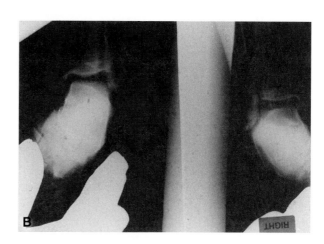

(A) Inversion stress test (talar tilt test) to check the integrity of the calcaneofibular ligament
(B) Radiograph of an inversion stress.

PATIENT POSITION	Lying or sitting with legs over the edge of a table
POSITION OF EXAMINER	In front of the patient One hand grasps the calcaneus and maintains the foot and ankle in neutral position The opposite hand stabilizes the lower leg; the thumb or forefinger is placed along the calcaneofibular ligament so that any gapping of the talus away from the mortise can be felt.
EVALUATIVE PROCEDURE	The hand holding the calcaneus provides an inversion stress by rolling the calcaneus medially, causing the talus to tilt
POSITIVE TEST	The talus tilts or gaps excessively, compared with the uninjured side; or pain is produced.
IMPLICATIONS	Involvement of the calcaneofibular ligament, possibly along with the anterior talofibular and posterior talofibular ligament

Box 5–6
EVERSION STRESS TEST (TALAR TILT)

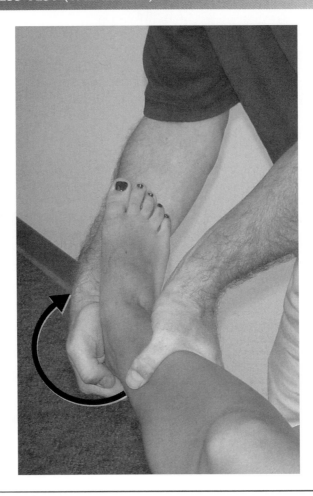

Eversion stress test to determine the integrity of the deltoid ligament, especially the tibiocalcaneal ligament.

PATIENT POSITION	Lying or sitting with legs over the edge of a table
POSITION OF EXAMINER	In front of the patient One hand grasps the calcaneus and maintains the foot in a neutral position.
EVALUATIVE PROCEDURE	The opposite hand stabilizes the lower leg. The thumb or forefinger may be placed along the deltoid ligament so that any gapping of the talus away from the mortise can be felt. The hand holding the calcaneus rolls it laterally, tilting the talus and causing a gap on the medial side of the ankle mortise.
POSITIVE TEST	The talus tilts or gaps excessively as compared with the uninjured side, or pain is described during this motion.
IMPLICATIONS	The deltoid ligament has been compromised.

Box 5–7
EXTERNAL ROTATION TEST (KLEIGER'S TEST)

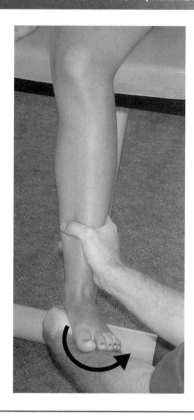

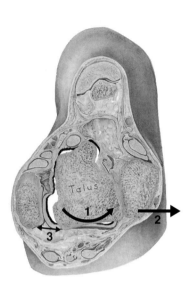

External rotation (Kleiger's) test for determination of rotatory damage to the deltoid ligament or the distal tibiofibular syndesmosis. The implication is based on the area of pain that is elicited. Externally rotating the talus **(1)** places a lateral force on the fibula **(2),** spreading the syndesmosis and stretching the deltoid ligament **(3).**

PATIENT POSITION	Sitting with legs over the edge of the table
POSITION OF EXAMINER	In front of the patient One hand stabilizes the lower leg in a manner that does not compress the distal tibiofibular syndesmosis. The other hand grasps the medial aspect of the foot while supporting the ankle in a neutral position.
EVALUATIVE PROCEDURE	The foot is externally rotated. To stress the syndesmosis, place the ankle in dorsiflexion. To stress the deltoid ligament, place the ankle in neutral position or slightly plantarflexed.
POSITIVE TEST	Deltoid ligament involvement: medial joint pain. The examiner may feel displacement of the talus away from the medial malleolus. Syndesmosis involvement: pain is described in the anterolateral ankle at the site of the distal tibiofibular syndesmosis.
IMPLICATIONS	Medial pain is indicative of trauma to the deltoid ligament. Pain in the area of the anterolateral ankle should be considered syndesmosis pathology unless determined otherwise (e.g., malleolus fracture)

Table 5–5
MECHANISMS OF INJURY OF THE COMMON PERONEAL NERVE

Mechanism	Causal Factor
Lesion	Fracture of the fibular head
Concussive	Contusion to the superior lateral portion of the lower leg
Compression	Knee braces or elastic wraps
Internal pressure	Prolonged squatting (e.g., baseball or softball catcher)
Entrapment	Exertional compartment syndromes
Traction	Varus stress to the knee, hyperextension of the knee, plantarflexion and inversion of the ankle

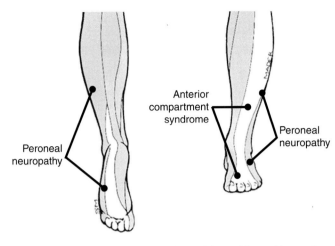

FIGURE 5–20. Local neuropathies of the ankle and lower leg. These findings should also be matched with those of a lower-quarter neurological screen.

Test for Ankle Syndesmosis Instability

Injury to the ankle syndesmosis, the anterior tibiofibular ligament, the interosseous membrane, and the posterior tibiofibular ligament may be determined through overpressure at the end of dorsiflexion ROM or through an external rotation force placed on the talus. During forced dorsiflexion, the anterior border of the talus is wedged into the talocrural joint, causing the fibula to move slightly away from the tibia. If the syndesmosis has been traumatized, pain will be elicited.

The external rotation test identifies syndesmosis pathology by forcing the talus and calcaneus against the lateral malleolus, causing it to be displaced laterally and posteriorly stressing the syndesmosis (See Box 5–7).

NEUROLOGIC TESTING

Neurologic dysfunction can occur secondary to compartment syndromes or direct trauma. The nerve most prone to trauma is the common peroneal nerve or its superficial or deep branches (Table 5–5). Figure 5–20 presents the distribution of neurologic symptoms around the ankle and foot. A lower quarter screen may also be required to rule out neurologic symptoms arising from the lumbar or sacral plexus (see Box 1–5).

 PATHOLOGIES AND RELATED SPECIAL TESTS

Although sprains are the predominant type of injury suffered by the lower leg and ankle, the evaluation process must not discount other potential injuries. Other acute injuries to this body area include fractures, dislocations, and tendon ruptures. Additionally, many overuse conditions affect the lower leg.

ANKLE SPRAINS

Most ankle sprains occur secondary to supination, causing trauma to the lateral ligament complex as a result of calcaneal inversion. A lesser yet significant percentage of ankle sprains involves the medial ankle ligaments and the distal tibiofibular syndesmosis. Because of the close association of many of the ankle ligaments with the joint capsule, ligament injury often results in trauma to the capsule. Ankle sprains may also be complicated by fractures of the ankle mortise, avulsion of the ligaments from their attachment site, dislocation of the talus, or nerve involvement.[10]

Lateral Ankle Sprains

The ankle complex (used here to describe the talocrural and subtalar joints) is least stable when it is in the *open-packed position* of plantarflexion and inversion. Most athletic skills require extreme amounts of supination, thereby predisposing the ankle to injury.

Sudden, forceful inversion of the ankle can lead to tearing of the lateral ligaments, and the specific structures involved depend on the position of the talocrural joint. Because it becomes taut when the ankle is supinated, the anterior talofibular ligament is the most commonly sprained ankle ligament. If the amount of supination is sufficient or if the ankle is near its neutral position, the calcaneofibular ligament also may be traumatized. A large amount of force is required to damage the posterior talofibular ligament. This structure limits inversion when the ankle is in its closed-packed position of dorsiflexion and eversion.

Open-packed position   The joint position at which its bones are maximally incongruent.

Anatomic and physiologic factors predisposing individuals to inversion ankle sprains include decreased proprioceptive ability, decreased muscular strength, and a lack of muscular coordination, all factors associated with a history of multiple ankle sprains. Tightness of the Achilles tendon or the triceps surae muscle group creates an increased risk of inversion sprain by placing the ankle complex in its open-packed position.

The frequency of ankle sprains has lead to the use of a number of prophylactic devices, including taping, soft and hard bracing, and various shoe designs, each with its own advantages, disadvantages, and levels of success.[11]

Moderate to severe ankle sprains result in re-incidence rates greater than 70 percent, with approximately 60 percent of those affected experiencing residual deficits on athletic performance.[12] Two theories have been suggested to account for this:[13] (1) the loss of the ligament's ability to passively support and protect the joint in conjunction with a reflex arc that is too slow to evoke a contraction in the peroneal muscles, limiting the force and speed of inversion;[14] and (2) decreased proprioceptive ability of the capsule, ligaments, and peroneal muscles.[15,16]

The primary clinical finding of an inversion ankle sprain is a history of inversion, plantarflexion, and/or rotation (see Table 5–3). A sensation of tearing or "popping" may also be described. Pain is localized along the lateral ligament complex and sinus tarsi. Because the anterior talofibular and posterior talofibular ligaments are capsular structures, tears of these ligaments can produce rapid, diffuse swelling. Being extracapsular, the calcaneofibular ligament produces relatively little edema when it is torn. Palpation elicits tenderness along the involved ligament. The associated joint capsule and the sinus tarsi may become tender.[8] Special attention must be paid to pain and crepitus elicited over the origin and insertion of the ligament, indicating a possible avulsion fracture (Table 5–6). Pain is demonstrated during the movements of inversion or plantarflexion, as described in the Range of Motion and the Ligamentous and Capsular Testing sections of this chapter.

Table 5–6
EVALUATIVE FINDINGS: Inversion Ankle Sprains

Examination Segment	Clinical Findings	
History	*Onset:*	Acute.
	Pain Characteristics:	Lateral aspect of the ankle around the area of the malleolus and sinus tarsi
	Mechanism:	Inversion, plantarflexion, or talar rotation in any combination
	Predisposing Conditions:	Achilles tendon and/or triceps surae tightness; tarsal coalition; a history of ankle sprains leading to decreased proprioceptive ability, decreased strength, or a lack of muscular coordination
Inspection	Findings include swelling around the lateral joint capsule, which may spread to the dorsum of the foot and into the sinus tarsi. Ecchymosis may be present around the lateral malleolus	
Palpation	Pain is elicited along the involved ligaments. The sinus tarsi may be sensitive to the touch Crepitus at the site of ligamentous origin or insertion may indicate an avulsion fracture	
Functional tests	*AROM:*	Pain on the lateral side of the ankle during plantarflexion and inversion indicates stretching of the lateral ligaments. Pain medially indicates a pinching of the medial structures
	PROM:	Motion produces pain along the ligaments, primarily: Inversion and plantarflexion: Anterior talofibular ligament, calcaneofibular ligament. Inversion, neutral position: Calcaneofibular ligament. Inversion and dorsiflexion: Posterior talofibular ligament.
	RROM:	Decreased strength or pain during most motions is found secondary to stretching of the ligaments or stretching or contraction of the peroneal muscles. Isometric contractions may not elicit pain.
Ligamentous Tests	Positive inversion stress test and/or anterior drawer test results	
Neurologic Tests	Sensory testing of the peroneal nerve distribution if neurological symptoms are present.	
Special Tests	Squeeze test to rule out a fracture of the distal fibula	
Comments	The clinician must be aware of an avulsion fracture of the lateral ligaments from the malleolus, impingement of the medial joint capsule, impingement of the structures beneath the medial malleolus, and possible fracture of the medial malleolus or base of the 5th MT. A chondral defect may be present in the articulating surfaces of the superior portion of the anteromedial talus and/or the inferior portion of the antermodial tibia. Adolescents displaying ankle instability should be referred for radiographic examination to rule out the possibility of an epiphyseal injury.	

AROM = active range of motion; PROM = passive range of motion; RROM = resisted range of motion; MT = metatarsal.

The severity and relative damage associated with moderate ankle sprains are often underestimated, and other trauma that is caused by the injury mechanism may be overlooked.[17] Excessive inversion can place compressive forces on the medial structures; exert a tensile force on the peroneal tendons and peroneal nerve; and involve the Achilles tendon, tibialis posterior, extensor digitorum brevis, and calcaneocuboid ligament.[10]

Inverting the talus can impinge the medial ligaments, medial joint capsule, and the structures passing beneath the medial malleolus, especially the tibialis posterior tendon. Excessive inversion of the talus and calcaneus can result in the fracture of the distal medial malleolus, base or styloid process of the fifth MT, or avulse the lateral ligaments from their site of origin or insertion (Fig. 5–21).

Chronic or severe inversion ankle sprains often result in a number of secondary conditions. After a tear of the anterior talofibular and calcaneofibular ligaments, the anterolateral capsule may develop a dense area of thickened connective tissue that becomes impinged between the lateral malleolus and calcaneus when the foot and ankle are dorsiflexed and everted.[18] "Bone bruises," accumulations of blood within the talus, nav-icular, and calcaneus, are also associated with inversion ankle sprains.[19]

Inversion sprains may produce an associated talar or tibial chondral lesion. These small fractures, not easily identified on standard radiographic examination, share a common trait of pain of unidentified origin and tenderness along the superior anteromedial (tibial) portion of the ankle mortise (Fig. 5–22). The use of magnetic resonance imaging (MRI) and bone scans has increased the frequency of diagnosis of this injury.[20,21] If this condition goes unrecognized, osteochondritis dissecans of the talocrural joint is likely to develop.[22]

Traction injuries to the peroneal nerve can affect the sensory and motor function of the lower leg and

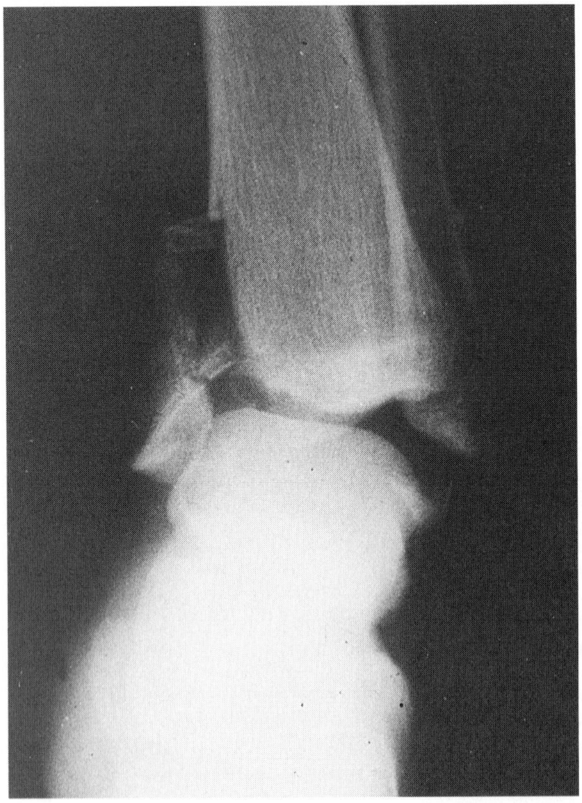

FIGURE 5–21. Fracture of the medial malleolus caused by excessive inversion of the ankle.

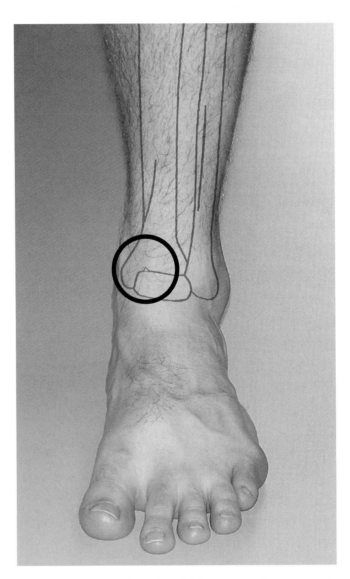

FIGURE 5–22. Location of a tibial osteochondral lesion following an inversion sprain. As the talus inverts, its supero-medial border may contact the tibia with sufficient force to cause a bony defect in either the tibia or talus.

FIGURE 5–23. Radiograph of a syndesmosis sprain. Note the wide gap between the tibia and fibula on the left image versus the image on the right. This injury results from the wide anterior border of the talus being forced into the mortise during hyperdorsiflexion, from external rotation of the foot, or both.

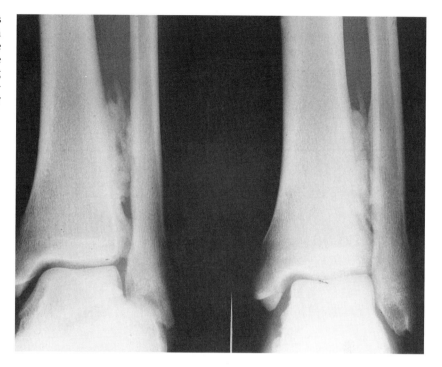

ankle. Decreased sensory function may be present in the involved ankle immediately after forceful plantarflexion and inversion. After a severe sprain, inhibition of sensory and motor function can extend as far as the hip.[23]

Added care is necessary when evaluating apparent ankle sprains in adolescents. Patients displaying excessive laxity require referral to a physician to rule out the presence of epiphyseal fractures.

Tape and braces have been used to prevent recurrence of ankle sprains. However, a complete rehabilitation program is required for all ankle sprains. Implementing early ROM exercises and other forms of mobilization has been shown to decrease pain and swelling while increasing overall ROM.[24,25] Early mobilization does result in more residual subjective complaints but has little long-term detrimental effect on athletic performance.[26]

Syndesmosis Sprains

Injury to the tibiofibular syndesmosis has been estimated to account for as much as 10 percent of all ankle sprains and as high as 18 percent in professional football players.[27] Although representing only a small percentage of all ankle sprains, syndesmotic ankle sprains are associated with significantly increased amounts of time lost from activity compared with other types of ankle sprains.

During excessive external rotation of the talus or forced dorsiflexion, the talus places pressure on the fibula, causing the distal syndesmosis to spread. The lateral displacement of the distal fibula can result in a sprain of the anterior and posterior tibiofibular ligaments, the interosseous membrane, and the crural interosseous ligament (Fig. 5–23).

Syndesmosis sprains, also referred to as "high ankle sprains," are often attributed to playing on artificial surfaces, but statistics do not substantiate this claim.[7] Other factors contributing to the occurrence of syndesmotic ankle sprains include *collision sports* in which the mechanism of injury involves planting the foot and "cutting" so that the talus is externally rotated and the foot is dorsiflexed. Another common mechanism is being fallen on while lying on the ground, causing dorsiflexion and external rotation of the foot. Syndesmotic and deltoid ligament sprains often occur concurrently.[7]

Pain is located primarily on the anterior aspect of the ankle and proximally along the interosseous membrane and is intensified during forced dorsiflexion, the external rotation test (see Box 5–7), or the **squeeze test** (Box 5–8).[28] Pain is often reported during palpation of the anterior and posterior tibiofibular ligaments (Table 5–7). The widening of the ankle mortise results in instability of the ankle as the talus is allowed a greater amount of glide within the joint.

Collision sports Individual or team sports relying on the physical dominance of one athlete over another. By their nature, these sports mandate violent physical contact.

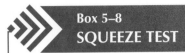

Box 5–8
SQUEEZE TEST

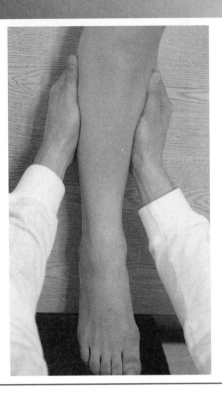

Squeeze test to identify fibular fractures or syndesmosis sprains. Pressure is applied transversely through the leg away from the site of pain.

PATIENT POSITION	Lying with the knee extended
POSITION OF EXAMINER	Standing next to, or in front of, the injured leg; the evaluator's hands cupped behind the tibia and fibula away from the site of pain
EVALUATIVE PROCEDURE	Gently squeeze (compress) the fibula and tibia, gradually adding more pressure if no pain or other symptoms are elicited. Progress toward the injured site until pain is elicited.
POSITIVE TEST	Pain is elicited, especially when it is away from the compressed area.
IMPLICATIONS	(A) Gross fracture or stress fracture of the fibula when pain is described along the fibular shaft (B) Syndesmosis sprain when pain is described at the distal tibiofibular joint
COMMENTS	Avoid applying too much pressure too soon into the test. Pressure should be applied gradually and progressively

When a syndesmotic sprain is suspected, palpate the entire length of the fibula for pain and crepitus. The forces required to produce a syndesmotic sprain may also be sufficient to fracture the fibula (Fig. 5–24). The fracture can occur in the proximal one third of the fibula, a **Maisonneuve fracture**.

Syndesmotic sprains require a longer recovery period than inversion sprains do. Patients also may benefit from a period of non-weight-bearing activity or immobilization.[7,27] Over time, *heterotopic ossification* or *synostosis* of the interosseous membrane may de-velop, prolonging pain during the push-off phase of gait.[7] If heterotopic ossification develops, surgery may be required.[29]

Heterotopic ossification Misplaced and unwanted development of calcium.

Synostosis The union of two bones though the formation of connective tissue.

Table 5–7
EVALUATIVE FINDINGS: Syndesmotic Ankle Sprains

Examination Segment	Clinical Findings	
History	*Onset:*	Acute
	Pain Characteristics:	Anterior portion of the distal tibiofibular syndesmosis
	Mechanism:	External rotation of the talus within the ankle mortise and/or dorsiflexion
Inspection	Swelling possibly present over the distal tibiofibular syndesmosis	
Palpation	Pain over the distal tibiofibular syndesmosis	
	Pain possibly elicited over the anterior and posterior tibiofibular ligaments	
	Palpation of the length of the fibula to rule out the presence of fibular fracture	
Functional Tests	*AROM:*	Motion is restricted and pain is elicited, especially with dorsiflexion and eversion, but pain is also present at the end ranges of plantarflexion and inversion. Any attempt at rotating the foot increases the pain anteriorly.
	PROM:	All motions are limited by pain with the greatest decreases noted in dorsiflexion and eversion
	RROM:	Resistance to the invertors and dorsiflexors of the foot and ankle may be weak and painful, although all resisted testing can be inhibited by pain in more severe syndesmotic sprains
Ligamentous Tests	Not applicable	
Neurologic Tests	Not applicable	
Special Tests	External rotation test; squeeze tests	
Comments	Heterotopic ossification or synostosis of the interosseous membrane may develop over time.	
	Syndesmosis sprains often occur concurrently with deltoid ligament sprains.	
	The presence of a Maisonneuve fracture of the fibula should be ruled out.	
	Syndesmotic sprains have an increased recovery time relative to other types of ankle sprains.	

AROM = active range of motion; PROM = passive range of motion; RROM = resisted range of motion.

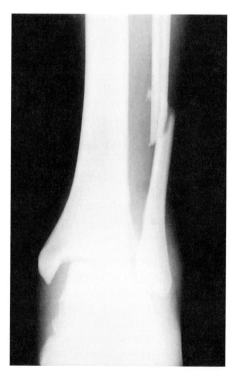

FIGURE 5–24. Fracture of the fibula concurrent with a sprain of the distal tibiofibular syndesmosis. When this fracture occurs more proximally on the fibula, it is termed a Maisonneuve fracture.

Medial Ankle Sprains

The strength of the deltoid ligament and the mechanical advantage of the longer lateral malleolus limit eversion. Because of the small amount of eversion (i.e., 5°) normally associated with the subtalar joint, the primary mechanism for damage to this ligament group is external rotation of the talus in the ankle mortise. These anatomic and biomechanical properties result in decreased trauma to the deltoid ligament, accounting for only 15 percent of all ankle sprains.[30] Because of its close association with the spring ligament, the stability of the medial longitudinal arch requires evaluation when a sprain of the deltoid ligament is suspected. The mechanism of injury of external rotation is similar for both eversion and syndesmotic sprains. Therefore both injuries must be ruled out because they may occur simultaneously.

Pain is present along the medial joint line and swelling tends to be more localized than that associated with lateral ankle sprains (Table 5–8). If an eversion mechanism is described, the lateral malleolus should be carefully evaluated for the presence of a "knock-off" fracture (Fig. 5–25).

Eversion may also cause an avulsion of the medial malleolus. A bimalleolar fracture (**Pott's fracture**) may be caused by a similar mechanism and carries with it the increased potential complication of a nonunion of the medial malleolus if surgical intervention is not performed. Interarticular trauma to the talus and tibia may also be present.

Table 5–8
EVALUATIVE FINDINGS: Eversion Ankle Sprains

Examination segment	Clinical Findings	
History	**Onset:**	Acute
	Pain Characteristics:	Medial border of the ankle and foot, radiating from the medial malleolus
	Mechanism:	Eversion and/or rotation
Inspection	Swelling around the medial joint capsule	
Palpation	Pain around the deltoid ligaments	
	Crepitus at the site of ligamentous origin or insertion may indicate an avulsion fracture	
Functional Tests	**AROM:**	Pain on the medial side of the ankle during plantarflexion indicates stretching of the anterior tibiotalar and/or or the tibionavicular ligaments. Pain during dorsiflexion indicates trauma to the posterior tibiotalar ligament. Lateral pain may indicate a pinching of the lateral ligaments and/or trauma to the lateral malleolus.
	PROM:	Motion produces pain along the ligaments, as described in the Ligamentous and Capsular Testing section of this chapter (also see Table 5–2)
	RROM:	Decreased strength or medial pain during most motions secondary to stretching of the medial ligaments
Ligamentous Tests	Positive eversion stress test and/or positive external rotation test results	
Neurologic Tests	Not applicable	
Special Tests	Squeeze test to rule out a fracture of the distal fibula.	
Comments	Excessive calcaneal eversion can result in a fracture of the lateral malleolus, talar dome, or disruption of the syndesmosis	
	A mechanism of external rotation warrants a careful evaluation of the syndesmosis as well as medial ankle structures.	

AROM = active range of motion; PROM = passive range of motion; RROM = resisted range of motion.

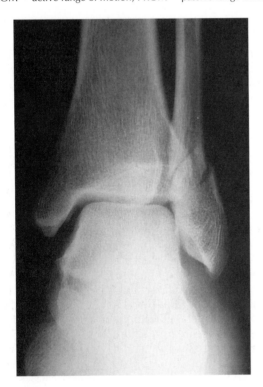

FIGURE 5–25. Fracture of the lateral malleolus caused by excessive eversion of the ankle. This type of fracture to the lateral malleolus is more common as it extends farther inferiorly than does the medial malleolus.

STRESS FRACTURES

Lower leg stress fractures involve the tibia, fibula, and talus and represent the accumulation of microtraumatic forces. Having symptoms of gradual onset, common complaints include pain along the shaft of the bone. In the case of fibular stress fractures, pain occurs proximal to the lateral malleolus and increases with activity and subsides with rest. During activity, decreased muscular strength and cramping may be reported. Palpation may reveal crepitus and point tenderness isolated to a single spot along the shaft of the bone. In many cases, the painful area is visually unremarkable (Table 5–9). A narrow tibial shaft, high degree of hip external rotation, and pes cavus are common predisposing factors for stress fractures.[31,32] Immature stress fractures, not visible on standard radiographic examination until bony callus formation has begun, typically around 3 weeks after the onset of injury, require the use of diagnostic techniques such as bone scans. Advanced stress fractures may be manifest through the squeeze test or through the **bump test** (Box 5–9). The signs and symptoms of stress fractures may mimic those of medial tibial stress syndromes and compartment syndromes (Table 5–10).

Pain guides the management of patients with stress fractures. Many individuals respond to rest and antiinflammatory medication. Advanced cases may require casting or a walker boot (Fig. 5–26).

Table 5–9
EVALUATIVE FINDINGS: Lower Leg Stress Fractures

Examination Segment	Clinical Findings	
History	*Onset:*	Insidious or chronic, secondary to repetitive running and/or jumping
	Pain Characteristics:	Along the shaft of the tibia or fibula; localized during or after exercise; may be described as a localized "ache" while at rest.
	Mechanism:	No definitive origin of pain. The history possibly indicates a sudden increase in the duration, frequency, or intensity of exercise or a change in playing surface or shoe wear.
	Predisposing Factors:	Individuals having a narrow tibial shaft, an externally rotated hip and/or pes cavus have a higher rate of injury.
Inspection	Normally unremarkable; however, localized swelling is possible in advanced stages.	
Palpation	Pain along the fracture site	
Functional Tests	All functional test results may be normal in the acute stages of stress fractures. In advanced cases or immediately after exercise, decreased strength may be evident owing to inflammation of the muscles near the site of the stress fracture.	
Ligamentous Tests	Not applicable	
Neurologic Tests	Not applicable	
Special Tests	The squeeze test is performed for advanced fibular stress fractures. The bump test is performed for advanced fibular, tibial, calcaneal, or talar stress fractures.	
Comments	Early stages of stress fractures may clinically resemble those of periosteitis. Early signs of stress fractures appear on bone scans. Stress fractures do not appear on standard radiographic examination for 4 to 6 wk after the onset of symptoms.	

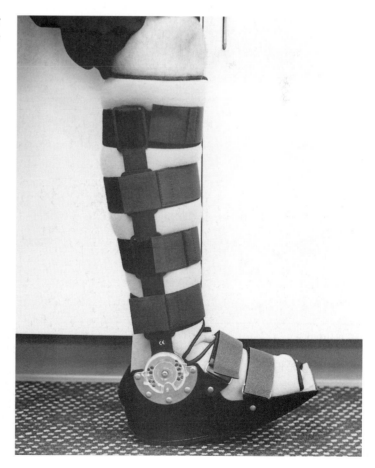

FIGURE 5–26. A walker boot. Walker boots allow for controlled range of motion, earlier stable weight bearing, and the ease of removal for rehabilitation.

Box 5–9
BUMP TEST FOR LOWER LEG STRESS FRACTURES

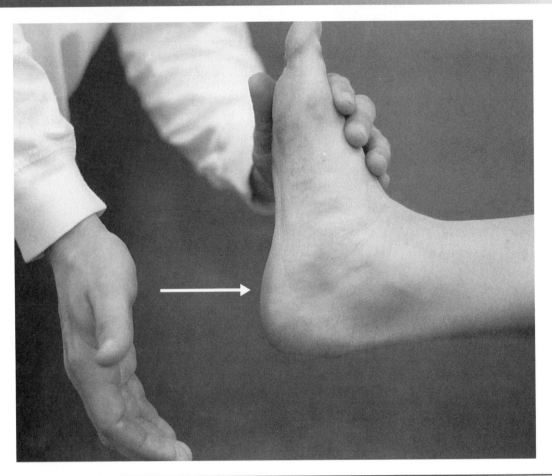

Bump test to identify stress fractures of the lower leg or talus. The examiner's hand is bumped against the patient's foot. The subsequent shock elicits pain in areas of stress fractures. Note that this test is not definitive.

PATIENT POSITION	Sitting with the involved leg off the end of the table and the knee straight, or lying supine The ankle in the neutral position
POSITION OF EXAMINER	Standing in front of the heel of the involved leg The posterior portion of the lower leg stabilized with the nondominant hand
EVALUATIVE PROCEDURE	Using the palm of the dominant hand, the examiner bumps the calcaneus with progressively more force until pain is elicited
POSITIVE TEST	Pain emanating from fracture of the calcaneus, talus, fibula, or tibia
IMPLICATIONS	Possible advanced stress fracture

Table 5–10
DIFFERENTIAL FINDINGS OF STRESS FRACTURES, MEDIAL TIBIAL STRESS SYNDROME, ACUTE COMPARTMENT SYNDROME, AND CHRONIC EXERTIONAL COMPARTMENT SYNDROME

Finding	Stress Fracture	Medial Tibial Stress Syndrome	Acute Compartment Syndrome	Chronic Exertional Compartment Syndrome
Pain characteristics	Localized over the involved area of the bone	More diffuse along the posteromedial border of the middle or distal one-third of the tibia.	Pain in the anterior compartment of the lower leg Numbness on the dorsum of the foot, especially the web space between the 1st and 2nd toes Dorsal pedis pulse may be diminished.	Pain in the anterior compartment of the lower leg Numbness on the dorsum of the foot, especially the web space between the 1st and 2nd toes Dorsal pedis pulse diminished
Onset	Following changes in footware or playing surfaces or increases in intensity, duration, or frequency of activity	Following changes in footware or playing surfaces or increases in intensity, duration, or frequency of activity	Acute following trauma to the anterior lower leg Acute during exercise but symptoms not decreasing with rest	Symptoms increasing in proportion to exercise Pain possibly limiting activity after symptoms begin
Pain influences	Increased with activity Decreased with rest Possibly progressing to constant pain	Initially, pain at the start of activity possibly diminishing with continued participation; pain possibly increasing again at the end of activity Pain decreasing with rest	Constant pain most likely prohibiting activity	Pain increasing with activity Pain decreasing with rest
Positive findings	Bump test may be positive	Pain with palpation over the posteromedial tibia Pain during toe raises Pain during resisted plantarflexion, inversion, or dorsiflexion	Pain with: AROM PROM RROM	Pain after or during exercise: AROM, PROM, RROM
Negative test results	AROM PROM RROM	AROM PROM		Most test results negative if the individual has not recently been exercising
Definitive diagnosis	Bone scan Radiograph MRI	Bone scan may show periosteal irritation	Increased intracompartmental pressure Pain that does not subside with rest	Increased intracompartmental pressure after activity Pain that subsides with rest

AROM = active range of motion; PROM = passive range of motion; RROM = resisted range of motion.

171

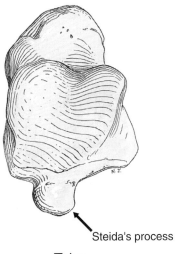

Talus
(superior view)

FIGURE 5–27. Steida's Process. A posterior projection off the talus.

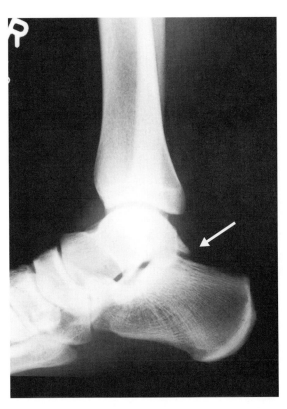

FIGURE 5–28. Radiograph of an os trigonum. The arrow indicates the location of the os trigonum, a fracture of Steida's process. A fracture line can be seen at the midpoint on the process.

OS TRIGONUM INJURY

An os trigonum is formed when **Steida's process** separates from the talus (Fig 5–27).[33, 34] Steida's process first appears between the ages of 8 to 13 years, normally fusing within 1 year after its appearance.[35, 36] Developmentally, an os trigonum is formed when the secondary center of ossification fails to fuse the process to the talus (Fig. 5–28). A traumatic os trigonum is formed by a nonunion fracture or stress fracture of Steida's process.[35, 36] An os trigonum is present in approximately 7 percent of the population. Athletes are at an increased risk of sustaining an injury to this structure.[35, 37, 38]

When an os trigonum impinges on surrounding tissues, symptoms occur. **Os trigonum syndrome** (also referred to as **"talarcompression syndrome"**) may involve: (1) an inflammation of the posterior joint, (2) inflammation of the ligaments surrounding the os trigonum, (3) a fracture of the os trigonum, or (4) pathology involving the Steida's process.[33] As the talocalcaneal unit moves into inversion and plantarflexion and the midtarsal joints pronate, the posterior talocalcaneal ligament tightens against the os trigonum or Steida's process. Eversion of the calcaneus, combined with subtalar and midtarsal joint pronation, causes the os trigonum or Steida's process to become compressed between the tibia and calcaneus.[33]

Inflammatory conditions of the os trigonum become symptomatic after activity, repetitive microtrauma, or other local inflammatory conditions.[39] Fractures of the os trigonum are characterized by the sudden onset of pain after forced plantarflexion or dorsiflexion. Swelling lateral or medial to the Achilles tendon may be noted. During palpation, tenderness is reported anterior to the Achilles tendon and posterior to the talus. Placing the ankle in plantarflexion may produce pain during ROM testing (Table 5–11). Plain film radiographs are used to identify the presence of an os trigonum.[40]

The treatment protocol is based on the patient's symptoms. A walker boot or cast with no weight bearing or partial weight bearing is used until the patient can ambulate without pain and a normal gait pattern. Patients can return to their activities after restoring full pain-free ROM and strength to the leg. The use of a viscoelastic heel insert may be helpful to absorb ground reaction forces. If the condition becomes chronic, the evaluation and use of a permanent orthotic to control foot motion may be warranted or surgical removal of the os trigonum may be required.

ACHILLES TENDON PATHOLOGY

Because of its dual association with the two prime plantarflexors, the gastrocnemius and the soleus, any injury to the Achilles tendon results in decreased plantarflexion strength. The decrease in plantarflexion strength may cause significant changes in gait, impairing the patient's ability to walk, run, and jump normally.

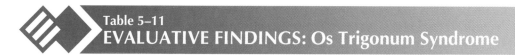

Table 5–11
EVALUATIVE FINDINGS: Os Trigonum Syndrome

Examination Segment	Clinical Findings	
History	*Onset:*	Acute or insidious; pain is increased with activity
	Acute:	Sudden onset of pain may suggest a fracture
	Location of Pain:	Posterior aspect of the talus, anterior to the Achilles tendon.
	Mechanism:	Acute: forced hyperpalantarflexion. Chronic or insidious: repetitive activity usually involving plantarflexion
	Predisposing Factors:	The presence of an nonunited lateral tubercle on the posterior aspect of the talus (os trigonum)
Inspection	Swelling possibly observed anteromedial and anterolateral to the Achilles tendon	
Palpation	Pain elicited when palpating the posterior talus, anterior to the Achilles tendon.	
Functional Tests	**AROM:** Pain with plantarflexion	
	PROM: Pain with forced plantarflexion	
	RROM: Pain with resistance on performing a heel raise.	
Ligamentous Tests	No significant findings	
Neurologic Tests	No significant findings	
Special Tests	Not applicable	
Differential Evaluation	Achilles tendonitis, tibialis posterior tendinitis, flexor hallicus longus tendinitis, peroneal tendon subluxation, lateral ankle instability, arthritis, tarsal tunnel syndrome, tarsal coalition, talus fracture.	
Comments	A definitive diagnosis is made with correlation of findings with the presence of an os trigonum on plain film radiographs or MRI.	

AROM = active range of motion; PROM = passive range of motion; RROM = resisted range of motion.

Achilles Tendinitis

The Achilles tendon is a poorly vascularized structure that receives limited blood supply from the posterior tibial artery. The distal avascular zone, 2 to 6 cm proximal to its insertion on the calcaneus, is the most common site of tendon pathology, including inflammation and rupture.[41, 42] The tendon's response to the inflammatory reaction is impeded by the poor blood supply in the area, causing delayed healing.

The poor vascular supply to the Achilles tendon brings into question if inflammation is even possible here, as the available blood supply may not be sufficient to provide a widespread inflammatory response. The tendon is, however, surrounded by a highly vascular structure, the **paratenon.** Inflammation of the paratenon, **peritendinitis,** produces pain and forms adhesions with the underlying tendon.[42, 43] *Tendinosis* is used to describe the degeneration of the tendon's substance. Although this breakdown is not always a precursor to a tendon rupture, tendinosis represents a progressive degeneration of the tendon:[42]

Peritendinitis → Tendinosis → Tendon rupture

Tendon ruptures are not always complete. Approximately 20 percent of peritendinitis cases are associated with a partial rupture of the Achilles tendon.[42]

Anatomic factors that may lead to the onset of Achilles tendon pathology include tibial varum, calcaneovalgus, hyperpronation, and tightness of the triceps surae and the hamstring muscle groups.[42] Factors such as running mechanics, duration and intensity of running, the type of shoe, and running surface, as well as the biomechanics of the foot and ankle, can result in inflammation of the Achilles tendon or its related structures. Achilles tendinitis may also have an acute onset resulting from a direct blow to the tendon. Certain antimicrobial medications such as fluoroquinolone have been associated with Achilles tendon pathology, including tendon ruptures.[44] Age and gender are the strongest predictors of Achilles tendon injury. As age increases, so does the risk of Achilles tendon pathology, especially in males who have three times the risk of developing symptoms than females.[45,46]

Individuals suffering from Achilles tendinitis (used collectively to describe peritendinitis and tendinosis) describe pain or "burning" radiating along the length

Tendinosis Lesions caused by decreased local blood flow (ischemia) secondary to peritendinitis.

of the tendon. The area is tender to the touch and crepitus may be elicited, particularly with active ROM. This condition may be the result of or may result in tightness of the triceps surae muscle group (Table 5–12). MRI is useful in definitively diagnosing the pathology leading to Achilles tendon pain and identifying the predisposition to ruptures.[44]

Most cases of Achilles tendonitis are traced to overuse syndromes and repeated eccentric loading of the tendon. Individuals with foot rigidity are predisposed to this condition because gait must be modified to compensate for a valgus or varus hindfoot. Improperly fitting footwear may cause friction between the heel counter and the tendon, and shoes with a rigid sole may not permit adequate ROM in the midfoot and forefoot, altering the biomechanics of the foot, ankle, and leg.

Oral antiinflammatory medications are often prescribed for those with acute or moderate inflammatory conditions, and a heel lift may be added to reduce the stresses placed on the Achilles tendon. In advanced cases, immobilization may be required, but the strength of the triceps surae muscle group is slow to return after this technique.[47] Corticosteroid injections may be used to control chronic or severe inflammation, but there is an increased risk of suffering an Achilles tendon rupture for 1 week after the injection.[46,48]

Stretching of the Achilles tendon and triceps surae is an important component of the therapeutic exercise program. The triceps surae can be strengthened as pain diminishes. A progressive return to activity includes instruction in the proper method of warming up, continued flexibility exercises, monitoring of shoewear and activity surfaces, and the application of ice after exercise.

Achilles Tendon Rupture

Forceful, sudden contractions, such as when a defensive back or basketball player changes direction or when a gymnast dismounts from a piece of apparatus, results in a large amount of tension developing within the Achilles tendon. If this tension becomes too great, the tendon fails, resulting in an Achilles tendon rupture.

Two theories attempt to account for onset of Achilles tendon ruptures: (1) chronic degeneration of the tendon and (2) failure of the inhibitory mechanism of the musculotendinous unit.[49] As described in the Achilles Tendinitis section, the Achilles tendon is poorly vascular-

Table 5–12
EVALUATIVE FINDINGS: Achilles Tendinitis

Examination Segment	Clinical Findings	
History	**Onset:**	Insidious or the result of trauma to the Achilles tendon
	Pain Characteristics:	Along the length of the Achilles tendon
	Mechanism:	Overuse or secondary to acute trauma, such as a blow to the Achilles tendon
		Improperly fitting shoe rubbing against the tendon may also activate the inflammatory response
	Predisposing Conditions:	Tibial varum; calcaneal valgum; hyperpronation or other forms of foot rigidity; tightness of the triceps surae muscle group; risk increases with age, especially in the male population
Inspection	Possible visible edema along the length of the tendon; the tendon on the involved leg may appear thicker than on the opposite leg	
Palpation	Pain elicited during palpation of the tendon	
	Crepitus may be evident with active motion	
Functional tests	**AROM:**	Pain and crepitus during plantarflexion and dorsiflexion
	PROM:	Pain during dorsiflexion, resulting from stretching the tendon
		Dorsiflexion range of motion possibly diminished secondary to Achilles tendon tightness
	RROM:	Pain and decreased strength present during plantarflexion
Ligamentous Tests	Not applicable	
Neurologic Tests	Not applicable	
Special Tests	None	
Comments	Approximately 20% of Achilles tendonitis cases also have a partial tear of the tendon	

AROM = active range of motion; PROM = passive range of motion; RROM = resisted range of motion.

FIGURE 5–29. Ruptured Achilles tendon. The patient's right (far) Achilles tendon has been ruptured. Note the depression proximal to the calcaneus and the involved swelling.

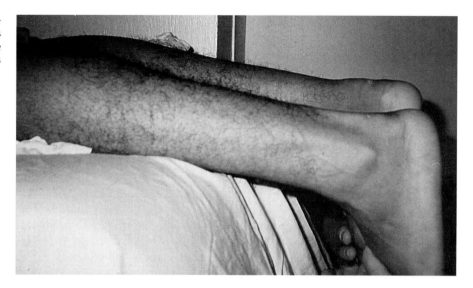

ized and the body is unable to keep pace with the tendon's breakdown (tendinosis). As a result, the tendon weakens. In the final stages of the degenerative process, a rupture occurs.[42,49] When the triceps surae's inhibitory mechanism fails, an excessive force (e.g., stepping in a hole) or a forceful muscle contraction (e.g., an explosive push-off) results in the rupture of the tendon. In both types of mechanisms, the rupture tends to occur in the tendon's avascular zone (the distal 2 to 6 cm).[49]

Although this injury can occur in either gender or in any age group, Achilles tendon ruptures tend to be most prominent in men older than age 30 years.[46] A complete rupture typically occurs in more sedentary individuals who perform episodic strenuous activity. Previous or current tendinosis, age-related changes in the tendon, and *deconditioning* may play roles in the onset of tendon ruptures.[50] Healthy and unhealthy tendons can be ruptured through direct trauma or by forceful concentric muscle contraction or eccentric loading of the tendon.[50]

The risk of tendon rupture is also increased for approximately 1 week after corticosteroid injections.[45,46] Although there are case reports of Achilles tendon rupture after corticosteroid injections in humans, there are no rigorous long-term studies that evaluate the risk of rupture with or without steroid injections.[51] Injections in the paratenon have been demonstrated to be effective without increasing the long-term rate of tendon rupture.[51,52]

Achilles tendon ruptures are characterized by the inability to push off with the injured leg during ambulation. The patient usually assumes a stiff-legged gait pattern characterized by external rotation of the extremity. The patient often has the sensation of being "kicked," followed by severe pain.[49] If the lesion oc-curs in the tendon's midsubstance, the defect may be observable or palpable. As swelling develops, the defect becomes difficult to palpate (Fig. 5–29). Although the tendon may be completely ruptured, the patient is still able to actively plantarflex the ankle through contraction of the peroneals, long toe flexors, and tibialis posterior muscles. However, the strength of the contraction is markedly diminished (Table 5–13). Clinically, the presence of a complete Achilles tendon rupture is confirmed through the **Thompson test** (Box 5–10).[9, 49] MRI can be used to identify partial tendon tears.[44]

Complete Achilles tendon ruptures are managed conservatively with casting or dorsiflexion night splints for a minimum of 8 weeks or through open or arthroscopic surgery.[53] The primary advantage of conservative care is the absence of wound problems and decreased medical costs. Disadvantages include an increased rate of rerupture, decreased muscle function, and patient dissatisfaction relative to surgical repair.[53–55]

The advantages of surgical repair include a reported rate of re-rupture less than 5 percent; a greater return to pre-injury activity; and a good return of plantarflexion strength, power, and endurance.[53–55] Most disadvantages are caused by surgical complications, including wound healing. The skin around the Achilles tendon is very thin with little subcutaneous tissue. Its limited blood supply makes the incision site prone to wound complications.

Deconditioning   The loss of once existing cardiovascular or muscular endurance and strength.

Table 5–13
EVALUATIVE FINDINGS: Achilles Tendon Rupture

Examination Segment	Clinical Findings	
History	***Onset:***	Acute
	Pain Characteristics:	Achilles tendon and/or lower portion of the gastrocnemius, the patient often reports the sensation of being kicked.
	Mechanism:	Forceful plantarflexion with eccentric loading, usually the result of eccentric loading or plyometric contraction of the calf musculature
	Predisposing Factor:	A possible relationship between a history of Achilles tendinitis and a rupture of the tendon
Inspection	A defect may be visible in the Achilles tendon or at the musculotendinous junction, but rapid swelling may obscure this; discoloration may be present around the tendon. The patient is unable to bear weight on the involved extremity because of pain.	
Palpation	A palpable defect in the Achilles tendon, although it may quickly become obscured by swelling Pain elicited along the tendon and lower gastrocnemius–soleus muscle group	
Functional Tests	***AROM:***	Plantarflexion may possibly still be present owing to the tibialis posterior, plantaris, peroneals, and long toe flexors, although the patient may complain of pain during this motion and during dorsiflexion (because of the stretching of the Achilles tendon).
	PROM:	Pain is elicited during dorsiflexion.
	RROM:	There is a weak or nonexistent ability to plantarflex.
Ligamentous Tests	Not applicable	
Neurologic Tests	Not applicable	
Special Tests	Positive Thompson test	
Comments	This injury tends to occur more frequently in males over age 30 years, but any age group is susceptible. The status of the dorsalis pedis pulse should be monitored.	

AROM = active range of motion; PROM = passive range of motion; RROM = resisted range of motion.

SUBLUXATING PERONEAL TENDONS

Forceful, sudden dorsiflexion and eversion or plantarflexion and inversion may stretch or rupture the superior peroneal retinaculum that holds the peroneal tendons behind the lateral malleolus. Extreme cases may also involve the inferior peroneal retinaculum (see Fig. 5–12). When these tendons lose their alignment from behind the lateral malleolus and slip anteriorly, the peroneals, which are normally plantarflexors, become dorsiflexors (Fig. 5–30). Anatomically, a flattened or convex fibular groove predisposes an individual to peroneal subluxations by lessening the bony channel through which the tendons pass.[56] Pes planus, hindfoot

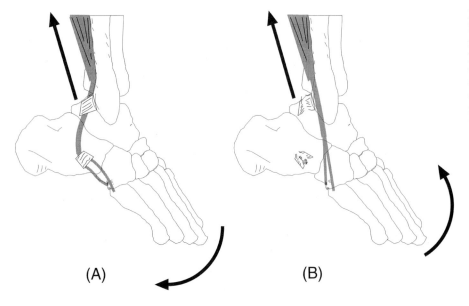

(A)   (B)

FIGURE 5–30. Illustration showing biomechanical changes with subluxating peroneal tendon. **(A)** When the peroneal retinacula is intact, the peroneals serve as plantarflexors of the foot. **(B)** Subluxating peroneal tendons, caused by the rupture or stretching of the retinacula, change the angle of pull to that of a dorsiflexor.

Box 5–10
THOMPSON TEST FOR ACHILLES TENDON RUPTURE

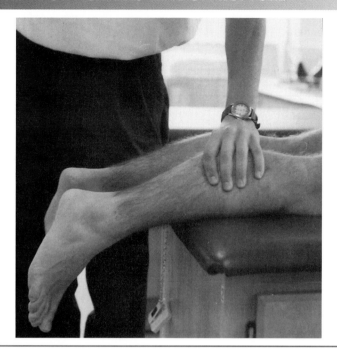

Thompson test for an Achilles tendon rupture. When the Achilles tendon is intact, squeezing the calf muscle results in slight plantarflexion. A positive Thompson test occurs when the calf is squeezed but no motion is produced in the foot, indicating a tear of the Achilles tendon.

PATIENT POSITION	Prone, with the foot off the edge of the table
POSITION OF EXAMINER	At the side of the patient with one hand over the muscle belly of the calf musculature
EVALUATIVE PROCEDURE	The examiner squeezes the calf musculature while observing for plantarflexion of the foot
POSITIVE TEST	When the calf is squeezed, the foot does not plantarflex
IMPLICATIONS	The Achilles tendon has been ruptured

valgus, recurrent ankle sprains, and laxity of the peroneal retinaculum all contribute to the onset of subluxating peroneal tendons.[9]

The peroneal tendons may dislocate from the groove behind the lateral malleolus, possibly being observed as they snap into and out of position during plantarflexion and dorsiflexion or active eversion.[9] This biomechanical change alters the biomechanics of the foot and ankle, resulting in pain and dysfunction (Table 5–14). Longitudinal tears may appear in the tendons, with the peroneus longus being the most frequently involved.[56–58] These ruptures contribute to future subluxations, dislocations, and peroneal tendinitis.[56–60] Ultrasonic images can be used to detect chronic subluxation, and kinematic MRIs can be used to identify positional subluxations.[61,62]

In cases in which the retinaculum is stretched, the degree of subluxation may be controlled by rehabilitation exercises, taping, and the use of a felt pad over the peroneal groove to assist in holding the tendons in place. However, after the retinaculum has been stretched, it does not return to its original length. When the retinacula have been completely disrupted or pain and dysfunction become great, surgery is required to deepen the fibular groove,[64] repair the involved retinaculum,[9,60] or both. Surgery to repair the soft tissue structures is usually necessary for patients with recurrent peroneal tendon dislocations.[63] If the subluxation is not reduced, chronic ankle instability, pain, and decreased strength impair ankle function.

NEUROVASCULAR DEFICIT

Disruption of the blood or nerve supply to or from the lower leg can result from acute trauma, overuse conditions, congenital defects, or surgery. A complete examination of the dermatomes, reflexes, and pulses of the

Table 5–14
EVALUATIVE FINDINGS: Subluxating Peroneal Tendons

Examination Segment	Clinical Findings	
History	***Onset:***	Acute or insidious
	Pain Characteristics:	Behind the lateral malleolus in the area of the superior peroneal retinaculum, across the lateral malleolus, length of the peroneal tendons, and, in some cases, at the site of the inferior peroneal retinaculum
	Mechanism:	Forceful dorsiflexion and eversion or plantarflexion and inversion
	Predisposing Conditions:	A flattened or convex fibular groove, pes planus, hindfoot valgus, recurrent ankle sprain, laxity of the peroneal retinaculum
Inspection	Swelling and ecchymosis may be isolated behind the lateral and inferior lateral malleolus (see functional tests).	
Palpation	Tenderness behind the lateral malleolus and perhaps over the site of the inferior peroneal retinaculum (see functional tests)	
Functional Tests	***AROM:***	The peroneal tendon may be seen, felt, or heard as it subluxates while the foot and ankle move from plantarflexion and inversion to dorsiflexion and eversion and back.
	PROM:	No significant clinical findings are noted.
	RROM:	Findings are the same as for AROM. The clinician should palpate the area behind the lateral malleolus to identify any abnormal movement of the peroneal tendons. The tendons may be seen to exhibit possible subluxation during resisted eversion.
Ligamentous Tests	No significant findings	
Neurologic Tests	Not applicable	
Special Tests	None	

AROM = active range of motion; PROM = passive range of motion; RROM = resisted range of motion.

lower leg and foot should be conducted to rule out the possibility of neurovascular involvement.

Anterior Compartment Syndrome

Resulting from increased pressure within the anterior compartment, anterior compartment syndrome threatens the integrity of the lower leg, foot, and toes by obstructing the neurovascular network (primarily the deep peroneal nerve and anterior tibial artery) contained within this compartment. The bony posterolateral border and dense fibrous fascial lining of the compartment possess poor elastic properties to accommodate for expansion of the intracompartmental tissues. When the compartment pressure exceeds *capillary perfusion pressure,* the local tissues do not receive an adequate supply of oxygen. The lack of oxygen leads to ischemia of the tissues and, if not treated, cell death.[65]

Anterior compartment syndromes are classified as being traumatic, acute exertional, or chronic exertional. Traumatic anterior compartment syndrome occurs from intracompartmental hemorrhage caused by a blow to the anterior or anterolateral portion of the lower leg. The subsequent bleeding and edema cause an increased pressure within the compartment, obstructing the neurovascular network to and from the dorsum of the foot. This results in ischemic destruction of the involved tissues.

Exertional compartment syndromes can have an acute or chronic onset, with symptoms occurring during or after exercise (or both). Chronic exertional compartment syndrome (CCS), also referred to as **recurrent compartment syndrome** or **intermittent** *claudication,* is an exertional condition that occurs secondary to anatomic abnormalities obstructing blood flow in exercising muscles. Many exertional compartment syndromes are related to an increased thickness of the fascia that inhibits venous outflow but not arterial inflow.[66] Other anatomic factors that predispose an individual to CCS include[67,68]

- Herniation of muscle, occluding the neurovascular network as it transverses the interosseous membrane
- Fascia's failing to accommodate the increase in muscle volume during exercise
- Excessive hypertrophy of the muscles within an otherwise normal fascial network
- Increased capillary permeability
- Postexercise fluid retention
- Decreased venous return

Capillary perfusion pressure Pressure within the capillaries that forces blood out into the surrounding tissues.

Claudication Pain arising in the lower leg as the result of inadequate venous drainage or poor arterial innervation.

The signs, symptoms, and pathology of acute and chronic exertional syndromes are similar. However, acute exertional compartment syndromes occur without prior symptoms and do not have a history of traumatic injury to the compartment.[65]

Compartmental syndromes have also been associated with tibial fractures,[69–71] anticoagulant therapy,[72] and diabetes.[73] The use of knee braces[74] and wearing high-heeled shoes or athletic shoes that have an increased heel height[75] have also been implicated in the onset of exertional compartment syndromes.

The "five P's" are used to describe the signs and symptoms of compartment syndromes; these are pain, pallor (redness), pulselessness, paresthesia, and paralysis.[65] Pain is localized within the affected compartment and is often disproportionate with the other findings of the examination. Numbness occurs in the web space between the first and second toes, possibly involving the dorsal and lateral aspects of the foot.[65] Pain is increased during active, passive, and resisted foot movement with decreased strength being noted during resisted dorsiflexion. A **drop foot gait** (see Chapter 9) may also be observed (Table 5–15).

The presence of the dorsalis pedis pulse must be established in the involved limb (Fig. 5–31). Because this pulse is not detectable in all individuals, both limbs must be examined. If the pulse is present in the uninvolved extremity but not in the involved extremity, then it can be deduced that blood flow to the foot has been compromised. The dorsalis pedis pulse will remain palpable in all but the most advanced cases of compartment syndromes. Although the blood pressure within the tibial artery may be sufficient to produce a palpable dorsalis pedis pulse, the pressure increase may be great enough to inhibit flow within the smaller vessels and capillaries.[67]

Compartment syndromes can be fully developed even though a patient still has normal pulses and full capillary refill. The tissue must be ischemic for approximately 1 hour before paresthesia and paralysis develop.

Table 5–15
EVALUATIVE FINDINGS: Anterior Compartment Syndrome

Examination Segment	Clinical Findings	
History	**Onset:**	Traumatic or exertional
	Pain Characteristics:	Numbness is possibly described in the dorsum of the foot, especially in the web space between the first and second toes
		Anterolateral portion of the lower leg, which is described as "achy," "sharp," or "dull"
		Other complaints such as muscle tightness, cramping, swelling, weakness, or the inability to exercise owing to pain
	Mechanism:	Traumatic: Direct blow to the anterolateral tibia
		Exertional: Symptoms reported during or after running or other prolonged activity
	Predisposing Conditions:	Anatomic factors that inhibit the expansion of the anterior compartment, tibial fracture, anticoagulant therapy, diabetes, prophylactic and functional knee braces, high-heeled shoes
Inspection	The anterior compartment may appear shiny and swollen. In advanced cases, possible discoloration of the dorsum of the foot may be present.	
Palpation	The anterior compartment is hard and edematous to the touch, the area is painful to the touch.	
	The presence of a normal dorsalis pedis pulse should be determined.	
Functional Tests	**AROM:**	Decreased (or absent) ability to dorsiflex the ankle or extend the toes. Drop foot gait may be observed.
	PROM:	Pain may be elicited during plantarflexion secondary to stretching of the tendons of tibialis anterior and the long toe extensors creating pressure within the compartment
	RROM:	Weakness is exhibited during dorsiflexion and toe extension.
Ligamentous Tests	Not applicable	
Neurologic Tests	Numbness may be present in the web space between the 1st and 2nd toes and possibly on the dorsum of the foot	
Special Tests	There are no clinician tests for these conditions. Anterior compartment syndrome is confirmed by measuring the intracompartmental pressure.	
Comments	The clinician should not apply a compression wrap during the treatment of anterior compartment syndrome because this technique increases the intracompartmental pressure and may exacerbate the condition.	
	Bilateral involvement in chronic anterior compartment syndromes is common.	

AROM = active range of motion; PROM = passive range of motion; RROM = resisted range of motion.

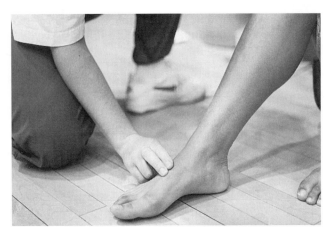

FIGURE 5–31. Locating the dorsalis pedis pulse. This pulse becomes diminished in the presence of anterior compartment syndrome or proximal joint dislocations. It is not always palpable and the findings of the involved limb should be compared to the uninvolved extremity.

The most important clinical finding of compartment syndromes is severe pain with passive stretching of the muscles within the compartment.[65] Compartment syndromes evoking decreased pulses, paresthesia, or paralysis of the involved muscles must be considered medical emergencies. The individual requires immediate referral for medical treatment. Chronic compartment syndromes usually present symptoms during exercise that subsequently subside with rest.

The diagnosis of compartment syndromes is based on the differential pressure (diastolic blood pressure minus intracompartmental pressure). A difference of 30 mm Hg may require a fasciotomy.[70,72] Compartmental pressures can also be monitored during exercise, an invasive technique performed in a medical facility. Increases of more than 15 mm Hg when resting, 30 mm Hg 1 minute after exercise, or 20 mm Hg 5 minutes post exercise are diagnostic signs of an exertional compartment syndrome.[65] An MRI may also be used to detect exertional compartment syndromes.[76]

After surgical fasciotomy of the compartments of the involved leg, the initial treatment and rehabilitation concerns involve adequate healing of the incision site because increased compartmental pressure and decreased blood flow may delay the healing process.[77] After wound healing has been established, therapeutic exercise to restore ROM and strength to the knee and ankle is begun. The patient is progressed with functional activities to return to full activity.

Deep Vein Thrombophlebitis

Thrombophlebitis, the inflammation of veins with associated blood clots, is most commonly found in postsurgical patients. However, is also may occur secondary to any trauma to the lower extremity. Patients with this condition complain of pain and tightness in the calf during walking. Inspection of the calf may reveal swelling. Palpation reveals warmth, tightness of the calf musculature, and pain. **Homan's sign** is used to clinically determine the possible presence of deep vein thrombosis (Box 5–11).

◆ ON-FIELD EVALUATION OF LOWER LEG AND ANKLE INJURIES

The goals of the on-field evaluation of patients with these injuries include ruling out fractures and dislocations, determining the athlete's weight-bearing status, and identifying the best method for removing the athlete from the field.

EQUIPMENT CONSIDERATIONS

The nature of competitive athletics brings with it ever more specialized footwear, braces, and types of tape. Although designed to protect athletes from injury while also improving performance, these devices may hinder the evaluation and management of acute injuries.

Footwear Removal

After a gross fracture or dislocation has been ruled out, the athlete's shoe must be removed so a thorough examination of the injury can be conducted after the athlete has reached the sideline. Most shoes may be easily removed by completely unlacing them, spreading the sides, and pulling the tongue down to the toes (Fig. 5–32). The athlete is asked to plantarflex the foot, if possible. The shoe is then removed by sliding the heel counter away from the foot and then lifting the shoe up and off the foot. Apprehensive athletes may be allowed to remove the shoe themselves. If a fracture or dislocation is suspected, the examiner should loosen the shoe enough to allow for palpation of the dorsalis pedis and posterior tibial pulses and transport the athlete with the shoe in place and the leg splinted.

Tape and Brace Removal

Prophylactic devices such as tape or ankle braces must be removed to allow for the complete examination of the foot and ankle. Braces tightened by laces or Velcro straps may be removed in a manner such as described for shoe removal. Ankle tape can be removed by cutting along a line parallel to the posterior portion of the malleolus on the side of the leg opposite the site of pain. The cut is then continued along the plantar aspect of the foot.

Box 5–11
HOMAN'S SIGN FOR DEEP VEIN THROMBOSIS

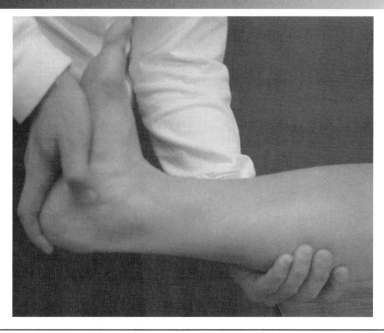

Homan's test for deep vein thrombosis. The calf is squeezed while the ankle is passively dorsiflexed. Indication of a positive result is a burning pain within the calf.

PATIENT POSITION	Sitting or supine with the knee extended
POSITION OF EXAMINER	At the end of the patient's leg with one hand on the plantar surface of the foot and the opposite hand grasping the calf.
EVALUATIVE PROCEDURE	The foot is passively dorsiflexed while the knee is kept extended. The examiner then squeezes the calf muscles.
POSITIVE TEST	Pain in the calf
IMPLICATIONS	Possible deep vein thrombophlebitis, this should be in agreement with other clinical findings of pain with deep palpation, swelling, heat, and dysfunction Ultrasonic imaging is used to make a definitive diagnosis of deep vein thrombosis
NOTE	A strain of the gastrocnemius or soleus may produce a false-positive result with this examination

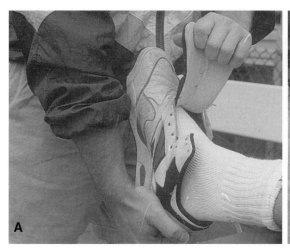
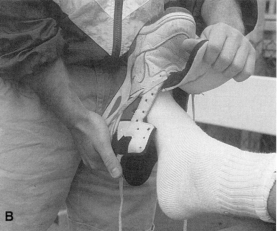

FIGURE 5–32. Removing the shoe following a foot or ankle injury. **(A)** After completely removing the laces, withdraw the tongue, and **(B)** slide the shoe from the foot.

ON-FIELD HISTORY

In the absence of gross deformity, the mechanism of injury and the associated sounds and sensations can help to identify the underlying pathology.

- **Mechanism of injury:** Identify the injurious forces placed on the ankle, keeping in mind that the injury may involve multiple forces (e.g., inversion and plantarflexion).

  - **Inversion:** Rolling the talus and calcaneus inward exerts tensile forces on the lateral aspect of the ankle and compressive forces on the medial aspect. Lateral ankle sprains, lateral ligament avulsions, and medial malleolar fractures are associated with this mechanism.
  - **Eversion:** Excessive eversion of the talus and calcaneus places tensile forces on the medial aspect of the ankle and compression on the lateral aspect. Syndesmotic ankle sprains and fractures of the lateral malleolus are also associated with this mechanism.
  - **Rotation:** Rotational forces can lead to syndemotic sprains or fracture of the tibia, fibula, or both.
  - **Dorsiflexion:** Forced dorsiflexion can strain or rupture the Achilles tendon or cause the distal tibiofibular syndesmosis to separate.
  - **Plantarflexion:** Although this mechanism is rare, forced plantarflexion can traumatize the extensor retinaculum and anterior joint capsule and its associated ligaments.

- **Associated sounds and sensations:** Ascertain for any sounds or sensations. A "snap" or "pop" may be associated with a ligament rupture or bony fracture. An audible snap or pop is also associated with an Achilles tendon rupture and may be described as being "kicked in the calf." Radiating pain or numbness in the anterior ankle and lower leg can indicate anterior compartment syndrome or trauma to the peroneal nerve.

ON-FIELD INSPECTION

During on-field inspection of ankle and lower leg injuries, any gross bony or joint injury must be ruled out before progressing to the other elements of the evaluation. Examine the contour and alignment of the lower leg, foot, and ankle, noting any discontinuity or malalignment of the structures that may indicate a fracture or dislocation.

ON-FIELD PALPATION

Assuming normal alignment of the lower leg, the evaluation proceeds to palpation of the bony structures and related soft tissue.

- **Bony palpation:** Begin by palpating the length of the tibia and fibula and continuing on to the talus, the remaining tarsals, and the MTs. Note any deformities, crepitus, or areas of point tenderness, especially in areas where pain is described. If a disruption of a long bone or joint is felt, splint the joint and transport the athlete to a hospital.
- **Soft tissue palpation:** Perform a quick yet thorough evaluation of the major soft tissues, emphasizing the ligamentous structures for point tenderness and the tendons for signs of rupture.

ON-FIELD RANGE OF MOTION TESTS

After the possibility of a gross fracture or dislocation has been ruled out, the athlete's ability to move the limb and subsequently bear weight must be established.

- **Willingness to move the involved limb:** If the athlete displays normal alignment of the limb, observe his or her willingness to move the injured body part through the full ROM. This task should be performed with a minimal amount of discomfort. If the athlete has no ability or is unwilling to move the involved limb, use assistance to remove the athlete from the field.
- **Willingness to bear weight:** If the athlete describes no pain and there are no signs of restriction in the ROM, assist the athlete to the standing position, bearing weight on the uninvolved leg. Assistance is provided by assuming position under the athlete's arm on the involved side, giving some support. The athlete should walk off the field, attempting to place as little weight as possible on the involved limb.

◆ INITIAL MANAGEMENT OF ON-FIELD INJURIES

This section describes the emergency management procedures for major trauma occurring to the ankle and lower extremity. Most ankle injuries (e.g., sprains, Achilles tendon ruptures) are managed on the sidelines or in athletic training rooms. On-field care involves ruling out the presence of a fracture or neurovascular deficit, keeping the injured body from bearing weight, and removing the athlete from the playing field.

ANKLE DISLOCATIONS

Resulting from excessive rotation combined with inversion or eversion, dislocations of the talocrural joint result in major disruptions of the joint capsule and associated ligaments. Associated fractures of the malleoli, long bones, or talus often occur. Resulting in immediate pain in the ankle and lower leg and loss of function, the patient may also report an audible snap or crack. The

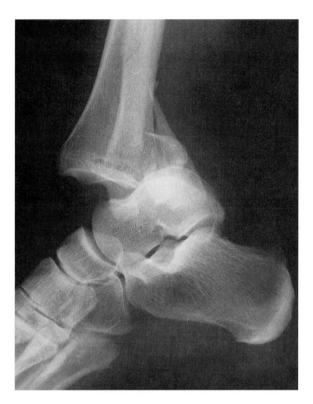

FIGURE 5–33. Posterior ankle dislocation. Often the talus displaces anteriorly relative to the tibia. This radiograph shows the talus being displaced posteriorly relative to the tibia. Note the fracture of the malleolus caused by the wide anterior talar border's being forced into the mortise.

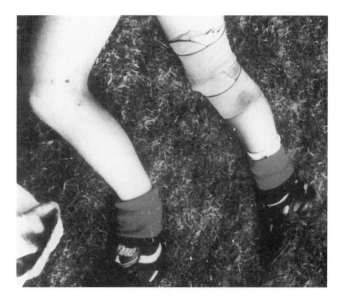

FIGURE 5–34. Obvious deformity caused by a lower leg fracture and possible ankle dislocation.

MANAGEMENT OF LOWER LEG FRACTURES AND DISLOCATIONS

Any obvious fracture or joint dislocation should immediately be immobilized using a moldable or vacuum splint (see Fig. 1–14). In most cases, it is recommended that the shoe be left in place while the athlete is being transported to the hospital. It may be more safely removed in the emergency room after further diagnostic tests, such as radiographic examination, to determine the full extent of the injury (Fig. 5–35). The laces and tongue of the shoe are loosened and the sock is cut to permit palpation of the dorsalis pedis and the posterior

foot and ankle may be grossly malaligned. If the defect is not visible, the superior portion of the talus may be palpated as it protrudes anteriorly from the ankle mortise (Fig. 5–33). The evaluation also must confirm the presence of the distal pulses and include a secondary survey of the ankle mortise and long bones for possible fracture.

LOWER LEG FRACTURES

Acute fractures and dislocations of the lower leg, especially those involving the tibial shaft, often exhibit obvious gross deformity (Fig. 5–34). In many instances, the patient and others in the vicinity of the injury report an audible snap (or crack) at the time of injury. Pain is reported along the fracture site, possibly radiating up the lower leg and extremity. Palpation may reveal crepitus or discontinuity along the bone shaft. If a bony defect is visible, palpation need not be performed. Although long bone fractures normally result in immediate dysfunction and an inability to bear weight, those suffering from fibular fractures may be capable of walking. In cases in which deformity or other signs of a gross fracture are absent, the squeeze test may be used to confirm a fibular fracture. The bump test may be used for calcaneal or talar fractures or hairline fractures of the tibia.

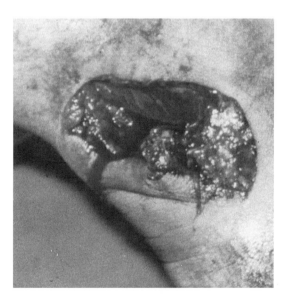

FIGURE 5–35. This apparent laceration is actually an open dislocation of the talus.

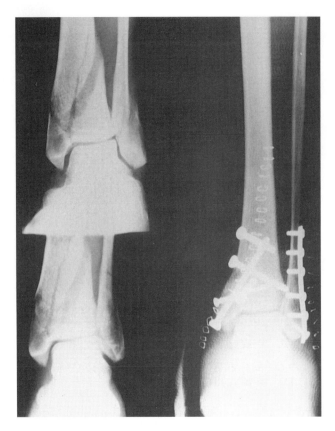

FIGURE 5–36. Radiograph showing screws and plates used to set a fracture of the ankle joint.

tibial pulses, which are then compared bilaterally and continually monitored.

Management of a compound fracture involves controlling bleeding and immobilizing the fracture. The area around the compound fracture should be packed with sterile bandages without causing any further disruption at the fracture site. After bleeding is controlled, the extremity can be immobilized in the position in which it is found, the pulses continually monitored, and the athlete transported to a medical facility.

Nondisplaced fibular or tibial fractures may be treated by simple casting. Comminuted or displaced fractures often require the use of internal or external fixation devices to realign and stabilize the fracture sites. A fracture of the distal fibula involving the syndesmosis may require an internal fixation device or a screw to maintain the alignment of the fibula with the tibia during the healing process and to prevent subsequent rotational instabilities of the talus (Fig. 5–36).[78]

ANTERIOR COMPARTMENT SYNDROME

Unlike other acute soft tissue injuries, suspected anterior compartment syndromes are not be treated with compression. The use of external compression devices, such as wraps or compression boots, increase the pres-

sure within the anterior compartment, thus exacerbating the condition. If acute gross hemorrhage is present or the dorsalis pedis pulse is absent, the athlete must be immediately referred for medical intervention. If, at the time of the injury, the athlete does not display signs of intracompartmental hemorrhage but there is reason to suspect such a response, provide the athlete with a list of the danger signs and symptoms (see Table 5–15) and instruct the athlete about contacting a physician if the symptoms worsen.

◆ REFERENCES

1. Campbell, DG, et al: Dynamic ankle ultrasonography. A new imaging technique for acute ankle ligament injuries. *Am J Sports Med* 22:855, 1994.
2. Garrick, JM: The frequency of injury, mechanism of injury, and epidemiology of ankle sprains. *Am J Sports Med* 5:241, 1971.
3. Garrick, JG, and Requa, RK: The epidemiology of foot and ankle injuries in sports. *Clin Sports Medicine* 7:29, 1988.
4. Takebe, K, et al: Role of the fibula in weight-bearing. *Clin Orthop* 184:2899, 1984.
5. Burks, RT, and Morgan, J: Anatomy of the lateral ankle ligaments. *Am J Sports Med* 22:72, 1994.
6. Norkin, CC, and Levangie, PK: The ankle-foot complex. In Norkin, CC, and Levangie, PK (eds): *Joint Structure and Function: A Comprehensive Analysis*, ed 2. Philadelphia, FA Davis, 1992, p. 383.
7. Doughtie, M: Syndesmotic ankle sprains in football: A survey of National Football League athletic trainers. *Journal of Athletic Training*, 34:15, 1999.
8. Breitenseher, MJ, et al: MRI of the sinus tarsi in acute ankle injuries. *J Comput Assist Tomogr*, 21:274, 1997.
9. Copeland, SA: Rupture of the Achilles tendon: A new clinical test. *Ann R Coll Surg Engl*. 72:270, 1990.
10. Fallat, L, Grimm, DL, and Saracco, JA: Sprained ankle syndrome: Prevalence and analysis of 639 acute injuries. *J Foot Ankle Surg*, 37:280, 1998.
11. Barrett, J, and Bilisko, T: The role of shoes in the prevention of ankle sprains. *Sports Med*, 20:277, 1995.
12. Yeung, MS, et al: An epidemiological survey on ankle sprains. *Br J Sports Med*, 28:112, 1994.
13. Johnson, MB, and Johnson, CL: Electromyographic response of peroneal muscles in surgical and nonsurgical injured ankles during sudden inversion. *J Orthop Sports Phys Ther*, 18:497, 1993.
14. Isalov, E: Response of peroneal muscles to sudden inversion of the ankle during standing. *Int J Sport Biomech*, 2:100, 1986.
15. Freeman, MAR: Treatment of ruptures of the lateral ligament of the ankle. *J Bone Joint Surg Br*, 47:661, 1965.
16. Freeman, MAR, et al: The etiology and prevention of functional instability of the foot. *J Bone Joint Surg Br*, 47:678, 1965.
17. Frey, C, et al: A comparison of MRI and clinical examination of acute lateral ankle sprains. *Foot Ankle Int*, 17:533, 1996.
18. Meislin, RJ, et al: Arthroscopic treatment of synovial impingement of the ankle. *Am J Sports Med*, 21:186, 1993.
19. Pinar, H, et al: Bone bruises detected by magnetic resonance imaging following lateral ankle sprains. *Knee Surg Sports Traumatol Arthrosc*, 5:113, 1997.
20. Taga, I: Articular cartilage lesions in ankles with lateral ligament injury: An arthroscopic study. *Am J Sports Med*, 21:120, 1993.
21. Loomer, R, et al: Osteochondral lesions of the talus. *Am J Sports Med*, 21:13, 1993.
22. Bassett, FH: A simple surgical approach to the posteromedial ankle. *Am J Sports Med*, 21:144, 1993.
23. Bullock-Saxton, JE: Local sensations and altered hip muscle function following severe ankle sprain. *Phys Ther*, 74:17, 1994.
24. Dettori, JR, et al: Early ankle mobilization, part I: The immediate effect on acute, lateral ankle sprains (a randomized clinical trial). *Mil Med*, 159:15, 1994.

25. Eiff, MP, Smith, AT, and Smith, GE: Early mobilization versus immobilization in the treatment of lateral ankle sprains. *Am J Sports Med*, 22:83, 1994.
26. Dettori, JR, and Basmania, CJ: Early ankle mobilization, part II: A one-year follow up of acute, lateral ankle sprains (a randomized clinical trial). *Mil Med*, 159:20, 1994.
27. Boytim, MJ, Fischer, DA, and Neumann, L: Syndesmotic ankle sprains. *Am J Sports Med*, 19:294, 1991.
28. Teitz, CC, and Harrington, RM: A biomechanical analysis of the squeeze test for sprains of the syndesmotic ligaments of the ankle. *Foot Ankle Int*, 19:489, 1998.
29. Veltri, DM, et al: Symptomatic ossification of the tibiofibular syndesmosis in professional football players: A sequela of the syndesmotic ankle sprain. *Foot Ankle Int*, 16:285, 1995.
30. Garrick, JG, and Requa, RK: Role of external support in the prevention of ankle sprains. *Med Sci Sports Exerc*, 5:200, 1973.
31. Giladi, M, et al: Stress fractures. Identifiable risk factors. *Am J Sports Med*, 19:647, 1991.
32. Saltzman, CL, Nawoczenski, DA, and Talbot, KD: Measurement of the medial longitudinal arch. *Arch Phys Med Rehabil*, 76:45, 1995.
33. Blake, RL, Lallas, PJ, and Ferguson, H: The os trigonum syndrome. A literature review. *J Am Podiatr Med Assoc*, 82:154, 1992.
34. Ihle, CL, and Cochran, KM: Fracture of the fused os trigonum. *Am J Sports Med*, 10:47, 1982.
35. Sarrafin, S: *Anatomy of the Foot and Ankle*. Philadelphia, J.B. Lippincott, 1983, p. 47.
36. Brodsky, AE, and Khalil, M: Talar compression syndrome. *Am J Sports Med*, 14:472, 1986.
37. Paulos, LE et al: Posterior compartment fracture of the ankles: A commonly missed athletic injury. *Am J Sports Med*, 11:439, 1983.
38. McDougall, A: The os trigonum. *J Bone Joint Surg Br*, 37:257, 1955.
39. Karasick, D, and Schweitzer, ME: The os trigonum syndrome: Imaging features. *AJR Am J Roentgenol*, 166:125, 1996.
40. Masciocchi, C, Catalucci, A and Barile, A: Ankle impingement syndromes. *Eur J Radiol*, 27(S1):S70, 1998.
41. Ahmed, IM, et al: Blood supply of the Achilles tendon. *J Orthop Res*, 16:591, 1998.
42. Scioli, MW: Achilles tendinitis. *Orthop Clin North Am*, 25:177, 1994.
43. Puddu, G, et al: A classification of Achilles tendon disease. *Am J Sports Med*, 4:145, 1976.
44. Gillet, P, et al: Magnetic resonance imaging may be an asset to diagnose and classify fluorouinolone-associated Achilles tendinitis. *Fundam Clin Pharmacol*, 9:52, 1995.
45. Astrom, M, and Rausing, A: Chronic Achilles tendinopathy. A survey of surgical and histopathic findings. *Clin Orthop*, Jul:151, 1995.
46. Astrom, M: Partial rupture in chronic Achilles tendinopathy. A retrospective analysis of 342 cases. *Acta Orthop Scand*, 69:404, 1998.
47. Alfredson, H: Achilles tendinosis and calf muscle strength. The effect of short-term immobilization after surgical treatment. *Am J Sports Med*, 26:166, 1998.
48. Shrier, I, Matheson, GO, and Kohl, HW 3rd: Achilles tendonitis: are corticosteroid injections useful or harmful? *Clin J Sport Med*, 6:245, 1996.
49. Leppilahti, J and Orava, S: Total achilles tendon rupture: A review. *Sports Med*, 25:79, 1998.
50. Saltzman, C, and Bonar, S: Tendon problems of the foot and ankle. In Lutter, LD, Mizel, MS, and Pfeffer, GB (eds): *Orthopaedic Knowledge Update: Foot and Ankle*. Rosemont, IL, American Academy of Orthopaedic Surgeons, 1994, p. 271.
51. Shrier, I, Matheson, GO, and Kohl, HW: Achilles tendonitis: Are corticosteroid injections useful or harmful? *Clin J Sports Med*, 6:245, 1996.
52. Read, MT: Safe relief of rest pain that eases with activity in achillodynia by intrabursal or peritendinous steroid injection: The rupture rate was not increased by these steroid injections. *Br J Sports Med*, 33:134, 1996.
53. Fierro, NL, and Sallis, RE: Achilles tendon rupture. Is casting enough? *Postgrad Med*, 98:145, 1995.
54. Troop, RL, et al: Early motion after repair of Achilles tendon ruptures. *Foot Ankle Int*, 16:705, 1995.
55. Nistor, L. Surgical and non-surgical treatment of the Achilles tendon rupture. *J Bone Joint Surg*, 63A:394–399, 1981.
56. Schweitzer, ME, et al: Using MR imaging to differentiate peroneal splits from other peroneal disorders. *AJR Am J Roentgenol*, 168:129, 1997.
57. Yao, L: MR Findings in peroneal tendonopathy. *J Comput Assist Tomogr*, 19:460, 1995.
58. Krause, JO, and Brodsky, JW: Peroneus brevis tendon tears: Pathophysiology, surgical reconstruction, and clinical results. *Foot Ankle Int*, 19:271, 1998.
59. Boles, MA, et al: Enlarged peroneal process with peroneus longus tendon entrapment. *Skeletal Radiol*, 26:313, 1997.
60. Mason, RB, and Henderson, JP: Traumatic peroneal tendon instability. *Am J Sports Med*, 24:652, 1996.
61. Magnano, GM, et al: High-resolution US of non-traumatic recurrent dislocation of the peroneal tendons: A case report. *Pediatr Radiol*, 28:476, 1998.
62. Shellock, FG, et al: Peroneal tendons: Use of kinematic MR imaging of the ankle to determine subluxation. *J Magn Reson Imaging*, 7:451, 1997.
63. Karlsson, J, Eriksson, BI, and Sward, L: Recurrent dislocation of the peroneal tendons. *Scand J Med Sci Sports*, 6:242, 1996.
64. Kollias, SL, and Ferkel, RD: Fibular grooving for recurrent peroneal tendon subluxation. *Am J Sports Med*, 25:329, 1997.
65. Sollsteimer, GT, and Shelton, WR: Acute atraumatic compartment syndrome in an athlete: A case report. *J Athletic Training*, 32:248, 1997.
66. Turnipseed, WD, Hurschler, C, and Vanderby, R Jr: The effects of elevated compartment pressure on tibial arteriovenous flow and relationship of mechanical and biochemical characteristics of fascia to genesis of chronic anterior compartment syndrome. *J Vasc Surg*, 21:810, 1995.
67. Pedowitz, RA, and Gershuni, DH: Diagnosis and treatment of chronic compartment syndrome. *Crit Rev Phys Rehabil Med*, 5:301, 1993.
68. Genuario, SE: Differential diagnosis: Exertional compartment syndromes, stress fractures, and shin splints. *Athletic Training: Journal of the National Athletic Trainers Association*, 24:31, 1989.
69. McQueen, MM, Christie, J, and Court-Brown, CM: Acute compartment syndrome in tibial diaphyseal fractures. *J Bone Joint Surg Br*, 78:95, 1996.
70. McQueen, MM, and Court-Brown, CM: Compartment monitoring in tibial fractures: The pressure threshold for decompression. *J Bone Joint Surg Br*, 78:99, 1996.
71. Heckman, MM, et al: Compartment pressure in association with closed tibial fractures. The relationship between tissue pressure, compartment, and the distance from the site of the fracture. *J Bone Joint Surg Am*, 76:1285, 1994.
72. McQueen, M: Acute anterior compartment syndrome. *Acta Chir Belg*, 98:166, 1998.
73. Chautems, RC, et al: Spontaneous anterior and lateral tibial compartment syndrome in a type I diabetic patient. *J Trauma*, 43:140, 1997.
74. Jerosch, J, et al: Secondary effects of knee braces on the intracompartmental pressure in the anterior tibial compartment. *Acta Orthop Belg*, 61:37, 1995.
75. Jerosch, J, et al: Influence on the running shoe sole on the pressure in the anterior tibial compartment. *Acta Orthop Belg*, 61:190, 1995.
76. Eskelin, MK, Lotjonen, JM, and Mantysaari, MJ: Chronic exertional compartment syndrome: MR imaging at 0.1 T compared with tissue pressure measurement. *Radiology*, 206:333, 1998.
77. Schepis, A, Gill, SS, and Foster, TA: Fasciotomy for exertional anterior compartment syndrome: Is lateral compartment release necessary? *Am J Sports Med*, 27:430, 1999.
78. Michelson, J: Controversies in ankle fractures. *Foot and Ankle*, 14:170, 1993.

The Knee

The knee complex, consisting of the tibiofemoral and patellofemoral joints, is tenuously constructed with little bony support and relies on soft tissue structures to control forces transmitted through the joint. Because the joint is located between the body's two longest lever arms, the femur and lower leg, extreme forces are placed on the knee's structures. This chapter discusses injury to the knee and related muscles. The patella, as it relates to the knee joint proper, is described in this chapter. Conditions that are exclusive to the patellofemoral articulation are described in Chapter 7, and injury to the quadriceps and hamstring muscle groups are addressed in Chapter 8.

◆ CLINICAL ANATOMY

The term "tibiofemoral joint" seems to imply that the knee involves only the articulation between the tibia and femur. In fact, it involves articulation among the femur, menisci, and tibia, all of which must function together. The patellofemoral mechanism must also be functioning properly to ensure adequate tibiofemoral mechanics. The superior tibiofibular syndesmosis, although not a part of the knee articulation, also influences knee function.

The length of the **femur,** the longest and strongest bone in the body, is approximately one quarter of the body's total height.[1] The femur's posterior aspect is demarcated by the **linea aspera,** a bony ridge spanning the length of the shaft (Fig. 6–1). As the femur reaches its distal end, the shaft broadens to form the medial and lateral condyles.

The **medial and lateral condyles** are convex structures covered with hyaline cartilage that articulate with the tibia. These structures have a discrete anteroposterior curvature that is convex in the **frontal plane.** The articular surface of the medial condyle is longer than that of the lateral condyle and flares outward posteriorly. The condyles share a common anterior surface, then diverge posteriorly, becoming separated by the deep **intercondylar notch.** An anterior depression

forms the **femoral trochlea** through which the patella glides as the knee moves in flexion and extension. The lateral and medial epicondyles arise off the condyles. The **lateral epicondyle** is wider and emanates from the femoral shaft at a lesser angle than the **medial epicondyle** does. The **adductor tubercle** arises off the superior crest of the medial epicondyle.

The **medial and lateral tibial plateaus** correspond to the femoral condyles. The medial tibial plateau is concave in both the frontal and sagittal planes. The lateral

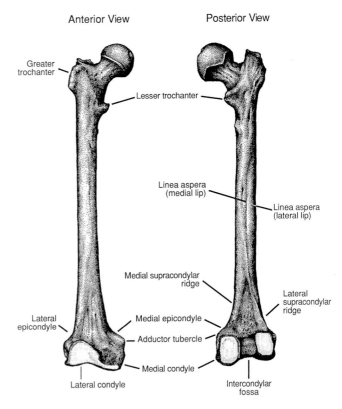

Anterior View   Posterior View

Greater trochanter

Lesser trochanter

Linea aspera (medial lip)

Linea aspera (lateral lip)

Medial supracondylar ridge

Lateral supracondylar ridge

Lateral epicondyle

Medial epicondyle

Adductor tubercle

Medial condyle

Lateral condyle

Intercondylar fossa

FIGURE 6–1. Anterior and posterior view of the femur. Note that the single anterior articular surface on the femur's condyles diverges posteriorly to form a lateral and medial compartment of the knee joint.

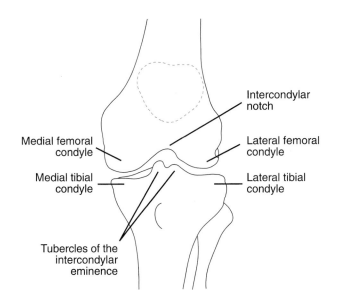

FIGURE 6–2. Articular structure of the knee. The articulation between the femoral and tibial condyles is enhanced by the menisci. The tubercles of the intercondylar eminence align with the intercondylar notch.

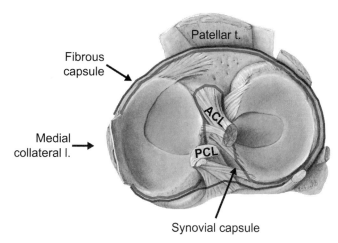

FIGURE 6–3. The knee's joint capsules. The fibrous capsular membrane completely envelops the bony surface of the knee. The synovial capsular membrane surrounds the medial and lateral articular surfaces but invaginates to exclude the cruciate ligaments.

articular plateau is concave in the frontal plane and convex in the sagittal plane. The medial tibial plateau is 50 percent larger than the lateral plateau to accommodate for the flare of the femur's medial condyle. Intercondylar eminences, raised areas between the tibial plateaus that match the femur's intercondylar notch, separate the two condyles (Fig. 6–2). On the anterior portion of the tibia is the **tibial tuberosity,** the site of the patellar tendon's distal attachment.

Two bones outside the tibiofemoral articulation directly affect the knee's function and stability. The **patella,** a sesamoid bone located in the patellar tendon (ligament), improves the mechanical function of the quadriceps during knee extension, dissipates the forces received from the *extensor mechanism,* and protects the anterior portion of the knee. Several of the soft tissues on the lateral aspect of the knee attach to the **fibular head.** Fracture of the proximal fibula or injury to the **proximal tibiofibular syndesmosis** can affect the stability of the knee.

ARTICULATIONS AND LIGAMENTOUS SUPPORT

The presence of the medial and lateral articular condyles classifies the tibiofemoral joint as a **double condyloid articulation,** capable of freedom of motion in two planes: (1) flexion and extension and (2) internal and external rotation. The other movements occurring between the tibia and femur, such as valgus and varus bending and anterior and posterior glide, are *accessory motions* attributed to the joint's anatomical structure. These motions can be increased after damage to one or more of the knee's ligaments or decreased by the formation of scar tissue.

Joint Capsule

A fibrous joint capsule surrounds the circumference of the knee joint. Along the medial, anterior, and lateral aspects of the joint, the capsule arises superior to the femoral condyles and attaches distal to the tibial plateau. Posteriorly, the capsule inserts on the posterior margins of the femoral condyles above the joint line, and inferiorly, to the posterior tibial condyle. The strength of the capsule is reinforced by the medial collateral ligament (MCL), patellofemoral ligaments, and retinaculum medially and laterally; the oblique popliteal ligament and arcuate ligaments posteriorly; and the patellar tendon anteriorly. Further reinforcement is gained from the muscles that cross the knee joint.

A **synovial capsule** lines the articular portions of the fibrous joint capsule. The synovium surrounds the articular condyles of the femur and tibia medially, anteriorly, and laterally. On the posterior portion of the articulation, the synovial capsule invaginates anteriorly along the femur's intercondylar notch and the tibia's intercondylar eminences, excluding the cruciate ligaments from the synovial membrane (Fig. 6–3).

Extensor mechanism The mechanism formed by the quadriceps and patellofemoral joint responsible for causing extension of the lower leg at the knee joint.

Accessory motion Motion that accompanies active movement and is necessary for normal motion but cannot be voluntarily isolated.

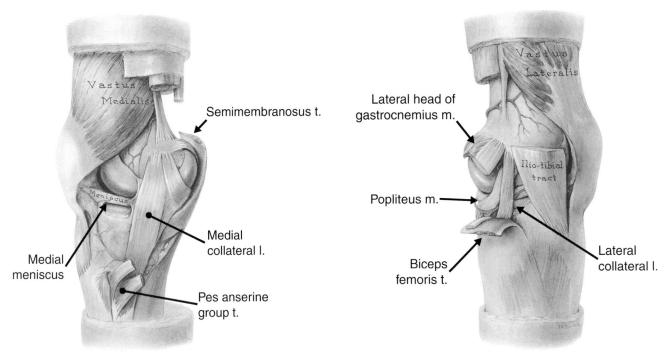

FIGURE 6–4. Medial collateral ligament. Arising from a broad band on the medial femoral epicondyle just below the adductor tubercle, it tapers inward to attach on the medial tibial plateau. Consisting of two layers separated by a bursa, the deep layer is continuous with the medial joint capsule and has an attachment on the medial meniscus.

FIGURE 6–5. Lateral collateral ligament. This ropelike structure originates from the lateral femoral epicondyle and attaches to the apex of the fibular head. The lateral collateral ligament is an extracapsular structure.

Collateral Ligaments

The **medial collateral ligament** (MCL) is the primary medial stabilizer of the knee. Formed by two layers, the **deep layer** is a thickening of the joint capsule and is attached to the medial meniscus. Separated from the deep layer by a bursa, the **superficial layer** arises from a broad band just below the adductor tubercle to insert on a relatively narrow site 7 to 10 cm below the joint line (Fig. 6–4). As a unit, the two layers of the MCL are tight in complete extension. As the knee is flexed to the midrange, its anterior fibers are taut; in complete flexion, the posterior fibers are tight. The MCL primarily acts to protect the knee against valgus forces while also providing a secondary restraint against external rotation of the tibia and anterior translation of the tibia on the femur, especially in the absence of an intact anterior cruciate ligament (ACL).

Unlike the MCL, the **lateral collateral ligament** (LCL) has no attachment to the joint capsule or meniscus. This cordlike structure arises from the lateral femoral epicondyle, sharing a common site of origin with the lateral joint capsule, and inserts on the proximal aspect of the fibular head (Fig. 6–5). The LCL is the primary restraint against varus forces when the knee is between full extension and 30 degrees of flexion. This structure also provides secondary restraint against internal and external rotation of the tibia on the femur.

Cruciate Ligaments

The cruciate ligaments, although intraarticular, are located outside of the synovial capsule (see Fig. 6–3). The ACL arises from the anteromedial intercondylar eminence of the tibia, travels posteriorly, and passes lateral to the posterior cruciate ligament (PCL) to insert on the medial wall of the lateral femoral condyle (Fig. 6–6). The ACL serves as a static stabilizer against:

1. Anterior translation of the tibia on the femur
2. Internal rotation of the tibia on the femur
3. External rotation of the tibia on the femur
4. Hyperextension of the tibiofemoral joint

The ACL has two discrete segments: an **anteromedial bundle** and a **posterolateral bundle**.[2] As the knee moves from extension into flexion, a juxtaposition of the ACL's attachment sites occurs. When the knee is fully extended, the femoral attachment of the anteromedial bundle is anterior to the attachment of the posterolateral bundle. When the knee is flexed, the relative positions are reversed, causing the ACL to wind upon itself (Fig. 6–7). This leads to varying portions of the ACL being taut as the knee moves through its range of motion (ROM). When the knee is fully extended, the posterolateral bundle is tight; when the knee is fully flexed, the anteromedial bundle is taut.

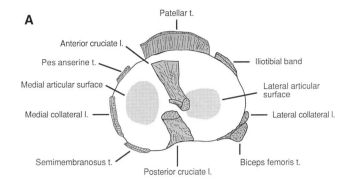

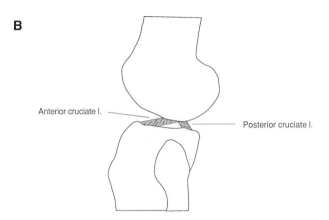

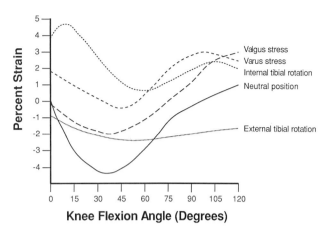

FIGURE 6–8. Strain placed on the anterior cruciate ligament through the passive range of motion. Altering the relative alignment of the tibia to the femur increases the strain on the ligament throughout the range of motion.

FIGURE 6–6. Cruciate ligaments. The ligaments are named according to their relative attachment on the tibia. **(A)** Superior view referencing the cruciate ligaments to each other and to other supportive structures about the knee. **(B)** Lateral view of the cruciate ligaments.

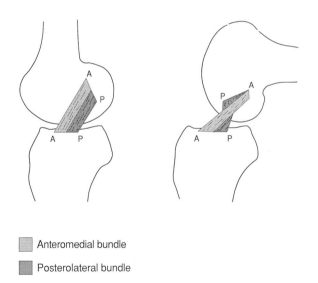

☐ Anteromedial bundle

■ Posterolateral bundle

FIGURE 6–7. Biomechanics of the anterior cruciate ligament. When the knee is fully extended, the femoral attachment site of the anteromedial bundle (A) is proximal to the attachment site of the posterolateral bundle (P). When the knee is flexed, these attachment sites juxtapose their positions, causing the anterior cruciate to wind upon itself.

The amount of strain placed on the ACL is influenced by the type of movement. During passive ROM (PROM), the amount of strain placed on the ACL is minimized when the tibia remains in the neutral position. In the final 15 degrees of extension, internally rotating the tibia greatly increases the strain placed on the ACL; externally rotating the tibia decreases the strain. Both valgus and varus stresses increase the strain placed in the ACL during PROM (Fig. 6–8).[3] During active ROM (AROM), the amount of strain placed on the ACL is greatest between 0 and 30 degrees of flexion.[4] Resisted ROM significantly increases the amount of strain between 0 and 45 degrees of flexion.[4]

The PCL arises from the posterior aspect of the tibia and takes a superior and anterior course, passing medially to the ACL, to attach on the lateral portion of the femur's medial condyle. The PCL, stronger and wider than the ACL, is considered the primary stabilizer of the knee.[5,6]

The PCL has three distinct components: the anterolateral, posteromedial, and meniscofemoral segments, each possessing unique biomechanical and anatomic properties.[7,8] As an entire unit, the PCL is the primary restraint against posterior displacement of the tibia on the femur and a secondary restraint against external tibial rotation.

Although the PCL offers significant support against posterior forces on the knee joint, its function is augmented by the posterolateral structures of the knee, specifically the popliteus complex.[9] A combined injury to the PCL and posterolateral structures results in greater posterior laxity than when either structure is affected alone.[10,11] When the knee is near extension, the primary restraint against posterior displacement of the tibia on the femur is obtained from the popliteus, posterior capsule, and other joint structures.[12] In the midrange of motion (40 to 120 degrees of flexion) the anterolateral bundle is the primary restraint against posterior tibial displacement; beyond 120 degrees of flexion, the posteromedial bundle also becomes taut.[12]

During the **screw home mechanism,** the PCL and ACL wind upon each other in flexion and unwind in extension. Damage to the PCL can result in an inherently unstable knee, not only in the frontal plane but also in the transverse plane because the axis of tibial rotation is removed.

Arcuate Ligament Complex

The **arcuate ligament complex,** formed by the arcuate ligament, LCL, oblique popliteal ligament, popliteus tendon, and lateral head of the gastrocnemius, provides support to the posterolateral joint capsule (Fig. 6–9). The oblique popliteal ligament arises off the tibia's medial condyle, traveling superiorly and laterally to attach on the middle portion of the posterior joint capsule, then merging into the semimembranosus tendon and arcuate ligament. Arising from the fibular head, the arcuate ligament passes over the popliteus muscle, where it diverges to insert on the intercondylar area of the tibia and the posterior aspect of the femur's lateral epicondyle. The arcuate ligament complex assists the cruciate ligaments in controlling posterolateral rotatory instability. Injury to this area results in increased external rotation of the tibia on the femur.

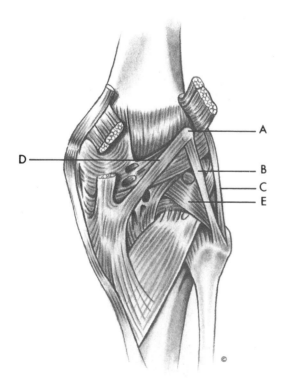

FIGURE 6–9. Structures of the posterolateral knee. (A) Fabella, (B) fabellofibular ligament, (C) lateral collateral ligament, (D) oblique popliteal ligament, and (E) arcuate ligament.

The fabella, when present, lies within the biceps femoris muscle. Although of little significance to the structure and function of the knee, when the fabella is present, a fabellofibular ligament attaches from the fabella to the fibular head, increasing the thickness of the tissues in the posterolateral corner of the knee.

Proximal Tibiofibular Syndesmosis

The proximal tibiofibular syndesmosis is more stable than the distal tibiofibular syndesmosis because of the alignment between the fibular head and the indentation on the proximal tibia. The superior tibiofibular joint is stabilized by the superior anterior and posterior tibiofibular ligaments and, to a lesser degree, by the interosseous membrane. Anterior displacement of the fibula is partially blocked by a bony outcrop from the tibia. Therefore, most fibular instabilities tend to occur posteriorly, possibly affecting the peroneal nerve.

THE MENISCI

The anatomic incongruence between the articular surfaces of the tibia and femur is somewhat remedied by the presence of the fibrocartilaginous medial and lateral menisci. The menisci serve to:

1. Deepen the articulation and fill the gaps that normally occur during the knee's articulation, increasing load transmission over a greater percentage of the joint surfaces
2. Improve lubrication for the articulating surfaces
3. Provide shock absorption
4. Increase the stability of the joint

When viewed in cross section, the menisci are wedge shaped, with their outer borders thicker than their inner rims. When viewed from above, this wedge creates a concave area on the tibia to accept the femur's articulating surfaces. Because of this geometry, the knee is more stable when it is bearing weight than when it is not.

Each meniscus is divided into an anterior, middle, and posterior third (Fig. 6–10). The anterior and posterior portions of the menisci are marked by the horns, the area of the menisci most frequently torn. The menisci have a narrow **vascular zone** along their outer rim and an **avascular zone** formed by the inner portion of the meniscus. Because of the presence of an active blood supply, meniscal tears occurring within the vascular zone have an improved chance of healing compared to tears in the avascular zone, which rely on nutrients' being delivered through the synovial fluid.

The **medial meniscus** resembles a half crescent, or C shape, that is wider posteriorly than it is anteriorly. The **lateral meniscus** is more circular in shape. Both menisci are attached at their peripheries to the tibia via the **coronary ligament.** The anterior horns of each meniscus are joined together by the **transverse liga-**

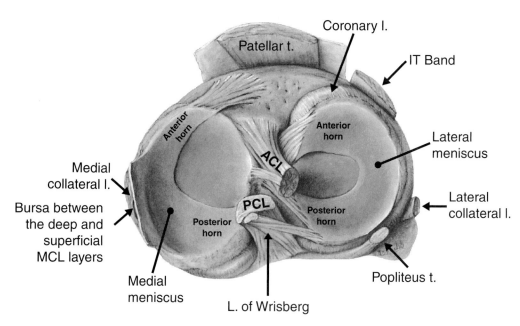

FIGURE 6–10. Superior view of the medial and lateral meniscus and their associated ligamentous structures. The peripheral border of the menisci is fixated to the tibia by the coronary ligament.

ment and connected to the patellar tendon via **patellomeniscal ligaments.**

The lateral meniscus, smaller and more mobile than the medial meniscus, attaches to the lateral aspect of the medial femoral condyle via the **meniscofemoral ligaments** (the **ligament of Wrisberg** and the **ligament of Humphrey**) and to the popliteus muscle via the joint capsule and coronary ligament. During knee extension, patellomensical ligaments pull the lateral meniscus anteriorly, distorting its shape in the anteroposterior plane. In the early degrees of flexion, the popliteus pulls the lateral meniscus posteriorly; in the later ROM, the meniscofemoral ligament pulls the posterior horn medially and anteriorly.[13]

MUSCLES OF THE KNEE

The muscles acting on the knee primarily serve to flex or extend it. The flexor musculature has the secondary responsibility of rotating the tibia. The flexors attaching on the tibia's medial side internally rotate it, and those attaching on the lateral side externally rotate it. The muscles acting on the knee, their origins, insertions, and innervation are presented in Table 6–1.

Anterior Muscles

Although its name implies the presence of four muscles, the **quadriceps femoris** muscle group is best described as five muscles, the **vastus lateralis, vastus intermedius, vastus medialis, vastus medialis oblique,** and **rectus femoris.** Each of the quadriceps femoris muscles has a common insertion on the tibial tuberosity

via the patellar tendon (Fig. 6–11). The vastus medialis has two discrete groups of fibers arising from the medial femoral condyle and the fascia of the adductor magnus. Separated by a fascial plane, the muscle is divided into the vastus medialis longus and the vastus

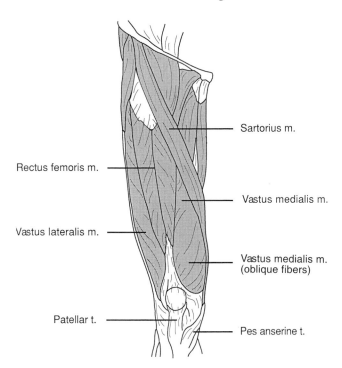

FIGURE 6–11. Anterior muscles acting on the knee. The vastus lateralis, rectus femoris, vastus intermedius (hidden beneath the rectus femoris), and vastus medialis share a common insertion via the patellar tendon.

Table 6–1
MUSCLES ACTING ON THE KNEE

Muscle	Action	Origin	Insertion	Innervation	Root
Biceps femoris	Knee flexion External tibial rotation Long head Hip Extension Hip external rotation	Long head Ischial tuberosity Sacrotuberous ligament Short head Lateral lip of the linea aspera Upper two-thirds of the supracondylar line	Lateral fibular head Lateral tibial condyle	Long head Tibial Short head Common peroneal	Long head S1, S2, S3 Short head L5, S1, S2
Gastrocnemius	Assists knee flexion Ankle plantarflexion	Medial head Posterior surface of the medial femoral condyle Adjacent portion of the femur and knee capsule Lateral head Posterior surface of the lateral femoral condyle Adjacent portion of the femur and knee capsule	To the calcaneus via the Achilles tendon	Tibial	S1, S2
Gracilis	Knee flexion Internal tibial rotation Hip adduction	Symphysis pubis Inferior ramus of the pubic bone	Proximal portion of the antero-medial tibial flare	Obturator (posterior)	L3, L4
Popliteus	Open chain Internal tibial rotation Knee flexion Closed chain External femoral rotation Knee flexion	Lateral femoral condyle Oblique popliteal ligament	Posterior tibia superior to the soleal line Fascia covering the soleus	Tibial	L4, L5, S1
Rectus femoris	Knee extension Hip flexion	Anterior inferior iliac spine Groove located superior to the acetabulum	To the tibial tubercle via the patella and patellar ligament	Femoral	L2, L3, L4

Muscle	Action	Origin	Insertion	Nerve	Root
Sartorius	Knee flexion Internal tibial rotation Hip flexion Hip abduction Hip external rotation	Anterior superior iliac spine	Proximal portion of the anteromedial tibial flare	Femoral	L2, L3
Semimembranosus	Knee flexion Internal tibial rotation Hip extension Hip internal rotation	Ischial tuberosity	Posteromedial portion of the tibia's medial condyle	Tibial	L5, S1
Semitendinosus	Knee flexion Internal tibial rotation Hip extension Hip internal rotation	Ischial tuberosity	Medial portion of the tibial flare	Tibial	L5, S1, S2
Vastus intermedius	Knee extension	Anterolateral portion of the upper two-thirds of the femur Lower one-half of the linea aspera	To the tibial tubercle via the patella and patellar ligament	Femoral	L2, L3, L4
Vastus lateralis	Knee extension	Proximal interochanteric line Greater trochanter Gluteal tuberosity Upper one-half of the linea aspera	To the tibial tubercle via the patella and patellar ligament	Femoral	L2, L3, L4

Vastus medialis	Knee extension
	Oblique portion
	Patellar stabilization
		Longus portion
		  Distal one-half of the intertrochanteric line
		  Medial portion of the linea aspera
		Oblique portion
		  Tendons from adductor longus and adductor magnus
			To the tibial tubercle via the patella and patellar ligament	Femoral	L2, L3, L4

medialis oblique (VMO). As a group, the quadriceps femoris extends the knee. The rectus femoris also serves as a hip flexor, especially when the knee is flexed. During knee extension, the VMO guides the patella medially.

Posterior Muscles

The **semitendinosus, semimembranosus,** and **biceps femoris** are collectively known as the **hamstring muscle group.** They act as a unit to flex the knee and extend the hip (Fig. 6–12). The biceps femoris serves to externally rotate the tibia while the semimembranosus and semitendinosus act to internally rotate the tibia. The hamstring muscles also decrease the shear forces that stress the ACL when the knee is flexed beyond 20 degrees.[14,15]

The posterolateral knee capsule is reinforced by the **popliteus** muscle (see Fig. 6–9). In an open kinetic chain, the popliteus causes internal rotation of the tibia on the femur; in a closed kinetic chain, the popliteus externally rotates the femur on the tibia. Responsible for unscrewing the knee from its locked position in extension, its remaining influence on knee flexion is slight.

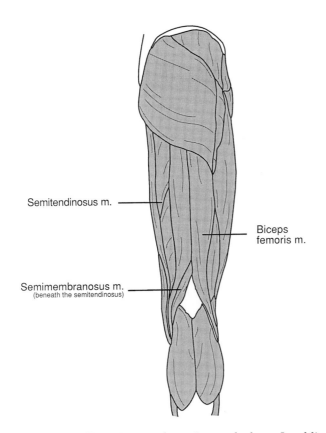

Semitendinosus m.

Biceps femoris m.

Semimembranosus m.
(beneath the semitendinosus)

FIGURE 6–12. Posterior muscles acting on the knee. In addition to flexing the joint, the biceps femoris externally rotates the tibia while the semimembranosus and semitendinosus internally rotate it.

However, when the patient is bearing weight with the knee partially flexed, the popliteus assists the PCL in preventing posterior displacement of the tibia on the femur.

A diamond-shaped **popliteal fossa** is formed by the leg's posterior musculature (Fig. 6–13). Although its inner boundaries are largely devoid of muscles (with the exception of the popliteus), the popliteal fossa contains the popliteal artery and vein; the tibial, common peroneal, and posterior femoral cutaneous nerve; and the small saphenous vein.

Pes Anserine Muscle Group

The **gracilis** and **sartorius** muscles, along with the **semitendinosus** muscles, form the **pes anserine** muscle group. In addition to flexing the knee, the pes anserine group internally rotates the tibia when the foot is not planted on the ground. When the foot is planted, the pes anserine externally rotates the femur on a fixed tibia.

The gracilis and semitendinosus muscles are relatively straightforward in their anatomic orientation. However, the **sartorius** muscle is an unusual one. Although its belly is located on the anterior aspect of the femur, it is a flexor of the knee joint (see Fig. 6–11). This occurs because the sartorius muscle crosses the knee posterior to its axis. Because of its origin proximal to the hip joint, the sartorius muscle also assists in hip flexion.

Iliotibial Band

The **tensor fasciae latae,** a small muscle originating from the anterior superior iliac crest inserts into the **iliotibial band (IT band).** The IT band travels down the lateral aspect of the femur to insert on **Gerdy's tubercle** on the anterolateral tibia and attaches to the lateral patellar retinaculum and the biceps femoris tendon through divergent slips.[16] Although the tensor fasciae latae and IT band make a relatively insignificant contribution to knee motion, the deep fibers of the IT band that attach to the lateral joint capsule function as an anterolateral knee ligament, playing a significant role in knee stability and patellofemoral pathology.[17]

The angle between the IT band and tibia varies according to the relative position of the lower leg, which, in turn, alters the knee's biomechanics. When the knee is fully extended, the IT band is anterior to or located over the lateral femoral condyle. When the knee is flexed beyond 30 degrees, the IT band shifts behind the lateral femoral condyle, giving it an angle of pull as if it were a knee flexor (Fig. 6–14). This posterior shift is greatly influenced by the biceps femoris, which has a fibrous expanse attaching to the IT band. During contraction of the biceps femoris, the IT band is drawn posteriorly.

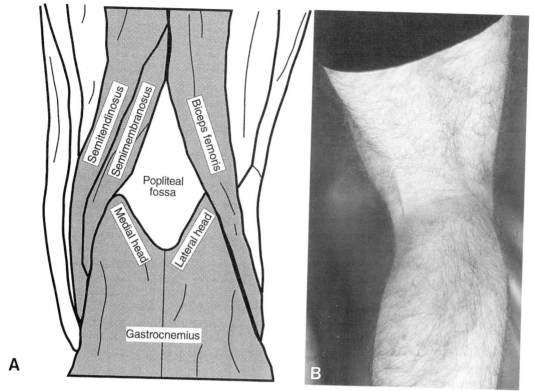

FIGURE 6–13. Popliteal fossa. **(A)** Anatomical reference and **(B)** surface anatomy.

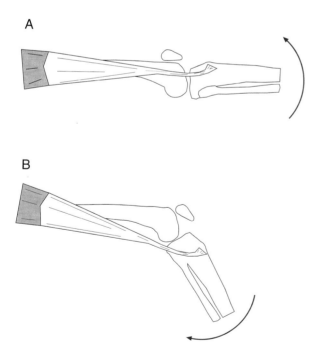

FIGURE 6–14. The iliotibial band's dynamic line of pull in flexion and extension. **(A)** When the knee is fully extended, the iliotibial band's angle of pull is that of a knee extensor. **(B)** When it is flexed past 30 degrees, it assumes an angle of flexor.

THE SCREW HOME MECHANISM

The unequal sizes of the femoral condyles and the tightening of the cruciate ligaments as they wind upon themselves during flexion necessitates a locking mechanism as the knee nears its final degrees of extension.[18] As the knee is extended to its terminal range, the lateral meniscus serves as a pivot point. The medial femoral condyle has a larger surface area than the lateral condyle. As the knee extends, the articular distance on the lateral femoral condyle is expended, and the medial articulation continues to glide, resulting in external rotation of the tibia with the lateral meniscus serving as the pivot point.

During extension of a non–weight-bearing knee, this mechanism occurs as 5 to 7 degrees of external rotation of the tibia on the femur. However, when bearing weight, the tibia is fixated so the terminal ROM is accomplished by a combination of the tibial external rotation and femoral internal rotation. To initiate flexion, the knee must be unlocked. When not bearing weight, this is accomplished by the popliteus muscle; when bearing weight, unlocking occurs by contraction of the popliteus, semimembranosus, and semitendinosus muscles.

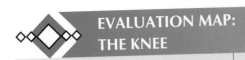

EVALUATION MAP: THE KNEE

1. HISTORY

Location of pain
Mechanism of injury
Foot fixation
Associated sounds or sensations
Onset of injury
Previous injury

2. INSPECTION

Girth measurements

Anterior structures
Alignment of patella
Patellar tendon
Quadriceps muscle group
Alignment of the femur on the tibia
Tibial tuberosity

Medial structures
Oblique fibers of vastus medialis

Lateral structures
Fibular head
Posterior tibial sag
Hyperextension

Posterior structures
Hamstring group
Popliteal fossa

3. PALPATION

Anterior structures
Patella
Patellar tendon
Tibial tuberosity
Quadriceps muscle group
Sartorius

Medial structures
Joint line/meniscus
Medial collateral ligament
Medial femoral condyle and
    epicondyle
Medial tibial plateau
Pes anserine tendon and bursa
Semitendinosus tendon
Gracilis

Lateral structures
Joint line/meniscus
Fibular head
Lateral collateral ligament
Popliteus tendon
Biceps femoris
Iliotibial band

Posterior structures
Popliteal fossa
Hamstring muscle group

**Determination of intracapsular versus
extracapsular swelling**
Sweep test
Ballotable patella

4. RANGE OF MOTION TESTS

Active motion
Flexion and extension
Internal and external rotation
    (screw home mechanism)

Passive motion
Flexion and extension

Resisted motion
Flexion and extension
Isolating the sartorius

5. LIGAMENTOUS TESTS

ACL instability
Anterior drawer test
Lachman's test
Modified Lachman's test

PCL instability
Posterior drawer test
Godfrey's test

MCL instability
Valgus stress test

LCL instability
Varus stress test

Proximal tibiofibular syndesmosis
Tibiofibular translation test

6. NEUROLOGIC TESTS

Peroneal nerve
Femoral nerve
Sciatic nerve
Lumbar nerve roots
Sacral nerve roots

7. SPECIAL TESTS

Rotary knee instabilities
Slocum drawer
Crossover test
Lateral pivot shift
Slocum ALRI
FRD test

Meniscal tears
McMurray's test
Apley's compression
Apley's distraction

ITB friction syndrome
Noble's compression test
Ober's test

ALRI = anterolateral rotatory instability; FRD = flexion–rotation drawer; IT = iliotibial; LCL = lateral collateral ligament; MCL = medial collateral ligament; PCL = posterior cruciate ligament.

CLINICAL EVALUATION OF KNEE AND LEG INJURIES

The patient is evaluated while wearing shorts to permit inspection and palpation of the muscles originating off the femur and pelvis. The patella is described in this section only as it relates to tibiofemoral function. Chapter 7 presents the detailed evaluation of patellofemoral conditions.

HISTORY

Blows to the knee place compressive forces on the joint structures at the point of the blow, tensile forces on the side opposite the blow, and shear forces across the joint. Rotatory forces about the knee, such as those experienced when an athlete cuts to change direction, place tensile forces about the joint capsule and cruciate ligaments. The menisci may also be torn by this mechanism secondary to impingement and shearing between the articular condyles.

- **Location of pain:** Tears of the collateral ligaments or the anteromedial or anterolateral capsule normally result in pain directly corresponding to the area of trauma. Pain arising from the ACL may be described as being "beneath the kneecap" or "inside the knee," and pain from the PCL may mimic that caused by a

strain of one of the gastrocnemius origins. Tears to the vascular zone of the menisci present with joint line pain. Tears in the avascular zone may be described as pain or, more commonly, as popping, clicking, or locking within the knee (Table 6–2).

- **Mechanism of injury:** Forces delivered to the knee in the frontal or sagittal plane when the knee is extended have less of a rotational component than blows received at an angle or when the knee is flexed. Forces delivered in a straight planar motion usually result in more isolated injuries to the ligamentous tissues. Rotational stresses may more commonly injure multiple ligamentous and meniscal tissues. A description of an acute, non-contact-related onset most likely reflects a rotational stress that was placed on the knee, as occurs when a person changes directions while running or pivoting (Table 6–3).
- **Weight-bearing status:** Rotational injuries may further be identified by establishing the weight-bearing status of the involved limb. A foot that was planted at the time of injury fixates the tibia, allowing the femur to rotate on it.
- **Associated sounds or sensations:** Determine the sensations and any associated sounds (e.g. "pop" or "snap") experienced at the time of the injury. After ruling out a patellar dislocation, subluxation, or fracture, these sounds may indicate a tear of one of the cruciate ligaments.[19] Patients often report the knee "giving way." With true giving way, the knee buckles

 Table 6–2
POSSIBLE TRAUMA BASED ON THE LOCATION OF PAIN

	Location of Pain			
	Lateral	**Anterior**	**Medial**	**Posterior**
Soft tissue	LCL sprain Lateral joint capsule sprain Superior tibiofibular syndesmosis sprain Lateral patellar retinaculum irritation* Biceps femoris strain Biceps femoris tendinitis Popliteal tendinitis IT band friction syndrome Lateral meniscus tear	ACL sprain (emanating from "inside" the knee) Patellar tendinitis* Patellar tendon rupture (partial or complete)* Patellar bursitis* Patellar maltracking— chondromalacia* Quadriceps contusion Fat pad irritation* Quadriceps tendon rupture*	MCL sprain Medial joint capsule sprain Medial patellar retinaculum irritation* Pes anserine bursitis or tendinitis Semitendinosus strain Semitendinosus tendinitis Semimembranosus strain Semimembranosus tendinitis Medial meniscus tear	PCL sprain Posterior capsule sprain Gastrocnemius strain Hamstring strain Popliteus tendinitis Popliteal cyst
Bony	Fibular head fracture Osteochondral fracture Osteochondritis dissecans Lateral femoral condyle contusion Lateral tibial plateau contusion	Patellar fracture Tibial plateau fracture Sinding-Johansen-Larsen disease* Osgood-Schlatter disease (in adolescents)* Patellar dislocation or subluxation* Chondromalacia	Osteochondral fracture Osteochondritis dissecans Medial femoral condyle contusion Medial tibial plateau contusion	

*Discussed in Chapter 7.

ACL = anterior cruciate ligament; IT = iliotibial; LCL = lateral collateral ligament; MCL = medial collateral ligament; PCL = posterior cruciate ligament.

Table 6–3
MECHANISM OF KNEE INJURIES AND THE RESULTANT SOFT TISSUE DAMAGE

Force Placed on the Knee	Tensile Forces	Compressive Forces
Valgus	Medial structures: MCL, medial joint capsule, pes anserine muscle group, medial meniscus	Lateral meniscus
Varus	Lateral structures: LCL, lateral joint capsule, IT band, biceps femoris	Medial meniscus
Anterior tibial displacement	ACL, IT band, LCL, MCL medial and lateral joint capsules	Posterior portion of the medial and lateral meniscus
Posterior tibial displacement	PCL, popliteus, medial and lateral joint capsules	Anterior portion of the medial and lateral meniscus
Internal tibial rotation	ACL, anterolateral joint capsule posteromedial joint capsule, posterolateral joint capsule, LCL	Anterior horn of the medial meniscus Posterior horn of the lateral meniscus
External tibial rotation	Posterolateral joint capsule, MCL, PCL, LCL, ACL	Anterior horn of the lateral meniscus Posterior horn of the lateral meniscus
Hyperextension	ACL, posterior joint capsule, PCL	Anterior portion of the medial and lateral meniscus
Hyperflexion	ACL, PCL	Posterior portion of the medial and lateral meniscus

ACL = anterior cruciate ligament; IT = iliotibial; LCL = lateral collateral ligament; MCL = medial collateral ligament; PCL = posterior cruciate ligament.

during weight bearing, likely indicating a meniscal injury or ligamentous instability. The sensation of giving way without actual buckling is usually related to quadriceps weakness or inhibition seen with patellofemoral joint disease.

True locking, the inability to fully extend the knee, indicates an unstable meniscal tear or loose body within the joint that wedges between the femur and tibia, locking joint. Patients may report catching or crepitation as locking. These symptoms often more accurately indicate patellofemoral joint disease.

- **Onset of injury:** Ligamentous injuries most often present with an acute onset related to a specific episode. Injuries having an insidious onset are most likely to involve inflammation of the muscles acting on the knee, may be the result of patellar maltracking, or may represent degenerative changes within the knee. As with chronic foot and ankle injuries, chronic knee pain may arise secondary to training errors, foot type, shoe type, postural deviations, and foot biomechanics. Meniscal injuries may be acute or have an insidious onset, as is often the case with the lateral meniscus.

- **Past history of injury:** A past history of injury for both the involved and uninvolved knee must be established. Previous injury can result in chronic inflammation secondary to internal derangement within the knee or biomechanical dysfunction. Nonsurgical ligament sprains may have healed with a great deal of scar tissue, restricting the ROM, or with excess laxity, both of which predispose the knee to reinjury. Surgical conditions involving grafts or repairs are also subject to reinjury.

INSPECTION

As much of the inspection process as possible is performed while the patient is weight bearing. Any observations of an antalgic gait or other gait deviations are also noted.

Girth Measurements

Chronic conditions or ongoing reevaluations of existing conditions must include a determination of the amount

FIGURE 6–15. Girth measurements of the knee. Measurements are taken over the joint line (0 inches) to measure for swelling. Measurements are then taken at 2-inch increments around the thigh to determine the presence of atrophy (1-inch increments are used for smaller patients). These findings are then compared with the opposite extremity.

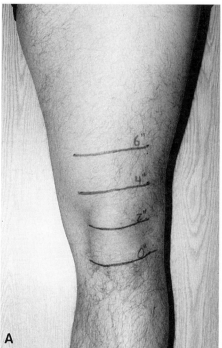 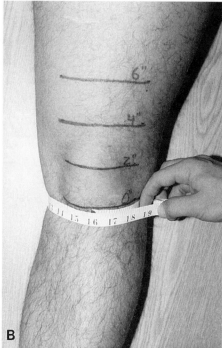

of swelling in and around the knee joint and atrophy of the quadriceps muscle groups. To be objective, these measurements must be made in a consistent and reproducible manner. Measurements are made around the joint line and then at consistent intervals up the quadriceps group (Fig. 6–15). The results of these findings are compared with those of the uninvolved limb and recorded in the medical file for future comparison. Note that the dominant thigh may naturally be hypertrophied relative to the nondominant thigh.

Inspection of the Anterior Structures

- **Alignment of patella:** Observe the patella, normally found resting above the femoral trochlea, evenly aligned with the medial and lateral aspects of the knee. Shifting of the patella away from its central position on the trochlea may indicate **patellar malalignment or dislocation.** Patellar dislocations normally occur laterally. A unilaterally high-riding patella, when accompanied by spasm of the quadriceps muscle group, indicates a **ruptured patellar tendon.** The actual tendon defect may be obliterated by swelling.
- **Patellar tendon:** Note any swelling over or directly around the patellar tendon, possibly indicating tendinitis or bursitis. Swelling on both sides that masks the definition of the tendon may indicate inflammation of the underlying fat pad.
- **Quadriceps muscle group:** Compare the mass and tone of the quadriceps muscle groups bilaterally and confirm any apparent deficits through girth mea-

surements. Note any discoloration, swelling, or loss of continuity within the quadriceps group.
- **Alignment of the femur on the tibia:** Observe the angle at which the tibia and femur articulate. The normal angle ranges from 180 to 195 degrees on the line formed by the lateral aspect of the knee. An angle of less than 180 degrees is termed **genu valgum** ("knock knees"); an angle greater than 195 degrees is described as **genu varum** ("bowlegs"). These conditions increase the tensile forces placed on structures located on the side of the joint line toward which the knee is bent, while placing compressive forces on the opposite side (Fig. 6–16).
- **Tibial tuberosity:** Look for possible enlargement of the tibial tuberosity. In adolescent patients, enlargement could indicate Osgood-Schlatter disease (see Chapter 7). A history of this condition may result in residual enlargement of the tibial tuberosity into adulthood (Fig. 6–17).

Inspection of the Medial Structures

- **Medial aspect:** Inspect the medial aspect of the knee joint, noting any swelling or discoloration along the tibia, knee joint line, femur, or pes anserine tendon.
- **Oblique fibers of vastus medialis:** Observe the VMO. The VMO should display normal muscle tone and girth compared with that of the opposite limb. This muscle group is the first to atrophy after injury, possibly as the result of disuse or an increase of intracapsular fluid that inhibits its normal function.[20]

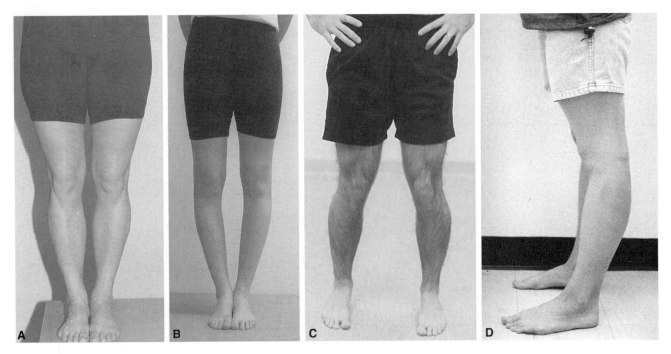

FIGURE 6–16. Alignment of the tibia on the femur. **(A)** Normal alignment, **(B)** genu varum (bow legs), **(C)** genu valgum (knock knees), and **(D)** genu recurvatum (hyperextension).

Inspection of the Lateral Structures

- **Lateral aspect:** Inspect the lateral aspect of the tibia, joint line, and femur for swelling or discoloration.
- **Fibular head:** Note the head of the fibula, normally aligned at an equal height compared with the opposite side. With the knee flexed, the biceps femoris tendon and LCL may be visible.
- **Posterior sag of the tibia:** With the patient lying supine and the knees flexed to 90 degrees, observe the relative positions of the tibia. In PCL-deficient knees, the tibia on the involved side drops or "sags"

posteriorly (Fig. 6–18). A straightedge placed along the patella and the anterior aspect of the tibia helps to identify the amount of sagging.
- **Hyperextension:** View the patient from the side while he or she stands with the knees fully extended. Hyperextension, or **genu recurvatum,** is indicated by the posterior bowing of the knee (see Fig. 6–16).

Inspection of the Posterior Structures

- **Hamstring muscle group:** Observe the length of the hamstring group for signs of contusions, indicating a

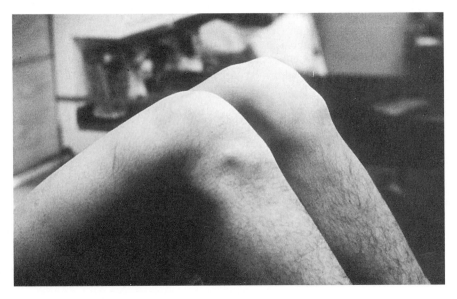

FIGURE 6–17. Residual enlargement of the tibial tuberosity caused by Osgood-Schlatter disease in youth.

FIGURE 6–18. **(A)** Posterior tibial sag indicating posterior cruciate ligament deficiency. Note the downward displacement of the tibia. **(B)** Illustration showing the posterior displacement of the tibia that is caused by tearing of the posterior cruciate ligament (the anterior cruciate ligament has been removed for clarity).

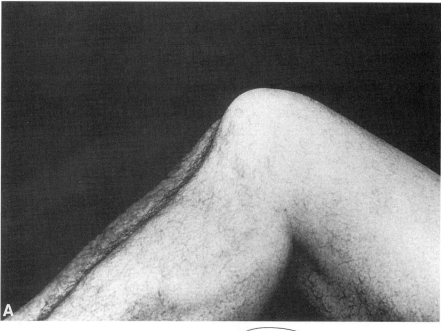

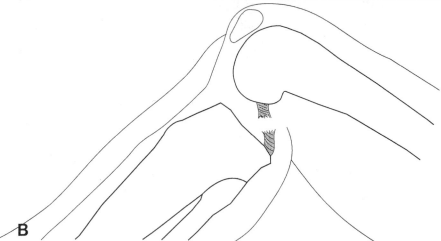

blow to this area, or ecchymosis, indicating a strain. Strains are described in Chapter 8.

- **Popliteal fossa:** Inspect the popliteal fossa for signs of swelling or discoloration that can indicate capsular trauma or tears of the distal hamstring tendons or the heads of the gastrocnemius muscle.

PALPATION

Palpation is performed to confirm the findings of the inspection portion of the evaluation process and further identify traumatized tissues, although many of the most often injured tissues cannot be palpated.

Palpation of the Anterior Structures

1. **Patella:** Begin palpating the patella at its superior patellar pole where the quadriceps muscle group inserts, noting for areas of point tenderness. Progress centrally down the patella to reach the inferior pole and the origin of the patellar tendon. Return to the starting point on the superior pole by palpating up the medial and lateral patellar borders.

    With the knee extended and the quadriceps relaxed, palpate the patella to ensure its proper alignment in the femoral trochlea and its freedom of movement. A rigid, displaced patella accompanied by the inability or unwillingness to extend the knee indicates a patellar dislocation.

2. **Patellar tendon:** Palpate the length of the patellar tendon from its insertion at the tibial tuberosity to the inferior aspect of the patella. The patellar tendon normally feels broad and ropelike. The tendon can also be palpated while the patient performs active ROM of the knee, noting any crepitus indicating patellar tendonitis.

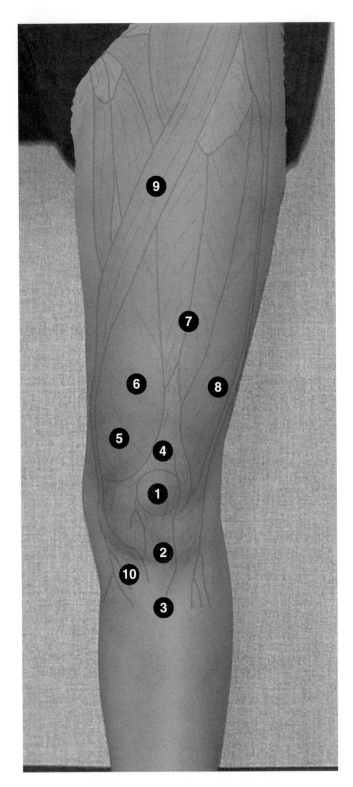

ease. Pain in mature patients may be caused by a contusion or inflammation.

4. **Quadriceps tendon:** From the superior aspect of the patella, palpate the quadriceps tendon as it attaches across the length of the patella's superior pole. Note that the suprapatellar pouch of the joint capsule and the suprapatellar fat pad lie deep to the quadriceps tendon.

5–8. **Quadriceps muscle group:** Palpate the vastus medialis oblique (5), the length of the vastus medialis (6), the rectus femoris (7), and the vastus lateralis muscles (8) (the vastus intermedius is not palpable), searching for point tenderness or spasm.

9. **Sartorius:** Palpate the sartorius muscle from its origin on the anterior superior iliac spine (ASIS) to its insertion as a part of the **pes anserine tendon** (10).

Palpation of the Medial Structures

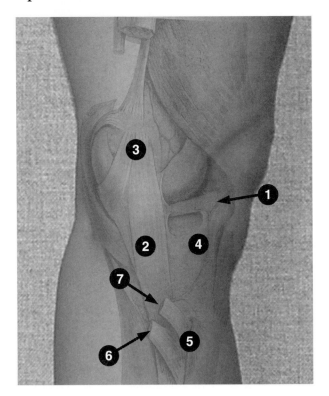

1. **Medial meniscus and joint line:** Place the knee in at least 45 degrees of flexion to locate the joint lines. Palpate on either side of the proximal aspect of the patellar tendon until the indentation formed by the femur and tibia is located. Palpate medially and posteriorly along the joint line, noting any crepitus or pain that may indicate possible meniscal, ligamentous, or capsular trauma. Externally rotating the lower leg makes the medial meniscus more palpable.

2. **Medial collateral ligament:** Palpate the length of the MCL from its origin on the medial femoral condyle, just below the adductor tubercle, progress-

3. **Tibial tuberosity:** Palpate the patellar tendon's attachment site on the tibia. The tibial tuberosity is normally a smooth, rounded protrusion. With adolescent patients, sensitivity and roughness of the tuberosity indicate an inflammation of the tibial tuberosity's growth center, **Osgood-Schlatter dis-**

ing inferiorly to its insertion on the medial tibial flare that can be located up to 7 cm distal to the joint line. The medial portion of the joint line is covered by the MCL.

3. **Medial femoral condyle and epicondyle:** Flex the knee beyond 90 degrees to expose the condyle immediately above the anteromedial joint line. Palpate this area posteriorly to the adductor tubercle. Injuries with rotational or loading type mechanisms may cause bone bruising or osteochondral fracture, causing pain in these structures.
4. **Medial tibial plateau:** Locate the medial tibial plateau inferior to the joint line. After palpating along its length, proceed inferiorly to locate the medial tibial flare.
5. **Pes anserine tendon and bursa:** Locate the medial tibial flare, the common site of attachment for the gracilis, sartorius, and semitendinosus muscles. Palpate the common insertion of these tendons and the overlying pes anserine bursa, located just medial to the tibial tuberosity, which may become inflamed because of direct blows or overuse.
6. **Semitendinosus tendon:** From the pes anserine attachment, palpate the semitendinosus tendon, the most medial tendon of the hamstring group, to its muscular belly.
7. **Gracilis:** Palpate the thin, ropelike gracilis, located immediately anterior to the semitendinosus tendon, from its insertion to the point that it is lost in the mass of the adductor group.

Palpation of the Lateral Structures

1. **Joint line:** Position the knee in at least 45 degrees of flexion to locate the anterolateral joint line. Begin palpating the joint line lateral to the patellar tendon and progress posteriorly. Pain along the joint line may indicate meniscal trauma. Internally rotating the lower leg makes the lateral meniscus more palpable.
2. **Fibular head:** Locate the fibular head below and slightly posterior to the lateral joint line. Two ropelike structures may be felt arising from the fibular head. The LCL projects off its superior portion; slightly posterior to this structure is the insertion of the biceps femoris tendon.
3. **Lateral collateral ligament:** Place the knee in 90 degrees of flexion and externally rotate and abduct the hip (i.e., cross the ankle of the involved leg over the opposite leg) to make the LCL more identifiable. Because it is a separate structure from the joint capsule, the LCL is easily identified as it arises from the fibular head and courses to the lateral femoral condyle.
4. **Popliteus:** Palpate a small portion of the anterior popliteus tendon, posterior to the LCL just above the joint line.
5. **Biceps femoris:** Flex the knee to 25 degrees and ask the patient to externally rotate the lower leg to make the biceps tendon easily palpable (note that as the

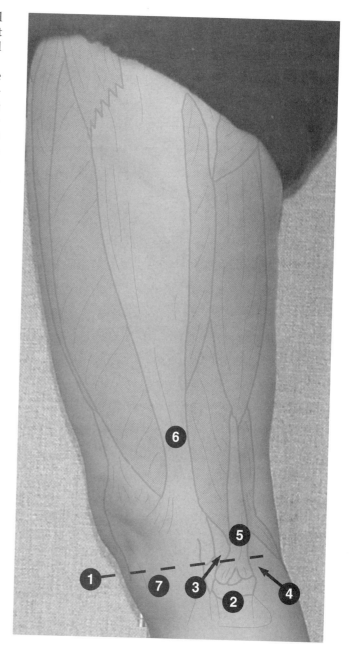

tendon crosses the joint line, it may become confused with the IT band). The biceps femoris tendon inserts on the fibular head, posterior to the insertion of the LCL. Continue palpating the biceps tendon to its muscular belly.
6. **Iliotibial band:** Palpate the IT band, located anterior to the biceps femoris tendon and arising from Gerdy's tubercle (7) just lateral to the tibial tuberosity, the IT band becomes more identifiable during resisted flexion past 30 degrees. Palpate the IT band upward to the tensor fasciae latae, noting any increased sensitivity, especially as it passes over the lateral femoral condyle, possibly indicating **iliotibial band friction syndrome.**

Palpation of the Posterior Structures

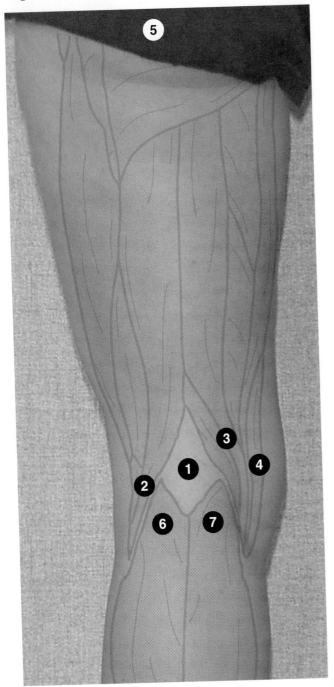

1. **Popliteal fossa:** Rupture of the knee's synovial membrane may cause fluid to escape from the capsule and accumulate in the popliteal fossa. After a period of time, this fluid is surrounded by a membranous sac, forming a popliteal cyst (Baker's cyst). These cysts are usually not grossly visible and typically require magnetic resonance imaging (MRI) for positive identification. Trauma to this area or edema within this space can occlude neurovascular structures, resulting in referred pain, inhibition of nerve transmission, or disruption of blood flow to or from the lower leg, possibly mimicking the signs and symptoms of thrombophlebitis.[21]

In younger patients, popliteal cysts most commonly form after meniscal tears, collateral ligament sprains, or trauma to the cruciate ligaments. In older adults, popliteal cysts often arise secondary to osteoarthritis or other inflammatory conditions.[21] With the patient prone, palpate the popliteal fossa for the presence of a cyst. The cyst is usually more prominent during palpation with the knee extended. It may feel as if it disappears when the knee is flexed. The cyst itself is usually not the cause of a patient's problem but is more indicative of pathology within the knee itself.

2–5. **Hamstring muscle group:** Palpate the length of the biceps femoris (2) on the lateral aspect of the knee and the semimembranosus (3) and semitendinosus (4) muscles on the medial side of the knee to their common insertion on the ischial tuberosity (5) noting for point tenderness, spasm, or deformity.

6–7. **Heads of the gastrocnemius:** Palpate the lateral (6) and medial heads (7) of the gastrocnemius muscle.

DETERMINATION OF INTRACAPSULAR VERSUS EXTRACAPSULAR SWELLING

Pathology to the knee can result in the formation of swelling within the joint capsule (intracapsular effusion) or outside of the capsule (extracapsular swelling). Joint effusion is identified by the ability to manually move ("milk") the fluid from one side of the knee to the other using the **Sweep test** (Box 6–1). Effusion inside the joint capsule can cause the patella to float over the femoral trochlea. With the patient's knee fully extended and the quadriceps relaxed, apply a downward pressure on the patella. A positive test result is demonstrated when the patella bounces back to its original position, a **Ballotable patella.**

Intracapsular joint effusion is caused by two different mechanisms. Acute injuries leading to intracapsular effusion usually indicate a torn ACL, a meniscus tear, a torn capsule possibly resulting from the dislocation of the patella, a fractured tibial plateau, or an osteochondral fracture. If aspirated, the fluid would most likely be dark red because of bleeding from these structures (**hemarthrosis**). In chronic conditions, the knee joint effusion may be caused by the inflammatory response producing excess synovial fluid such as in arthritic knees, a mensical tear in the avascular zone, or with chondromalacia patella.

Extracapsular edema is often caused by inflammation of the soft tissues surrounding the joint, possibly indicating inflamed bursae or a contusion. Venous in-

---

Hemarthrosis Blood within a joint cavity.

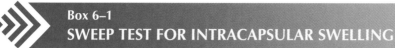

Box 6–1
SWEEP TEST FOR INTRACAPSULAR SWELLING

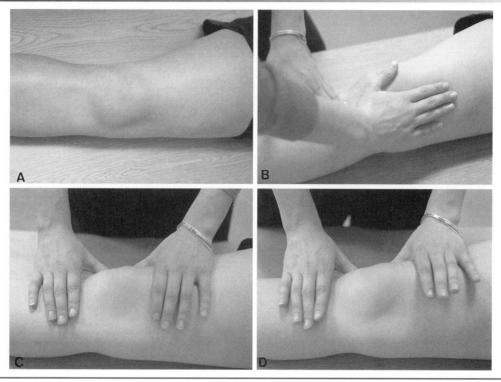

Sweep test to determine the presence of intracapsular swelling.

PATIENT POSITION	Lying supine with the knee extended
POSITION OF EXAMINER	Standing lateral to the patient
EVALUATIVE PROCEDURE	Assuming that the initial pocket of edema is on the medial side of the knee (**A**): (**B**) The edema is stroked ("milked") proximally and laterally. (**C**) The normal contour of the knee is restored. (**D**) When pressure is applied on the lateral aspect of the knee, a fluid bulge immediately appears on the medial aspect.
POSITIVE TEST	Reformation of edema on the medial side of the knee when pressure is applied to the lateral aspect.
IMPLICATIONS	Swelling within the joint capsule, indicating possible anterior cruciate ligament trauma, osteochondral fracture, synovitis, meniscal lesion, or patellar dislocation.
MODIFICATION	If swelling is more prevalent on the lateral aspect of the knee, the steps are performed on the lateral side of the knee joint.

sufficiencies may affect the knee in addition to the entire lower extremity, causing the build-up of edema.

RANGE OF MOTION TESTING

The only voluntary movements available at the knee joint are flexion and extension and tibial internal and external rotation. The motions of flexion and extension are easily measured and quantified, but tibial rotation is less accurately measured. The use of a goniometer to measure knee flexion and extension is described in Box 6–2.

Active Range of Motion

- **Flexion and extension:** The arc of motion for knee flexion and extension is 135 to 145 degrees, with the majority of the motion occurring as flexion (Fig. 6–19). A fully extended knee normally is at 0 degrees, but in certain cases may be as great as 10 degrees beyond 0 (genu recurvatum). Knee flexion may be limited by tightness of the quadriceps group, especially in the rectus femoris, and a fully extended hip can limit the amount of flexion available at the knee.

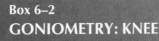

Box 6–2
GONIOMETRY: KNEE

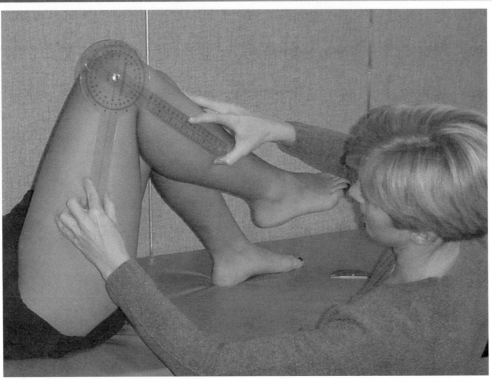

PATIENT POSITION	Lying supine. Knee flexion and extension may also be measured with the patient supine and a bolster placed under the distal femur.

GONIOMETER ALIGNMENT

FULCRUM	Centered over the lateral femoral epicondyle
STATIONARY ARM	Centered over the midline of the femur, aligned with the greater trochanter
MOVEMENT ARM	Centered over the midline of the fibula, aligned with the lateral malleolus

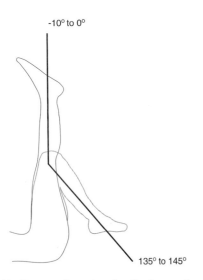

-10° to 0°

135° to 145°

FIGURE 6–19. Range of motion for flexion and extension of the knee.

- **Internal and external rotation:** To allow for full ROM during knee flexion and extension, the tibia must internally and externally rotate on the femur. Observe and bilaterally compare the rotation of the tibial tuberosity to estimate the amount of internal and external rotation that occurs during active knee flexion and extension.

Passive Range of Motion

- **Extension:** Extension is measured with the tibia slightly elevated by placing a *bolster* under the distal tibia with the patient in the supine position. Extension produces a firm end-feel because the poste-

Bolster A support used to maintain the position of a body part.

rior capsule and the cruciate ligaments stretch. Tightness of the hamstring group may limit extension, especially in cases in which the knee has been flexed for extended periods because of stiffness, swelling, immobilization, or flexion contracture.

- **Flexion:** Flexion is measured with the patient lying supine to remove the influence of excessive rectus femoris tightness. Restrictions in the flexion ROM in the supine position suggest joint capsule adhesions. Flexion measured in the prone position with the rectus femoris stretched over the hip and knee joints more closely reflects the affect of muscular tightness on the joint. The normal end-feel for flexion is soft because of the approximation of the gastrocnemius group with the hamstrings or the heel striking the buttock.

Resisted Range of Motion

During resisted knee flexion, obvious internal or external rotation of the tibia can identify weakness in the medial or lateral hamstrings, especially if this rotation is greater than that observed during testing of the uninvolved side (Box 6–3). Excessive internal rotation indicates biceps femoris weakness. External rotation indicates semimembranosus or semitendinosus pathology (or both).

TESTS FOR JOINT STABILITY

Ligamentous stability of the knee may occur in one plane, either as anteroposterior instability in the frontal plane or as valgus-varus instability in the sagittal plane. It may also occur as a multidirectional rotatory instability. This section presents tests for uniplanar instabilities. Tests for rotatory instabilities are discussed in the

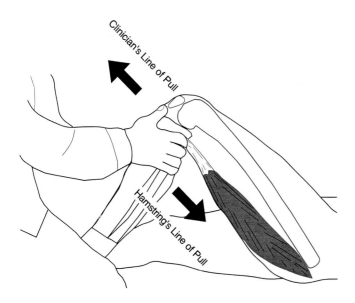

FIGURE 6–20. Masking a potentially positive anterior drawer test. Contraction of the hamstring group pulls the tibia posteriorly, the direction opposite the line of pull.

Pathologies and Related Special Tests section of this chapter.

Tests for Anterior Cruciate Ligament Instability

Two basic tests are used to determine the relative stability of the ACL by attempting to displace the tibia anteriorly on the femur. The ACL provides 86 percent of the restraint against this motion.[22] In the case of a complete ACL disruption, further displacement is limited by the posterior capsule, the deep layer of the MCL, and the arcuate ligament complex.

The **anterior drawer test** involves placing the knee in 90 degrees of flexion and attempting to displace the tibia anteriorly (Box 6–4). In this position, the anterior drawer test is particularly sensitive to tears in the ACL's anteromedial bundle.[23–26] The line of pull from the hamstrings complements the function of the ACL, possibly masking an otherwise positive test result (Fig. 6–20). The hamstrings, however, do not replicate the function of the ACL as the knee nears extension.[15]

Common pitfalls of the anterior drawer test include:

1. The need to overcome the effects of gravity while moving the tibia anteriorly
2. Guarding by the hamstring group, masking anterior displacement of the tibia on the femur
3. Effusion within the capsule, providing resistance to movement or the inability to flex the knee to 90 degrees
4. The geometry of the articular condyles, causing the triangular shape of the menisci to form a block against anterior movement of the tibia, similar to a doorstop's wedging against the bottom of a door
5. Flexing the knee to 90 degrees, causing anterior displacement of the tibia, masking the amount of further displacement during the drawer test[27]
6. Because the knee is placed in 90 degrees of flexion, the anterior drawer test may be more sensitive to lesions localized within the anteromedial bundle[28]

A modification of the anterior drawer test, the **Lachman's test,** tends to isolate the posterolateral bundle of the ACL because the knee is flexed to 20 degrees (Box 6–5 and see Fig. 6–8). This test is considered to be more reliable than the anterior drawer test for determining ACL damage.

Performing Lachman's test requires a firm grasp to manipulate the tibia and femur. In many cases, athletes or other large patients have heavy, muscular legs, making it difficult to perform this test. In these cases, the femur may be rested on a tightly rolled towel or stabilized by an assistant.[29] Another method is to abduct the patient's leg off the side of the table and flex the knee to 25 degrees. One hand stabilizes the femur on the table and the foot is supported between the examiner's legs.[30]

Box 6–3
RESISTED KNEE RANGE OF MOTION

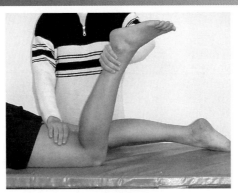

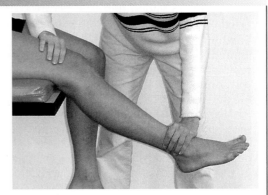

	Flexion	Extension
STARTING POSITION	The patient is prone and the knee is extended	The patient is seated with the knee flexed
STABILIZATION	Distal hamstrings	Distal quadriceps
RESISTANCE	Over the Achilles tendon	Proximal to the talocrural joint
MODIFICATION	Isometric break tests may be applied when the knee is flexed to 10°, 45°, and 90° unless this protocol is contraindicated by the patient's postoperative condition or other clinical findings.	Isometric break tests may be applied with the knee flexed to 15°, 45°, 90°, and 120° unless this protocol is contraindicated by the patient's postoperative condition or other clinical findings.
MUSCLES TESTED	Semimembranosus, semitendinosus, biceps femoris, sartorius, gastrocnemius, gracilis, popliteus	Rectur femoris, vastus lateralis, vastus intermedius, vastus medialis

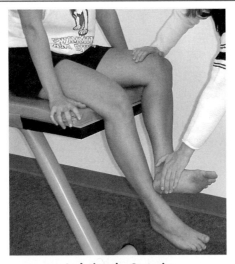

Isolating the Sartorius

STARTING POSITION	The heel of the leg being tested is positioned over the anterior talocrural joint with the patient sitting over the edge of the table.
RESISTANCE	Grasping the distal lower leg and over the distal quadriceps muscle.
MOTION	The patient attempts to slide the heel up the opposite tibia while resisting hip flexion, knee flexion, and femoral external rotation.

Box 6–4

ANTERIOR DRAWER TEST FOR ANTERIOR CRUCIATE LIGAMENT LAXITY

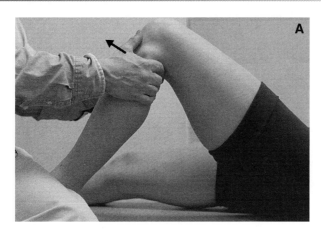

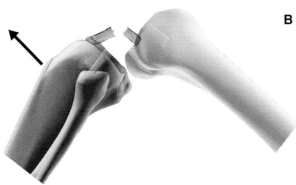

The anterior drawer test for anterior cruciate laxity (**A**). Schematic representation of tibial displacement in a positive test (**B**).

PATIENT POSITION	Lying supine Hip flexed to 45° and the knee to 90°
POSITION OF EXAMINER	Sitting on the examination table in front of the involved knee, grasping the tibia just below the joint line of the knee. Thumbs are placed along the joint line on either side of the patellar tendon. The index fingers are used to palpate the hamstring tendons to ensure that they are relaxed.
EVALUATIVE PROCEDURE	The tibia is drawn anteriorly.
POSITIVE TEST	An increased amount of anterior tibial translation compared with the opposite (uninvolved) limb or the lack of a firm end-point
IMPLICATIONS	A sprain of the anteromedial bundle of the ACL or a complete tear of the ACL
COMMENTS	The hamstring muscle group must be relaxed to ensure proper test results.

ACL = anterior cruciate ligament.

Box 6–5
LACHMAN'S TEST FOR ANTERIOR CRUCIATE LIGAMENT LAXITY

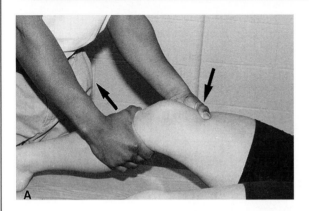

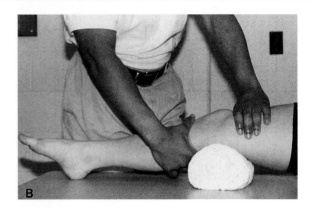

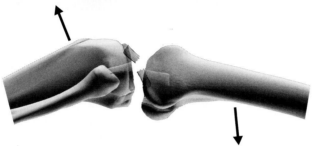

C

The Lachman's test **(A)** and modification of the Lachman's test **(B)**. Schematic representation of tibiofemoral translation in the presence of ACL deficiency **(C).**

PATIENT POSITION	Lying supine The knee passively flexed to 20 to 25°
POSITION OF EXAMINER	One hand grasps the tibia around the level of the tibial tuberosity and the other hand grasps the femur just above the level of the condyles
EVALUATIVE PROCEDURE	While the examiner supports the weight of the leg and the knee is flexed to 20°, the tibia is drawn anteriorly while a posterior pressure is applied to stabilize the femur.
POSITIVE TEST	An increased amount of anterior tibial translation compared with the opposite (uninvolved) limb or the lack of a firm end-point
IMPLICATIONS	Sprain of the ACL
MODIFICATION	As shown in **B** above, the femur may be stabilized by placing a rolled towel beneath the knee to assist in stabilizing the femur.
COMMENTS	See Box 6–6, The Alternative Lachman's Test

ACL = anterior cruciate ligament.

FIGURE 6–21. Instrumented testing of the anterior cruciate ligament using the KT-1000TM arthrometer.

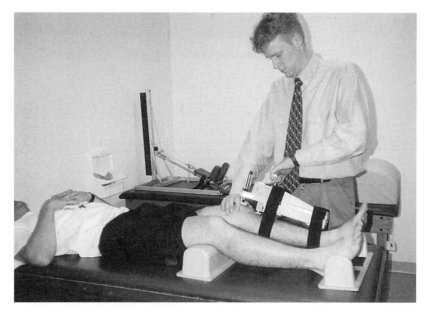

In each of these modifications, the tibia is drawn forward in a way similar to the drawer test procedure. The art of manual ACL and PCL testing is being augmented and quantified by instrumented **arthrometers** (Fig. 6–21). These devices measure the amount of tibial translation in a more accurate, quantitative, reproducible manner and are less prone to the physical limitation faced by the clinician when performing the anterior drawer or Lachman's test.[31–35] However, as with other clinical testing procedures, the reliability of instrumented arthrometers is correlated with the skill and experience of the individual performing the test.[36]

Any knee having an apparently positive anterior drawer or Lachman's test result also needs to be screened for PCL insufficiency. If the PCL is deficient, tests for ACL insufficiency may appear positive as the tibia is relocated anteriorly from its posteriorly subluxed position on the femur.[37,38]

The **alternate Lachman's test** can be used to differentiate abnormal tibiofemoral glide caused by tears of the ACL from that caused by PCL deficiencies.[37] This test places the patient in the prone, rather than the supine, position, preventing the posterior tibial sag resulting from the supine position (Box 6–6).

Tests for Posterior Cruciate Instability

Tests for damage of the PCL attempt to determine the amount of posterior displacement of the tibia on the femur relative to the uninvolved side. This motion places stress primarily on the PCL, followed by the arcuate ligament complex and the anterior joint capsule.

A posterior sag of the tibia may be evidenced when the flexed knee is viewed from the lateral side (see Fig. 6–18). Using the same positioning as the anterior drawer, the **posterior drawer test** attempts to displace the tibia posteriorly (Box 6–7). **Godfrey's test** uses gravity to extenuate the posterior sag as noted during the inspection process (Box 6–8). The following grading system is used for PCL sprains:[39,40]

Grade	Clinical Signs	Posterior Displacement
I	Palpable but diminished step-off between tibia and femur	0 to 5 mm
II	Step off is lost; the tibia cannot be pushed beyond the medial femoral condyle	5 to 10 mm
III	Step off is lost; the tibia can be pushed beyond the MFC	>10mm

Tests for Medial Collateral Ligament Instability

When the knee is fully extended, the MCL is assisted in limiting valgus stress by the posterior oblique ligament, posteromedial capsule, cruciate ligaments, and the muscles crossing the medial joint line. When the knee is flexed to 25 degrees, the MCL is the primary structure for resisting valgus forces.[41]

The **valgus stress test** is performed once with the knee fully extended and again when the knee is flexed to 25 degrees (Box 6–9). Valgus laxity demonstrated on a fully extended knee indicates a major disruption of the medial supportive structures. Placing the knee in approximately 25 degrees of flexion isolates the stress to the MCL.

The **varus stress test** is used to determine the integrity of the LCL, lateral joint capsule, IT band, arcuate ligament complex, and lateral musculature when it is performed in complete extension (Box 6–10). When the knee is flexed to 25 degrees and the varus stress reapplied, the LCL is better isolated. A positive varus stress test result when the knee is fully extended may indicate trauma to the other lateral or internal structures or both.

Box 6–6
ALTERNATE LACHMAN'S TEST

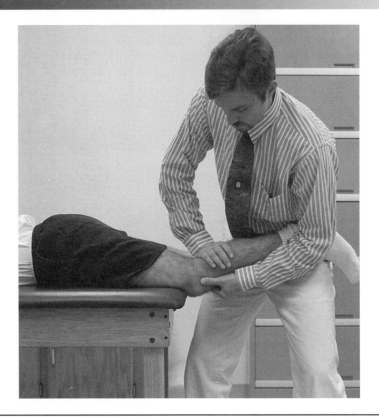

Alternate Lachman's test to differentiate between anterior tibial glide caused by ACL versus PCL laxity.

PATIENT POSITION	Prone The knee passively flexed to 30°
POSITION OF EXAMINER	Positioned at the legs of the patient so that the examiner supports the ankle The examiner's hand palpates the anterior joint line on either side of the patellar tendon
EVALUATIVE PROCEDURE	A downward pressure placed on the proximal portion of the posterior tibia as the examiner notes any anterior tibial displacement.
POSITIVE TEST	Excessive anterior translation relative to the uninvolved knee indicates a sprain of the ACL.
IMPLICATIONS	Positive test results found in the anterior drawer and/or Lachman's test and in the alternate Lachman's test indicate a sprain of the ACL A positive anterior drawer test and/or Lachman test result and a negative alternate Lachman's test result implicate a sprain in the PCL.

ACL = anterior cruciate ligament; PCL = posterior cruciate ligament.

Box 6–7

POSTERIOR DRAWER TEST FOR POSTERIOR CRUCIATE LIGAMENT INSTABILITY

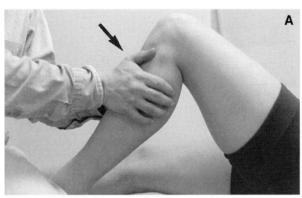

A

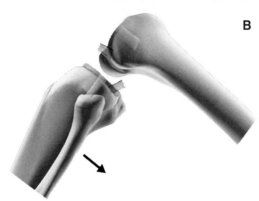

B

Posterior drawer test for PCL instability. **(A)** The tibia is moved posteriorly relative to the femur. **(B)** Translation of the tibia on the femur in the presence of a PCL tear.

PATIENT POSITION	Lying supine The hip flexed to 45° and the knee flexed to 90°
POSITION OF EXAMINER	Sitting on the examination table in front of the involved knee The patient's tibia stabilized in the neutral position
EVALUATIVE PROCEDURE	The examiner grasps the tibia just below the joint line of the knee with the fingers placed along the joint line on either side of the patellar tendon. The proximal tibia is pushed posteriorly.
POSITIVE TEST	An increased amount of posterior tibial translation compared with the opposite (uninvolved) limb or the lack of a firm end-point
IMPLICATIONS	A sprain of the PCL

PCL = posterior cruciate ligament.

Box 6–8
GODFREY'S TEST FOR POSTERIOR CRUCIATE LIGAMENT INSTABILITY

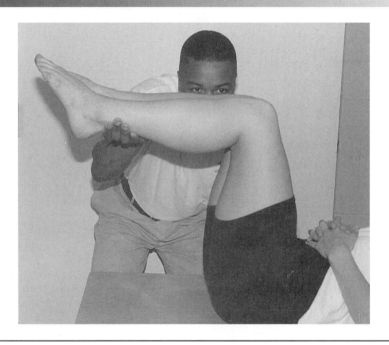

Godfrey's Test for posterior cruciate ligament laxity. Note the downward displacement of the left (facing) tibia

PATIENT POSITION	Lying supine with the knees extended and legs together
POSITION OF EXAMINER	Standing next to the patient
EVALUATIVE PROCEDURE	Lift the patient's lower legs and hold them parallel to the table so that the knees are flexed to 90°. Observe the level of the tibial tuberosities.
POSITIVE TEST	A unilateral posterior (downward) displacement of the tibial tuberosity
IMPLICATIONS	A sprain of the PCL
COMMENTS	The lower leg must be stabilized as distally as possible; supporting the tibia proximally prevents it from sagging posteriorly. An assistant may be used to hold the distal legs.

PCL = posterior cruciate ligament.

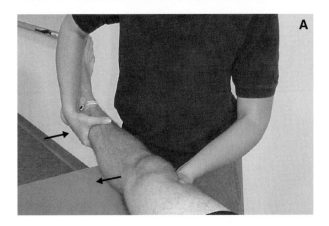

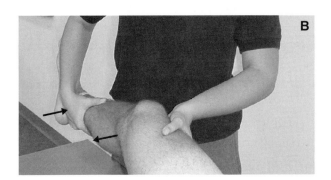

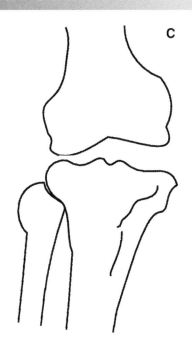

Valgus stress test **(A)** in full extension to determine the integrity of medial capsular restraints, **(B)** with the knee flexed to 25° to isolate the medial collateral ligament, and schematic representation of the opening of the medial joint line **(C)**.

PATIENT POSITION	Lying supine with the involved leg close to the edge of the table
POSITION OF EXAMINER	Standing lateral to the involved limb One hand supports the medial portion of the distal tibia while the other hand grasps the knee along the lateral joint line. To test the entire medial joint capsule, the knee is kept in complete extension. To isolate the MCL, the knee is flexed to 25°.
EVALUATIVE PROCEDURE	A medial (valgus) force is applied to the knee while the distal tibia is moved laterally.
POSITIVE TEST	Increased laxity, decreased quality of the end-point, and pain compared with the uninvolved limb
IMPLICATIONS	In complete extension: a sprain of the MCL, medial joint capsule, and possibly the cruciate ligaments In 25° flexion: a sprain of the MCL
MODIFICATION	To promote greater relaxation of the patient's musculature, the thigh may be left on the table with the knee flexed over the side.
COMMENTS	When testing the knee in full extension, it is recommended that the thigh be left on the table, preventing shortening of the hamstring muscle group. The apprehension test (see Chapter 7) should be performed before valgus stress testing in patients who have a history of patellar dislocations or subluxations.

MCL = medial collateral ligament.

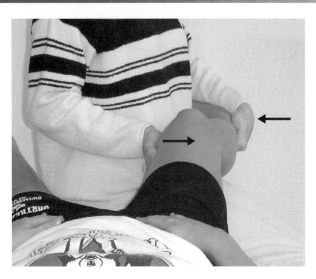
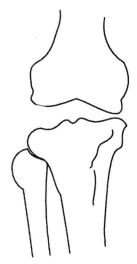

PATIENT POSITION	Lying supine with the involved leg close to the edge of the table
POSITION OF EXAMINER	Sitting on the table One hand supports the lateral portion of the distal tibia, while the other hand grasps the knee along the medial joint line. To test the entire lateral joint capsule, the knee is kept in complete extension. To isolate the LCL, the knee is flexed to 25°.
EVALUATIVE PROCEDURE	A lateral (varus) force is applied to the knee while the distal tibia is move inward.
POSITIVE TEST	Increased laxity, decreased quality of the end-point, or pain compared with the uninvolved limb
IMPLICATIONS	In complete extension: a sprain of the LCL, lateral joint capsule, cruciate ligaments, and related structures, indicating possible rotatory instability of the joint In 25° of flexion: a sprain of the LCL
COMMENTS	When testing the knee in full extension, it is recommended that the thigh be left on the table, preventing shortening of the hamstring muscle group.

LCL = lateral collateral ligament.

Tests for Stability of the Proximal Tibiofibular Syndesmosis

The proximal tibiofibular syndesmosis is of concern because of the attachment of the LCL and biceps femoris to the fibular head. Instability of the syndesmosis most commonly caused by a "glancing" blow to the superior fibula results in altered biomechanics and decreased lateral stability secondary to abnormal movement between the fibula and tibia (Box 6–11).

NEUROLOGIC TESTING

A neurologic examination is required when referred pain to the knee is suspected, the proximal tibiofibular joint displays laxity, or after a dislocation of the tibiofemoral joint. Neurologic involvement may also be associated with swelling within the popliteal fossa or lateral joint line. Additionally, local or distal neurologic involvement may occur after surgery (Fig 6–22). (Refer to Box 1–5 for a lower quarter screen.)

◆ PATHOLOGIES AND RELATED SPECIAL TESTS

Trauma to the knee may result from a contact-related mechanism, through rotational forces placed on the knee while bearing weight, or secondary to overuse. Knee injuries suffered by school-aged athletes (including college students) are most likely to be the result of a

Box 6–11
TIBIOFIBULAR TRANSLATION TEST

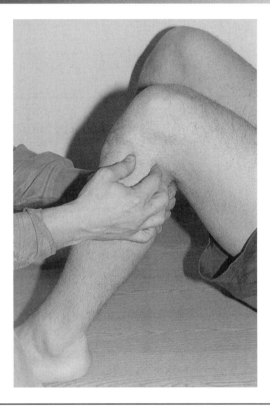

PATIENT POSITION	Lying supine with the knee passively flexed to approximately 90°
POSITION OF EXAMINER	Standing lateral to the involved side
EVALUATIVE PROCEDURE	One hand stabilizes the tibia while the other hand grasps the fibular head. While stabilizing the tibia, the examiner attempts to displace the fibular head anteriorly and then posteriorly.
POSITIVE TEST	Any perceived movement of the fibula on the tibia compared with the uninvolved side or pain elicited during the test
IMPLICATIONS	An anterior fibular shift indicates damage to the proximal posterior tibiofibular ligament; posterior displacement reflects instability of the anterior tibiofibular ligament of the proximal tibiofibular syndesmosis.

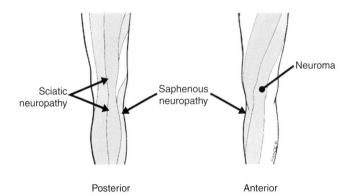

FIGURE 6–22. Local neuropathies of the knee. These findings should also be correlated with a lower quarter neurological screen.

single traumatic episode. A small portion of this population and a larger percentage of older athletes are likely to suffer from degenerative changes within the knee.

UNIPLANAR KNEE SPRAINS

Uniplanar knee sprains present with instability in only one of the body's cardinal planes. Damage to the MCL or LCL leads to valgus or varus instability in the frontal plane. Trauma to the ACL or PCL results in instability in the sagittal plane where the tibia shifts anteriorly or posteriorly relative to the femur. This type of injury involves damage that is isolated to a single structure. When multiple structures are involved (e.g., the ACL and lateral joint capsule), a multiplanar or rotatory instability results.

Medial Collateral Ligament Sprains

The MCL is damaged from valgus tensile forces, most commonly caused by a blow to the lateral aspect of the knee. Noncontact valgus loading or a rotational force being placed on the knee can also injure the MCL. When the knee is fully extended, the valgus force is dissipated by the superficial and deep layers of the MCL, the anteromedial and posteromedial joint capsule, and the tendons of the pes anserine group. When the knee is flexed beyond 20 degrees, the superficial layer of the MCL becomes more responsible for resisting valgus forces.

Medial collateral ligament sprains may occur in isolation, but because of the deep layer's communication with the medial joint capsule and medial meniscus, concurrent injury to these structures must always be suspected. Rotational forces placed on the knee at the time of injury may also lead to the involvement of the ACL.[42] Fractures of the distal femoral physis can mimic a third-degree MCL sprain in growing patients (Table 6–4).[43] As described in Chapter 7, patellar dislocations

can occur secondary to a valgus force placed on the knee. Therefore, all MCL sprains must include an evaluation of the patella for lateral dislocation before stress testing.[44]

Most MCL injuries are managed nonoperatively, even when surgical repair of other structures, including the ACL, is warranted.[45,46] The ligament lies within the soft tissue matrix of the medial aspect of the knee and enjoys an adequate blood supply for healing. An aggressive functional rehabilitation program provides long-term stability against valgus forces.[45] Successful nonoperative rehabilitation of the MCL includes protecting the joint from valgus stress while healing, providing an optimal healing environment within the MCL through a controlled restoration of ROM, and adequate strengthening and proprioceptive training of the lower extremity. Use of a knee brace with the ability to limit ROM may be indicated in grade II and III injuries to control further injurious stress and provide the restoration of motion without compromising healing within the ligament.[47,48]

Operative treatment for injuries of the MCL has been shown to have a high complication rate, including postoperative stiffness and patellofemoral dysfunction.[49] Clinicians need to be aware of these potential complica-

---

Table 6–4
EVALUATIVE FINDINGS: Medial Collateral Ligament Sprain

Examination Segment	Clinical findings	
History	*Onset:*	Acute
	Pain Characteristics:	Medial aspect of the knee, especially along the joint line
	Mechanism:	A valgus force to the knee or, less commonly, external rotation of the tibia
Inspection	Immediate inspection of an MCL injury may produce unremarkable findings	
	Over time, swelling may be present along the medial aspect of the knee	
Palpation	Tenderness along the length of the MCL from its origin below the adductor tubercle to the insertion on the medial tibial flare	
Functional tests	*AROM:*	Pain with possible loss of motion during the terminal ranges of flexion and extension; greater loss of range of motion when the MCL is torn proximal to the joint line because of greater capsular involvement[42]
	PROM:	Pain and possible loss of motion during the terminal ranges of flexion and extension.
	RROM:	Decreased strength secondary to pain.
Ligamentous tests	Valgus laxity in complete extension indicates involvement of the MCL, medial capsular structures and possibly the cruciate ligaments.	
	Valgus laxity in 25° of flexion indicates involvement of the MCL	
Neurologic tests	Not applicable	
Special tests	Slocum drawer test for laxity of the anteromedial capsule	
Comments	Adolescent patients displaying the valgus laxity should be referred to a physician to rule out the possibility of trauma to the epiphyseal plate	
	If a rotational force is suspected, laxity is displayed in complete extension, or the Slocum drawer test result is positive, pathology to the ACL and PCL should be ruled out	
	The patella should be checked for lateral stability prior to valgus stress testing	
	An associated bone bruise or OCD may occur secondary to lateral compressive forces	

ACL = anterior cruciate ligament; AROM = active range of motion; MCL = medial collateral ligament; OCD = osteochondral defect; PCL = posterior cruciate ligament; PROM = passive range of motion; RROM = resisted range of motion.

tions whenever treating a patient after surgical repair of the MCL so any symptoms found during the evaluation can be properly treated.

Lateral Collateral Ligament Sprains

Caused by a blow to the medial knee that places tensile forces on the lateral structures or by internal rotation of the tibia on the femur, LCL sprains result in varus laxity of the knee. The extracapsular nature of the LCL gives it a normally "springy" end-feel. A varus stress test result that feels empty when compared with the contralateral side should be considered a positive result for an LCL sprain (Table 6–5).

Because a varus force with concurrent internal tibial rotation can cause damage to the lateral capsular structures and the ACL, anterolateral rotatory instability (ALRI) must be suspected in patients suffering from LCL trauma. Because of the relative proximity of the peroneal nerve, patients suspected of having suffered an injury to the lateral or posterolateral aspect of the knee require careful evaluation of distal function of the common and superficial peroneal nerve.

Although the LCL is an extracapsular and extraarticular structure, the ligament still relies on synovial fluid for much of its nutrition.[50] The LCL's relatively poor

healing properties and the ligament's importance in providing rotational stability to the knee often necessitate early surgical repair or late reconstruction.[51]

Anterior Cruciate Ligament Sprains

Injury to the ACL results from a force causing an anterior displacement of the tibia relative to the femur (or the femur being driven posteriorly on the tibia), from noncontact-related rotational injuries, or from hyperextension of the knee. Unlike injury to the body's other ligaments, the majority of ACL sprains arise from noncontact-related torsional stress, such as what occurs when an athlete cuts or pivots.[23, 24]

The rotatory forces placed on the knee make "isolated" trauma to the ACL unlikely. Instability of the knee is greatly increased when trauma also damages one or more of the other ligaments or the menisci.[33] As is described in the Rotatory Instabilities section of this chapter, the degree of anterior displacement of the tibia is increased and an anterior subluxation of the tibial condyles results when the anteromedial or anterolateral joint capsules, pes anserine, biceps femoris, or IT band are also traumatized.

Several intrinsic and extrinsic factors predisposing factors to ACL injuries have been suggested (Table

Table 6–5
EVALUATIVE FINDINGS: Lateral Collateral Ligament Sprain

Examination Segment	Clinical Findings	
History	**Onset:**	Acute
	Pain characteristics:	Lateral joint line of the knee and fibular head
	Mechanism:	Varus force placed on the knee or excess internal tibial rotation
Inspection	Swelling, if present, is likely to be diffuse, especially when trauma is isolated to the LCL, because it is an extracapsular structure	
Palpation	Palpation eliciting tenderness along the length of the LCL and possibly the lateral joint line	
Functional tests	**AROM:**	Pain and loss of motion may be experienced during flexion and at the terminal extension
	PROM:	Pain and loss of motion may be experienced during the terminal ROMs, although lack of such pain does not conclusively rule out LCL trauma
	RROM:	Same as for PROM
Ligamentous tests	Varus laxity in complete extension indicates involvement of the lateral capsular structures and possibly the cruciate ligaments Varus laxity in 25° of flexion isolates the LCL	
Neurologic tests	Not applicable	
Special tests	Slocum drawer test for laxity of the anterolateral capsule	
Comments	The LCL has a normal "spring" when a varus force is applied Adolescent patients displaying varus laxity require a referral to a physician to rule out possible epiphyseal plate trauma For patients who have reported a rotatory mechanism of injury or who display LCL laxity through either a varus stress or a positive Slocum drawer test result, anterolateral rotatory instability must be suspected	

ACL = anterior cruciate ligament; AROM = active range of motion; MCL = medial collateral ligament; PCL = posterior cruciate ligament; PROM = passive range of motion; RROM = resisted range of motion.

Table 6–6
FACTORS PREDISPOSING INDIVIDUALS TO ANTERIOR CRUCIATE LIGAMENT INJURY

Extrinsic to the Knee	Intrinsic to the Knee
Sport-specific body motions[52]	Joint laxity[52]
Muscle strength[52]	Limb alignment[52]
Muscular coordination[52]	Small intercondylar notch[52,61,62]
Athletic skill coordination[52]	Small size of the ACL[52]
The shoe–surface interface[52]	Genu recurvatum[55,57]
Hyperpronation of the foot (navicular drop)[53–55]	
Weakness or rupture of the tibialis posterior[56]	
Anterior pelvic tilt[57]	
Anteverted hips[57]	
Menstrual cycle[58–60]	

ACL = anterior cruciate ligament.

6–6).[52] Most predisposing factors share the common trait of causing internal tibial rotation, thus placing an additional stress on the ACL.

Associated with the injury mechanism, the patient may describe hearing or sensing a "pop" within the knee joint and an immediate loss of knee function. Swelling occurs rapidly secondary to trauma of the medial geniculate artery, the ACL's primary blood supply. Normally this hemarthrosis remains within the fibrous capsule, but trauma to the capsule results in diffuse swelling that may *extravasate* distally over time. Intracapsular swelling combined with the tension placed on the ACL limits the ROM (see Fig. 6–8). Laxity of the ACL may be confirmed through Lachman's test and the anterior drawer test. However, clinical laxity is not a strong predictor of functional ability (Table 6–7).[63]

Because PCL deficiency can replicate positive test results for ACL involvement as the tibia is returned to its normal position, tests for PCL tears need to be performed to rule out such false-positive results.

The term "partially torn ACL" is a functional misnomer. Because the bands of the ACL wind upon each other, even partial trauma to an individual band results in biomechanical dysfunction, instability, and increased stress on the remaining fibers, predisposing them to future injury. Knees with partial tears of the ACL, typically involving the anteromedial bundle, may initially appear stable during manual stress testing but degrade to demonstrate signs of clinical instability as the remaining ligament fibers adaptively lengthen secondary to increased stress loads.[28]

The early onset of degenerative arthritis is thought to be one possible consequence of an ACL-deficient knee. If the patient has functional instability, repeated episodes of instability may lead to further injury of the joint. The menisci are especially vulnerable in symptomatic ACL deficient knees. Patients who perform phys-

ical activities that do not involve cutting or pivoting on a planted foot may not experience pain or dysfunction.

The rehabilitation program focuses on restoring ROM, lower extremity strength, and proprioception. The use of a functional knee brace may be helpful, although the *efficacy* of these devices has not been substantiated.

Anterior cruciate ligament deficient patients who perform activities involving cutting and pivoting most likely benefit from ACL reconstruction. Several donor tissue options are available, including *autografts* and *allografts*. The use of an accelerated rehabilitation program involving early return of ROM, early weight bearing, and restoration of muscular function has been found to decrease the time lost after surgery.[64] Accelerated programs have also been found to decrease surgical morbidity, including postoperative stiffness and patellofemoral pain.[65]

Anterior Cruciate Ligament Injuries in Females

The increased popularity of women's athletics has attracted a large number of female athletes into the world of sports. Although the expected increase in participation of female athletes would normally give rise to an increased number of injuries, female athletes have experienced a disproportionately high rate of noncontact ACL injuries relative to their male counterparts.[57,66,67]

Although women normally have an increased amount of anterior tibial translation compared with men, this fails to account for the high incidence rate.[14] The intrinsic and extrinsic factors presented in Table 6–6 that preload the ACL and predispose individuals to ACL injuries also hold true for women. In particular, subtalar joint pronation or navicular drop, genu recurvatum, anterior pelvic tilt, and anteverted hips seem to account for much of the discrepancy in injury rates.[55,57] Also, females, on average, have narrower intercondylar notch widths, which may partially account for the higher noncontact ACL injury rate in female athletes.[62]

Anterior cruciate ligament laxity has also been traced to the different phases of the menstrual cycle. Laxity has been associated with surging levels of estrogen and

Extravasate Fluid escaping from vessels into the surrounding tissue.

Efficacy The ability of a protocol to produce the intended effects.

Autograft The tissues used to replace the ligament harvested from the patient's body (e.g., bone-patellar tendon-bone, hamstring tendon).

Allograft The tissues used to replace the ligament obtained from a cadaver.

Table 6–7
EVALUATIVE FINDINGS: Anterior Cruciate Sprain

Examination Segment	Clinical Findings	
History	*Onset:*	Acute
	Pain characteristics:	Within the knee joint, sometimes described as "pain" or a "pop" under the kneecap
	Mechanism:	Rotation of the knee while the foot is planted (tensile forces), a blow that drives the tibia anterior relative to the femur or the femur posterior relative to the tibia (shear force), or hyperextension
	Predisposing conditions:	See Table 6–6
Inspection	Rapid effusion, usually forming within hours after the onset of injury	
Palpation	For isolated ACL injuries, pain is not normally reported during palpation (other than that resulting from a contusion caused by the traumatic force) The sweep and ballotable patella test results are positive if intracapsular swelling is present	
Functional tests	*AROM:*	Pain or intracapsular swellng may prohibit any meaningful ROM tests; pain is expected to be greatest at the extremes of the ROM
	PROM:	Pain likely throughout the ROM (especially at the extremes) and possibly intensified when the tibia is internally or externally rotated
	RROM:	Pain and limitation in the ROM possibly precluding this portion of the examination's being conducted in the acute stage of injury
Ligamentous tests	Lachman's test, alternate Lachman's test, and anterior drawer test	
Neurologic tests	Not applicable	
Special tests	None for isolated ACL sprains (see anteromedial and anterolateral instability)	
Comments	The anterior drawer and Lachman's tests may not produce positive test results in the hours after the onset of the injury because of muscle guarding Trauma to the PCL may produce false-positive results for ACL insufficiency	

ACL = anterior cruciate ligament; AROM = active range of motion; PCL = posterior cruciate ligament; PROM = passive range of motion; ROM = range of motion; RROM = resisted range of motion.

progesterone; laxity is most increased during the luteal phase of the menstrual cycle. Increased laxity was also demonstrated during the follicular phase.[58] The risk of sustaining an ACL injury appears to be increased during the week before or after the start of the menstrual period, when the ACL is most lax.[59,60]

Posterior Cruciate Ligament Sprains

Uniplanar PCL injury results from the tibia's being driven posteriorly on the femur or from hyperflexion or hyperextension of the knee when the joint is distracted (e.g., when the heel steps in a hole). Landing on the anterior tibia while the knee is flexed can drive the tibia posteriorly, stressing the PCL (Fig. 6–23).

Immediately after the onset of injury, the patient may be relatively asymptomatic or may display the signs and symptoms of a strain of the medial head of the gastrocnemius or a sprain of the posterior capsule.[68] Over time, symptoms such as pain in the posterior

knee, weakness of the hamstring and quadriceps muscle groups, and reduced ROM during flexion become evident. The posterior drawer and sag tests are highly reliable and sensitive in identifying the presence of chronic PCL sprains (Table 6–8).[69] Instability is greatest when there is concurrent damage to both the PCL and the posterolateral structures of the knee.[10,11] The presence of a partial or complete tear of the PCL can be identified through MRI.[69]

Statically, joint loading, joint congruency, and muscular activity can compensate for PCL deficiency. The strength of the quadriceps muscle group soon returns after a PCL sprain to assist the popliteus in providing muscular compensation against posterior tibial displacement.[9,38,70] Actual posterior laxity does not always result in knee dysfunction.[71] Nonoperative patients can regain full function and independence and may often return to athletic competition unhindered by the ligamentous deficit.[71] However, over time PCL deficiency can result in changes in the structure and function of the ACL, leading to chronic joint instability.[70,72]

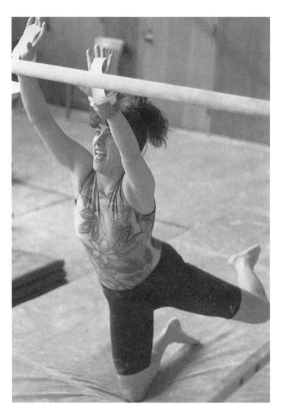

FIGURE 6–23. Mechanism for posterior cruciate ligament (PCL) trauma. Landing on a bent knee and plantarflexed foot forces the tibia posteriorly relative to the femur.

ROTATIONAL KNEE INSTABILITIES

Unlike uniplanar knee instabilities, rotatory (multiplanar) instabilities involve abnormal internal or external rotation at the tibiofemoral joint. The types of instabilities are named based on the relative direction in which the tibia subluxates on the femur. When this type of instability occurs, the axis of tibial rotation is shifted in the direction opposite that of the subluxation (Fig. 6–24). The four categories of rotatory instability are presented in Table 6–9.

Rotatory instabilities result when multiple structures are traumatized, often as the result of rotational forces placed on the knee. The tests for laxity of the individual structures may produce only mildly positive results. However, when the combined laxity of each structure is summed, the degree of instability is marked.

Any injury to the knee's ligaments is suspect for causing rotatory instability. Therefore, any injury to the cruciate or collateral ligaments, the IT band, the joint capsule, or the biceps femoris must be presumed as potentially resulting in rotational instability.[16] Clinically, patients suffering from rotatory instability report the feeling of the knee "giving way," decreased muscle strength, diminished performance, and a lack of confidence in the stability of the joint. Tests for rotatory instability must not be performed as part of an on-field examination. These tests will often only produce positive results when the patient is under anesthesia.

◢◢◢ **Table 6–8**
EVALUATIVE FINDINGS: Posterior Cruciate Ligament Sprain

Examination Segment	Clinical Findings	
History	*Onset:*	Acute
	Pain characteristics:	Within the knee joint radiating posteriorly, although pain may not be experienced
	Mechanism:	Posterior displacement of the tibia on the femur (effect magnified when the foot is plantarflexed)
		Hyperflexion of the knee
		Hyperextension of the knee
Inspection	The involved knee displaying a posterior sag of the tibia; effusion formation possible over time	
Palpation	Tenderness may be elicited in the popliteal fossa if the sprain involves the posterior capsular structures or popliteus muscle; otherwise, no pain or abnormalities are usually noted.	
Functional tests	*AROM:*	Acutely, normal ROM present; pain and restrictions possible as the knee nears full flexion
	PROM:	Pain produced as the knee nears 90° of flexion and with overpressure during flexion, especially in the presence of a partial PCL tear
	RROM:	Normal strength during extension; pain as the knee nears terminal flexion
Ligamentous tests	Posterior drawer test; Godfrey's sign, external rotation test	
Neurologic tests	Not applicable	
Special tests	None	
Comments	Acutely, PCL sprains may resemble strains of the medial head of the gastrocnemius or a sprain of the posterior capsule	

AROM = active range of motion; PCL = posterior cruciate ligament; PROM = passive range of motion; RROM = resisted range of motion.

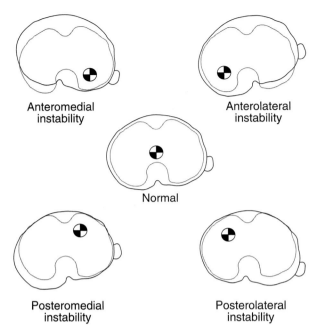

FIGURE 6–24. Classification of rotatory instabilities. The tibial articulating surface is shown in solid lines, the femoral articular surfaces in shaded lines. The type of instability is described based on the displacement of the tibia relative to the femur. Note that the axes of rotation are approximated.

Anterolateral Rotatory Instability

Involving trauma to the ACL and the anterolateral capsular restraints, anterolateral rotary instability (ALRI) results in a greater displacement of the tibia because of the injury to the lateral extraarticular restraints.[73] Disruption of the LCL, IT band, biceps femoris, and lateral meniscus accentuates the amount of anterior tibial displacement and internal tibial rotation, especially when combined with a tear of the ACL. Many special tests exist for determining the presence of ALRI, each with its own merits

and limitations. The large number of tests probably reflects their relatively low reliability.

Three tests specific to this pathology are discussed here: the lateral pivot shift, the Slocum ALRI test, and the flexion-rotation drawer. In addition, two tests, the Slocum drawer test and the crossover test, may be used to determine the presence of either ALRI or anteromedial rotatory instability (AMRI). A positive result for any one of the following techniques is sufficient to warrant further examination by an orthopedic physician.

A derivation of the anterior drawer test, the **Slocum drawer test** attempts to isolate either the anteromedial or the anterolateral joint capsule (Box 6–12). Internally rotating the tibia checks for the presence of ALRI; externally rotating it checks for AMRI.

The **crossover test** is a semifunctional test used to determine the rotational stability of the knee (Box 6–13). This test is not as exacting as other tests for ligamentous instability, but it has the advantage of replicating a sport-specific skill. Although primarily used to determine the presence of ALRI, the crossover test may be modified to test for AMRI by stepping behind with the uninvolved leg.

Used to evaluate ALRI, the **pivot shift test** (also known as the lateral pivot shift) duplicates the anterior subluxation and reduction that occurs during functional activities in ACL-deficient knees (Box 6–14). The tibia is internally rotated and a valgus force is applied to the joint while the knee is moved from extension into flexion. In the presence of a torn ACL, the femur is displaced posteriorly when the knee is placed in 10 to 20 degrees of flexion. As the knee continues into flexion, the IT band changes its angle of pull from that of an extensor to that of a flexor. When the knee reaches the range of 30 to 40 degrees of flexion, the IT band causes the tibia to relocate, resulting in an appreciable "clunk." The pivot shift has been documented as a sensitive test for acute and chronic ACL injuries.[74] However, the presence of a negative pivot shift test result does not rule out the possibility of a partial ACL tear.[75]

Table 6–9
CLASSIFICATION OF ROTATIONAL KNEE INSTABILITIES

Instability	Tibial Displacement	Pathologic Axis	Structural Instability
Anteromedial	Medial tibial plateau subluxates anteriorly	Posterolateral, resulting in abnormal external tibial rotation	ACL, anteromedial capsule, MCL, pes anserine, medial meniscus, posteromedial capsule
Anterolateral	Lateral tibial plateau subluxates anteriorly	Posteromedial, resulting in abnormal internal tibial rotation	ACL, anterolateral capsule, LCL, IT band, biceps femoris, lateral meniscus, posterolateral capsule
Posteromedial	Medial tibial plateau subluxates posteriorly	Anterolateral, resulting in abnormal internal tibial rotation	Posterior oblique ligament, MCL, semimembranosus, anteromedial capsule
Posterolateral	Lateral tibial plateau subluxates posteriorly	Anteromedial, resulting in abnormal external tibial rotation	Arcuate ligament complex, LCL, biceps femoris, posterolateral capsule

ACL = anterior cruciate ligament; IT = iliotibial; LCL = lateral collateral ligament; MCL = medial collateral ligament.

Box 6–12
SLOCUM DRAWER TEST FOR ROTATIONAL KNEE INSTABILITY

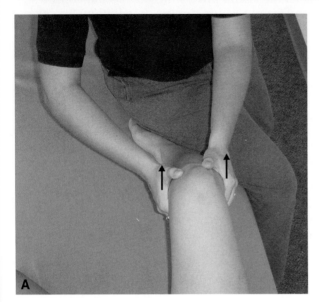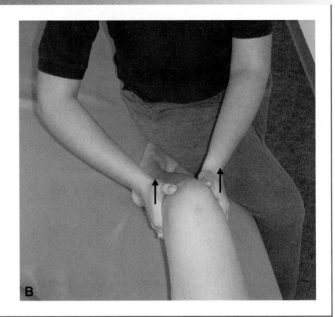

Slocum drawer test with the tibia internally rotated to isolate the lateral capsular structures **(A)** and with the tibia externally rotated to isolate the medial capsule **(B).**

PATIENT POSITION	Lying supine with the knee flexed to 90°
POSITION OF EXAMINER	Sitting on the patient's foot: **(A)** The tibia is internally rotated to 25° to test for anterolateral capsular instability. **(B)** The tibia is externally rotated to 15° to test for anteromedial capsular instability.
EVALUATIVE PROCEDURE	The tibia is drawn anteriorly.
POSITIVE TEST RESULT	An increased amount of anterior tibial translation compared with the opposite (uninvolved) limb or the lack of a firm end-point
IMPLICATIONS	**(A)** Test for anterolateral instability: damage to the ACL, anterolateral capsule, LCL, IT band, popliteus tendon, posterolateral capsule **(B)** Test for anteromedial instability: damage to the MCL, anteromedial capsule, ACL, posteromedial capsule

ACL = anterior cruciate ligament; IT = iliotibial; LCL = lateral collateral ligament; MCL = medial collateral ligament.

Box 6–13
CROSSOVER TEST FOR ROTATIONAL KNEE INSTABILITY

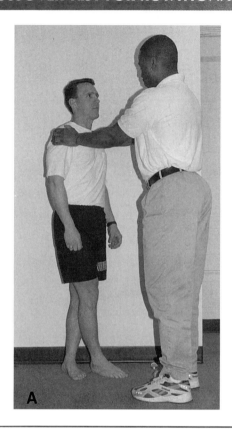

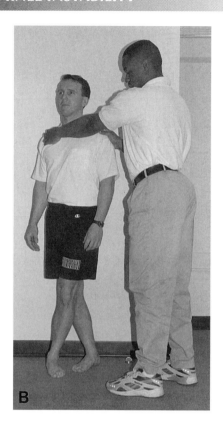

Crossover test: Stepping in front of the injured leg determines the presence of anterolateral rotatory instability **(A)**. Stepping behind the injured leg determines anteromedial rotatory instability **(B)**. Note that patient's left leg is being tested.

PATIENT POSITION	Standing with the weight on the involved limb
POSITION OF EXAMINER	Standing in front of the patient
EVALUATIVE PROCEDURE	**(A)** ALRI: The patient steps across and in front with the uninvolved leg, rotating the torso in the direction of movement. The weight-bearing foot remains fixated. **(B)** AMRI: The patient steps across and behind with the uninvolved leg rotating the torso in the direction of movement. The weight-bearing foot remains fixated.
POSITIVE TEST	Patient reports pain, instability, or apprehension
IMPLICATIONS	**(A)** ALRI: Instability of the lateral capsular restraints **(B)** AMRI: Instability of the medial capsular restraints

ALRI = anterolateral rotatory instability; AMRI = anteromedial rotatory instability.

Box 6–14

LATERAL PIVOT SHIFT TEST FOR ANTEROLATERAL KNEE INSTABILITY

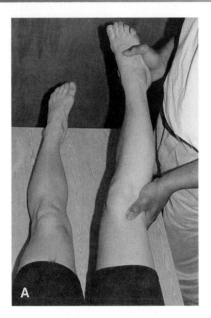 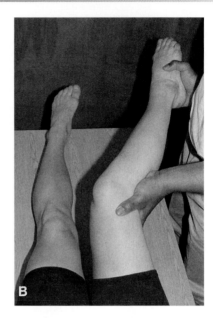

PATIENT POSITION	Lying supine with the hip passively flexed to 30°
POSITION OF EXAMINER	Standing lateral to the patient, the distal lower leg and/or ankle is grasped, maintaining 20° of internal tibial rotation. The knee is allowed to sag into complete extension (**A**). The opposite hand grasps the lateral portion of the leg at the level of the superior tibiofibular joint, increasing the force of internal rotation.
EVALUATIVE PROCEDURE	While maintaining internal rotation, a valgus force is applied to the knee while it is slowly flexed (**B**). To avoid masking any positive test results, the patient must remain relaxed throughout this test.
POSITIVE TEST	The tibia's position on the femur reduces as the leg is flexed in the range of 30° to 40°. During extension, the anterior subluxation is felt.
IMPLICATIONS	Tear of the ACL, posterolateral capsule, arcuate ligament complex, or the IT band
COMMENTS	Meniscal involvement may limit ROM to produce a false-negative test result. Muscle guarding can produce a false-negative result. This test is most reliable when performed by a physician while the patient is under anesthesia.

ACL = anterior cruciate ligament; IT = iliotibial; ROM = range of motion.

During the **Slocum ALRI test**, The patient's body weight is used to fixate the femur while the knee is flexed and a simultaneous valgus force is applied (Box 6–15). As the knee reaches 30 to 50 degrees, a subluxation of the tibia is reduced. This test is not as sensitive as the lateral pivot shift but is useful when dealing with large or heavy patients.

The **flexion-rotation drawer test (FRD)** involves the stabilization of the tibia, resulting in the relative subluxation of the femur (Box 6–16). In the presence of

ALRI, lifting and supporting the distal lower leg causes the femur to displace posteriorly and rotate externally. The test then identifies the subsequent reduction of the femur relative to the tibia.

Anteromedial Rotatory Instability

O'Donohue described a triad injury involving the ACL, MCL, and medial meniscus, resulting in AMRI. Recently this definition has been revised, with the lat-

Box 6–15

SLOCUM ANTEROLATERAL ROTATORY INSTABILITY (ALRI) TEST

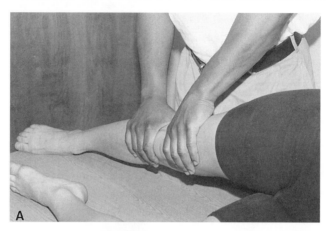

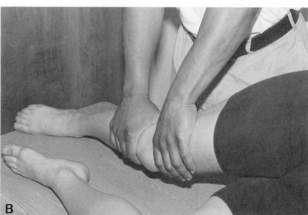

PATIENT POSITION	**(A)** Lying on the uninvolved side Uninvolved leg flexed at the hip and knee, moving it anterior to the involved extremity Involved hip externally rotated Involved leg extended with the medial aspect of the foot resting against the table to provide stability
POSITION OF EXAMINER	Standing behind the patient, grasping the knee on the distal aspect of the femur and the proximal fibula
EVALUATIVE PROCEDURE	A valgus force is placed on the knee, causing it to move into 30° to 50° of flexion **(B)**.
POSITIVE TEST	An appreciable "clunk" or instability as the lateral tibial plateau subluxates or pain or instability is reported
IMPLICATIONS	Tear of the ACL, LCL, anterolateral capsule, arcuate ligament complex, biceps femoris tendon and/or IT band.

ACL = anterior cruciate ligament; IT = iliotibial; LCL = lateral cruciate ligament.

eral meniscus being involved in this type of injury more frequently than in the medial one.[76] As described in the ALRI section, the variants of the Slocum drawer test and the crossover test may be used to determine the presence of AMRI. Additionally, isolated tests for ACL and MCL insufficiency yield positive test results.

Posterolateral Rotatory Instability

Posterolateral rotatory instability involves the anterior displacement of the lateral femoral condyle relative to the tibia (the tibia externally rotating relative to the femur). The amount of external tibial rotation varies greatly from person to person and increases with the

Box 6-16

FLEXION-REDUCTION DRAWER TEST FOR ANTEROLATERAL ROTATORY INSTABILITY

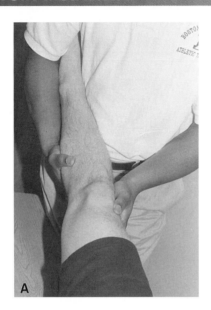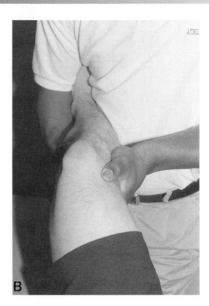

PATIENT POSITION	Lying supine The clinician lifts the calf and ankle so that the knee is flexed to approximately 25°. Heavier patients may require that the tibia be supported between the examiner's arm and torso.
POSITION OF EXAMINER	Standing lateral and distal to the involved knee
EVALUATIVE PROCEDURE	The tibia is depressed posteriorly to the femur. A valgus stress and axial compression along the tibial shaft are applied as the knee is slowly flexed.
POSITIVE TEST	The femur's relocating itself on the tibia by moving anteriorly and internally rotating on the tibia
IMPLICATIONS	Tear of the ACL, LCL, anterolateral capsule, arcuate ligament complex, biceps femoris tendon and/or IT band.

ACL = anterior cruciate ligament; IT = iliotibial; LCL = lateral cruciate ligament.

amount of knee flexion.[77] This motion is produced when the axis of rotation is moved medially over the medial meniscus.

The patient often reports a history of external tibial rotation or knee hyperextension and describes knee instability. Pain is localized to the posterolateral aspect of the knee, but distraction of these structures may produce pain in the medial knee secondary to compression of the structures.[78] The patient may describe the sensation of the knee's giving way during activity or static stance. Pain and instability make participation in strenuous activities difficult or impossible. Gross swelling is often not present. Non–weight-bearing ROM is not affected, but pain may be described medially. Tests for valgus and varus instability typically yield negative results (Table 6–10). The **External Rotation Test for Posterolateral Rotatory Instability** may produce positive findings (Box 6–17).[79,80]

MENISCAL TEARS

Historically, the majority of meniscal tears were believed to involve the medial meniscus. However, contemporary research has reversed this thought.[81,82] Many lateral meniscal tears, often asymptomatic, are associated with ACL sprains. Improved diagnostic tests such as MRIs are now detecting lateral meniscal tears that once may have gone undetected.

Acute meniscal tears result from rotation and flexion of the knee, impinging the menisci between the articular condyles of the tibia and femur. Because of its greater mobility, the lateral meniscus may develop tears secondary to repeated stress, presenting with an insidious onset.

Two evaluative tests, **McMurray's test** (Box 6–18) and **Apley's compression and distraction test** (Box 6–19), may be used to determine the presence of meniscal tears.

Table 6–10
EVALUATIVE FINDING: Posterolateral Rotatory Instability

Examination Segment	Clinical Findings	
History	**Onset:**	Most have an acute onset, although chronic cases are possible.
	Pain characteristics:	Along the posterolateral knee and popliteal area
		Possibly evolving to an ache throughout the knee
	Mechanism:	Most commonly, a direct blow to the posterolateral aspect of the knee; rotational force
Inspection	Possible effusion with ACL or PCL involvement; swelling possibly more diffuse because of tearing in the capsule	
Palpation	Tenderness possible along the posterolateral capsule, lateral knee, and popliteal fossa	
Functional tests	**AROM:**	Acutely, normal ROM; pain and restrictions possible as the knee nears full flexion
	PROM:	Pain produced as the knee nears 90° of flexion and with hyperextension
	RROM:	Ability to resist possibly inhibited by pain, especially as the knee moves back into a flexed position
Ligamentous tests	Posterior drawer test, Godfrey's sign, external rotation test; other tests for rotatory instability may also show positive results	
	Tests for assessing the instability of other injured ligaments as needed	
Neurologic tests	Peroneal nerve distribution should be assessed	
Special tests	None	
Comments	Posterolateral instability is typically found concurrently with a tear of the anterior or posterior cruciate ligament.	

ACL = anterior cruciate ligament; AROM = active range of motion; PCL = posterior cruciate ligament; PROM = passive range of motion; ROM = range of motion; RROM = resisted range of motion.

The patient's functional status, combined with the associated signs and symptoms, may be the best criteria for determining trauma to these structures and disability caused by the injury. Classic symptoms of meniscal tears involve "locking" or "clicking" (or both) in the knee, pain along the joint line, and the knee's "giving way" during activity. Patients noting "locking" of their knee should be further questioned about the nature of this phenomenon. Patients may describe a rotational mechanism combined with flexion and a valgus or varus stress (Table 6–11). It should be noted that pain may not be described if the tear occurs in the avascular zone of the meniscus. Meniscal lesions may mimic the symptoms of patellofemoral dysfunction. Chapter 7 discusses the differential evaluation between these two conditions.

Meniscal cysts are frequently associated with meniscal tears. After a longitudinal tear along the periphery of the meniscus, breaches are formed in the joint capsule that fill with synovial fluid. Meniscal cysts, typically painless and immobile, are often found coincidentally during MRI scanning or arthroscopic examination.[21]

OSTEOCHONDRAL DEFECTS

Osteochondral defects (OCDs) are fractures of the articular cartilage and underlying bone that are typically caused by compressive and shear forces (Fig. 6–25). Eighty percent of knee OCDs involve the medial femoral condyle. The lateral femoral condyle, tibial articulating surface, and patella are also susceptible to OCDs.[83] Males are affected three times more frequently than females.[83]

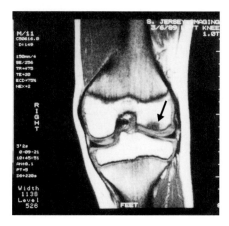

FIGURE 6–25. MRI of an osteochondral defect. The arrow points to an OCD on the lateral femoral condyle.

Box 6–17
EXTERNAL ROTATION TEST FOR POSTEROLATERAL KNEE INSTABILITY

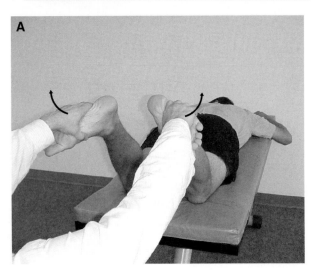

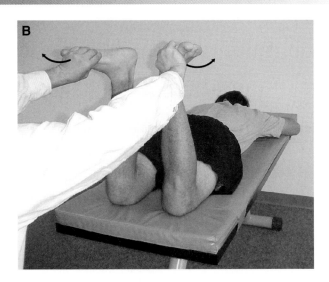

The external rotation test for posterolateral knee instability at 30° of the knee flexion **(A)** and at 90° of knee flexion **(B)**.

PATIENT POSITION	Prone or supine
POSITION OF EXAMINER	Standing at the patient's feet
EVALUATIVE PROCEDURE	The knee is flexed to 30° Using the medial border of the foot as a point of reference, the examiner forcefully externally rotates the patient's lower leg. The position of external rotation of the foot relative to the femur is assessed and compared with the opposite extremity. The knee is then flexed to 90° and the test repeated.
POSITIVE TEST	An increase of external rotation greater than 10° compared with the opposite side[79]
IMPLICATIONS	Difference at 30° of knee flexion but not at 90°: injury isolated to the arcuate ligament complex and the posterolateral structures of the knee Difference at 30° *and* 90° of knee flexion: trauma to the PCL, posterolateral knee structures, and the arcuate ligament complex Difference at 90° of knee flexion but not at 30°: isolated PCL sprain
COMMENTS	This test can also be performed with the patient in the supine position. Normal variations for rotation are expected. The results of one extremity must be compared with those of the opposite leg.

PCL = posterior cruciate ligament.

Box 6–18
MCMURRAY'S TEST FOR MENISCAL LESIONS

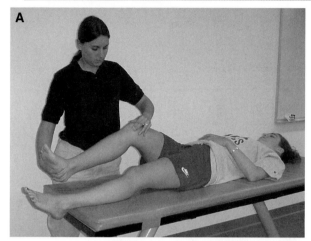
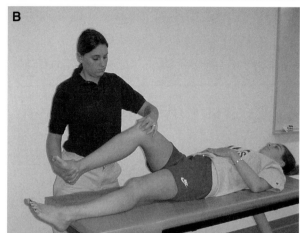
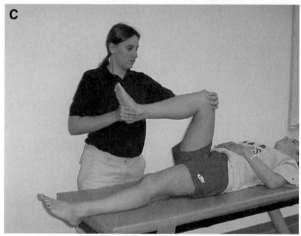
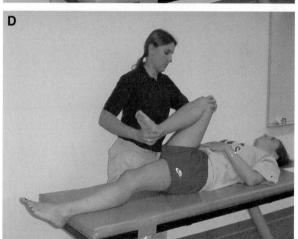

PATIENT POSITION	Lying supine
POSITION OF EXAMINER	Standing lateral and distal to the involved knee One hand supporting the lower leg while the thumb and index finger of the opposite hand positioned in the anteromedial and anterolateral joint line on either side of the patellar tendon (**A**).
EVALUATIVE PROCEDURE	(**B**) Pass one: With the tibia maintained in its neutral position, a valgus stress is applied while the knee is flexed through its available ROM. A varus stress is then applied as the knee is returned to full extension. (**C**) Pass two: The examiner internally rotates the tibia and applies a valgus stress while the knee is flexed through its available ROM. A varus stress is then applied as the knee is returned to full extension. (**D**) Pass three: With the tibia externally rotated, the examiner applies a valgus stress while the knee is flexed through its available ROM. A varus stress is then applied as the knee is returned to full extension.
POSITIVE TEST	A popping, clicking, or locking of the knee; pain emanating from the menisci; or a sensation similar to that experienced during ambulation
IMPLICATIONS	A meniscal tear on the side of the reported symptoms
COMMENTS	In acute injuries, the available ROM may not be sufficient to perform this test. Full flexion is required to isolate the posterior horns of the meniscus. Chondromalacia patellae or improper tracking of the patella may produce a click resembling that is associated with a meniscal tear.

ROM = range of motion.

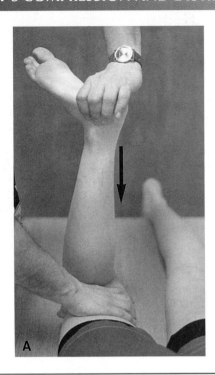
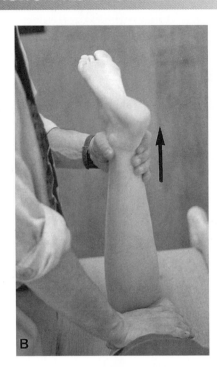

During the compression segment, pain may be caused by the menisci being caught between the tibia and femur **(A)**. During the distraction segment, the joint's ligaments are stressed **(B)**. Also, pain exhibited during compression should be reduced as the tibia is distracted from the femur.

PATIENT POSITION	Lying prone with knee flexed to 90°
POSITION OF EXAMINER	Standing lateral to the involved side
EVALUATIVE PROCEDURE	**(A)** Compression test: the clinician applies pressure to the plantar aspect of the heel, applying an axial load to the tibia while simultaneously internally and externally rotating the tibia. **(B)** Distraction test: the clinician grasps the lower leg and stabilizes the knee proximal to the femoral condyles. The tibia is distracted away from the femur while internally and externally rotating the tibia.
POSITIVE TEST	Pain experienced during compression that is reduced or eliminated during distraction
IMPLICATIONS	Meniscal tear
COMMENTS	Pain that is experienced only during distraction or during both compression and distraction may indicate trauma to the collateral ligaments, joint capsule, or cruciate ligaments.

Table 6–11
EVALUATIVE FINDINGS: Meniscal Tears

Examination Segment	Clinical Findings	
History	*Onset:*	Acute; patients with involving accumulated microtrauma often still present as having an acute onset
	Pain Characteristics:	Along the medial or lateral joint line with possible posterior knee pain; the patient may report episodes of the knee "giving out"
	Mechanism:	Tibial rotation combined with flexion and a varus or valgus stress
	Predisposing condition:	Over time, repetitive motion can degrade the lateral meniscus
Inspection	Inspection of a patient with an acutely torn meniscus normally does not present any conclusive findings.	
	Over time, or in the case of a peripheral tear of the meniscus, swelling may be seen along the joint or in the popiliteal fossa.	
	Joint effusion may develop over 24 to 48 hours.	
	A torn meniscus may prevent the patient from fully extending the knee, thus carrying it in a flexed position.	
Palpation	Pain along the joint line	
Functional tests	The ROM available may be limited owing to a mechanical block formed by a defect in the meniscus	
	AROM:	Possible decrease in ROM
	PROM:	Pain is present near the extremes of flexion or extension
	RROM:	Pain or locking is revealed as the torn portion of the meniscus passes beneath the femur's articular surface
Ligamentous tests	The integrity of all the knee ligamentous structures must be established	
	The presence of any ligamentous injury to the knee limits the ability to determine meniscal pathology during the clinical examination	
Neuroligic tests	Not applicable	
Special tests	Positive McMurray's test result or positive Apley's compression/distraction test result	
Comments	All suspected ACL and MCL injuries should be suspected of involving a meniscal tear until proven otherwise	

ACL = anterior cruciate ligament; AROM = active range of motion; PCL = posterior cruciate ligament; PROM = passive range of motion; ROM = range of motion; RROM = resisted range of motion.

The signs and symptoms of OCDs are often masked by those of a concurrent injury, although the OCD itself is often asymptomatic. Symptomatic OCDs are characterized by complaints of diffuse pain within the knee, a "locking" sensation, and the knee's giving way. A "clunking" sensation may also be described. Pain is increased during weight-bearing activities. Additionally, an increase in pain and a decrease in strength are noted in closed kinetic chain activities relative to open chain motions. **Wilson's test** can be used as a clinical evaluation tool for the presence of OCDs on the knee's articular surface (Box 6–20). A definitive diagnosis must be made with radiographic examination or MRI.

Osteochondral defects can be managed conservatively. Activity is modified to reduce painful stresses placed on the knee. When conservative treatment fails, surgical repair of the defect may be required. Surgical intervention can include simple debridement or procedures such as abrasion arthroplasty, subchondral drilling, or microfracture techniques to stimulate fibrocartilage formation in the defect. Newer surgical interventions include autogenous chondrocyte transplantation, or osteoarticular transplantation (OATs procedure). The goals of these techniques are to place newly grown articular cartilage within the defect or to transplant healthy articular cartilage from one area of the knee into the defect.[84]

After surgery, a 4- to 6-week period of protected weight-bearing activities may be necessary to reduce shearing stresses on the implant. Continuous passive motion (CPM) is advocated to assist in delivery of nutrients to the healing tissues. Aquatic therapy can be used in the early active ROM period to provide ROM and strengthening while decreasing weight-bearing stresses through the joint. After the early protection phase of rehabilitation, strength, ROM, and proprioceptive exercises are advanced to restore normal function to the knee.

Box 6–20
WILSON'S TEST FOR OSTEOCHONDRAL DEFECTS OF THE KNEE

A

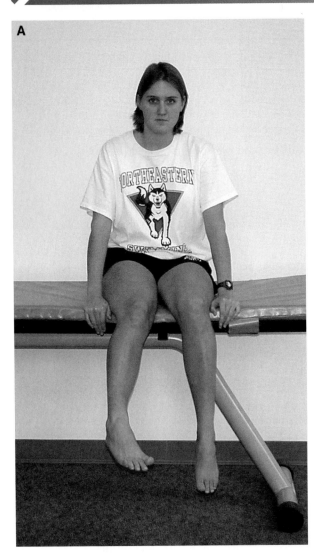

B

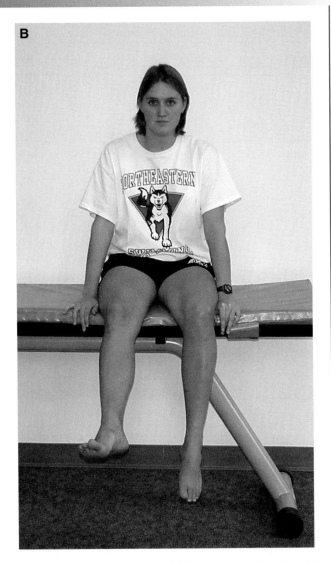

While the tibia is internally rotated, the patient extends the knee **(A)**. When pain is experienced, the patient externally rotates the tibia **(B)**. In the presence of some OCDs, pain is relieved during the external rotation.

PATIENT POSITION	Sitting with the knee flexed to 90°
POSITION OF EXAMINER	In front of the patient to observe any reactions secondary to pain
EVALUATIVE PROCEDURE	**(A)** The patient actively extends the knee while maintaining the tibia in internal rotation. The patient is told to stop the motion and hold the knee in the position in which pain is experienced. **(B)** If pain is experienced, the patient is instructed to externally rotate the tibia while the knee is held at its present point of flexion.
POSITIVE TEST	Pain experienced during extension with internal tibial rotation that is relieved by externally rotating the tibia
IMPLICATIONS	OCD or osteochondritis dissecans on the intercondylar area of the medial femoral condyle

OCD = osteochondral defect.

Table 6–12
EVALUATIVE FINDINGS: Iliotibial Band Friction Syndrome

Examination Segment	Clinical Findings	
History	*Onset:*	Insidious
	Pain characteristics:	Pain over the lateral femoral condyle proximal to the joint line that may radiate distally; pain increased when running downhill
	Mechanism:	Activities involving repeated knee flexion and extension
	Predisposing condition:	Tightness of the iliotibial band; genu varum, pronated feet, leg length discrepancy
Inspection	The patient may present with one or more of the following bony alignments: Genu Varum Excessive pronation during gait Leg length discrepancy	
Palpation	In advanced cases, pain elicited over the lateral femoral condyle, about 2 cm above the joint line	
Functional tests	*AROM:*	ROM is normal
	PROM:	ROM is normal
	RROM:	Pain may be described as the knee passes 30° during flexion and extension (representing the point where the IT band shifts over the lateral femoral condyle)
Ligamentous tests	None	
Neuroligic tests	Not applicable	
Special tests	Positive Noble's compression test result	
Comments	IT band tightness should be confirmed with Ober's test	

AROM = active range of motion; IT = iliotibial; PROM = passive range of motion; ROM = range of motion; RROM = resisted range of motion.

ILIOTIBIAL BAND FRICTION SYNDROME

Resulting from friction between the IT band and the lateral femoral condyle, IT band friction syndrome tends to occur in athletes who are participating in sports that require repeated knee flexion and extension, such as running, rowing, and cycling. Secondary to overuse, a bursa located between the distal IT band and the lateral femoral condyle becomes inflamed. This condition may progress to involve periosteitis of the condyle. The bursa cushioning the IT band from the lateral femoral condyle is not a primary bursa, but rather, a continuation of the knee joint capsule.[85,86]

Several factors may predispose IT band friction syndrome.[87–89] Genu varum may project the lateral femoral condyle laterally, increasing the friction as the IT band passes over it. Pronated feet, leg length differences, and other conditions resulting in internal tibial rotation alter the angle at which the IT band approaches its attachment on Gerdy's tubercle, increasing pressure at the lateral femoral condyle. Finally, a large lateral femoral condyle may result in increased irritation of the IT band as it passes over the condyle.

The patient typically describes a "burning" pain over the lateral femoral condyle that may radiate distally.

Point tenderness is displayed at the point where the IT band passes over the condyle. Pain may be described during resisted ROM testing as the knee approaches 30 degrees of flexion. However, no pain may be described during active ROM (AROM) or passive ROM (PROM) testing (Table 6–12). Pain may also be described while running down hills secondary to an increased stride length causing more pressure over the condyle. The presence of IT band friction syndrome may be confirmed through The **Noble compression test** as the IT band passes over the lateral femoral condyle (Box 6–21). Iliotibial band tightness can be identified by the **Ober's test** (Box 6–22).

The initial treatment approach for IT band syndrome is to correct any biomechanical faults such as the use of orthotics to correct hyperpronation or alterations in training during athletic activities. The use of nonsteroidal antiinflammatory medication and local modalities to decrease the inflammation at the bursa and IT band as it passes over the lateral epicondyle are usually helpful. Stretching of the tensor fascia latae, the IT band, and any other tight musculature is also warranted. As with any lower extremity injury, the full return of strength to the leg is required to send the patient back to full pain-free activity.

Box 6-21
NOBLE'S COMPRESSION TEST FOR ILIOTIBIAL BAND FRICTION SYNDROME

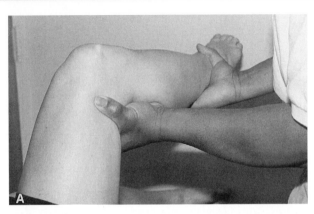

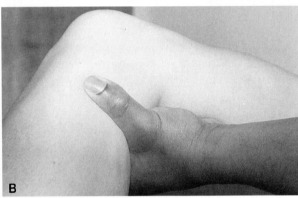

The examiner attempts to compress the distal portion of the IT band against the lateral femoral condyle during passive motion of the knee. In the presence of IT band inflammation, pain will be elicited.

PATIENT POSITION	Lying supine with the knee flexed
POSITION OF EXAMINER	Standing lateral to the side being tested The knee supported above the joint line with the thumb over or just superior to the lateral femoral condyle (**A**). The opposite hand controlling the lower leg
EVALUATIVE PROCEDURE	While applying pressure over the lateral femoral condyle, the knee is passively extended and flexed (**B**).
POSITIVE TEST	Pain under the thumb, most commonly as the knee approaches 30°
IMPLICATIONS	Inflammation of the IT band, its associated bursa, or inflammation of the lateral femoral condyle

IT = iliotibial.

Box 6–22
OBER'S TEST FOR ILIOTIBIAL BAND TIGHTNESS

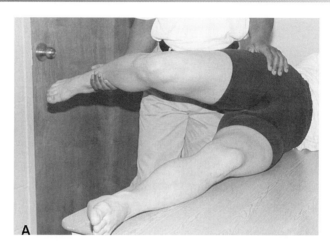

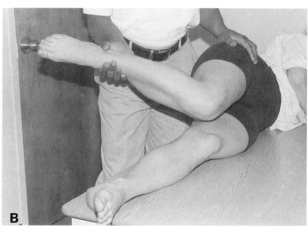

To eliminate false-positive test results, the tensor fasciae latae must first clear the greater trochanter. A positive test result occurs when the knee does not adduct past parallel.

PATIENT POSITION	Lying on the side opposite that being tested with the tested knee in flexion The opposite leg (i.e., the bottom leg) may be flexed to 90° at the knee and hip to stabilize the torso and pelvis.
POSITION OF EXAMINER	Standing behind the patient The leg grasped along the medial aspect of the proximal tibia
EVALUATIVE PROCEDURE	The examiner abducts and extends the hip to allow the tensor fasciae latae to clear the greater trochanter **(A).** The hip is then allowed to passively adduct to the table with the knee kept straight.
POSITIVE TEST	The leg is unable to adduct past parallel **(B).**
IMPLICATIONS	Tightness of the IT band, predisposing the individual to IT band friction syndrome and/or lateral patellar malalignment.
COMMENTS	With the involved knee flexed to 90°, the examiner should be aware that this position places tension on the femoral nerve (see Femoral Nerve Traction Test in Chapter 10) and on the medial structure of the knee. To avoid these complications, the Ober test may be performed with the knee in extension.

IT = iliotibial.

Table 6–13
EVALUATIVE FINDINGS: Popliteus Tendinitis

Examination Segment	Clinical Findings	
History	**Onset:**	Insidious
	Pain characteristics:	Pain in the popliteal fossa radiating along the length of the popliteus tendon anterior to the LCL; increased when running downhill
	Mechanism:	Overuse
	Predisposing conditions:	Hyperpronated feet
Inspection	In acute conditions, inspection is unremarkable; in chronic conditions, swelling may be noted along the lateral joint line	
	Inspect the feet for excessive pronation during gait, a predisposing factor for popliteus tendinitis	
Palpation	Palpation is best performed in the figure-4 position (see Fig. 6–26)	
	Pain and crepitus elicited along the tendon anterior to the LCL	
Functional tests	**AROM:** ROM full and normal	
	PROM: ROM full and normal	
	RROM: Pain possible during resisted flexion from full extension as the popliteus "unscrews" the tibia	
Ligamentous tests	None	
Neuroligic tests	Not applicable	
Special tests	None	
Comments	The findings for popliteus tendinitis are similar to those of IT band friction syndrome, except for the location of the pain	

AROM = active range of motion; LCL = lateral collateral ligament; PROM = passive range of motion; ROM = range of motion; RROM = resisted range of motion.

POPLITEUS TENDINITIS

Tendinitis arises secondary to other biomechanical changes in the knee or lower extremity or secondary to repetitive stress. The popliteus muscle is often injured in conjunction with other knee injuries.[90] Popliteus tendinitis manifests itself similarly to IT band friction syndrome. The exception is the location of the pain. Individuals suffering from popliteus tendinitis describe pain in the proximal portion of the tendon, immediately posterior to the LCL. Similar to IT band friction syndrome, patients who excessively pronate their feet are predisposed to this condition, which worsens when

running downhill (Table 6–13). The popliteus acts to prevent a posterior shift of the tibia on the femur during midstance, and running downhill places excessive strain on the tendon.[91] Palpation of the popliteus tendon is most easily conducted when the foot of the involved leg is placed on the uninvolved knee in the figure-4 position, a position that may produce pain in and of itself (Fig. 6–26).

The function of the popliteus muscle changes, albeit slightly, in knees that are ACL deficient[92] and more significantly when the PCL is absent.[9] Because the popliteus helps retract the lateral meniscus during knee flexion, inhibition or dysfunction of this muscle may alter

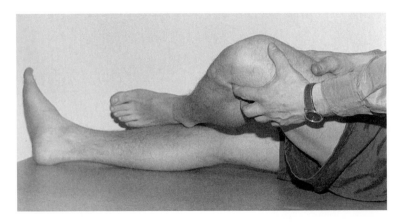

FIGURE 6–26. "Figure 4" position for palpating the popliteus tendon, located just posterior to the lateral collateral ligament.

the biomechanics of the lateral meniscus, possibly resulting in an increased loading on the cartilage.[13] As with other tendinitis conditions, correction of abnormal biomechanics, the use of nonsteroidal antiinflammatory agents, and the use of local modalities to decrease inflammation are needed to return the patient to full activity.

 ## ON-FIELD EVALUATION OF KNEE INJURIES

The process used during the on-field evaluation of knee injuries is similar to that described for the ankle. The presence of a gross fracture or dislocation of the tibiofemoral joint or the patellofemoral joint (see Chapter 7) must be ruled out before a finite examination is performed. Question the athlete about the mechanism of injury, the fixation of the foot, and any associated sounds and sensations.

EQUIPMENT CONSIDERATIONS

Protective devices around the knee include both stabilizing and prophylactic braces, neoprene sleeves, and padding, all of which must be removed before evaluating the knee and patella.

Football Pants

The pants worn for practice and competition in football are tight fitting but, fortunately, are elastic. Expose the knee by reaching under the anterior portion of the pant and locating the kneepad. Hold down the kneepad while the pant leg is pulled up and over the knee or the pad is removed from the pocket. Then remove the pad and flip the pouch up and out of the way (Fig. 6–27). If the pants are extraordinarily tight fitting or inelastic or if a brace is worn beneath the pants, making the preceding procedure difficult, cut the pant leg along one of the seams.

Knee Brace Removal

Both prophylactic and stabilizing knee braces greatly hinder the on-field evaluation of knee injuries. After the pant leg has been pulled over the brace, prophylactic knee braces can be removed by loosening the lower strap holding it in place or cutting the tape. To remove the upper support, slide a hand under the strap or tape while pulling downwardly on the brace (see Fig. 6–27).

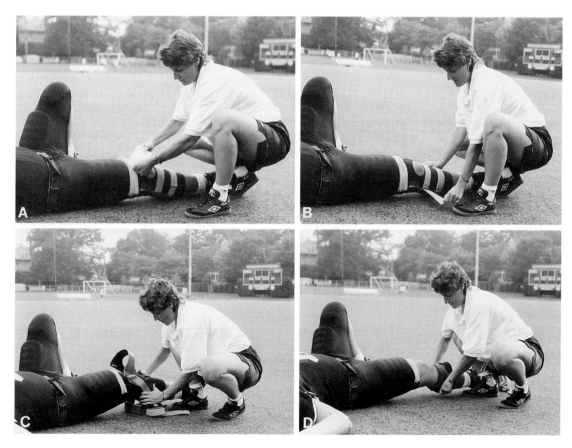

FIGURE 6–27. Removing a knee brace. **(A)** Remove the knee pad and flip its pouch upward. **(B)** Remove the Velcro straps. **(C)** Displace the distal (tibial) portion of the brace and slide the proximal portion from beneath the pant. **(D)** Remove any underlying padding.

Because of the complexity of many of the stabilizing knee braces, it is usually easiest to remove or detach all of the tibial straps first and then detach the femoral ones. If the athlete does not experience pain during knee flexion, slightly flex the knee to allow the lower (tibial) portion of the brace to move away from the leg and then lift the upper portion up and downward, away from the knee.

ON-FIELD HISTORY

- **Location of the pain:** Inquire about the location of any pain. Pain localized to the joint line can indicate meniscal tears. Diffuse pain can indicate trauma to the MCL or joint capsule. Pain described as arising from within the knee joint, from "under the knee cap," or in the posterior aspect of the knee is associated with cruciate ligament sprains.
- **Mechanism of injury:** Identify the forces exerted on the knee, keeping in mind that the injury may involve multiple forces (e.g., valgus stress with tibial rotation). To cross-reference the injury mechanism with the possible trauma, refer to Table 6–3.
- **History of injury:** Ascertain if the athlete has suffered any significant prior ligamentous injury that may influence the findings of the current examination.
- **Associated sounds and sensations:** Question the patient about any sounds or sensations. A "snap" or "pop" may be associated with a ligament rupture, most commonly associated with the ACL. True locking of the knee can be associated with an unstable meniscal tear that has lodged between the knee's articular surfaces. A snapping, popping, or giving-way sensation may also be associated with a patellar dislocation or subluxation (discussed in Chapter 7).
- **Associated neurologic symptoms:** Inquire about any neurologic symptoms. Reports of parasthesia distal to the knee or the inability to dorsiflex the foot indicate trauma to the common peroneal nerve. In the presence of these symptoms, suspect a dislocated tibiofemoral joint until this condition can be ruled out.

ON-FIELD INSPECTION

- **Patellar position:** Ensure that the patella is properly seated within the femoral trochlea.
- **Alignment of the tibofemoral joint:** Through concurrent inspection and palpation, identify that the tibia and femur are properly aligned.

ON-FIELD PALPATION

- **Extensor mechanism:** Palpate the length of the patellar tendon, patella, quadriceps tendon, and distal quadriceps for incongruity and point tenderness, noting the overall integrity of the extensor mechanism.

- **Medial collateral ligament and medial joint line:** Note any point tenderness along the joint line, indicating meniscal pathology.
- **Lateral collateral ligament and lateral joint line:** Palpate the LCL, an extracapsular structure, for areas of defect or point tenderness. As with the medial meniscus, lateral joint line pain can indicate pathology of the lateral meniscus.
- **Fibular head:** Palpate the fibular head to rule out the presence of a fracture and determine the stability of the proximal tibofibular syndesmosis.

ON-FIELD RANGE OF MOTION TESTS

In the absence of gross deformity, suspected fracture, or joint dislocation, have the athlete actively flex and extend the knee throughout the ROM. The inability to perform this motion signifies that the patient should be transported from the field to the sideline for futher evaluation. If ligamentous damage is suspected, ligamentous tests may be performed before removing the athlete from the field so the tests can be conducted before muscle guarding sets in. Resisted and passive ROM tests may not be indicated during the on-field assessment.

ON-FIELD LIGAMENTOUS TESTS

If a ligamentous injury is suspected, valgus stress testing, varus stress testing, Lachman's test, and if possible, a posterior draw test may be carried out before moving the athlete and the onset of reflexive muscle guarding. If the athlete cannot be properly assessed on the field, transport the individual to the sideline in a non–weight-bearing position. Because of the awkward position that an examiner is placed in when performing on-field ligamentous tests, repeat these tests for accuracy when the athlete has been moved to the sideline.

 ## ON-FIELD MANAGEMENT OF KNEE INJURIES

TIBIOFEMORAL JOINT DISLOCATIONS

True dislocations of the tibiofemoral joint present with severe pain, muscle spasm, and obvious deformity of the joint. Although the joint can dislocate perpendicular to the long axis of the femur, most tibiofemoral dislocations occur with the tibia's sliding anteriorly over the femur, resulting in a shortening of the involved leg (Fig. 6–28). Consider a tibiofemoral joint to be dislocated or having been dislocated and then spontaneously reduced when distal neurovascular symptoms are present. Because of the trauma to the neurovascular structures, this condition is considered a medical emergency.

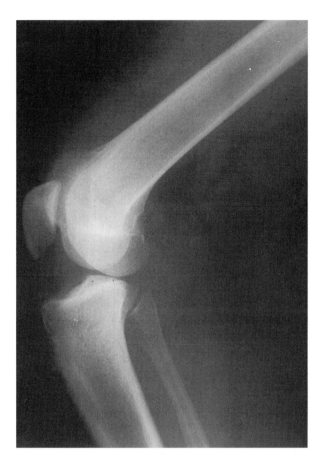

FIGURE 6–28. Radiograph view of a tibiofemoral dislocation. Note the anterior displacement of the tibia relative to the femur.

Management of this condition consists of immobilizing the limb, establishing the presence of a distal pulse (e.g., dorsalis pedis), treating the athlete for shock, and activating the emergency medical system for immediate physician intervention.

COLLATERAL AND CRUCIATE LIGAMENT SPRAINS

While the athlete is still on the playing field or court, only uniplanar ligamentous stress tests are performed. This sequence should consist of valgus and varus stress testing for the collateral ligaments, Lachman's test for ACL deficiency, and the posterior drawer test for PCL laxity. For the basis of comparison and if the situation permits, also evaluate the uninvolved knee at this time. Laxity in the involved knee warrants the athlete's being removed from the field in a non–weight-bearing manner, such as a two-person assist.

After removing the patient to the sideline and, if significant laxity or pain are demonstrated, treat the knee with ice, compression, and elevation. Place the knee in an immobilizer and refer the athlete to a physician.

MENISCAL TEARS

The on-field determination of the possibility of a meniscal tear is based on the athlete's description of the injury mechanism. Until otherwise ruled out, suspect a meniscal tear in athletes who describe a "locking" or "giving way" at the time of the injury or are hesitant to move the knee. Likewise, assume any rotational mechanism or possible ACL or MCL sprain to involve the meniscus. The use of McMurray's test is not recommended during the on-field evaluation of possible meniscal injuries.

◆ REFERENCES

1. Moore, KL: The lower limb. In Moore, KL: *Clinically Oriented Anatomy*, ed 2. Baltimore, Williams & Wilkins, 1985, p. 403.
2. Fu, F, et al: Biomechanics of knee ligaments. Basic concepts and clinical application. *J Bone Joint Surg Am*, 75:1716, 1993.
3. Arms, SW, et al: The biomechanics of anterior cruciate ligament rehabilitation and reconstruction. *Am J Sports Med*, 12:8, 1984.
4. Beynnon BD, et al. Anterior cruciate ligament strain behavior during rehabilitation exercises in vivo. *Am J Sports Med*, 23:24, 1995.
5. Van Dommelen, BA, and Fowler, PJ: Anatomy of the posterior cruciate ligament. A review. *Am J Sports Med*, 17:24, 1989.
6. Harner, CD, et al: Comparative study of the size and shape of human anterior and posterior cruciate ligaments. *J Orthop Res*, 13:429, 1995.
7. Harner, CD, et al: The human posterior cruciate ligament complex: An interdisciplinary study. Ligament morphology and biomechanical evaluation. *Am J Sports Med*, 23:736, 1995.
8. Kusayama, T, Harner, CD: Anatomical and biomechanical characteristics of the human meniscofemoral ligaments. *Knee Surg Sports Traumatol Arthrosc*, 2:234, 1994.
9. Harner, CD, et al: The effects of a popliteus muscle load on in situ forces in the posterior cruciate ligament and on knee kinematics. A human cadaveric study. *Am J Sports Med*, 26:669, 1998.
10. Gollenhon, DL, Torzilli, PA, and Warren, RF: The role of the posterolateral and cruciate ligaments in the stability of the human knee. A biomechanical study. *J Bone Joint Surg*, 69A:233, 1987.
11. Grood, ES, Stowers, SF, and Noyes, FR: Limits of movement in the human knee. Effect of sectioning the posterior cruciate ligament and posterolateral structures. *J Bone Joint Surg*, 70A:88, 1988.
12. Race, A, and Amis, AA: Loading of the two bundles of the posteior cruciate ligament: An analysis of bundle function in a-P drawer. *J Biomech*, 29:873, 1996.
13. Jones, CD, Keene, GC, and Christie, AD: The popliteus as a retractor of the lateral meniscus of the knee. *Arthroscopy*, 11:270, 1995.
14. Rosene, JM, and Fogarty, TD: Anterior tibial translation in collegiate athletes with normal anterior cruciate integrity. *J Athletic Training*, 34:93, 1999.
15. Pandy, MG, and Shelburne, KB: Dependence of cruciate-ligament loading on muscle forces and external load. *J Biomech*, 30:1015, 1997.
16. Terry, GC, and LaPrade, RF: The biceps femoris muscle complex at the knee: Its anatomy and injury patterns associated with acute anterolateral-anteromedial rotatory instability. *Am J Sports Med*, 24:2, 1996.
17. Terry, GC, et al: How iliotibial tract injuries of the knee combine with acute anterior cruciate ligament tears to influence abnormal anterior tibial displacement. *Am J Sports Med*, 21:55, 1993.
18. Soderberg, GL: Kinesiology: *Application to Pathological Motion*. Baltimore, Williams & Wilkins, 1986, p. 207.
19. Reid, DC: Knee ligament injuries: Anatomy, classification, and examination. In Reid, DC (ed): *Sports Injury: Assessment and Rehabilitation*. New York, Churchill Livingstone, 1992, p. 449.

20. Voight, M, and Weider, D: Comparative reflex response times of vastus medialis oblique and subjects with extensor mechanism dysfunction. *Am J Sports Med*, 19:131, 1991.

21. Yu, WD, and Shapiro, MS: Cysts and other masses about the knee. Identifying and treating common and rare lesions. *Phys Sports Med*, 27:59, 1999.

22. Blair, DF, and Willis, RP: Rapid rehabilitation following anterior cruciate ligament reconstruction. *Athletic Training: Journal of the National Athletic Trainers Association*, 26:32, 1991.

23. Johnson, BC, and Cullen, MJ: The anterior cruciate ligament: Injuries and functions in anterolateral rotatory instability. *Athletic Training: Journal of the National Athletic Trainers Association*, 17:79, 1982.

24. DiStefano, VJ: The enigmatic anterior cruciate ligament. *Athletic Training: Journal of the National Athletic Trainers Association*, 16:244, 1981.

25. Girgis, FG, Marshall, JL, and Al Monajem, ARS: The cruciate ligaments of the knee joint. Anatomical, functional, and experimental analysis. *Clin Orthop*, 106:216, 1975.

26. Furman, W, Marshall, JL, and Girgis, FG: The anterior cruciate ligament: A functional analysis based on post mortem studies. *J Bone Joint Surg Am*, 58:178, 1976.

27. More, RC, et al: Hamstrings-an anterior cruciate ligament protagonist. *Am J Sports Med*, 21:231, 1993.

28. Lintner, DM, et al: Partial tears of the anterior cruciate ligament. Are they clinically detectable? *Am J Sports Med*, 23:111, 1995.

29. Whitehill, WR, Wright, KE, and Nelson, K: Modified Lachman test for anterior cruciate ligament instability. *J Athletic Training*, 29:256, 1994.

30. Adler, GG, Hoekman, RA, and Beach, DM: Drop leg Lachman test: A new test of anterior knee laxity. *Am J Sports Med*, 23:320, 1995.

31. Harter, RA, et al: A comparison of instrumented and manual Lachman test results in anterior cruciate ligament-reconstructed knees. *Athletic Training: Journal of the National Athletic Trainers Association*, 25:330, 1990.

32. Barber-Westin, SD, and Noyes, FR: The effect of rehabilitation and return to activity on anterior-posterior knee displacements after anterior cruciate ligament reconstruction. *Am J Sports Med*, 21:264, 1993.

33. Sgaglione, NA, et al: Arthroscopically assisted anterior cruciate ligament reconstruction with the pes anserine tendons. *Am J Sports Med*, 21:249, 1993.

34. Cross, MJ, et al: Acute repair of injury to the anterior cruciate ligament. A long-term followup. *Am J Sports Med*, 21:128, 1993.

35. Webright, WG, Perrin, DH, and Gansneder, BM: Effect of trunk position on anterior tibial displacement measured by the KT-1000 in uninjured subjects. *J Athletic Training*, 33:233, 1998.

36. Berry, J, et al: Error estimates in novice and expert raters for the KT-1000 arthrometer. *J Orthop Sports Phys Ther*, 29:49, 1999.

37. Draper, DO, and Schulthies, S: A test for eliminating false positive anterior cruciate ligament injury diagnoses. *J Athletic Training*, 28:355, 1993.

38. Jonsson, H, and Karrholm, J: Three-dimensional knee kinematics and stability in patients with a posterior cruciate ligament tear. *J Orthop Res*, 17:185, 1999.

39. Covey, DC, and Sapega, AA: Injuries to the posterior cruciate ligament. *J Bone Joint Surg*, 75A:1376, 1993.

40. Covey, DC, and Sapega, AA: Anatomy and function of the posterior cruciate ligament. *Clin Sports Med*, 13:509, 1994.

41. Norkin, CC, and Levangie, PK: The knee complex. In Norkin, CC, and Levangie, PK (eds): *Joint Structure and Function: A Comprehensive Analysis*, ed 2. Philadelphia, FA Davis, 1992, p. 348.

42. Robbins, AJ, Newman, AP, and Burks, RT: Postoperative return of motion in anterior cruciate ligament and medial collateral ligament injuries. The effects of medial collateral ligament rupture location. *Am J Sports Med*, 21:20, 1993.

43. Veenema, KR: Valgus knee instability in an adolescent. Ligament sprain or physeal fracture? *The Physician and Sportsmedicine*, 27:62, 1999.

44. Clancy, WG, and Bosanny, JJ: Functional treatment and rehabilitation of quadriceps contusions, patella dislocations and "isolated" medial collateral ligament injuries. *Athletic Training: Journal of the National Athletic Trainers Association*, 17:249, 1982.

45. Reider, B: Medial collateral ligament injuries in athletes. *Sports Med*, 21:147, 1996.

46. Hillard-Sembell, D: Combined injuries of the anterior cruciate and medial collateral ligaments of the knee. Effect of treatment on stability and function of the joint. *J Bone Joint Surg Am*, 78:169, 1996.

47. Reider B, et al: Treatment of isolated medial collateral ligament injuries with early functional rehabilitation: A five-year follow-up study. *Am J Sports Med*, 22:470–477, 1993.

48. Indelicato, PA. Isolated medial collateral ligament injuries of the knee. *J Am Acad Ortho Surgeons*, 3:9–14,1995.

49. Noyes, FR, and Barber-Westin, SD: The treatment of acute combined ruptures of the anterior cruciate and medial ligaments of the knee. *Am J Sports Med*, 23:380, 1995.

50. Murakami, Y, et al: Quantitative evaluation of nutritional pathways for the posterior cruciate ligament and the lateral collateral ligament in rabbits. *Acta Physiol Scand*, 162, 447, 1998.

51. Latimer, HA, et al: Reconstruction of the lateral collateral ligament of the knee with patellar tendon allograft. Report of a new technique in combined ligament injuries. *Am J Sports Med*, 26:656, 1998.

52. Arendt, E, and Dick, R: Knee injury patterns among men and women in collegiate basketball and soccer: NCAA data and review of literature. *Am J Sports Med*, 23:694, 1995.

53. Beckett, ME, et al: Incidence of hyperpronation in the ACL injured knee: A clinical perspective. *J Athletic Training*, 27:58, 1992.

54. Woodford-Rogers, B, Cyphert, L, and Denegar, CR: Risk factors for anterior cruciate ligament injury in high school and college athletes. *Journal of Athletic Training*, 29:343, 1994.

55. Loundon, JK, Jenkins, W, and Loundon, KL: The relationship between static posture and ACL injuries in female athletes. *J Orthop Sports Phys Ther*, 24:91, 1996.

56. Supple, KM, et al: Posterior tibial dysfunction. *Semin Arthritis Rheum*, 22:106; 1992.

57. Loudon, JK, Jenkins, W, and Loudon, KL: The relationship between static posture and ACL injury in female athletes. *J Orthop Sports Phys Ther*, 24:91, 1996.

58. Heitz, NA, et at: Hormonal changes throughout the menstrual cycle and increased anterior cruciate ligament laxity in females. *J Athletic Training*, 34:144, 1999.

59. Wojtys, EM, et al: Association between the menstrual cycle and anterior cruciate ligament injuries in female athletes. *Am J Sports Med*, 26:614, 1998.

60. Myklebust, G, et al: A prospective study of anterior cruciate ligament injuries in elite Norwegian team handball. *Scand J Med Sci Sports*, 8:149, 1998.

61. Schickendantz, MS, and Weiker, GG: The predictive value of radiographs in the evaluation of unilateral and bilateral anterior cruciate injuries. *Am J Sports Med*, 21:110, 1993.

62. Shelbourne, KD, Davis, TJ, and Klootwyk, TE: The relationship between intercondylar notch width of the femur and the incidence of anterior cruciate ligament tears. *Am J Sports Med*, 26:402, 1998.

63. Snyder-Mackler, L, et al: The relationship between passive joint laxity and functional outcome after anterior cruciate ligament surgery. *Am J Sports Med*, 25:191, 1997.

64. Shelbourne KD, Nitz P. Accelerated rehabilitation after anterior cruciate ligament reconstruction. *Am J Sports Med*, 18:292–299, 1990.

65. Shelbourne, KD, and Gray, T: Anterior cruciate ligament reconstruction with autogenous patellar tendon graft followed by accelerated rehabilitation: A two to nine year followup. *Am J Sports Med*, 25:786, 1997.

66. Arendt, EA, Agel, J and Dick, R: Anterior cruciate ligament injury patterns among collegiate men and women. *J Athletic Training*, 34:86, 1999.

67. Ireland, ML: Anterior cruciate ligament injury in female athletes: Epidemiology. *J Athletic Training*, 34:150, 1999.

68. Sauers, RJ: Isolated posterior cruciate tear in a college football player. *Athletic Training: Journal of the National Athletic Trainers Association*, 21:248, 1986.

69. Rubinstein, RA, et al: The accuracy of the clinical examination in the setting of posterior cruciate ligament injuries. *Am J Sports Med*, 22:550, 1994.

70. Keller, PM, et al: Nonoperatively treated isolated posterior cruciate ligament injuries. *Am J Sports Med*, 21:132, 1993.

71. Shelbourne, KD, Davis, TJ, and Patel, DV: The natural history of acute, isolated, nonoperatively treated posterior cruciate ligament injuries. A prospective study. *Am J Sports Med*, 27:276, 1999.

72. Ochi, M, et al: Isolated posterior cruciate ligament insufficiency induces morphological changes of anterior cruciate ligament collagen fibrils. *Arthroscopy*, 15:292, 1999.

73. Wroble, RR, et al: The role of the lateral extraarticular restraints in the anterior cruciate ligament-deficient knee. *Am J Sports Med*, 21:257, 1993.

74. Katz, JW, and Fingeroth, RJ: The diagnostic accuracy of ruptures of the anterior cruciate ligament comparing the Lachman test, the anterior drawer sign, and the pivot shift test in acute and chronic knee injuries. *Am J Sports Med*, 14:88, 1986.

75. Lucie, RS, Wiedel, JD, and Messner, DG: The acute pivot shift: Clinical correlation. *Am J Sports Med*, 12:189, 1984.

76. Shelbourne, KD, and Nitz, PA: The O'Donoghue triad revisited. Combined knee injuries involving anterior cruciate and medial collateral ligament tears. *Am J Sports Med*, 19:474, 1991.

77. Cooper, DE: Tests for posterolateral instability of the knee in normal subjects. Results of examination under anesthesia. *J Bone Joint Surg*, 73(A):30, 1991.

78. Ferrari, DA, Ferrari, JD, and Coumas, J: Posterolateral instability of the knee. *J Bone Joint Surg*, 76-B:187, 1994.

79. Loomer, RL: A test for posterolateral rotatory instability. *Clin Orthop*, 235, 1995.

80. Cooper, DE: Tests for posterolateral instability of the knee in normal subjects: Results of examinations under anesthesia. *J Bone Joint Surg*, 70-A:386, 1991.

81. Krinskey, MB, et al: Incidence of lateral meniscus injury in professional basketball players. *Am J Sports Med*, 20:17, 1992.

82. Scriber, K, and Mathney, M: Knee injuries in college football: An 18 year report. *Athletic Training: Journal of the National Athletic Trainers Association*, 25:233, 1990.

83. Ralston, BM, et al: Osteochondritis dissecans of the knee. *The Physician and Sportsmedicine*, 24:73, 1996.

84. Minas T, Nehrer S. Current concepts in the treatment of articular cartilage defects. *Orthopedics*, 20:525, 1997.

85. Muhle, C, et al: Iliotibial band friction syndrome: MR imaging findings in 16 patients and MR arthrographic study of six cadaveric knees. *Radiology*, 212:103, 1999.

86. Nemeth, WC, and Sanders, BL: The lateral synovial recess of the knee: Anatomy and role in chronic Iliotibial band friction syndrome. *Arthroscopy*, 12:574, 1996.

87. Lebsack, D, Gieck, J, and Saliba, E: Iliotibial band friction syndrome. *Athletic Training: Journal of the National Athletic Trainers Association*, 25:356, 1990.

88. Lucas, CA: Iliotibial band friction syndrome exhibited in athletes. *J Athletic Training*, 27:250, 1992.

89. Olsen, DW: Iliotibial band friction syndrome. *Athletic Training: Journal of the National Athletic Trainers Association*, 21:32, 1986.

90. Brown, TR, et al: Diagnosis of popliteus injuries with MR imaging. *Skeletal Radiol*, 24:511, 1995.

91. Davis, M, Newsam, CJ and Perry, J: Electromyograph analysis of the popliteus muscle in level and downhill walking. *Clin Orthop*, Jan:211, 1995.

92. Weresh, MJ, Gabel, RH, Brand, RA, and Tearse, DS: Popliteus function in ACL-deficient patients. *Scand J Med Sci Sports*, 7:14, 1997.

The Patellofemoral Articulation

The patellofemoral articulation is an integral part of the knee. These two areas are separated in this text because of the differences in the mechanisms and onset of injury. With only a few exceptions, injury to the patellofemoral articulation is the result of overuse, congenital malalignment, or structural insufficiency.

 ### CLINICAL ANATOMY

Lying within the patellar tendon, the patella is the largest sesamoid bone in the body. The patella's anatomical design allows for increased efficiency of the quadriceps muscle group, protection of the anterior portion of the knee joint, and the absorption and transmission of the patellofemoral *joint reaction forces.* In both the frontal and sagittal planes, the patella is triangular. In the frontal plane, the superior portion is wider than its inferior apex; in the sagittal plane, it is marked with an anterior, nonarticulating surface and a narrower posterior articulating surface (Fig. 7–1).

The articular surface of the patella is composed of three distinct facets, each covered with up to a 5-mm thickness of hyaline cartilage. The medial and lateral facets have superior, middle, and inferior articular surfaces. The odd facet, lying medial to the medial facet, has no articular subdivisions (Fig. 7–2).

The patella tracks medially during the range of 45 to 18 degrees as the knee moves from flexion to extension. Then, during the final 18 degrees of extension, the

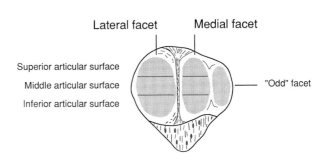

FIGURE 7–2. Posterior view of the left patella. The lateral and medial facets may be conceptualized as having superior, middle, and inferior articular surfaces. The odd facet has no such subdivisions.

patella tracks laterally. During flexion, the patella increases its angle of horizontal tilt, which then decreases during extension.[1]

During the movements of flexion and extension, the patella tracks within the femoral trochlear groove, an area between the two femoral condyles lined with articular cartilage. When the knee is fully extended, the patella rests anterior to the distal portion of the femoral shaft, just proximal to the femoral groove. During flexion, the patella makes initial contact with the groove at 10 to 20 degrees of flexion and becomes seated within the groove as the knee approaches 20 to 30 degrees.[2] At this point, the lateral border of the trochlea becomes prominent, forming a strong barrier against lateral patellar movement. Patellar tracking is enhanced when the leg is bearing weight.[3]

Distinct portions of the patella become involved in the articulation as the knee progresses through the range of motion (Table 7–1). The average patellofemoral contact area varies throughout the range of

---

Joint reaction forces Forces that are transmitted through a joint's articular surfaces.

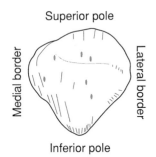

FIGURE 7–1. Anterior view of the left patella.

Superior pole

Medial border

Lateral border

Inferior pole

Table 7–1
ARTICULATION OF THE PATELLOFEMORAL JOINT

Position (Flexion), degrees	Patellar Facets in Contact with the Femoral Trochlear Groove
0	Patella resting on the suprapatellar fat pad on the distal femoral shaft
20	Inferior portion of facets
45	Medial and lateral facets
90	Largest contact area across the medial and lateral facets
135	Odd facet

motion, with the greatest amount of surface area reported between 60 and 90 degrees of flexion.[4-6] Compressive forces are placed on the patella as it moves through the femoral trochlea. These forces range from 0.5 times body weight when walking on a level surface to 3.3 times body weight when walking up and down stairs or running on hills.[7] The maximum compressive force placed on the patella occurs at 30 degrees of flexion.[4,8]

The patella's position is maintained throughout the arc of motion by the patellar retinaculum (Fig. 7–3). The **lateral retinaculum** originates off the vastus lateralis and the iliotibial band and inserts on the patella's lateral border. The **medial retinaculum** originates from the distal portion of the vastus medialis and adductor magnus and inserts on the medial border of the patella. The superior portion of the knee's fibrous capsule thickens and inserts on the patella's superior border forming the **medial and lateral patellofemoral ligaments.**

MUSCULAR ANATOMY AND RELATED SOFT TISSUES

The quadriceps femoris muscles specifically affect the patella's function. During flexion, the patella is pulled inferiorly by the patellar tendon's attachment to the tibial tuberosity. During extension, the quadriceps femoris and its tendon pull the patella superiorly.

Normally the length of the patellar tendon is approximately the same length as the long axis of the patella ($\pm 10\%$) (Fig. 7–4).[9] Abnormally long or short tendons alter the mechanics, and therefore the strength, of the extensor mechanism.

The **vastus lateralis** is the primary muscle pulling the patella laterally. Medially, the **oblique fibers of the vastus medialis (VMO)** approach the patella at a 55 degree angle, guiding the patella medially and preventing lateral patellar subluxation.[10] The adductor magnus, serving as part of the origin of the VMO and medial retinaculum, may have a secondary function in limiting the amount of lateral patellar tracking.[11,12] Tightness of the iliotibial (IT) band can accentuate the lateral tracking of the patella, resulting in subluxations or patellar malalignment.

In healthy individuals, the VMO contracts simultaneously with or before vastus lateralis contraction. With patellofemoral pain syndromes, an inhibitory feedback mechanism, initiated by pain or swelling, causes latent VMO contraction timing.[13] A buildup of 20 to 30 mL of excess fluid within the capsule neurologically inhibits the VMO, compared with 50 to 60 mL of fluid for the rest of the extensor mechanism.[14]

The alignment of the foot and normal flexibility of the triceps surae and hamstring muscle groups are needed to provide adequate knee range of motion and normal patellofemoral mechanics. Tightness of the gastrocnemius or soleus muscle may prohibit the 10 degrees of dorsiflexion required while walking and the 15 degrees of dorsiflexion required when running. The most common compensation for a lack of dorsiflexion is pronation of the foot. Likewise, increased foot pronation increases the amount of internal tibial rotation, affecting the relationship of the extensor mechanism by rotating the tibial tuberosity toward the midline.

BURSA OF THE EXTENSOR MECHANISM

Individual anatomical differences and varying biomechanics result in varying numbers of bursae being directly involved with the extensor mechanism. However, four bursae are consistently found throughout the

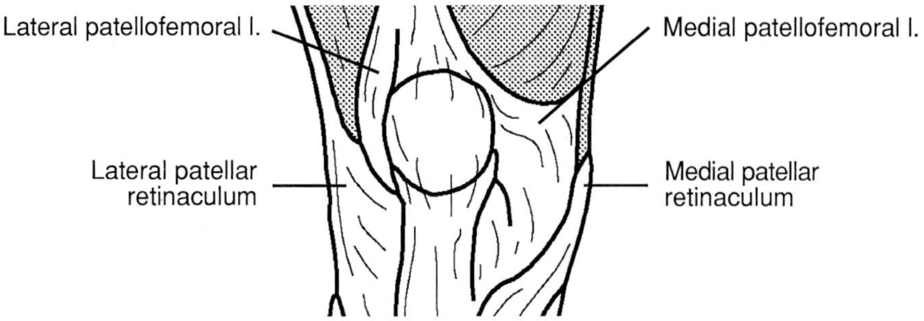

FIGURE 7–3. Patellar retinaculum and medial and lateral patellofemoral ligaments (partially hidden by the quadriceps muscle).

Lateral patellofemoral l.

Medial patellofemoral l.

Lateral patellar retinaculum

Medial patellar retinaculum

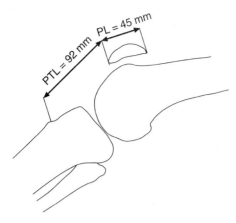

FIGURE 7–4. Calculation of the length of the patellar tendon (drawn from a radiograph). PTL = patellar tendon length; PL = patellar length. Note that this figure depicts patella alta.

population (Fig. 7–5). Lying deep at the distal end of the quadriceps femoris muscle group and allowing free movement over the distal femur, the **suprapatellar bursa** is an extension of the knee's joint capsule. This bursa is held in place by the articularis genus muscle. The **prepatellar bursa** overlies the anterior portion of the patella and allows the patella to move freely beneath the skin. The distal portion of the patellar tendon receives protection against friction and blows by the **subcutaneous infrapatellar bursa,** overlying the tibial

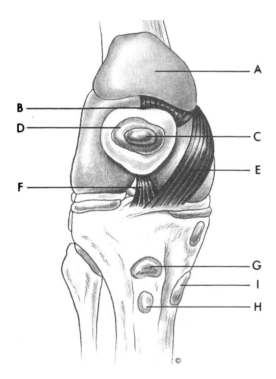

FIGURE 7–5. Bursae about the knee joint: **(A)** Suprapatellar pouch, **(B)** suprapatellar plica, **(C)** superficial prepatellar bursa, **(D)** deep prepatellar bursa, **(E)** medial plica, **(F)** infrapatellar bursa, **(G)** deep infrapatellar bursa, **(H)** superficial infrapatellar bursa, and **(I)** pes anserine bursa.

tuberosity, and the **deep infrapatellar bursa,** located between the tendon and the tibia. The **infrapatellar fat pad** separates the patellar tendon and the deep infrapatellar bursa from the joint capsule of the knee.

◆ CLINICAL EVALUATION OF THE PATELLOFEMORAL JOINT

Dysfunction of joints superior to or inferior to the knee may manifest themselves as patellofemoral pain. Findings of the patellofemoral joint evaluation may necessitate adjunct evaluation of the hip, lower leg, ankle, foot, and related body areas. To meet this need, have the patient dress in shorts and bring his or her casual and competitive footwear to the evaluation.

HISTORY

Many patellofemoral joint injuries are the result of overuse stresses, structural abnormalities, or biomechanical deficiencies of the lower leg. However, several acute, traumatic conditions can affect the patella and the extensor mechanism.

- **Mechanism and onset of injury:** Determine whether the chief complaint is the result of a single traumatic episode or if it stems from an insidious onset.
  - **Acute onset:** Contusions and fractures may result from direct blows. Strains or ruptures of the patellar tendon can be caused by dynamic overload of the musculotendinous unit. A dislocated patella has an acute onset, but repeated subluxations are most likely the result of chronic conditions.
  - **Chronic or insidious onset:** Low-energy trauma, such as that associated with walking and running, can exacerbate patellar maltracking problems and lead to tendinitis, bursitis, fat pad syndrome, or subtle subluxations (Box 7–1).

- **When pain occurs:** For chronic conditions, questions focus on when the pain occurs, which activities cause its onset, and how these symptoms affect the level of activity. Activities such as ascending or descending stairs or open chain knee extension exercises increase compressive forces of the patella on the knee. Pain occurring after prolonged periods of sitting, the "movie sign" ("theater sign"), may describe pain arising from prolonged pressure being placed on one or more facets. Descriptions of the knee as "locking" or "giving way" require follow up for more details to determine the underlying event. A distinction must be made between true locking of the knee and "clicking" beneath the patella. True locking of the knee is not indicative of patellofemoral pathology but, rather, of meniscal tears. Reports of the knee's giving way may be the result of patellar subluxation or of internal derangement of the knee itself.

Box 7–1

CHONDROMALACIA PATELLA

Although often referred to and treated as a discernible ailment, chondromalacia patella (CP) is best thought of as a symptom. Chondromalacia patella is the softening and subsequent wearing away of the patella's hyaline cartilage. This malady presents itself as grinding beneath the patella and may cause related swelling and pain. It is confirmed only through visual inspection during arthroscopy. CP is nebulous in nature because it is often found incidentally in otherwise normal knees.[15] Likewise, many individuals describing these symptoms before surgery have no signs of CP at the time of arthroscopy.[16–18]

Chondromalacia patella is most often, if not always, the result of biomechanical changes affecting the lower extremity. As such, chondromalacia may be treated symptomatically, but the key to its remedy is determining and correcting the underlying pathology.

- **Location of the pain:** Pain radiating medially or laterally from the patella may indicate pathological glide within the trochlea or an abnormal patellar tilt. Posterior knee pain is a common complaint associated with synovitis, but the pain may radiate to any area of the knee. Pain may also be referred to the anterior knee secondary to **Legg-Clavé-Perthes disease** or a **slipped capital femoral epiphysis** (see Chapter 8).[19]

- **Level of activity:** Any changes in the level of activity, a change in the surface on which the activity occurs, or a change of footwear or equipment (e.g., as occurs in changing from playing first base to playing catcher or from bicycling to running) must be determined. Each of these may place excessive or unaccustomed forces on the patellofemoral joint.

- **Prior surgery:** Knee surgery can result in inflammation, adhesion, or entrapment of the patella's restraints, resulting in painful movement and reduced range of motion.[20]

- **Relevant past history:** Prior injuries to the lower leg commonly alter the biomechanics of the extensor mechanism. Question the patient and review the medical file to identify conditions such as foot pathologies, recurrent ankle sprains, Achilles tendon pathology, knee sprains, injury to the hip, or conditions involving the lumbar spine. Injury to the opposite limb may result in compensation by the currently involved knee.

INSPECTION

Examine the entire knee complex for signs of gross deformity, including patellar malalignment, dislocation, and the integrity of the patellar tendon.

- **Patellar alignment:** With the knee fully extended and the patient bearing weight, observe the patella for alignment, at approximately the center of the femur, with the inferior pole located at the upper margin of the femoral trochlea (Fig. 7–6).

- **Patellar malalignment:** Look for possible malalignment. Several types of patellar malalignments may be demonstrated when the lower extremity is bearing weight (Box 7–2). Clinically, patella alta—a high-riding patella—may be identified through the camel sign (Fig. 7–7).

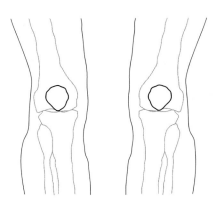

FIGURE 7–6. Normal patellar alignment with the knee extended.

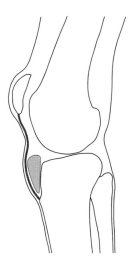

FIGURE 7–7. "Camel sign," a clinical indication of patella alta. The high-riding patella exposes the fat pad, forming a "double hump" when viewed from the lateral side.

Box 7–2
PATELLAR POSITION

	Patella Alta	Patella Baja	Squinting Patellae	"Frog Eyed" Patella
Description	High-riding patellae; the camel sign may be present (see Figure 7–7)	Low-riding patellae	Patellae positioned medially	Patellae high riding and positioned laterally
Potential causes	Abnormally long patellar tendon	Abnormally short patellar tendon Arthrofibrosis after surgery or injury	Hip **anteverson,** internal femoral rotation, internal tibial rotation, arthrofibrosis after surgery or injury	Hip retroversion, external rotation, external tibial rotation
Consequences	Increased patellar glide, decreased quadriceps strength, increased patellofemoral compressive forces when the knee is flexed	Decreased patellar glide, decreased tibiofemoral range of motion, decreased quadriceps strength, increased patellofemoral compressive forces when the knee is flexed	Increased Q angle, tight medial retinaculum, maltracking of the patella, altered patellofemoral compressive forces	Increased lateral patellar glide, tight lateral retinaculum, patellar maltracking decreased quadriceps strength, increased patellofemoral compressive forces where the knee is flexed

- **Posture of the knee:** Inspect the knee for the presence of the following alignments, which are also described in Chapter 3:
  - **Genu varum** places an increased compressive force on the lateral patellar facets.
  - **Genu valgum** causes excessive lateral forces, increasing the pressure on the medial and odd facets.
  - **Genu recurvatum** places additional pressure on the superior articular surfaces.

  The effects of the surrounding soft tissues on patellar position occurs in three dimensions. Changing the tibiofemoral angle causes the patella to rotate about its long axis. A varus alignment causes lateral rotation, causing increased pressure between the lateral facet and the lateral femoral trochlea. A valgus alignment causes medial rotation and increased pressure on the odd and medial facets.

- **Q angle:** Determine the approximate tracking of the patella through the measurement of the Q angle, the relationship between the line of pull of the quadriceps and the patellar tendon. This measurement should be performed once with the knee extended and then again with the knee flexed to 90 degrees to account for increased lateral movement of the patella during flexion and for external rotation during non–weight-bearing knee extension. With the knee extended, the normal Q angle is 13 degrees for men and 18 degrees for women (Box 7–3). When the knee is flexed to 90 degrees, the Q angle should be 8 degrees for both genders (Box 7–4).[21] Increased Q angles increase the forces placed on the medial patellar facet, medial patellar retinaculum, and lateral border of the femoral trochlea secondary to an increased lateral glide of the patella.

  Q angle measurements reflect a functional position when they are taken when the patient is standing. Likewise, isometrically contracting the quadriceps muscle tends to decrease the Q angle and more accurately reflects the biomechanics of patellar motion.[22]

- **Tubercle sulcus angle:** With the patient sitting off the examination table and the lower legs hanging freely, observe the relationship between the tibial tuberosity and the inferior patellar pole. If the tuberosity is more than 10 degrees lateral to the inferior pole, the patient is predisposed to lateral patellar tracking.[19]

- **Leg length difference:** Structural or functional leg length differences can affect the extensor mechanism and influence patellar tracking. Refer to Chapter 3 for methods of determining the presence of structural and functional leg length differences.

- **Foot posture:** Observe the position of the foot. While the patient is weight bearing, the foot should maintain a neutral or slightly pronated position. Excessive pronation results in internal tibial rotation, and excessive supination results in external tibial rotation. Pronation of one foot and supination of the other indicates a leg length discrepancy, with the supinated foot representing the shorter leg. A standing leg length difference can be resolved by supinating the pronated foot to bring the anterior superior iliac spines to an equal level.

- **Areas of scars:** Examine for any scars from previous injury such as lacerations or abrasions or prior surgeries for medial collateral ligament (MCL), lateral collateral ligament (LCL), meniscal, or cruciate ligament trauma. These areas may develop a keloid (see Fig. 1–4) or result in the formation of a neuroma, each of which may serve as the source of the pain.

PALPATION

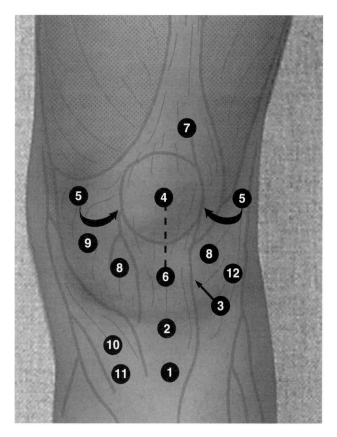

The complete palpation of the patellofemoral articulation must include the bony and soft tissue structures of the tibiofemoral articulation to rule out pathology of these structures. Extra caution is necessary when moving the patella. Patients who have a history of patellar dislocations or subluxations may become fearful or apprehensive about the patella being displaced as it is moved during the examination process.

continued on page 252

Anteversion   A forward bending or angulation of a bone or organ.

Box 7–3

Q ANGLE MEASUREMENT WITH THE KNEE EXTENDED

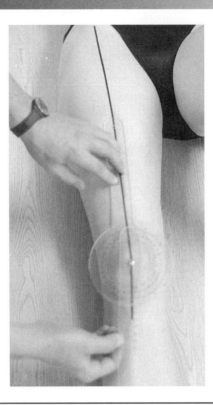

Measurement of the Q angle with the knee extended in a non–weight-bearing position; the anatomic landmarks of the ASIS, center of the patella, and the tibial tuberosity are used to align the goniometer

PATIENT POSITION	Lying supine with the knee fully extended
POSITION OF EXAMINER	Standing on the side of the limb to be measured
EVALUATIVE PROCEDURE	The examiner identifies and marks the ASIS, the midpoint of the patella, and the tibial tuberosity. A goniometer is placed so that the axis is located over the patellar midpoint, the center of the stationary arm is over the line from the ASIS to the patella, and the moving arm is placed over the line from the patella to the tibial tuberosity.
POSITIVE TEST	A Q angle greater than 13° in men or 18° in women
IMPLICATIONS	Increased lateral forces leading to a laterally tracking patella
MODIFICATION	These steps may be repeated with the patient standing. Re-measure the Q angle with the quadriceps isometrically contracted. Differences between the two measures may provide insight to patellar tracking deficits.[22]

ASIS = anterior superior iliac spine.

Box 7–4
Q ANGLE MEASUREMENT WITH THE KNEE FLEXED

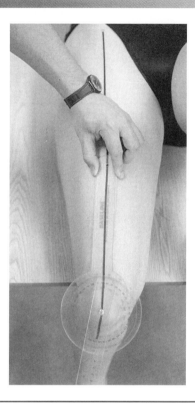

Measurement of the Q angle with the knee flexed to 90°; the anatomic landmarks of the ASIS, center of the patella, and the tibial tuberosity are used to align the goniometer.

PATIENT POSITION	Sitting with legs over the edge of the table with the knees flexed to 90°
POSITION OF EXAMINER	Standing on the side of the limb to be measured
EVALUATIVE PROCEDURE	The examiner identifies and marks the ASIS, the midpoint of the patella, and the tibial tuberosity. A goniometer is placed so that the axis is located over the patellar midpoint, the center of the stationary arm parallels the line from the ASIS to the patella, and the moving arm is placed over the line from the patella to the tibial tuberosity.
POSITIVE TEST VAULT	A Q angle greater than 8°[22]
IMPLICATIONS	Increased lateral tracking during knee flexion, predisposing the patient to lateral patellar subluxations or dislocations

ASIS = anterior superior iliac spine.

continued from page 249

This section describes palpation of the knee and patella only as it relates to patellar dysfunction.

1. **Tibial tuberosity:** Palpate the tibial tuberosity, identified by the insertion of the patellar tendon. The tibial tuberosity can become tender secondary to patellar tendinitis or a contusion. Tenderness and enlargement of the tuberosity in adolescent patients indicates the possibility of Osgood-Schlatter disease.

2. **Patellar tendon and bursae:** Palpate the tendon at the level of the infrapatellar pole moving distally to the tendon's midsubstance on through to its insertion at the tibial tuberosity. Pain elicited at the infrapatellar pole through the midsubstance may indicate patellar tendinitis; pain localized in the midsubstance may reflect a strain of this structure or tendinitis. Palpate the **subcutaneous infrapatellar bursa** and **deep infrapatellar bursa** for tenderness, swelling, and the skin's ability to glide freely over the tibial tuberosity.

3. **Fat pads:** Place the knee in extension to squeeze the fat pads beneath the patellar tendon out to either side, masking the deep infrapatellar bursa from palpation. Palpate these fat pads for signs of inflammation as they exit from behind, medially, and laterally to the patellar tendon. Because these structures are highly innervated, they are prone to hypersensitivity during inflammatory conditions.

4. **Patella and bursae:** During palpation of the patella, be alert for pain arising from the bone itself to distinguish it from pain arising from the soft tissue. Palpate the patellar body to rule out the presence of fracture, indicated by pain, roughening, discontinuity, or crepitus. Continue to palpate along the periphery of the four borders, attempting to elicit tenderness secondary to inflammatory conditions. If pain is present at the superior border, palpate up the length of the quadriceps group, noting the point at which the pain disappears. In some instances, the patella may be in two pieces, either from previous trauma or congenital defect (Fig. 7–8). This condition, a **bipartite patella,** reduces the efficiency of the extensor mechanism. The **prepatellar bursa** overlies the patella. Ensure that the skin over the patella moves freely and is not painful. The prepatellar bursa may become irritated and inflamed from overuse; from a contusing force to the anterior patella; or from prolonged periods of kneeling, as is seen with wrestlers. This bursa is also a common site of bacterial or staphylococcal infection.

5. **Patellar articulating surface:** With the knee extended, move the patella laterally to expose the outer portion of the lateral articular facet and medially to expose the odd facet. The exposed facets are palpated for signs of tenderness.

6. **Femoral trochlea:** In the patella's resting position on an extended knee, palpate the medial and lateral femoral trochlear borders for tenderness, keeping in mind that the lateral border is more exposed than the medial border is. Moving the patella medially and laterally exposes more of the femoral articular surface.

7. **Suprapatellar bursa:** Locate the suprapatellar bursa under the quadriceps group approximately 3 inches (four fingers' breadth) above the patella. With the ex-

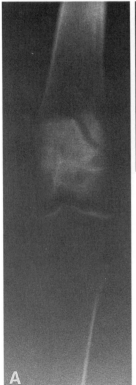
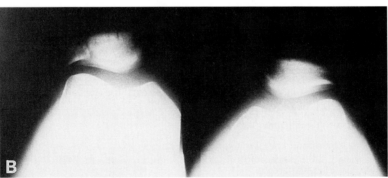

FIGURE 7–8. (A) Anterior view of a bipartite patella of the left knee. **(B)** "Merchant view" of the patella. Note the discrepancy in the continuity of the left and right patellae.

ception of puncture wounds, the suprapatellar bursa is rarely injured by direct trauma. It may, however, become inflamed or enlarged secondary to effusion in, or inflammation of, the knee joint capsule.

8. **Retinacular and capsular structures:** Palpate the medial and lateral retinacula, patellofemoral ligaments, and capsule for pain. The retinaculum and the associated structures may become painful with excessive movement of the patella.

9. **Synovial plica:** Palpate the anteromedial and anterolateral joint capsule for bands of thickened or folded tissue, denoting a synovial plica. These areas may become irritated and inflamed from being rubbed across bony structures or other tissues.

10–12. **Related structures:** The pes anserine muscle group and its associated bursae in the area of the medial tibial flare are common sites of inflammation (10). Hypersensitivity of one or more nerves can result in pain radiating through the knee and lower extremity. Neuroma, most commonly occurring from laceration of nerves during surgery involving the infrapatellar branch of the saphenous nerve, may be confirmed via a test for Tinel's sign over the medial aspect of the knee (11). Determine the flexibility of the IT band because tightness of this structure serves to increase the amount of lateral patellar tracking. Trigger points can be found in the IT band, causing tightness along its entire length (12).

Grinding beneath the patella while it is compressed and moved against the femur suggests the presence of chondromalacia. Although this condition occurs in a significant portion of the population, its presence may reflect biomechanical changes in the extensor mechanism or elsewhere in the lower extremity. The presence of chondromalacia may further be substantiated through Clarke's sign (Box 7–5).

Box 7–5
CLARKE'S SIGN FOR CHONDROMALACIA PATELLA

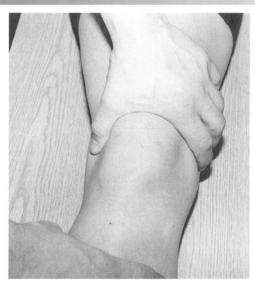

Clarke's sign for chondromalacia patella; this test elicits a great deal of pain and elicits a positive result in otherwise asymptomatic knees.

PATIENT POSITION	Lying supine with the knee extended
POSITION OF EXAMINER	Standing lateral to the limb being evaluated; one hand is placed proximal to the superior patellar pole, applying a gentle downward pressure
EVALUATIVE PROCEDURE	The patient is asked to contract the quadriceps muscle while pressure is maintained on the patella, pushing it into the femoral trochlea.
POSITIVE TEST	The patient experiences patellofemoral pain and the inability to hold the contraction.
IMPLICATIONS	Possibly chondromalacia patella The Clarke's sign is an unreliable test, producing false-positive results in otherwise asymptomatic knees.
MODIFICATION	The test may be performed with the knee flexed to various angles to assess different areas of patellofemoral contact.

RANGE OF MOTION TESTING

Unrestricted movement of the patella is required for the lower leg to achieve its full range of motion. The normal and abnormal movement of the patella as the knee moves from flexion to extension is discussed here. The complete range of motion testing of the knee joint is described in Chapter 6.

- **Active range of motion:** As the knee moves from flexion into extension, the patella normally glides superiorly and tracks somewhat laterally. Tightness of the lateral structures accentuates the lateral displacement of the patella. During flexion, the patella glides inferiorly and medially as it situates itself in the femoral trochlea.
- **Resisted range of motion:** Pain at the patella during movement may indicate a malalignment, resulting in soft tissue stretch as well as compressive forces on the articular facets, more so on the medial side. Resistive range of motion is performed in both the open and closed kinetic chain to determine the effect of introducing body weight on patellar motion. Isokinetic knee testing for patients suffering from acute patellofemoral pain may not be indicated because of the increased compressive forces placed on the patella at slower speeds.[23]
- **Lower extremity flexibility:** The relative flexibility of the quadriceps, hamstrings, IT band, and triceps surae is determined. Tightness in these muscle groups can result in decreased functional range of motion in the knee, force the quadriceps to exert more pressure on the patella, or cause patellar tracking deficits.

LIGAMENTOUS TESTING

Evaluate all major knee ligaments for normal integrity, as described in Chapter 6. Laxity of the knee joint can result in abnormal patellar tracking secondary to uniplanar or rotatory shifting of the tibia or femur, causing patellofemoral pain.

The ligamentous and capsular stability of the patella is based on the presence of patellar tilt and the amount of glide available to the patella. Glide tests are performed to assess the laxity or tightness of the retinacula by measuring how far the patella can be moved passively from its resting position in the trochlea.

The following description of the assessment of patellar glide and tilt have been adapted from the American Academy of Orthopaedic Surgeons' guidelines.[24]

- **Patellar glide:** To determine the amount of glide, visualize the patella as having four quadrants. Place the knee on a bolster so that it is flexed to 30 degrees. The patient must be fully reclined to relax the quadriceps muscles (Fig. 7–9). To ensure accuracy during the measurements, avoid tilting the patella as it is glided medially and laterally (Box 7–6).
- **Patellar tilt:** Patellar tilt, the rotation of the patella about its midsagittal axis, evaluates the tension within the lateral retinaculum, lateral capsule, IT band, and vastus lateralis tendon. The evaluation is performed with the patient lying supine with the knee extended and the femoral condyles parallel to the table (Box 7–7).
- **Synthesis of findings:** The relationship between patellar glide and patellar tilt needs to be considered to determine the functional limitations of the patellofemoral articulation and subsequently to determine a treatment regimen. A hypomobile medial glide in the presence of a positive tilt test result tends to respond favorably to conservative treatment. A negative patellar tilt test result combined with a hypomobile medial glide may require the surgical release of the lateral retinacular structures to permit proper glide within the trochlea. A negative preoperative patellar tilt result has been positively correlated with a successful outcome of the release of the lateral structures.[24]

NEUROLOGIC TESTING

The assessment of the sensory, motor, and reflex function for the patellofemoral joint is the same as described for the knee in Chapter 6.

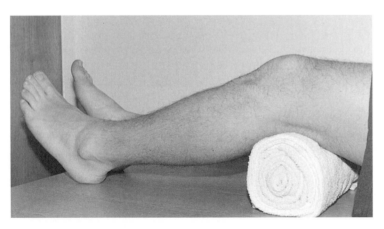

FIGURE 7–9. Positioning of the patient during the patellar glide tests. The knee is flexed to 30° and the individual is encouraged to keep the quadriceps musculature relaxed.

Box 7–6
PATELLAR GLIDE TESTS

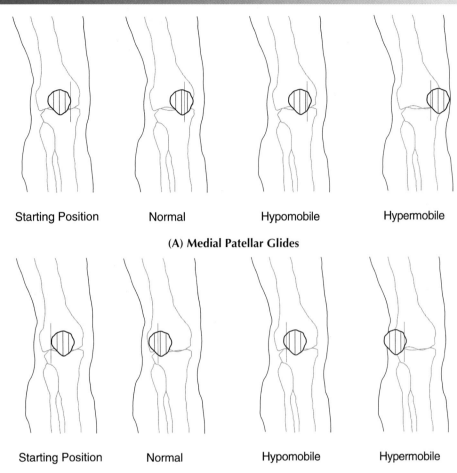

Starting Position Normal Hypomobile Hypermobile

(A) Medial Patellar Glides

Starting Position Normal Hypomobile Hypermobile

(B) Lateral Patellar Glides

During medial **(A)** and lateral **(B)** patellar glide tests, the patella is viewed as having four quadrants. The amount of glide is based on the movement relative to the quadrants.

PATIENT POSITION	Supine with a bolster placed under the knee so that it is flexed to 30°
POSITION OF EXAMINER	Standing lateral to the patient
EVALUATIVE PROCEDURE	**(A)** Medial glide: Move the patella medially, placing stress on the lateral retinaculum and other soft tissue restraints. **(B)** Lateral glide: Move the patella laterally, placing stress on the medial retinaculum, VMO, and medial capsule.
POSITIVE TEST	Medial glide: The patella should glide one to two quadrants (approximately half its width) medially. Movement of less than one quadrant is hypomobile medial glide. Movement more than two quadrants is hypermobile medial glide. Lateral glide: Normal lateral motion is 0.5 to 2.0 quadrants of glide. Less than that is hypomobile lateral glide; greater than two quadrants is hypermobile lateral glide.
IMPLICATIONS	Medial glide: Hypomobile glide is the result of tightness of the lateral retinaculum or IT band. Hypermobile medial glide indicates laxity of the lateral restraints. Lateral glide: Hypomobile lateral glide is caused by tightness of the medial restraints. Laxity of the medial restraints results in hypermobile lateral glide, a predisposition to patellar dislocations.
COMMENT	The patient may be apprehensive during lateral glide tests, fearful that the motion could result in the patella dislocation.

IT = iliotibial; VMO = oblique fibers of the vastus medialis.

> **Box 7–7**
> ## PATELLAR TILT TEST

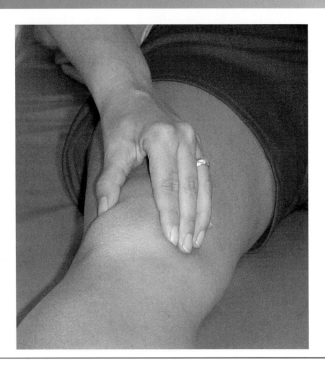

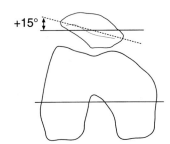

The patellar tilt test evaluates rotation of the patella around its midsagittal axis.

PATIENT POSITION	Supine with the knee extended and the femoral condyles parallel to the table
POSITION OF EXAMINER	Standing lateral to the patient
EVALUATIVE PROCEDURE	Grasp the patella with the forefinger and thumb, elevating the lateral border and depressing the medial border.
POSITIVE TEST RESULT	A normal result is the lateral border raising between 0° and 15°. More than 15° is hypermobile lateral tilt; less than 0° is a hypomobile lateral tilt.
IMPLICATIONS	A tilt of less than 0° indicates tightness of the lateral restraints and often occurs in the presence of a hypomobile medial glide.[25] A tilt of more than 15° may predispose the individual to anterior knee pain.

 ## PATHOLOGIES AND RELATED SPECIAL TESTS

The terms "patellofemoral dysfunction" and "patellofemoral pain syndrome" are used to describe a wide range of symptoms occurring around the knee and patella. These symptoms range from pain being described as dull to sharp and in locations including the anterior (prepatellar) and posterior (retropatellar) portions of the patella, as well as its four borders. The onset of symptoms may occur during periods of inactivity, especially when the patient is sitting (theater sign) and during or after activity. This section describes the possible causes for this wide range of symptoms so that an adequate treatment and rehabilitation plan may

be constructed to relieve the pain and also correct the cause of the symptoms.

Pain and dysfunction arising from the patellofemoral complex often mimic the symptoms of meniscal trauma. Table 7–2 presents subjective findings that may be used to differentiate between injuries of the two structures.

PATELLOFEMORAL PAIN SYNDROME

Patellofemoral pain syndrome and patellofemoral joint dysfunction are all-inclusive diagnoses for pain in and around the patellofemoral joint that cannot be explained by a specific pathology. Typically having an in-

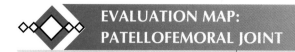

EVALUATION MAP: PATELLOFEMORAL JOINT

1. HISTORY

Mechanism of injury
Onset of injury
When pain occurs
Location of the pain
Level of activity
Prior surgery
Relevant past history

2. INSPECTION

Patellar alignment

Patella malalignment
  Patellar tendon length
  Patella baja
  Patella alta
  Squinting patellae
  "Frog-eyed" patellae
Tibiofemoral alignment

Q angle
  Knee extended
  Knee flexed

Standing leg length difference
Foot posture
Areas of scars

3. PALPATION

Tibial tuberosity
Patellar tendon
Patellar tendon bursae
Patellar fat pads
Patella
Patellar bursae
Patellar articulating surface
Femoral trochlea
Suprapatellar bursa
Retinacular and capsular structures
Synovial plica
Related structures

4. RANGE OF MOTION TESTS

Active knee range of motion
Resisted knee range of motion
Lower extremity flexibility

5. LIGAMENTOUS TESTS

Patellar glide
  Medial glide
  Lateral glide
  Patellar tilt

6. NEUROLOGICAL TESTS

Peroneal nerve
Femoral nerve
Sciatic nerve
Lumbar nerve roots
Sacral nerve roots

7. SPECIAL TESTS

Patellar dislocation
  Apprehension test

Synovial plica
  Test for medial synovial plica
  Stutter test

Table 7–2

SUBJECTIVE FINDINGS IN THE DIFFERENTIATION OF MENISCAL AND PATELLAR PAIN

History	Meniscus	Patella
Onset	Usually acute twisting injury	Occasionally direct anterior knee blow but usually insidious related to overuse and training errors
Symptom site	Localized medial or lateral joint line	Diffuse, most commonly anterior
Locking	Frank transient locking episodes with the knee unable to fully terminally extend	Catching without locking, stiffness after immobility, but not true locking
Weight bearing	Pain sharp and simultaneous with loaded weight bearing	Pain possibly coming on during weight bearing but often continuing into the evening and night
Cutting sports	Pain with loaded twisting maneuvers	Some pain possible, but not sharp and clearly related to cutting
Squatting	Pain at full squat; inability to "duck walk"	Pain when extensors used to rise from a squat
Kneeling	Not painful because meniscus is not weight loaded	Pain from patellar compression
Jumping	Weight loaded without torque or twist tolerated	Extensors heavily stressed, causing pain on descent impact
Stairs or hills	Pain often going upstairs with loaded knee flexion, causing squatlike meniscal compression	More patellar loading and pain going downstairs because gravity-assisted impact increases patellofemoral stress
Sitting	No pain	Stiffness and pain from lack of the distraction–compression effect on abnormal articular cartilage

sidious onset, patellofemoral joint disease is occasionally precipitated by direct trauma to the joint or by overuse. The patient's primary complaint of anterior knee pain is initially caused by activity. Over time, the pain may become constant.

Complaints of pain are usually associated with stair climbing, sitting for long periods of time, and other activities in which the knee is flexed for prolonged periods. Mild swelling may be present. Pain is increased with active and resisted extension of the knee and during the end range of passive flexion. Clarke's sign may be positive. The integrity of the tissues surrounding the patellofemoral joint are evaluated for tightness and hyperlaxity by assessing patellar glide and tilt. Along with the active contractions of the surrounding musculature, the integrity of the surrounding static stabilizers affect patellar tracking. Subtalar joint pronation has also been implicated as a biomechanical cause of patellar pain.[26]

Treatment of patients with patellofemoral pain syndrome usually begins by modifying activity to avoid pain and the use of nonsteroidal anti-inflammatory medications. The use of ice, especially after activity, may be helpful. If tightness is assessed in the surrounding capsule and retinacular tissues, patella mobilization and passive stretching may be helpful. Therapeutic exercise for improving flexibility of lower extremity musculature and strengthening the hip and thigh muscles to improve patellar tracking is also useful.

The use of shoe orthotics as an adjunct to exercise has been shown to reduce patellofemoral pain.[27] Patellar taping is useful in reducing subjective reports of pain and improving extensor mechanism function[28,29] and may alter the activation of the VMO oblique and vastus lateralis muscles.[30] Patellar taping may only be helpful in patients with patellar tracking problems.[8]

PATELLAR MALTRACKING

The onset of patellofemoral dysfunction has historically been attributed solely to an increased Q angle. However, patellofemoral function is based on a number of individual variables, each influencing the extensor mechanism.[31,32] Normal tracking of the patella within the femoral trochlea depends on the relationships between the alignment of the femur on the tibia; the Q angle; the integrity of the patella's soft tissue restraints; foot mechanics; and the flexibility of the triceps surae, quadriceps, hamstring muscle groups, and IT band (Table 7–3).

Many of the predisposing conditions to patellar tracking disorders are congenital. However, injury to the patella or knee may cause a change in one of the variables. For example, a lateral dislocation of the patella results in tearing of the medial restraints, causing increased laxity. Likewise, an injury to the knee can cause atrophy of the VMO, increasing the amount of lateral patellar glide with subsequent shortening of the

Table 7–3
STRUCTURAL ABNORMALITIES AND THEIR RESULTANT FORCES AND BIOMECHANICAL CHANGES

Alignment	Resulting Forces and Biomechanical Changes
Genu varum	Increased compressive forces on the medial tibiofemoral articulating surfaces
	Tensile forces on the lateral tibiofemoral ligaments
	Quadriceps exerting medially directed forces on the patella
	Compressive forces on the lateral facet
	Stretching of the lateral patellar restraints
Genu valgum	Increased compressive forces on the lateral tibiofemoral articulating surfaces
	Tensile forces on the medial tibiofemoral ligaments
	Quadriceps exerting laterally directed forces on the patella
	Compressive forces on the odd and medial facets
	Stretching of the medial patellar restraints
Increased Q angle or lax medial restraints	Lateral tracking of the patella
	Compressive forces on the lateral facet
	Stretching of the medial patellar restraints
Decreased Q angle or lax lateral restraints	Medial tracking of the patella
	Compressive forces on odd and medial facets
	Stretching of the lateral patellar restraints
Genu recurvatum	Decreased compressive forces in terminal knee extension

lateral restraints. Other variables affecting the equation are increased body weight and gait mechanics.[33]

Patients suffering from patellar tracking conditions describe a gradual onset with symptoms related to increased activity. Redistribution of forces along the patellar facets can result in pain during activities of daily living (ADLs), such as prolonged periods of sitting or walking up and down the stairs. The lack of appropriate muscle length and excessive pronation contribute to patellar maltracking.

PATELLAR SUBLUXATION AND DISLOCATION

Acute, chronic, or congenital laxity of the medial patellar restraints or abnormal tightness of the lateral retinaculum results in an increased lateral glide of the patella, predisposing patients to subluxations and dislocations. Patellar subluxations may occur without the person's knowledge, producing symptoms described as the knee "giving out" during weight-bearing. True dislocation of the patella causes it to shift laterally and lock out of place, resulting in obvious gross deformity and spasm of the quadriceps group as it guards the injury (Fig. 7–10).

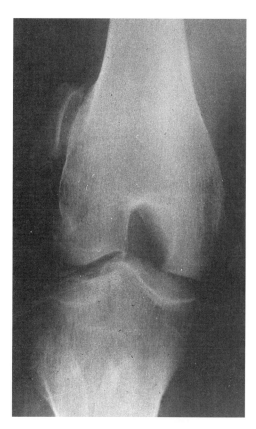

FIGURE 7–10. A radiograph of a laterally dislocated patella. This view, taken from the knee's posterior aspect, shows the patella resting on the lateral femoral condyle.

The patella is most apt to dislocate or subluxate when the maximum strain is placed on the lateral patellar restraints, normally within the range of 20 to 30 degrees of knee flexion or after a valgus blow to the knee.[34] Dislocations caused by blunt trauma may also result in a fracture of the patella.[35] Noncontact dislocations may result in osteochondral damage, patellar bone bruises, or osteochondritis dissecans.[36,37] Multiple dislocations or subluxations result in a wearing of the articular cartilage. However, the incidence of true osteoarthritis is reduced in this population relative to those having normal tightness in the patellar restraints.[38]

Several factors predispose an individual to patellar subluxations and dislocations. Those with hypomobile medial glide have an increased tendency for subluxations than those persons with hypermobile lateral glide.[39] The tightness of the lateral restraints serves to pull the patella laterally during knee extension. A flattened posterior (articulating) patellar surface increases the likelihood of spontaneous (non-contact-related) patellar dislocation.[40] Factors such as external tibial rotation and hyperpronated feet increase the Q angle, causing the patella to track laterally.[41] A family history of patellar dislocations or subluxations also increases the risk of injury.[42]

Both acute patellar dislocations and subtle subluxations result in large, bloody effusions within 24 hours after the onset of the injury. A complete dislocation seldom occurs without tearing of the VMO from the patella or from its origin near the adductor tubercle or the adjacent intermuscular septum.[42] The insertion of the medial patellar retinaculum is often avulsed from the patella.[35] For this reason, palpation of the medial patellar retinaculum and the VMO at either its origin or insertion produces pain (Table 7–4). Patients suffering from chronic patellar instability also produce a positive **apprehension test,** which should be performed before testing for patellar mobility and before performing a valgus stress test (Box 7–8). Radiographic examination is obtained for all dislocations or subluxations to rule out osteochondral fractures of the patella and femur. The mechanism for patellar dislocations and subluxations is similar to that of an MCL sprain, and the possibility of this injury must be ruled out.

The use of prophylactic or rehabilitational braces has little effect on preventing the reoccurrence of patellar dislocations or subluxations.[43] Conservative treatment includes casting, posterior splinting, and functional bracing. Of these methods, the use of posterior splints has the lowest recurrence rate, but operative treatment frequently yields the best results.[44] The most common surgical technique involves shifting the patellar tendon attachment to correct patellar tracking problems.[45]

PATELLAR TENDINITIS

Common in individuals participating in jumping activities, running sports, and weight lifting, patellar tendinitis most often has an insidious onset. Acute tendinitis

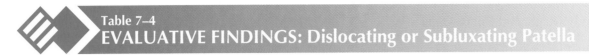

Table 7–4
EVALUATIVE FINDINGS: Dislocating or Subluxating Patella

Examination Segment	Clinical Findings	
History	**Onset:**	Acute or recurrent
	Pain characteristics:	Medial joint capsule, indicating trauma to the medial patellar restraints as well as pain reported beneath the patella
	Mechanism:	During extension of the knee or an eccentric contraction of the quadriceps group within the last 30° of the range of motion; a valgus force may also be associated with the onset of injury
	Predisposing factors:	Lateral patellar tracking; increased Q angle; tight lateral restraints; lax medial restraints; family history of patellar dislocation/subluxation
Inspection	Unreduced patellar dislocations exhibit obvious deformity. Effusion of the knee occurs within 24 hours after the onset of the injury.	
Palpation	Pain is produced over the medial retinaculum and lateral articular facet. Complete dislocations reveal pain at the origin of the VMO at the adductor tubercle or intermuscular septum or at its insertion on the patella, secondary to tearing of this structure.	
Functional tests	These tests must not be performed on unreduced patellar dislocations. The following assume the patella has relocated and no obvious deformity exists:	
	AROM:	Pain occurring during the first 30° of flexion or terminal extension
	PROM:	Pain may arise secondary to stretching of the retinaculum, especially as the knee enters into flexion
	RROM:	Decreased strength during extension when the knee is flexed between 0° and 30°
Ligamentous tests	Hypermobile lateral glide usually associated with a positive patellar tilt test result	
Neurological tests	Not applicable	
Special tests	Positive patellar apprehension test result	
Comments	Dislocations or subluxations of the patella may result in osteochondral fractures to the lateral femoral condyle or posterior surface of the patella. If the presence of a valgus force is determined during the history-taking process, the integrity of the MCL should be established	

AROM = active range of motion; MCL = medial collateral ligament; PROM = passive range of motion; RROM = resisted range of motion; VMO = vastus medialis oblique.

also can occur as the result of a blow to the tendon. Repetitive motions on a biomechanically malaligned extensor mechanism can result in unequal loads on the extensor tendon.[46,47] Microtearing of the fibers results in the formation of excess connective tissues and endothelial cells, increased vascularity, and the alteration of the tendon's normal cellular structure.[47,48] A tendinosis may also develop around the tendon.[49] The proximal portion of the posterior middle and central thirds of the patellar tendon are the most frequently inflamed portions of the tendon.[47,50] Prolonged patellar tendon inflammation can result in an elongation of the inferior patellar pole[50] and *morphologic* changes in the medal patellar retinaculum.[51]

The most common site of pain associated with patellar tendinitis is the inferior pole of the patella. Pain may also be described at the superior pole in the case of quadriceps tendinitis (jumper's knee), in the midsubstance of the tendon, or at the tendon's attachment to the tibial tuberosity. (Table 7–5). Resisted knee extension may increase pain to the point that strength is in-

hibited. The end range of passive knee flexion, performed with the patient in the prone position, elicits pain in the patellar tendon and may result in decreased quadriceps flexibility. Commonly, athletes should be able to passively flex the knee so that the heel of the foot can touch, or almost touch, the buttocks. Crepitus can be palpated in tendons during active or resisted movements. Pain that is elicited from either side of the patellar tendon indicates **fat pad syndrome.** Magnetic resonance imaging (MRI) is useful in identifying the presence of patellar tendinitis.[47,49,50]

If conservative treatment (as described in the section on patellofemoral pain syndrome) fails, surgical intervention may be needed.[48] Surgical care involves debridement of the tendon.

Morphologic   Changes in form and structure with regard to function.

Box 7–8
APPREHENSION TEST FOR A SUBLUXATING/DISLOCATING PATELLA

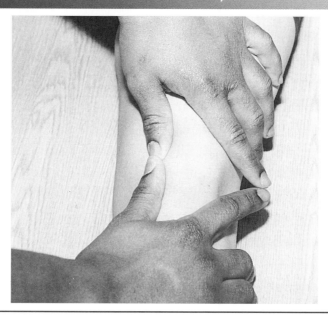

The apprehension test for patellar dislocation. The examiner glides the patella laterally. A positive test is indicated by the patient's contracting the muscle, describing pain, or otherwise showing apprehension (anticipation) of an impending dislocation.

PATIENT POSITION	Lying supine with the knee extended.
POSITION OF EXAMINER	Standing lateral to the involved side.
EVALUATIVE PROCEDURE	The examiner attempts to move the patella as far laterally as possible, taking care not to cause it to actually dislocate.
POSITIVE TEST	Forcible contraction of the quadriceps by the patient to guard against dislocation of the patella. The patient may also demonstrate apprehension verbally or through facial expression.
IMPLICATIONS	Laxity of the medial patellar retinaculum, predisposing the patient to patellar subluxations or dislocations.

PATELLAR TENDON RUPTURE

Mechanical failure of the patellar tendon is uncommon in otherwise healthy individuals. Diseases such as rheumatoid arthritis, diabetes, *lupus,* chronic renal disease, or gout as well as chronic inflammation of the patellar tendon or the use of corticosteroid medications may predispose patellar tendon ruptures.[52–54] Tension developed within the quadriceps unit overloads the patellar tendon, resulting in the rupture of its midsubstance or avulsion from the patella or patellar tuberosity. This muscular load most commonly occurs secondary to hyperflexion of the knee or powerful knee extension from a weight-bearing position.[55]

Patellar tendon ruptures cause immediate gross deformity as the patella is displaced proximally on the femur, exposing the condyles. During palpation, a depression is noted in the infrapatellar region.[55] Because of the severity of the trauma, gross swelling rapidly accumulates. The ability to actively extend the lower leg is lost and the individual is unable to perform a straight leg raise on the affected side. However, the patient is still able to contract the quadriceps (Table 7–6). Although the ligaments of the involved knee may have been compromised at the time of injury, no ligamentous stability tests are performed before the patient is examined by a physician.

Lupus A systemic disease affecting the internal organs, skin, and musculoskeletal system.

Table 7–5
EVALUATIVE FINDINGS: Patellar Tendinitis

Examination Segment	Clinical Findings	
History	*Onset:*	Insidious onset in most cases, but inflammation is possible secondary to contusive forces to the tendon.
	Pain characteristics:	Inferior patellar poles, midsubstance of the tendon, or the tendon's point of insertion on the tibial tuberosity
	Mechanism:	Repeated activity involving resisted knee extension (e.g., jumping) or secondary to contusive forces on the patella
	Predisposing factors:	Patellar maltracking; overuse
Inspection	The patellar tendon and inferior patellar pole may appear inflamed. Swelling may be localized around the patellar tendon.	
Palpation	Tenderness of the patellar tendon, especially at its insertion on the infrapatellar pole Crepitus in advanced cases	
Functional tests	*AROM:* Pain during active knee extension possible in advanced cases *PROM:* Pain during the end range of knee flexion *RROM:* Pain throughout resisted knee extension	
Ligamentous tests	Not applicable	
Neurologic tests	Not applicable	
Special tests	Not applicable	
Comments	There may be an associated tightness of the quadriceps musculature.	

AROM = active range of motion; PROM = passive range of motion; RROM = resisted range of motion.

Table 7–6
EVALUATIVE FINDINGS: Patellar Tendon Rupture

Examination Segment	Clinical Findings	
History	*Onset:*	Acute
	Pain characteristics:	Patellar tendon, patella, and quadriceps muscle group
	Mechanism:	Dynamic overload of the extensor mechanism secondary to extending the knee against resistance or a forceful eccentric contraction of the quadriceps muscle
	Predisposing factors:	A history of a chronically inflamed patellar tendon; history of repeated local corticosteroid injections; rheumatoid arthritis; diabetes; gout; lupus
Inspection	Gross deformity caused by the patella riding high on the femur, exposing both femoral condyles and a defect in the patellar tendon Obvious anterior soft tissue swelling, possibly masking the underlying deformity	
Palpation	A palpable defect in the patellar tendon, along with exposed femoral condyles Rapid, gross swelling possibly masking palpation findings	
Functional tests	*AROM:* The patient is able to contract the quadriceps but is unable to extend the knee against gravity. The patient is unable to perform straight leg raises, accentuating the visible defects about the knee. *PROM:* An empty end-feel during flexion or a soft end-feel owing to the approximation of the hamstrings and gastrocnemius; PROM not performed acutely in the presence of an obvious tendon rupture *RROM:* Not advised because further damage to the extensor mechanism may result.	
Ligamentous tests	Not performed during the initial evaluation and management of a suspected tendon rupture, although damage to the knee ligaments suspected	
Neurologic tests	Lower leg dermatomes checked to rule out secondary trauma to the peroneal or tibial nerve	
Special tests	Not applicable	
Comments	Patellar tendon ruptures tend to occur in men younger than age 40 years, although any segment of the population is susceptible.	

AROM = active range of motion; PROM = passive range of motion; RROM = resisted range of motion.

FIGURE 7–11. Photograph of a grossly swollen prepatellar bursa of the left knee.

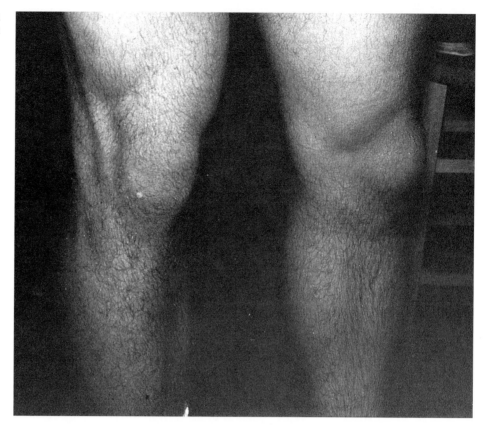

Patients suffering from patellar tendon ruptures require immediate immobilization and transportation to the hospital (see the On-field Management of Patellar Tendon Ruptures section). Surgical intervention within 7 to 10 days of the injury and appropriate rehabilitation can fully restore function to the knee. Most athletes are able to progress to a full return to activity approximately 12 months after surgery.[56] Delaying surgery significantly decreases the functional outcome.[55]

PATELLAR BURSITIS

The extensor mechanism's bursa may be inflamed secondary to a single traumatic force, repeated low-intensity blows, overuse, or infection (e.g., with **Staphylococcus**). The superficial prepatellar bursa and the subcutaneous infrapatellar bursa are most often injured secondary to direct trauma, resulting in localized swelling (Fig. 7–11).[57] The suprapatellar and deep infrapatellar bursae become inflamed secondary to overuse. Pain caused by bursitis usually remains localized and the infrapatellar fat pads often become sympathetically tender (Table 7–7). Those conditions with a sudden onset and no history of trauma or overuse with associated redness and warmth about the knee require referral to a physician to rule out infection. Treatment of patellar bursitis consists of modifying activity to reduce painful stresses and controlling inflammation.[57]

SYNOVIAL PLICA

A synovial plica is a fold of the fibrous membrane that projects into the joint cavity. This congenital abnormality is a remnant of folds formed during the embryologic stage of development. During maturation, these folds are absorbed into the joint capsule; however, in the majority of the population, either a thickened area or a crease within the membrane remains.[58] Normally a synovial plica remains asymptomatic until the area is traumatized by a direct blow to the capsule or is inflamed secondary to stretching and friction caused by the plica bow-stringing across the femoral condyle during flexion, resulting in two reservoirs for synovial fluid: a suprapatellar reservoir and the cavity of the knee joint itself.[59–61] Although the onset of symptoms occurs most commonly in adolescents, plical syndromes may afflict patients of all ages at all stages of developmental maturity.[62] Synovial plica syndrome most commonly involves the medial joint capsule, but this condition can involve the lateral capsule.[63]

When the plica becomes symptomatic, it loses its elastic qualities and alters the biomechanics of patellar gliding mechanism. Prolonged inflammation of the plica leads to fibrosis and chronic disturbances within the knee. The symptoms presented by synovial plica syndrome may mimic those of chondromalacia patella, meniscal tears, patellar subluxation, and patellar mal-tracking syndromes (Table 7–8).[61,64] Longitudinal tears

Table 7–7
EVALUATIVE FINDINGS: Prepatellar Bursitis

Examination Segment	Clinical Findings	
History	*Onset:*	Acute or chronic
	Pain characteristics:	Localized to a specific bursa and possibly the infrapatellar fat pads
	Mechanism:	Direct trauma to the bursa or overuse
	Predisposing factors:	Other local inflammatory conditions (e.g., patellar tendinitis); weight bearing on the knees (e.g., wrestling)
Inspection	Localized swelling possible if a superficial bursa involved	
Palpation	Point tenderness may be experienced when directly palpating the bursa or the area over the bursa; tenderness over the infrapatellar fat pads may also be described.	
Functional tests	*AROM:*	In chronic or severe cases, pain may be described within a specified range or throughout the entire ROM.
	PROM:	Pain is experienced at a specific point in the ROM.
	RROM:	Decreased strength and pain occur throughout the ROM.
Ligamentous tests	Not applicable	
Neurologic tests	Not applicable	
Special tests	Not applicable	
Comments	The specific bursa involved is based on the specific location of pain.	
	Patients with no relevant history for the onset of bursitis or who have superficial wounds over the bursa should be referred to a physician to rule out the possibility of infection.	

AROM = active range of motion; PROM = passive range of motion; ROM = range of motion; RROM = resisted range of motion.

Table 7–8
EVALUATIVE FINDINGS: Synovial Plica Syndromes

Examination Segment	Clinical Findings	
History	*Onset:*	Insidious
	Pain characteristics:	Pain is located in the anterior portion of the knee; the patient may describe clicking, popping, psuedolocking of the knee, or the knee's "giving way." Symptoms are often described as being worse in the morning, with a gradual decrease as the day progresses.
	Mechanism:	Friction caused by the plica's rubbing across a femoral condyle
	Predisposing factors:	Congenitally large or thickened plica; the likelihood of onset decreasing with increasing age
Inspection	No visual findings.	
Palpation	Symptomatic plica possibly felt as a thickened, bandlike structure that is tender to the touch	
	Plica affect the anteromedial capsule more so than the anterolateral capsule.	
	Swelling possibly noted during palpation	
Functional tests	*AROM:*	Pain experienced as the plica crosses the femoral condyle, with possible clicking or "catching" described by the patient; a snapping heard by the examiner and felt by palpating the joint capsule
	PROM:	A clicking or pseudolocking as the knee is flexed and extended over the point at which the plica rubs or catches on the femoral condyle
	RROM:	Pain as described for AROM
Ligamentous tests	Lateral patellar glide may be decreased.	
Neurologic tests	Not applicable	
Special tests	Positive medial synovial plica test or stutter test result	
Comments	The symptoms of synovial plica may mimic that of a meniscal tear, subluxating patella, or chondromalacia that has been caused by biomechanical changes in the knee.	
	Longitudinal tears within the plica can result in pseudolocking of the knee.	

AROM = active range of motion; PROM = passive range of motion; RROM = resisted range of motion.

Box 7–9
TEST FOR MEDIAL SYNOVIAL PLICA

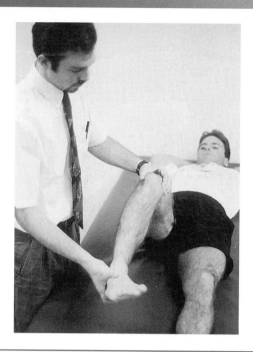
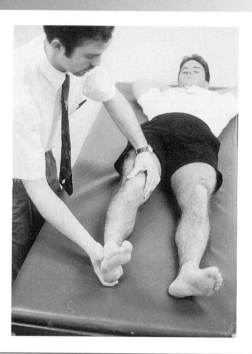

A positive test reproduces the patient's symptoms and the examiner may feel the plica as it crosses the medial femoral condyle.

PATIENT POSITION	Lying supine with the knee flexed or with the patient seated.
POSITION OF EXAMINER	Standing on the side being tested.
EVALUATIVE PROCEDURE	With the knee flexed to 90° and the tibia internally rotated, the examiner passively moves the patella medially while palpating the anteromedial capsule. The knee is then extended and flexed from 90° to 0° while the tibia is internally rotated.
POSITIVE TEST	Reproduction of the symptoms is described by the patient. The clinician may feel the plica as it crosses the medial femoral condyle, especially in the range of 60° to 45° of flexion.
IMPLICATIONS	Symptomatic medial synovial plica.

of the plica can result in pseudolocking of the knee.[61] The presence of medial plica syndrome may be confirmed through either the **test for medial plica syndrome** (Box 7–9) or **the stutter test** (Box 7–10).[65] A medial synovial plica can be confirmed using MRI.[66,67]

Initial management of a symptomatic synovial plica includes modifying activity to reduce the irritating stresses and controlling the inflammatory response. Strengthening the VMO may lessen the symptoms by reducing the tensile forces placed on the plica.[61]

OSGOOD-SCHLATTER DISEASE

Osgood-Schlatter disease is an adolescent inflammatory condition that strikes the tibial tuberosity's growth plate where the patellar tendon attaches. Its onset is traced to repeated avulsion fractures of the tendon from its attachment and is caused by rapid growth, increased strength of the quadriceps, or both. These forces result in osteochondritis of the tubercle (Fig. 7–12). The symptoms of Osgood-Schlatter disease are similar to those of patellar tendinitis. However, differentiation is made by the patient's age (i.e., in adolescents) and the pain's being localized to the tibial tuberosity and distal portion of the patellar tendon (Table 7–9). A history of Osgood-Schlatter disease may lead to residual enlargement of the tibial tuberosity. In the adult population, enlargement of the tibial tuberosity may be caused by a history of apophysitis.

Osgood-Schlatter disease is managed conservatively by modifying activity to reduce antagonistic stresses on

Box 7–10
STUTTER TEST FOR A MEDIAL SYNOVIAL PLICA

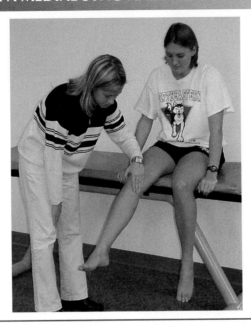

The examiner palpates the patella for irregular movement (stutter) as the patient extends the knee. When a plica snags against the medial femoral condyle, it may cause a momentary disruption in patellar motion.

PATIENT POSITION	Sitting with the knee flexed over the edge of the table.
POSITION OF EXAMINER	Standing lateral to the involved side, lightly cupping one hand over the patella, being careful not to compress the articular surfaces.
EVALUATIVE PROCEDURE	The patient slowly extends the knee.
POSITIVE TEST	Irregular motion or stuttering between 40° and 60° as the plica passes over the medial condyle.
IMPLICATIONS	Medial synovial plica.

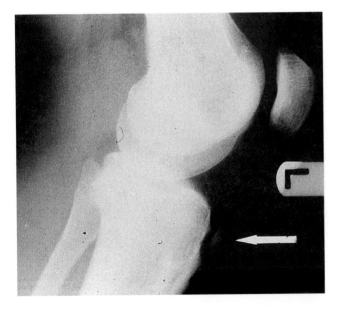

FIGURE 7–12. Radiograph of Osgood-Schlatter disease showing the bony outgrowth.

Table 7–9
EVALUATIVE FINDINGS: Osgood-Schlatter Disease

Examination Segment	Clinical Findings	
History	*Onset:*	Insidious
	Pain characteristics:	Radiating up the distal one third of the patellar tendon
	Mechanism:	Stress placed on the tibial tuberosity's growth plate by forceful contraction or passive tension of the extensor mechanism; onset often associated with a rapid growth spurt or overtraining
	Predisposing factors:	Rapid muscular development during adolescence
Inspection	Swelling or deformity of the tibial tuberosity	
Palpation	Tenderness and perhaps crepitus over the tibial tuberosity and patellar tendon	
Functional tests	*AROM:*	Pain possibly experienced over the tibial tuberosity during active knee extension, especially when bearing weight
	PROM:	Pain over the tibial tuberosity during the end range of knee flexion secondary to strain placed on the patellar tendon
	RROM:	Pain and weakness during knee extension
Ligamentous tests	Not applicable	
Neurologic tests	Not applicable	
Special tests	Not applicable	
Comments	The signs and symptoms of Osgood-Schlatter disease may mimic those of patellar tendinitis, but the symptoms are localized to the tibial tuberosity. These findings in postadolescent patients may indicate a history of apophysitis.	

AROM = active range of motion; PROM = passive range of motion; RROM = resisted range of motion.

the tibial tuberosity and controlling inflammation. Surgical excision of the tibial tuberosity avulsion may be required if conservative treatment fails.[68]

SINDING-LARSEN-JOHANSSON DISEASE

Sinding-Larsen-Johansson Disease is found at the attachment of the patellar tendon into the inferior patellar pole or, less commonly, at the quadriceps tendon attachment at the proximal pole of the patella.[69,70] As with Osgood-Schlatter disease, Sinding-Larsen-Johansson disease is caused by a stress fracture or avulsion because of the repetitive forces associated with running and jumping. Continued traction forces on the growth areas of the patella lead to the disruption of the epiphysis.

Sinding-Larsen-Johansson disease typically affects males more often than females and is most common in the 10- to 14-year age group.[71] Complaints of pain and swelling at the affected pole of the patella are usually accompanied by an antalgic gait. Physical examination reveals point tenderness at the lesion site, pain with quadriceps stretching, and pain with active and resisted quadriceps function. Radiographs typically reveal the fragmentation at the superior or inferior pole of the patella. As with Osgood-Schlatter Disease, the fragmentation may cause a visible or palpable deformity at the lesion site (Table 7–10).

Treatment focuses on the symptoms and also on the possible causes. A 4- to 8-week period of rest, including immobilization in a cast or long leg immobilizer, helps to decrease the inflammatory process. Use of a long leg immobilizer allows the patient to receive *palliative* treatments such as ice or iontophoresis with anti-inflammatory medications if needed. As the symptoms of pain and swelling decrease, a program of stretching and strengthening of the quadriceps is initiated.

Similar to patients with other growth injuries, those with Sinding-Larsen-Johansson disease may remain periodically symptomatic until skeletal maturation is reached. In this case, patients need to respect the symptoms and rest as needed from the aggravating activities. They may even have to cease performing certain motions, especially those involving jumping.

Palliative   Serving to relieve or reduce symptoms without curing.

Table 7–10
EVALUATIVE FINDINGS: Sinding-Larsen-Johansson Disease

Examination Segment	Clinical Findings	
History	**Onset:**	Insidious
	Pain characteristics:	Superior or inferior patellar pole point tenderness, beginning as activity-related pain and progressing to pain at all times
	Mechanism:	Repetitive stresses from running and jumping
	Predisposing conditions:	A tight quadriceps muscle group; repetitive stress
Inspection	Antalgic gait; a deformity possibly present at the affected pole of the patella	
Palpation	Point tenderness at the affected pole of the patella	
Functional tests	**AROM:**	Full, with pain experienced at the end range of flexion and with knee extension
	PROM:	Knee flexion limited by pain
	RROM:	Pain with knee extension
Ligamentous tests	Not applicable	
Neurologic tests	Not applicable	
Special tests	Not applicable	
Comments	Sinding-Larsen-Johansson disease may remain periodically symptomatic until skeletal maturation is reached.	

AROM = active range of motion; PROM = passive range of motion; RROM = resisted range of motion.

PATELLAR FRACTURE

Blunt trauma to the patella, such as when an ice hockey player is being driven into the boards, can result in a fracture. Although this force may result in the rupture and immediate swelling of the prepatellar bursae, palpation may reveal crepitus over the body of the patella and one or more false joints (Fig. 7–13). The risk of patellar fracture may be increased following bone-patellar tendon-bone autograft anterior cruciate ligament reconstruction.[72,73] Active knee extension (if possible) and passive knee flexion produce severe pain. Resistive knee extension cannot be performed because of pain secondary to the pressures placed on the patella.[74]

ON-FIELD EVALUATION OF PATELLOFEMORAL INJURIES

Acute, traumatic injuries of the patellofemoral articulation mainly involve the patellar tendon, tracking of the patella within the femoral trochlea, and, on rare occasions, the bone itself. This type of trauma tends to produce gross deformity and loss of knee function.

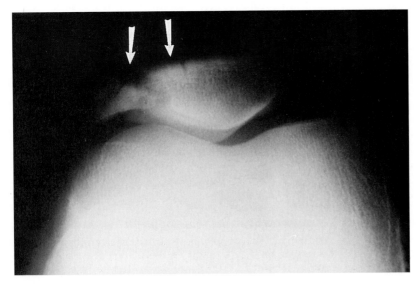

FIGURE 7–13. A "sunrise" radiograph of a fractured patella.

EQUIPMENT CONSIDERATIONS

Refer to Chapter 6, The Knee, for a discussion of the removal of knee equipment.

ON-FIELD HISTORY

Unless the nature of the athlete's condition is obviously apparent, the location of pain, mechanism of injury, and any associated sounds or other descriptors of the injury must be established. Initially it may be difficult to differentiate trauma to the patellofemoral joint from tibiofemoral injury.

Inspect the patella to ensure that it assumes its normal position on the femur and has a normal shape. The patellar tendon should be visible as it runs from the tibial tuberosity to the infrapatellar pole. Rupture of this tendon results in violent spasm of the quadriceps muscle, causing it to "ball up" on the femur. In the event of an obvious injury, a secondary screen must be performed to rule out any less obvious injury. Confirm any suspicions of injury obtained during the history-taking or inspection process through palpation. Any indication of a patellar dislocation, fracture, or patellar tendon rupture warrants the termination of the evaluation and immediate immobilization and transportation for further medical evaluation.

ON-FIELD PALPATION

Begin by palpating the patellar tendon for tenderness, indicating a possible strain or aggravation of existing inflammation, from the tibial tuberosity to its insertion on the infrapatellar pole. Continue to palpate up the quadriceps muscles, paying close attention to the tone of muscle and tenderness over the VMO. Spasm of the quadriceps muscle may indicate a patellar dislocation, especially if the knee remains flexed. Tenderness may be elicited over the VMO secondary to tearing of the fibers during lateral dislocation of the patella.

From the VMO palpate inferiorly to locate the medial joint capsule, which is tender after a lateral patellar dislocation. Palpate the lateral joint capsule for tenderness, indicating possible medial displacement of the patella.

ON-FIELD FUNCTIONAL TESTS

After the possibility of major disruption to the patellofemoral joint has been ruled out, an assessment of the athlete's functional status may begin. Some of these movements may have been voluntarily performed by the athlete during the earlier portions of the examination.

- **Willingness to move the involved limb:** Ask the athlete to fully flex and extend the involved limb. An unwillingness or inability to complete this task is a sign that the athlete must be assisted off the field or court. If the athlete is able to complete the full range of motion, break pressure may be applied with the knee near full extension and again in partial flexion to obtain a gross determination of muscular strength.
- **Willingness to bear weight:** If the preceding tests show normal or near normal results, possibly allow the athlete to bear weight by assisting the athlete to the standing position and letting him or her bear weight on the uninvolved limb. The athletic trainer then assumes a position under the involved side to help support the athlete's body weight, if needed.

 ## INITIAL MANAGEMENT OF ON-FIELD INJURIES

The primary concerns for the on-field management of patients with patellofemoral injuries involve the rupture of the patellar tendon, fractures of the patella, or an unreduced patellar dislocation. The following protocol is suggested for the initial management of patients with these conditions. It should be noted that the management of a fractured patella and that of a patellar tendon rupture are essentially the same.

PATELLAR TENDON RUPTURE

Sudden overloading of the musculotendinous unit of the quadriceps can result in a rupture of the tendon in its midsubstance or an avulsion from its attachment on the patella's inferior pole or the tibial tuberosity. This injury results in immediate loss of function and gross deformity as the quadriceps contracts, possibly pulling the patella up the femur. Splint the knee in extension and immediately transport the athlete for further medical attention.

PATELLAR DISLOCATION

Dislocation of the patella is marked by obvious deformity in which the patella is shifted laterally. On-field reduction of a dislocated patella should not be attempted. However, spontaneous reductions may occur if the athlete relaxes the quadriceps group and gravity causes the knee to extend. All cases of patellar dislocation require referral to a physician so that fractures to the patella's and femur's articulating surfaces may be ruled out.

Splint known patellar subluxations or dislocations that have spontaneously reduced with the knee fully extended or slightly flexed. An unreduced dislocation must be splinted in the position in which the knee was found. This is most easily accomplished using a long moldable aluminum splint, bending one end to serve as a truss between the femur and lower leg (Fig. 7–14).

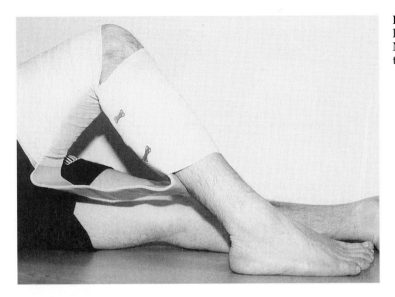

FIGURE 7–14. Splinting of the leg for an acutely dislocated patella, using a moldable aluminum splint. Note that part of the splint serves as a truss to maintain the current position of the knee.

◆ REFERENCES

1. Powers, CM, Shellock, FG, and Pfaff, M: Quantification of patellar tracking using kinematic MRI. *J Magn Reson Imaging,* 8:724, 1998.
2. Goodfellow, J, Hungerford, DS, and Zindel, M: Patellofemoral joint mechanics and pathology: Functional anatomy of the patellofemoral joint. *J Bone Joint Surg* Br, 58:287, 1976.
3. Doucette, SA, and Child, DD: The effect of open and closed chain exercise and knee joint position on patellar tracking in lateral patellar compression syndrome. *J Orthop Sport Phys Ther,* 23:104, 1996.
4. D'Agata, S, et al: An in vitro analysis of patellofemoral contact areas and pressures following procurement of the central one-third patellar tendon. *Am J Sports Med,* 21:212, 1993.
5. Hubert, HH, and Hayes, WC: Patellofemoral contact pressures: The influence of Q-angle and tibiofemoral contact. *J Bone Joint Surg Am,* 66:715, 1984.
6. Hubert, HH, et al: Force ratios in the quadriceps tendon and ligamentum patellae. *J Orthop Res,* 2:49, 1984.
7. Rintala, P, and Lic, P: Patellofemoral pain syndrome and its treatment in runners. *Athletic Training: Journal of the National Athletic Trainers Association,* 25:107, 1990.
8. Reilly, DT, and Mantens, M: Experimental analysis of the quadriceps muscle force and patellofemoral joint reaction force for various activities. *Acta Orthop Scand,* 43:126, 1972.
9. Insall, J, Goldberg, V, and Saluati, ER: Recurrent dislocation and the high-riding patella. *Clin Orthop,* 88:67, 1972.
10. Lieb, FJ, and Perry, J: Quadriceps function: An anatomical and mechanical study using amputated limbs. *J Bone Joint Surg Am,* 50:1535, 1968.
11. Brownstein, BA, Lamb, RL, and Mangine, RE: Quadriceps torque and integrated electromyography. *J Orthop Sport Phys Ther,* 6:309, 1985.
12. Hanten, WP, and Schultheis, SS: Exercise effect on electromyographic activity of the vastus medialis oblique and vastus lateralis muscles. *Phys Ther,* 70:561, 1990.
13. Voight, M, and Weider, D: Comparative reflex response times of vastus medialis oblique and subjects with extensor mechanism dysfunction. *Am J Sports Med,* 19:131, 1991.
14. Spencer, JD, Hayes, KC, and Alexander, IJ: Knee joint effusion and quadriceps reflex inhibition in man. *Arch Phys Med Rehabil,* 65:171, 1984.
15. Casscells, W: Gross pathological changes in the knee joint of the aging individual. A study of three hundred cases. *J Bone Joint Surg Am,* 57:1033, 1975.
16. Bentley, G, and Dowd, G: Current concepts of etiology and treatment of chondromalacia patella. *Clin Orthop,* 189:209, 1984.
17. Metcalf, R: An arthroscopic method for lateral release of the subluxating or dislocating patella. *Clin Orthop,* 167:9; 1982.
18. McGinty, J, et al: 1991 AAOS Instructional Course Lecture on Patellofemoral Pain. American Academy or Orthopaedic Surgeons, Chicago, 1991.
19. Post, WR: Patellofemoral pain. Let the physical exam define treatment. *Physician and Sportsmedicine,* 26:68, 1998.
20. Tomaro, JE: Prevention and treatment of patellar entrapment following intra-articular ACL reconstruction. *Athletic Training: Journal of the National Athletic Trainers Association,* 26:11, 1991.
21. Fulkerson, JP: Patellofemoral pain disorders: evaluation and management. *J Am Acad Orthop Surg,* 2:124, 1994.
22. Guerra, JP, Arnold, MJ and Gajdosik, RL: Q angle: Effects of isometric quadriceps contraction and body postion. *J Orthop Sport Phys Ther,* 19:200, 1992.
23. Bennett, G, and Stauber, W: Evaluation and treatment of anterior knee pain using eccentric exercise. *Med Sci Sports Exerc,* 18:526, 1986.
24. Kolowich, P, et al: Lateral release of the patella: Indications and contraindications. *Am J Sports Med,* 18:359, 1990.
25. Fulkerson, J, et al: 1991 AAOS Instructional Course Lecture on Patellofemoral Pain, American Academy of Orthopaedic Surgeons, 1991.
26. Powers, CM; Maffucci, R, and Hampton, S: Rearfoot posture in subjects with patellofemoral pain. *J Orthop Sports Phys Ther,* 22:155, 1995.
27. Eng, JJ, and Pierrynowski, MR: Evaluation of soft foot orthotics in the treatment of patellofemoral pain syndrome. *Phys Ther,* 73:6, 1993.
28. Ernst, GP, Kawaguchi, J and Saliba, E: Effect of patellar taping on knee kinetics of patients with patellofemoral pain syndrome. *J Orthop Sports Phys Ther,* 29:661, 1999.
29. Powers, CM, et al: The effects of patellar taping on stride characteristics and joint motion in subjects with patellofemoral pain. *J Orthop Sports Phys Ther,* 26:286,1997.
30. Gilleard, W, McConnel, J, and Parsons, D: The effect of patellar taping on the onset of vastus medialis obliquus and vastus lateralis muscle activity in persons with patellofemoral pain. *Phys Ther,* 78:25, 1998.
31. Caylor, D, Fites, R, and Worrell, TW: The relationship between quadriceps angle and anterior knee pain syndrome. *J Orthop Sports Phys Ther,* 17:11, 1993.
32. Shelton, GL, and Thigpen, LK: Rehabilitation of patellofemoral dysfunction: A review of literature. *J Orthop Sports Phys Ther,* 14:234, 1991.

33. Moss, RI, DeVita, P, and Dawson, ML: A biomechanical analysis of patellofemoral stress syndrome. *J Athletic Training*, 27:64, 1992.

34. Luo, ZP, et al: Tensile stress of the lateral patellofemoral ligament during knee motion. *Am J Knee Surg*, 10:139, 1997.

35. Burks, RT, et al: Biomechanical evaluation of lateral patellar dislocations. *Am J Knee Surg*, 11:24, 1998.

36. Stanitski, CL, and Paletta, GA: Articular cartilage injury with acute patellar dislocation in adolescents. Arthroscopic and radiographic correlation. *Am J Sports Med*, 26:52, 1998.

37. Sallay, PI, et al: Acute dislocation of the patella. A correlative pathoanatomic study. *Am J Sports Med*, 24:52, 1996.

38. Maenpaa, H, and Lehto, MU: Patellofemoral osteoarthritis after patellar dislocation. *Clin Orthop*, Jun:156, 1997.

39. Stanitski, CL: Articular hypermobility and chondral injury in patients with acute patellar dislocation. *Am J Sports Med*, 23:146, 1995.

40. Maenpaa, H, Huhtala, H, and Lehto, MU: Recurrence after patellar dislocation. Redislocation in 37/75 patients followed for 6–24 years. *Acta Orthop Scand*, 68:424, 1997.

41. Cameron, JC, and Saha, S: External tibial torsion: An underrecognized cause of recurrent patellar dislocation. *Clin Orthop*, Jul:177, 1996.

42. Maenpaa, H, and Lehto, MU: Surgery in acute patellar dislocation: Evaluation of the effect of injury mechanism and family occurrence on the outcome of treatment. *Br J Sports Med*, 29:239, 1995.

43. Muhle, C, et al: Effect of a patellar realignment brace on patients with patellar subluxation and dislocation. Evaluation with kinematic magnetic resonance imaging. *Am J Sports Med*, 27:350, 1999.

44. Maenpaa, H, and Lehto, MU: Patellar dislocation. The long-term results of nonoperative management in 100 patients. *Am J Sports Med*, 25:213, 1997.

45. Bellemans, J, et al: Anteromedial tibial tubercle transfer in patients with chronic anterior knee pain and a subluxation-type patellar malalignment. *Am J Sports Med*, 25:375, 1997.

46. Verheyden, F, Geens, G and Nelen, G: Jumper's knee: Results of surgical treatment. *Acta Orthop Belg*, 63:102, 1997.

47. Yu, JS, et al: Correlation of MR imaging and pathologic findings in athletes undergoing surgery for chronic patellar tendinitis. *AJR Am J Roentgenol*, 165:115, 1995.

48. Griffiths, GP and Selesnick, FH: Operative treatment and arthroscopic findings in chronic patellar tendititis. *Arthroscopy*, 14:836, 1998.

49. Popp, JE, Yu, JS and Kaeding, CC: Recalcitrant patellar tendinitis. Magnetic resonance imaging, histologic evaluation, and surgical treatment. *Am J Sports Med*, 25:218, 1997.

50. McLoughlin, RF, et al: Patellar tendinitis: MR imaging features, with suggested pathogenesis and proposed classification. *Radiology*, 197:843, 1995.

51. Grossfeld, SL and Engebresten, L: Patellar tendinitis—A case report of elongation and ossification of the inferior pole of the patella. *Scand J Med Sci Sports*, 5:308, 1995.

52. Podesta, L, Sherman, MF, and Bonamo, JR: Bilateral simultaneous rupture of the infrapatellar tendon in a recreational athlete. A case report. *Am J Sports Med*, 19:325, 1991.

53. Rosenberg, JM, and Whitaker, JH: Bilateral infrapatellar tendon rupture in a patient with jumper's knee. *Am J Sports Med*, 19:94, 1991.

54. Clark, SC, et al: Bilateral patellar tendon rupture secondary to repeated local steroid injection. *J Accid Emerg Med*, 12:300, 1995.

55. Levine, RJ: Patellar tendon rupture. The importance of timely recognition and repair. *Postgrad Med*, 100:241, 1996.

56. Enad, JG: Patellar tendon ruptures. *South Med J*, 92:563, 1999.

57. Yu, WD, and Shapiro, MS: Cysts and other masses about the knee. Identifying and treating common and rare lesions. *Physician and Sportsmedicine*, 27:59, 1999.

58. Hardaker, TW, Whipple, TL, and Bassett, FH: Diagnosis and treatment of the plica syndrome of the knee. *J Bone Joint Surg Am*, 62:221, 1980.

59. Patel, D: Plica as a cause of anterior knee pain. *Orthop Clin North Am*, 17:273, 1986.

60. Amatuzzi, MM, Fazzi, A, and Varella, MH: Pathologic synovial plica of the knee. Results of conservative treatment. *Am J Sports Med*, 18:466, 1990.

61. Gerbino, PG II, and Micheli, LJ: Bucket-handle tear of the medial plica. *Clin J Sport Med*, 6:265, 1996.

62. Kim, SJ, Min, BH and Kim, HK: Arthroscopic anatomy of the infrapatellar plica. *Arthroscopy*, 12:561, 1996.

63. Kurosaka, M, et al: Lateral synovial plica syndrome. A case report. *Am J Sports Med*, 20:92, 1992.

64. Johnson, DP, et al: Symptomatic synovial plicae of the knee. *J Bone Joint Surg Am*, 75:1485, 1993.

65. Noble, BA, Hajek, MR, and Porter, M: Diagnosis and treatment of iliotibial band tightness in runners. *Physician and Sportsmedicine* 10:67, 1982.

66. Kosarek, FJ and Helms, CA: The MR appearance of the infrapatellar plica. *AJR Am J Roentgenol*, 172:481, 1999.

67. Jee, WH, et al: The plica syndrome: Diagnostic value of MRI with arthroscopic correlation. *J Comput Assist Tomogr*, 22:814, 1998.

68. Flowers, MJ, and Bhadreshwar, DR: Tibial tuberosity excision for symptomatic Osgood-Schlatter disease. *J Pediatr Orthop*, 15:292, 1995.

69. Medlar, RC and Lyne, ED: Sinding-Larsen-Johansson disease. *J Bone Joint Surg*, 60A:1113, 1978.

70. Batten, J and Menelaus, MB: Fragmentation of the proximal pole of the patella. *J Bone Joint Surg*, 67B:249, 1985.

71. Ogden, JA: *Sinding-Larsen-Johansson Disease in Skeletal Injury in the Child*. W.B. Saunders Co., Philadelphia, 765–768, 1990.

72. Viola, R, and Vianello, R: Three cases of patella fracture in 1,320 anterior cruciate ligament reconstructions with bone-patellar tendon-bone autograft. *Arthroscopy*, 15:93, 1999.

73. Simonian, PT, Mann, FA, and Mandt, PR: Indirect forces and patellar fracture after anterior cruciate ligament reconstruction with the patellar ligament. Case Report. *Am J Knee Surg*, 8:60, 1995.

74. Exler, Y: Patellar fracture: Review of the literature and five case presentations. *J Orthop Sports Phys Ther*, 13:177, 1991.

8 The Pelvis and Thigh

The pelvic girdle forms the structural base of support between the lower extremity and the trunk. A relatively immobile structure, the pelvis is formed by pairs of three fused bones joined anteriorly by the pubic symphysis. The posterior portion of the pelvis is formed by the sacrum's wedging itself between the two halves of the pelvis. The hip articulation, formed by the femoral head and the acetabulum, is the strongest and most stable of the body's joints. However, this benefit is gained at the expense of range of motion (ROM).

◆ CLINICAL ANATOMY

The anterior and lateral portion of the pelvis is formed by two **innominate bones,** each consisting of the ilium, the ischium, and the pubis (Fig. 8–1). The posterior junction of the pelvic girdle is formed by its articulation with the **sacrum,** a broad, thick bone that fixates the spinal column to the pelvis. The sacrum is responsible for stabilizing the pelvic girdle.

On the lateral aspect of the pelvis, the **acetabulum,** a downwardly and outwardly directed depression, accepts the femoral head within its fossa. The acetabulum's superior wall is formed by the ilium, the inferior wall by the ischium, and the internal (medial) wall by the pubis. A depression for the **ligamentum teres** is centered within the fossa. The **labrum,** a thick ring of fibrocartilage, lines the outer rim of the acetabulum and deepens the articular area. The labrum is thicker and stronger superiorly than inferiorly (Fig. 8–2).

The **femoral head** is globular, with an articular surface that is slightly over a 180 degree arc in diameter. Its articulating surface is thickly covered with hyaline

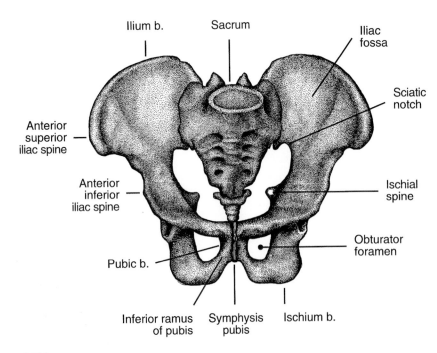

Ilium b. Sacrum Iliac fossa

Anterior superior iliac spine

Sciatic notch

Anterior inferior iliac spine

Ischial spine

Obturator foramen

Pubic b.

Inferior ramus of pubis Symphysis pubis Ischium b.

FIGURE 8–1. Anterior view of the bony pelvis. A total of seven bones form the pelvis: Two ischial, two pubic, and two ilial bones form each half, and the posterior border is formed by the sacrum.

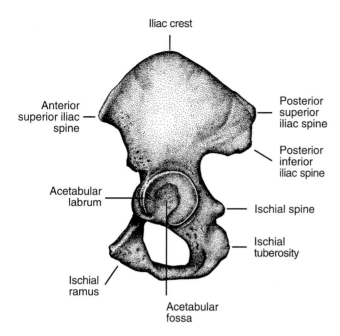

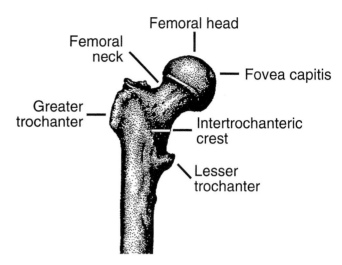

FIGURE 8–3. Femoral neck and head.

FIGURE 8–2. Lateral view of the pelvis showing the acetablum. The acetabular fossa is bordered by the fibrocartilaginous glenoid labrum.

cartilage except for a central depression that accepts the ligamentum teres. Connected to the femur's shaft by the **femoral neck,** the head is angled at approximately 125 degrees in the frontal plane (Fig. 8–3). This relationship, known as the **angle of inclination,** changes as an individual grows and develops. The angle of inclination is slightly decreased in women (Fig. 8–4). In the transverse plane, the relationship between the femoral head and femoral shaft is the **angle of torsion,** normally an angle of 15 degrees (Fig. 8–5).

On the proximal portion of the femoral shaft, the **greater trochanter** projects laterally and the **lesser trochanter** projects medially. The trochanters are the attachment sites for many of the pelvic and hip muscles.

ARTICULATIONS AND LIGAMENTOUS SUPPORT

The pelvic bones articulate anteriorly at a relatively immobile joint, the **pubic symphysis** (see Fig. 8–1). Formed by the fibrocartilaginous interpubic disk, a small degree of spreading (distraction), compression, and rotation between the two halves of the pelvic girdle occurs here.

Posteriorly, each ilium articulates with the sacrum at the **sacroiliac (SI) joints.** A combination of synovial and syndesmotic joints, these joints vary considerably in their shapes and sizes. The surfaces of each bone are a collection of concave and convex areas with the concavities of one bone corresponding to convexities of the opposing bone. The resulting articulation is very sturdy with a limited ROM.

The hip articulation, the **coxofemoral joint,** is a ball-and-socket joint possessing three degrees of freedom of movement: flexion and extension; abduction

FIGURE 8–4. Deviations of the hip in the frontal plane. The femoral head normally assumes a 125° angle with the long axis of the femur (**A**). An increase in this angle is termed coxa valga (**B**); a decrease, coxa vara (**C**).

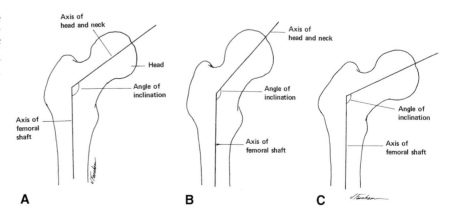

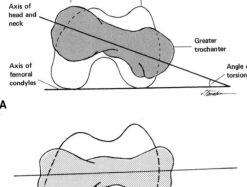

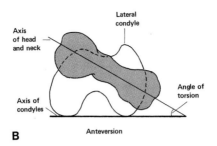

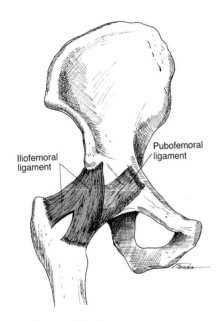

FIGURE 8–5. Deviations of the hip in the transverse plane. **(A)** Normal hip angulation, approximately 15°; **(B)** an increased angle, anteversion; **(C)** A decreased angle between the femoral condyles and femoral head is termed retroversion

FIGURE 8–6. External hip ligaments.

and adduction; and internal and external rotation. The depth of the acetabulum, the relative strength of the ligaments, and the strong muscular support limit the hip's ROM in all planes.

Surrounding the joint, a strong, dense synovial capsule arises from the acetabular rim and runs to the distal aspect of the femoral neck. Accessory bands, or ligaments, associated with the capsule assist in reinforcing the joint (Fig. 8–6).

The Y-shaped **iliofemoral ligament** (also referred to as the "Y ligament of Bigelow") originates from the anterior inferior iliac spine. Its central fibers split, with one band inserting on the distal aspect of the anterior intertrochanteric line and the other band inserting on the proximal aspect of the anterior intertrochanteric line and the femoral neck. This strong structure reinforces the anterior portion of the joint capsule, thus limiting hyperextension. Its superior fibers limit adduction and its inferior fibers limit abduction. The fibrous arrangement of the iliofemoral ligament allows us to stand upright with a minimal amount of muscular activity.

Also reinforcing the anterior capsule is the **pubofemoral ligament.** Emerging from the pubic *ramus* and inserting on the anterior aspect of the intertrochanteric fossa, this ligament limits abduction and hyperextension of the hip.

Posteriorly the joint is augmented by the **ischiofemoral ligament.** This triangular ligament has an origin spanning from the posterior acetabular rim with upwardly spiraling fibers attaching to the joint capsule and the inner surface of the greater trochanter. The spiraling nature of this ligament results in it limiting hip extension.

Within the joint, the **ligamentum teres** (also referred to as the "ligament of the head of the femur") serves as a conduit for the medial and lateral circumflex arteries. It has little function in stabilizing the hip (Fig. 8–7).[1] However, trauma to this structure through axial compression of the femoral head or dislocation of the joint may result in disruption of these arteries.

The **inguinal ligament** originates off the anterior superior iliac spine (ASIS) and inserts at the pubic symphysis. This ligament serves to contain the soft tissues as they course anteriorly from the trunk to the lower extremity. This structure demarcates the superior border of the femoral triangle.

Ramus   A division of a forked structure.

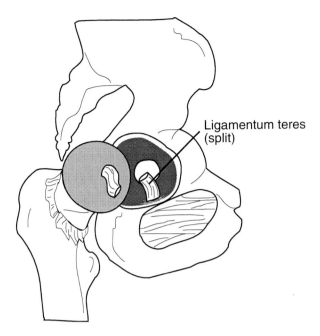

FIGURE 8–7. Ligamentum teres (shown split). This structure serves little, if any, role in supporting the hip. It serves primarily as a conduit for the passage of the medial and lateral circumflex arteries.

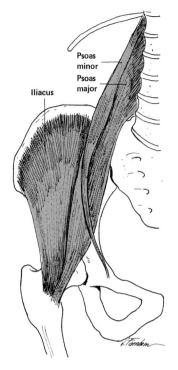

FIGURE 8–8. Iliopsoas group formed by the iliacus, psoas major, and psoas minor muscles.

MUSCULAR ANATOMY

Movements of the hip joint are controlled by groups of large extrinsic and small intrinsic muscles. The large muscle groups act primarily to flex, extend, and internally rotate the hip. The smaller intrinsic hip muscles serve to externally rotate it. During activities such as running and cutting, the hip abductors and adductors act to stabilize the hip rather than generate mechanical power.[2] The muscles acting on the hip, along with their origins, insertions, and innervations, are presented in Table 8–1.

Anterior Musculature

Crossing the anterior portion of both the knee joint and the hip, the **rectus femoris**, part of the **quadriceps femoris group,** is a powerful flexor of the hip, providing the greatest contribution to hip flexion when the knee is also flexed. The **sartorius,** in addition to flexing the knee, contributes to flexion, abduction, and external rotation of the hip. The psoas major, psoas minor, and iliacus, collectively known as the **iliopsoas group,** are the primary hip flexors when the knee is extended, working in concert with the rectus femoris when the knee is flexed (Fig. 8–8).

The rectus femoris, sartorius, and iliacus all anteriorly rotate the pelvis on the sacrum as they contract. Tightness in these muscles can cause increased stress on the sacroiliac joint, also causing the pelvis to rotate anteriorly on the sacrum.

Medial Musculature

The medial muscles acting on the hip joint adduct and internally rotate the femur. The bulk of the inner thigh is formed by the **adductor group,** consisting of the adductor longus, adductor magnus, and adductor brevis. This muscle group's action is supplemented by the pectineus (Fig. 8–9). One additional adductor, the **gracilis,** is described in Chapter 6.

Lateral Musculature

The most superficial of the lateral muscles are the **gluteus medius** and the **tensor fasciae latae** (Fig. 8–10). A prime abductor of the hip joint, the gluteus medius is also important in maintaining the horizontal position of the pelvis and the torso's upright posture during gait. For example, weakness of the right gluteus medius causes the pelvis to lower on the left side when the left leg is not bearing weight. The torso compensates for the unequal position of the pelvis by leaning to the right. This compensating movement is termed **Trendelenburg's gait pattern.** Through its insertion on the iliotibial (IT) tract, the tensor fasciae latae is an abductor and internal rotator of the hip.

Table 8–1
MUSCLES ACTING ON THE HIP

Muscle	Action	Origin	Insertion	Innervation	Root
Adductor brevis	Hip adduction Hip internal rotation	• Pubic ramus	• Pectineal line • Medial lip of linea aspera	Obturator	L2, L3, L4
Adductor longus	Hip adduction Hip internal rotation	• Pubic symphysis	• Middle one third of medial linea aspera	Obturator	L2, L3, L4
Adductor magnus	Hip adduction Hip internal rotation	• Inferior pubic ramus • Ramus of ischium • Ischial tuberosity	• Line spanning from the gluteal tuberosity to the adductor tubercle of the medial femoral condyle	Obturator Sciatic	L2, L3, L4 L4, L5, S1
Biceps femoris	Hip extension Hip external rotation Knee flexion External rotation of the tibia	Long head • Ischial tuberosity • Sacrotuberous ligament Short head • Lateral lip of the linea aspera • Upper two thirds of the supracondylar line	• Lateral fibular head • Lateral tibial condyle	Long head Tibial Short head Common peroneal	Long head S1, S2, S3 Short head L4, L5, S1
Gemellus inferior	Hip external rotation	• Tuberosity of ischium	• Greater trochanter of femur via the obturator internus tendon	Sacral plexus	L4, L5, S1
Gemellus superior	Hip external rotation	• Spine of ischium	• Greater trochanter of femur via the obturator internus tendon	Sacral plexus	L4, L5, S1
Gluteus maximus	Hip extension Hip external rotation Hip adduction (lower fibers) Hip adduction (upper fibers)	• Posterior gluteal line of ilium • Posterior sacrum • Posterior coccyx	• Gluteal tuberosity of femur • Through a fibrous band to the iliotibial tract	Inferior gluteal	L5, S1, S2
Gluteus medius	Hip abduction Anterior fibers Hip flexion Hip internal rotation Posterior fibers Hip extension Hip external rotation	• External surface of superior ilium • Anterior gluteal line • Gluteal aponeurosis	• Greater trochanter of femur	Superior gluteal	L4, L5, S1

Muscle	Action	Origin	Insertion	Innervation	Nerve Roots
Gluteus minimus	Hip abduction Hip internal rotation Hip flexion	• Lower portion of ilium • Margin of greater sciatic notch	• Greater trochanter of femur	Superior gluteal	L4, L5, S1
Gracilis	Hip adduction Knee flexion	• Symphysis pubis • Inferior pubic ramus	• Medial tibial flare	Obturator	L3, L4
Iliacus	Hip flexion	• Superior surface of the iliac fossa • Internal iliac crest • Sacral ala	• Lateral to the psoas major, distal to the lesser trochanter	Lumbar plexus	L1, L2, L3, L4
Obturator externus	Hip external rotation	• Pubic ramus	• Trochanteric fossa of femur	Obturator	L3, L4
Obturator internus	Hip external rotation	• Obturator membrane • Margin of obturator foramen • Pelvic surface of ischium	• Greater trochanter of femur	Sacral plexus	L5, S1, S2
Pectineus	Hip adduction	• Superior symphysis pubis	• Pectineal line of femur	Obturator	L3, L4
Piriformis	Hip external rotation	• Pelvic surface of sacrum • Rim of greater sciatic foramen	• Greater trochanter of femur	Sacral plexus	S1, S2
Psoas major and minor	Hip flexion	• Transverse process of T12 and all lumbar vertebrae	• Lesser trochanter of femur	Lumbar plexus	L1, L2, L3, L4
Quadratus femoris	Hip external rotation	• Tuberosity of ischium	• Intertrochanteric crest of femur	Sacral plexus	L4, L5, S1
Rectus femoris	Hip flexion Knee extension	• Anterior inferior iliac spine • Groove located superior to the acetabulum	• To the tibial tuberosity via the patella and patellar ligament	Femoral	L2, L3, L4
Sartorius	Hip flexion Hip abduction Hip external rotation Knee flexion Internal tibial rotation	• Anterior superior iliac spine	• Proximal portion of the anteromedial tibial flare	Femoral	L2, L3
Semimembranosus	Hip extension Hip internal rotation Knee flexion Internal tibial rotation	• Ischial tuberosity	• Posteromedial portion of the medial condyle of the tibia	Tibial	L5, S1
Semitendinosus	Hip extension Hip internal rotation Knee flexion Internal tibial rotation	• Ischial tuberosity	• Medial portion of the tibial flare	Tibial	L5, S1, S2
Tensor fasciae latae	Hip flexion Hip internal rotation Hip abduction	• Anterior superior iliac spine • External lip of the iliac crest	• Iliotibial tract	Superior gluteal	L4, L5, S1

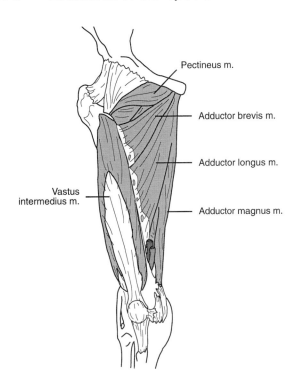

FIGURE 8–9. Adductors of the hip. The only muscle of this group that is uniquely identifiable is the adductor longus, which becomes visible during resisted adduction.

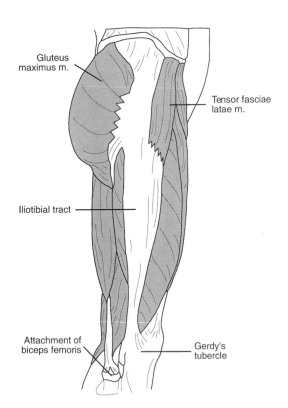

FIGURE 8–10. Superficial lateral and posterior hip muscles. The tensor fasciae latae muscle attaches to Gerdy's tubercle via the iliotibial tract. The remaining lateral muscles, the gluteus medius and gluteus minimus, lie hidden beneath the gluteus maximus, tensor fasciae latae, and iliotibial tract.

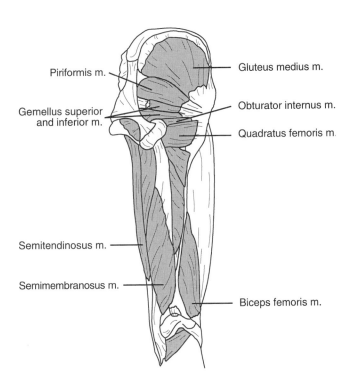

FIGURE 8–11. Intrinsic hip muscles. The intrinsic muscles serve primarily to externally rotate the hip

Six intrinsic muscles form a posterolateral cuff around the femoral head (Fig. 8–11). The **piriformis, quadratus femoris, obturator internus, obturator externus, gemellus superior,** and **gemellus inferior** all primarily function to externally rotate the hip.

Posterior Musculature

The mass of the buttocks is formed by the **gluteus maximus,** a powerful extensor of the hip, especially when the knee is flexed (see Fig. 8–10). When the knee is extended, the **hamstring muscle group** also acts as a hip extensor. In addition, the hamstring group is responsible for decelerating knee extension and hip flexion during running through an eccentric contraction. The hamstrings can also cause posterior rotation of the pelvis on the sacrum from their attachment on the ischial tuberosity.

FEMORAL TRIANGLE

Formed by the inguinal ligament superiorly, the sartorius laterally, and the adductor longus medially, the femoral triangle represents a clinically significant landmark (Fig. 8–12). Portions of the **femoral nerve, femoral artery,** and **femoral vein** are located within this area. The femoral pulse is palpable as it crosses the crease between the thigh and abdomen. Likewise, the triangle contains lymph nodes that may become enlarged with an infection or active inflammation in the lower extremity.

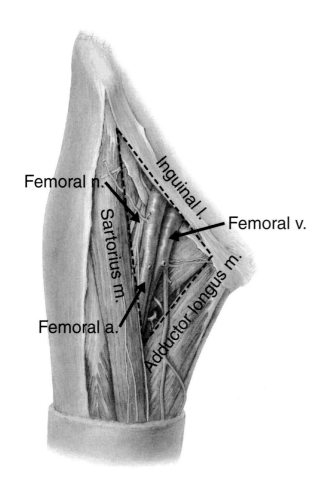

FIGURE 8–12. Femoral triangle. This anatomical area is formed by the sartorius muscle laterally, the adductor longus medially, and the inguinal ligament superiorly. The femoral neurovascular bundle passes through this area.

BURSAE

Three primary bursae are found in the hip and pelvic region, each serving to decrease friction between the gluteus maximus and its adjacent bony structures. The **trochanteric bursa** lubricates the site at which the gluteus maximus passes over the greater trochanter. The **gluteofemoral bursa** separates the gluteus maximus from the origin of the vastus lateralis. The **ischial bursa** serves as a weight-bearing structure when an individual is seated, cushioning the ischial tuberosity where it passes under the gluteus maximus.

 ## CLINICAL EVALUATION OF PELVIS AND THIGH

Serving as the anatomical and mechanical interface between the lower extremity and spinal column, the pelvis influences and is influenced by these areas. A complete evaluation of the pelvis and thigh may also include a thorough evaluation of the lower extremity, spinal column, and posture.

To permit the complete examination of these areas, the patient typically is dressed in shorts and a t-shirt. Use discretion when evaluating areas around the genitalia. Attempt to recruit a clinician of the same gender as the patient to perform the evaluation. The evaluation should always be done in the presence of a witness.

HISTORY

The majority of pelvic girdle and hip injuries in active individuals tend to be of a chronic or overuse origin, increasing the importance of a complete and accurate history of the injury.

- **Location of symptoms:** Deep hip joint pain can originate in the coxofemoral joint itself or be referred from the lumbar spine, sacroiliac joint, or both. A strain to the hip adductors or hip flexors causes pain in the pubic region or anterior hip, respectively. Greater trochanteric bursitis is a common hip pathology that usually results in pain in the posterior aspect of the greater trochanter (Table 8–2).
- **Onset:** Most pelvic girdle and hip pathology tends to be chronic or caused by overuse. The date of onset of the patient's symptoms must be correlated to any changes in training techniques such as surface changes, footwear, or alterations in training techniques or intensity.
- **Training techniques:** Recent changes in training techniques can lead to overuse injuries, including greater trochanteric bursitis or hip flexor tendinitis, especially if the history of the patient's running regimen includes training on a banked surface or the addition of hills. Development of stress fractures may be related to recent increases in training intensity, frequency, or duration.
- **Mechanism of injury:** A direct blow to the iliac crest may lead to a contusion (**hip pointer).** Blows to the buttocks, such as from a fall, can lead to a contusion of the coccyx or ischium or to sacroiliac pathology. A sudden pain, especially during an eccentric contraction of a muscle, usually indicates a strain of that muscle. Pain that gradually builds over time may indicate a stress fracture or tendinitis.
- **Prior medical conditions:** Congenital or childhood abnormalities of the hip can result in altered biomechanics of the hip, knee, or ankle during adulthood. *Legg-Calvé-Perthes disease* can lead to residual flattening of the proximal femoral epiphysis, resulting in decreased hip internal rotation and abduction.[3] A

Legg-Calvé-Perthes disease Avascular necrosis occurring in children age 3 to 12 years, causing osteochondritis of the proximal femoral epiphysis and potentially decreasing the range of hip motion in adult life.

EVALUATION MAP: PELVIS AND THIGH

1. HISTORY

Location of symptoms
Onset
Training techniques
Mechanism of injury

2. INSPECTION

Hip angulations
Angle of inclination
Angle of torsion

Medial structures
Adductor group

Anterior structures
Hip flexors

lateral structures
Iliac crest
Nélaton's line

Posterior structures
Gluteus maximus
Posterior superior iliac spine
Median sacral crests

Leg length discrepancy
Functional leg length discrepancy
True leg length discrepancy
Apparent leg length discrepancy

3. PALPATION

Medial structures
Pubic bone
Adductor muscle group

Anterior structures
Anterior superior iliac spine
Anterior inferior iliac spine
Sartorius
Rectus femoris

Lateral structures
Iliac crest
Greater trochanter
Gluteus medius
Tensor fasciae latae

Posterior structures
Median sacral crests
Posterior superior iliac spine
Ischial tuberosity
Gluteus maximus
Hamstring muscles
Ischial bursa
Sciatic nerve

4. RANGE OF MOTION TESTS

AROM
Flexion
Extension
Adduction
Abduction
Internal rotation
External rotation

PROM
Flexion
Extension
Adduction
Abduction
Internal rotation
External rotation

RROM
Flexion
Iliopsoas
Rectus femoris
Sartorius
Extension
Hamstrings
Gluteus maximus
Adduction
Abduction
Internal and external rotation
Thomas test for tightness of the hip flexors
Trendelenburg's test

5. LIGAMENTOUS TESTS

Capsular testing
Flexion
Extension
Internal rotation
External rotation

6. NEUROLOGICAL TESTS

Sciatic nerve compression
Lower quarter screen

7. SPECIAL TESTS

Muscle weakness or tightness
Trendelenburg test
Thomas Test
Degenerative hip changes
Hip scouring
Piriformis syndrome

---

slipped capital femoral epiphysis can lead to excessive external rotation of the hip and restricted or painful internal rotation.[4]

The history-taking process may be expanded based on the patient's responses in the preceding categories.

INSPECTION

Inspection of most acute injuries is difficult because of the bony, muscular, and ligamentous arrangement of the hip and pelvis. With the exception of contusions to the iliac crest and hip dislocations, most trauma to this area cannot be visualized. Therefore, the focus of the inspection phase is to identify secondary signs of pathology or determine the presence of conditions that may alter the biomechanics of the hip and lower extremity, predisposing the patient to injury.

Slipped capital femoral epiphysis Displacement of the femoral head relative to the femoral shaft; common in children age 10 to 15 years and especially prevalent in boys.

Table 8–2
POSSIBLE TRAUMA BASED ON THE LOCATION OF PAIN*

	Location of Pain			
	Medial	**Anterior**	**Lateral**	**Posterior**
Soft tissue	Adductor strain Gracilis strain	Rectus femoris strain Iliopsoas strain Sartorius strain Symphysis pubis sprain Rectus femoris or iliopsoas tendinitis Iliofemoral bursitis Lymphatic edema	Trochanteric bursitis Gluteus medius strain Gluteus minimus strain	Ischial bursitis Hamstring strain Gluteus maximus strain
Bony	Adductor avulsion fracture Stress fracture	Pubic bone fracture Arthritis	Iliac crest contusion Hip joint dysfunction	Sacroiliac pathology

*excluding gross injury.

Inspection of Hip Angulations

- **Angle of inclination:** The angular relationship of the femoral head and the femoral shaft may be roughly determined by observing the relationship between the femur and tibia (see Fig. 6–16). Abnormalities at the epiphysis, trochanteric, or subtrochanteric regions can result in significant deviations in the angle of inclination, especially when the deformity develops during childhood.[5,6] An increase in the angle of inclination, **coxa valga,** may be manifested through either genu varum or a laterally positioned patellae. Decreases in this angle, **coxa vara,** may lead to genu valgum or a medially positioned "squinting" patellae (see Box 7–2). In each case, the mechanical advantage of the gluteus medius is reduced by altering its line of pull on the femur. Radiographic examination is necessary to definitively determine the angle of inclination.

- **Angle of torsion:** Similar to the angle of inclination, the angle of torsion must be definitively measured through the use of radiographs. However, the accuracy of this method is subject to question.[7,8] Box 8–1 presents a method for clinically estimating the angle of torsion.

  ○ **Anteverted hips:** Increases greater than 15 degrees in the angle of torsion, **anteversion,** result in internal femoral rotation, squinting patellae, and a toe-in (pigeon-toed) gait. In patients with anteverted hips, an increase in internal femoral rotation and a decrease in external rotation occurs.

  ○ **Retroverted hips:** When the angle of torsion is less than 15 degrees, **retroversion,** the femur externally rotates, resulting in a toe-out (duck-footed) position of the feet. The patella is laterally positioned with a decrease in hip internal rotation and an increase in external rotation. The amount of retroversion demonstrated in early adolescence tends to diminish with age.[9]

Inspection of the Medial Structures

- **Adductor group:** Observe the area overlying the adductor muscle group for signs of swelling or ecchymosis, indicating a strain of these structures or a contusion to the area.

Inspection of the Anterior Structures

- **Hip flexors:** Observe the area of the hip flexors distal to the ASIS for swelling or ecchymosis, indicating a strain of these structures.

Inspection of the Lateral Structures

- **Iliac crest:** Inspect the iliac crest, located immediately beneath the skin. This area is vulnerable to contusions that initiate a very active inflammatory process. These contusions, or **hip pointers,** result in pain, disability, and discoloration (Fig. 8–13).

- **Nélaton's line:** Draw an imaginary line from the ASIS to the ischial tuberosity. Nélaton's line is a quick screen to help determine the presence of coxa vara (Fig. 8–14).[10] Location of the greater tuberosity well superior to this line indicates coxa vara. As with all tests, the results should be compared with those of the uninvolved side.

Inspection of Posterior Structures

- **Posterior superior iliac spine:** If visible, compare the skin indentations bilaterally for symmetry. This should include height of the posterior superior iliac spine (PSIS) from the floor and identification of localized swelling.

Box 8–1
CLINICAL DETERMINATION OF THE ANGLE OF TORSION

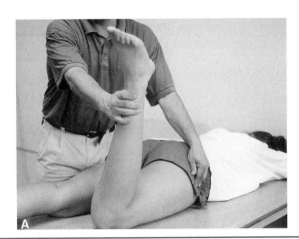

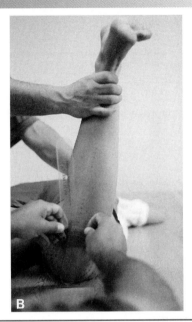

This procedure is most easily performed by two clinicians, one to manipulate the leg and the other to goniometrically measure the angle of the lower leg perpendicular to the table.

PATIENT POSITION	Prone with the knee of the leg being evaluated flexed to 90°
POSITION OF EXAMINER	The use of two examiners is recommended. Examiner 1: On the contralateral side to that being tested; one hand palpates the greater trochanter and the other hand manipulates the lower extremity. Examiner 2: Holding a goniometer distal to the flexed knee with the stationary arm perpendicular to the tabletop.
EVALUATIVE PROCEDURE	**(A)** Examiner 1 internally rotates the femur by moving the lower leg inward and outward until the greater trochanter is maximally prominent. This represents the point at which the femoral head is parallel with the tabletop. **(B)** Examiner 2 then measures the angle formed by the lower leg while the knee remains flexed to 90°.
POSITIVE TEST	Angles less than 15° represent femoral retroversion; angles greater than 15° represent anteversion.
IMPLICATIONS	As described in Positive Test above.

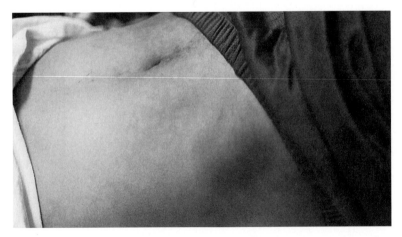

FIGURE 8–13. Contusion to the iliac crest. This injury, the so-called "hip pointer," results in gross discoloration, swelling, pain, and loss of function.

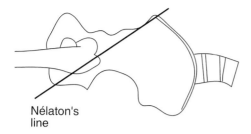

FIGURE 8–14. Nélaton's line. This clinical sign is used to determine the presence of coxa vara. An imaginary line is drawn from the anterior superior iliac spine to the ischial tuberosity. If the greater tuberosity is located superior to this line, coxa vara should be suspected.

- **Gluteus maximus:** Inspect the gluteals for bilateral symmetry. Atrophy of the muscle group could indicate an L5-S1 nerve root pathology.
- **Hamstring muscle group:** Inspect the length of the hamstring muscles, noting for deformity or discoloration that indicates a muscular tear (Fig. 8–15).
- **Median sacral crests:** Observe the sacral area. Although injury to this area is rare, **pilonidal cysts,** an infection over the posterior aspect of the *median* sacral crests, cause severe pain and disability. As the cyst matures, it protrudes from the gluteal crease and appears violently red. Patients suspected as suffering

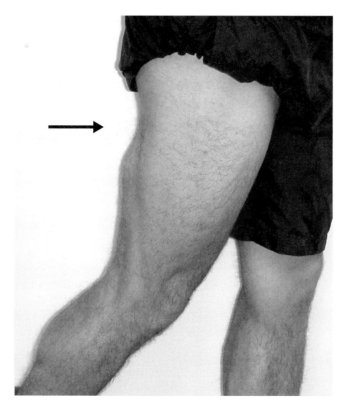

FIGURE 8–15. A tear of the biceps femoris muscle. Note the indentation on the proximal portion of the posterolateral thigh.

from a pilonidal cyst require an immediate referral to a physician.

Inspection of Leg Length Discrepancy

Pain emanating from the foot, lower leg, knee, hip, and spine or deficits in gait may be related to leg lengths of greater than 2 cm.[11] Refer to Chapter 3 for information on the various means of determining leg length differences.

PALPATION

The hip and thigh are characterized by areas of subcutaneous bone and other areas of large muscle mass. When performing palpation, use discretion, maintaining the patient's modesty and privacy at all times.

Palpation of the Medial Structures

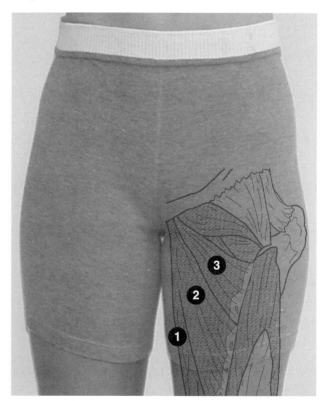

1. **Adductor longus:** Abduct the hip to place the adductor muscles on stretch, making the adductor longus muscle visibly prominent at the point that it arises from the symphysis pubis. Using discretion, palpate close to the origin of the adductor group for any tenderness or defect indicating an avulsion fracture.

Median Along the body's midline.

2. **Adductor magnus:** Locate the adductor magnus superior and lateral to the adductor longus. This muscle makes up the bulk of the inner thigh.

3. **Adductor brevis:** Locate the bulk of the adductor brevis under the quadriceps muscle. Continue to palpate superiorly to locate the **pectineus.**

Palpation of the Anterior Structures

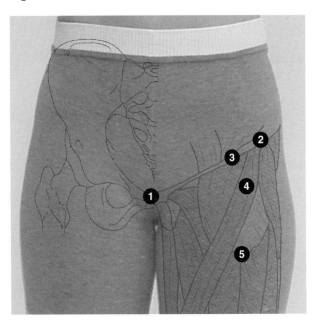

1. **Pubic bone:** Use discretion palpating this area. Follow the femoral creases downward toward the pubic bone, located under the pubic fat pad (mons pubis) superior to the genitalia. These bones, as well as the symphysis pubis, may be injured secondary to a blunt force such as when a gymnast strikes his or her pubic bone against the horse, balance beam, or bars. The pubic symphysis can become inflamed secondary to overuse injuries and sheer forces, leading to **osteitis pubis.**

2. **Anterior superior iliac spine:** Follow the iliac crest anteriorly to locate the ASIS. This structure is easily palpable in thin patients but may become obscured in muscular or obese individuals. With the patient standing, palpate the ASISs bilaterally. These structures should be of equal height; any difference indicates a functional or true leg length discrepancy.

3. **Anterior inferior iliac spine:** From the ASIS, continue to palpate downward to locate the anterior inferior iliac spine (AIIS). This structure is not always identifiable.

4. **Sartorius:** Palpate the sartorius from its insertion on the ASIS to where it crosses the femoral crease. In some patients, the sartorius may be palpable along its entire length.

5. **Rectus femoris:** Keep in mind that both heads of the rectus femoris lie under the sartorius and therefore are not palpable. However, when the knee is flexed and the hip forced into extension, the resulting tension may cause a strain of the rectus femoris or an avulsion

of its origin. The length of the muscle belly becomes palpable just distal and lateral to the sartorius and should be palpated to its insertion on the patella.

Palpation of the Lateral Structures

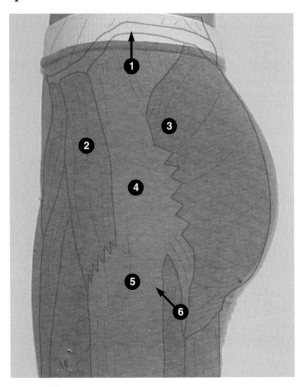

1. **Iliac crest:** Find the iliac crest, usually easily located on most patients, and palpate along its length from the ASIS to the PSIS. After a contusion, the iliac crest becomes swollen and tender to the touch. Crepitus also may be present.

2. **Tensor fasciae latae:** Locate this area below the anterior third of the iliac crest. The tensor fasciae latae is not easily distinguished from the gluteus medius.

3. **Gluteus medius:** To isolate the gluteus medius, position the patient in a sidelying position with the upper hip actively abducted 10° to 15°. The length of the muscle is palpable from its origin just inferior to the iliac crest to its insertion on the superior portion of the greater trochanter (Fig. 8–16). The inability to maintain this position during the examination may indicate gluteus medius weakness, which is then confirmed through the **Trendelenburg's test.**

4. **IT band:** Palpate the length of the IT band from its origin from the tensor fasciae latae to its insertion on Gerdy's tubercle. The IT band is a common site of trigger points and may become adhered to the underlying tissues.

5. **Greater trochanter:** Locate the greater trochanter at approximately the midline on the lateral thigh 6 to 8 inches below the iliac crest. The greater trochanter becomes more identifiable as the femur is internally and externally rotated and its posterior aspect becomes exposed. This area becomes tender secondary to tendinitis of the gluteus medius or IT band tightness.

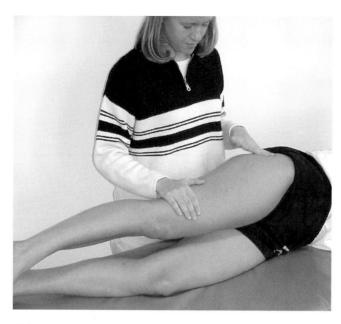

FIGURE 8–16. Positioning of the patient to isolate the gluteus medius during palpation. Slightly abducting the hip makes the gluteus medius palpable.

6. **Trochanteric bursa:** Overlying the posterior aspect of the greater trochanter, the trochanteric bursa is not directly palpable. Inflammation of this bursa causes it to feel thick and elicits pain at the posterior aspect of the greater trochanter.

Palpation of the Posterior Structures

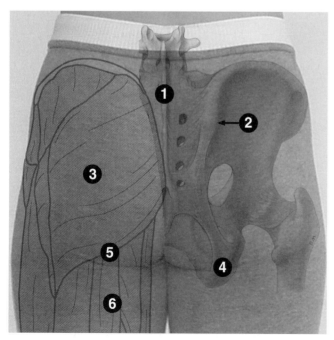

1. **Median sacral crests:** Palpate the fused remnants of the sacral spinous processes from below the L5 vertebra to the midportion of the gluteal crease.

2. **Posterior superior iliac spine:** Locate the PSIS at the inferior portion of the gluteal dimples. Under normal circumstances, these bony landmarks are palpable and align at the same level. Tenderness may indicate sacroiliac pathology.

3. **Gluteus maximus:** Palpate the bulk of the gluteus maximus. This structure is easily palpable and may be made more identifiable by having the patient squeeze the buttocks together or extend the hip.

4. **Ischial tuberosity and bursa:** Position the patient in the sidelying position with the non–weight-bearing hip flexed. The ischial tuberosity can be identified by locating the gluteal fold and palpating deeply at approximately the midline of the gluteal fold. Tenderness at this site may indicate an avulsion fracture or hamstring tendinitis. Similar to the trochanteric bursa, the ischial bursa cannot be identified unless it is inflamed, at which time it is tender to the touch.

5. **Sciatic nerve:** Although the sciatic nerve is not directly palpable, attempt to palpate its approximate course for tenderness. Begin palpation of this structure by locating the ischial tuberosity and the greater trochanter. The sciatic nerve is found as a cord midway between these two structures. An irritated sciatic nerve is exquisitely tender when compared with the contralateral side.

6. **Hamstring muscles:** Locate the common origin of the hamstring group on the ischial tuberosity. Palpate the semitendinosus and semimembranosus down the medial side of the posterior femur. Also palpate the biceps femoris down the lateral border, noting any tenderness, spasm, defects, or pain.

RANGE OF MOTION TESTING

The ROM available to the hip joint is limited by its bony and soft tissue restraints. The position of the knee also can further limit the hip's ROM. A fully flexed knee can limit the amount of extension at the hip because the rectus femoris is stretched to its limits. An extended knee with stretched hamstrings can limit the amount of hip flexion available. The muscles acting on the hip in each of its motions are presented in Table 8–3. Goniometric evaluation of hip ROM is presented in Box 8–2.

There is no true active range of motion (AROM) at the sacroiliac joints. Any motion is accessory in nature and is minimal in the absence of pathology.

Active Range of Motion

- **Flexion and extension:** The arc of motion available to the hip with the knee flexed ranges from 130 to 150 degrees. The majority of this motion (120 degrees to 130 degrees) occurs during flexion (Fig. 8–17). Extending the knee limits the amount of flexion available to the hip by placing the hamstring muscle group on stretch.
- **Adduction and abduction:** AROM for abduction of the hip is approximately 45 degrees from the neutral position and for adduction, 20 to 30 degrees after the opposite limb is cleared from the movement (Fig. 8–18).

Table 8–3
MUSCLES ACTING ON THE HIP ACCORDING TO MOTION

Flexion	Abduction	Internal Rotation
Gluteus medius (anterior fibers)	Gluteus maximus (lower fibers)	Adductor brevis
Gluteus minimus	Gluteus medius	Adductor longus
Iliacus	Gluteus minimus	Adductor magnus
Psoas major	Sartorius	Gluteus medius (anterior fibers)
Psoas minor		Gluteus minimus
Rectus femoris		
Sartorius		

Extension	Adduction	External Rotation
Biceps femoris	Adductor brevis	Biceps femoris
Gluteus maximus	Adductor longus	Gemellus inferior
Gluteus medius (posterior fibers)	Adductor magnus	Gemellus superior
Semimembranosus	Gluteus maximus (upper fibers)	Gluteus maximus
Semitendinosus	Gracilis	Gluteus medius (posterior fibers)
	Pectineus	Obturator extremus
		Obturator internus
		Piriformis
		Quadratus femoris
		Sartorius

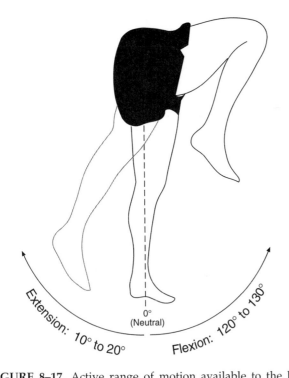

FIGURE 8–17. Active range of motion available to the hip during flexion and extension. The range for hip flexion is decreased when the knee is extended secondary to tightness of the hamstring muscles and is limited during extension when the knee is flexed because of tightness of the rectus femoris.

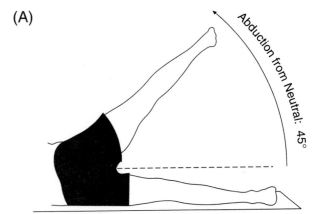
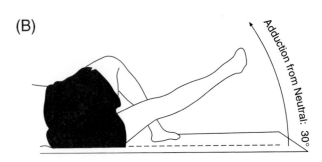

FIGURE 8–18. Active hip abduction **(A)** and adduction **(B)**.

Box 8–2
GONIOMETRY: Hip

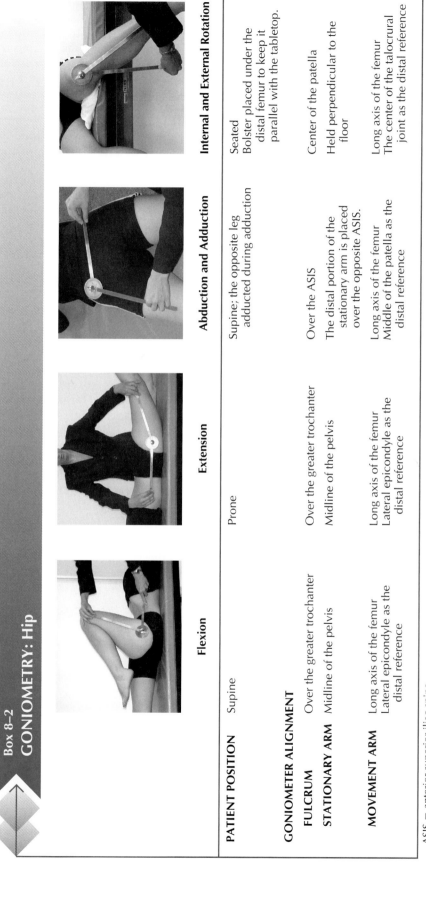

	Flexion	Extension	Abduction and Adduction	Internal and External Rotation
PATIENT POSITION	Supine	Prone	Supine; the opposite leg adducted during adduction	Seated Bolster placed under the distal femur to keep it parallel with the tabletop.
GONIOMETER ALIGNMENT				
FULCRUM	Over the greater trochanter	Over the greater trochanter	Over the ASIS	Center of the patella
STATIONARY ARM	Midline of the pelvis	Midline of the pelvis	The distal portion of the stationary arm is placed over the opposite ASIS.	Held perpendicular to the floor
MOVEMENT ARM	Long axis of the femur Lateral epicondyle as the distal reference	Long axis of the femur Lateral epicondyle as the distal reference	Long axis of the femur Middle of the patella as the distal reference	Long axis of the femur The center of the talocrural joint as the distal reference

ASIS = anterior superior iliac spine.

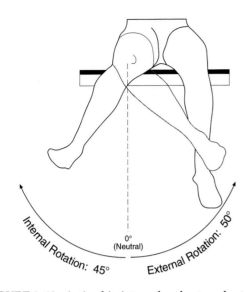

FIGURE 8–19. Active hip internal and external rotation. Note that, in the seated position, the lower leg moves in a direction opposite that of the femur (e.g., during internal femoral rotation the lower leg rotates outwardly).

- **Internal and external rotation:** With the hip in the flexed position, such as when a patient is sitting with legs bent at the end of a table, external rotation ranges from 40 to 50 degrees from the neutral position. Internal rotation is slightly less, approximately 45 degrees from the neutral position (Fig. 8–19). Extending the hip reduces the ROM available in each direction.

Passive Range of Motion

- **Flexion and extension:** To measure passive flexion of the hip, the patient is in the supine position. The pelvis is stabilized by either grasping the iliac crest or placing the hand under the lumbar spine to eliminate compensation by pelvic rotation. As the hip is flexed, the knee is allowed to flex from tension placed on the hamstring muscles and gravity. With pressure applied proximal to the knee joint (i.e., without forcing knee extension), the normal end-feel for hip flexion is soft owing to the approximation of the quadriceps group with the abdomen. When the knee is forced to remain in extension during hip flexion, the end-feel is firm because of the stretching of the hamstring muscle groups (Fig. 8–20).

Tightness of the hip flexors can result in an increased lordotic curvature of the lumbar spine. The **Thomas test** is used to differentiate between tightness of the iliopsoas muscle group and tightness of the rectus femoris muscle (Box 8–3). The testing procedures for isolating the sartorius are described in Box 6–3.

During passive hip extension ROM measurements, the patient is prone and the knee is kept extended. The pelvis is stabilized to prevent it from being lifted off the table. The normal end-feel for hip extension is firm because of the stretching of the anterior joint capsule and the iliofemoral, ischiofemoral, and pubofemoral ligaments. If extension is measured with the knee flexed, a firm end-feel is obtained from tension within the rectus femoris muscle (Fig. 8–21).

- **Adduction and abduction:** The patient is in the supine position with the knee extended for the measurement of both passive adduction and abduction. The leg opposite that being tested is abducted to permit unrestricted adduction of the extremity being tested. To isolate the hip joint, the pelvis is stabilized

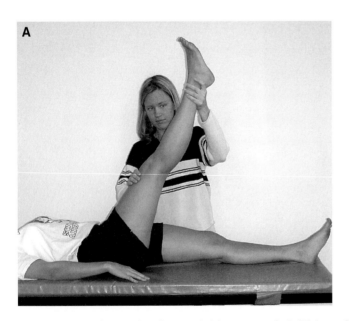
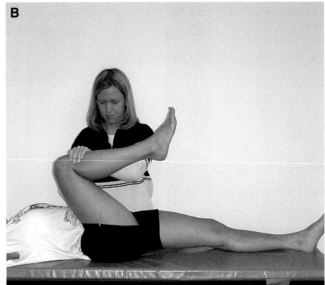

FIGURE 8–20. Passive hip flexion: **(A)** knee extended; **(B)** knee flexed.

> **Box 8–3**
> ## THOMAS TEST FOR HIP FLEXOR TIGHTNESS

A
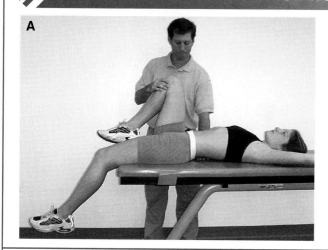

B
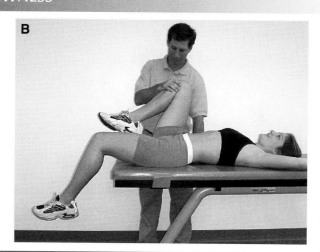

Thomas test for hip flexor tightness. The patient's left (forward) leg is tested. **(A)** Tightness of the left rectus femoris muscle; **(B)** tightness of the left iliopsoas group.

PATIENT POSITION	Lying supine with the knees bent at the end of the table.
POSITION OF EXAMINER	Standing beside the patient.
EVALUATIVE PROCEDURE	The examiner places one hand between the lumbar lordotic curve and the tabletop. One leg is passively flexed to the patient's chest, allowing the knee to flex during the movement. The opposite leg (the leg being tested) rests flat on the table.
POSITIVE TEST	**(A)** The lower leg moves into extension. **(B)** The involved leg rises off the table.
IMPLICATIONS	**(A)** Tightness of the rectus femoris. **(B)** Tightness of the iliopsoas muscle group.
COMMENTS	The patient may passively flex the hip and knee by using the arms to pull the leg to the chest. The amount of lumbar flattening can be determined by placing a hand under the lumbar spine.

A
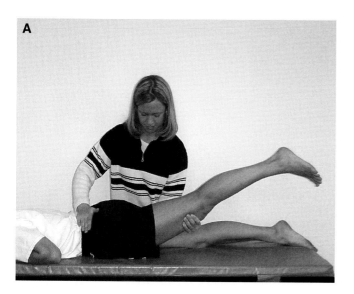

B
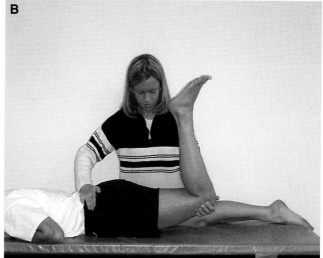

FIGURE 8–21. Passive hip extension: **(A)** knee extended; **(B)** knee flexed.

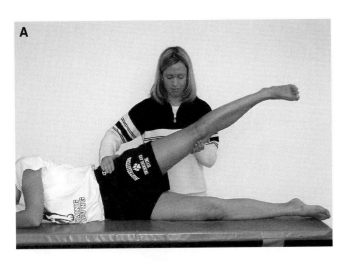
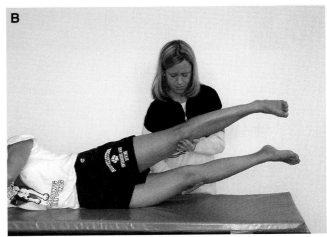

FIGURE 8–22. **(A)** Passive hip abduction. **(B)** Passive hip adduction.

to prevent lateral tilting during the motion (Fig. 8–22). The normal end-feel during adduction is firm owing to tension produced in the lateral joint capsule, the IT band, and the gluteus medius muscle. During abduction, a firm end-feel is obtained because of the tightness in the medial joint capsule and in the pubofemoral, ischiofemoral, and iliofemoral ligaments.

- **Internal and external rotation:** The patient is supine with the hip and knee flexed to 90 degrees. The clinician stabilizes the distal femur with one hand and manipulates the distal lower leg to rotate the femur (Fig. 8–23).

When the knees are flexed, the lower leg rotates in the direction opposite that of the femur (e.g., when the femur is internally rotated, the lower leg rotates out-

wardly). The end-feel is firm in both directions. Internal femoral rotation is limited by tension in the posterior joint capsule and the intrinsic external hip rotators. External femoral rotation is limited by the anterior joint capsule and the iliofemoral and pubofemoral ligaments. Internal rotation may be increased with patients having anteverted hips and decreased in the presence of retroverted hips. External rotation may be increased in individuals with retroverted hips and decreased in those with anteverted hips.

Resisted Range of Motion

Resisted range of motion (RROM) testing is highlighted in Box 8–4. In addition to the standard RROM testing for the hip muscles, postural muscles of the pelvic girdle

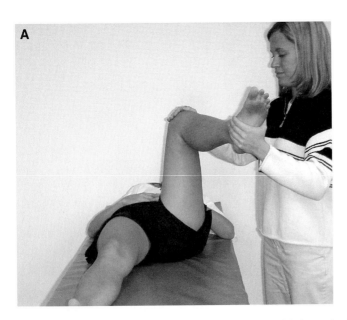
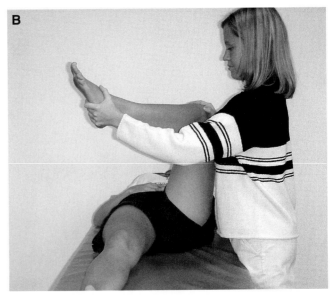

FIGURE 8–23. **(A)** Passive hip internal rotation, and **(B)** passive hip external rotation.

The Pelvis and Thigh **291**

Box 8–4
RESISTED RANGE OF MOTION: Hip

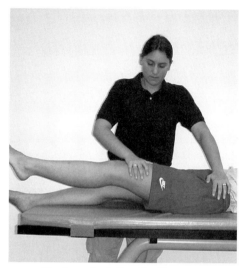

Flexion—Isolating the Iliopsoas

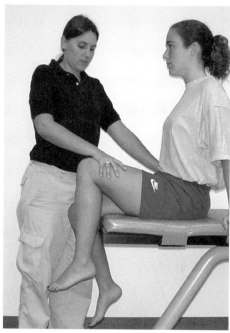

Flexion—Isolating the Rectus Femoris

STARTING POSITION	Supine or seated with the knee extended.	Seated with the knee flexed over the edge of the table.
STABILIZATION	Over the ASIS.	Pelvis stabilized.
RESISTANCE	Anterior aspect of the distal femur.	Anterior aspect of the distal femur.

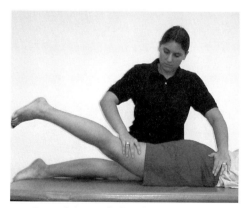

Extension—Isolating the Hamstrings

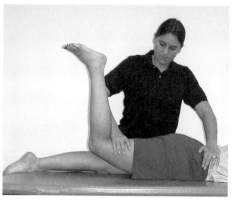

Extension—Isolating the Gluteus Maximus

STARTING POSITION	Prone with the knee extended.	Prone with the knee flexed to 90°.
STABILIZATION	Posterior pelvis.	Posterior pelvis.
RESISTANCE	Proximal to the popliteal fossa.	Posterior aspect of the distal femur.

(continued)

Box 8–4
RESISTED RANGE OF MOTION: Hip *(continued)*

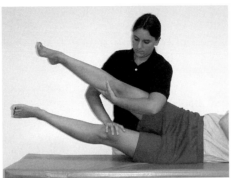

Adduction

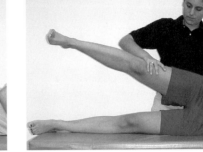

Abduction

STARTING POSITION	Sidelying on the side being tested with the knee extended. The opposite (nontested) leg supported by the examiner.	Sidelying on the opposite side being tested with the knee flexed slightly.
STABILIZATION	The pelvis and torso are actively stabilized by the patient.	The pelvis and torso are actively stabilized by the patient.
RESISTANCE	Over the medial femur, proximal to the knee	Over the lateral femoral condyle
MUSCLES TESTED	Adductor magnus, adductor longus, adductor brevis, gluteus maximus (lower fibers), gracilis, pectineus	Gluteus medius, gluteus maximus (upper fibers), gluteus minimus, sartorius

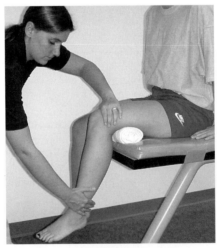

Internal and External Rotation

STARTING POSITION	Seated with the knees flexed over the edge of the table. A bolster placed under the distal femur to keep it parallel with the tabletop.
STABILIZATION	The patient's arms extended and supporting the torso on the table.
RESISTANCE	On the side of the distal lower leg opposite the motion being tested.
MUSCLES TESTED	Internal rotation (shown): Adductor longus, adductor magnus, adductor brevis, gluteus medius, gluteus minimus, semimembranosus, semitendinosus
	External rotation: Biceps femoris, gluteus maximus, piriformis, sartorius, gemellus inferior and superior, obturator internus and externus, quadratus femoris

ASIS = anterior superior iliac spine.

may also be assessed during gait. Patients suffering from weakness of, or trauma, to the gluteus medius tilt the pelvis to the side opposite the insufficiency, displaying **Trendelenburg's gait.** Weakness of the gluteus medius muscle is demonstrated through the **Trendelenburg's test** (Box 8–5). Trendelenburg's gait is discussed in detail in Chapter 9.

LIGAMENTOUS TESTING

No specific tests exist to determine the integrity of the hip's ligaments. Any dysfunction in the mechanics of these structures is determined through testing the passive movement of the joint. Hyperextension of the hip places the iliofemoral, pubofemoral, and ischiofemoral

Box 8–5
TRENDELENBURG'S TEST FOR GLUTEUS MEDIUS WEAKNESS

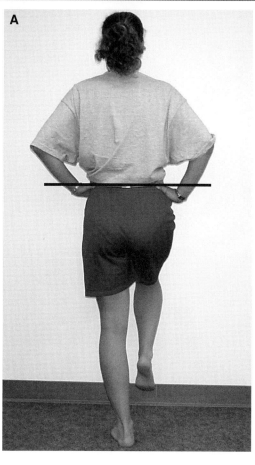
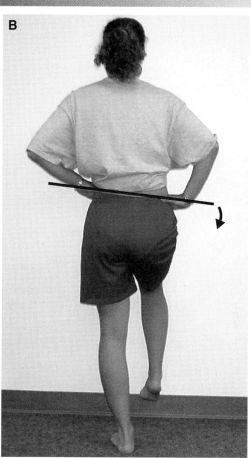

The patient is asked to stand on the affected leg **(A)**. In the presence of gluteus medius weakness, the pelvis lowers on the opposite side of the affected leg **(B)**.

PATIENT POSITION	Standing with the weight evenly distributed between both feet. The patient's shorts are lowered to the point at which the iliac crests or posterior superior iliac spines are visible.
POSITION OF EXAMINER	Standing, sitting, or kneeling behind the patient.
EVALUATIVE PROCEDURE	The patient lifts the leg opposite the side being tested.
POSITIVE TEST	The pelvis lowers on the non–weight-bearing side.
IMPLICATIONS	Insufficiency of the gluteus medius to support the torso in an erect position, indicating weakness in the muscle or decreased innervation.

ligaments on stretch. Adducting the hip stresses the superior fibers of the iliofemoral ligament, while abducting the hip places a strain on the pubofemoral ligament and the lower fibers of the iliofemoral ligament.

NEUROLOGIC TESTING

Pain, paresthesia, and inhibition of muscular innervation may be referred through the hip and into the lower extremity from impingement of the lumbar or sacral plexus or their associated nerve roots. A complete lower quarter screen should be performed for pathology involving the femoral or sciatic nerve (see Box 1–5). Impingement of the sciatic nerve from spasm of the piriformis muscle, **piriformis syndrome,** is discussed in the Pathologies and Related Special Tests section of this chapter.

 ## PATHOLOGIES AND RELATED SPECIAL TESTS

Most often, trauma to the hip and pelvis and the related muscles occurs acutely in the form of contusions or strains. Chronic conditions often result from improper biomechanics stemming from poor posture, leg length discrepancies, or overuse syndromes. Injury to the hip joint itself is rare in athletes, but the amount of force needed to acutely traumatize this structure makes any injury to it a potential medical emergency.

MUSCLE STRAINS

Muscle strains most frequently occur secondary to a dynamic overload during an eccentric muscle contraction. Many times these injuries are typified by pain at the muscular insertion into the bone or at the musculotendinous junction. The iliopsoas, quadriceps, adductors, or hamstrings are commonly injured secondary to an overstretching of the fibers or dynamic overload during an eccentric contraction. Patients suffering from strains of the proximal rectus femoris may obtain relief of the pain experienced when walking up and down stairs by turning around and carefully walking backward.[12] Table 8–4 presents an overview of the mechanisms and ROM deficits common to muscular strains of the hip and thigh.

Table 8–4
CHARACTERISTICS OF MUSCULAR STRAINS OF THE HIP AND THIGH

		Pain or Deficit Elicited During Range of Motion Testing		
Muscle	**Force**	**Active**	**Passive**	**Resisted**
Rectus femoris	Hyperextension of the hip and flexion of the knee Dynamic overload; isometric contraction	Hip flexion, knee extension	Hip extension, knee flexion	Hip flexion with an extended knee Knee extension
Iliopsoas	Hyperextension of the hip Resisted hip flexion	Hip flexion	Hip extension	Hip flexion with a flexed knee
Quadriceps strain (other than rectus femoris)	Hyperflexion of the knee Dynamic overload; resisted knee extension	Knee extension with a flexed hip	Knee flexion	Knee extension
Hamstring strain	Dynamic overload; eccentric contraction Tensile force; overstretching the muscle	Knee flexion Hip extension with an extended knee	Knee extension Hip flexion	Knee flexion Hip extension with an extended knee
Gluteus maximus	Dynamic overload; eccentric contraction; isometric contraction	Hip extension with a flexed knee	Hip flexion with a flexed knee	Hip extension with a flexed knee
Adductor group	Tensile; overstretching the muscle Dynamic overload; eccentric contraction; isometric contraction	Hip adduction	Hip abduction	Hip adduction

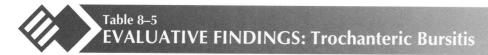

Table 8–5
EVALUATIVE FINDINGS: Trochanteric Bursitis

Examination Segment	Clinical Findings	
History	*Onset:*	Acute or insidious
	Pain characteristics:	Over the greater trochanter, radiating posteriorly to the buttock; pain increased when the patient climbs stairs.
	Mechanism:	Acute: Direct blow to the greater trochanter.
		Chronic: Irritation from the IT band passing over the bursa.
	Predisposing conditions:	Increased Q angles (above the norm for the patient's gender) possibly predisposing him or her to overuse forces being placed on the trochanteric bursa; leg length discrepancy
Inspection	The area over the greater trochanter is usually unremarkable.	
Palpation	Palpation reveals tenderness over the trochanteric bursa.	
	Crepitus may also be experienced during active movement of the hip.	
Functional tests	Flexion and extension and internal and external rotation, either actively or passively, causing pain as the IT band passes over the greater trochanter, resulting in decreased ROM.	
	RROM: Pain occurring during resisted hip extension.	
	Pain occurring during resisted hip adduction.	
Ligamentous tests	Not applicable.	
Neurologic tests	Not applicable.	
Special tests	Ober's test for IT band tightness.	
Comments	Chronic trochanteric bursitis may result in "snapping hip" syndrome.	
	The signs and symptoms of trochanteric bursitis may mimic those of a femoral neck stress fracture.	
	Pain may be referred from the sacroiliac joint or low back.	

IT = iliotibial; ROM = range of motion; RROM = resisted range of motion.

BURSITIS

Resulting from increased friction between a muscle or tendon and bone, bursitis in the hip region usually is isolated to the greater trochanteric, ischial, or iliopsoas bursae. The onset of these conditions may be related to biomechanical factors, congenital influences, or environmental conditions such as prolonged periods of sitting. Septic infection has also been cited as a cause of inflammation of the hip bursae.[13] A definitive diagnosis of these conditions can be made through ultrasonic imaging, computed tomography scans, or magnetic resonance imaging.[13]

Trochanteric Bursitis

Irritation of the trochanteric bursa may result from a single blow. However, more commonly, it may be caused by friction from the IT band as it crosses over this structure during the movements of flexion, extension, internal rotation, and external rotation. A history of a rapid increase in the frequency, intensity, or duration of training is often associated with this condition. Women may be predisposed to this condition because of an increased Q angle (Table 8–5).

Chronic inflammation of the trochanteric bursa is one of the possible causes of **"snapping hip" syndrome,** in which an audible snap occurs as the IT band passes over the greater trochanter. Greater trochanteric bursitis commonly results in reduced hip ROM, especially in flexion and extension and internal and external rotation secondary to pain located directly posterior to the greater trochanter. Trochanteric bursitis can mimic or mask the signs and symptoms of a femoral neck stress fracture.[14]

Ischial Bursitis

Movement of the buttocks while the patient is weight bearing in the seated position, such as the rocking motion associated with rowing or biking, can cause friction to irritate the ischial bursa. These structures can also be traumatized secondary to a direct blow, such as a fall. Ischial bursitis can be further irritated by prolonged periods of sitting, as occurs during bus or airplane trips. Point tenderness at the ischial tuberosity is characteristic of ischial bursitis. A careful history is necessary to rule out the possibility of a hamstring strain or an avulsion of its attachment, both of which have signs and symptoms similar to those of ischial bursitis (Table 8–6). Use of an inflatable doughnut pad for sitting during prolonged periods to lessen the weight-bearing forces placed on these structures may be helpful.

Table 8–6
EVALUATIVE FINDINGS: Ischial Bursitis

Examination Segment	Clinical Findings	
History	**Onset:**	Acute or insidious.
	Pain characteristics:	Over the ischial tuberosity in the vicinity of the gluteal fold.
	Mechanism:	Acute: Direct blow to the ischial tuberosity, such as falling on it.
		Chronic: Repeated shifting and moving while weight bearing in the seated position (e.g., rowing).
	Predisposing conditions:	Tightness of the hamstring muscle group, prolonged sitting and rocking, especially on a hard surface (i.e., bike seat, scull seat).
Inspection	Unremarkable	
Palpation	Tenderness over the ischial tuberosity; the bursa feels thick and crepitus may be present.	
Functional tests	**AROM:** Pain during active hip flexion.	
	PROM: Pain at the end of passive hip flexion.	
	RROM: Pain during resisted hip extension with the knee flexed to isolate the gluteus maximus.	
Ligamentous tests	Not applicable.	
Neurologic tests	Prolonged irritation of the ischial bursa possibly placing pressure on the sciatic nerve, requiring the evaluation of the sensory and motor nerves of the posterior lower leg.	
Comments	Prolonged periods of sitting may cause an increase in symptoms.	

AROM = active range of motion; PROM = passive range of motion; RROM = resisted range of motion.

Iliopsoas Bursitis

Inflammation of the iliopsoas bursa, seldom occurring as an isolated event, may be associated with rheumatoid arthritis or osteoarthritis of the hip.[15] Pain in the anterior hip is often the only symptom of iliopsoas bursitis. However, a mass may be palpated in the groin or around the inguinal ligament.[15,16] This condition has also been implicated as another cause of snapping hip syndrome.[13,17–19] Strengthening the hip rotators can resolve the symptoms associated with both the inflamed bursa and snapping hip syndrome.[20]

DEGENERATIVE HIP CHANGES

Age, repetitive trauma, acute trauma, or improper bony arrangements of the hip can result in degeneration of the articular surfaces of the femur and acetabulum. In athletes, these conditions most commonly include arthritis, osteochondritis dissecans, acetabular labrum tears, and *avascular necrosis.* All share the common characteristic of further degeneration if left undetected and untreated. Chronic hip degeneration occurs with age, commonly affecting people older than age 50 years. Younger patients may develop degenerative hip changes secondary to acute trauma.

The primary complaint associated with the early stages of hip degeneration is pain only during weight bearing. As the degeneration continues, the pain becomes more constant. The location of this pain may lead to the suspicion of lumbar spine or sacroiliac pathology because pain may be referred to the low back and distally into the anterior thigh, knee, or adductor group.

Physical evaluation reveals a loss of motion in all of the hip's planes, with rotational motions being lost first, followed by abduction. Strength assessment with manual muscle testing may be inconclusive secondary to pain. **Hip scouring** causes the two articular surfaces to compress and rub over one another, resulting in pain (Box 8–6). Radiographic evaluation provides conclusive evidence of deterioration of the hip's articular surfaces.

PIRIFORMIS SYNDROME

Recall that the sciatic nerve passes under or through the piriformis muscle as the nerve travels across the posterior pelvis. Spasm or hypertrophy of the piriformis places pressure on the sciatic nerve, mimicking the signs and symptoms of lumbar nerve root compression or sciatica in the buttock and posterior leg.[21] The resulting symptoms, piriformis syndrome, are six times more common in women than men.[22] Improved diagnostic tests for lumbar nerve root impingement and intervertebral disk disease have decreased the frequency and popularity of the diagnosis of piriformis syndrome.[23]

Avascular necrosis Death of cells secondary to lack of an adequate blood supply.

> **Box 8–6**
> **HIP SCOURING TEST**

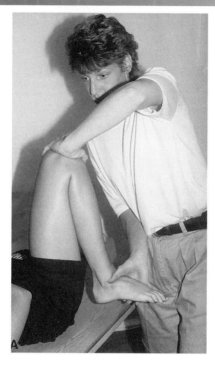
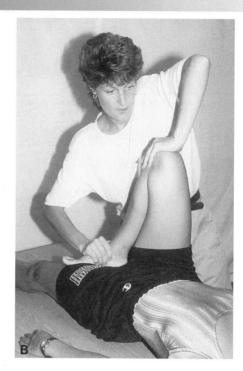

PATIENT POSITION	Supine
POSITION OF EXAMINER	At the side of the patient, fully flexing the patient's hip and knee.
EVALUATIVE PROCEDURE	The examiner applies pressure downward along the shaft of the femur to compress the joint surfaces. The femur **(A)** internally and **(B)** externally rotated with the hip in multiple angles of flexion.
POSITIVE TEST	Pain described or symptoms in the hips reproduced.
IMPLICATIONS	A possible defect in the articular cartilage of the femur or acetabulum (e.g., obsteochondral defects, arthritis).
COMMENTS	This test may also produce pain in the presence of a labral tear.

Although the signs and symptoms of piriformis syndrome are similar to those caused by other lumbopelvic maladies, piriformis syndrome remains relatively undefined and confusing.[24] Complaints include burning, pain, numbness, or paresthesia that are increased with contraction of the piriformis or during palpation or prolonged sitting.[21] However, little commonality in the factors leading to these symptoms is noted.[25] Symptoms may be heightened by the straight leg raising test on the involved side, passive hip internal rotation, and resisted external rotation with the patient seated (Table 8–7). Resisted hip abduction with the patient seated may also increase the symptoms (Fig. 8–24). These symptoms may also be caused by entrapment of the sciatic nerve by the hamstring muscles, termed **hamstring syndrome.**[26]

Treatment of piriformis syndrome includes stretching, strengthening, and possible injection of the piriformis

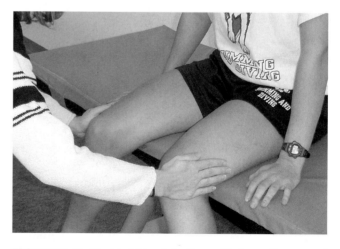

FIGURE 8–24. Resisted hip abduction with the patient seated to duplicate pain caused by piriformis syndrome.

Table 8–7
EVALUATIVE FINDINGS: Piriformis Syndrome

Examination Segment	Clinical Findings	
History	***Onset:***	Acute Insidious onsets possibly related to hypertrophy of the piriformis or biomechanical changes in the hip, pelvis, or sacrum; in most cases, time of onset is not discernible.
	Pain characteristics:	Pain deep in the posterior aspect of the hip, radiating into the buttock and down the posterior aspect of the leg; increases upon standing and often decreases with the patient lying supine and the knees flexed.
	Mechanism:	Few common traits are associated with the onset of piriformis syndrome; factors such as a blow to the buttock, hyperinternal rotation of the femur, or other trauma may cause spasming of the piriformis muscle.
	Predisposing conditions:	Anatomical deviation in which the sciatic nerve passes through the piriformis muscle; females have an increased risk of acquiring piriformis syndrome.
Inspection	The patient may present with an antalgic gait. In chronic conditions, atrophy of the gluteus maximus may be noted.	
Palpation	Tenderness during palpation of the sciatic notch; also, an associated increase in symptoms may be reported.	
Functional tests	***AROM:***	Pain may be experienced during external rotation owing to the piriformis muscle's contracting and placing pressure on the sciatic nerve.
	PROM:	Increased symptoms with passive internal rotation of the hip while patient supine; symptoms reduced with passive external rotation.
	RROM:	Pain elicited or symptoms increased during resisted external hip rotation with the patient in the seated position (see Fig. 8–23); pain also possible during resisted hip abduction.
Ligamentous tests	Not applicable.	
Neurologic tests	The L2 through L4 dermatomes require evaluation for numbness or paresthesia.	
Special tests	Positive straight leg raise test result or resisted hip abduction in the seated position.	
Comments	The signs and symptoms of piriformis syndrome closely replicate those of other lumbopelvic disorders. A definitive diagnosis by a physician is required.	

AROM = active range of motion; PROM = passive range of motion; RROM = resisted range of motion.

muscle. Surgical release of the piriformis muscle may be indicated in cases that do not respond to conservative care.[27]

 ## ON-FIELD EVALUATION OF PELVIS AND THIGH INJURIES

Trauma to the coxofemoral joint is rare in sports. The bony and muscular anatomy is normally well padded in collision sports, such as football and ice hockey, which mandate the use of protective padding over the anterior thigh, ilium, and sacrum. However, when trauma does occur, it is usually severe. More commonly, injuries to this region involve muscular strains, contusions, and sprains of the SI joint.

Upon arriving at the scene, note whether the athlete is moving the involved leg. If the leg is moving, a gross dislocation of the hip or fracture of the femur may be ruled out. However, a subluxation of the hip must still

be considered. A fixed, immobile, awkwardly positioned, or noticeably shortened leg may indicate a dislocation of the hip joint or a fracture of the femoral neck. The shaft of the femur is inspected for normal contour.

The mechanism of injury and other factors surrounding the onset of the injury must be ascertained as soon as possible in the history-taking process. Relevant questions include determining the injurious force, associated sounds and sensations, and any pertinent history of injury.

After a hip dislocation or subluxation and femoral fracture have been ruled out, AROM of both the knee and the hip is initiated. This is easily performed by having the athlete flex the thigh to the chest and straightening the leg back out again. This procedure is then repeated for passive and resisted motion. If the athlete is unable to fully bear weight, a decision needs to be made on how to remove the athlete from the playing arena. These techniques are described in Chapter 1.

INITIAL EVALUATION AND MANAGEMENT OF ON-FIELD INJURIES

On-field management of hip and thigh injuries is needed primarily for contusions or muscle strains. However, hip dislocations and femur fractures represent medical emergencies requiring astute management to limit the scope of trauma and increase the athlete's chances for a full recovery.

ILIAC CREST CONTUSION

Contusions to the iliac crest, "hip pointers," result in a seemingly disproportionate amount of pain, swelling, discoloration, and subsequent loss of function (see Fig. 8–13). The key to reducing the amount of time lost because of this injury lies in the recognition of its signs and symptoms (Table 8–8) and its immediate management.

Athletes suspected of sustaining a significant contusion of the iliac crest require immediate removal from competition, treatment with ice packs, and placement on crutches to avoid weight-bearing stresses. If the injury is minor and occurs during a game situation, the athlete may be allowed to return to competition, provided that full lower extremity and torso function is demonstrated. In this case, the injured area is padded to protect against further injury. Additionally, the athlete must be treated immediately after the game.

QUADRICEPS CONTUSION

Even mild contusive forces transmitted to the quadriceps group can result in the death of muscle fibers. As the severity of the impact increases, so does the proportion of muscle fiber death that occurs. Contusions to the quadriceps group result in decreased force during knee extension. Associated pain and spasm limit the amount of flexion available to the joint. The extremity is often grossly discolored, and the traumatized area is painful to the touch. Intramuscular hematoma gives the muscle a hardened feel in the area and increases the girth of the muscle. Over time, the contour of the quadriceps group is lost secondary to atrophy. The risk of myositis ossificans is increased when a sympathetic effusion of the knee joint occurs (Fig. 8–25).[28]

The first 24 hours after the injury are critical to the long-term management and rehabilitation of athletes suffering from quadriceps contusions. Athletes who describe pain during active knee or hip or knee flexion who have weakness during manual muscle testing of these motions are to be removed from competition for immediate management of their injury. After the determination of the injury has been made, ice packs are applied to the area and flexion of the knee joint, as much as pain allows, is encouraged. As the treated area becomes numb, the amount of knee flexion is gradually increased to tolerance (Fig. 8–26). Maintaining the knee's ROM decreases the possibility of myositis ossificans formation.

Table 8–8
EVALUATIVE FINDINGS: Iliac Crest Contusion (Hip Pointer)

Examination Segment	Clinical Findings	
History	**Onset:**	Acute.
	Pain characteristics:	Iliac crest, possibly radiating into the internal and external oblique muscles.
	Mechanism:	Direct blow to an unprotected ilium.
Inspection	Rapid onset of swelling and redness; ecchymosis developing over time.	
Palpation	Crepitus felt during palpation of the iliac crest. Point tenderness elicited along the iliac crest and associated muscles. Spasm of the associated muscles may also be present.	
Functional tests	All muscles having an origin or insertion along the iliac crest may be affected by this injury. In most cases, the internal and external obliques elicit pain when the trunk is flexed away from the involved side. In more severe instances, hip flexion and abduction and movement of the trunk in any direction also cause pain.	
Ligamentous tests	Not applicable.	
Neurologic tests	A complete sensory and vascular check of the involved lower leg is necessary to rule out trauma to the neurovascular structures about the hip.	
Special tests	Not applicable.	
Comments	Radiography may be required to rule out the possibility of an iliac fracture.	

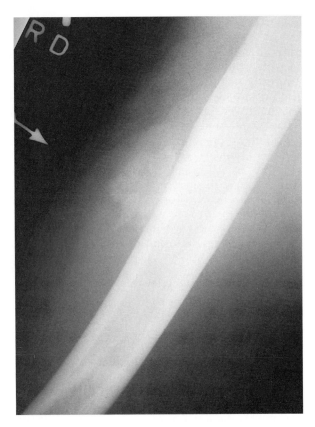

FIGURE 8–25. Femoral myositis ossificans resulting from a quadriceps contusion.

HIP DISLOCATION

Because of the hip's strong ligamentous and bony arrangement, dislocations are rare. However, their occurrence represents a medical emergency requiring immediate care. The majority of hip dislocations involve posterior displacement of the femoral head.[29] Fractures to the femoral neck or the acetabulum (or both) may also result. Most dislocations occur when the hip is in flexion and adduction and an axial force is delivered to the femur, displacing it posteriorly and causing the head to be driven through the posterior capsule.[30]

Athletes suffering from a hip dislocation complain of immediate, intense pain within the joint and buttock, possibly describing the sensation of the hip's "going out." The femur and lower leg are often positioned in internal rotation and adduction so that the involved knee rests against the knee of the opposite side (Fig. 8–27).[31] AROM is impossible or results in severe pain. Although no attempt is made to reduce the dislocation on the field, the examiner must perform a sensory and vascular check of the involved extremity. Integrity of the motor nerves can be determined by asking the athlete to extend and flex the toes. These results are documented for reference by the emergency room staff. Immediate immobilization of the hip and lower leg and transport to an emergency facility is necessary to allow rapid reduction of the dislocation with the patient under anesthesia.[29]

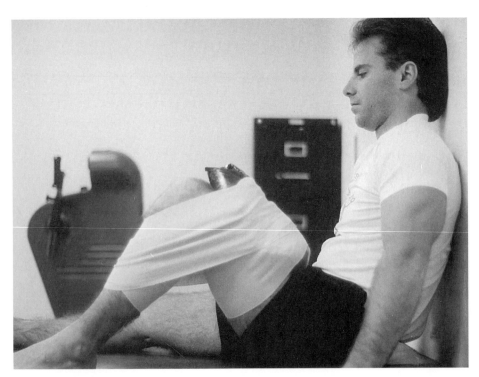

FIGURE 8–26. Method of managing a quadriceps contusion. The quadriceps is flexed to the point that pain is experienced and then extended to the point that the pain disappears. Ice is applied and the process is repeated when the patient reports numbness.

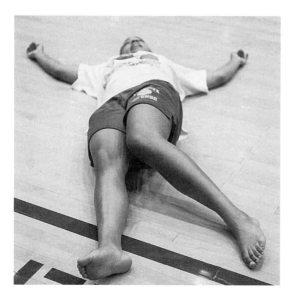

FIGURE 8–27. Position of the lower leg following a posterior hip dislocation: adduction and internal rotation of the hip.

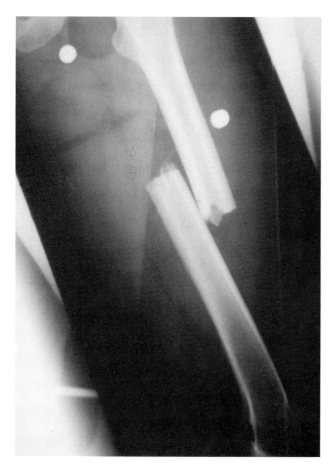

FIGURE 8–28. Radiograph of a complete fracture of the femoral shaft. This type of injury results in obvious deformity of the thigh.

FEMORAL FRACTURE

Resulting from a torsional or shear force to the shaft, femoral fractures are relatively rare in athletes. This fact is based on the "weak link" principle, in which these forces are more likely to result in trauma to the ankle, lower leg, or knee. Because they result in immediate loss of function, pain, and deformity, complete fractures of the femur are easily recognizable (Fig. 8–28).

The femoral shaft and neck may also be the site of a stress fracture, a pathology difficult to diagnose because of the similarity in symptoms to those of a chronic hip flexor strain or tendinitis of the muscles in the area. Initially, the athlete complains of pain only during activity and may then progress to pain at rest. A definitive diagnosis is made through a bone scan. The most commonly prescribed treatment is rest to prevent the stress fracture from progressing to full-fledged femoral fracture.

◆ REFERENCES

1. Norkin, CC, and Levangie, PK: The hip complex. In Norkin, CC, and Levangie, PK (eds): *Joint Structure and Function: A Comprehensive Analysis,* ed 2. Philadelphia, FA Davis, 1992, p 310.
2. Neptune, RR; Wright, IC, and van den Bogert, AJ: Muscle coordination and function during cutting movements. *Med Sci Sports Exerc,* 31:294, 1999.
3. Fisher, R: An epidemiological study of Legg-Perthes disease. *J Bone Joint Surg Am,* 54:769, 1972.
4. Jacobs, B: Diagnosis and history of slipped capital femoral epiphysis. In *American Academy of Orthopaedic Surgeons: Instructional Course Lectures,* vol 21. St Louis, CV Mosby, 1972.
5. Beals, RK: Coxa vara in childhood: Evaluation and management. *J Am Acad Orthop Surg,* 6:93, 1998.
6. Shim, JS, et al: Genu valgum in children with coxa vara resulting from hip disease. *J Pediatr Orthop,* 17:225, 1997.
7. Sugano, N, Noble, PC, and Kamaric, E: A comparison of alternative methods of measuring femoral anteversion. *J Comput Assist Tomogr,* 22:610, 1998.
8. Hermann, KL, and Egund, N: Measuring anteversion in the femoral neck from routine radiographs. *Acta Radiol,* 39:410, 1998.
9. Matovinovic, D, et al: Comparison in regression of femoral neck anteversion in children with normal, intoeing and outtoeing gait: Prospective study. *Coll Antropol,* 22:525, 1998.
10. Adams, MC: *Outline of Orthopaedics.* London: E and S Livingstone, 1968.
11. Brand, RA, and Yack, HJ: Effects of leg length discrepancies on the forces at the hip joint. *Clin Orthop,* Dec:172, 1996.
12. Johnson, GE: Personal communication. August 19, 1994.
13. Ginesty, E, et al: Iliopsoas bursopathies. A review of twelve cases. *Rev Rhum Engl Ed,* 65:181, 1998.
14. Jones, DL, and Erhard, RE: Diagnosis of trochanteric bursitis versus femoral neck stress fracture. *Phys Ther,* 77:58, 1997.
15. Fortin, L, and B'elanger, R: Bursitis of the iliopsoas: Four cases with pain as the only clinical indicator. *J Rheumatol,* 22:1971, 1995.
16. Flanagan, FL, et al: Symptomatic enlarged iliopsoas bursae in the presence of a normal plain hip radiograph. *Br J Rheumatol,* 34:365, 1995.
17. Johnston, CA, et al: Iliopsoas bursitis and tendinitis. A review. *Sports Med,* 25:271, 1998.
18. Vaccaro, JP, Sauser, DD, and Beals, RK: Iliopsoas bursa imaging: Efficacy in depicting abnormal iliopsoas tendon motion in patients with internal snapping hip syndrome. *Radiology,* 197:853, 1995.

19. Janzen, DL, et al: The snapping hip: Clinical and imaging findings in transient subluxation of the iliopsoas tendon. *Can Assoc Radiol J*, 47:202, 1996.
20. Johnston, CA, Lindsay, DM, and Wiley, JP: Treatment of iliopsoas syndrome with a hip rotation strengthening program: A retrospective case series. *J Orthop Sports Phys Ther*, 29:218, 1999.
21. Parziale, JR, Hudgins, TH, and Fishman, LM: The piriformis syndrome. *Am J Orthop*, 25:819, 1996.
22. Keskula, DR, and Tamburell, M: Conservative management of piriformis syndrome. J *Athletic* Training, 27:102, 1992.
23. Hughes, SS, et al: Extrapelvic compression of the sciatic nerve. An unusual cause of pain about the hip: Report of five cases. *J Bone Joint Surg Am*, 74:1553, 1992.
24. Silver, JK, and Leadbetter, WB: Piriformis syndrome: Assessment of current practice and literature review. *Orthopedics*, 21:1133, 1998.
25. Carter, AT: Piriformis syndrome: A hidden cause of sciatic pain. *Athletic Training: Journal of the National Athletic Trainers Association*, 23:243, 1988.
26. Woodhouse, ML: Sciatic nerve entrapment: A cause of proximal posterior thigh pain in athletes. *Athletic Training: Journal of the National Athletic Trainers Association*, 25:351, 1990.
27. Hanania, M, and Kitain, E: Perisciatic injection of steroid for the treatment of sciatica due to piriformis syndrome. *Reg Anesth Pain Med*, 23:223, 1998.
28. Clancy, WG, and Bosanny, JJ: Functional treatment and rehabilitation of quadriceps contusions, patellar dislocations and "isolated" medial collateral ligament injuries. *Athletic Training: Journal of the National Athletic Trainers Association*, 17:249, 1982.
29. Parris, HG, Sallis, RE, and Anderson, DV: Traumatic hip dislocation. Reducing complications. *Physician and Sportsmedicine*, 21:67, 1993.
30. Gieck, J, et al: Fracture dislocation of the hip while playing football. *Athletic Training: Journal of the National Athletic Trainers Association*, 21:124, 1986.
31. O'Donoghue, DH: Injuries of the pelvis and hip. In O'Donoghue, DH (ed): *Treatment of Injuries to Athletes*, ed 3. Philadelphia, WB Saunders, 1976, p 497.

CHAPTER 9

Evaluation of Gait

MONIQUE BUTCHER, PhD, ATC
AND PETER ZULIA, PT, ATC

Walking can be described as a series of narrowly averted catastrophes.[1] First the body falls forward. Then, to prevent the catastrophe of falling, the legs move under the body and establish a new base of support with the feet. Watching a toddler walk across the room, struggling to control balance against the force of gravity, demonstrates the intricacy of this chain of events. As motor development and coordination develops, walking becomes a subconscious effort.

The coordination of muscle action during gait is amazing to behold and complex to analyze. Gait analysis is the functional evaluation of a person's walking or running style.[2] An organized approach to this analysis provides a systematic method of identifying specific deviations in the gait pattern and determining their cause and implications.

The goals of gait analysis vary depending on the limitation and need of each patient. Minor injuries may require limited analysis, gait training, and rehabilitation, but more serious problems require more extensive measures. The goals of gait analysis vary from establishing safe gait to improving gait until it becomes *functional* or *cosmetic*.[3]

Dysfunctional or *antalgic gait* can arise from acute or chronic injury or improper biomechanics. Consider, for example, an athlete who limps off the basketball court after suffering an ankle sprain. The trauma to the stabilizing ligaments combined with pain prohibits the ankle from normal weight bearing. The foot compensates for this dysfunction by altering the weight-bearing surfaces. This, in turn, alters the mechanics of the knee, the hip, and possibly the lumbar spine. Theoretically, when acute trauma heals normally, normal gait should return. Chronic injuries (e.g., peroneal tendonitis) or congenital abnormalities (e.g., tarsal coalition) can alter the gait pattern permanently. This altered gait further influences the stresses placed on the joint surfaces, bones, and soft tissue structures, thus predisposing the patient to additional injury to the foot and proximally along the kinetic chain.

Abnormal gait caused by improper lower extremity biomechanics redistributes the forces across the joint surfaces, potentially resulting in injury. In this case, a correction of the biomechanics must be attempted through a combination of therapeutic intervention, new footwear, prophylactic support, or orthoses. The purpose of the subsequent rehabilitation program is to alleviate the symptoms and correct the underlying pathology.

 ## OBSERVATION TECHNIQUES

Observation is the process of gathering, organizing, and interpreting sensory information about human motor performances.[3] In this case, motor performance refers to producing an efficient means of walking or running. Detailed observation is best obtained by using stop-action video. The speed of the video can be decreased and replayed, allowing careful breakdown of the phases of the gait cycle. When combined with specialized computer software programs, video can be used to quantify specific *kinetic* and *kinematic* parameters:

- Limb position
- Range of motion (ROM)
- Speed of motion
- Force production
- Timing of each event in the gait cycle

Functional gait   A walking or running pattern that has been corrected so that activities of daily living or sport can be performed; this does not imply a cosmetic gait.

Cosmetic gait   A walking or running pattern that has been corrected so that it has aesthetic quality for the patient.

Antalgic gait   Abnormal or irregular walking or running pattern that has resulted from a biomechanical deviation or injury.

Kinetic   The forces being analyzed; the causes of joint action.

Kinematic   The characteristics of movement related to time and space (e.g,. range of motion, velocity, and acceleration); the effects of joint action.

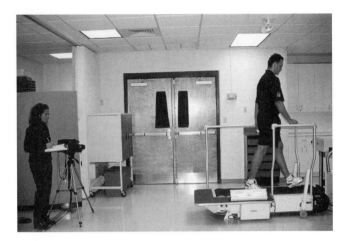

FIGURE 9–1. Setup for gait observation

Video analysis is also useful because it serves as a permanent record of the patient's gait that can be used to gauge the patient's progress.

A treadmill can also be used to analyze gait at various speeds and inclines with regular or high-speed cameras positioned to the side, back, and front of the patient, thus providing a more thorough analysis (Fig. 9–1). If only one camera is available, it can be moved from view to view. Label the videotapes with the date, treadmill speeds, camera speed, and other pertinent information. A written analysis of the gait on each tape is kept in the patient's file. The patient needs to be familiar with walking or running on the treadmill and the examiner must be aware of the subtle differences between ambulating on a treadmill versus a regular surface. Unfamiliarity of walking on a treadmill, decreased *stride length,* and an unnatural gait cycle caused by concentrating on the task of walking can produce artificial results on the treadmill. Therefore, it is best to observe the patient on both surfaces.

An adequate amount of time must be allotted to allow for a complete analysis of gait and to observe the detail and timing of the motion. Preplan when, where, and with what materials you will observe the patient. The guidelines for observational gait analysis are as follows:

1. Prepare the area and materials ahead of time.
2. Avoid clutter in the viewing background.
3. Have the patient wear clothing that does not restrict viewing of joints.
4. Ensure that the patient is at a normal walking pace; otherwise, gait will be altered.
5. Position yourself in a position to view the individual segments (i.e., if you are observing for forefoot pronation and supination, then squat down so your eyes are in line with the patient's feet).
6. Observe the subject from multiple views (anterior, posterior, and both lateral views) but not from an oblique angle.

7. Look at the individual body parts first, then the whole body, then the individual parts again.
8. Conduct multiple observations or trials.
9. Conduct the analysis with and without the patient wearing shoes.
10. Label all videotapes (if used) with pertinent data.

Good observation is not limited to the visual inspection of gait. Auditory information about the rhythm, or *cadence,* of the patient's gait also offers clues for intervention.

Analysis of gait also provides relevant information regarding the nature of the patient's present condition and the predisposing conditions contributing to the injury or possibly inhibiting recovery. The findings of the visual gait analysis must be correlated to the findings of an orthopedic evaluation of the lower extremity and a postural evaluation (Fig 9–2).

 GAIT CYCLE

The gait cycle represents the combined function of the lower extremity, pelvis, and spinal column. During gait, the arms swing to help maintain balance. Each segment of the gait cycle, its role in the absorption and distribution of forces, and its relationship to the other phases of gait must be understood to fully comprehend and apply the information gained during the analysis.

Walking involves a cyclical motion with progressive, alternate leg action. The bipedal position of humans permits rapid initiation of this motion. The *center of gravity* is easily displaced in the desired direction because (1) it is positioned high, at approximately the second sacral segment, over a relatively small base of support, and (2) the greater portion of the body weight is located in the trunk, head, and shoulders, rather than in the lower extremities (Fig. 9–3).[4]

The components of normal walking gait do not transfer to most athletic activites. Sport-specific skills such as sidestepping in soccer, crossover steps in volleyball, and lunge-type movements in sports or work activities do not adhere to the traditional definitions of gait. Force distribution across the foot, muscle actions, joint motions, and the center of gravity are unique to the specific motion being produced.

Stride length   The distance traveled between two successive initial contacts of the same extremity

Cadence   The number of steps per unit of time (i.e., steps per minute).

Center of gravity   The point inside or outside the body where all things are equally balanced or where gravitational pull is concentrated.

OXFORD PHYSICAL THERAPY & REHABILITATION

LOWER EXTREMITY BIOMECHANICAL EVALUATION

I. HISTORY

Name _____ Age _____ Date _____ Diagnosis _____

Occupation _____

Chief Complaint _____

Onset of Symptoms _____ When Does Pain Occur _____

Amount of Participation _____

Physical History _____

II. PRONE

A. STJ	R	L		B. Forefoot	R	L		C. Flexibility	R	L
Valgus	___	___		Valgus	___	___		Gastroc	___	___
Varus	___	___		Varus	___	___		Soleus	___	___
Neutral	___	___						Rectus femoris	___	___
Inversion	___	___						Hip flexors	___	___

D. Callus Formation   E. PSIS   R   L   F. Palpation _____
_____   Med/Lat   Med/Lat   _____
_____   Inf/Sup   Inf/Sup   G. Resistive Testing _____
                             Post/Ant Post/Ant   _____
                             Level

III. SUPINE

A. 1st Ray

  R   Plantarflex Dorsiflex   Neutral
  L   Plantarflex Dorsiflex   Neutral

B. 1st Ray ROM

  R ↑ Plantarflex   ↑ Dorsiflex   Equal
  L ↑ Plantarflex   ↑ Dorsiflex   Equal

C. MTP ROM	R	L
Dorsiflexion	_____	_____
Plantarflexion	_____	_____

D. Midtarsal ROM (O-oblique/L-longitudinal)

_____

_____

E. Talar Rock   R   +   -   L   +   -

F. Passive Spring Test   R   +   -   L   +   -

G. Superior Tibiofibular Joint   R ↓ Anterior ↓ Posterior   Equal
                                 L ↓ Anterior ↓ Posterior   Equal

H. Femoral Torsion Test   R   Neutral   IR/ER   IR ___ ER ___
                                 L   Neutral   IR/ER   IR ___ ER ___

I. ASIS   R   L
                                 Med/Lat   Med/Lat   equal
                                 Inf/Sup   Inf/Sup
                                 Post/Ant   Post/Ant

A

FIGURE 9–2. An example of documentation used during the physical evaluation of gait.

III. **SUPINE** (Continued)

J. Piriformis Flexibility   R   Tight   Normal   L   Tight   Normal

K. Hamstring Flexibility   R   Tight   Normal   L   Tight   Normal

IV. **SITTING**

A. Resistive Testing _____

B. Palpation _____

C. Tibial Torsion   R _____   L _____

V. **STANDING**

A. Toe Raise

	B. 1/4 Squats	
R ↓ Rearfoot Supination Rearfoot Supination	R ↓ Rearfoot Pronation	Rearfoot Pronation
R ↓ Forefoot Pronation Forefoot Pronation	R ↓ Forefoot Pronation	Forefoot Supination
L ↓ Rearfoot Supination Rearfoot Supination	L ↓ Rearfoot Pronation	Rearfoot Pronation
L ↓ Forefoot Pronation Forefoot Pronation	L ↓ Forefoot Pronation	Forefoot Supination

C. Standing Rotation _____

D. Tib/fib Rotation Test   R   L   E. Rearfoot Position   R   L
    Anterior Glide   ___ ___   Pronated   ___ ___
    Posterior Glide   ___ ___   Supinated   ___ ___
                                             Neutral   ___ ___

F. Supro Test _____   G. Knee Position _____

H. Iliac Crest   Level   R   Low   L   Low

J. Gait _____

VII. **ASSESSMENT** _____

VIII. **TODAY'S TREATMENT**

A. Modalities _____

B. Orthotics/Shoe Lift _____

C. Pelvic Girdle _____

D. Cross Friction Massage _____

IX. **HOME EXERCISE PROGRAM**

	SETS	REPS	TIME		SETS	REPS	TIME
Heel Raises	___	___	___	Gastroc/soleus	___	___	___
Toe Raises	___	___	___	Hamstring	___	___	___
Windshield Wiper	___	___	___	IT Band	___	___	___
Theraband inversion	___	___	___	Piriformis	___	___	___
eversion	___	___	___	Plantar fascia	___	___	___
dorsiflexion	___	___	___				
plantarflex	___	___	___				

X. **PLAN** _____

XI. **NEXT MD VISIT** _____

B

FIGURE 9–2. *(continued)*

FIGURE 9–3. Path of the center of gravity during gait. The body's center of gravity, typically located near the L5/S1 joint, moves approximately 2 cm in the frontal plane and 4 cm in the transverse plane during normal gait.

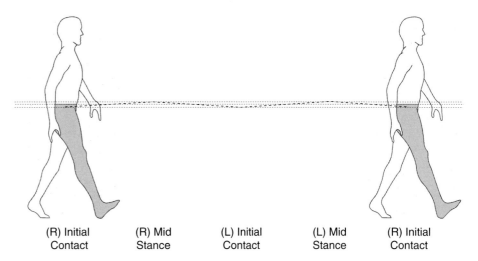

(R) Initial Contact	(R) Mid Stance	(L) Initial Contact	(L) Mid Stance	(R) Initial Contact

NORMAL GAIT

To detect and correct gait anomalies, an examiner must first know what normal gait looks and sounds like. The normal cadence for walking in adults is 107 $+/-$ 2.7 steps per minute, with women having an increased cadence than men.[5] The normal step or stride length for the right and left stride is 75 plus or minus 1.6 cm.[5] Therefore, when observing walking gait, the examiner can listen as the limb makes contact with the surface for a symmetrical and uninterrupted rhythm.

The terminology used in this chapter has been established by the Rancho Los Amigos Medical Center.[6] A comparison between traditional terminology and that used by the Rancho Los Amigos method is presented in Table 9–1. The joint positions, muscle activity, and weight-bearing surfaces of the foot presented in this section are based on normative values for a healthy population. Gait is affected by intrinsic factors such as joint ROM, muscle strength, body type, and gender. Extrinsic factors affecting gait include the relative incline of the surface, the surface type, and footwear.

Table 9–1
COMPARISON OF GAIT TERMINOLOGY

Traditional	Rancho Los Amigos
Heel strike	Initial contact
Heel strike to foot flat	Loading response
Foot flat to midstance	Midstance
Midstance to heel-off	Terminal stance
Toe-off	Preswing
Toe-off to acceleration	Initial swing
Acceleration to midswing	Midswing
Midswing to deceleration	Terminal swing

GAIT PHASES

In walking, the *stance phase* begins with the initial contact of the heel on the ground and ends as the toe breaks contact with the surface (toe-off). The period between toe-off and the next initial contact is termed the *swing phase,* the open kinetic chain or non–weight-bearing period during which the limb repositions itself (Fig. 9–4). During walking, while one leg is in the stance phase, the other is in the swing phase. At two points in the gait cycle, midstance and terminal stance, the body is supported by a single limb. Efficient walking has minimal upward and side-to-side motion and maximal forward motion. Rotation of the pelvis in the transverse plane adds to the step length.

Stance Phase

Advancement of the body over the supporting limb occurs in the stance phase, constituting approximately 60 percent of the gait cycle. A closed kinetic chain is created in the lower extremity during weight bearing, allowing forces from the lower extremity to be transferred to the ground, thereby producing movement.[7] The stance phase is the high-energy portion of gait because the descending leg decelerates just before and at the time of the initial contact, thus preventing injury to the heel. The shock absorption through the kinetic chain that enables the body to be balanced and then to push off also requires energy.[4] Five distinct periods occur during the stance phase: initial contact, loading

Stance phase   The weight-bearing phase of gait, beginning on initial contact with the surface and ending when contact is broken.

Swing phase   The non–weight bearing phase of gait; beginning at the instant the foot leaves the surface and ending just before initial contact.

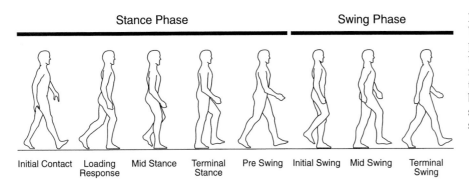

Stance Phase | Swing Phase

Initial Contact | Loading Response | Mid Stance | Terminal Stance | Pre Swing | Initial Swing | Mid Swing | Terminal Swing

FIGURE 9–4. Phases of the gait cycle. With the right (facing) limb as an example, two distinct phases occur—the weight-bearing stance phase and the non–weight-bearing swing phase. With the exception of the dual phases of double limb support, one limb is in the stance phase and the other is in the swing phase and vice versa.

response, midstance, terminal stance, and preswing (Box 9–1).

Initial Contact

Initial contact begins with the instant that the foot touches the supporting surface. Contact should be through the lateral aspect of the plantar surface of the heel as the stance phase of the opposite limb is ending with toe-off. The subtalar joint of the contact foot is supinated approximately 5 degrees and the talocrural joint is dorsiflexed. During this period, both limbs are in contact with the ground at the same time. This double-support period represents approximately 20 percent of the total gait cycle.

Loading Response

Immediately after initial contact, the loading response occurs. Here, the limb reacts to absorbing the impact of the body weight by initiating flattening of the foot. The talocrural joint plantarflexes and the subtalar joint pronates, resulting in calcaneal eversion.[8] Subtalar pronation unlocks the midtarsal joints, allowing the foot to become flexible, accommodate to uneven surfaces, and absorb ground reaction forces (GRFs). Tibial internal rotation results because of the subtalar pronation that creates increased medial forces at the foot, leg, and knee. During this time, the tibialis posterior eccentrically contracts, decelerating the rate of pronation. The eccentric action of the tibialis anterior decelerates plantarflexion.[7] The hip maintains a flexed position during this time. This period lasts until the opposite extremity has left the surface and the double limb support has ended.

Midstance

Midstance begins as the body weight moves directly over the stationary support limb and concludes when the center of gravity is directly over the foot. The foot is evenly distributed on the supporting surface. The talocrural joint continues to dorsiflex, but the subtalar joint now supinates, increasing calcaneal inversion. Supination of the subtalar joint locks the midtarsal joints, stiffening the foot into a rigid lever and preparing the limb to be more efficient during propulsion at toe-off. Subtalar joint supination and tibial external rotation occurs as the knee and hip joints move into extension.

Terminal Stance

The terminal stance begins as the center of gravity passes over the foot and ends just before the contralateral limb makes initial contact with the ground. The body moves ahead of the supporting foot and moves forward with the weight shift over the metatarsal heads until the contralateral limb provides a new base of support. The toes are extended with the weight-bearing forces placed on the first metatarsophalangeal (MTP) joint. The subtalar joint is supinated approximately 5 degrees and the tibia is externally rotated. In preparation for the swing phase, the knee and hip continue to flex.

Preswing

The final period of the stance phase is preswing. Preswing is the transitional period of double support during which the limb is rapidly unloaded from the ground and prepared to swing. It begins with the initial contact of the contralateral limb and ends with the toe-off of the stance limb. This is the second of the two periods with double limb support in a normal walking gait cycle.

Swing Phase

The low-energy phase of the gait cycle occurs during the acceleration portion, or swing phase, and represents approximately 38 percent of the gait cycle.[7] The swing phase begins as soon as the toes leave the surface and terminates when the limb next makes contact with the surface. Gravity is working in favor of the pendulum swing of the limb by pulling the leg mass down toward the surface. The momentum gained at toe-off helps carry the leg through the swing phase. This takes considerably less energy than that expended in the stance phase.[4] Three distinct periods occur during the swing phase: initial swing, midswing, and terminal swing (Box 9–2).

Initial Swing

Initial swing begins at the point when the toes leave the ground and continues until the knee reaches its maximum range of flexion, approximately 60 degrees. The femur is advanced, toe clearance is insured by the ankle dorsiflexors, and a propulsion force is developed. Pronation occurs at the subtalar joint.

Midswing

During midswing, the knee extends from the point of maximum flexion to the point at which the tibia reaches a vertical position perpendicular to the surface. The thigh continues to advance, toe clearance is ensured, and the propulsion force continues to be developed. The talocrural joint is dorsiflexed into a neutral position or into slight dorsiflexion.

Terminal Swing

The final period of the swing phase is the terminal swing, which occurs from the end of the midswing to the initial contact period of the stance phase. The trunk is erect, the thigh decelerates for heel contact, and the knee extends to create a *step length* for heel contact. Supination occurs at the subtalar joint in preparation for intial contact.

QUALITATIVE OBSERVATION OF GAIT

The joint actions at the hip, knee, ankle, and foot provide the major forces in propelling the center of gravity in walking while other joints contribute to the total movement. To lengthen the stride, the pelvis rotates on the supporting femur because of the internal rotation at the hip joint. At the same time, the swinging limb is rotated externally at the hip to keep the foot aligned with the direction of movement. In addition, the torso is rotated by the spine to keep the shoulders perpendicular to the line of motion.

During initial contact, the body weight is placed on the lateral aspect of the heel. Then it moves forward toward the lateral edge of the foot through the loading response and midstance phases and finally diagonally toward the undersurface of the great toe at terminal stance. At preswing, body weight is under the first MTP joint. Although similarities can be found among individuals, each pressure pattern is unique to each individual.[4]

The rise and fall of the body in a vertical direction is approximately 5 cm. The path of the center of gravity is that of a sinusoidal, or a smooth curve. No sharp braking force is evident. There is a slight amount of lateral motion in the horizontal plane. The more efficient the walking gait is, the less horizontal motion is present. As the speed of walking increases, the rotation of the spine is aided by shoulder action, with the right arm moving forward as the left foot advances. In fast walking, the stance phase and swing phases are commonly equal. In slow walking, gravitational force contributes less. Hip flexion and step length also decrease.

In general, the following questions should be addressed during gait analysis.[9] Very specific instances may be evaluated using the forms presented later in this chapter.

1. Does the center of gravity remain within a relatively small horizontal distance?
2. Does the trunk remain upright with only small amounts of flexion and extension?
3. Does the head bob up and down unnecessarily?
4. Is there an appropriate ROM of the limbs during the movement?
5. Does the lateral aspect of the heel strike the surface?
6. Does the subject toe in or toe out during the walking movement?
7. Do the arms move equally in opposition to the legs?
8. Do the arms have a rhythmic pendulum-type swinging action?
9. Does the movement flow continuously, or are there momentary pauses in the movement?
10. Does the cadence sound symmetrical?
11. Do the legs appear symmetrical during similar phases of gait?
12. Does the pelvis rotate properly?

RUNNING GAIT

Running involves a series of smoothly coordinated jumps executed from one foot to the other foot.[10] The purpose of running is to displace the body from one position to another at a moderate to fast speed.[9] Similar to walking, running uses a cyclical motion of the lower legs, but the arms also swing through an arc and in opposition to the movement of the legs. As the speed of the run increases, various aspects of the technique, such as arm swing ROM, stride length, cadence, and knee flexion ROM, change in proportion to the speed. Muscular force and speed of contraction requirements change, particularly with the eccentric contractions required to achieve control of pronation during the loading response and initiate supination prior to preswing.[11] Less upward and downward motion of the total body also accompanies faster speeds.

RUNNING GAIT CYCLE

As in walking, the running gait cycle begins with the initial contact of the limb in the stance phase. The loading response and the midstance period occur more rapidly during running gait. The end of the stance phase is a significant biomechanical sequence necessary to generate quick, forceful forward propulsion.

Step length   The distance traveled between the initial contacts of the right and left foot.

Box 9–1
STANCE PHASE OF GAIT

	Initial Contact	Loading Response	Midstance	Terminal Stance	Preswing
Weight-bearing surface					
Subtalar joint	5° of supination	10° pronation	5° pronation, supinating toward neutral	5° supination	10° supination
Talocrural joint	Neutral moving to 10° of dorsiflexion	15° plantarflexion	0° to 5° dorsiflexion	5° to 10° dorsiflexion moving toward plantarflexion	0° to 20° plantarflexion
Knee	0° of flexion: Tibia externally rotated	15° flexion: Tibia internally rotates, tibia begins to externally rotate as the knee extends	15° flexion to 0°: Tibia externally rotating	5° flexion to 0°: Tibia externally rotates	0° to 30° flexion: Tibia externally rotates
Hip	30° of flexion: Femur externally rotated	30° flexion: Femur internally rotating to neutral	25° flexion to 0°: Femur internally rotated	0° to 10° extension: Femur externally rotates and adducts	20° extension to 0° extension: Femur externally rotates with slight abduction

Muscle activity					
Foot intrinsics Isometric stabilization	Eccentric	Concentric	Concentric	Concentric	Concentric
Plantarflexors Silent	Eccentric	Eccentric	Eccentric to concentric	Concentric	Concentric
Dorsiflexors Eccentric	Eccentric	Concentric, but momentum can carry the talocrural joint through its range of motion.	Isometric	Concentric to silent	Concentric to silent
Quadriceps Concentric	Eccentric	Silent	Silent	Eccentric to silent	Eccentric to silent
Hamstrings Eccentric	Isometric stabilization	Isometric	Concentric	Concentric	Concentric
Hip adductors Eccentric	Eccentric	Isometric	Isometric	Eccentric to control the pelvis	Eccentric to control the pelvis
Gluteus maximus Isometric to eccentric	Concentric	Silent	Isometric	Isometric	Isometric
Gluteus medius and minimus Eccentric	Isometric or concentric	Concentric	Concentric	Isometric	Isometric
Iliopsoas Eccentric	Isometric stabilization	Eccentric	Eccentric	Concentric	Concentric

Box 9–2
SWING PHASE OF GAIT

	Initial Swing	Midswing	Terminal Swing
Limb position			
Weight-bearing surface			
Subtalar joint Pronating	Neutral	Neutral	5° supination
Talocrural joint 20° dorsiflexion	Neutral	Neutral	Neutral
Knee 30° to 60° flexion: Tibia internally rotates		30° to 0° flexion: Tibia externally rotates	0°: Tibia externally rotates
Hip 0° to 20° flexion: Femur externally rotates to neutral		20° to 30° flexion: Femur externally rotates	30° flexion: Femur externally rotates

Muscle Activity			
Foot intrinsics	Isometric stabilization	Isometric	Isometric stabilization
Plantarflexors	Concentric, reducing muscular activity	Concentric	Isometric
Dorsiflexors	Concentric until the foot is clear of the ground, then isometric	Isometric	Isometric
Quadriceps	Concentric	Silent—Momentum carries the limb through the ROM	Concentric to stabilize the knee
Hamstrings	Concentric to eccentric	Eccentric	Eccentric
Hip adductors	Concentric	Isometric	Eccentric
Gluteus maximus	Isometric	Eccentric	Eccentric
Gluteus medius and minimus	Isometric	Isometric	Isometric
Iliopsoas	Concentric	Concentric or silent	Isometric

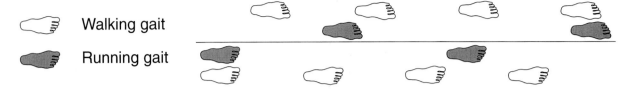

Walking gait

Running gait

FIGURE 9–5. Comparison of strides between walking and running gaits. Running requires greater range of motion, balance, and strength compared with walking. Notice the increased stride length and decreased stride width associated with running.

At initial contact, the hip is flexed to approximately 50 degrees. From this point, the hip moves towards extension during the remainder of the stance phase. The knee, flexed approximately 40 degrees at initial contact, reaches a maximum range of 60 degrees of flexion during the loading response and then moves into extension through the rest of the stance phase.

The talocrural joint is dorsiflexed to a maximum range of 25 degrees at the point of initial contact. The subtalar joint is supinated at initial contact, then pronates to allow for adaptation to uneven surfaces and absorption of forces. As the limb continues from midstance to preswing, the talocrural joint plantarflexes and the subtalar joint supinates to form a rigid lever for the athlete to push off.

The swing phase clears the non–weight-bearing limb over the ground and positions the foot to accept weight bearing, allowing the individual to perform as efficiently as possible. Because weight-bearing forces are not involved, the probability of injury during the swing phase is decreased when compared with that of the weight-bearing stance phase. Most injuries occurring during the swing phase of the running cycle involve the lower extremity muscles that are needed to decelerate and control the limb.

During the initial swing phase, the hip is at an angle of 10 degrees of extension. The hip then flexes during the remainder of the swing period, reaching approximately 50 to 55 degrees of flexion during the terminal swing period.

The knee moves through its greatest ROM during the swing phase. While fully extended at initial swing, the knee can reach 125 degrees of flexion during midswing. Knee flexion varies given the type of run being performed (i.e., jog or sprint). Extreme knee flexion is characteristic of sprinters. By increasing the knee flexion angle, the length of the radius of rotation is decreased, reducing the *moment of inertia,* thus making it easier to rotate the limb about the hip joint. In walking or distance running, in which less angular acceleration of the legs is required, flexion at the knee during the swing phase remains relatively small and the leg's moment of inertia with respect to the hip is relatively large. In terminal swing, the knee extends to approximately 40 degrees of flexion in preparation for initial

contact. Initially during the swing period, the talocrural joint is at 25 degrees of plantarflexion but proceeds rapidly to 20 degrees of dorsiflexion, where it remains until initial contact during the stance phase.

The gait cycle, as described in this chapter, does not apply to all athletic motions. Lateral movements, back peddling, and changing directions alter the weight distribution and muscle actions of the lower extremity, torso, and upper extremity.

WALKING VERSUS RUNNING GAIT

Running is a modification of walking, but with two distinct differences: (1) there is the presence of a flight phase during which neither foot is in contact with the supporting surface, and (2) at no time are both feet in contact with the surface at the same time. During walking, the stance phase accounts for 62 percent of the total gait cycle; during running, it accounts for approximately one third of the cycle (depending on the speed of running) (Fig. 9–5).[1] Although differences in the degrees of joint motion and timing of actions exist, the same joints are used in running as in walking.

 GROUND REACTION FORCES

During gait, every contact of the foot with the surface generates an upward reaction force. These ground reaction forces (GRFs) are measured in analyzing differences in gait patterns across the life span and among individuals with various conditions. Researchers have studied the GRFs sustained with every foot strike during running to investigate factors related to performance and running related injuries. The magnitude of the vertical component of the GRF during running is generally two to three times that of the runner's body weight, with the pattern of force sustained during

---

Moment of inertia The amount of force needed to overcome a body's or body part's present state of rotatory motion.

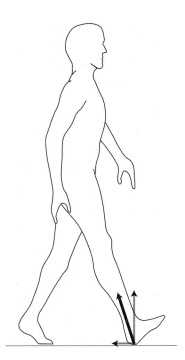

FIGURE 9–6. Ground reaction forces with horizontal, vertical, and resultant components during walking.

ground contact varying with running style. Runners are classified as rearfoot, midfoot, or forefoot strikers, according to the portion of the shoe first making contact with the ground. Typical vertical GRF patterns for rearfoot strikers are shown in Fig. 9–6. Factors influencing GRF patterns include running speed, running style, ground surface, and grade of incline.[12] The running shoes worn and the use of orthotics are other factors that can affect GRF patterns.[13]

Overstriding can be counterproductive. GRFs with larger retarding horizontal components are generated. Also, with longer strides, muscles crossing the knee absorb more of the shock that is transmitted upward through the musculoskeletal system, which may translate to additional stress being placed on the knees.[14]

The following questions are addressed during the observation of running gait..[9] Specific instances may be evaluated using the forms presented earlier in this chapter.

1. Does the body appear to glide across the surface with minimal upward and downward motion?
2. Does flexion at the hip, knee, and ankle vary appropriately with the intended speed of the run?
3. Does the support leg fully extend at takeoff?
4. Does the foot land directly under the body?
5. Does the trunk lean slightly forward in level-surface running?
6. Do the arms swing slightly toward the midline of the body with bent elbows and in opposition with the legs?
7. Does the patient eliminate any exaggerated rotary or twisting action around the trunk and hips?
8. Does the cadence sound symmetrical?

 PATHOLOGIES AFFECTING THE GAIT CYCLE

With an understanding of the events that occur during the normal gait cycle, now it is possible to examine pathological gait. Using the Ranchos Los Amigos gait sheet and key analysis questions cited earlier, the presence or absence of the critical events in the gait cycle can be determined. When preparing for your analysis, refer to the observational analysis guidelines cited earlier.

Evaluation of gait after an injury or surgical procedure is often complicated because people compensate for a dysfunction. Because the body is a kinetic chain system, other parts of the body appear to be dysfunctional as they assume compensatory roles (Box 9–3). These deviations result without conscious effort by the patient. Rather, they represent the body's protecting itself after injury or from further injury. These observations must not be a substitute for a complete examination of the involved areas.

ACUTE LOWER EXTREMITY STRAINS AND SPRAINS

In general, if an athlete is limping off to the sidelines with the majority of weight bearing on the toes or ball of the foot, the person has most likely injured the structures surrounding the knee joint. Injury to the knee ligaments or surrounding musculature usually results in an absence of initial contact by the heel, making it possible to avoid terminal knee extension, a position that usually exacerbates pain during gait. It also significantly shortens the stance phase on the injured side.

A varus, or lateral, thrust, in which the knee joint opens or bows laterally during stance phase, has been described in patients with combination posterior cruciate and lateral collateral ligament tears.[15] Patients with anterior cruciate ligament (ACL) tears have altered gait patterns as well.[16] These patients have larger maximum impact forces while running when compared with those of healthy runners. They also exhibit a greater extensor torque at the hip and ankle and a reduced extensor torque at the knee during the stance phase of running.[17] In an apparent attempt to stabilize the knee, increased hamstring activity and reduced quadriceps activity are also produced by patients with ACL tears.[18,19] Surgical intervention causes patients to walk in a more flexed knee and hip position, particularly at initial contact and mid stance.[16,20] However, shortly after surgery, the overly flexed walking pattern begins to recover significantly to what is was before surgery.

A flat-footed gait most likely indicates an ankle sprain or gastrocnemius or soleus strain. Usually, an absence of initial contact with the heel is observed. Athletes often move the center of gravity quickly over the foot, making contact with a flat foot instead. Plantarflexion at the ankle is avoided in the terminal stance and preswing phases as the limb is quickly brought

Box 9–3
COMPENSATORY GAIT DEVIATIONS

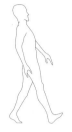

Gluteus maximus gait
At initial contact, the thorax is thrust posteriorly to maintain hip extension during the stance phase, often causing a lurching of the trunk.
Cause: Weakness or paralysis of the gluetus maximus muscle.

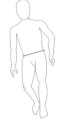

Trendelenburg's gait (gluteus medius gait)
During the stance phase of the affected limb, the thorax lists toward the involved limb. This serves to maintain the center of gravity and prevent a drop in the pelvis on the affected side.
Cause: Weakness of the gluteus medius muscle.

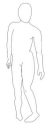

Psoatic limp
To compensate during the swing phase, lateral rotation and flexion of the trunk occurs with hip adduction. The trunk and pelvic movements are exaggerated.
Cause: Weakness or *reflex inhibition* of the psoas major muscle (Legg-Perthes disease).

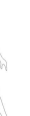
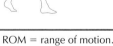

Steppage gait (dropfoot)
The foot slaps at initial contact, owing to foot drop. During the swing phase the affected limb demonstrates increased hip and knee flexion to avoid toe dragging, producing a "high-step" pattern.
Cause: Weakness or paralysis of the dorsiflexors.

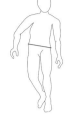

Stiff knee or hip gait
In the swing phase, the affected extremity is lifted higher than normal to compensate for knee or hip stiffness. To accomplish this, the uninvolved extremity demonstrates increased plantarflexion.
Cause: Knee or hip pathology that results in a decrease in the ROM.

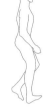

Calcaneal gait
During the stance phase, increased dorsiflexion and knee flexion occur on the affected side, resulting in a decreased step length.
Cause: Paralysis or weakness of the plantarflexors or painful weight bearing on the forefoot or toes.

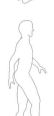

Short leg gait
Increased pronation occurs in the subtalar joint of the long leg, accompanied by a shift of the trunk toward the longer extremity.
Cause: True (anatomical) leg length discrepancy; the right (facing) leg is longer.

ROM = range of motion.

into swing phase. Shortening the stance phase helps keep weight bearing to a minimum. In addition, because the body is a kinetic chain system, the examiner may also note compensatory reactions to the knee and hip motion, trunk lean, arm swing, and possibly to motions of the uninvolved limb. Adductor strains usually result in a gait with an internally rotated hip; slightly flexed knee; slightly plantarflexed ankle; and limitations in hip extension, a result of muscle guarding of the adductor group. These positions at the hip and knee keep the adductors from being placed on stretch; the plantarflexion exhibited at the ankle is a compensatory reaction to the hip and knee motion. A shortened stance phase is observed on the involved limb with the possibility of associated motions at the trunk, arms, and uninvolved limb.

OVERUSE INJURIES

Overuse injuries such as iliotibial (IT) band syndrome, medial tibial stress syndrome (MTSS), Achilles tendinitis, and peroneal tendinitis also cause deviations in gait (Table 9–2). When pain is present, a gait limitation will occur. For example, when pain is experienced with MTTS, an examiner may note a quick move from dorsiflexion to plantarflexion in the stance phase. This is in an attempt to decrease the eccentric stress on the tibialis

Reflex inhibition A reflex arc prohibiting the contraction of a specific muscle or muscle group (term is discussed in Box 9–3)

Table 9–2
EFFECTS OF PREDISPOSING CONDITIONS ON THE STANCE PHASE OF THE GAIT CYCLE

Pathology	Initial Contact	Loading Response	Midstance	Terminal Stance
Decreased dorsiflexion		Increased subtalar pronation Forefoot abduction		Decreased ability to toe-off Premature heel rise
Decreased motion: first MTP joint		Increased midtarsal joint pronation		Decreased ability to toe-off Premature heel rise
Extrinsic leg or thigh muscle weakness		Altered position	Increased subtalar joint pronation Increased tibial rotation Inability to supinate	Incomplete resupination Decreased ability to toe-off
Hip rotator muscle weakness		Toe-out gait	Increased rotation of femur and tibia	
Neurologic impairment	Inability to dorsiflex	Multiple compensatory changes		Inability to plantarflex
Rearfoot valgus	Increased subtalar pronation Increased medial leg or foot stresses	Excessive pronation	Impaired resupination	Incomplete resupination with decreased force at toe-off
Rearfoot varus	Decreased shock absorption	Decreased subtalar pronation: Heel approaching the vertical position	Decreased ability to accommodate to uneven surfaces	Decreased ability to supinate
Hypomobile first ray	Altered midfood and forefoot position	Instability in midtarsal joints and forefoot	Altered distribution of ground reaction forces	Pain or decreased force at toe-off
Plantarflexed first ray	First ray contacts the ground	Decreased subtalar pronation	Decreased ability to absorb shock	Increased force on first ray
Forefoot varus		Toe-out gait	Increased pronation	
Forefoot valgus		Decreased ability to absorb shock	Decreased subtalar joint motion	Decreased force at toe-off
Tarsal coalition			Decreased subtalar joint motion	
Tibial torsion		Increased compensatory subtalar joint pronation		
Femoral torsion			Toe-in gait	
Leg length discrepancy		Increased subtalar joint pronation secondary to internal tibial rotation Compensatory pronation of the longer leg with compensatory supination of the shorter leg		
Rapid or prolonged pronation of subtalar joint		Increased medial foot or leg forces Increased internal tibial rotation		Decreased ability to toe-off

MTP = metatarsophalangeal.

posterior muscle as it attempts to eccentrically control pronation during the stance phase. Patients with peroneal tendinitis may avoid supination during the initial contact phase and exhibit contact on the medial heel to decrease the eccentric stress on the ankle everters. Achilles tendinitis causes a flat-footed gait with an early lift off to avoid stretching the tendon as the ankle goes into dorsiflexion and plantarflexion during terminal stance and preswing.

LEG LENGTH DISCREPANCIES

Anatomical asymmetry between the right and left lower extremities greater than 0.5 inches often results in gait problems caused by pronation of the longer limb and supination of the shorter limb (see Fig. 3–8). A significant increase in GRFs and lower extremity joint angles occurred after a heel lift was inserted on the shorter leg. Increases were observed in the maximum vertical forces for both legs with the lift present. A significant increase in maximum side-to-side (medial) force was found for the short leg, in both no-lift and lift conditions.[21] Such medial and lateral differences indicate compensatory mechanisms acting to stabilize the body during ambulation. Patients with leg length discrepancies often exhibit an asymmetrical gait pattern with the shorter leg's spending less time in the stance phase. These discrepancies may create an abnormal sounding cadence during the gait cycle.

FUNCTIONAL BRACING

Applying a brace to a leg with an ACL injury significantly reduces rotation during low load athletic maneuvers such as running. Unfortunately, many patients do not wear their brace when running because they claim it is too cumbersome. Wearing a functional knee brace increases knee flexion just before initial contact in walking, and hip extensor and ankle plantarflexor torques during running. Even when tested on uninjured individuals, a functional knee brace can cause individuals to perform with the same kinetics and energy demands as those observed in ACL-injured patients.[17,18] Wearing a brace does have consequences. Some ACL braces can weigh up to 2 lbs, and the added weight increases energy consumption that could have an impact on the endurance of the limb. Also, by reducing its energy reserves, use of the brace could place the limb at risk for re-injury during a sporting event.[19]

The effect of tape and orthoses application at the ankle has been studied for changes in ROM, strength and functional performance.[22] Taping and bracing may affect the available ROM at the ankle and theoretically alter functional activity.[23] Vertical jumping height with the ankle taped or braced may decrease if there are restrictions of dorsiflexion and plantarflexion at the ankle.[24,25] Taping and bracing that allow near normal dorsiflexion and plantarflexion, even if they restrict inversion, do not adversely effect performance of functional activities such as jumping, running, and agility drills.[26,27]

REFERENCES

1. Steindler, A: *Kinesiology of the Human Body Under Normal and Pathological Conditions*. Charles C. Thomas, Springfield, 1955.
2. Nuber, GW: Biomechanics of the foot and ankle during gait. *Clin Sports Med*, 7:1, 1988.
3. Knudson, DV, and Morrison, CS: *Qualitative Analysis of Human Movement*. Champaign, IL Human Kinetics, 1997.
4. Adrian, MJ, and Cooper, JM: *Biomechanics of Human Movement*, ed 2. Dubuque, IA, WCB Brown & Benchmark, 1995.
5. Murray, MP: Walking patterns of men with Parkinsonism. *Am J Phys Med*, 57:278–294, 1978.
6. *Normal and Abnormal Gait Syllabus*. Physical Therapy Department, Rancho Los Amigos Hospital, Downey, CA, 1989.
7. Root, ML, Orient, WP, and Weed, JH: Normal and abnormal function of the foot. *Clinical Biomechanics*, vol II. Los Angeles, Clinical Biomechanics Corp, 1977.
8. Donatelli, R, et al: Biomechanical foot orthotics: A retrospective study. *J Orthop Sports Phys Ther*, 10:205, 1988.
9. Phillip, JA, and Wilkerson, JD: *Teaching Team Sports: A Coeducational Approach*. Champaign, IL, Human Kinetics, 1990.
10. Slocum, D, and James, S: Biomechanics of running. *JAMA*, 205:97–104, 1968.
11. Donatelli, R: *The Biomechanics of the Foot and Ankle*, ed 2. Philadelphia, FA Davis, 1996.
12. Cavanagh PR, and Lafortune MA: Ground reaction forces in distance running. *J Bio*, 13:397, 1980.
13. Putnam, CA, and Kozey, JW: Substantive issues in running. In Vaughan CL (ed): *Biomechanics of Sport*. Boca Raton, FL, CRC Press, 1989.
14. Derrick, TR, Hamill, J, and Caldwell, GE: Energy absorption of impacts during running at various stride lengths. *Med Sci Sports Exerc*, 30:128, 1998.
15. Barrett, G: Posterior cruciate ligament: Anatomy, diagnosis, surgical treatment. Presented at the Annual Symposium of the Southeast Athletic Trainers' Association, Atlanta, GA, April 1, 2000.
16. Ernst, GP, et al: Lower extremity compensations following anterior cruciate ligament reconstruction. *Phys Ther*, 80:251, 2000.
17. DeVita, P, Blankenship, P, and Skelly, W: Effects of a functional knee brace on the biomechanics of running. *Med Sci Sports Exerc*, 24:797–806, 1992.
18. De Vita, P, Torry, M, Glover, K, and Speroni, D: A functional knee brace alters joint torque and power patterns during walking and running. *J Biomechanics*, 29:583–588, 1996.
19. Branch, T, and Hunter, R: Functional analysis of anterior cruciate ligament braces. *Clin Sports Med*, 9:771–797, 1992.
20. DeVita, P, et al: Gait adaptations before and after anterior cruciate ligament reconstruction surgery. *Med Sci in Sports and Exerc*, 853–859, 1997.
21. Schuit, D: The effects of heel lifts on ground reaction force patterns and lower extremity joint angles in subjects with structural leg length discrepancies. PhD dissertation, University of Illinois at Urbana-Champaign, IL, 1988.
22. Ryan, J, and Krajewski, P: Ankle taping and orthoses: A review of the literature. *J Back Musculoskel Rehabil*, 2:63, 1992.
23. McIntyre, DR, Smith, MA, and Denniston, NL: The effectiveness of strapping techniques during prolonged dynamic exercises. *Athletic Training*; 18:52, 1983.
24. Juvenal, JP: The effects of ankle taping on vertical jumping ability. *Athletic Training*, 7:146, 1972.
25. Mayhew, JL: Effects of ankle taping on motor performance. *Athletic Training*, 7:10, 1972.
26. Wiley, JP, and Nigg, BM. The effect of an ankle orthosis on ankle range of motion and performance. *J Orthop Sports Phys Ther*, 23:362, 1996.
27. Gross, MT, et al: Effect of ankle orthoses on functional performance for individuals with recurrent lateral ankle sprains. *J Orthop Sports Phys Ther*, 25:245, 1997.

C H A P T E R

10

The Thoracic and Lumbar Spine

Formed by 33 vertebral segments and divided into four distinct portions, the spinal column and its associated muscles provide postural control to the torso and skull, while also protecting the spinal cord. The contradictory needs for range of motion (ROM) versus protection of the spinal cord are met in varying degrees throughout the various regions of the spine (Fig. 10–1).

The cervical spine provides the greatest ROM, but here the spinal cord is the most vulnerable. The thoracic spine provides the greatest protection of the spinal cord but does so at the expense of ROM. The

lumbar spine provides a more equal balance between protection of the spinal cord and available ROM. The sacrum and coccyx are composed of fused bone. The sacrum functions to affix the spinal column to the pelvis and serve as a site for muscle attachment. At this level, the spinal cord has exited the column.

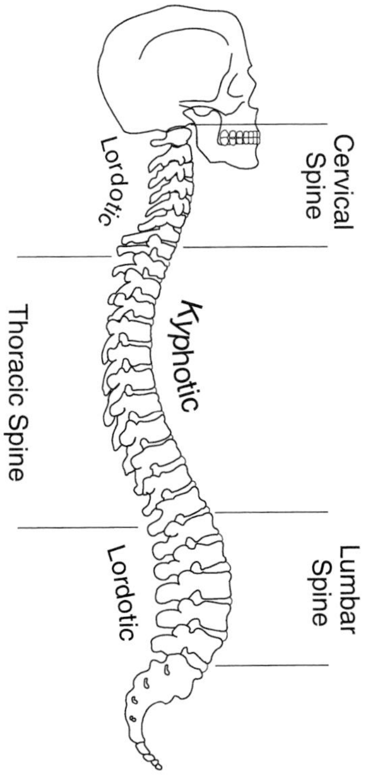

Injury to the spine during athletic competition accounts for an estimated 10 to 15 percent of all spinal injuries, with 6 to 10 percent of these injuries resulting in trauma to the spinal cord or spinal nerve roots.[1] In the general population, 60 to 80 percent of people experience back pain during their lives that is sufficient enough to seek medical attention.[1] This chapter discusses conditions affecting the spine that are most likely to be evaluated away from practice and competition. On-field recognition and management of cervical, thoracic, and lumbar spinal injuries are discussed in Chapter 18.

◆ CLINICAL ANATOMY

Figure 10–2 compares the relative sizes of the cervical (n = 7), thoracic (n = 12), and lumbar (n = 5) vertebrae and identifies the bony landmarks. The body's weight is transmitted primarily along the spinal column via the vertebral body, whose size is related to the amount of force it transmits. Carrying only the weight of the head, the vertebral bodies of the cervical vertebrae are much smaller than those of the lumbar vertebrae, which are required to transmit and absorb the weight of the entire torso.

BONY ANATOMY

The **neural arch,** formed by the pedicle and lamina on each side, serves as the protective tunnel through which the spinal cord passes. The laterally projecting **transverse processes** provide an attachment site for the spine's intrinsic ligaments and muscles, increasing the muscles' mechanical leverage. The prominent posterior

FIGURE 10–1. The three segments of the mobile spinal column with their normal curvature noted.

319

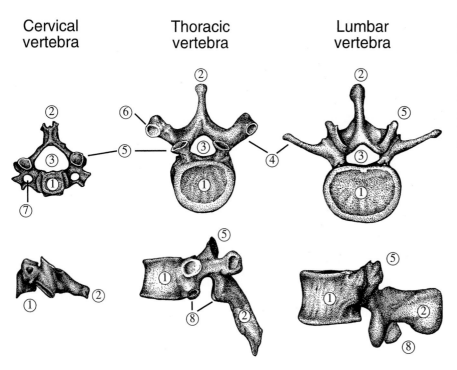

Cervical vertebra

Thoracic vertebra

Lumbar vertebra

FIGURE 10–2. Comparative anatomy of the cervical, thoracic, and lumbar spine. Note the presence of a "Scotty dog" in the lateral view of the lumbar vertebra. (1) Vertebral body, (2) spinous process, (3) vertebral foramen, (4) transverse process, (5) superior articular facet, (6) costotransverse facet, (7) transverse foramen, (8) inferior articular facet.

projections, the **spinous processes,** act as attachment sites for muscles and ligaments. Their angulation relative to the other vertebrae serves to limit extension of the spine.

Two sets of articular processes arise from the superior and inferior surfaces of the lamina. The vertebrae's superior facets articulate with the inferior facets of the vertebrae immediately above, forming synovial *facet joints* (zygapophyseal joints). The bony arrangement of these joints is such that the lateral portion of the superior facet articulates with the medial portion of the inferior facet. These joints contribute significantly to spinal motion and decrease the weight-bearing stress through the vertebral body and disc by creating two additional areas for load transmission. The facet joints, transmit-

ting 20 percent of the weight-bearing forces through the spine, significantly contribute to load transmission.[2] The area between the superior and inferior facets of a vertebra, the **pars interarticularis,** is a common site of stress fractures in the lumbar spine.

The anterior portions of each pedicle contain vertebral notches, concave depressions along the inferior surfaces and superior portions of the bone. The vertebral notch on the inferior portion of one pedicle is matched with the vertebral notch on the superior portion of the pedicle below, forming the **intervertebral foramen,** the space where spinal nerve roots exit the vertebral column (Fig. 10–3).

The relative sizes of the vertebral body and the transverse and spinous processes vary according to their function at each of the spinal levels (Table 10–1). The cervical spine, the most mobile of the vertebral segments, has the smallest vertebral bodies. Refer to Chapter 11 for a description of the cervical spine.

In the thoracic segment of the spinal column, the vertebral bodies begin to widen and thicken to assist in managing the weight of the torso. The spinous processes project downward to limit extension and provide a strong attachment site for the thoracic muscles and ligaments. The transverse processes thicken to articulate with the ribs forming the **costotransverse joints** in ribs one through 10. Ribs 11 and 12 do not articulate with the transverse processes, so these joints do not exist at these levels. In addition to articulating with the

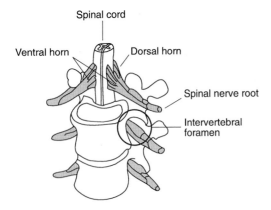

Spinal cord

Ventral horn

Dorsal horn

Spinal nerve root

Intervertebral foramen

FIGURE 10–3. Nerve roots exiting between the vertebrae. The pedicle of the superior and inferior vertebrae align to form the intervertebral foramen, allowing the spinal nerves to exit the vertebral column.

Facet joints An articulation of the facets between each contiguous part of vertebrae in the spinal column.

Table 10–1
STRUCTURAL ADAPTATIONS OF VERTEBRAL ANATOMY AT THE DIFFERENT SPINAL LEVELS

	Bony Anatomy			
Level	**Vertebral Body**	**Transverse Process**	**Spinous Process**	**Facet Joints**
Cervical	Small; view in the frontal plane is wider than in the sagittal plane. Vertebral body is absent in C1; the remaining bodies progressively increase in size.	Short; processes contain the transverse foramen for passage of the vertebral artery.	Small and short, except for C7, which has characteristics of a thoracic vertebra.	C0 and C1: Ellipsoid joint C1 and C2: Positioned in the transverse plane C3 to C7: Approximately 45° from transverse plane in the frontal plane
Thoracic	Diameter and thickness increase as the spine continues inferiorly. Demifacets are present to accept the head of the ribs.	Solid configuration allows for the attachment of muscles and costo-vertebral ligaments. The processes of T1 through T12 have articular surfaces for the ribs.	Long and slender; their downward projections result in an overlap of spinous process of the vertebra below; the spinous processes of the lower thoracic vertebrae gradually thicken and straighten to resemble those of the lumbar vertebrae.	Oblique, but lying primarily in the frontal plane
Lumbar	Vertebral bodies are broad in both the frontal and sagittal planes.	Long for leverage; thin in the cross section.	The superior borders are posteriorly projected with a large inferior flare.	The facet joints of L1 through L3 are located in the sagittal plane; the facets of L4 and L5 are frontally oriented.

transverse processes, a **costovertebral joint** is formed between each rib and the vertebral bodies. The joints formed on the T1 and T10 through T12 vertebral levels articulate with a single rib on each side. The remaining ribs articulate with two vertebrae at the **superior costal** and **inferior costal facets** and the associated interverte-bral disc on each side.

Molded by five fused vertebrae, the sacrum is a broad, thick, triangular bone that fixates the spinal column to the pelvis and is responsible for stabilizing the pelvic girdle (Fig. 10–4). The weight of the torso and skull is transmitted through the **sacroiliac (SI) joints** to the lower extremity. Ground reaction forces from the lower extremities are transmitted through the SI joints up the spinal column.

The sacrum's laterally projecting articular surfaces have an irregular shape that, when matched to the iliac's facets, form the very stable SI joint. Its anterior and posterior surfaces are roughened to permit firm at-tachment of muscles acting on the femur and pelvis. Four pairs of foramina perforate the bone to permit the passage of the dorsal and ventral primary divisions of the nerves of the sacral plexus from their posterior ori-gin into the pelvic cavity.

Lumbarization occurs when the first sacral vertebra fails to unite with the remainder of the sacrum, forming a separate vertebra having characteristics similar to those of the lumbar spine, essentially becoming a sixth lumbar vertebra. **Sacralization,** on the other hand, occurs when

the fifth lumbar vertebra becomes fused to the sacrum (Fig. 10–5). This may occur unilaterally or bilaterally, re-sulting in complete fusion of these segments. Except for radiographic diagnosis, these conditions are virtually un-detectable and typically asymptomatic. However, pa-tients may demonstrate decreased lumbar ROM.

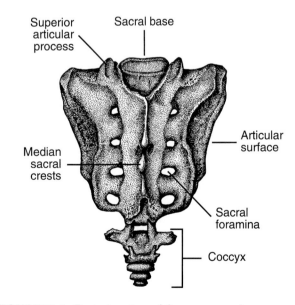

FIGURE 10–4. Posterior view of the sacrum and coccyx.

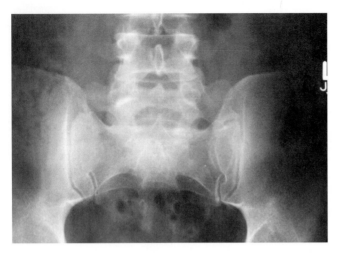

FIGURE 10–5. Sacralized L5 vertebrae. The L5 and S1 vertebra are fused together.

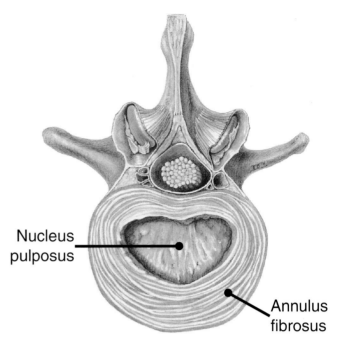

FIGURE 10–6. Illustration of an intervertebral disc. The firm, outer annulus fibrosus surrounds the pliable nucleus pulposus.

The distal end of the spinal column is formed by the **coccyx.** Formed by the fusion of three or four rudimentary bony pieces, the coccyx provides an attachment site for some of the muscles of the pelvic floor and, sometimes, portions of the gluteus maximus.

INTERVERTEBRAL DISCS

Found in varying thicknesses between the cervical, thoracic, and lumbar vertebrae, intervertebral discs act to increase the total ROM available to the spinal column. The discs also serve as shock absorbers of longitudinal and rotational stresses placed on the column through compression. Each disc is formed by a tough, dense outer layer, the **annulus fibrosus,** surrounding a flexible inner layer, the **nucleus pulposus** (Fig. 10–6).

Twenty-three intervertebral discs are found along the spinal column. No disc is found between the skull and the first cervical vertebra (C0–C1) or between the first and second cervical vertebrae (C1–C2). Individual discs are referenced by the vertebrae between which they are found. For instance, the disc located between the fourth and fifth lumbar vertebrae is known as the L4–L5 intervertebral disc.

The annulus fibrosus consists of multilayered fibers that cross from opposite directions, forming an X pattern. This arrangement leaves some portion of the disc taut regardless of the position of the vertebral column and increases the overall strength of the tissue. When viewed in cross-section, the annulus fibrosus is thinner posteriorly than anteriorly. A vertebral endplate, an expanse of fibrocartilage from the annulus fibrosus, inserts on the vertebra above and below to secure the disc to the spinal column.

The core of the disc, the nucleus pulposus, is a highly elastic, semigelatinous substance that is 60 to 70 percent

water.[3] The high water content makes the nucleus pulposus resistant to being compressed while still allowing it to be deformable. During the course of the day, the nucleus pulposus becomes dehydrated from the body weight placed on it, compressing water out of its core. During sleep or other long periods of reclining, the compressive forces placed on the discs are eliminated, allowing the nucleus pulposus to become rehydrated. Physical activity such as running compresses the intervertebral discs between T7–L1 and L5–S1, resulting in a decreased ROM in the lumbar spine after activity.[4]

Permanent dehydration also occurs through the aging process. Until the age of approximately 40 years, the disc is fully hydrated. After this age, dehydration begins. By age 60 years, the discs have reached their maximum state of dehydration, resulting in decreased ROM and a slight narrowing of the intervertebral foramen.[5]

The annulus fibrosus and the posterior longitudinal ligament are richly innervated by sensory nerves.[6] This nerve supply can account for much of the pain associated with disc degeneration or herniation. This type of pain is referred to as **discogenic pain.**

The amount of stress placed on the lumbar intervertebral discs is influenced by the position of the trunk. In the supine position, the disc is under a load of approximately 75 kg of pressure. When an individual stands up, the load increases to 100 kg. When sitting and leaning forward, the total load increases to 275 kg.[7]

FIGURE 10–7. Accessory vertebral motions. In addition to the cardinal spinal movements of flexion and extension, rotation, and lateral bending, the facet joints allow for anterior and posterior translation, lateral translation, and compression and distraction of contiguous vertebrae.

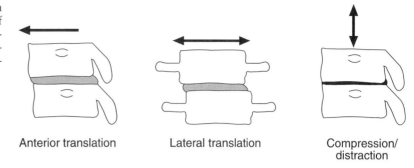

Anterior translation   Lateral translation   Compression/distraction

ARTICULATIONS AND LIGAMENTOUS ANATOMY

The spinal column allows for three degrees of freedom of movement: (1) flexion and extension, (2) rotation, and (3) tilting, resulting in lateral bending. The accessory motions occurring at the facet joints allowing these physiologic motions to occur include (1) anterior and posterior glide, or flexion; (2) lateral glide, or extension; and (3) compression and distraction, or side bending and rotation (Fig. 10–7). The amount of movement between any two vertebrae is rather limited, but the sum of these motions provides a large amount of ROM for the spinal column as a whole.

The articulation between each pair of vertebrae is formed by cartilaginous and synovial joints. The union between an intervertebral disc and the superior and inferior vertebrae forms the *cartilaginous joint,* and the facet joints represent the synovial articulations. The exception to this is the joint formed between the first and second cervical vertebrae.

The entire length of the spinal column is reinforced by the **anterior and posterior longitudinal ligaments** (Fig. 10–8). The broader, thicker anterior longitudinal ligament (ALL) spans the length of the vertebral column from the occiput to the sacrum, attaching to both the vertebral bodies and the intervertebral discs. The fibrous arrangement of this ligament strengthens the anterior portion of the intervertebral discs and vertebrae, functioning to limit extension of the spine and is the thinnest in the lumbar spine.

The posterior longitudinal ligament (PLL) originates from the occiput as a thick structure but gradually thins as it progresses down the vertebral column. Lining the anterior portion of the vertebral canal, the PLL fans out and thickens as it passes over the intervertebral discs, only attaching to their margins to allow the passage of blood vessels. This ligament serves primarily to limit flexion of the spine.

Running the length of the spinal column, the **supraspinous ligament** attaches to the posterior apex of each spinous process. In the cervical spine, the supraspinous ligament becomes the **ligamentum nuchae.** Two ligaments are intrinsic to the adjoining vertebrae. Filling the space formed between the spinous processes, the **interspinous ligaments** limit flexion and rotation of the spine. The posterior margin of the vertebral canal is formed by the **ligamentum flavum,** a pair of elastic ligaments connecting the lamina of one vertebra to the lamina of the vertebra above it. The ligamentum flavum reinforces the facet joints, and its unusual elastic property assists the trunk in returning from flexion to the neutral position.

Sacroiliac Joint

A series of ligaments serve to bind the sacrum to the pelvis. The **interosseous sacroiliac ligaments** are formed by strong fibers spanning the anterior portion of the ilium and the posterior portion of the sacrum, filling the void behind the articular surfaces of these bones (Fig. 10–9). The anterior and posterior surfaces of the articulation are strengthened by the **dorsal and ventral sacroiliac ligaments.** The dorsal SI ligament is made of fibers that run transversely to join the ilium to the upper portion of the sacrum and vertical fibers connecting the lower sacrum to the posterior superior iliac spine (PSIS). Lining the anterior portion of the pelvic cavity, the ventral SI ligaments attach to the anterior

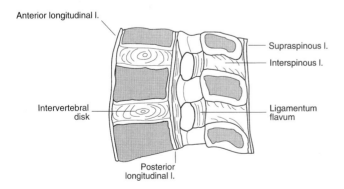

Anterior longitudinal l.
Intervertebral disk
Posterior longitudinal l.
Supraspinous l.
Interspinous l.
Ligamentum flavum

FIGURE 10–8. Cross-sectional view of the ligaments of the vertebral column.

Cartilaginous joint A relatively immobile joint in which two bones are fused by cartilage.

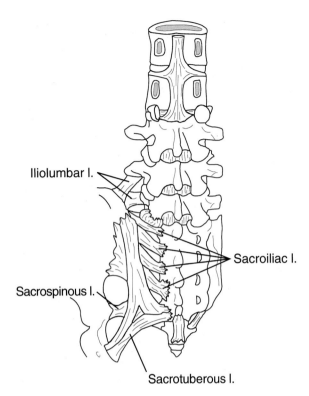

FIGURE 10–9. Posterior sacroiliac ligaments. The strong ligamentous configuration of the sacroiliac joint permits only slight movement.

RELATIONSHIP BETWEEN SPINAL AND VERTEBRAL SEGMENTS

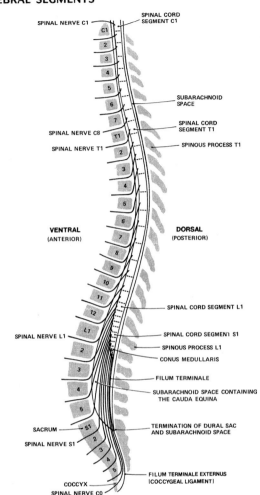

FIGURE 10–10. Relationship between the vertebrae and spinal nerve roots showing anatomical relationships.

portion of the sacrum. Two accessory ligaments assist in maintaining the stability of the SI joint. The **sacrotuberous ligament** arises from the ischial tuberosity to blend with the inferior fibers of the dorsal SI ligaments. Indirectly supporting the sacrum, the **sacrospinous ligament** originates from the sacrum's ischial spine and attaches to the coccyx.

The SI joints are more mobile in young individuals and become less mobile with age. In *postpartum* females, the stresses of athletics can injure the structurally weakened SI joints. At the time of birth, the hormone **relaxin** is released into the mother's system. Relaxin increases the extensibility of the ligamentous structures in and around the birth canal.[8] These hormones affect the ligaments of the SI joint, resulting in increased pelvic motion and increasing the risk of pathology at the SI joint.

LUMBAR AND SACRAL PLEXUS

A nerve plexus is best described as a network formed by a consecutive series of spinal nerves. These systems are formed by both *convergent* and *divergent* pathways, causing an intermixing of sensory and motor impulses. Although the root of a plexus may be supplied by one spinal nerve, the nerves exiting the plexus contain fibers from more than one spinal nerve root.[9]

A total of 31 pairs of nerve roots exit the spinal column (Fig 10–10). The thoracic and lumbar spine have a pair of nerves exiting below the corresponding vertebra (e.g., the T1 nerve root exits below the body of the first thoracic vertebra). There are 12 pairs of thoracic nerves and five pairs of lumbar nerves. Although there are seven cervical vertebrae, eight pairs of nerve roots exit in this area. The first seven cervical nerves exit above the vertebrae. The "odd" cervical nerve, C8, exits below the seventh cervical vertebra (between the seventh cervical and first thoracic vertebrae).

Postpartum	After childbirth.
Convergent	Two nerves combining together to form a single nerve.
Divergent	One nerve splitting to form two individual nerves.

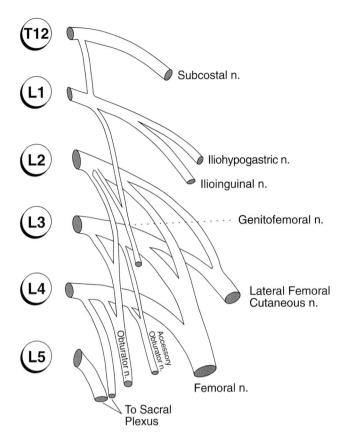

FIGURE 10–11. Lumbar plexus. Note that the lower portion of the lumbar plexus merges with the upper portion of the sacral plexus.

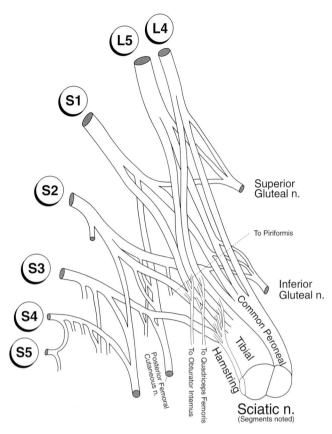

FIGURE 10–12. Sacral plexus. This nerve package supplies the lower leg, ankle, and foot through the tibial and common peroneal nerves.

Several pairs of nerve plexus are formed by the sacral, lumbar, thoracic, cervical, and cranial nerve roots. This chapter addresses the lumbar plexus and sacral plexus. The brachial plexus is described in Chapter 11, and the cranial plexus is presented in Chapter 18. Note that few texts agree on the actual nerve roots forming each plexus.

Lumbar Plexus

Formed by the twelfth thoracic nerve root and the L1 through L5 nerve roots, the lumbar plexus innervates the anterior and medial muscles of the thigh and the dermatomes of the medial leg and foot. The posterior branches of the L2, L3, and L4 nerve roots converge to form the **femoral nerve,** and their anterior branches merge to form the obturator nerve (Fig. 10–11).

Sacral Plexus

A portion of the L4 nerve root, the L5 nerve root, and the lumbosacral trunk courses downward to form the superior portion of the sacral plexus (Fig. 10–12). This plexus supplies the muscles of the buttocks and, through the sciatic nerve, innervates the muscles of the

posterior femur and the entire lower leg. The sciatic nerve can be conceptualized as having three distinct sections: (1) the **tibial nerve,** formed by the anterior branches of the upper five nerve roots; (2) the **common peroneal nerve,** formed by the posterior branches of the upper four nerve roots; and (3) a slip of the tibial nerve that innervates the hamstring muscles.

MUSCULAR ANATOMY

A complex network of muscles acts on the spinal column. These muscles, interwoven with the fibers of other muscles, function in an orchestrated manner to provide the support needed for static posture and the dynamic control needed for motion.

Two groups of muscles influence the movement of the spinal column. **Extrinsic muscles** primarily function to provide respiration and movement associated with the upper extremity and scapula, indirectly influencing the spinal column. **Intrinsic muscles** lie close to the spinal column and directly influence its motion.

No muscles act directly to affect the movement at the SI joint, but movement can be indirectly influenced

Table 10–2

EXTRINSIC MUSCLE ACTING ON THE SPINAL COLUMN

Muscle	Action	Origin	Insertion	Innervation	Root
Rectus abdominis	Flexion of the lumbar spine against gravity Posterior rotation of the pelvis	• Pubic crest • Pubic symphysis	• Costal cartilage of the 5th through 7th ribs • Xiphoid process of sternum	Ventral rami	T5–T12
External oblique	**Bilateral contraction:** Flexion of the lumbar spine Posterior rotation of the pelvis **Unilateral contraction:** Rotation of the lumbar spine to the opposite side Lateral bending of the lumbar spine to the same side	• 5th through 8th ribs (anterior fibers) • 9th through 12th ribs (lateral fibers)	• Via an aponeurosis to the linea alba (anterior fibers) • Anterior superior iliac spine, pubic tubercle, and the anterior portion of the iliac crest (lateral fibers)	Iliohypogastric Ilioinguinal Ventral rami	T1–T12
Internal oblique	**Bilateral contraction:** Support of the abdominal viscera Posterior rotation of the pelvis Flexion of the lumbar spine **Unilateral contraction:** Rotation of the lumbar spine to the same side Lateral bending of the lumbar spine to the same side	• Lateral two thirds of the inguinal ligament (lower fibers) • Anterior one third of the iliac crest (upper fibers) • Middle one third of the iliac crest (lateral fibers)	• Crest of pubis, pectineal line (lower fibers) • 10th through 12th ribs (lateral fibers) • Linea alba (all portions)	Iliohypogastric Ilioinguinal Ventral rami	T7–T12
Latissimus dorsi	Extension of the spine Anterior rotation of the pelvis (also see shoulder function) Stabilization of the lumbar spine via the thoracodorsal fascia	• Spinous processes of T6 through T12 and the lumbar vertebrae via the thoracodorsal fascia • Posterior iliac crest	• Intertubercular groove of the humerus	Thoracodorsal	C6, C7, C8
Trapezius (middle one third)	Retraction of scapula Fixation of thoracic spine	• Lower portion of the ligamentum nuchae • Spinous processes of the 7th cervical vertebra and T1 through T5	• Acromion process • Spine of the scapula (superior, lateral border)	Accessory	Cranial nerve XI
Trapezius (lower one third)	Depression of scapula Retraction of scapula Upward rotation of the scapula Fixation of thoracic spine	• Spinous processes and supraspinal ligaments of T8 through T12	• Spine of the scapula (medial portion)	Accessory	Cranial nerve XI
Rhomboid major	Retraction of scapula Elevation of scapula Downward rotation of scapula Fixation of thoracic spine	• Spinous processes of T2, T3, T4, and T5	• Vertebral border of scapula (lower two thirds)	Dorsal scapular	C5
Rhomboid minor	Retraction of scapula Elevation of scapula Downward rotation of scapula Fixation of thoracic spine	• Inferior portion of the ligamentum nuchae • Spinous processes C7 and T1	• Vertebral border of scapula (upper one third and superior angle)	Dorsal scapular	C5

Table 10–3
MOTIONS PRODUCED BY THE INTERNAL AND EXTERNAL OBLIQUE MUSCLES

Muscle	Bilateral Contraction	Unilateral Contraction
External oblique	Flexion of the lumbar spine Posterior pelvic rotation Compression of the abdominal viscera Depression of the thorax Assistance in respiration	Contralateral rotation of the trunk Ipsilateral lateral flexion of the trunk Rotation of the pelvis
Internal oblique	Flexion of the lumbar spine Compression of the abdominal viscera Depression of the thorax Assistance in respiration	Ipsilateral rotation of the trunk Ipsilateral lateral flexion of the trunk

through two means: (1) the muscles originating on the sacrum that function to control the hip joint and (2) any musculature attaching to the pelvic bones that can cause rotation of the pelvis.

Extrinsic Muscles

The posterior muscles acting on the spinal column are the **latissimus dorsi, levator scapulae, rhomboid major and minor,** and **trapezius.** Serving to connect the upper extremity to the axial skeleton, these muscles primarily influence humeral and scapular motion (Table 10–2). These muscles are described in Chapter 11.

Anteriorly and laterally, the rectus abdominis, internal oblique, and external oblique function to flex, rotate, or laterally bend the spinal column. The primary flexor of the spine, the **rectus abdominis** also influences spinal posture by rotating the pelvis posteriorly, flattening the lumbar spine. When the **internal and exter-**nal obliques on the same side of the trunk contract, the torso bends to that side. Contraction of the internal oblique and the external oblique muslces on the opposite side of the body result in the torso's rotating toward the side of the internal oblique muscle (Table 10–3). The **transverse abdominis** assists in stabilizing the lumbar spine by acting like a corset.

The muscles of the hip and pelvis, as described in Chapter 8, influence the spine by anteriorly or posteriorly rotating the pelvis and create a firm foundation or support for muscle attachment.

Intrinsic Muscles

The intrinsic spinal muscles are divided into superficial, intermediate, and deep layers (Fig. 10–13). The superficial layer of the lumbar and thoracic spine muscles is presented in Table 10–4 The intrinsic muscles acting on the cervical spine are discussed in Chapter 11.

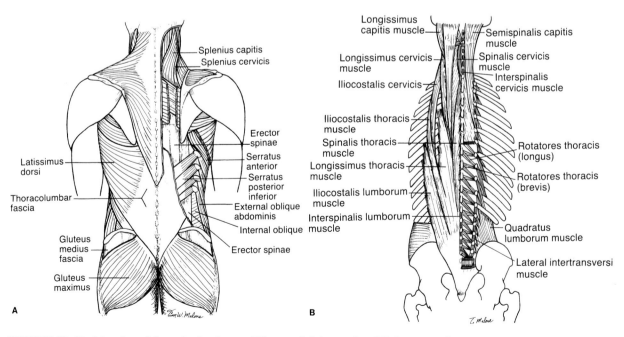

FIGURE 10–13. Muscles of the spinal column: **(A)** superficial muscles, **(B)** deep muscles.

Table 10–4
INTRINSIC MUSCLES ACTING ON THE SPINAL COLUMN

Muscle	Action	Origin	Insertion	Innervation	Root
Iliocostalis lumborum	**Bilateral contraction:** Extension of spinal column **Unilateral contraction:** Lateral bending of spinal column to the same side	• Posterior aspect of the iliac crest	• Inferior angles of ribs 6 through 12	Posterior primary divisions of the spinal nerves	Multiple roots, segmentally along the length of the muscle
Iliocostalis thoracis	**Bilateral contraction:** Extension of spinal column **Unilateral contraction:** Lateral bending of spinal column to the same side	• Ribs 6 though 12	• Ribs 1 through 6 • Transverse process of C7	Posterior primary divisions of the spinal nerves	Multiple roots, segmentally along the length of the muscle
Longissimus thoracis	**Bilateral contraction:** Extension of spinal column **Unilateral contraction:** Lateral bending of spinal column	• Common erector spinae tendon	• Transverse process of T3 through T21 • Ribs 3 through 12	Posterior primary divisions of the spinal nerves	Multiple roots, segmentally along the length of the muscle
Spinalis thoracis	**Bilateral contraction:** Extension of the spine **Unilateral contraction:** Lateral bending of the spine to the same side	• Common erector spinae tendon	• Spinous processes of upper thoracic spine	Posterior primary divisions of the spinal nerves	Multiple roots, segmentally along the length of the muscle
Semispinalis thoracis	**Bilateral contraction:** Extension of thoracic and cervical spine **Unilateral contraction:** Rotation to the opposite side	• Transverse process	• Travel upwardly and medially to attach to a spinous process 5 or 8 vertebrae above the origin	Posterior primary divisions of the spinal nerves	Multiple roots, segmentally along the length of the muscle
Multifidus (or multifidi)	**Bilateral contraction:** Stabilization of vertebral column **Unilateral contraction:** Rotation of spine to the opposite side	Lumbar region • Superior aspect of sacrum Thoracic region • Transverse processes Cervical region • Articular processes	• Spinous process	Posterior primary divisions of the spinal nerves	Multiple roots, segmentally along the length of the muscle
Rotatores	**Bilateral contraction:** Extension of spine Stabilization of vertebral column **Unilateral contraction:** Rotation of spine	• Transverse process	• Spinous process of the vertebra immediately above the origin	Posterior primary divisions of the spinal nerves	Multiple roots, segmentally along the length of the muscle

Forming the intermediate layer of the intrinsic muscles, the **erector spinae** is composed of three pairs of muscles; from lateral to medial, these are the **iliocostalis**, the **longissimus**, and the **spinalis**. Each of these muscles is then divided into three individual elements, the iliocostalis, formed by the **lumborum, thoracis**, and **cervicis** portions; and the longissimus and spinalis muscles, consisting of the **thoracis, cervicis,** and **capitis** portions. Small bundles of muscle fibers overlap to the point that every vertebra and rib has both a muscular attachment and insertion on it. The erector spinae muscle group is the primary mover for spinal extension and controls the rate of spinal flexion against gravity through eccentric contractions. The erector spinae group also assists in the movements of lateral flexion and rotation of the trunk.

The deep intrinsic layer is collectively known as **transversospinal muscles** because the fibers run from one transverse process to the spinous process superior to them.[10] Individually, this group is formed by the **semispinalis, multifidus,** and **rotatores** muscles. The multifide muscles play an important role in the dynamic, segmental stabilization of the lumbar spine.

The semispinalis muscle is divided into **thoracis, cervicis,** and **capitis** segments. These muscles act primarily to contralaterally rotate the spinal column, especially above the lumbar level. They also contribute slightly to spinal extension and ipsilateral lateral flexion.

 ## CLINICAL EVALUATION OF THE THORACIC AND LUMBAR SPINE

Because of its important role in protecting the spinal cord and spinal nerve roots, injury to the vertebrae can have catastrophic results. In acute trauma, the primary role of the initial evaluation is to rule out the presence of trauma that has, or can, jeopardize the integrity of the spinal cord or nerve roots. Chapter 18 discusses these evaluative procedures. Many spinal pain syndromes are associated with improper foot mechanics, muscular tightness of the lower extremity, and imbalances of the pelvic and abdominal muscles (see Chapter 3).[11] The techniques presented in this chapter assume that significant vertebral fractures or dislocations have been ruled out.

HISTORY

Pain produced during activities of daily living (ADLs) provides valuable information about the cause of the pain and other activities that may reproduce or decrease the pain (Table 10–5). Pain that occurs during certain times of the day can indicate a postural position that irritates the involved nerve root (or roots) or other soft tissue structures.

- **Location of the pain:** Pain radiating into the extremity or peripheral paresthesia or numbness is the re-

Table 10–5
RAMIFICATIONS OF SPINAL PAIN EXHIBITED DURING THE ACTIVITIES OF DAILY LIVING

Activity	Ramifications
Bending	Pain may be initially worsened with flexion exercises.
Sitting	Pain may be initially worsened with flexion exercises.
Rising from sitting	This motion causes changes in the interdiscal forces. Sharp pain suggests derangement of the disc.
Standing	The spine is placed in extension. Pain may be initially experienced with extension exercises.
Walking	The amount of spinal extension increases as the speed of gait increases.
Lying prone	The spine is placed in or near full extension.
Lying supine	When lying supine on a hard surface, the amount of extension is maintained. When lying on a soft surface, the spine falls into flexion.

sult of impingement or pressure on a nerve root exiting the intervertebral foramen or dural irritation proximal to the site of pain. Unlike other anatomical areas, low back pain is often ambigious as to the exact location and underlying cause of the pain.[12] Sacroiliac pathology usually causes pain around the PSIS of the affected side or radiating into the hip and groin. Spasm of the piriformis muscle can replicate the symptoms of sciatic nerve dysfunction.

- **Onset of the pain:** The patient's description of the onset of the pain, such as a description of acute, chronic, or insidious onset of pain, along with other symptoms is important. Although patients may describe a single incident that acutely initiated the pain, the trauma is probably an accumulation of repetitive stresses and macrotrauma developed during the episode described.

- **Mechanism of injury:** Any known mechanism of injury (e.g., flexion, extension, lateral bending, or rotation) can be used to possibly identify the involved structures. A direct blow to the lumbar or thoracic area may cause a contusion of the involved structures, the kidneys, or other internal organs. Sports (e.g., gymnastics, blocking in football, cheerleading) in which the spine is regularly placed in hyperextension place increased compressive stress on the pars interarticularis and other posterior spinal structures. Offensive linemen in football place enormous compressive and shear forces on the lumbar spine and therefore are particularly predisposed to injury.[13] Frequently, patients are unable to identify a specific episode of injury.

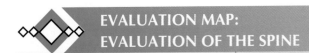

EVALUATION MAP: EVALUATION OF THE SPINE

1. HISTORY

Location of the pain
Onset of the pain
Mechanism of injury
Consistency of the pain
Paresthesia
Activities or positions that alter the
    level of symptoms
Bowel or bladder signs
History of spinal injury

2. INSPECTION

General inspection
    Frontal curvature
        Test for scoliosis
    Sagittal curvature
        Lordotic and kyphotic curves
    Observation of gait
    Skin markings

Thoracic spine
    Breathing patterns
    Bilateral comparison of skinfolds

Lumbar spine
    General movement and posture
    Lordotic curve
    Standing posture

3. PALPATION

Thoracic spine
    Spinous processes
    Supraspinous ligaments
    Costovertebral junction
    Trapezius
    Scapular muscles
    Paravertebral muscles

Lumbar spine
    Spinous processes
    Step-off deformity
    Paravertebral muscles

Sacrum and pelvis
    Median sacral crests
    Iliac crests
    Posterior superior iliac spine
    Gluteals
    Ischial tuberosity
    Greater trochanter
    Sacral nerve
    Pubic symphysis

4. RANGE OF MOTION TESTS

AROM
    Flexion
    Extension
    Lateral bending
    Rotation

PROM
    Flexion
    Extension
    Rotation
    Side gliding

RROM
    Flexion
    Extension
    Rotation

5. LIGAMENTOUS TESTS

Spring test for facet joint mobility

6. NEUROLOGICAL TESTS

Beevor's sign–thoracic nerve
    inhibition
Lower motor neuron lesions
    Upper quarter screen
    Lower quarter screen
Sciatic nerve compression

7. SPECIAL TESTS

Herniated disc
    Valsalva test
    Milgram test
    Kernig's test/Brudzinski test
    Well straight leg raising test
    Quadrant test

Nerve Root Impingement
    Quadrant test
    Femoral nerve stretch test

Sciatic Nerve Involvement
    Straight leg raise
    Slump test
    Tension sign/Bowstring test

Dural sheath irritation
    Kernig's test/Brudzinski test

Spondylolysis/Spondylolisthesis
    Single leg stance test

Sacroiliac Joint Dysfunction
    Sacroiliac compression/distraction
        test
    FABERE test
    Gaenslen's test
    Long sit test

Hoover test

AROM = active range of motion; PROM = passive range of motion; RROM = resisted range of motion.

- **Consistency of the pain:** The frequency and consistency of the patient's pain can serve as an indication of the type of pathology that is involved.

    o **Constant pain:** Pain that is unyielding and does not increase or subside based on the position of the patient's spine is indicative of chemically induced pain, such as that relating to inflammation of the dural sheath.

    o **Intermittent pain:** Symptoms that increase or decrease based on the position of the spine (e.g., flexion, extension, lateral bending) indicate pain of a mechanical origin. Placing the body in one position may cause compression or stretching of a nerve root. Likewise, relief (or a decrease in symptoms) can be obtained by moving the spine into a specific position that lessens the pressure on the involved structure, a posture that the patient will try to maintain.

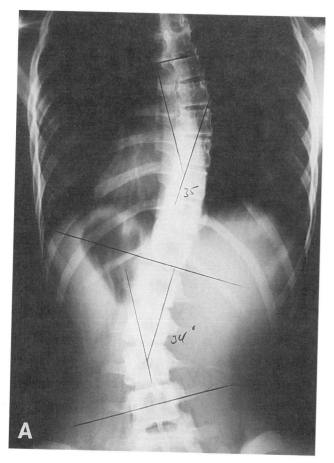

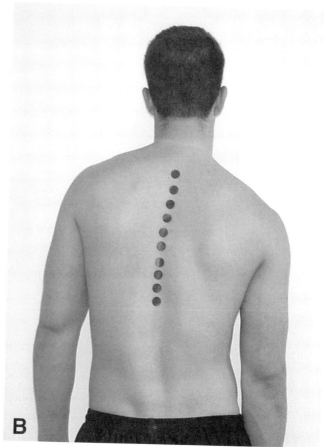

FIGURE 10–14. Scoliosis, lateral bending of the spinal column in the frontal plane. **(A)** A radiograph of moderate to severe scoliosis. **(B)** Dots have been placed over the spinous processes.

- **Bowel or bladder signs:** Is the person experiencing any bowel or bladder problems? *Incontinence* or urinary retention may indicate lower nerve root lesions **(cauda equina syndrome)** or spinal cord injury, a medical emergency warranting immediate referral to a physician.

- **History of spinal injury:** Any pertinent history that may lead to structural degeneration or predispose the patient to chronic problems is important. The current symptoms may be the result of the formation of scar tissue that is impinging or restricting other structures.

- **Changes in activity:** Changes in the level, intensity, or duration of activity or changes in running surfaces, footwear, beds, and so on can redistribute the forces transmitted to the spinal column. (Refer to Chapter 3 for more information on how these changes can affect posture and cause pain.)

INSPECTION

A general inspection of the entire spinal column is necessary to determine the alignment in the sagittal and

frontal planes. The muscles of the spinal column and torso require inspection to determine the presence of spasm or atrophy, each indicating a possible irritation of one or more spinal nerve roots. Last, finite inspection of each spinal segment as well as the individual vertebra may provide an indication of a malalignment of one vertebra relative to the ones above and below it. The patient's general posture, as described in Chapter 3, also must be assessed.

General Inspection

- **Frontal curvature:** Inspect the alignment of the lumbar, thoracic, and cervical vertebrae with the patient lying prone and while he or she is standing. Normally this alignment should be straight. Lateral curvature of the spinal column, **scoliosis,** generally afflicts the thoracic or lumbar spine (or both) in the frontal plane (Fig. 10–14). Scoliosis may be visible

---

Incontinence   A loss of bowel or bladder control.

Box 10–1

TEST FOR SCOLIOSIS

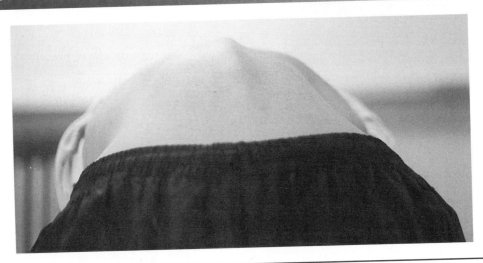

Posterior view of the spinal column while the patient flexes the spine; note the presence of a hump over the left thoracic spine, suggesting scoliosis.

PATIENT POSITION	Standing with hands held in front with the arms straight.
POSITION OF EXAMINER	Seated in front of or behind the patient.
EVALUATIVE PROCEDURE	The patient bends forward, sliding the hands down the front of each leg.
POSITIVE TEST	An asymmetrical hump is observed along the lateral aspect of the thoracolumbar spine and rib cage.
IMPLICATIONS	If scoliosis is present but disappears during flexion, then functional scoliosis is suggested. Scoliosis that is present while the patient is standing upright and while forwardly flexed indicates structural scoliosis.

when the patient is bearing weight, not bearing weight, or both. Functional and structural scoliosis may be detected by having the patient flex the spine segmentally in a slow, controlled manner while bearing weight (Box 10–1). Functional scoliosis is marked by the curvature's disappearance during forward flexion; in structural scoliosis, the curve is still present in this position. Individuals who are suspected of having previously undiagnosed scoliosis need to be referred to a physician for further evaluation. Those who have been previously diagnosed need monitoring on a regular basis for increases in the amount of curvature.

- **Sagittal curvature:** From the side, observe the patient's lordotic cervical, kyphotic thoracic, lumbar lordotic, and sacral kyphotic curves. Changes in any of these curves may produce stress on spinal structures, leading to pain and dysfunction. Muscular spasm, as seen in patients with acute injuries, usually serves to flatten these curves.

- **Observation of gait:** Note the patient's gait. Spinal pain may grossly influence walking and running gait. Common gait deviations resulting from spinal pain include a slouched, shuffling, or shortened gait. Chapter 9 provides detailed discussion regarding gait analysis. Additionally, a patient's unwillingness to move the body as a whole after injury to the spinal region may become evident during ambulation.

- **Skin markings:** Note the presence of any darkened areas of skin pigmentation. **Café-au-lait spots** (Fig. 10–15) may be normally occurring skin discolorations or may represent collagen disease or *neurofibromatosis 1*.[14,15]

Neurofibromatosis 1 Increased cell growth of neural tissues; normally a benign condition; pain possible secondary to pressure on the local nerves.

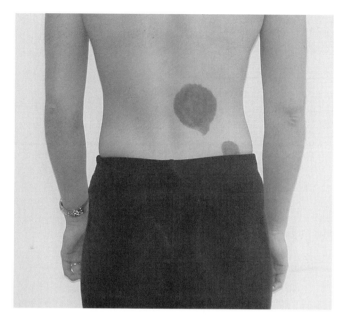

FIGURE 10–15. Café-au-lait spots. These skin discolorations could potentially represent a collagen disorder, neurofibromatosis 1, or can be normally occurring.

Inspection of the Thoracic Spine

- **Breathing patterns:** Injury to the thoracic vertebrae, pressure on the thoracic nerve roots, or trauma to the ribs or costal cartilage may result in pain during respiration, resulting in irregular or shallow breathing patterns.
- **Bilateral comparison of skin folds:** The natural folds of the patient's torso are compared for symmetry. Unevenness or asymmetry of these folds could be caused by a bilateral muscle imbalance, increased or decreased kyphosis, scoliosis, or disease.
- **Shape of the chest:** The chest should be shaped symmetrically from side to side. An advanced scoliosis may cause a noticeable "rib hump" as the vertebrae rotate and also sidebend as the disease progresses. The vertebral rotation causes the ribs to become prominent in the posterior aspect of the spine.

Inspection of the Lumbar Spine

- **General movement and posture:** Observe the patient for poor postural movement habits such as improper standing or sitting postures and improper lifting mechanics (e.g., bending instead of squatting to lift objects).
- **Lordotic curve:** Note the patient's lordotic curve. The lordotic curve can be either accentuated or reduced in patients suffering from low back pain or trauma. Reduction of the lordotic curve may be attributed to acute pain, muscle spasm, or tightness of the hamstring muscle group. Increased lordosis may be traced to tightness in the hip flexor muscle groups or weakness in the abdominal musculature.

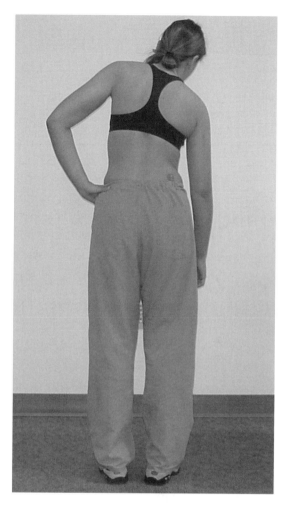

FIGURE 10–16. Compensatory posture for nerve root impingement. The patient will naturally shift the body to lessen the pressure on the nerve root. The posture is labeled for the side of the patient's body. This would be a right compensatory posture.

- **Standing posture:** While observing the patient from behind, observe for a lateral shift in the trunk and pelvis, indicating possible impingement of a nerve root. In this case, the patient instinctively shifts the upper trunk to reduce the amount of pressure on the nerve (Fig. 10–16). The shift is named for the direction the upper trunk moves relative to the patient.
- **Erector muscle tone:** Inspect the paraspinal muscles for equal tone. A unilaterally hypertrophied or atrophied muscle could indicate instability or poor or abnormal posture.
- **Faun's beard:** Observe the sacrum and lower lumbar spine for a tuft of hair, **Faun's beard,** possibly indicating *spina bifida occulta.*

Spina bifida occulta   Incomplete closure of the spinal vertebrae.

Table 10–6
BONY LANDMARKS DURING PALPATION

Structure	Landmark
Cervical vertebral bodies	On the same level as the spinous processes
C1 transverse process	One finger's breadth inferior to the mastoid process
C3–C4 vertebrae	Posterior to the hyoid bone
C4–C5 vertebrae	Posterior to the thyroid cartilage
C6 vertebra	Posterior to the cricoid cartilage; moves during flexion and extension of the cervical spine
C7 vertebra	Prominent posterior spinous process
Thoracic spinal bodies	Underlying the spinous processes of the superior vertebra
T1 vertebra	Prominent protrusion inferior to the cervical spine; does not disappear during extension
T2 vertebra	Posterior from the jugular notch of the sternum
T3 vertebra	Even with the medial border of the scapular spine
T7 vertebra	Even with the inferior angle of scapula
Lumbar spinal bodies	Upper portion of the spinous processes overlying the inferior half of the same vertebra
L3 vertebra	In normal body build, posterior from the umbilicus
L4 vertebra	Level with the iliac crest
L5 vertebra	Typically demarcated by bilateral dimples, but variable from person to person
S2	At the level of the posterior superior iliac spine

PALPATION

Table 10–6 presents a list of landmarks used to orient the location of specific spinal structures. The ease of palpation of these structures depends on the patient's body mass.

Palpation of the Thoracic Spine

1. **Spinous processes:** Palpate the spinous processes along the length of the thoracic spine. The spinous process of T3 normally aligns with the medial border of the scapular spine, and T7 aligns with the inferior

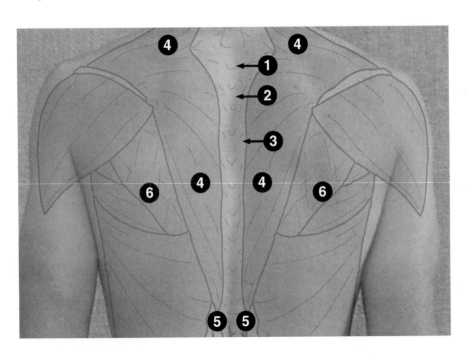

Table 10–7
RELATIVE ALIGNMENT OF THE THORACIC SPINOUS PROCESSES (RULE OF 3'S)

Level	Spinous Process Alignment
T1–T3	At the same level as the transverse processes and the vertebral body
T4–T6	Midway between the transverse processes of the originating vertebra and the transverse processes of the one below
T7–T9	At the same level as the transverse processes of the inferior vertebra
T10	At the level of the T11 vertebral body
T11	Halfway between T11 and T12
T12	At the same level as the T12 vertebral body

angle of the scapula. Use the "Rule of 3's" (Table 10–7) to help orient yourself to the spinous processes relative to the vertebral body.

2. **Supraspinous ligaments:** Identify the supraspinous ligament as it fills the space between the spinous processes. Other ligamentous structures of the spinal column can be palpated lateral to this structure.

3. **Costovertebral junction:** Keep in mind that the articulation of the ribs and thoracic vertebrae are not directly palpable when they are covered by large paravertebral muscles but can be palpated on individuals with slender to normal builds.

4. **Trapezius:** Palpate the middle and lower portions of both trapezius muscles from their origin on the spinous processes to their insertions on the scapular spines. The rhomboid major and minor and the levator scapulae lie underneath the middle and upper

trapezius. Tenderness of these muscles, including the presence of trigger points, may be elicited during palpation.

5. **Paravertebral muscles:** Palpate the paravertebral muscles as they become prominent in the area of the scapula along their length to the pelvis (actual muscle group not shown in this figure).

6. **Scapular muscles:** Palpate the muscles acting on the scapula to identify areas of tenderness, spasm, or other abnormality.

Palpation of the Lumbar Spine

1. **Spinous processes:** Palpate the spinous processes along the entire length of the lumbar spine, with the L4 process at approximately the same level as the iliac crests. The L5 spinous process is relatively smaller and rounder than the other spinous processes and normally disappears when the hip is passively extended.

2. **Step-off deformity:** During palpation of the lumbar spinous process, note whether one process is located more anteriorly than the one below it. Step-off deformities indicate *spondylolisthesis*, which most commonly occurs between the L4 and L5 or L5 and S1 vertebrae.

3. **Paravertebral muscles:** From the thoracic spine, continue to palpate the length of the paravertebral muscles along the length of the lumbar spine. Tightness of these muscles increases the amount of lordosis in the lumbar spine.

Spondylolisthesis   The forward slippage of a vertebra on the one below it.

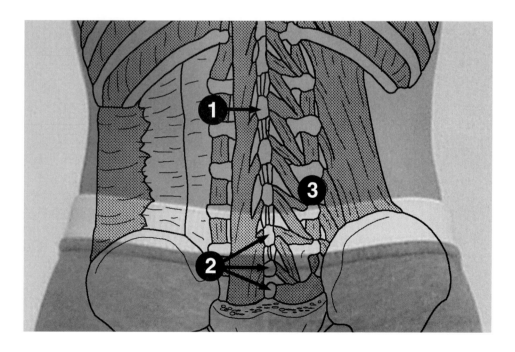

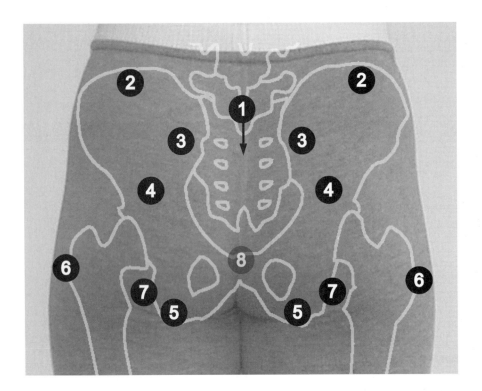

Palpation of the Sacrum and Pelvis

1. **Median sacral crests:** Attempt to palpate the fused remnants of the sacral spinous processes from below the L5 vertebra to the midportion of the gluteal crease.

2. **Iliac crests:** Palpate laterally from the PSIS to find the iliac crests and anteriorly to locate the anterior superior iliac spine (ASIS) and check for level and symmetry (see Fig. 3–9).

3. **Posterior superior iliac spine:** Locate the PSIS near the inferior portion of the gluteal dimples (Fig. 10–17). Under normal circumstances, these bony landmarks are palpable and align at the same level (see Figure 3–12). Tenderness may indicate sacroiliac pathology.

4. **Gluteals:** Posteriorly, locate the gluteus maximus, the most prominent muscle mass. From this point, palpate laterally to identify the gluteus medius as it emerges from beneath the iliac crest. Atrophy of the gluteals can indicate nerve pathology.

5. **Ischial tuberosity:** Locate the ischial tuberosity at the proximal aspect of the hamstrings. The ischial tuberosity may become irritated secondary to high hamstring strains, ischial bursitis, or contusive forces.

6. **Greater trochanter:** Palpate the lateral femur to locate the greater trochanter, which should be bilaterally level. During active or passive internal and external hip rotation, the greater trochanter can be felt as it rolls beneath the fingers. Identify localized pain that may be caused by inflammation of the gluteus medius attachment or by greater trochanteric bursitis versus radiating spinal pain.

7. **Sciatic nerve:** Palpate the sciatic nerve by placing the thumb on the ischial tuberosity and the third finger on the PSIS. The second finger will fall into the sciatic notch. The nerve is at its most superficial point as it passes by the ischial tuberosity. Tenderness on one tuberosity and not on the other may indicate sciatic nerve inflammation.

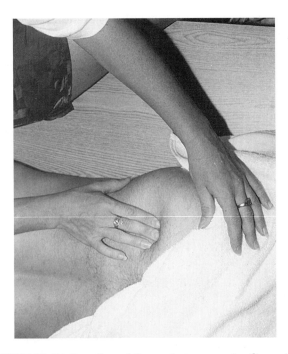

FIGURE 10–17. Location of the posterior superior iliac spine.

8. Pubic symphysis: Locate the symphysis pubis on the anterior portion of the pelvis, just superior to the genitalia at the midline of the body. This structure may become subluxed secondary to a hard jarring injury such as a fall. Use discretion and provide privacy when palpating this area.

RANGE OF MOTION TESTING

Although various forms of goniometers and protractors are available to assess the ROM available in the spine, in actual practice, gross observation of the ROM is typically used and the grade is expressed as a percentage of the total possible normal ROM. Similar to what occurs with the body's other joints, spinal ROM is graded quantitatively as well as qualitatively, noting any pain produced during or at the end of the movement.

A set of 10 repetitions of any particular motion can be used to determine the effect of repeated movement on the quantity and location of pain. In general, repeated movements in one direction that result in pain radiating distally are to be avoided during the rehabilitation program. Motions resulting in the centralization of pain should be incorporated in the rehabilitation program. This latter concept forms the basis of the *McKenzie exercises* and rehabilitation protocol.[16]

When gravity assists the active motion, such as spinal flexion when standing, document that the measurement was conducted with the patient in a gravity-assisted position. ROM testing, as described in this section, is contraindicated for patients with acute injuries until the possibility of a vertebral fracture or dislocation has been ruled out.

The total motion produced by the thoracic and lumbar spines is difficult to isolate into its individual segments. The motions of these two areas are evaluated as a single unit, the trunk. In addition, it is difficult to isolate passive motion in a gravity-dependent position, so active and passive ROM testing often occurs concurrently when the techniques described in the "Active Range of Motion" section are used.

Techniques for testing passive ROM (PROM) against gravity are included for completeness. Quantifiable ROM testing techniques are presented in Box 10–2.

Active Range of Motion

• **Flexion and extension:** Active trunk flexion is measured with the patient standing. To aid in documenting the available motion and the progression of this motion over time, the distance from the fingertips to the floor can be measured (the accuracy of this measurement is affected by tightness of the hamstrings and calf muscles and scapular protraction). Even though this position allows gravity to assist the movement, it is a more accurate indication of available motion than is the *hook-lying position*. Testing in the hook-lying position requires the abdominal muscles to overcome the weight of the trunk, limit-

ing the apparent amount of motion. To avoid motion initiating at the hips and ensure that spinal flexion is being observed, forward flexion is begun by bending the patient's chin to the chest and then rolling the flexion down the vertebral column until hip flexion is seen or felt (Fig. 10–18).

Normally, the abdominal muscles receive concurrent innervation from the T5 through T12 nerve roots. **Beevor's sign** (Box 10–3), a modified sit-up, can indicate pathology to the lower thoracic nerve roots.

Extension is also measured with the patient standing with his or her feet shoulder width apart and his or her hands on the hips while the spine is slowly extended. The clinician should stand in back of the patient to assist the patient, if needed (see Fig. 10–18).

• **Lateral bending:** The patient stands with the feet shoulder width apart and the hand opposite the direction of the movement resting on the ilium. The patient then bends the trunk laterally, attempting to touch the fingertips to the ground as the clinician stabilizes the pelvis to prevent lateral tilt. The distance between the ground and the fingertips is measured, recorded, and compared bilaterally (Fig. 10–19).

• **Rotation:** The patient is placed in the sitting position to stabilize the pelvis and lower extremity. The patient then rotates the shoulder girdles and spinal column as if looking behind the back (Fig. 10–20) Rotation of the trunk occurs primarily in the thoracic spine. The amount of rotation should be equal in each direction.

Passive Range of Motion

• **Flexion:** With the patient in the hook-lying position, the examiner brings the knees to the chest by lifting under the knees and thighs and flexing the hip and thoracic spine (Fig. 10–21A). Flexion in the thoracic area is limited by the rib articulations, with the exception of T11 and T12, both of which are relatively mobile.

• **Extension:** The patient is placed in the prone position with the hands flat on the table at shoulder level in a position to perform a push-up. The patient then extends the arm, lifting the torso while the hips and legs remain flat on the table (Fig. 10–21B). This motion is limited by the spinous process' making contact with the one below it.

McKenzie exercises A protocol of exercises involving spinalflexion and extension used during the treatment and rehabilitation of back injuries, for improving range of motion and strengthening the spine.

Hook-lying position Lying supine with the hips and knees flexed and the feet flat on the table.

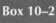

Box 10–2
GONIOMETRY: TRUNK RANGE OF MOTION TESTING

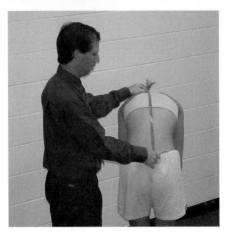
Flexion

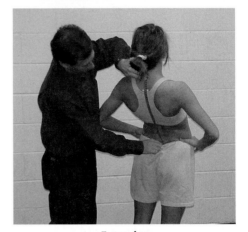
Extension

PATIENT POSITION	Standing with knees extended and the spine in the neutral position
PROCEDURE	The procedure is the same for flexion and extension.
INITIAL MEASUREMENT	Using a tape measure, the distance (in cm) between the C7 and S1 vertebrae is determined.
MOTION	The trunk is fully flexed or extended. Observe the pelvis for rotation that indicates compensation for spinal motion.
FINAL MEASUREMENT	The distance between the C7 and S1 vertebrae is determined. The difference between the initial and final measurement is calculated and the value recorded.

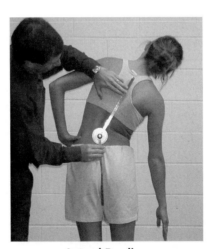
Lateral Bending

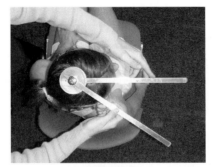
Rotation

PATIENT POSITION	Standing with the knees extended and the spine in the neutral position	Seated Feet placed firmly on the floor
GONIOMETER ALIGNMENT		
FULCRUM	Aligned over the S1 spinous process	Aligned over the center of the patient's head
STATIONARY ARM	Aligned over the median sacral crest	Parallel to the line formed by the iliac crests
MOVEMENT ARM	Aligned with the C7 vertebrae	Parallel to the line formed by the two acromion processes.

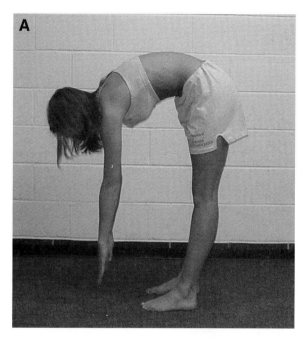

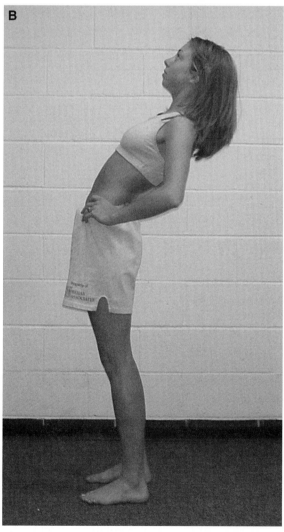

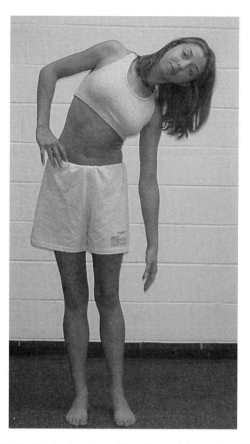

FIGURE 10–19. Active lateral bending with gravity. The patient attempts to touch the fingers to the floor. Observe for the normal segmental motion.

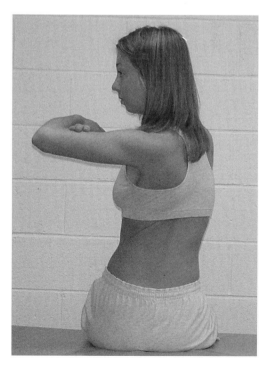

FIGURE 10–18. Active trunk **(A)** flexion and **(B)** extension.

FIGURE 10–20. Active trunk rotation. This motion occurs primarily in the thoracic spine.

BEEVOR'S SIGN FOR THORACIC NERVE INHIBITION

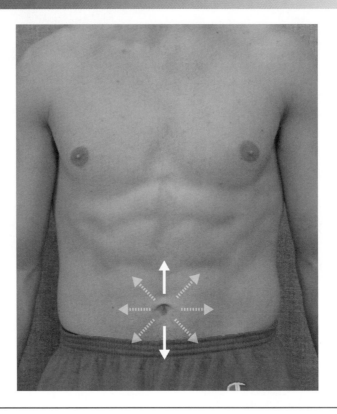

Lateral movement of the umbilicus can indicate inhibition of the nerves innervating the abdominal muscles.

PATIENT POSITION	Hook-lying
POSITION OF EXAMINER	At the side of the patient
EVALUATIVE PROCEDURE	The patient performs an abdominal curl (partial sit-up)
POSITIVE TEST	The umbilicus moves up, down, or to one side
IMPLICATION	Segmental involvement of the nerves innervating the rectus abdominis (T5 through T12); this should draw suspicion to the paraspinal muscles innervated by the same nerve roots.
COMMENT	Normally the umbilicus should not move at all during this test, but will move toward the stronger muscle group in the presence of pathology.

- **Rotation:** From the hook-lying position, the patient's legs and pelvis are rotated to bring the lateral portion of the knee toward the table while the shoulders remain flat (Fig. 10–22). The amount of motion available is compared in each direction. This movement is limited by the alignment of the facet joints. Virtually no rotation occurs between the L1 to L4 vertebrae.

- **Side gliding:** With the patient standing, the clinician braces his or her shoulder against the patient's outer portion of the upper arm. While reaching around the patient with both arms and interlocking the fingers at the iliac crest, the upper and lower trunk is glided, returning the shifted spine into a neutral position. A

modification of this procedure is shown in Figure 10–23. This test is repeated on each side. Side gliding is considered significant for nerve root compression if the motion alters the quantity or location of the pain. This only needs to be performed in the presence of a laterally shifted spine or with radiating pain.

Resisted Range of Motion

The procedure for checking resisted ROM (RROM) for the thoracic and lumbar spine is presented in Box 10–4. RROM testing of flexion and rotation also checks the strength of the muscles responsible for lateral bending.

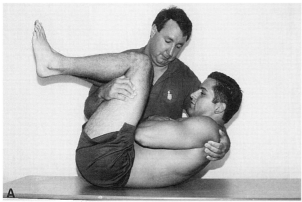

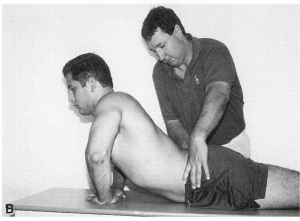

FIGURE 10–21. Passive trunk **(A)** flexion and **(B)** extension.

LIGAMENTOUS TESTING

There are no tests to check the integrity of single isolated ligaments. Clues as to the presence of ligamentous pathology arise during the passive testing of the spine's ROM (Table 10–8). However, these results may easily be confused with pain caused by intervertebral

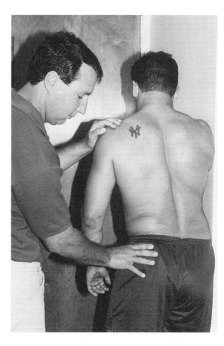

FIGURE 10–23. Passive lateral glide of the trunk. The patient's shoulder is stabilized against the wall while the examiner forces the pelvis laterally.

disc lesions or pathology to the nerve roots or peripheral nerves.

Sprains to the spinal ligaments usually occur more frequently in the cervical spine because of its increased ROM. The conclusion of a ligamentous sprain is generally derived by excluding the possibility of other pathologies. The history of a mechanism that would stress the spinal ligaments, pain along the spinal column and at the end of PROM, and static pain when the muscles are relaxed and the ligaments are acting as the only static stabilizers, can lead to the conclusion of a

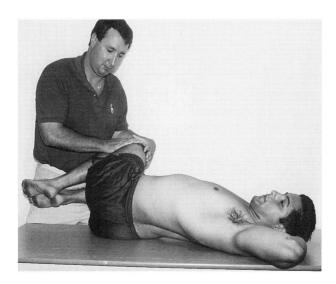

FIGURE 10–22. Passive trunk rotation.

Table 10–8 **SPINAL LIGAMENTS STRESSED DURING PASSIVE RANGE OF MOTION TESTING**	
Motion	**Ligaments Stressed**
Flexion	Posterior longitudinal ligament
	Supraspinous ligament (thoracic and lumbar spine)
	Interspinous ligament
	Ligamentum flavum
Extension	Anterior longitudinal ligament
Rotation	Interspinous ligament
	Ligamentum flavum
Lateral bending (these tests are usually inconclusive)	Interspinous ligament
	Ligamentum flavum

Box 10–4
RESISTED RANGE OF MOTION FOR THE TRUNK

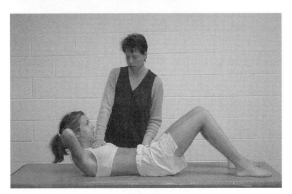

Flexion

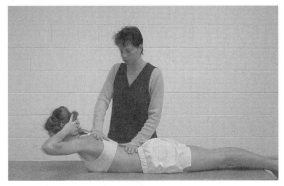

Extension

STARTING POSITION	Supine with the knees flexed and the feet flat on the table The patient's hands interlocked behind the head	Prone with the arms outstretched above the head, at the side, or interlocked behind the head
STABILIZATION	Pelvis	Lower lumbar region
RESISTANCE	Resistance is applied to the superior sternum as the patient lifts the scapulae off the table.	Resistance is applied to the upper thoracic spine as the patient lifts the head, chest, and arms off the table.
MUSCLES TESTED	Rectus abdominis, internal oblique, external oblique	Iliocostalis lumborum, iliocostalis thoracis, longissimus thoracis, spinalis thoracis, semispinalis thoracis, rotatores, latissimus dorsi

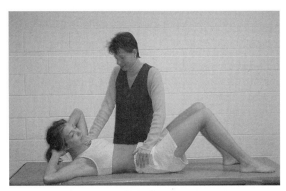

Rotation

STARTING POSITION	Supine. The patient's hands interlocked behind the head
STABILIZATION	Opposite ASIS
RESISTANCE	Resistance is applied over the anterior aspect of the shoulder as it is rotated off the table. This procedure is repeated for the opposite side.
MUSCLES TESTED	Internal oblique, external oblique (opposite side), rotatores, multifidi (opposite side)

ASIS = anterior superior iliac spine.

Box 10–5
SPRING TEST FOR FACET JOINT MOBILITY

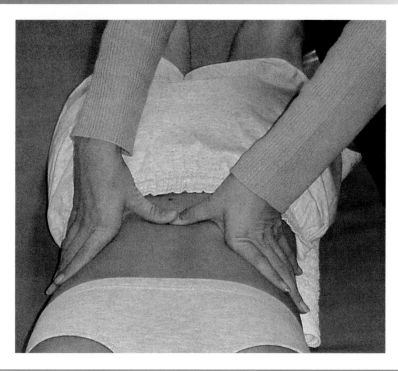

PATIENT POSITION	Prone
POSITION OF EXAMINER	Standing over the patient with the thumbs placed over the spinous process to be tested
EVALUATIVE PROCEDURE	The examiner carefully pushes the spinous process anteriorly, feeling for the springing of the vertebrae.
POSITIVE TEST	The vertebra does not move ("spring") or pain is elicited.
IMPLICATIONS	Hypomobility of the vertebrae, especially at the facet joints or a sprain

sprain. This assumes that all other possible pathologies have been ruled out.

The total ROM available to the spinal column is equal to the sum of the motions between any two contiguous vertebrae. Although it is difficult to check the amount of motion that occurs at each individual spinal segment, the accessory movement of the segment can be grossly determined. The **spring test** (Box 10–5) is used to determine hypomobility of a vertebral segment caused by facet joint dysfunction. Hypomobility or hypermobility of these joints can potentially cause pain along the spinal column.

SPECIAL TESTS

Several special tests are commonly incorporated into all spinal evaluations. These are presented in this section and the remaining special tests are described in their appropriate locations in the "Pathologies and Related Special Tests" section of this chapter.

Test for Nerve Root Impingement

Impingement of spinal nerve roots may result from a narrowing of the intervertebral foramen caused by stenosis, facet joint degeneration, herniated intervertebral discs, or other space-occupying lesions. Increased *intrathecal* pressure can increase the patient's symptoms by forcing the annulus pulposus outward, compressing the nerve root and causing *radicular pain*. The **Valsalva test** (Box 10–6) and the **Milgram Test** (Box 10–7) are used clinically to identify the effect of increased intrathecal pressure, but the patient may self-report increased symptoms while bearing down during bowel movements or while lifting weights.

Intrathecal   Within the spinal canal.

Radicular pain   A sharp, shooting pain that tends to remain within a specific dermatome.

Box 10–6
VALSALVA TEST

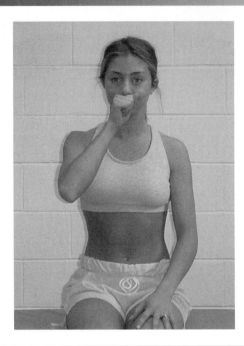

The Valsalva test attempts to increase intrathecal pressure, duplicating nerve-root pain that may be elicited while coughing or with bowel movements.

PATIENT POSITION	Sitting
POSITION OF EXAMINER	Standing within arms' reach in front of the patient
EVALUATIVE PROCEDURE	The patient takes and holds a deep breath while bearing down similar to performing a bowel movement.
POSITIVE TEST	Increased spinal or radicular pain
IMPLICATIONS	Increase in intrathecal pressure causes pain secondary to a space-occupying lesion such as a herniated disc, tumor, or osteophyte anywhere along the spinal column.
MODIFICATION	If the patient is embarrassed or apprehensive about simulating a bowel movement, he or she may be instructed to blow into a closed fist as if inflating a balloon.
COMMENTS	This can be performed for any level of the spine. The test increases intrathecal pressure, resulting in a slowing of the pulse, decreased venous return, and increased venous pressure, all of which may cause fainting.

Box 10–7
MILGRAM TEST

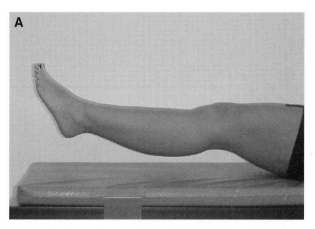

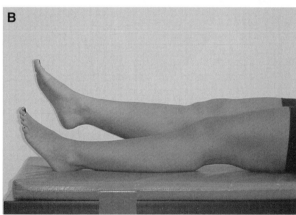

PATIENT POSITION	Supine
POSITION OF EXAMINER	At the feet of the patient
EVALUATIVE PROCEDURE	**(A)** The patient performs a bilateral straight leg raise to the height of 2 to 6 inches and is asked to hold the position for 30 seconds.
POSITIVE TEST	**(B)** The patient is unable to hold the position, cannot lift the leg, or experiences pain with the test.
IMPLICATIONS	Intrathecal or extrathecal pressure causing an intervertebral disc to place pressure on a lumbar nerve root.

> **Box 10–8**
> **KERNIG'S TEST**

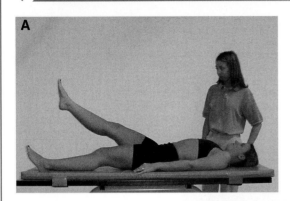

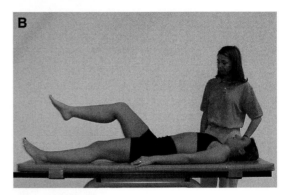

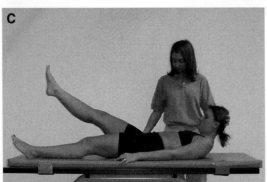

PATIENT POSITION	Supine
POSITION OF EXAMINER	At the side of the patient
EVALUATIVE PROCEDURE	The patient performs a unilateral active straight leg raise with the knee extended until pain occurs (**A**). After pain occurs, the patient flexes the knee (**B**).
POSITIVE TEST	Pain is experienced in the spine and possibly radiating into the lower extremity. This pain is relieved when the patient flexes the knee.
IMPLICATIONS	Nerve root impingement secondary to a bulging of the intervertebral disc or bony entrapment; irritation of the dural sheath; or irritation of the meninges.
MODIFICATION	In the absence of pain during the active straight leg raise, the examiner may further elongate the spinal cord and increase the tension on the dural sheath by passively flexing the patient's cervical spine (**Brudzinski's test**) and repeating the test (**C**).

Kernig's test (Box 10–8) is also used to identify bulging intervertebral discs but also presents positive results in the presence of inflammation of the nerve or its dural sheath.

The **straight leg raise test** (Box 10–9) is used to identify either sciatic nerve irritation or a herniated intervertebral disc that is irritating the nerve root. The **well straight leg raise** (Box 10–10) can be used to discriminate between the two conditions.[18–20]

The **quadrant test** (Box 10–11) is used to determine dural irritation and facet joint compression, and the **slump test** (Box 10–12) can be used to identify possible compression of the lumbar nerve roots.

Test for Patient Malingering

By their very nature, lumbopelvic disorders are difficult to objectively evaluate, forcing the clinician to rely on subjective information gained from the history of the injury. On occasion, a person may overstate the quantity of pain and dysfunction associated with an injury or may be malingering. The **Hoover test** (Box 10–13) is a classic procedure used to determine whether the individual is malingering during the performance of functional and special tests.[21–23]

Box 10–9
STRAIGHT LEG RAISE TEST

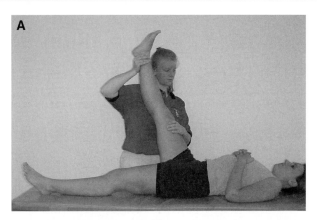

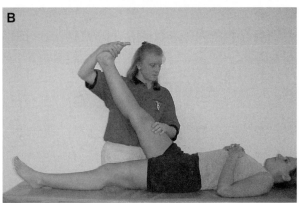

(A) The involved leg is flexed at the hip until symptoms are experienced. **(B)** The involved leg is extended approximately 10° (until symptoms subside) and the ankle is then passively dorsiflexed. A return of the symptoms indicates a stretching of the dural sheath.

PATIENT POSITION	Supine
POSITION OF EXAMINER	At the side to be tested; one hand grasps under the heel while the other is placed on the anterior knee to keep it in full extension during the examination.
EVALUATIVE PROCEDURE	While keeping the knee in extension, the examiner raises the leg by flexing the hip until discomfort is experienced or the full ROM is obtained.
POSITIVE TEST	The patient complains of pain before the end of the normal ROM (70°). The pain may be described as radiating distally along the tested leg, usually in the posterior thigh, radiating into the calf and perhaps the foot.
IMPLICATIONS	Sciatic nerve irritation Pain described before the hip reaches 70° of hip flexion may indicate discal involvement.[17]
MODIFICATION	After pain is experienced, the leg is lowered to the point at which the pain stops. The examiner passively dorsiflexes the ankle and/or has the patient flex the cervical spine. Serving to stretch the dural sheath, this flexion recreates the symptoms. If the patient's prior pain was caused by tight hamstrings, this modification does not elicit pain.

ROM = range of motion.

Box 10–10
WELL STRAIGHT LEG RAISING TEST

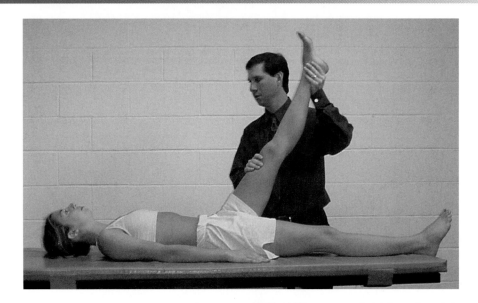

The well straight leg raise test differs from the straight leg raise test in that the unaffected leg is elevated.

PATIENT POSITION	Supine
POSITION OF EXAMINER	At the side to be tested (the extremity not suffering the symptoms); one hand grasps under the heel while the other is placed on the anterior thigh just superior to the knee to stabilize the leg in extension.
EVALUATIVE PROCEDURE	Keeping the knee in extension, the examiner raises the leg by flexing the hip until discomfort is reported.
POSITIVE TEST	Pain is experienced on the side opposite that being raised.
IMPLICATIONS	A large space-occupying lesion such as a herniated intervertebral disc.

Box 10–11
QUADRANT TEST

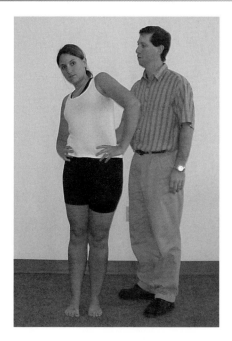
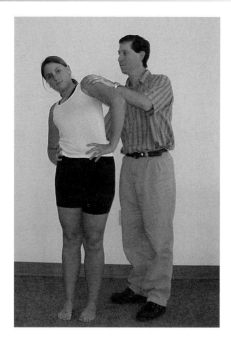

PATIENT POSITION	Standing with the feet shoulder width apart
POSITION OF EXAMINER	Standing behind the patient, grasping the patient's shoulders
EVALUATIVE PROCEDURE	The patient extends the spine as far as possible, then sidebends and rotates to the affected side. The examiner provides overpressure through the shoulders, supporting the patient as needed.
POSITIVE TEST	Reproduction of the patient's symptoms
IMPLICATIONS	Radicular pain indicates compression of the intervertebral foramina that impinges on the lumbar nerve roots Local (nonradiating) pain indicates facet joint pathology Symptoms isolated to the area of the PSIS; may also indicate SI joint dysfunction.

PSIS = posterior superior iliac spine; SI = sacroiliac.

Box 10–12
SLUMP TEST

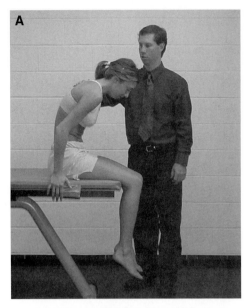

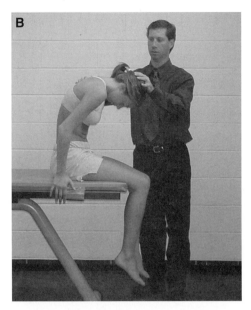

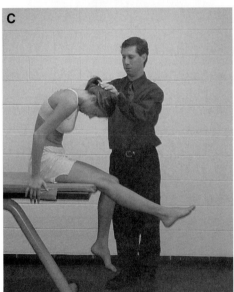

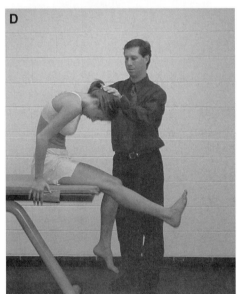

PATIENT POSITION	Sitting over the edge of the table
POSITION OF EXAMINER	At the side of the patient
EVALUATIVE PROCEDURE	The following sequence is followed until symptoms are provoked: **1.** The patient slumps forward along the thoracolumbar spine, rounding the shoulders while keeping the cervical spine in neutral **(A)**. **2.** The patient flexes the cervical spine. The clinician then holds the patient in this position **(B)**. **3.** The knee is actively extended **(C)**. **4.** The ankle is actively dorsiflexed **(D)**. **5.** Repeat steps 2 through 4 on the opposite side.
POSITIVE TEST	Sciatic pain or reproduction of other neurologic symptoms
IMPLICATIONS	Impingement of the dural lining, spinal cord, or nerve roots

> **Box 10–13**
> **HOOVER TEST**

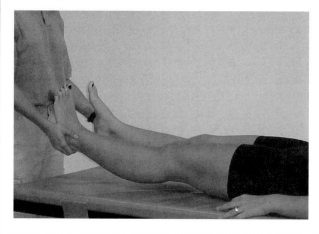 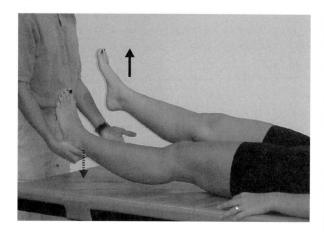

PATIENT POSITION	Supine
POSITION OF EXAMINER	At the feet of the patient with the evaluator's hands cupping the calcaneus of each leg
EVALUATIVE PROCEDURE	The patient attempts an active straight leg raise on the involved side
POSITIVE TEST	The patient does not attempt to lift the leg and the examiner does not sense pressure from the uninvolved leg pressing down on the hand as should instinctively happen.
IMPLICATION	The patient is not attempting to perform the test (i.e., malingering).

NEUROLOGIC TESTING

Because of the close involvement of the spinal column to the spinal cord and its nerve roots, many of the maladies affecting the spine may result in decreased neurologic function in the extremities as well as the trunk. Clinically, this involvement can be determined through the use of manual muscle tests, deep tendon reflexes, and sensory testing. Chapter 18 discusses the management of acute spinal injuries.

Tests for Lower Motor Neuron Lesions

Lower motor neuron trauma to the spinal nerve roots or the peripheral nervous system results in *hyporeflexia,* flaccidity of the muscles, and denervation atrophy. This condition most often results from compression or stretching of the nerves. Temporary hyporeflexia, sensory deficit, or muscle weakness may indicate nerve root impingement or transient quadriplegia (see Chapter 18).

Lower motor neuron injuries include neurapraxia, axonotmesis, and neurotmesis. Refer to Chapter 18 for a description of upper motor neuron lesions.

The upper and lower quarter screens provide an efficient evaluation for neurologic function in the extremities. The screens use manual muscle testing, sensory testing, and deep tendon reflexes to assess neurologic function (Box 10–14). Upper quarter screens are presented in Chapter 11.

◆ PATHOLOGIES AND RELATED SPECIAL TESTS

The structure and function of the spinal column exposes it and its supportive structures to almost constant stress during ADLs. These stresses are further increased during heavy labor or athletic competition. In addition to the contact forces related to athletic competition, movement of the torso results in shear forces across the column. Sitting or standing upright places an axial load on these structures. Even lying down can result in dysfunction if the surface is too hard or too soft. Regardless, the spinal column displays an enormous capability to adapt to the forces placed on it. When the spinal column is unable to adapt, injury occurs. Dysfunction of the SI joint can occur acutely secondary to a dynamic overload or insidiously from an unknown cause.

Hyporeflexia   A diminished or absent reflex response.

Box 10–14
LOWER QUARTER NEUROLOGICAL SCREEN

Nerve Root Level	Sensory Testing	Motor Testing	Reflex Testing
L1		Lumbar plexus	None
L2		Lumbar plexus	Partial
L3		Femoral n.	Partial
L4		Deep peroneal n.	Patellar t.
L5		Deep peroneal n.	Patellar t.
S1		Tibial n.	Achilles t.
S2	P. femoral cutaneous n.	Intrinsic foot/toe muscles Lateral plantar n.	Achilles t.

The evaluation of back injuries relies on a thorough, accurate history that provides the examiner with a reasonable expectation of any pathology present in the patient. A standardized physical evaluation is used to corroborate the findings from the patient's history. The idiopathic and inconsistent behavior of low back pain makes identifying the underlying pathology difficult. The treatment and rehabilitation implications of the pathology are equally uncertain. A system that classifies low back pathology based on the treatment approach has been proposed.[24–26] This system groups patients based on the evaluation findings to determine the treatment approach (Table 10–9). For example, patients who demonstrate pain during flexion and pain relief during extension are grouped into the "extension" category, and this motion is emphasized during the initial rehabilitation protocol.

Table 10–9

CLASSIFICATION CATEGORIES OF LOW BACK INJURY BASED ON THE TREATMENT APPROACH

Classification (Treatment Approach)	Evaluation Findings
Extension	Flexion activities such as sitting and bending increase symptoms Pain exhibited or radiating during trunk flexion ROM testing Pain decreased during extension activities such as when standing or walking Pain reduced or centralized with extension ROM testing
Flexion	Extension motions such as standing and walking increase symptoms Pain exhibited or radiating during trunk extension ROM testing Pain decreased with flexion activities such as sitting and bending Pain reduced or centralized with flexion ROM testing
Mobilization	Pain with positive sacroiliac tests (sacroiliac mobilization) Pain with lumbar opening or closing patterns with ROM testing (lumbar mobilization)
Lateral shift	Shifting of trunk laterally relative to the pelvis Unequal lateral bending ROM Symptoms improving with pelvic translocation Symptoms worsening with opposite pelvic translocation
Traction	Radicular pain Symptoms worsening with most ROM tests Symptoms not improving with any tests

ROM = range of motion.

ERECTOR SPINAE MUSCLE STRAIN

Strains of the spinal erector muscle group may be one of the most common orthopedic maladies seen for treatment. Although this condition is common, it is also often self-limiting. Similar to sprains of the spinal ligaments, muscle strain is usually diagnosed after the exclusion of all other possible problems. Commonly, the patient presents with a history of heavy or repetitive lifting and complaints of aching pain centralized to the low back. Pain increases with passive and active flexion as well as resisted extension. Lower quarter screens show negative results.

FACET JOINT DYSFUNCTION

The lumbar facet joints give the spine rigidity and protect the intervertebral discs against rotational injury.[27,28] Pathology of the facet joints can account for as much as 40 percent of all chronic low back pain.[29] The signs and symptoms of facet joint dysfunction are vague and often resemble other low back pathologies, including strains and spasm of the paraspinal muscles, nerve root impingement, and disc degeneration.

Facet joint pathology may involve dislocation or subluxation of the facet, **facet joint syndrome** (inflammation), or degeneration of the facet itself (e.g., arthritis). Over time, the presence of one of these conditions can lead to the other. A dislocated or subluxated facet joint tends to "lock" the involved spinal segment, causing the vertebrae to become hypomobile (see Box 10–5, Spring test for vertebral mobility). The patient may report a history of extension, rotation, or lateral bending of the spine with pain that tends to be localized over the affected facet. Unlike with other spinal conditions, the patient may describe a decrease in symptoms with an increase in activity.

Facet joint syndrome occurs from repetitive stress to the facet joint through movement or loading. The pain is usually localized to the spinal level that is irritated and does not radiate unless the nerve root is secondarily involved. The pain may become more diffuse if several levels of facets are involved. Localized muscle spasm may be present in the paravertebral musculature. (Table 10–10). Any motion that loads the facet joint, especially extension, hyperextension, rotation, and side bending to the involved side, reproduces symptoms.

Degeneration of the facet joint has an undefined history of injury. If the degeneration is significant, the size of the intervertebral foramen will decrease, potentially impinging the associated nerve root and causing radicular pain. Nerve entrapment can be reduced by the patient's assuming a posture that decreases pressure on the nerve root, usually caused by flexion reducing the size of the intervertebral foramen. A definitive diagnosis of facet joint degeneration is made using radiographs or magnetic resonance imaging (MRI) or by a physician's injecting the facet with an anesthetic and

Table 10–10
EVALUATIVE FINDINGS: Facet Joint Dysfunction

Examination Segment	Clinical Findings	
History	**Onset:**	Insidious
	Pain characteristics:	Localized over the involved facets and the surrounding musculature
	Mechanism:	Extension, rotation, or lateral bending of the vertebrae
	Predisposing conditions:	Repeated motions of spinal extension, rotation, or lateral bending
Inspection	The patient may assume a posture that lessens the pressure on the affected facets.	
Palpation	Possible local muscle spasm is noted in the paravertebral muscles.	
Functional tests	Motions of extension, rotation, and lateral bending to the involved side all produce pain.	
Ligamentous tests	Spring test may cause pain or reveal decreased motion.	
Neurologic tests	Not applicable unless secondary nerve root impingement occurs.	
Special tests	Quadrant test may be positive. Tests for intervertebral disc lesions are negative.	
Comments	Continued degeneration of the facet joint may reduce the size of the intervertebral foramen and result in compression of the spinal nerve root.	

noting the subsequent change in symptoms.[27–29] Prolonged dysfunction of the facet joint or *facetectomy* can accelerate the degeneration of the intervertebral discs or predispose the discs to injury.[27]

Initial treatment of patients with facet joint pathologies involves the use of nonsteroidal anti-inflammatory drugs (NSAIDs) to decrease joint inflammation. The patient should be instructed to avoid postures and movements that irritate the facet and increase pain. Local therapeutic modalities such as moist heat, electrical stimulation, or ice may be helpful to decrease subsequent muscle spasm. The use of mobilization is helpful early on to assist in reducing pain in the area.

These patients must also be thoroughly evaluated for muscle imbalances that may be contributing to their facet joint dysfunction. The trunk and pelvic musculature must be assessed for tightness and weakness. A program of stretching and strengthening helps in decreasing pain and maintaining good health in the back. The mechanics and postures that the patient assumes should be evaluated as possible contributory causes of the facet joint pathology and corrected as needed.

INTERVERTEBRAL DISC LESIONS

The degeneration of intervertebral discs involves the loss of water from the nucleus pulposus, decreasing the protein content and altering the chemical structure. Biochemical changes associated with the aging process further extenuate the loss of water, causing an increased stress load to be placed on the annulus fibrosus and leading to the bulging of the nucleus pulposus (Fig. 10–24).

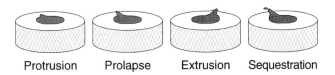

Protrusion   Prolapse   Extrusion   Sequestration

FIGURE 10–24. Classifications of intervertebral disc lesions.

Disc herniation is the extrusion of the nucleus pulposus through a weakened region in the annulus fibrosus with subsequent impingement on one or more lumbar nerve roots. A complete herniation typically results in pressure of the nerve root exiting below the affected disc (Fig. 10–25). For example, a herniation of the L4–L5 disc places pressure on the L5 nerve root. The lesion can involve any protrusion of the nuclear material into the annulus, even if it has not herniated through the entire structure. The worst-case scenario involves the nuclear material's breaking away from the rest of the disc and becoming *sequestrated.* Note that MRIs have demonstrated that many disc protrusions remain asymptomatic.[30]

The signs and symptoms of an intervertebral disc herniation are primarily that of nerve root compression that results in pain in the lumbar spine and radicular pain aggravated by activity (Table 10–11).[17] The patient

Facetectomy   The surgical resection of a vertebral facet.

Sequestrated   Pertaining to a necrotic fragment of tissue that has become separated from the surrounding tissue.

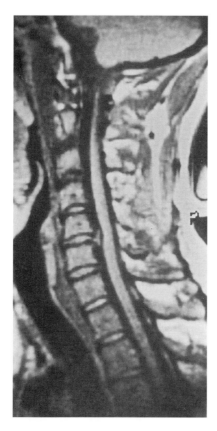

FIGURE 10–25. Myelogram of a disc herniation. Notice the narrowing of the spinal canal.

typically describes an insidious onset, but the pain may be related to a single specific episode. Often, the breakdown of the disc is related to repetitive stress, but the episode resulting in the symptoms reflects the final failure in the annulus fibrosus to contain the nucleus pulposus. Changes in body position (e.g., sitting to standing or standing to lying) are painful as the changes in disc pressure increase pressure on the structures. On inspection, the patient may be noted as having a slow, deliberate gait and, in the acute and subacute stages, a flattened lumbar spine. In an attempt to decrease the pressure on the nerve root, the patient may stand with a lateral shift, usually away from the side of the leg pain. If the patient demonstrates a leg length discrepancy, the pain usually occurs on the side of the body with the shorter leg.[31]

Question the patient to determine the exact location (or locations) of pain. Typically, the pain is in the low back and buttocks. However, it also can radiate into the posterior thigh, calf, heel, and foot, depending on the level of the nerve root irritation. The pain patterns stemming from disc lesions may be inconsistent, with changes in the position of the lumbar spine reducing the pressure on the nerve root causing a decrease in symptoms. A precise neurologic evaluation is needed to determine the spinal levels that are involved. A lower quarter neurologic screen is used to evaluate strength, deep tendon reflexes, and sensation. Findings of bilateral leg pain, absent deep tendon reflexes, or changes in bowel and bladder function warrant

Table 10–11
EVALUATIVE FINDINGS: Lumbar Disc Degeneration

Examination Segment	Clinical Findings	
History	*Onset:*	Insidious
	Pain characteristics:	Pain localized to the affected vertebra; compression of the spinal nerve root leading to pain in the low back and buttocks possibly radiating into the thigh, calf, heel, and foot
	Mechanism:	Repetitive loading of the intervertebral disc over time
	Predisposing conditions:	History of lumbar spine trauma
Inspection	Slow gait Flattened lumbar spine Changes in position are guarded and painful.	
Palpation	Spasm of the musculature possible	
Functional tests	ROM limited by pain in all directions. Determination by examiner if motion in any one direction increases or decreases the symptoms. Motion that decreases symptoms possibly useful in the treatment of the patient.	
Ligamentous tests	Not applicable.	
Neurologic tests	Lower quarter screen	
Special tests	Straight leg raising, well straight leg raising, Milgram test, sciatic and femoral nerve tension tests	
Comments	Standard lumbar spine radiographs are reliable for making a definitive diagnosis of lumbar disc degeneration. It should be noted that all discs tend to begin degenerating by the fourth decade of life and may be a concurrent finding with other spine pathology.	

ROM = range of motion.

immediate referral for evaluation of **cauda equina syndrome.**

Special tests are used to confirm the findings identified during the history, inspection, and neurologic screening portions of the evaluation. The Valsalva test (see Box 10–6), Milgram test (see Box 10–7), straight leg raise (see Box 10–9), the well straight leg raise (see Box 10–10), and the **femoral nerve stretch test** (Box 10–15) are commonly used to identify intervertebral disc lesions.

The evaluation of disc changes through diagnostic imaging is made more effective with MRI scans. Standard radiographic examinations are effective only in measuring secondary changes associated with disc degeneration (i.e., a narrowing of the intervertebral space). Because of its ability to directly measure a structure's water content, MRI scans are effective in the early detection of disc degeneration.[32]

Initially, rehabilitation exercises consist of those motions that localize the pain toward the involved disc **(centralization),** usually extension motions and core stability and pelvic stabilization exercises. Because of the stress placed on the disc during flexion and rotation of the lumbar spine, some advocate avoiding these exercises until the symptoms decrease.[17] Rehabilitation can also include the use of a support to maintain lumbar curvature while sitting and anti-inflammatory medications.[6] Disc ruptures that do not respond to conservative care may require surgery to remove the involved section of the intervertebral disc and fuse the superior and inferior vertebra.[6]

SCIATICA

Sciatica, a general term for any inflammation involving the sciatic nerve, does not describe the actual condition that is insulting the nerve and causing the inflammation. Whenever possible, this term should be avoided and the source of the irritation should be determined so that an appropriate treatment plan can be developed. Causes of sciatica include lumbar disc herniation,

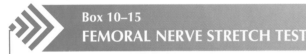

Box 10–15
FEMORAL NERVE STRETCH TEST

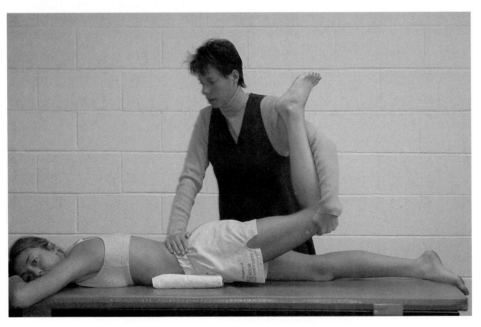

PATIENT POSITION	Prone with a pillow under the abdomen or sidelying
POSITION OF EXAMINER	At the side of the patient
EVALUATIVE PROCEDURE	The examiner passively extends the hip while keeping the patient's knee flexed to 90°.
POSITIVE TEST	Pain is elicited in the anterior and lateral thigh.
IMPLICATION	Nerve root impingement at the L2, L3, or L4 level
COMMENT	The examiner should attempt to fully flex the knee with the hip in the neutral position to determine any strain of the quadriceps muscle that may also cause pain.

sacroiliac joint dysfunction, scar tissue formation around the nerve root, nerve root inflammation, spinal stenosis, synovial cysts, cancerous or noncancerous tumors, and other disease states.[33–39]

The signs and symptoms of sciatica are similar to those described for lumbar disc ruptures that place pressure on one or more nerve roots. Pain radiates along the involved dermatome (or dermatomes) and muscular weakness may be described in the posterior muscles. In advanced cases, nerve conduction velocity and the Achilles tendon reflex may be diminished.[40,41] Special tests are used to determine if tension of, or pressure on, the sciatic nerve reproduces the patient's symptoms.[18,42–46] The two most commonly used special tests to determine sciatic nerve pathology are the **straight leg raise test** (Lasegue's test) (see Box 10–9) and the **tension sign** (Box 10–16).

The treatment and rehabilitation protocol focus on resolving the pathology that is irritating the sciatic nerve. Oral anti-inflammatory medications or corticosteroids provide symptomatic relief of the condition.[47] Bed rest has not been proven to be an effective treatment approach for patients with sciatic nerve conditions.[48] These symptoms should not be elicited during treatment. Rehabilitation exercise should not cause or exacerbate the symptoms. Exercises for strength and ROM are added as they are tolerated by the patient. Modifications of exercise or positioning are often useful in taking tension off the sciatic nerve.

SPONDYLOPATHIES

Bony disorders of the spinal column, **spondylopathies,** can afflict patients of any age and athletes in any sport, but they tend to be more prevalent in those who hyperextend their lumbar spines during activity. A genetic, congenital weakness in the pars interarticularis can predispose this structure to a stress fracture.[49] The cause may be traced to hypermobility of the spine, disease state, or acute trauma. However, a stress reaction leading to a fracture is the most prevalent bony injury to the spine in athletes.[50] These defects are caused by repetitive forced hyperextension such as that experienced by football linemen, gymnasts, and cheerleaders. Spondylopathies most

---

Box 10–16
TENSION SIGN

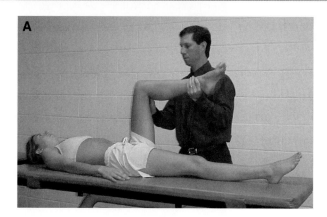
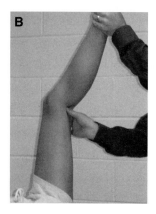

PATIENT POSITION	Supine
POSITION OF EXAMINER	At the patient's side that is to be tested; one hand grasps the heel while the other grasps the thigh.
EVALUATIVE PROCEDURE	The hip is flexed to 90°, with the knee flexed to 90°. The knee is then extended as far as possible with the examiner palpating the tibial portion of the sciatic nerve as it passes through the popliteal space **(A)**.
POSITIVE TEST	Exquisite tenderness with possible duplication of sciatic symptoms, as compared with the opposite side.
IMPLICATIONS	Sciatic nerve irritation
MODIFICATION	The **Bowstring test** is a variation of this technique **(B)**. The examiner extends the patient's knee until radiating symptoms are experienced. The knee is then flexed approximately 20° or until the symptoms are relieved. The examiner then pushes on the tibial portion of the sciatic nerve to reestablish the symptoms.

Table 10–12
CLASSIFICATION OF SPONDYLOPATHIES

Term	Description
Spondylalgia	Pain arising from the vertebrae
Spondylitis	Inflammation of the vertebrae
Spondylizema	Downward (inferior) displacement of a vertebra caused by the degeneration of the one below it
Spondylolisthesis	Forward slippage of a vertebra on the one below it (may occur secondary to spondylolysis, in which the fracture of the pars interarticularis results in the anterior displacement of the vertebral body)
Spondylolysis	Degeneration of a vertebral structure secondary to repetitive stress, most commonly affecting the pars interarticularis but with no displacement of the vertebral body
Spondylopathy	Any disorder of the vertebrae
Spondylosis	Arthritis or osteoarthritis of the vertebrae; results in pressure's being placed on the vertebral nerve roots

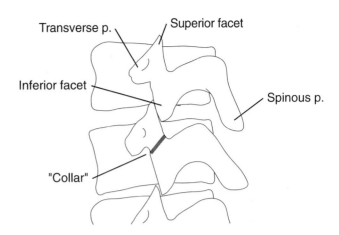

FIGURE 10–26. "Collared Scotty dog" deformity. On a radiograph, the presence of a collar on the Scotty dog indicates a nondisplaced stress fracture on the pars interarticularis, spondylolysis.

the affected vertebra and the one below it is lost, resulting in the superior vertebra's sliding anteriorly, and possibly inferiorly, on the one below it (Fig. 10–27). A radiographic examination of this condition reveals a "decapitated Scotty dog" deformity, in which the head of the dog, the anterior element of the vertebra, has be-

commonly occur at the L4–L5 or L5–S1 levels but may develop anywhere along the vertebral column.[49,51] Table 10–12 presents an encapsulated description of common spondylopathies.

Spondylolysis

Spondylolysis is a defect in the pars interarticularis, the area of the vertebral arch between the inferior and superior articular facets, usually brought on by repetitive stress. It can occur bilaterally or unilaterally. Bilateral defects in the pars interarticularis result in **listhesis,** the posterior portion of the vertebra, the laminae, inferior articular surfaces, and spinous process' separating from the vertebral body.[52] This defect, when seen on an oblique radiographic view, appears as a "collared Scotty dog" deformity, with the area of the stress fracture representing the dog's collar (Fig. 10–26).

The patient presents with localized low back pain that is increased during and after activity. During observation, spinal alignment is usually normal. Active ROM is normal for flexion, but pain restricts extension. Results of special tests and neurologic tests are normal. The evaluative findings of advanced spondylolysis resemble those of spondylolisthesis.

Spondylolisthesis

Spondylolysis may progress to spondylolisthesis, in which the defects in both elements of the pars interarticularis result in the separation of the vertebra into two uniquely identifiable structures. The fixation between

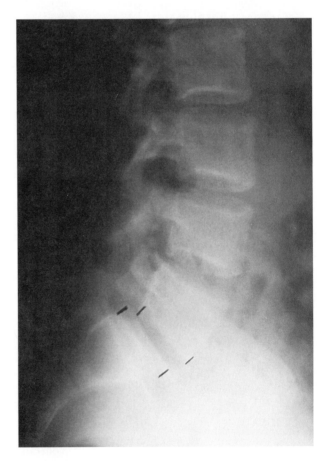

FIGURE 10–27. Spondylolisthesis of the L5-S1 junction. Notice that the L5 vertebra is anteriorly displaced relative to S1.

Table 10–13
EVALUATIVE FINDINGS: Spondylolysis and Spondylolisthesis

Examination Segment	Clinical Findings	
History	**Onset:**	Insidious; the pain begins as an ache and evolves to constant pain
	Pain characteristics:	Pain in the lumbar spine, possibly radiating into the buttocks and upper portion of the posterolateral thighs; the intensity of pain increases as the condition worsens.
	Mechanism:	Current thought suggests that the pars interarticularis suffers a stress fracture secondary to repetitive stress caused by the spine's going into extension.
	Predisposing conditions:	Imbalances in trunk muscular strength, endurance, and flexibility; activities that repetitively place the lumbar spine into hyperextension; females have a higher incidence rate than males.
Inspection	Gross inspection of the spinal curvatures may reveal hyperlordosis in the lumbar spine. The patient may walk with a short stride and remain stiff legged.	
Palpation	A palpable "step-off" deformity may be detected at the involved lumbar level. Possible spasm of the paraspinal muscles may be noted.	
Functional tests	**AROM:**	ROM during trunk flexion is restricted but pain free. Pain is described as the patient returns to an upright posture and during active extension of the spine. Pain may also be elicited during lumbar rotation and lateral rotation.
	PROM; RROM:	Hip flexion may indicate tightness of the hamstring muscles. Weakness of the spinal erector muscles.
	Other:	Tightness of the hamstrings or weakness of the abdominal muscles may be noted. Refer to Chapter 3 and Appendix B for muscle length assessment techniques.
Ligamentous tests	Spring test may reveal pain.	
Neurologic tests	Lower quarter screen is used to rule out involvement of one or more lumbar nerve roots. Results of this are typically negative, but the presence of positive neurologic signs can indicate that the vertebrae is slipping, requiring immediate physician referral.	
Special tests	Single leg stance; straight leg raises may produce a pain that is worse than that normally caused by tightness of the hamstring group.	
Comments	Radiographic examination, CT scan, or MRI is required to differentiate between spondylolysis and spondylolisthesis.	

AROM = active range of motion; CT = computed tomography; MRI = magnetic resonance imaging; PROM = passive range of motion; ROM = range of motion; RROM = resisted range of motion.

come detached from the body, the posterior element (Fig. 10–28). The severity of the spondylolisthesis is determined by the relative amount of anterior displacement of the vertebra. After the fracture occurs, the displacement of the vertebra usually does not progress under the normal daily stresses.[51] However, the stresses of sports and other exertive activities may increase the amount of anterior displacement. True healing of the fracture site rarely occurs.[49]

Spondylolisthesis is most prevalent in adolescents and in women. Also, young gymnasts have an incidence of pars interarticularis defects four times higher than that of the average population.[32] Patients with spondylolisthesis have a history and physical presentation that is very similar to that of spondylolysis (Table 10–13). The pain may be more intense and is likely to be more constant. On observation and with palpation, an actual step-off deformity may be identified, as the normal continuity of the lumbar spine is lost when the vertebra shifts forward. More severe cases of spondylolisthesis

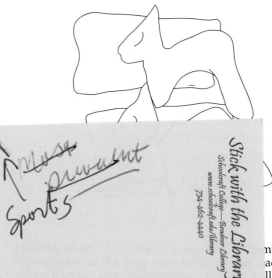

nity. Further ad to a dis- llared Scotty anteriorly.

Box 10-17
SINGLE LEG STANCE TEST

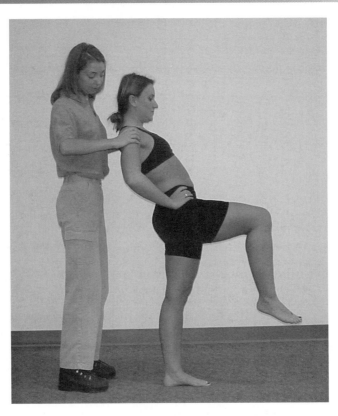

PATIENT POSITION	Standing with the body weight evenly distributed between the two feet
POSITION OF EXAMINER	Standing behind the patient, ready to provide support if the patient begins to fall
EVALUATIVE PROCEDURE	The patient lifts one leg, then places the trunk in hyperextension. The examiner may assist the patient during this motion. The procedure is then repeated for the opposite leg.
POSITIVE TEST	Pain is noted in the lumbar spine or SI area.
IMPLICATION	Shear forces are placed on the pars interarticularis by the iliopsoas pulling the vertebra anteriorly, resulting in pain.
COMMENTS	When the lesion to the pars interarticularis is unilateral, pain is evoked when the opposite leg is raised. Bilateral pars fractures result in pain when either leg is lifted. This test may exhibit pain specifically at the area of the PSIS secondary to SI joint irritation.

PSIS = posterior superior iliac spine; SI = sacroiliac.

result in a flattening of the buttocks when viewed laterally and more severe limitations in ROM. Similarly to intervertebral disc pathologies, pain may be described in the lumbar region when the patient returns to a standing posture.

Results of special tests and neurologic tests may become positive if the slippage of the vertebra is great enough to impinge on the neurologic structures. Pain associated with spondylolysis and early stages of spondylolisthesis tends not to radiate.[51] Although not a definitive test, a suspicion of spondylolysis or spondy-

lolisthesis may be reinforced by the **single leg stance test** (Box 10-17).

The treatment of patients with spondylolysis and spondylolisthesis is primarily based on the patient's symptoms. Rehabilitation exercises should resolve muscular tightness and strength deficit problems, but extension exercises that place stress on the pars interarticularis are avoided in the early stages.[49,51] Posture awareness is emphasized. The patient is taught how to control pelvic position and instructed about ways to avoid placing the lumbar spine in extension. The most

Table 10–14
EVALUATIVE FINDINGS: Sacroiliac Dysfunction

Examination Segment	Clinical Findings	
History	*Onset:*	Acute or insidious
	Pain characteristics:	Over one or both SI joints; pain possibly radiating to the buttock, groin, or thigh
	Mechanism:	No one mechanism leads to the onset of SI joint dysfunction, but it may be related to prolonged stresses placed across the sacroiliac joint by soft tissues.
	Predisposing conditions:	Postpartum women may be predisposed to SI joint pathology because relaxin released at the time of birth increases the extensibility of the ligaments surrounding the SI joints. Hormonal changes before menstrual period may increase the laxity of the SI ligaments, causing SI pain.
Inspection	The levels of the iliac crests, ASIS, and PSIS are observed for symmetry.	
Palpation	Tenderness may be elicited over the SI joint and the PSIS.	
Functional tests	Trunk flexion, either actively or passively, with the knees extended may cause sufficient movement of the sacrum on the ilia to cause pain.	
Ligamentous tests	See special tests section	
Neurologic tests	A complete lower quarter screen of the sensory, motor, and reflex distributions to rule out lumbar nerve root involvement.	
Special tests	Long sit test; SI compression and distraction; straight leg raising, fabere test; Gaenslen's test; quadrant test	
Comments	The pain distribution may mimic lumbar nerve root involvement. A combination of findings from multiple special tests is more reliable than the results of a single test.	

ASIS = anterior superior iliac spine; PSIS = posterior superior iliac spine; SI = sacroiliac.

conservative form of treatment, the use of a lumbar brace, is attempted if other forms of rehabilitation fail to produce the desired results.

SACROILIAC DYSFUNCTION

Although the SI joints are relatively immobile, a slight amount of accessory movement, rotation, or translation of the ilium on the sacrum occurs here. When these motions become extreme, the ilium rotates to the point that it subluxates on the sacrum. Injury to or degeneration of the pubic symphysis can also lead to SI dysfunction.[53] The resulting pain and dysfunction often resemble those associated with lumbar nerve root compression. Single tests for sacroiliac dysfunction are not reliable measures of the presence of pathology in this region (Table 10–14).[54] Combining the results of a series of these tests, however, does improve reliability.[55,56]

With an inflamed SI joint, compression or distraction of the two halves of the pelvis causes motion at the SI joint, resulting in a duplication of the patient's symptoms (Box 10–18). A positive compression or distraction test result does not indicate the nature of the pathology, but only shows that a form of pathology is present.

The **fabere sign** (Box 10–19), or Patrick's test, is used to elicit pain in the SI joints as well as the hip. The term *fabere* is used as a mnemonic describing the position of

the hip during testing: Flexion, **AB**duction, External Rotation, and Extension. The **Gaenslen's test** (Box 10–20), is used to place a rotatory stress on the joint by forcing one hip into hyper...

When viewed ... clock-wise ... ior mo... ilium ... the ... pearing the pa... sition, relative occurre... indicating lateral si...

Altern... rotate pos... ing a posi... may be a ca... typified by... be shorter ti... supine. As th... sit position, the rotated ilium ... to move from a relatively shorter positio... a longer one. This occurrence is a positive long sit test result, indicating a posterior rotation of the SI joint on the ipsilateral side as the leg moves from a shorter to a longer position.

Box 10–18
SACROILIAC JOINT COMPRESSION AND DISTRACTION TESTS

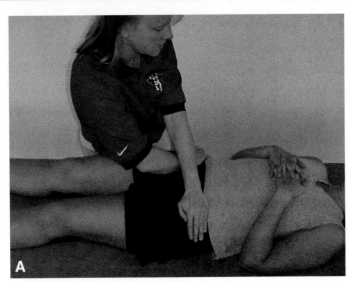
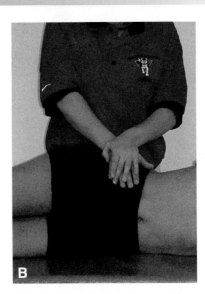

(A) Sacroiliac joint compression test. Spreading the ASIS compresses the SI joint. **(B)** Sacroiliac joint distraction test. Compressing the ASIS distracts the SI Joints. The distraction test should be performed on both sides.

PATIENT POSITION	Compression: Supine Distraction: Sidelying
POSITION OF EXAMINER	Compression: At the side of the patient with the hands placed over the opposite ASIS bilaterally Distraction: Behind the patient with both hands over the lateral aspect of the pelvis.
EVALUATIVE PROCEDURE	Compression: The examiner applies pressure to spread the ASIS, thus compressing the SI joints. Distraction: The examiner applies pressure down through the anterior portion of the ilium, spreading the SI joints.
POSITIVE TEST	Pain arising from the SI joint
IMPLICATIONS	Sacroiliac pathology

ASIS = anterior superior iliac spine; PSIS = posterior superior iliac spine; SI = sacroiliac.

Box 10–19
FABERE TEST

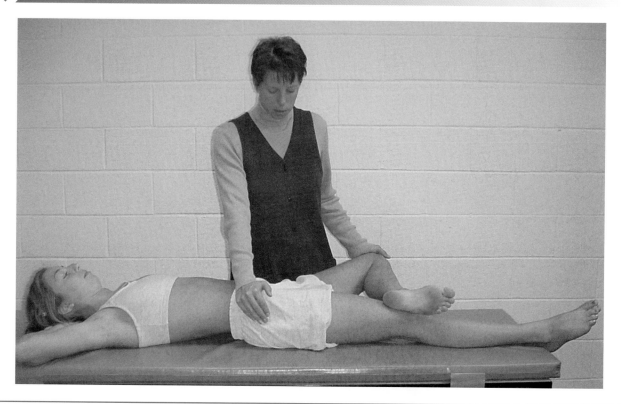

Fabere (flexion, abduction, external rotation, and extension) test for hip or sacroiliac pathology.

PATIENT POSITION	Supine, with the foot of the involved side crossed over the opposite thigh
POSITION OF EXAMINER	At the side of the patient to be tested with one hand on the opposite ASIS and the other on the medial aspect of the flexed knee
EVALUATIVE PROCEDURE	The extremity is allowed to rest into full external rotation followed by the examiner's applying overpressure at the knee and ASIS
POSITIVE TEST	Pain in the sacroiliac joint or hip
IMPLICATIONS	Pain in the inguinal area anterior to the hip may indicate hip pathology. Pain during the application of overpressure in the SI area may indicate SI joint pathology.

ASIS = anterior superior iliac spine; SI = sacroiliac.

Box 10–20
GAENSLEN'S TEST

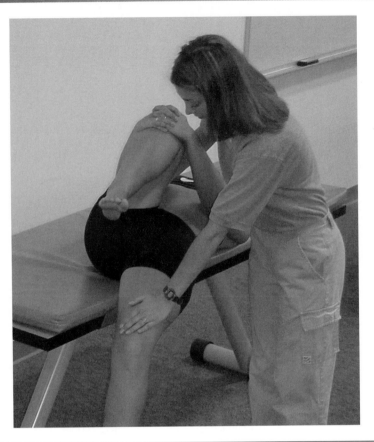

Gaenslen's test places a rotational force on the SI joints.

PATIENT POSITION	Supine, lying close to the side of the table
POSITION OF EXAMINER	Standing at the side of the patient
EVALUATIVE PROCEDURE	The examiner slides the patient close to the edge of the table. The patient pulls the far knee up to the chest. The near leg is allowed to hang over the edge of the table.
POSITIVE TEST	While stabilizing the patient, the examiner applies pressure to the near leg, forcing it into hyperextension. The lumbar spine should not go into extension during this test. Pain in the SI region
IMPLICATIONS	SI joint dysfunction

SI = sacroiliac.

Box 10–21
LONG SIT TEST

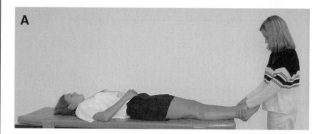

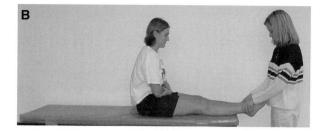

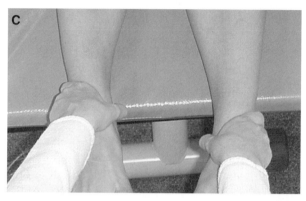

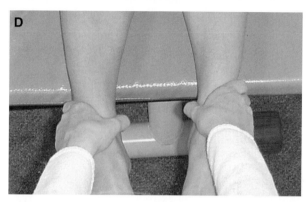

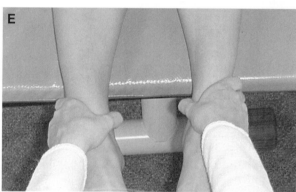

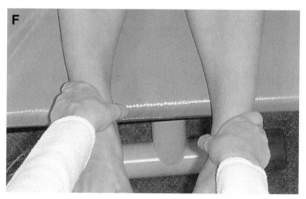

(A) Starting position. (B) Finishing position.
(C) Left leg is longer when supine and becomes shorter when assuming a sitting position.
(D) Signifying anterior rotation of the ilium.
(E) Left leg is shorter when supine and becomes longer when assuming a sitting position.
(F) Signifying posterior rotation of the ilium.

PATIENT POSITION	Supine with the heels off the table.
POSITION OF EXAMINER	Holding the feet with the thumbs placed over the medial malleoli.
EVALUATIVE PROCEDURE	The examiner provides slight traction on the legs while the patient arches and lifts the buttocks off the table. The patient then rests supine on the table. The patient then moves from a supine to a long sit position. The examiner must pay close attention to the position of the malleoli at all times throughout the test. This test is done actively if possible, without assistance provided by the upper extremities.
POSITIVE TEST	The movement of the medial malleoli is observed. If the involved leg (painful side) goes from a longer to a shorter position, there is an anterior rotation of the ilium on that side. If the involved side goes from a shorter to a longer position, posterior rotation of the ilium on the sacrum is indicated.
IMPLICATIONS	Rotated ilium as noted above.

◆ ON-FIELD EVALUATION OF THORACIC AND LUMBAR SPINE INJURIES

All injuries to the spinal column requiring an on-field evaluation must be treated as being catastrophic in nature until determined otherwise. Bilateral symptoms in the upper extremities or symptoms in the lower extremities should alert the examiner to the potential of spinal cord involvement. Chapter 18 discusses the evaluation and management of potentially catastrophic spinal cord injuries.

ON-FIELD HISTORY

- **Location of pain:** Pain that is localized to the vertebral column can indicate a disc rupture, sprain, or facet pathology. Pain running parallel to the vertebral column may indicate spasm of the paravertebral muscles. Pain radiating into the extremities may indicate trauma to one or more spinal nerve roots.
- **Peripheral symptoms:** Pain, weakness, or numbness that radiates into the extremity is usually the result of nerve root impingement.
- **Mechanism of injury:** External forces that produce rotation of the spine may result in facet joint dislocation or subluxation, disc trauma, or ligamentous sprains. Eccentric contractions may result in a muscular strain.

ON-FIELD INSPECTION

- **Position of the athlete:** Observe the athlete's position. Is the athlete prone or supine? If the athlete is supine and trauma to the vertebra, spinal cord, nerve roots, or spinal musculature is suspected, these structures cannot be palpated without moving the athlete. If spinal cord involvement is suspected, the athlete must be managed according to the procedures described in Chapter 18.
- **Posture:** Note the presence of abnormal posture, including flexion or extension posturing of the extremities or flaccidity of the muscles possibly indicating spinal cord involvement. The patient may also assume a posture that decreases the amount of pressure placed on the involved structure (e.g., disc, facet joints) or the posture may be influenced by muscle spasm.
- **Willingness to move:** Assume that a motionless athlete is unconscious until otherwise ruled out. Disc lesions, vertebral fractures, facet dislocations, or muscle spasm may cause the athlete to move in a guarded manner.

ON-FIELD NEUROLOGIC TESTS

If the athlete describes symptoms that radiate into the extremities, the following on-field neurologic assessments is necessary. If these tests show positive results (or if there is reason to suspect a vertebral fracture or dislocation), then the athlete must be managed as described in Chapter 18.

- **Sensory tests:** Bilaterally check the anterior, posterior, medial, and lateral aspects of the extremities to assure equal sensory function within the dermatomes. Absent or diminished sensation in one or more extremity can indicate serious spinal cord trauma.
- **Motor tests:** Ask the athlete to wiggle the feet and hands and bend the knees and elbows. The inability to perform these tasks may indicate spinal cord trauma.

ON-FIELD PALPATION

If the athlete is in the prone position, the majority of the lumbar and thoracic spine can be easily palpated, although portions of the back may be covered by protective equipment. Do not roll an athlete who is supine to perform palpation if the possibility of spinal cord involvement or vertebral fracture exists.

- **Bony palpation:** Palpate the spinous processes of the lumbar and thoracic spine (typically easily palpable [refer to Tables 10–6 and 10–7 for the approximate location of the spinous processes]). The transverse processes may be masked by the paravertebral muscles, but their location can be palpated for tenderness.
- **Paraspinal muscles:** Palpate the paraspinal muscles to identify areas of spasm. If the trauma was caused secondary to a direct blow, the area may be tender to the touch.

◆ ON-FIELD MANAGEMENT OF THORACIC AND LUMBAR SPINE INJURIES

This section describes the on-field management of thoracic and lumbar spine injuries. Athletes suspected of having vertebral fractures or dislocations in these areas of the spinal column should be spine boarded as described in Chapter 18.

THORACIC SPINE

Forced flexion or lateral bending of the thoracic spine places compressive forces on the anterior aspect of the vertebral bodies in the lower thoracic spine. The upper thoracic spine can be compressed by an axial load's being placed on the cervical spine.[57,58] In most instances, neurologic function is normal, leaving the on-field determination of a possible fracture to be based on the mechanism of injury and point tenderness over the affected vertebra.[59] If the fracture goes unrecognized, pain and stiffness in the thoracic region and pain during deep inspiration may be reported.[57] Although it is a rare occurrence, fractured thoracic vertebra may puncture the esophagus[60] or the aorta.[61]

Although most thoracic spine fractures are stable, athletes suspected of suffering from this pathology must be spine boarded and transported to undergo further medical evaluation.[59] Radiographs are used to confirm the presence of the fracture.

LUMBAR SPINE

Catastrophic injury to the lumbar spine is relatively rare because of the decreased ROM of this area and the extremely high forces needed to cause this injury. However, this fact should not allow the athletic trainer or physician to become complacent during the evaluation process. As with all spinal injuries, the evaluation of the lumbar spine must be approached as if a catastrophic injury exists until it has been ruled out.

The athlete must be questioned for a history of symptoms, including pain and paresthesia. Pain localized over a spinous process may indicate a compression or burst fracture. This alone is reason for immediate referral. Any symptoms suggesting neurologic involvement must be investigated. An athlete reporting bilateral symptoms must be treated as having a spinal cord injury, immobilized on a spine board, and properly transported to a medical facility.

Direct blows to the lumbar or thoracic region may result in trauma to the kidneys, ribs, or other internal organs. The evaluation of these conditions is discussed in Chapter 12.

◆ REFERENCES

1. Tall, RL, and DeVault, W: Spinal injury in sport: Epidemiologic consideration. *Clin Sports Med*, 12:441, 1993.
2. Nachemson, A, and Eifstrom, G: Intravital dynamic measurements in lumbar discs. *Scand J Rehabil Med* (suppl):1, 1960.
3. Oegema, TR: Biochemistry of the intervertebral disc. *Clin Sports Med*, 12:419, 1993.
4. Carrigg, SY, and Hillemeyer, LE: The effect of running-induced intervertebral disc compression on thoracolumbar vertebral column mobility in young, healthy males. *J Orth Sports Phys Ther*, 16:19, 1992.
5. Naylor, A, and Shentall, R: Biochemical aspects of intervertebral discs in aging and disease. In Jayson, M (ed): *The Lumbar Spine and Back Pain*. New York, Grune and Stratton, Inc, 1976, pp 317–326.
6. Hanley, ED, and David, SM: Lumbar arthrodesis for the treatment of back pain. *J Bone Joint Surg*, 81(A):716, 1999.
7. Nachemson, A, and Morris, JM: In vivo measurements of intradiscal pressure. *J Bone Joint Surg*, 46(A):1077, 1964.
8. MacLennan, AH: The role of the hormone relaxin in human reproduction and pelvic girdle relaxation. *Scand J Rheumatol*, 20(suppl 88):7, 1991.
9. Hollinshead, WH, and Jenkins, DB: The organs and organ systems. In Hollinshead, WH, and Jenkins, DB (eds): *Functional Anatomy of the Limbs and Back*. Philadelphia, WB Saunders, 1981, p 55.
10. Moore, KL: The back. In Moore, KL (ed): *Clinically Oriented Anatomy*, ed 2. Baltimore, Williams & Wilkins, 1985, p 599.
11. Massie, DL, and Haddox, A: Influence of lower extremity biomechanics and muscle imbalances on the lumbar spine. *Athletic Therapy Today*, March:46, 1999.
12. Boissonnault, W, and DiFabio, RP: Pain profile of patients with low back pain referred to physical therapy. *J Orthop Sport Phys Ther*, 24:180, 1996.
13. Gatt, CJ, et al: Impact loading of the lumbar spine during football blocking. *Am J Sports Med*, 25:317, 1997.
14. Landau, M, and Krafchik, BR: The diagnostic value of café-au-lait macules. *J Am Acad Dermatol*, 40:877, 1999.
15. Abeliovich, D, et al: Familial café-au-lait spots: A variant of neurofibromatosis type 1. *J Med Genet*, 32:985, 1995.
16. McKenzie, RA: The lumbar spine: *Mechanical Diagnosis and Therapy*. Waikanae, New Zealand, Spinal Publications, 1981.
17. Fritz, JM: Lumbar intervertebral disc injuries in athletes. *Athletic Therapy Today*, March:27, 1999.
18. Scham, SM, and Taylor, TKF: Tension signs in lumbar disc prolapse. *Clin Orthop*, 75:195, 1971.
19. Hudgens, WR: The crossed-straight-leg-raising test. *N Engl J Med*, 297:1127, 1977.
20. Woodhall, R, and Hayes, GJ: The well-leg-raising test of Fajersztajn in the diagnosis of ruptured lumbar intervertebral disc. *J Bone Joint Surg Am*, 32:786, 1950.
21. Hoover, CF: A new sign for the detection of malingering and functional paresis of lower extremities. *JAMA*, 51:746, 1908.
22. Archibald, AC, and Wiechec, F: A reappraisal of Hoover's test. *Arch Phys Med Rehabil*, 51:234, 1970.
23. Arieff, AJ, et al: The Hoover sign: An objective sign of pain and/or weakness in the back or lower extremities. *Arch Neurol*, 5:673, 1961.
24. Fritz, JM: Use of a classification approach to the treatment of 3 patients with low back syndrome. *Phys Ther*, 78:766, 1998.
25. Delitto, A, Erhard, RE, and Bowling, RW: A treatment-based classification approach to low back syndrome: Identifying and staging patients for conservative treatment. *Phys Ther*, 75:740, 1995.
26. Fritz, JM, Erhard, RE and Vignovic, M: A nonsurgical treatment approach for patients with lumbar spinal stenosis. *Phys Ther*, 77:963, 1997.
27. Natarajan, RN, et al: Study on effect of graded facetectomy on change in lumbar motion segment torsional flexibility using three-dimensional continuum contact representation for facet joints. *J Biomech Eng*, 121:215, 1999.
28. Boden, SD, et al: Orientation of the lumbar facet joints: association with degenerative disc disease. *J Bone Joint Surg*, 78(A):403, 1996.
29. Dreyer, SJ, and Dreyfuss, PH: Low back pain and the zygapophysial (facet) joints. *Arch Phys Med Rehabil*, 77:290, 1996.
30. Jensen, MC, et al: Magnetic imaging of the lumbar spine in people without back pain. *N Engl J Med* 331:69, 1994.
31. ten Brinke, A, et al: Is leg length discrepancy associated with the side of radiating pain in patients with a lumbar herniated disc? *Spine*, 24:684, 1999.
32. Tertti, M, et al: Disc degeneration in young gymnasts: A magnetic resonance imaging study. *Am J Sports Med*, 18:206, 1990.
33. Jonsson, B, and Stromqvist, B: Clinical characteristics of recurrent sciatica after lumbar discectomy. *Spine*, 21:500, 1996.
34. Benyahya, E, et al: Sciatica as the first manifestation of a leiomyosarcoma of the buttock. *Rev Rheum Engl Ed*, 64:135, 1997.
35. Amundsen, T, et al: Lumbar spinal stenosis. Clinical and radiological features. *Spine*, 20:1178, 1995.
36. Maheshwaran, S, et al: Sciatica in degenerative spondylolisthesis of the lumbar spine. *Ann Rheum Dis*, 54:539, 1995.
37. Spencer, DL: The anatomical basis of sciatica secondary to herniated lumbar disc: A review. *Neurol Res*, 21(suppl 1):S33, 1999.
38. Zwart, JA, Sand, T and Unsgaard, G: Warm and cold sensory thresholds in patients with unilateral sciatica: C fibers are more severely affected than a-delta fibers. *Acta Neurol Scand*, 97:41, 1998.
39. Tomaszewski, D: Vertebral osteomyelitis in a high school hockey player: A case report. *J Athletic Training*, 34:29, 1999.
40. Long, DM, et al: Persistent back pain and sciatica in the United States: Patient characteristics. *J Spinal Disord*, 9:40, 1996.

41. Zabelis, T, Karandreas, N, and Lygidakis, C: The tendon reflexes in the electrodiagnosis of sciatica. *Electromyogr Clin Neurophysiol,* 35:175, 1995.

42. Charnley, J: Orthopedic signs in the diagnosis of disc protrusion with special reference to the straight-leg-raising test. *Lancet,* 1:156, 1951.

43. Edgar, MA, and Park, WM: Induced pain patterns on passive straight-leg-raising in lower lumbar disc protrusion. *J Bone Joint Surg Br,* 56:658, 1974.

44. Goddard, BS, and Reid, JD: Movements induced by straight-leg-raising in the lumbo-sacral roots, nerves, and plexus and in the intrapelvic section of the sciatic nerve. *J Neurol Neurosurg Psychiatr,* 28:12, 1965.

45. Urban, LM: The straight-leg-raising test: A review. *J Orthopedic Sports Phys Ther,* 2:117, 1981.

46. Wilkins, RH, and Brody, IA: Lasegue's sign. *Arch Neurol,* 21:219, 1969.

47. Watts, RW, and Silagy, CA: A meta-analysis on the efficacy of epidural corticosteroids in the treatment of sciatica. *Anaesth Intensive Care,* 23:564, 1995.

48. Voormen, PC, et al: Lack of effectiveness of bed rest for sciatica. *N Engl J Med,* 340:418, 1999.

49. Motley, G, et al: The pars interarticularis stress reaction, spondylolysis, and spondylolisthesis progression. *J Athletic Training,* 33:351, 1998.

50. Jackson, D, et al: Stress reactions involving the pars interarticularis in young athletes. *Am J Sports Med,* 9:305, 1981.

51. Pezzullo, DJ: Spondylolisthesis and spondylolysis in athletes. *Athletic Therapy Today,* March:36, 1999.

52. Moore, KL: The perineum and pelvis. In Moore, KL (ed): *Clinically Oriented Anatomy.* Baltimore, Williams & Wilkins, 1985, p 389.

53. Major, NM, and Helms, CA: Pelvic stress injuries: the relationship between osteitis pubis (symphysis pubis stress injury) and sacroiliac abnormalities in athletes. *Skeletal Radiol,* 26:711, 1997.

54. Potter, NA, and Rothstein, JM: Intertester reliability for selected clinical tests of the sacroiliac joint. *Phys Ther,* 65:1671, 1985.

55. Cibulka, MT, Delitto, A, and Koldehoff, RM: Changes in innominate tilt after manipulation of the sacroiliac joint in patients with low back pain: An experimental study. *Phys Ther,* 68:1359, 1988.

56. Broadhurst, NA, and Bond, MJ: Pain provocation tests for the assessment of sacroiliac joint dysfunction. *J Spinal Disord,* 11:341, 1998.

57. Elattrache, N, Fadale, PD and Fu, FH: Thoracic spine fracture in a football player. A case report. *Am J Sports Med,* 21:157, 1993.

58. Kifune, M, et al: Fracture pattern and instability of throacolumbar injuries. *Eur Spine J,* 4:98, 1995.

59. McHugh-Pierzina, VL; Zillmer, DA, and Giangarra, CE: Thoracic compression fracture in a basketball player. *J Athletic Training,* 30:163, 1995.

60. Brouwers, MA, Veldhuis, EF, and Zimmerman, KW: Fracture of the thoracic spine with paralysis and esophageal perforation. *Eur Spine J,* 6:211, 1997.

61. Bakker, FC, Patka, P, and Haarman, HJ: Combined repair of a traumatic rupture of the aorta and anterior stabilization of a thoracic spine fracture: a case report. *J Trauma,* 40:128, 1996.

11

The Cervical Spine

The cervical spine provides the greatest range of motion (ROM) among the segments of the spinal column. However, the spinal cord is the most vulnerable in this location of the spinal column. Because of its important role in protecting the spinal cord and spinal nerve roots, injury to the cervical vertebrae can have catastrophic results.

This chapter describes the clinical evaluation of cervical spine pathology. Chapter 18 describes the on-field evaluation and management of patients with potentially catastrophic cervical spine trauma. The procedures described in this chapter assume that the possibility of spinal fracture and dislocation have been ruled out.

 ## CLINICAL ANATOMY

Carrying only the weight of the head, the vertebral bodies of the cervical vertebrae are much smaller than the other sections of the spinal column. The first two vertebrae of the cervical spine are unique. The first cer-

vical vertebra, the **atlas,** has no vertebral body and supports the weight of the skull through two concave facet surfaces, forming the **atlanto-occipital joint.** The primary movement at the junction between the atlas and the skull (the C0-C1 articulation) is flexion and extension, such as when nodding the head "yes." A slight amount of lateral flexion also occurs at the C0-C1 articulation. At the C1 vertebrae, the transverse processes are exceptionally long and no true spinous process exists. The second cervical vertebra, the **axis,** has a small body with a superior projection, the **dens.** The articulation between the anterior arch of the atlas and the dens forms the **atlanto-axial joint,** providing the majority of rotational motion of the skull on the spinal column, as when shaking the head "no" (Fig. 11–1). Moving inferiorly along the rest of the cervical vertebrae, the dimensions of the bone increase to provide the stability needed to support the increasing loads and larger muscle masses attaching at these levels. The cervical vertebrae are unique because the transverse processes contain the **transverse foramen,** through which the vertebral arteries pass.

As with the lumbar spine, the cervical spine's facet joints are formed by the lateral portion of the superior facet that articulates with the medial portion of the inferior facet. Refer to Chapter 10 for more information about these joints.

The intervertebral discs in the cervical spine, as throughout the rest of the spine, are formed by the dense outer annulus fibrosus surrounding the flexible interdiscal tissue, the nucleus pulposus (see Chapter 10). In this region, the discs are smaller because they have less weight to support. Because of the unique anatomical features of the first two cervical vertebrae, intervertebral disks are not located at the C0-C1 and C1-C2 articulations.

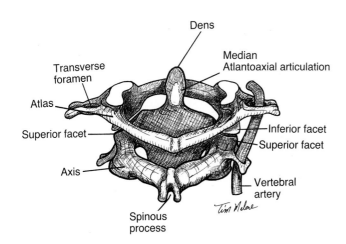

FIGURE 11–1. Atlanto-axial joint formed between the first and second cervical vertebrae. The dens serves as the axis of rotation for the skull's movement on the vertebral column.

LIGAMENTOUS ANATOMY

Extending from the cervical spine to the lumbar spine, **anterior** and **posterior longitudinal ligaments** reinforce the spinal column (Fig. 11–2). The anterior longi-

369

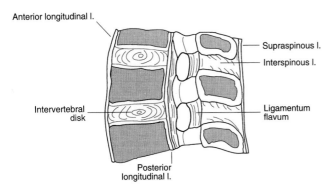

FIGURE 11–2. Cross-sectional view of the ligaments of the vertebral column.

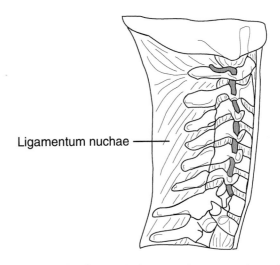

FIGURE 11–3. In the cervical spine, the supraspinous ligament thickens to form the ligamentum nuchae.

tudinal ligament strengthens the anterior portion of the intervertebral discs and vertebrae and limits extension of the spine.

The posterior longitudinal ligament is the densest in the cervical spine, gradually thinning as it progresses down the vertebral column. This ligament primarily limits flexion of the spine and reinforces the posterior aspect of the intervertebral disc.

In the cervical spine, the supraspinous ligament becomes the **ligamentum nuchae,** a triangular septum that serves as a broad area for muscle attachment. The ligamentum nuchae restricts flexion in the cervical spine (Fig. 11–3).

The **interspinous ligaments,** which occupy the space between the spinous processes, limit flexion and rotation of the spine. The posterior margin of the vertebral canal is formed by the **ligamentum flavum,** a pair of elastic ligaments connecting the lamina of one vertebra to the lamina of the vertebra above it. The ligamentum flavum limits flexion and rotation of the spine.

BRACHIAL PLEXUS

Although there are seven cervical vertebrae, eight pairs of nerve roots exit in this area. The first seven cervical nerves exit above the corresponding vertebrae. The "odd" cervical nerve, C8, exits below the seventh cervical vertebra (between the seventh cervical and first thoracic vertebrae) (Fig. 11–4).

Supplying innervation to portions of the shoulder, the length of the arm, and hand, the brachial plexus is formed by the C5 through C8 and the T1 nerve roots. The C4 or T2 nerve roots (or both) also may be included (Fig. 11–5). The brachial plexus is best conceptualized as having five segmental areas: roots, trunks, divisions, cords, and branches.

FIGURE 11–4. Pairing of the cervical nerve roots.

RELATIONSHIP BETWEEN SPINAL AND VERTEBRAL SEGMENTS

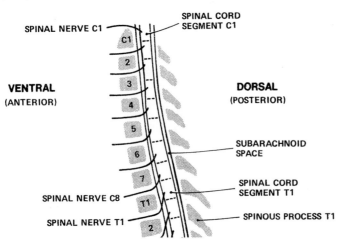

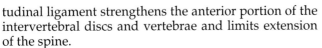

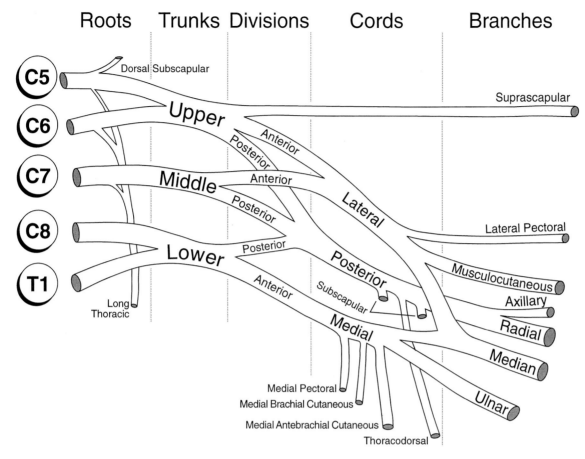

FIGURE 11–5. Brachial plexus formed by the C5 through C8 and T1 spinal nerve roots. Note that some texts include the C4 and/or T2 nerve roots as a part of the brachial plexus.

The C5 and C6 nerve roots converge to form the upper trunk. The C7 nerve root forms the middle trunk. The C8 and T1 nerve roots merge to form the lower trunk. Each trunk then diverges into anterior and posterior divisions. The posterior divisions of each trunk converge to form the posterior cord; the anterior division of the upper and middle trunks merge to form the lateral cord, and the anterior division of the lower cord forms the medial cord.

Each cord diverges to form the terminal branches of the brachial plexus. The lateral cord diverges into the lateral pectoral nerve, the muscultaneous nerve, and sends a branch that partially innervates the median nerve. The posterior cord splits into the axillary and radial nerves. One portion of the medial cord forms the ulnar nerve, and one portion converges with a division of the lateral cord to form the median nerve. These terminal branches innervate the arm, forearm, and hand. The nerves arising from the medial and lateral cords are routed to the pectoral muscles and the flexor muscles originating on the anterior portion of the arm (relative to the *anatomical position*). The nerves emerging from the posterior cord innervate the muscles of the shoulder itself and the extensor muscles originating on

the posterior aspect of the arm. In Figure 11–5, the other nerves that arise from the brachial plexus are identified.

MUSCULAR ANATOMY

Many of the spinal muscles discussed in Chapter 10 also act on the cervical spine. With bilateral contraction, the cervical spine muscles extend or flex the cervical spine and head. Unilateral contractions primarily result in side bending and contribute to cervical rotation. When coupled with the contractions of other muscles contralateral to themselves, these muscles primarily work to rotate the spine.

The superficial layer of the cervical musculature is formed by the **splenius capitis** and **splenius cervicis** muscles. These muscles, when acting bilaterally, extend

Anatomical position   The position that the body assumes when standing upright with the feet and palms facing anteriorly.

A

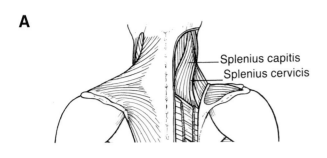

- Splenius capitis
- Splenius cervicis

B

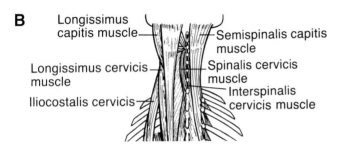

- Longissimus capitis muscle
- Longissimus cervicis muscle
- Iliocostalis cervicis
- Semispinalis capitis muscle
- Spinalis cervicis muscle
- Interspinalis cervicis muscle

FIGURE 11–6. Muscles of the spinal column: **(A)** superficial muscles, **(B)** deep muscles.

the head and neck. When acting alone, they laterally flex and rotate the head and cervical spine to the same side as the muscle (Fig. 11–6). The intrinsic muscles (those originating and attaching on the spinal column) acting on the cervical spine are presented in Table 11–1.

Many of the muscles acting on the cervical spine are superficial and, depending on the fixation of the origin or insertion, act on the shoulder, cervical spine, or head. The extrinsic muscles (those originating away from the spinal column) are presented in Table 11–2.

When its insertion on the scapula is fixed, the upper one third of the **trapezius** (discussed in Chapter 13) bilaterally acts to extend the cervical spine and skull. When the trapezius works unilaterally with other musculature, it laterally bends and rotates the cervical spine and skull. The **sternocleidomastoid (SCM)** is responsi-

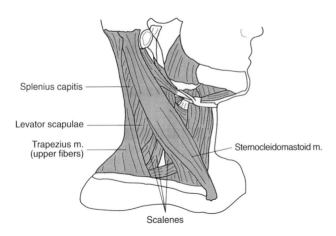

- Splenius capitis
- Levator scapulae
- Trapezius m. (upper fibers)
- Sternocleidomastoid m.
- Scalenes

FIGURE 11–7. Cervical musculature.

ble for rotating the skull to the opposite side and for lateral bending of the cervical spine to the same side as the contracting muscle (Fig. 11–7). The anterior, middle, and posterior **scalene** muscles laterally flex the cervical spine. When the cervical spine is fixated, the scalenes elevate the rib cage to assist in inspiration. The scalene group is significant because the brachial plexus passes between its anterior and middle portions. Spasm or tightness of the scalenes can place pressure on the neurovascular structures of the upper extremities, causing **thoracic outlet syndrome.**

◆ CLINICAL EVALUATION OF CERVICAL SPINE

The spinal cord and its nerve roots are vulnerable in the cervical spine. When the magnitude of the trauma is severe, catastrophic results may ensue. This chapter describes the evaluation of patients with noncatastrophic trauma to the cervical spine and assumes that vertebral fractures and dislocations have been ruled out. Chapter 18 describes the on-field evaluation and management of patients with cervical spine injuries.

HISTORY

The onset and identification of functional activities causing the symptoms may assist in determining the underlying pathology.

- **Location of the pain:** Is the pain localized or does it radiate? Pain that is localized to the cervical spine may indicate a muscle strain, ligament sprain, vertebral fracture or dislocation, or facet syndrome. Radiating symptoms are a strong indication that trauma has occurred to the cervical nerve root or spinal cord.

- **Onset of the pain:** Does the patient describe an acute, chronic, or insidious onset of pain and other symptoms? Although acute injuries usually are related to specific mechanisms of injury, chronic and insidious onsets typically occur with mechanisms related to overuse and postural considerations.

- **Mechanism and onset of injury:** Does the patient describe an acute onset of injury or did the symptoms gradually occur?
  - **Insidious onset:** Symptoms that occur with a gradual or insidious onset usually warrant a thorough postural evaluation to determine a cause-and-effect relationship.
  - **Acute onset:** When an acute onset of injury is described, the mechanism of injury can provide clues to the trauma (Table 11–3). When the report of an axial load being placed on the cervical spine is described, a possible vertebral fracture must be considered until ruled out with radiographic examination.

Table 11–1
INTRINSIC MUSCLES ACTING ON THE CERVICAL SPINAL COLUMN

Muscle	Action	Origin	Insertion	Innervation	Root
Splenius capitis	Lateral bending of the cervical spine	• Lower half of the ligamentum nuchae	• Mastoid process of the temporal bone and adjacent occipital bone (capitis portion)	Branches of cervical nerves (CN)	C4–C8
Splenius cervicis	Rotation of the face toward the same side Extension of the cervical spine	• Spinous processes of C7 through T6 vertebrae	• Transverse processes of C2 through C4 vertebrae (cervicis portion)	Branches of CN	C4–C8
Iliocostalis cervicis	Extension of spinal column Lateral bending of spinal column	• Ribs 3 through 6	• Transverse processes of C4 through C6	Branches of CN	C4–C8
Longissimus thoracis	Extension of spinal column Lateral bending of spinal column	• Common erector spinae tendon	• Transverse process of T3 through T12 • Ribs 3 through 12	Branches of CN	C4–C8
Longissimus cervicis	Extension of spinal column Lateral bending of spinal column	• Transverse processes of T1 through T5	• Transverse processes of C2 through C6	Branches of CN	C4–C8
Longissimus capitis	Extension of skull and cervical spine Rotation of the face toward the same side	• Articular processes of C5 through C7	• Mastoid process of skull	Branches of CN	C4–C8
Spinalis cervicis	Extension of the spine Lateral bending of the spine	• Upper thoracic and lower cervical spinous processes	• Ligamentum nuchae	Branches of CN	C4–C8
Spinalis capitis	Extension of the spine Lateral bending of the spine	• Upper thoracic and lower cervical spinous processes	• Ligamentum nuchae	Branches of CN	C4–C8
Semispinalis thoracis	Extension of thoracic and cervical spine Rotation to the opposite side	• Transverse process	• Travel upwardly and medially to attach to a spinous process 5 or 8 vertebrae above the origin	Deeper stratum of CN	C4–C8
Semispinalis cervicis	Extension of thoracic and cervical spine Rotation to the opposite side	• Transverse process	• Travel upwardly and medially to attach to a spinous process 5 or 8 vertebrae above the origin	Deeper stratum of CN	C4–C8
Semispinalis capitis	Extension of skull Rotation to the opposite side	• Transverse process	• Travel upwardly and medially to attach to a spinous process 5 or 8 vertebrae above the origin	Deeper stratum of CN	C4–C8
Multifidus (or multifidi)	Rotation of spine to the opposite side Stabilization of vertebral column	• Articular processes	• Spinous process	Deeper stratum of CN	C4–C8
Rotatores	Extension of spine Rotation of spine Stabilization of vertebral column	• Transverse process	• Spinous process of the vertebrae immediately above the origin	Deeper stratum of CN	C4–C8

CN = cervical nerve.

Table 11–2
EXTRINSIC MUSCLES ACTING ON THE CERVICAL SPINAL COLUMN

Muscle	Action	Origin	Insertion	Innervation	Root
Trapezius (upper one-third)	Cervical extension Cervical side bending Elevation of scapula Upward rotation of scapula Rotation of the cervical spine to the opposite side	• Occipital protuberance • Nuchal line of the occipital bone • Upper portion of the ligamentum nuchae	• Lateral one third of clavicle • Acromion process	Spinal Accessory	CN XI
Levator scapulae	Elevation of the scapula Downward rotation of the scapula Extension of cervical spine	• Spinous process of C7 • Transverse processes of cervical vertebrae C1 through C4	• Superior medial border of scapula	Dorsal subscapular	C3, C4, C5
Sternocleidomastoid	Flexion of the cervical spine Rotation of the skull to the opposite side Lateral bending of the cervical spine Elevation of the clavicle and sternum	• Medial clavicular head • Superior sternum	• Mastoid process of the skull	Spinal accessory	CN XI C2, C3
Scalene, anterior	Lateral bending of the cervical spine Elevation of the rib cage	• Anterior portion of the transverse processes of C3 to C6	• Sternal attachment of the 1st rib	Dorsal rami	C4, C5, C6
Scalene, middle	Lateral bending of the cervical spine Elevation of the rib cage	• Anterior portion of the transverse processes of C2 to C7	• Lateral to the insertion of the anterior scalene on the 1st rib	Dorsal rami	C3, C4, C5, C6, C7, C8
Scalene, posterior	Lateral bending of the cervical spine Elevation of the rib cage	• Anterior portion of the transverse processes C5 and C6	• Medial portion of the 2nd rib	Dorsal rami	C6, C7, C8

CN = cranial nerve.

374

EVALUATION MAP: CERVICAL SPINE

1. HISTORY

Location of the pain
Onset of the pain
Mechanism of injury
Consistency of the pain
History of spinal injury

2. INSPECTION

Forward head posture
Position of the head on the shoulders
Bilateral soft tissue comparison
Level of the shoulders

3. PALPATION

Anterior cervical spine
  Hyoid bone
  Thyroid cartilage
  Cricoid cartilage
  Sternocleidomastoid
  Scalenes
  Carotid artery
  Lymph nodes

Posterior cervical spine
  Occiput/superior nuchal line
  Transverse processes
  Spinous processes
  Trapezius

4. RANGE OF MOTION TESTS

Cervical spine
AROM
  Flexion
  Extension
  Lateral Flexion
  Rotation
PROM
  Flexion
  Extension
  Lateral flexion
  Rotation
RROM
  Flexion
  Extension
  Lateral flexion
  Rotation

5. LIGAMENTOUS TESTS

Spring test (see Chapter 10)

6. NEUROLOGICAL TESTS

Upper motor neuron lesions
  Babinski test
  Oppenheim test

Lower motor neuron lesions
  Upper quarter screen
  Lower quarter screen

7. SPECIAL TESTS

Brachial plexus pathology
  Brachial plexus traction test

Cervical nerve root impingement
Shoulder abduction test
  Cervical compression test
  Spurling's test
  Cervical distraction test

Vertebral artery test

AROM = active range of motion; PROM = passive range of motion; RROM = resisted range of motion.

Table 11–3
POSSIBLE PATHOLOGY BASED ON THE MECHANISM OF INJURY

Mechanism	Pathology
Flexion	Compression of the anterior vertebral body and intervertebral disc Sprain of the supraspinous, interspinous, and posterior longitudinal ligaments and ligamentum flavum Sprain of the facet joints Strain of the posterior cervical musculature
Extension	Sprain of the anterior longitudinal ligament Compression of the posterior vertebral body and intervertebral disc Compression of the facet joints Fracture of the spinous processes
Lateral bending	On the side towards the bending: 　Compression of the cervical nerve roots 　Compression of the vertebral bodies and intervertebral disc 　Compression of the facet joints On the side opposite the bending: 　Stretching of the cervical nerve roots 　Sprain of the lateral ligaments 　Sprain of the facet joints 　Strain of the cervical musculature
Rotation	Disc trauma Ligament sprain Facet sprain or dislocation Vertebral dislocation
Axial load	Compression fracture of the vertebral body Compression of the intervertebral disc

- **Consistency of the pain:** Is the pain constant or intermittent? Chemically induced pain, such as that relating to inflammation, is more constant with no change in symptoms as the cervical spine changes position. Mechanical pain, caused by compression of a nerve root, tends to vary in intensity, and relief (or a decrease in symptoms) can be obtained by moving the spine into a specific position, such as tilting the head away from the involved side, which lessens the pressure on the involved structure.
- **History of spinal injury:** Does the patient have a history of spinal injury? Identify any pertinent history that may lead to structural degeneration or predispose the patient to chronic problems. The current symptoms may be the result of scar tissue formation's impinging or restricting other structures, a previously injured disc, or the formation of osteophytes within the intervertebral foramina.

INSPECTION

A general inspection of the entire spinal column is necessary to determine proper posture in the sagittal and frontal planes.

Inspection of the Cervical Spine

- **Cervical curvature:** Observe for the presence of a lordotic curve, typical of the cervical spine. A flattening of the cervical curvature or lateral bending may indicate posturing to decrease pressure on the nerve roots (usually on the side away from the bend). An increased lordotic curve can lead to a forward head posture. Flattening of the lordotic curve can indicate spasm of the cervical muscles.
- **Position of the head on the shoulders:** Note the position of the head. The head should be seated symmetrically on the cervical spine with the shoulders held in an upright position. Unilateral spasm of the cervical muscles results in lateral flexion of the head toward the involved side. The rotation of the chin opposite the side of the tilt may indicate **torticollis** ("wry neck"), a congenital or acquired spasm of the SCM muscle. A forward head posture can be caused by long-standing postural changes in chronic conditions, muscle spasm, or weakness.
- **Bilateral soft tissue comparison:** Inspect the contour and tone of the trapezius and the other cervical musculature for equality of mass, tone, and texture. The trapezius of the dominant side may be hypertrophied relative to the opposite side. The posterior scapular muscles and the deltoids are inspected for normal muscle mass, tone, and texture. Atrophy of these muscles may result from impingement of a cervical nerve root or from brachial plexus trauma.
- **Level of the shoulders:** Standing in front of the patient, observe the level of the patient's shoulders. The height of the acromioclavicular joints, the deltoid, and clavicles should be level; the dominant shoulder is often slightly depressed relative to the nondominant shoulder.

Table 11–4 **BONY LANDMARKS FOR PALPATION**	
Structure	**Landmark**
Cervical vertebral bodies	On the same level as the spinous processes
C1 transverse process	One finger's breadth inferior to the mastoid process
C3-C4 vertebrae	Posterior to the hyoid bone
C4-C5 vertebrae	Posterior to the thyroid cartilage
C6 vertebrae	Posterior to the cricoid cartilage; movement during flexion and extension of the cervical spine
C7 vertebra	Prominent posterior spinous process

PALPATION

Table 11–4 presents a list of landmarks that can be used to orient the location of specific cervical spine structures.

Palpation of the Anterior Cervical Spine Structures

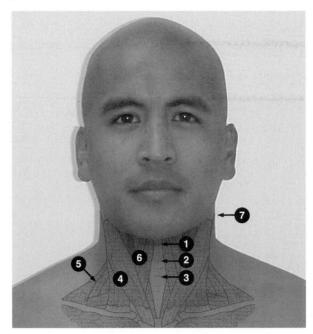

1. **Hyoid bone:** Located across from the C3 vertebra, palpate the hyoid bone for tenderness. While gently palpating this structure, request that the patient swallow, noting the superior and inferior movement of the hyoid bone.

2. **Thyroid cartilage:** Locate the thyroid cartilage, found at the level of the fourth and fifth cervical vertebrae. The thyroid cartilage is a fibrous shield protecting the anterior surface of the larynx. This structure gently shifts laterally and, similar to the hyoid bone, raises and lowers during the act of swallowing.

3. **Cricoid cartilage:** Identify the cricoid cartilage, which lies at the level of the sixth cervical vertebra. The cricoid cartilage demarcates the location where the pharynx joins the esophagus and the larynx joins the trachea. The cartilage is identified by the thickened rings that can be palpated along its anterior surface.

4. **Sternocleidomastoid:** Palpate the cordlike SCM along its length from its origin on the mastoid process and superior nuchal line to its insertion on the sternum and clavicle. Rotating the head causes the SCM on the side opposite the movement to become more prominent during palpation.

5. **Scalenes:** Palpate the scalene muscles just posterior to the SCM muscle at about the C3 to C6 level. Tightness or spasm of this muscle group may cause abnormal cervical posture or lead to **thoracic outlet syndrome.**

6. **Carotid artery:** Palpate the carotid pulse between the thyroid cartilage and the SCM.

7. **Lymph nodes:** Within the upper trapezius and beneath the mandible, palpate the lymph nodes lying within the SCM. Lymph nodes become enlarged secondary to infection, illness, or inflammation.

Palpation of the Posterior and Lateral Spine Structures

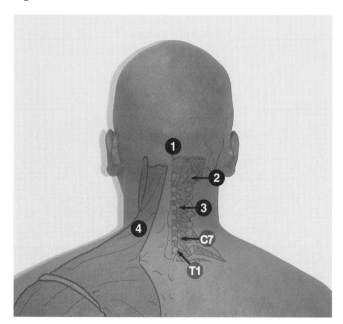

1. **Occiput and superior nuchal line:** The occipital bone, the most posterior aspect of the skull, is located at the apex of the cervical spine. Palpate this area for tenderness because it is the site of attachment for the cervical musculature.

2. **Transverse processes:** Located approximately one finger's breadth inferior to the mastoid processes, the transverse processes of C1 are the only processes of the cervical spine that are palpable. The area overlying the remaining transverse processes are palpated at the same level as the spinous processes for tenderness or crepitus.

3. **Spinous processes:** The spinous processes are more easily palpated when the cervical spine is slightly flexed. Locate the area where the cervical and thoracic spines meet slightly above the superior angle of the scapula. Here two spinous processes are more prominent than the rest. The lower protrusion is the spinous process of T1, and the superior protrusion is the C7 spinous process. From here, palpate the spinous processes of C6, C5, and, possibly, C4 and C3. Above the C5 level, the spinous processes begin to be masked by the soft tissue but the area overlying the remaining processes should be palpated for tenderness or crepitus. Each of these processes should be aligned immediately superior to the one below it.

4. **Trapezius:** Beginning at the occiput and superior nuchal line, the upper portion of the trapezius is palpated inferiorly to its insertion on the lateral clavicle, acromion process, and spine of the scapula. The thickness of this muscle is easily palpated as it spans from the cervical spine to the acromion process. Most of the remaining cervical musculature lies beneath the trapezius and is not directly palpable.

RANGE OF MOTION TESTING

Cervical ROM can be quantified by using a tape measure to note the distance of the chin from the jugular notch of the sternum or the ear to the acromion process (Fig 11–8).

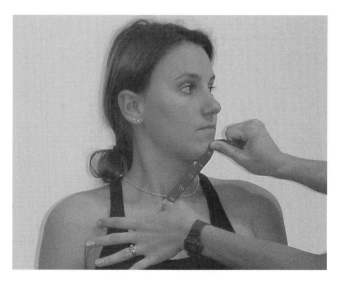

FIGURE 11–8. Measuring cervical range of motion with a tape measure. The distance from the jugular notch on the sternum to the point of the chin is measured and recorded for each motion. Cervical rotation is demonstrated in this photograph.

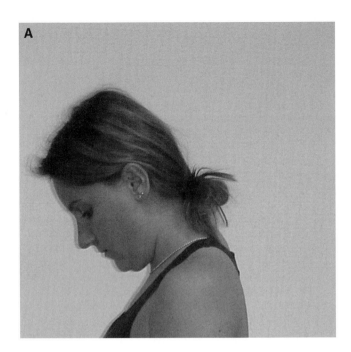

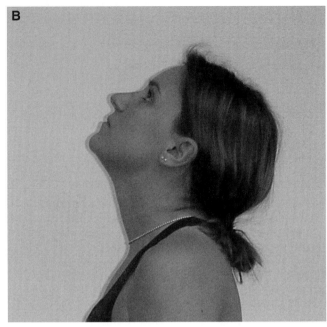

FIGURE 11–9. Active **(A)** flexion and **(B)** extension of the cervical spine. The patient may attempt to compensate for a lack of cervical flexion by rounding the shoulders and compensate for a lack of extension by retracting the scapulae.

Active Range of Motion

- **Flexion and extension:** Test for flexion and extension while the patient is standing or in a sitting position. Most of the flexion and extension motion that occurs in the cervical spine takes place at the atlanto-occipital joint (capitol flexion and extension) (Fig 11–9A). Flexion is performed by asking the patient to touch the chin to the chest, noting for rotation of the skull that indicates substitution by the SCM on the side opposite to the rotation. Extension is tested by having the patient look up toward the ceiling (Fig. 11–9B).

- **Lateral flexion:** With the patient seated, determine if the ROM of the head toward each shoulder is equal and pain free (Fig 11–10). This motion occurs primarily in the upper vertebrae, producing approximately 45 degrees of motion in each direction.

- **Rotation:** With the patient seated and the head held upright and facing forward, observe the amount of rotation as the patient attempts to look over each shoulder (Fig 11–11). This motion, occurring primarily at the atlanto-axial joint, normally is equal and pain free in each direction.

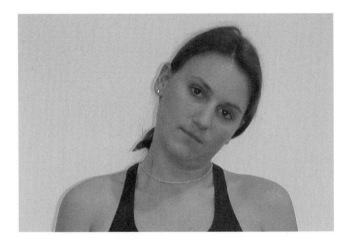

FIGURE 11–10. Active left lateral bending of the cervical spine. The patient may attempt to compensate for decreased cervical ROM by elevating the shoulder girdle.

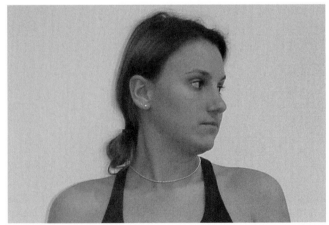

FIGURE 11–11. Active left rotation of the cervical spine. The patient may compensate for a lack of cervical rotation by rotating the torso in the direction opposite that of the cervical movement.

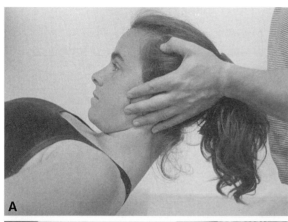

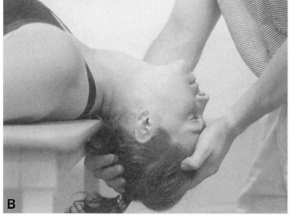

FIGURE 11–12. Passive **(A)** flexion and **(B)** extension of the cervical spine.

Passive Range of Motion

- **Flexion:** With the patient in the supine position, grasp the patient's head under the occiput and attempt to bring the chin to the chest (Fig. 11–12A). The normal end-feel for this movement is firm owing to the chin striking the chest. Spasm in the posterior cervical muscles results in a pathological firm end-feel; mechanical blockage of the atlanto-occipital joint or the vertebrae causes a premature, hard end-feel.

- **Extension:** Measure passive ROM (PROM) with the patient supine so that the head is off the end of the table and the neck is allowed to move into extension (Fig. 11–12B). The normal end-feel for this motion is hard as the occiput makes contact with the rest of the cervical spine.

- **Lateral flexion:** Continuing in the supine position, keep the patient's cervical spine in the neutral position between flexion and extension. Using one hand under the occiput, tilt the head and neck to bring the ear toward the shoulder (Fig. 11–13). Stabilize the contralateral shoulder with the opposite hand if needed. The normal end-feel for lateral flexion is firm owing to soft tissue stretch.

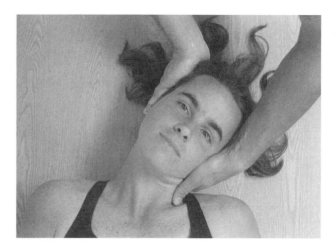

FIGURE 11–13. Passive left lateral flexion of the cervical spine.

- **Rotation:** With the patient supine, grasp the patient's forehead and occiput to maintain the cervical spine in its neutral position. Then apply pressure to rotate the skull and neck (Fig. 11–14). The skull and spine should be rotated together. A firm end-feel is expected from stretching of the SCM muscle and intrinsic neck ligaments.

Resisted Range of Motion

Resisted ROM (RROM) is highlighted in Box 11–1.

LIGAMENTOUS TESTING

There are no specific ligamentous tests for the cervical spine. The end range of PROM testing, in the absence of muscular tightness or contractions, stresses the spinal ligaments (Table 11–5).

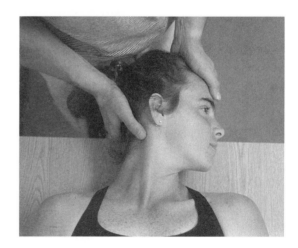

FIGURE 11–14. Passive left rotation of the cervical spine.

Box 11–1
RESISTED RANGE OF MOTION FOR THE CERVICAL SPINE

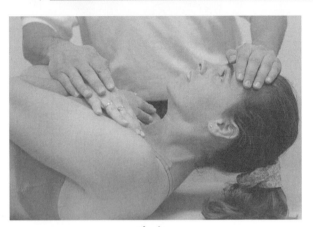

Flexion

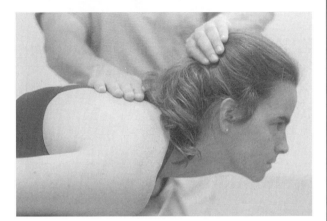

Extension

	Flexion	Extension
STARTING POSITION	Seated or supine with the cervical spine and head in the neutral position	Seated or prone with the cervical spine and head in the neutral position
STABILIZATION	Over the superior aspect of the sternum	Superior aspect of the thoracic spine (e.g., T2–T9)
RESISTANCE	To the forehead	To the skull over the occiput
MUSCLES TESTED	Sternocleidomastoid, anterior scalene	Trapezius (upper one third, levator scapulae, cervical paraspinal muscles (see Table 11–1)

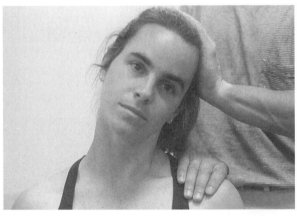

Lateral Flexion

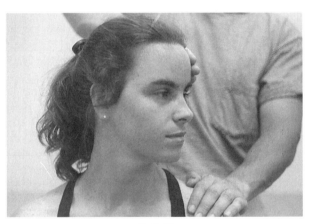

Rotation

	Lateral Flexion	Rotation
STARTING POSITION	Seated with the cervical spine and head in the neutral position	Seated with the cervical spine and head in the neutral position
STABILIZATION	Over the acromioclavicular joint on the side toward the motion	Over the anterior shoulder on the side toward the rotation.
RESISTANCE	Over the temporal and parietal bones on the side toward the motion	Over the temporal bone on the side toward the motion.
MUSCLES TESTED	Sternocleidomastoid, scalenes, paraspinal muscles on the side being tested	Sternocleidomastoid (opposite side), multifidus (opposite side), rotatores, upper trapezius (opposite side)

Table 11–5
CERVICAL SPINE LIGAMENTS STRESSED DURING PASSIVE RANGE OF MOTION TESTING

Motion	Ligaments Stressed
Flexion	Posterior longitudinal ligament Ligamentum nuchae Interspinous ligament Ligamentum flavum
Extension	Anterior longitudinal ligament
Rotation	Interspinous ligament Ligamentum flavum
Lateral bending (these tests are usually inconclusive)	Interspinous ligament Ligamentum flavum

NEUROLOGIC TESTING

Because of the mobility and relative lack of protection of the cervical spine, lower motor neuron lesions in this area are common. An upper quarter neurological screen is used to determine trauma to the C5 through T1 nerve roots. Spinal cord involvement also requires a lower quarter screen (see Box 1–5).

Upper Quarter Neurologic Screen

Box 11–2 highlights the areas of an upper quarter neurologic screen.

Upper Motor Neuron Lesions

Trauma to the brain or spinal cord can result in *hyperreflexia*, spasticity, and hypertonicity of muscles; weakness of the muscles innervated distal to the lesion; loss of sensation; and ataxia. Other clinical findings of this condition may include muscle tremor and uncontrollable involuntary movement. In athletes, upper motor neuron lesions most often are the result of head injury. The **Babinski test** (Box 11–3) and the **Oppenheim test** (Box 11–4) are used to evaluate for an upper motor neuron lesion. A positive Babinski or Oppenheim test result after traumatic injury should be treated as a potentially catastrophic head and spinal cord injury. Additionally, the loss of bowel and bladder control can be a sign of upper motor neuron lesions.

 ## CERVICAL SPINE PATHOLOGIES AND RELATED SPECIAL TESTS

Acute injuries to the cervical spine occur in contact and collision sports when the spine is compressed or forced past its normal ROM. The "whiplash" type of injury occurs as the head is moving in one direction and the cervical muscles eccentrically contract to counter this motion. Chronic conditions develop from poor postural habits, repetitive movements, decreased flexibility, and

muscular insufficiency. These conditions worsen with time secondary to the adaptive shortening of tissues, resulting in increased pain and spasm. Certain disease states such as viral infections (e.g., meningitis), allergic reactions to medication, and other diseases may mimic the symptoms of traumatic injury to the cervical spine, especially if they are creating swelling and pain within the lymphatic glands in the area.[1]

The first step when evaluating cervical pathologies is to rule out the presence of any potentially catastrophic injuries. Examiners must be thorough in evaluating the local cervical structures and determining any effect that the pathology may be causing distally through the radiation of signs and symptoms.

BRACHIAL PLEXUS PATHOLOGY

Acute trauma to the brachial plexus, often referred to as a "burner" or "stinger," is common in contact sports. The onset of this injury may be caused by a traction force placed on the brachial plexus itself (brachial plexus stretch) or an impingement of the cervical nerve roots (brachial plexus compression). In football players, the brachial plexus may be traumatized by compression of the brachial plexus between the shoulder pad and the superior medial scapula and is more common in defensive players.[2,3] This site, **Erb's point** (Fig. 11–15), is located 2 to 3 cm above the clavicle in front of the transverse process of the sixth cervical vertebra and represents the most superficial passage of the brachial plexus.

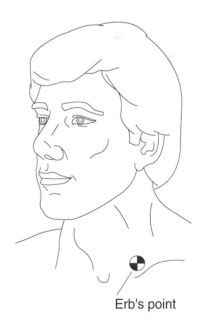

Erb's point

FIGURE 11–15. Erb's point, representing the most superficial passage of the brachial plexus. Pressure to this area can result in pain and paresthesia radiating into the upper extremity.

Hyperreflexia Increased action of the reflexes.

Box 11–2
UPPER QUARTER NEUROLOGIC SCREEN

Nerve Root Level	Sensory Testing	Motor Testing	Reflex Testing
C5	Axillary n.	Axillary n.	Biceps brachii
C6	Musculocutaneous n.	Musculocutaneous n.(C5 & C6)	Brachioradialis
C7	Radial n.	Radial n.	Triceps brachii
C8	Ulnar n. (mixed)	Median & palm. interosseous n.	None
T1	Med. brachial cutaneous n.	None	None

Box 11–3
BABINSKI TEST FOR UPPER MOTOR NEURON LESIONS

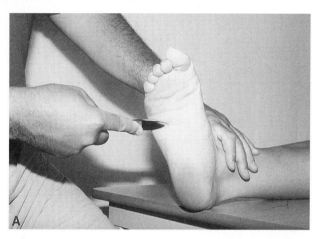

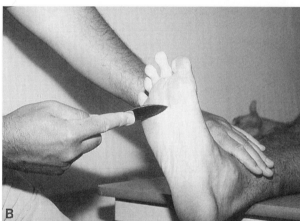

The Babinski test is most commonly performed during the evaluation of an acute head or cervical spine injury to determine the presence of an upper motor neuron lesion.

PATIENT POSITION	Supine.
POSITION OF EXAMINER	At the foot of the patient; a blunt device, such as the handle of a reflex hammer or the handle of a pair of scissors, is needed.
EVALUATIVE PROCEDURE	The examiner runs the device up the plantar aspect of the foot, making an arc from the calcaneus medially to the ball of the great toe (A).
POSITIVE TEST	The great toe extends and the other toes splay (B).
IMPLICATIONS	Upper motor neuron lesion, especially in the pyramidal tract, caused by brain or spinal cord trauma or pathology
COMMENTS	The Babinski reflex occurs normally in newborns and should spontaneously disappear shortly after birth.

Box 11–4
OPPENHEIM TEST FOR UPPER MOTOR NEURON LESIONS

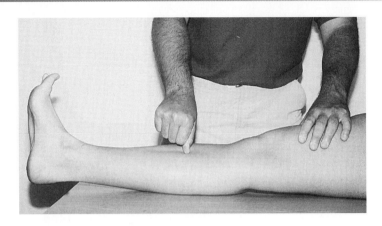

The Oppenheim test is most commonly performed during the evaluation of a patient with acute head or cervical spine injury to determine the presence of an upper motor neuron lesion.

PATIENT POSITION	Supine
POSITION OF EXAMINER	At the patient's side
EVALUATIVE PROCEDURE	The examiner's fingernail is run along the crest of the anteromedial tibia.
POSITIVE TEST	The great toe extends and the other toes splay or the patient reports hypersensitivity to the test.
IMPLICATIONS	Upper motor neuron lesion caused by brain or spinal cord trauma or pathology

Stretching of the brachial plexus occurs when the head is forced laterally while the opposite shoulder is depressed, such as when tackling in football (Fig. 11–16). The resulting force places traction on the nerves on the side opposite the lateral bending of the neck. Any of the cervical nerve roots may be affected by a traction mechanism, but the lateral and posterior cords that are innervated by the C5 and C6 nerve roots (suprascapular, lateral pectoral, musculocutaneous, and axillary nerves) are most commonly involved when the mechanism involves side bending of the head and depression of the shoulder (see Figure 11–5).[4] Forced abduction of the arm can involve the C8 and T1 nerve roots. Repeated low-intensity traction of the brachial plexus can hinder the local microcirculation of the plexus and cause ischemic changes in the nerves.[5]

A brachial plexus compression occurs on the side toward the bending of the neck when the nerve roots are impinged between the vertebrae. The likelihood of the impingement mechanism is increased by the narrowing of the intervertebral foramen (**spinal stenosis**).[6] A positive Spurling test result (described later in this chapter) is evidence of a mechanical narrowing of the intervertebral foramen by spinal stenosis, degenerative disc disease, or an asymmetric disc bulge.[7]

The signs and symptoms of any type of brachial plexus pathology are similar. Immediate pain, often reported as "burning" or "an electrical shock" radiating through the upper extremity, is typically described. Characteristically, the athlete leaves the field with the involved arm dangling limply at the side or the person may be shaking the hand and arm as to regain feeling. Manual muscle testing for the muscles innervated by the involved cervical nerve root reveals decreased strength on the involved side along with paresthesia in the dermatomes innervated by the same nerve roots (Table 11–6). These signs and symptoms normally subside within minutes.[4] Repeated or severe brachial plexus injuries may produce signs and symptoms that diminish much more slowly.

Athletes must not be allowed to return to competition until all symptoms have cleared; they must have full ROM, a full return of sensation, and normal strength throughout the affected extremity. Athletes suffering from chronic brachial plexus pathology display a dropped shoulder and atrophy of the shoulder and cervical musculature on the involved side and note a decrease in bench press weight.[2]

Despite the presence of a common set of symptoms, examiners must not become complacent to the possibil-

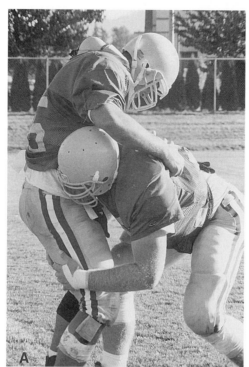

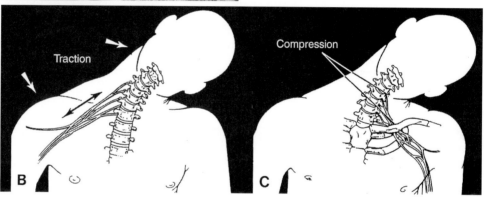

FIGURE 11–16. Mechanism for a brachial plexus injury. **(A)** The cervical spine is forced laterally and the opposite shoulder is depressed, resulting in elongation of the trapezius and brachial plexus. **(B)** Elongation of the trapezius muscle with concurrent depression of the shoulder can result in a traction injury to the brachial plexus. **(C)** Compression (impingement) of the brachial plexus can result on the side toward which the head is tilted.

ity of more severe cervical trauma. A thorough examination of the cervical spine must be undertaken to rule out the presence of a cervical fracture or dislocation. After these conditions have been ruled out, the **Brachial plexus traction test** may be used to duplicate the mechanism of injury and reproduce the patient's symptoms (Box 11–5). Many of the special tests described in the section on cervical nerve root impingement also produce positive results in the presence of brachial plexus pathology. Computed tomography (CT) scans, MRIs, and electromyographic (EMG) analysis can be used to identify local trauma to the nerves or nerve roots.[8]

The treatment and management of patients with brachial plexus trauma is discussed in the section on on-field management in this chapter. Rehabilitation of patients with brachial plexus trauma includes strengthening of the cervical musculature, biofeedback exercises, functional exercise programs, and cervical ROM exercises and re-educating the upper extremity muscles that may have been affected.[9] This set of exercises should also be used to prevent the onset of brachial plexus trauma and other cervical spine injuries.

CERVICAL NERVE ROOT IMPINGEMENT

Degenerative disc changes, acute disc trauma, a unilaterally dislocated cervical facet joint, a degenerated facet joint, exostosis of the intervertebral foramina, or inflammation may result in pressure's being placed on one or more cervical nerve roots.[10] The resulting pressure produces pain and spasm in the cervical region with possible pain and paresthesia in the affected dermatome, muscular weakness, altered reflexes, and atrophy in the region supplied by the involved root (Table 11–7). In

Table 11–6

EVALUATIVE FINDINGS: Brachial Plexus Trauma

Examination Segment	Clinical Findings	
History	**Onset:**	Acute
	Pain characteristics:	Pain in the trapezius and deltoid, radiating into the arm
	Mechanism:	**Brachial plexus stretch:** Lateral bending of the cervical spine and depression of the opposite shoulder, resulting in tension on the brachial plexus; symptoms occur on the **side opposite** the lateral bend.
		Brachial plexus compression: Lateral bending of the cervical spine, resulting in the entrapment of the cervical nerve roots; symptoms occur on the **side toward** the lateral bend.
	Predisposing conditions:	History of repeated brachial plexus trauma; stenosis of the intervertebral foramen
Inspection	The involved arm hangs limply at the patient's side. Inspection of the cervical spine is necessary for signs of a cervical fracture or dislocation.	
Palpation	Palpation of the cervical spine is necessary to rule out the possibility of a vertebral fracture or dislocation.	
Functional Tests	Initially, AROM of the limb is diminished; the patient is unable to complete a manual muscle test. Return of motor function usually begins minutes after the onset of injury. RROM possibly demonstrating weakness throughout the musculature innervated by the plexus. Strength begins to return within minutes after the onset of injury.	
Ligamentous tests	Not applicable	
Neurologic Tests	A complete upper quarter screen is necessary to identify the involved cervical nerve roots. All sensory, motor, and reflex test results must be normal and equal before allowing athletes to return to competition.	
Special Tests	Brachial plexus stretch tests, cervical compression and distraction tests, and Spurling test	
Comments	The presence of a cervical fracture or dislocation must be ruled out before initiating the tests for brachial plexus pathology.	

AROM = active range of motion; RROM = resisted range of motion.

Table 11–7

EVALUATIVE FINDINGS: Cervical Nerve Root Compression

Examination Segment	Clinical Findings	
History	**Onset:**	Acute or chronic
	Pain characteristics:	Commonly the lower cervical vertebrae (C4 to C7); symptoms possibly radiating into the trapezius, scapula, shoulder, arm, wrist, and hand
	Mechanism:	Compression or irritation of the associated nerve root (or roots).
	Predisposing conditions:	Disc pathology, narrowing of the intervertebral foramen, facet degeneration, prior trauma to the cervical spine
Inspection	Head and cervical spine are postured to relieve pressure on the involved nerve root.	
Palpation	Point tenderness may be noted at the involved vertebral level.	
Functional tets	**AROM:** Pain experienced during extension, lateral bending toward the involved side, and rotation	
	PROM: Pain experienced during extension, lateral bending toward the involved side, and rotation	
	RROM: Pain and weakness possible for all motions	
Ligamentous tests	Not applicable	
Neurologic tests	Upper quarter screen may reveal muscle weakness, paresthesia, and diminished reflexes specific to the involved nerve root.	
Special tests	Cervical compression test (increases symtpoms), cervical distraction tests (decreases symptoms), Spurling test, vertebral artery test, shoulder abduction test	
Comments	Acute onset of symptoms associated with a traumatic force should be suspected of involving a cervical fracture, dislocation, or sprain.	

AROM = active range of motion; PROM = passive range of motion; RROM = resisted range of motion.

Box 11–5
BRACHIAL PLEXUS TRACTION TEST

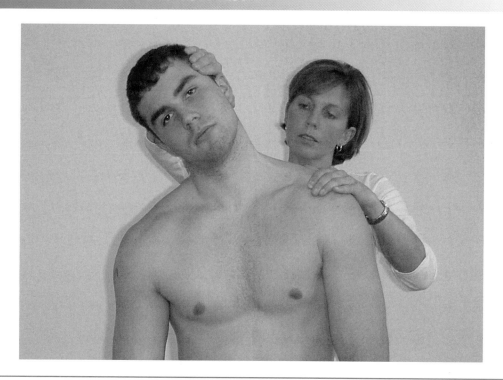

The examiner attempts to duplicate the mechanism of injury and replicate the patient's symptoms. Pain radiates down the patient's left shoulder when a traction injury exists and down the patient's right shoulder when a compression injury exists. This test should be duplicated in each direction and should not be performed until the possibility of cervical spine fracture or instability has been ruled out

PATIENT POSITION	Seated or standing
POSITION OF EXAMINER	Standing behind the patient
EVALUATIVE PROCEDURE	One hand placed on the side of the patient's head; the other hand placed over the acromioclavicular joint The cervical spine is laterally bent and the opposite shoulder depressed.
POSITIVE TEST	Pain radiating through the upper arm.
IMPLICATIONS	**Radiating pain on the side opposite the lateral bending:** Tension (stretching) of the brachial plexus **Radiating pain on the side toward the lateral bending:** Compression of the cervical nerve roots between two vertebrae
COMMENTS	This test should not be performed until the possibility of a cervical fracture or dislocation has been ruled out.

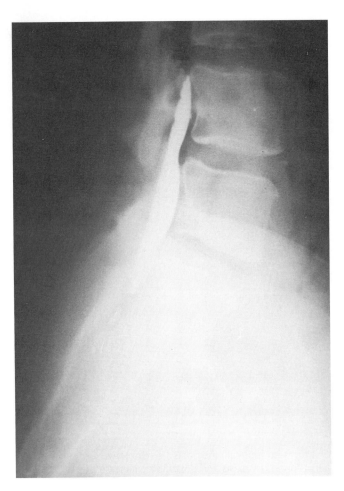

FIGURE 11–17. Myelogram of a disc herniation compressing the spinal cord and associated nerve roots.

the presence of disc *herniations* and vertebral impingement, the patient's pain is often influenced by the position of the head and cervical spine (Fig. 11–17). In addition to cervical disc dysfunction, refer to "Intervertebral Disc Lesions" in this chapter for more information.

Unyielding pain may signify an intervertebral disc rupture or the presence of a tumor.[11] Pain that does not subside during treatment or has an unknown cause requires a physician's diagnosis. In the case of tumor, symptoms increase as the size of the tumor increases, possibly leading to paraplegia, quadriplegia, or death.

The special tests that are described in this section must not be performed if the possibility of a cervical fracture, cervical dislocation, or other instability of the vertebrae exists.

The majority of cervical disc herniations involve the C5-C6 or C6-C7 intervertebral discs.[12] The patient describes pain when the cervical spine is placed in a position that forces the disc's nucleus pulposus outwardly

towards the involved nerve root. The **shoulder abduction test** is a clinical test used for the presence of a herniated disc and may be a position that the patient describes using to decrease the symptoms (Box 11–6).[13] Other special tests for narrowing of the intervertebral foramen also show positive results if the disc is herniated. The presence of disc herniations is confirmed through the use of MRI.[12,14,15] Conservative therapy consisting of cervical traction, muscular strengthening, patient education, and anti-inflammatory medications can produce satisfactory relief of the symptoms.[16,17] The results of conservative care are best achieved when the protrusion is less than 4 mm and does not place pressure on the spinal cord.[16] A physician is responsible for determining the patient's acceptable level of activity.

Narrowing of the intervertebral foramen secondary to exostosis of the vertebrae, enlargement or irritation of the dural sheath surrounding the cervical nerve root, and degeneration of the facet joints can be confirmed with the **cervical compression test** (Box 11–7). The **Spurling test** (Box 11–8), a modification of the cervical compression test, is useful in differentiating symptoms that radiate to the upper extremity from local pathology to that extremity such as those seen in patients with shoulder pathologies.

The underlying cause of constant pain can be determined by the **cervical distraction test** (Box 11–9). Manual traction to the skull separates the cervical vertebrae, relieving any pressure placed on the nerve roots. This indicates that the pain is caused by mechanical pressure arising from entrapment of the nerve root or pressure caused by a disc herniation. The distraction is also used as a gross determinant of an individual's response to traction therapy.

The same mechanisms that produce cervical nerve root symptoms may also impinge the vertebral artery. A test for *patency* of the vertebral artery, the **vertebral artery test** (Box 11–10) determines whether there is the potential for claudication and interruption of the blood flow to the brain. Dizziness, confusion, or *nystagmus* are signs and symptoms of an impingement of the vertebral arteries.[18] A positive test result precludes further evaluation and treatment of the cervical spine until the patient is properly evaluated by a physician for occlusion of the vertebral arteries.

Herniation   The protrusion of a tissue through the wall that normally contains it.

Patency   The state of being freely open.

Nystagmus   An uncontrolled side-to-side movement of the eyes.

Box 11–6
SHOULDER ABDUCTION TEST

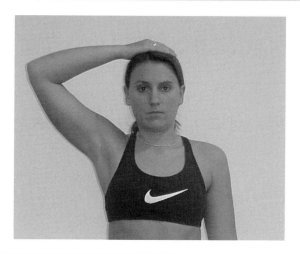

Because of its pain relieving qualities, the patient may assume this posture on his or her own.

PATIENT POSITION	Seated or standing
POSITION OF EXAMINER	Standing in front of the patient
EVALUATIVE PROCEDURE	The patient actively abducts the arm so that the hand is resting on top of the head.
POSITIVE TEST	Decrease in the patient's symptoms secondary to decreased tension on the involved nerve root
IMPLICATIONS	Herniated disc or nerve root compression

ON-FIELD EVALUATION AND MANAGEMENT OF CERVICAL SPINE INJURIES

All injuries to the spinal column requiring an on-field evaluation must be treated as possibly life threatening until spinal cord involvement and serious injury have been ruled out. Bilateral symptoms in the upper extremities or symptoms in the lower extremities should alert the examiner to the potential of spinal cord involvement. Chapter 18 discusses the evaluation and management of patients with potentially catastrophic spinal cord injuries.

BRACHIAL PLEXUS INJURY

Typically, athletes with a brachial plexus injury leave the field of play under their own power, with the in-volved arm dangling limp at the side. The head may be held in a position to relieve any stress placed on the brachial plexus as the result of spasm of the trapezius muscle. The athlete's signs and symptoms (see Table 11–6) are usually transient in nature. After a thorough evaluation to rule out the possibility of trauma to the cervical vertebrae, the cervical spine can be treated with ice packs to decrease pain and spasm.

The athlete should demonstrate a normal neurologic examination without weakness and with full pain-free ROM before returning to activity. Any continuation of the signs and symptoms precludes further participation until the athlete is cleared to return to play by a physician. Repeated episodes of brachial plexus trauma may result in scar tissue formation over one or more nerve roots. Also, a pathological narrowing of the foramen may occur.

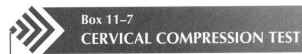

Box 11–7
CERVICAL COMPRESSION TEST

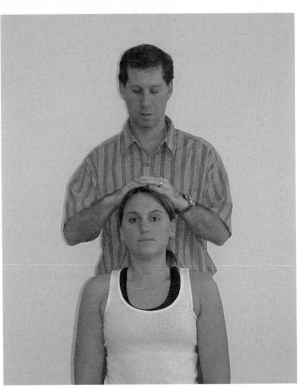

The cervical compression test attempts to duplicate the patient's symptoms by increasing pressure on the cervical nerve roots. This test should not be performed until cervical fracture, dislocation, or instability has been ruled out.

PATIENT POSITION	Sitting
POSITION OF EXAMINER	Standing behind the patient with hands interlocked over the top of the patient's head
EVALUATIVE PROCEDURE	The examiner presses down on the crown of the patient's head.
POSITIVE TEST	The patient experiences pain in the upper cervical spine, upper extremity, or both.
IMPLICATIONS	Compression of the facet joints and narrowing of the intervertebral foramen resulting in pain
COMMENTS	This test should not be performed until the possibility of a cervical fracture or instability has been ruled out.

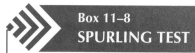

Box 11–8
SPURLING TEST

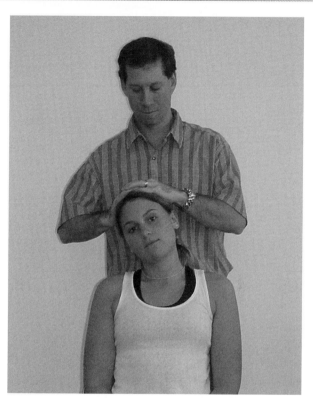

Similar to the cervical compression test, Spurling's test attempts to compress one of the cervical nerve roots. This test should not be performed until the possibility of a cervical fracture, dislocation, or instability has been ruled out.

PATIENT POSITION	Seated
POSITION OF EXAMINER	Standing behind the patient with the hands interlocked over the crown of the patient's head
EVALUATIVE PROCEDURE	The patient extends and laterally bends the cervical spine. A compressive force is then placed along the cervical spine.
POSITIVE TEST	Pain radiating down the patient's arm
IMPLICATIONS	Nerve root impingement by narrowing of the neural foramina
COMMENTS	This test should not be performed until the possibility of a cervical fracture or dislocation has been ruled out.

Box 11–9
CERVICAL DISTRACTION TEST

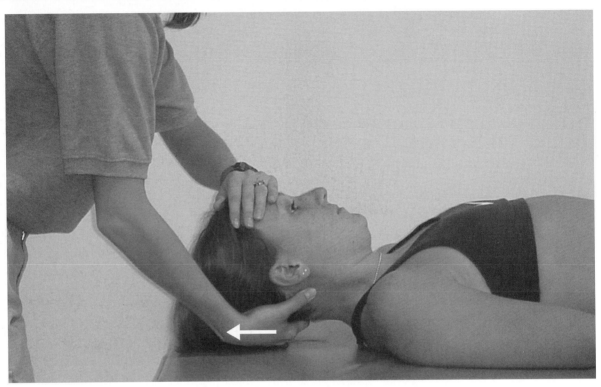

The cervical distraction test attempts to relieve the patient's symptoms by decreasing pressure on the cervical nerve roots. This test should not be performed until cervical fracture, dislocation, or instability has been ruled out.

PATIENT POSITION	Supine to relax the postural muscles of the cervical spine
POSITION OF EXAMINER	At the head of the patient with one hand under the occiput and the other on top of the forehead, stabilizing the head
EVALUATIVE PROCEDURE	The examiner applies traction on the patient's head, causing distraction of the cervical spine.
POSITIVE TEST	The patient's symptoms are relieved or reduced.
IMPLICATIONS	Compression of the cervical facet joints and/or stenosis of the neural foramina.
COMMENTS	This test should not be performed until the possibility of a cervical fracture or dislocation has been ruled out.

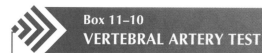

Box 11–10
VERTEBRAL ARTERY TEST

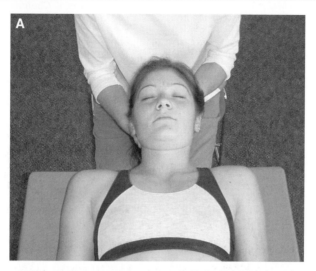

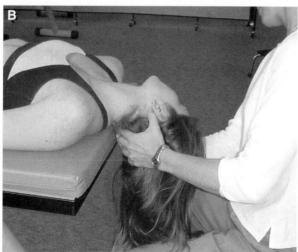

The vertebral artery test is performed to assure the competency of the vertebral artery prior to initiating treatment or rehabilitation techniques that may compromise a partially occluded artery. This test should not be performed until the presence of a cervical fracture, dislocation, or instability has been ruled out.

PATIENT POSITION	Supine
POSITION OF EXAMINER	Seated at the head of the patient with the hands placed under the occiput to stabilize the head
EVALUATIVE PROCEDURE	The examiner passively extends and laterally flexes the cervical spine **(A)**. The head is then rotated toward the laterally flexed side and held for 30 s **(B)**. During this procedure, the examiner must monitor the patient's pupillary activity.
POSITIVE TEST	Dizziness, confusion, nystagmus, unilateral pupil changes, nausea
IMPLICATIONS	Occlusion of the cervical vertebral arteries
COMMENTS	Patients with a positive test result should be referred to a physician before any other evaluative tests are performed or a rehabilitation plan is implemented and before being allowed to return to competition.

REFERENCES

1. Yang, SS, and Hershman, EB: Idiopathic brachial plexus neuropathy: A review. *Crit Rev Musculoskel Med,* 5:193, 1993.
2. Markey, KL, Di Benedetto, M, and Curl, WW: Upper trunk brachial plexopathy: The stinger syndrome. *Am J Sports Med,* 21:650, 1993.
3. Vereschagin, KS, et al: Burners. Don't overlook or underestimate them. *The Physician and Sportsmedicine,* 19:96, 1991.
4. Speer, KP, and Bassett, FH: The prolonged burner syndrome. *Am J Sports Med,* 18:591, 1990.
5. Kitamura, T, et al: Brachial plexus stretching injuries: Microcirculation of the brachial plexus. *J Shoulder Elbow Surg,* 4:118, 1995.
6. Meyer, SA, et al: Cervical spinal stenosis and stingers on collegiate football players. *Am J Sports Med,* 22:158, 1994.
7. Reilly, PJ, and Torg, JS: Athletic injury to the cervical nerve roots and brachial plexus. *Operative Techniques in Sports Medicine,* 1:231, 1993.
8. Walker, AT, et al: Detection of nerve rootlet avulsion on CT myelography in patients with birth palsy and brachial plexus injury after trauma. *AJR Am J Roentgenol,* 167:1283, 1996.
9. Bajuk, S, Jelnikar, T, and Ortar, M: Rehabilitation of patient with brachial plexus lesion and break in axillary artery. Case Study. *J Hand Ther,* 9:399, 1996.
10. Shapiro, S, et al: Outcome of 51 cases of unilateral locked cervical facets: interspinous braided cable for lateral mass plate fusion with interspinous wire with iliac crests. *J Neuorsurg,* 91:19, 1999.
11. D'Haen, B, et al: Chordoma of the lower cervical spine. *Clin Neurol Neurosurg,* 97:245, 1995.
12. Bucciero, A, Vizioli, L, and Cerillo, A: Soft cervical disc herniation. An analysis of 187 cases. *J Neurosurg Sci,* 42:125, 1998.
13. Davidson, RI, Dunn, EJ, and Metzmaker, JN: The shoulder abduction test in the diagnosis of radicular pain in cervical extradural compressive monoradiculopathies. *Spine,* 6:441, 1981.
14. van de Kelft, E, and van Vyve, M: Diagnostic imaging algorithm for cervical soft disc herniation. *Acta Chir Belg,* 95:152, 1995.
15. Saal, JS: Magnetic resonance neurography for cervical radiculopathy: a preliminary report. *Neurosurgery,* 38:488, 1996.
16. Saal, JS, Saal, JA, and Yurth, EF: Nonoperative management of herniated cervical intervertebral disc with radiculopathy. *Spine,* 21:1877, 1996.
17. Humphreys, SC, et al: Flexion and traction effect on C5-C6 foraminal space. *Arch Phys Med Rehabil,* 79:1105, 1998.
18. Maitland, GD: Vertebral manipulation. Budderworth Publishing, London, 1973.

12

The Thorax and Abdomen

The internal organs—the heart, lungs, spleen, and kidneys—responsible for maintaining the body's homeostasis lie well protected within the thoracic and abdominal cavities. However, extraordinary forces can result in damage to these structures, endangering the individual's life. Although less well protected than the organs in the thorax, the abdominal organs, liver, digestive system, and lower urinary tract, are more resilient to trauma because they are less firmly attached, increasing their ability to absorb shock. With the exception of the liver, the abdominal organs tend to be hollow, thus providing additional shock-absorbing capabilities.

Injury to the body's *visceral* organs can range from the mundane to the catastrophic. A keen awareness of the internal systems of the body, the factors predisposing these organs to injury, and the signs and symptoms of trauma are needed for proper recognition and management of these conditions. The progressive nature of the symptoms makes early identification and repeated examination and evaluation critical parts of athletic health care.

◆ CLINICAL ANATOMY

With the sternum anteriorly, the vertebrae posteriorly, and the ribs connecting the two, the thorax forms a protective shell around the torso's upper internal organs (Fig. 12–1). The **sternum** consists of three sections: the **manubrium** superiorly, the central **body,** and the inferiorly projecting **xiphoid process.** The sternal body and the manubrium are connected by a fibrocartilaginous joint that fuses during adolescence to form a single, solid bone.

The upper seven ribs are classified as **true ribs** because they articulate with the sternum through their own **costal cartilages.** Ribs eight through 10 articulate with the sternum through a conjoined costal cartilage. Thus, they are termed **false ribs.** Ribs 11 and 12, the **floating ribs,** do not have an anterior articulation. An anomalous **cervical rib** may project off the seventh cervical vertebra. Although this structure is often benign,

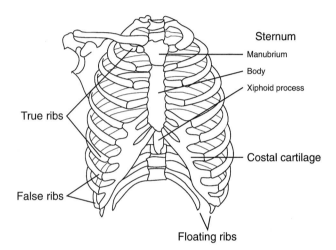

FIGURE 12–1. Illustration of the thorax. The rib cage formed by the true ribs (1 through 7), false ribs (8 through 10), and floating ribs (11 and 12); the sternum (manubrium, body, and xiphoid process); and the costal cartilage. The posterior margin of the thorax is formed by the thoracic and vertebrae.

it can be a source of compression on the brachial plexus, the subclavian artery, or the subclavian vein, predisposing the individual to **thoracic outlet syndrome** (see Chapter 13).

The abdominal region has no anterior or lateral bony protection and receives only slight protection on its posterior surface from the thoracic and lumbar vertebrae and the floating ribs. The inferior portion of the abdomen is protected by the sacrum posteriorly and the ilia laterally.

Located within the thorax and abdomen are numerous internal organs. Many of the internal organs come in pairs. Reference to these organs is relative to the pa-

---

Visceral   Pertaining to the internal organs contained within the thorax and abdomen.

---

tient; thus, the right kidney is on the examiner's left side when facing the patient from the front.

MUSCULAR ANATOMY

Many of the muscles acting on the thorax and abdomen have been previously discussed and are only referenced in this chapter. Additionally, those muscles arising from the thorax to act on the scapula and humerus also influence the thorax (these muscles are discussed in Chapters 10 and 13).

Muscles of Inspiration

The **diaphragm** is a muscular membrane that separates the thoracic cavity from the abdominal cavity. Innervated by the **phrenic nerve,** as the diaphragm contracts, it moves downward, creating a vacuum in the thorax pulling air into the lungs. The diaphragm is interrupted at several points by portals through which the major vessels pass into the torso and lower legs.

The rib cage's intrinsic skeletal muscles are collectively referred to as the **intercostal muscles.** Spanning from rib to rib, these muscles assist in the respiratory process. Inspiration is also assisted by the **scalene muscles** elevating the first and second ribs. The sternocleidomastoid, trapezius, serratus anterior, pectoralis major and minor, and latissimus dorsi all function as secondary muscles of inspiration, used when breathing becomes difficult.

Muscles of Expiration

The abdominal muscles—the **rectus abdominis, internal oblique,** and **external oblique** (discussed in Chapter 10)—are supported across the abdomen by the **transverse abdominis.** In addition to flexing and rotating the lumbar and thoracic spine, the contraction of these muscles creates a positive pressure gradient across the diaphragm, resulting in the expiration of air.

RESPIRATORY TRACT ANATOMY

The **trachea,** connecting the larynx to the bronchioles, is a membranous tube formed by muscle and connective tissue. Its anterior border is protected from crushing forces by a series of cartilaginous semicircular rings. The trachea diverges into two principal **bronchi.** The left bronchus divides into two **segmental bronchi,** and three segmental bronchi are formed on the right side, each matching the number of lobes on the corresponding lung (Fig. 12–2). Each segmental bronchus then subdivides into the **bronchioles.**

In the lungs, carbon dioxide is exchanged for oxygen. The right lung has three lobes (i.e., upper, middle, and lower), while the left lung has only an upper and lower

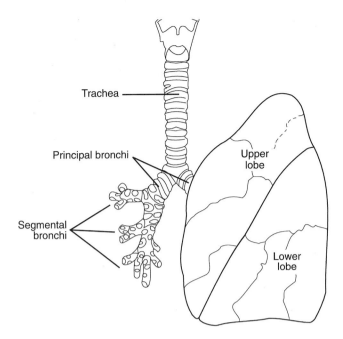

FIGURE 12–2. Respiratory tract. The trachea, principal bronchi, the segmental bronchi, and the left lung (relative to the patient). The right lung has been removed to view the bronchial segments. The left lung is formed by two lobes, whereas the right lung has a third, or middle, lobe between the upper and lower ones.

lobe, each matching with a segmental bronchus. The thoracic cavity is encased with pleural linings. The **parietal pleura** lines the thoracic wall, and the **visceral pleura** surrounds the lungs, forming a **pleural cavity** between the two. As the chest cavity expands during inspiration, a negative pressure is formed within the pleural cavity, causing an expansion of the lungs and the subsequent inflow of air for breathing.

The actual exchange of gases occurs at the level of the **alveoli,** the terminal branches of the bronchioles. The alveolar walls contain the capillary system, which receives deoxygenated blood from the right side of the heart via the **pulmonary arteries.** After the exchange of gases, the oxygenated blood returns to the left side of the heart via the **pulmonary veins.**

The trachea and its conducting airways are lined with **mucosal cells.** Mucus, formed in the submucosa by glands, is excreted to the mucosal lining. Here, the mucus acts as a filtration system, working like millions of little sponges absorbing airborne pollutants, dust, and other unwanted substances. Normally the contaminated mucus is routed upward by **ciliary cells** to the pharynx, where it is unconsciously swallowed. When an excess demand is placed on the mucosal system, the mucus is routed up, through, and out the nasal passage.

The upper portions of the respiratory system—the nose, mouth, larynx, and pharynx—are discussed in Chapter 17.

Table 12–1
THE CHAMBERS OF THE HEART

Heart Chamber	Function
Right atrium	Receives deoxygenated blood via: • Superior vena cava from the head, neck, and upper extremities • Inferior vena cava from the trunk and lower extremities Delivers blood to the right ventricle through the right artrioventicular (tricuspid) valve.
Right ventricle	Receives deoxygenated blood from the right atrium. Delivers blood through the semilunar valve (pulmonic valve) to the lungs via the left and right pulmonary arteries
Left atrium	Receives oxygenated blood from the lungs via the right and left pulmonary veins Delivers blood to the left ventricle through the left atrioventicular (mitral) valve
Left ventricle	Delivers oxygenated blood through the semilunar valve (aortic valve) to the ascending aorta

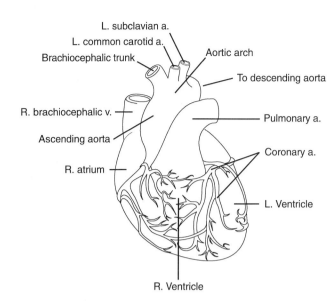

FIGURE 12–3. Anterior view of the heart. Blood supply to the body is delivered through the aorta. The left atrium is hidden in this view.

CARDIOVASCULAR ANATOMY

Under normal circumstances, the **heart** beats at a rate that equals the metabolic needs of the body, delivering oxygen and nutrients to the body's tissues. As the tissues' demands for these nutrients increase, so does the heart rate.

The heart is divided into four chambers, with the right-side chambers handling deoxygenated blood and the left-side chambers handling oxygenated blood (Table 12–1). The **aorta** exits the heart, carrying oxygenated blood to the body. Soon after leaving the heart, the aorta takes a sharp bend inferiorly, forming the **aortic arch.** From this arch, many other arteries diverge from the aorta, including the **brachiocephalic trunk, the left common carotid artery,** and the **left subclavian artery.** The brachiocephalic branches into the **right subclavian** and **right common carotid arteries,** delivering blood to the right upper extremity, the brain, and the head. Continuing *caudally* from its arch, the aorta forms the **descending thoracic aorta** and when passing through the diaphragm, **becomes the abdominal aorta,** supplying blood to the torso and lower extremity (Fig. 12–3).

In addition to supplying the rest of the body with oxygenated blood, the heart must also pump blood to itself through the right and left **coronary arteries.** The right coronary artery branches into the right marginal artery and the posterior interventricular artery. The left coronary artery branches into the anterior interventric-

ular artery and the circumflex artery, which then leads to the left marginal artery.

DIGESTIVE TRACT ANATOMY

Solids and liquids enter the digestive tract through the mouth and travel through the **esophagus** to enter the stomach. After they are in the stomach, the ingested food substances form a **bolus,** which is routed into the **small intestine** through the **pylorus.** The small intestine is divided into the **duodenum, jejunum,** and **ileum.** After passing through the small intestine, the bolus enters the **large intestine (colon),** proceeding through the **cecum, ascending colon, transverse colon, descending colon, sigmoid,** and **rectum** to its exit from the body via the **anus** (Fig. 12–4). The **appendix** projects off the cecum. Its mucus membrane lining can become inflamed or infected, leading to **appendicitis.**

The **liver,** the largest organ in the body, takes up the entire right side of the torso inferior to the diaphragm and is protected by the lower ribs and the costal arch of the false ribs (Fig. 12–5). Through its connection with the **gallbladder** and common **bile duct,** the liver introduces **bile** into the stomach to assist in the digestion of fats. The liver also acts as a warehouse for storing glucose, the body's immediate fuel system, and is a repository for the metabolism of intrinsic and extrinsic

Caudal (caudally)   Moving inferiorly (towards the tail).

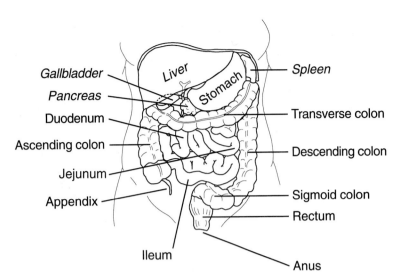

FIGURE 12–4. Stomach and intestine. The liver, gallbladder, pancreas, and spleen are presented for reference purposes.

chemical substances. The liver's many tasks require a large blood supply. Injury to this organ results in massive amounts of blood being lost into the abdominal cavity.

In addition to the liver's function as a digestive organ, it also functions to filter toxins and wastes out of the blood and produces mediators for blood clotting.

LYMPHATIC ORGAN ANATOMY

Located on the left side of the body at the level of the ninth through eleventh ribs, the **spleen** is a solid, fragile organ that is supported by ligaments attaching it to the kidney, colon, stomach, and diaphragm (Fig. 12–6). The largest of the lymphatic organs, its primary function is to produce and destroy blood cells during times of systemic infection. During certain disease states,

such as *mononucleosis,* the spleen becomes engorged with blood, causing it to protrude below the ribs' protective bony cover, increasing the risk of injury. When the spleen is traumatized, surgical removal may be necessary. If the spleen is removed, its functions are assumed by the liver and bone marrow.

URINARY TRACT ANATOMY

The kidneys, also responsible for filtering toxins from the blood, regulate the body's *electrolyte* levels by maintaining the balance of water, sodium, and potassium. The kidneys lie on each side of the vertebral col-

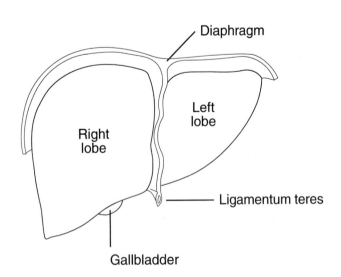

FIGURE 12–5. Anterior view of the liver. This structure is supported by ligaments arising from the inferior surface of the diaphragm.

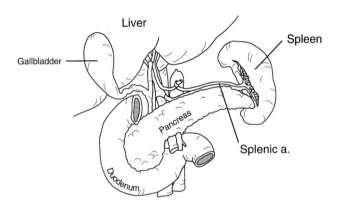

FIGURE 12–6. Spleen. During illness the spleen may become enlarged, causing it to become vulnerable to injury.

Mononucleosis   A disease state caused by an abnormally high number of mononuclear leukocytes in the blood stream.

Electrolyte   Ionized salts, including sodium, potassium, and chloride, found in blood, tissue fluids, and cells.

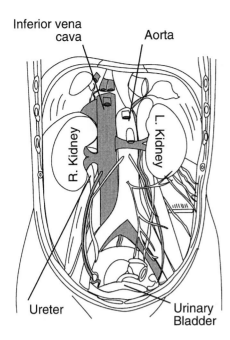

FIGURE 12–7. Relative location of the kidneys. Note that the right kidney is located inferior to the left kidney, exposing its inferior border to direct trauma from blows to the posterolateral thorax.

umn at the level of the T12 to L3 vertebrae, with the right kidney lying slightly lower than the left (Fig. 12–7). The lower portion of each kidney is unprotected by the ribs, thus increasing the susceptibility to trauma secondary to direct blows to the low back.

The kidney's filtrate, **urine,** exits through small, muscular tubes, the **ureters.** Well protected by the posterior wall of the abdomen, these structures are rarely injured. Both ureters deposit their contents into a central **urinary bladder,** located posterior to the pubic symphysis, within the pelvic cavity. As the bladder fills, the smooth muscle reacts to parasympathetic stimuli, triggering the urge to urinate. From the bladder, urine exits the body through the **urethra.**

REPRODUCTIVE TRACT ANATOMY

In both men and women, the essential organs of reproduction are located in the lower abdomen. The male **testes** have the dual function of producing sperm and the male sex hormone, testosterone. The **epididymis,** a coiled tube on the posterior aspect of the testes, stores sperm (Fig. 12–8). The external location of the male reproductive organs increases the incidence of injury, most often occurring secondary to a direct blow.

The female organs of reproduction, the paired **ovaries** and **fallopian tubes** and a singular hollow **uterus,** are attached by ligaments to the pelvic wall and sit relatively well protected (Fig. 12–9). The ovaries, endocrine glands, are the source of estrogen and proges-

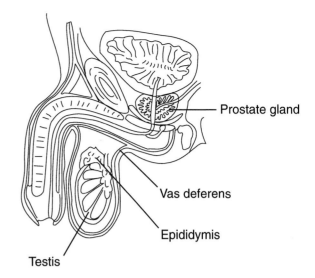

FIGURE 12–8. Male reproductive system. The external location of the testicles predisposes them to injury from direct blows.

terone, the female sex hormones. They also house the reproductive eggs that are released for fertilization in the fallopian tubes and then implanted into the uterus.

◆ CLINICAL EVALUATION OF THE THORAX AND ABDOMEN

Injuries to the internal organs and ribs usually follow a high-velocity blow to the affected area, resulting in trauma to the area beneath the impact. Structures on the side opposite of the impact may also be injured as they rebound off bony structures, a *contrecoup* injury. These conditions may not be evident immediately after the injury but can quickly progress to life-threatening conditions, thereby necessitating frequent re-examination.

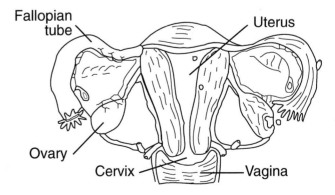

FIGURE 12–9. Female reproductive system. The internal location of these organs provides excellent protection against most traumatic forces.

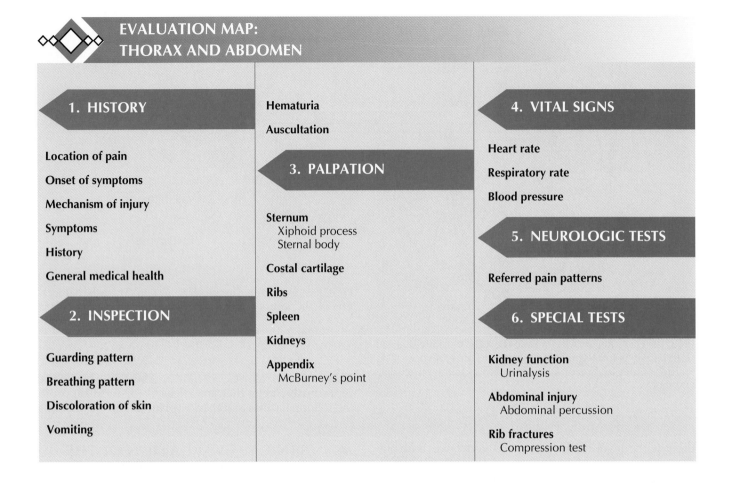

EVALUATION MAP: THORAX AND ABDOMEN

1. HISTORY

Location of pain

Onset of symptoms

Mechanism of injury

Symptoms

History

General medical health

2. INSPECTION

Guarding pattern

Breathing pattern

Discoloration of skin

Vomiting

Hematuria

Auscultation

3. PALPATION

Sternum
　Xiphoid process
　Sternal body

Costal cartilage

Ribs

Spleen

Kidneys

Appendix
　McBurney's point

4. VITAL SIGNS

Heart rate

Respiratory rate

Blood pressure

5. NEUROLOGIC TESTS

Referred pain patterns

6. SPECIAL TESTS

Kidney function
　Urinalysis

Abdominal injury
　Abdominal percussion

Rib fractures
　Compression test

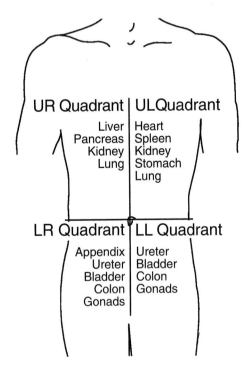

UR Quadrant | UL Quadrant

Liver | Heart
Pancreas | Spleen
Kidney | Kidney
Lung | Stomach
　 | Lung

LR Quadrant | LL Quadrant

Appendix | Ureter
Ureter | Bladder
Bladder | Colon
Colon | Gonads
Gonads |

FIGURE 12–10. Abdominal quadrant reference system. The sagittal quadrants are relative to the athlete. Therefore, the right kidney is on the athlete's right-hand side.

The thoraco-abdominal region is referenced on a quadrant system, dividing the torso into left and right upper and lower quadrants relative to the umbilicus (Fig. 12–10). The evaluation process is eased by the clinician's knowledge of the organs housed in each of these quadrants and their normal functions. Additionally, as discussed in the section on neurologic testing in this chapter, pain of visceral origin may be referred to the body's periphery.

HISTORY

- **Location of pain:** The location of the pain must be determined as closely as possible. Musculoskeletal injuries to the ribs, costal cartilage, or abdominal muscles are usually tender at the site of the injury. Injury to the internal organs may result in a more diffuse pain at rest. However, these areas can be more specifically localized as the patient moves or the area is palpated. Blows to the low back may result in a kidney contusion, especially on the patient's right side (see Fig. 12–7). Pain in the thorax, abdomen, shoulder, or arm can be referred from the visceral organs. Pain in the upper left quadrant and shoulder, **Kehr's sign,** may indicate a ruptured spleen that is irritating the diaphragm.

- **Onset of symptoms:** With an internal injury, the onset of pain may be gradual, taking hours to develop as internal bleeding accumulates within the cavity. The pain associated with a musculoskeletal injury can be acute or may initially go unnoticed or undernoticed. When the rib cage or abdominal muscles are injured, pain may be provoked by breathing, coughing, or sneezing. Distance runners may be affected by stomach or abdominal cramping during competition. Causes of this condition may be irregular breathing patterns, gastrointestinal upset, bloating, gas, nausea, heartburn, dehydration, constipation, or *dysmenorrhea*.[1]

- **Mechanism of injury:** Injury to the thoracic, abdominal, and pelvic organs usually results from a direct blow to the area, such as being hit by a competitor or colliding with a piece of equipment or the ground. Suspicion of trauma to the ribs or internal organs is increased when the blow is received to an unprotected area.

- **Symptoms:** The chief complaints may include pain or difficulty breathing, diffuse abdominal pain, nausea, dizziness, or vomiting of blood. The patient should also be questioned regarding the presence of blood in the urine or stool. Because of the associated metabolic changes, injury to the abdominal organs increases the individual's thirst beyond that which is expected after competition.

- **Medical history:** Because of the acute nature of these injuries, the patient typically does not have a history of injury. With certain asthmatic conditions, a history of disease may be documented, but athletes with *exercise-induced asthma* may not have been previously diagnosed. Other illnesses may predispose specific internal organs to acute internal injury. For example, mononucleosis can enlarge the spleen and expose it to an increased incidence of injury. Viral *pericarditis* can cause chest pains or predispose an individual to cardiac arrest.

- **General medical health:** The use of medications and other medical treatments now allows individuals to compete with conditions that once would have excluded them from competition. Athletes can compete with conditions such as *cystic fibrosis*, asthma, spastic colitis, renal disease, hypertension, and undescended testicles. Although these conditions should be identified during the pre-participation physical examination, a prudent evaluation involves questions regarding the existence of any underlying medical conditions.

INSPECTION

The inspection process begins with observation of the patient's overall posture. Leaning of the thorax to one side may indicate that the patient is stretching a cramping muscle; flexing of the trunk may indicate cramping. The individual may also be splinting the painful area by grasping the torso or abdomen. A person suffering from a significant internal injury is often unwilling to move, preferring to remain in the fetal position or lie supine with the knees flexed.

- **Throat:** Observe the trachea and larynx for their normal positions through the midline of the cervical spine. Deviations from this position could indicate trauma to these structures or the presence of a **pneumothorax**.

- **Breathing pattern:** Note any abnormalities in the breathing pattern. Difficulty in breathing may have many causes that include asthma, allergies, cardiac contusion, injury to the ribs or costal cartilage, lung trauma (e.g., pneumothorax, hemothorax, or pulmonary contusion), or other injury to the internal organs. Observe respirations for rate, depth, and quality. Internal injuries can cause breathing to become rapid and shallow because deep breaths may cause pain. Observe the chest wall movement in those having trouble breathing. The ribs should rise and fall in a symmetrical pattern; any deviations in this pattern could be the result of fractured ribs or a pneumothorax. Subcutaneous emphysema may indicate lung trauma.

- **Nail beds:** Observe for normal capillary refill in the nail beds. Disruption of the cardiac or pulmonary systems would result in cyanosis of the nail beds, fingers, and toes. (Fig. 12–11).

- **Muscle tone:** Observe the tone of the abdominal muscles. As time progresses, the injured area may become distended secondary to bleeding.

- **Discoloration of skin:** Note the location of any contusions, wounds, or abrasions. These discolorations serve to warn of possible injury to the underlying internal organs.

- **Vomiting:** Observe the patient for and question about any vomiting after the injury because it is common after many internal injuries or injury to the male genitals. Blood in the vomitus may signify injury to the stomach, esophagus, pulmonary trauma, or chronic conditions such as ulcers.

- **Hematuria:** Obtain a urine sample from the patient, if possible, and note its appearance. Also question the patient about the presence of blood in the urine, or hematuria. This symptom denotes significant injury to the kidneys and warrants immediate referral

---

Dysmenorrhea Pain during menstruation.

Exercise-induced asthma Bronchospasm caused by exercise.

Pericarditis Inflammation of the lining surrounding the heart.

Cystic fibrosis A congenital condition of the exocrine glands that affects the pancreas, respiratory system, and other systems.

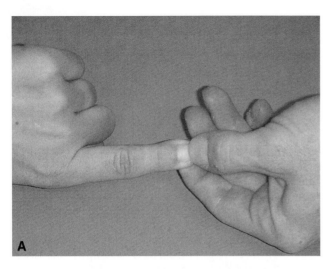
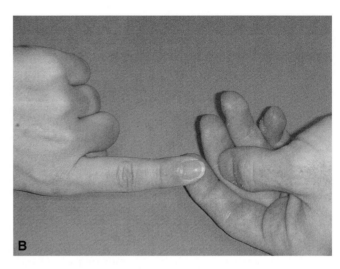

FIGURE 12–11. Checking capillary refill of the fingernail. **(A)** When compressed, the skin beneath the nail will turn a lighter shade. **(B)** In the presence of proper refill, the natural color will rapidly return.

to a physician. Any patient suspected of having an internal injury must be instructed to observe the color of the urine upon the next voiding. Immediately after the injury, blood may not be visible to the unaided eye but can be detected using a microscope or chemically with specially formulated chemical strips dipped into the urine. Note that hematuria may normally be present after certain athletic events such as long-distance running or in *menstruating* women (Box 12–1).

• **Normal and abnormal sounds:** Perform auscultation, listening to sounds with a stethoscope, to help establish the presence of internal injury (Fig. 12–12). Auscultate breath sounds over all the lobes of each lung. Inhalation typically reveals a dry, smooth, unobstructed sound that is equal throughout each lobe. The absence of breath sounds may indicate a col-

lapsed lung such as might occur with a pneumothorax. Pneumonia or other build-up of fluid within the lungs may produce rales, a localized moist sounding movement of air.

The abdomen typically makes an occasional "gurgling" sound as *peristalsis* occurs. After injury, the peristaltic mechanism may be inhibited or may sympathetically shut down. In either case, the bowel

---

Menstruation (menstruating)   The period of bleeding during the menstrual cycle.

Peristalsis   A progressive smooth muscle contraction producing a wavelike motion that moves matter through the intestines.

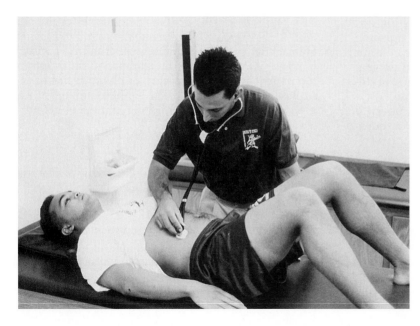

FIGURE 12–12. Auscultation of the abdomen. The integrity of the abdomen and its hollow organs can be assessed through listening to the bowel sounds. Although the abdomen typically makes a gurgling sound, abdominal trauma reduces or eliminates this noise.

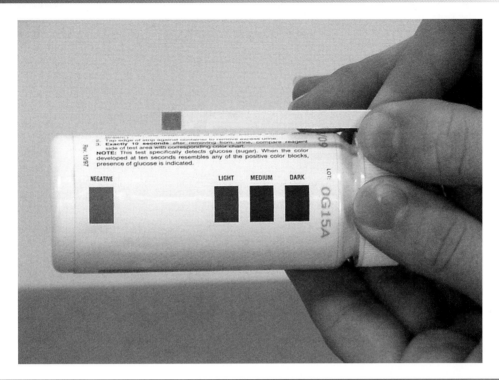

EVALUATIVE PROCEDURE	The external urethra and surrounding area is cleansed using soap and water and then rinsed.
	To clear the urethra, the initial flow of urine is into a toilet bowl or "dirty" collection container.
	One to 2 oz of urine are then collected in a clean specimen cup.
	The dipstick is then immersed into the specimen cup.
	The manufacturer's recommendations for immersion time and interpretation times are followed.
TEST RESULTS	The colors produced on the dipstick are matched to the values provided by the manufacturer.

IMPLICATIONS

Element	Normal	Interpretation
Specific gravity	1.006 to 1.030	**Low reading**: Diabetes mellitus, excessive hydration, renal failure **High reading**: Dehydration; heart or renal failure
pH	4.6 to 8.0	**Low reading**: Chronic obstructive pulmonary disease, diabetic ketoacidosis **High reading**: Renal failure, urinary tract infection
Glucose, g/d	<0.5	Diabetes, stress
Ketones	0	Anorexia, poor nutrition, alcoholism, diabetes mellitus
Protein	0	Congestive heart failure, polycystic kidney disease
Hemoglobin	0	Urinary tract infection, kidney disease or trauma
RBC	0	Kidney disease or trauma, kidney stones, bladder infection, urinary tract infection

COMMENTS	The above interpretations are partial lists. High or low readings should be interpreted by a physician.
	Factors such as diet and the level of exercise can alter the urinalysis readings.

RBC = red blood cell.

sounds are absent. The exact placement of the stethoscope over specific portions of the bowel is not crucial because these sounds resound throughout the cavity. Auscultation is conducted before palpation of the abdomen because manipulation of the abdomen during palpation may falsely produce normal bowel sounds.

PALPATION

The findings of the history-taking process are reinforced and supplemented by the findings obtained during the palpation phase. Because there are few special tests for assessing thoracic and abdominal injuries, knowledge of the underlying anatomy is needed so that a specific palpation assessment may be performed.

1–3. **Sternum:** Begin palpating the rib cage at the manubrium, continuing inferiorly to include the sternal body **(2)**, and xiphoid process **(3)** and noting for tenderness and deformity. Injury to the upper sternum may involve the sternoclavicular joint (see Chapter 11).

4. **Costal cartilage and rib:** Palpate the costal cartilage and ribs as a whole, with any specific areas of tenderness then being isolated. Palpate the costal cartilage and rib from anterior to posterior, noting any pain, crepitus, and deformity. Any suspicion of a rib fracture requires full evaluation by a physician.

5. **Spleen:** Palpate for an enlarged spleen under the left rib cage. Having the patient raise the arms above the head will make the spleen more prominent and more easily palpated.

6. **Kidneys:** Locate the kidneys under the posterolateral portion of the rib cage. The left kidney is relatively well protected within the rib cage. The right kidney rests more inferior.

7. **McBurney's point:** Note any tenderness at McBurney's point, located one third of the way between the right anterior superior iliac spine and the navel, possibly indicating acute appendicitis (Fig. 12–13).

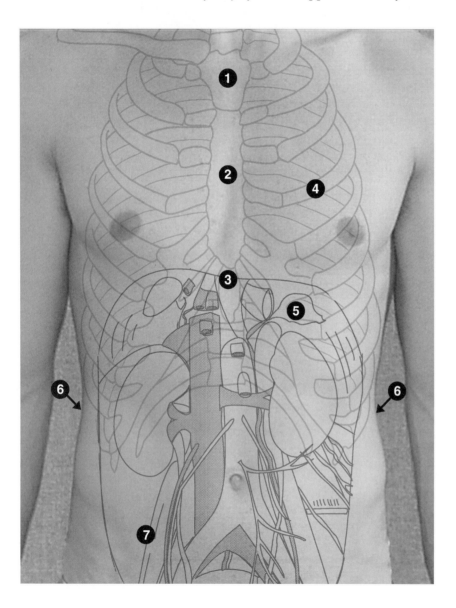

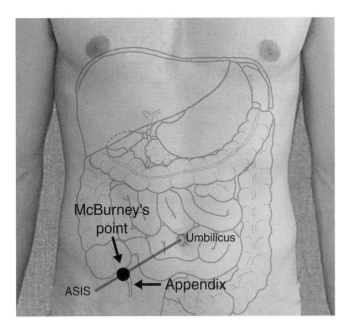

FIGURE 12–13. McBurney's point, located approximately one-third of the way between the ASIS and the umbilicus. This point becomes tender in the presence of appendicitis.

Palpation of the Abdomen

The patient should be in the hook-lying position to relax the abdominal muscles (Fig. 12–14). The abdomen is palpated relative to the four quadrants depicted in Figure 12–10.

- **Rigidity:** Abdominal rigidity may occur secondary to muscle guarding or with blood accumulating in the abdomen. The presence of guarding alone indicates internal injury, which necessitates further evaluation by a physician.
- **Areas of pain:** Pain caused by palpation is another cause of concern. An awareness of the approximate location of the organs within the abdomen assists in detecting possible injury.

- **Rebound tenderness:** An inflamed peritoneum is sensitive to stretching. Pressure applied over the injured site gradually stretches the peritoneum in a relatively pain-free manner. However, pain experienced when the pressure is suddenly released indicates inflammation of the peritoneum.
- **Tissue density:** Percussing over specific organs can be used to determine the density of the underlying tissues (Box 12–2). Internal bleeding may fill the abdominal cavity, causing the abdomen to feel and sound solid.
- **Quadrant analysis:** The abdomen is palpated in the quadrant format as presented in Figure 12–10. Correlations of tenderness include the following:

Quadrant Segment (Relative to the Patient)		
	Right	**Left**
Upper	**Liver:** Pain is associated with *cholecystitis* or liver laceration. **Gallbladder:** Pain without the history of trauma indicates gallbladder disease.	**Spleen:** Rigidity under the last several ribs indicates trauma to the spleen.
Lower	**Appendix:** Rebound tenderness indicates appendicitis. **Colon:** Colitis or diverticulitis may cause pain. **Pelvic inflammation** results in diffuse tenderness.	**Colon:** Colitis or diverticulitis may cause pain. **Pelvic inflammation** results in diffuse tenderness.

Other less specific symptoms include pain in the upper abdomen arising from the pancreas, heart, diaphragm, or esophagus or pain in the lower middle

Cholecystitis   Inflammation of the gallbladder.

FIGURE 12–14. Positioning of the athlete during palpation of the abdomen. The "hook-lying" position relaxes the abdominal muscles, easing palpation of the underlying structures.

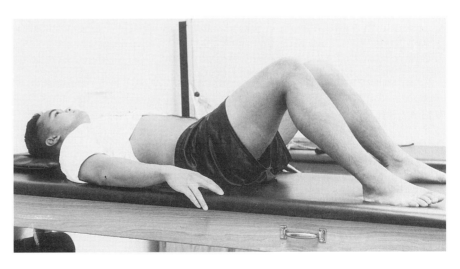

Box 12–2
ABDOMINAL PERCUSSION

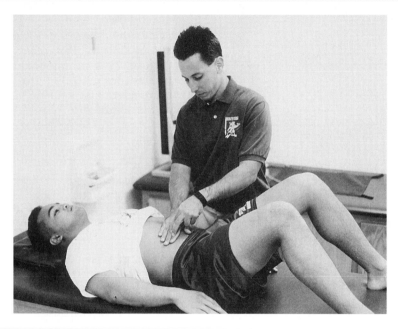

PATIENT POSITION	Hook lying
POSITION OF EXAMINER	Standing to the patient's side The examiner lightly places one hand palm down over the area to be assessed The index and middle fingers of the opposite hand tap the DIP joints of the hand placed over the athlete's abdomen
EVALUATIVE PROCEDURE	The fingertips of the top hand quickly strike the middle phalanges of the bottom hand in a tapping motion. The sound of the echo within the abdomen is noted. Areas over solid organs have a dull thump associated with them. Hollow organs make a crisper, more **resonant** sound.
POSITIVE TEST	A hard, solid sounding echo over areas that should normally sound hollow.
IMPLICATIONS	Internal bleeding filling the abdominal cavity.

DIP = distal interphalangeal.

abdomen in the area of the femoral creases from bladder or *gonad* pathology. The low back may be painful and have increased tenderness with palpation owing to kidney contusions, *kidney stones,* or infection.

VITAL SIGNS

Previous chapters have examined a joint's range of motion (ROM) as an indicator of its functional ability. This chapter uses the vital signs to assess the function of the internal abdominal and thoracic organs. The examiner requires skill, practice, and knowledge in assessing the vital signs and interpreting the significance of these findings. This assessment is important for any injury, especially in case of internal injury or shock (Table 12–2). During the evaluation and management of a pa-

tient with an injury or illness, the values obtained for each of these tests are recorded and periodically reevaluated to note trends in the vital signs.

- **Heart rate:** The heart rate is determined by identifying the carotid pulse. However, the radial, femoral, or brachial pulses may be used as well (Box 12–3). An athlete's resting heart rate typically ranges from

Resonant Producing a vibrating sound or percussion.

Gonad An organ producing gender-based reproductive cells; the ovaries or testicles.

Kidney stones A crystal mass formed in the kidney that is passed through the urinary tract.

Table 12–2
SIGNS AND SYMPTOMS OF SHOCK

Rapid, weak pulse
Decreased blood pressure
Rapid, shallow breathing
Excessive thirst
Nausea and vomiting
Pale, bluish skin
Restlessness or irritability
Drowsiness or loss of consciousness

60 to 100 beats per minute (BPM). Highly conditioned athletes have lower heart rates. Older or recreational athletes have heart rates at the higher end of the scale. When assessing the heart rate of an athlete who has just stopped exercising, an increased heart rate caused by the demands of exercise should be considered. After an internal injury, the athlete displays a rapid heart rate, or tachycardia.

- **Respiratory rate:** At rest, normal respiration ranges from 12 to 20 breaths per minute, with well-conditioned athletes falling on the lower end of the range. Abnormal breathing patterns and the possible causes of their onset include:

  ○ **Rapid, shallow breaths:** Internal injury; shock

  ○ **Deep, quick breaths:** Pulmonary obstruction; asthma

  ○ **Noisy, raspy breaths:** Airway obstruction

- Any *sputum* that may be produced as the person coughs should be checked for the presence of blood. Pink or bloody sputum indicates internal bleeding requiring emergency treatment.

- **Blood pressure:** A measurement of the pressure exerted by the blood on the arterial walls, blood pressure is affected by a decrease in blood volume (severe bleeding or dehydration), a decreased capacity of the vessels, shock, or a decreased ability of the heart to pump blood (cardiac arrest). Decreased blood pressure indicates a decreased ability to deliver blood, with its nutrients and oxygen, to the organs of the body. Organs are highly susceptible to *anoxia* and can be severely damaged secondary to a decrease in blood pressure.

High blood pressure, or hypertension, is commonly seen in the general population. A dangerous precursor to cardiovascular problems, high blood pressure can exert extreme pressure on the blood vessels, particularly in the smaller vasculature of the brain. Excessive pressure causes these vessels to rupture, resulting in a **cerebrovascular accident** (CVA) or "stroke." The presence of high blood pressure warrants referral to a physician for further evaluation (Box 12–4).

NEUROLOGIC SIGNS

Illness and trauma to the internal organs often manifest themselves by symptoms radiating to the upper extremity, chest, and low back. These patterns of referred pain from the viscera tend to radiate to the part of the body served by the somatic sensory fibers associated with the segment of the spinal cord receiving sensory information (Fig. 12–15).

Sputum   A substance formed by mucus, blood, or pus expelled by coughing or clearing the throat.

Anoxia   The absence of oxygen in the blood or tissues.

FIGURE 12–15. Referred pain patterns from the viscera. Pain from the internal organs tends to radiate along the corresponding somatic sensory fibers.

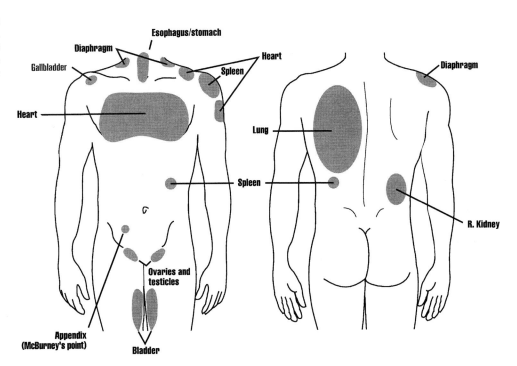

Box 12–3
DETERMINATION OF HEART RATE USING THE CAROTID PULSE

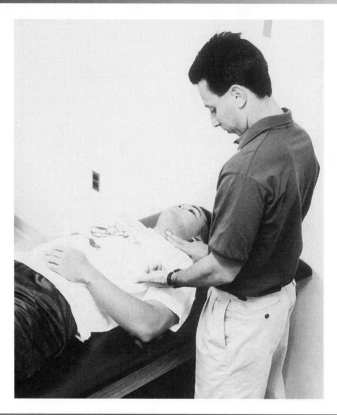

PATIENT POSITION	Seated or lying down
POSITION OF EXAMINER	Using the index and middle fingers to locate the thyroid cartilage, move the fingers laterally in either direction to find the common carotid artery between the thyroid cartilage and the sternocleidomastoid muscle.
EVALUATIVE PROCEDURE	Count the number of pulses in a 15-s interval and multiply that number by 4 to determine the number of beats per minute. The examiner also attempts to determine the quality of the pulse: strong (bounding) or weak.
POSITIVE TEST	Not applicable
IMPLICATIONS	The quality and quantity of the heart rate established. **Normal (general population)**: 60 to 100 bpm **Well-trained athletes**: 40 to 60 bpm **Tachycardia**: Greater than 100 bpm **Bradycardia**: Less than 60 bpm
COMMENTS	The baseline heart rate should be recorded and rechecked at regular intervals.

Box 12–4
BLOOD PRESSURE ASSESSMENT

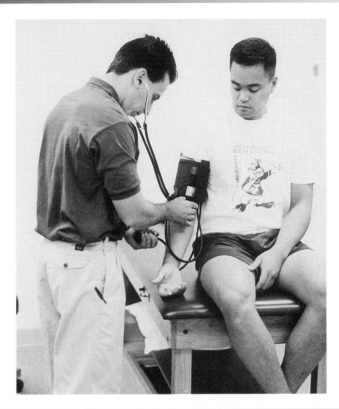

PATIENT POSITION	Seated or lying supine
POSITION OF EXAMINER	In front of or beside the patient in a position to read the gauge on the BP cuff.
EVALUATIVE PROCEDURE	The cuff is secured over the upper arm. Many cuffs have an arrow that must be aligned with the brachial artery. The stethoscope is placed over the brachial artery. The cuff is inflated to 180 to 200 mm Hg. The air is slowly released from the cuff. While reading the gauge, note the point at which the first pulse sound, the systolic pressure, is heard. Continuing to slowly release the air from the cuff, note the value at which the last pulse, the diastolic value, is heard.
POSITIVE TEST	A systolic value below 100 mm Hg or above 140 mm Hg A diastolic value below 65 mm Hg or above 90 mm Hg
IMPLICATIONS	Low BP may indicate shock or internal hemorrhage High BP indicates hypertension
COMMENTS	The athlete's baseline BP should be obtained annually during the preparticipation physical examination and should be compared with the current readings. Larger patients may require the use of a larger BP cuff. A cuff that is too small erroneously increases the BP.

BP = blood pressure.

◆ PATHOLOGIES OF THE THORAX AND ABDOMEN AND RELATED SPECIAL TESTS

Almost all injuries to the thorax and abdomen have an acute onset, but an underlying disease state or illness may predispose an organ to trauma. Many of these conditions have no visible signs or symptoms, causing the assessment, management, and referral to be based on the findings obtained during the history and palpation section of the examination. When the nature of the condition is in doubt, it is best to err on the side of safety and refer the patient to a physician.

INJURIES TO THE THORAX

The mechanism of injury of the thorax may involve the superficial tissues, ribs, heart, or lungs. Likewise, the signs and symptoms of injury to the superficial tissues may mask trauma to the underlying structures.

Rib Fractures

The lateral and anterior portions of the fifth through ninth ribs are most commonly fractured. The upper two ribs are protected by the clavicle and the mass of the pectoralis major muscle. The upper six or seven ribs are protected on their posterior aspect by the scapula, lessening the incidence of rib trauma in these areas. The floating ribs have only a posterior attachment on the vertebrae, allowing them to bend and absorb the force of an impact. Additionally, in sports such as football, the upper ribs are protected by shoulder pads and the

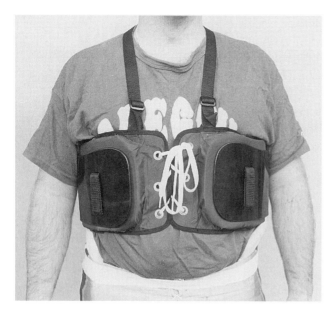

FIGURE 12–16. Flak jacket. These devices may be used to protect the ribs, kidneys, and spleen from traumatic forces.

lower ribs by a "flak jacket" type of padding (Fig. 12–16). Most rib fractures are the result of a single traumatic blow, but repetitive stresses and explosive muscle contractions may also lead to rib fractures.[2]

In cases of a rib fracture, the chief complaint is pain directly at the fracture site that worsens and radiates with deep inspirations, coughing, sneezing, and movement of the torso. The patient may assume a comfortable posture by leaning toward the side of the fracture and may actively splint the fracture site by holding the painful area to limit the amount of chest wall movement during inspiration. Respirations are usually shallow and rapid to minimize the amount of chest movement. Palpation of the area produces pain over the site of the injury, and deformity of the bone or crepitus may also be noted (Table 12–3). The suspicion of a rib fracture can be confirmed through the **rib compression test** (Box 12–5).

A blow in the anteroposterior direction usually results in an outward dispersion of forces along the ribs, forcing the fractured rib segments outward as well. Blows to the lateral rib cage have a higher incidence of inwardly projecting fractures, possibly leading to a pneumothorax or hemothorax.[3] Fractures of the first and second ribs, often associated with cervical trauma, may occlude the underlying vasculature.[3] Unrecognized rib fractures can result in a nonunion, seriously impairing the patient's ability to move the trunk.[4]

The ribs are also subject to stress fractures, especially in sports such as rowing, swimming, and golf.[5–9] Most commonly occurring in the posterolateral portion of the fourth through ninth ribs, stress fractures are the result of sudden increases in training or improper biomechanics. The signs and symptoms of rib stress fractures cause them to be misidentified as erector spinae muscle strains.[8]

The possible complications warrant that all patients with suspected rib fractures be referred to a physician for further evaluation and a definitive diagnosis. Rib fractures are managed by controlling the inflammatory response. Pain may be addressed with ice, medication, or both. A rib belt or tape strapping can be used to limit the amount of rib and chest motion that accompanies breathing and other activities of daily living. If deep breathing has been impaired, rehabilitation may involve the use of a spirometer (see Chapter 20).[3]

Flail Chest

Flail chest occurs when four or more ribs are fractured in two places, causing the segment of the chest wall between the fracture sites to collapse instead of expanding with inspiration (paradoxical respiratory movements) (Fig. 12–17). Exhalation causes the chest segment to protrude as the rest of the chest wall contracts, making flail chest easily recognizable during observation. The inability to inspire air is attributed to a collapsed lung under the flail segment and the pain experienced with breathing.

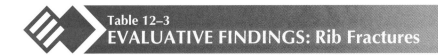

Table 12–3
EVALUATIVE FINDINGS: Rib Fractures

Examination Segment	Clinical Findings	
History	***Onset:***	Acute
	Pain Characteristics:	Over a discrete area of the ribs
	Mechanism:	Direct blow; when the force occurs in the anteroposterior direction, the fracture has the tendency to displace outwardly. A blow from the lateral side results in the fractured ribs being displaced inwardly, threatening the lungs and other internal organs.
Inspection	Possible splinting posture; the patient holds the injured area or leans toward the injured side. Discoloration and swelling may be visible over the injury site. Respirations are shallow and rapid to minimize chest movement.	
Palpation	Point tenderness over the area of impact Deeper palpation may reveal crepitus or identification of the fracture.	
Functional Tests	Movement of the torso—either through active motion or from deep respiration, coughing, or sneezing—produces pain along the fracture site; also possible limited torso movement.	
Ligamentous Tests	Not applicable	
Neurologic Tests	Not applicable	
Special Tests	Rib compression test (contraindicated in the presence of an obvious fracture or lung trauma)	
Comments	Bony fragments that are displaced inward may jeopardize the integrity of the lungs and other internal organs. The signs and symptoms of rib fractures and costochondral injury closely resemble each other.	

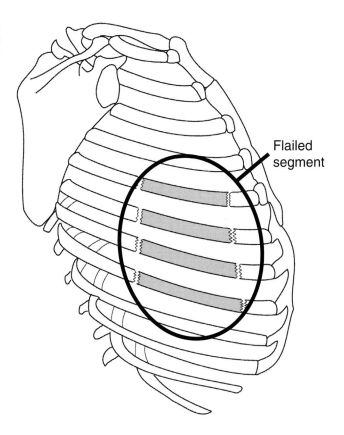

FIGURE 12–17. Flail chest. The flailed segment moves paradoxically to the normal breathing pattern. During inhalation the segment depresses within the rib cage, during exhalation it protrudes from the rest of the thorax.

Flailed segment

Box 12–5
COMPRESSION TEST FOR RIB FRACTURES

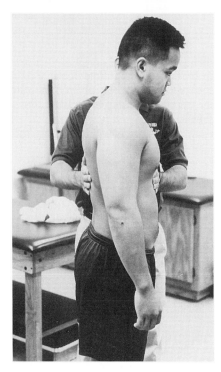 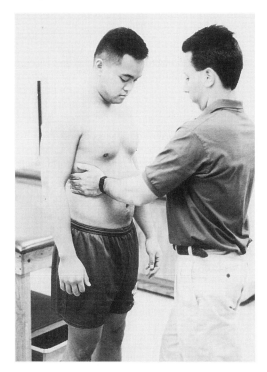

PATIENT POSITION	Seated or standing
POSITION OF EXAMINER	Standing in front of the patient with the hands on opposite sides of the rib cage.
EVALUATIVE PROCEDURE	The examiner compresses the rib cage in an anterior-posterior direction and quickly releases the pressure. The rib cage is then compressed from the patient's side and the pressure is quickly released.
POSITIVE TEST	Pain in the rib cage
IMPLICATIONS	Damage to the rib cage, including the possibility of a fracture, contusion, or costochondral separation.

Costochondral Injury

A costochrondral injury is usually caused by overstretching the costochondral junction as the arm is forced into hyperflexion and horizontal abduction, potentially separating the costocartilage from the ribs. The signs of costochondral injury are similar to those of rib fractures, but the pain is anteriorly located at the costal—cartilage junction (see Table 12–3). The patient has immediate pain at the injury site and may report hearing a "snap" or "pop" at the time of injury. Pain is increased with deep breathing, coughing, sneezing, and movement. As with rib fractures, the patient guards the area through body positioning and splinting with the hands. Swelling is often present and palpation reveals point tenderness over the site of the trauma as well as deformity if the rib has separated from the cartilage.

Patients with costochondral injuries are managed similarly to those with rib fractures, with the protocol focused on decreasing pain, controlling inflammation, and eliminating unnecessary movement of the rib cage.

Pneumothorax

A pneumothorax is the accumulation of air in the pleural cavity that disrupts the lung's ability to expand and draw in oxygen. The decrease in inspired oxygen decreases the amount of oxygen absorbed into the bloodstream, resulting in hypoxia and the development of respiratory distress.

Table 12–4
EVALUATIVE FINDINGS: Pneumothorax

Examination Segment	Clinical Findings	
History	**Onset:**	Acute or insidious
	Pain Characteristics:	Upper left or right quadrant; diaphragm. In some cases, the patient is unable or unwilling to speak.
	Mechanism:	Rupture of a bleb, causing air to enter the pleural cavity or an object or rib puncturing the pleural cavity
	Predisposing Condition:	The presence of a fragile bleb within the lung.
Inspection	Difficulty breathing	
	A guarding posture possibly with the patient clutching the chest and ribs	
	In an acute spontaneous pneumothorax, no visible signs present over the rib cage.	
	Acute traumatic pneumothorax possibly showing trauma at the point of impact	
	Possible cyanosis	
	Progression of a traumatic pneumothorax to the point that the tissue between the clavicle and ribs and the neck veins becomes distended	
	Possible tracheal deviation away from the side of the injury	
	Auscultation of the involved lung revealing absent breath sounds	
Palpation	If of a traumatic onset, the affected area is tender secondary to a contusion, fracture, or costalcartilage separation	
	Percussion of the affected side of the chest producing a hollow sound when compared with the opposite lung	
Vital Signs	Respiration labored and shallow	
	Blood pressure dropping rapidly	
Ligamentous Tests	Not applicable	
Neurologic Tests	Not applicable	
Special Tests	Not applicable	
Comments	An open pneumothorax is characterized by a penetrating wound into the chest cavity. Air can be heard rushing in and out of the wound during respiration.	
	Oxygen must be administered to decrease the amount of respiratory distress.	

A pneumothorax can be either open or closed. A **spontaneous pneumothorax** occurs when *blebs* rupture and allow air to leak into the pleural cavity. It also may result from inflammatory changes in the distal airways.[10] A spontaneous pneumothorax can result secondary to a blow to the rib cage or a penetrating rib cage injury; occur without a history of mechanical force; or arise after surgery.[11,12] Improper breathing patterns during strenuous activities such as weightlifting may also lead to a spontaneous pneumothorax.[13]

When a spontaneous pneumothorax fails to spontaneously close, a **tension pneumothorax** develops. In this case, the air within the pleural cavity continues to build up, placing pressure on the lung and causing it to collapse. If this condition goes unchecked, the subsequent pressure affects the opposite lung, the heart, and the major arteries, leading to death.

Respiratory distress is a common finding in patients with these conditions. The patient may complain of pain and shortness of breath or may be unable to speak, appearing agitated or anxious. Labored and shallow respirations accompany a rapidly decreasing blood pressure. Breath sounds, as assessed during auscultation, may be decreased or completely absent on the affected side. The skin may appear to be *cyanotic.* In extreme cases, the tissues between the ribs and clavicle are distended (Table 12–4). The trachea deviates away from the side of the trauma.

Penetrating wounds through the chest wall and into the pleural cavity from a foreign object or a rib fracture result in an open pneumothorax. Air is allowed to leak in and out of the pleural cavity, disabling the normal respiratory mechanism. This injury is also referred to as a "sucking chest wound" because of the sound made

Bleb A large, loose blood vessel having the potential to rupture.

Cyanotic Dark blue or purple tint to the skin and mucous membranes caused by a decreased oxygen supply.

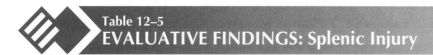

Table 12–5
EVALUATIVE FINDINGS: Splenic Injury

Examination Segment	Clinical Findings	
History	**Onset:**	Acute, although the onset of symptoms may take hours
	Pain Characteristics:	Pressure experienced in the upper left quadrant, discrete area of referred pain in the anterior and posterior portions of the lower left quadrant, and the upper left shoulder (**Kehr's sign**)
	Mechanism:	Blow to the abdomen or thorax, compressing or jarring the spleen
	Predisposing Conditions:	Mononucleosis, systemic infection
Inspection	The impact site possibly showing signs of a contusion or rib fracture Nausea and vomiting possible	
Palpation	Cold and clammy skin with the onset of shock Tenderness in area over the impact site Distention of upper left quadrant	
Functional Tests	Pain in the upper left quadrant and shoulder aggravated by movement. Blood pressure low	
Ligamentous Tests	Not applicable	
Neurologic Tests	Not applicable	
Special Tests	Not applicable	
Comments	Athletes suffering from mononucleosis or other systemic infections are predisposed to spleen injury secondary to the enlargement and hardening of this organ.	

when the patient inhales. Refer to the "On-Field Management" section of this chapter for a description of the initial care of patients with this condition.

Hemothorax

A hemothorax is similar to—and often occurs concurrently with—a pneumothorax. In a hemothorax, respiratory distress is caused by a collection of blood in the pleural cavity. Bleeding occurs from an internal chest wound (e.g., a fractured rib lacerating a lung) or from the rupture of a blood vessel within the chest cavity. The signs and symptoms of a hemothorax are very similar, if not identical, to those of a pneumothorax. However, with a hemothorax, the person may cough up bloody sputum, hemoptysis (see Table 12–4). Refer to the "On-Field Management" section of this chapter for a description of the initial care of patients with this condition.

PATHOLOGY OF THE ABDOMINAL AND URINARY ORGANS

Most of the abdominal organs lie relatively unprotected inferior to the ribs, but their ability to absorb mechanical blows is enhanced by their hollow structure. The lymphatic organs tend to be more solid in nature but are somewhat protected by the lower portion of the rib cage.

Splenic Injury

The spleen may be injured when the abdomen receives a blunt blow such as when a person falls on a ball or other object. The subsequent force delivered to the spleen can result in possible contusion or laceration. An inflamed spleen, which can occur in patients with mononucleosis, pneumonia, or other systemic infections, is predisposed to injury because of the organ's increased mass and decreased elasticity.[14] In patients with advanced disease states, such as mononucleosis, the spleen may spontaneously rupture without a history of blunt force.[15] Likewise, the time between physical trauma to the spleen and the onset of symptoms may be delayed for weeks, days, or years.[16]

The signs and symptoms of shock soon develop after acute spleen trauma. The telltale indicator of a ruptured spleen is the **Kehr's sign,** pain in the upper left quadrant and left shoulder. These symptoms are aggravated by movement, and the patient may vomit or describe being nauseated (Table 12–5). The vital signs are key indicators of *hemodynamic* changes.

If the patient vomits, attempt to observe the discharge to determine if it is undigested food, red from

Hemodynamic   The process of blood circulating through the body.

blood, or greenish from bile. Advise the patient with abdominal injury not to eat or drink because doing so may worsen the symptoms or complicate any surgical procedure that may need to be performed. Various imaging techniques, such as magnetic resonance imaging and computed tomography (CT) scans, are used to identify splenic trauma.[17] Patients suspected of a splenic injury require referral to a physician for immediate evaluation, observation, and treatment.

Kidney Pathologies

The kidneys sit well protected behind the lower ribs and spinal musculature. Forces of sufficient magnitude to traumatize the kidneys are often associated with concurrent injury to the lower ribs, lower thoracic vertebrae, upper lumbar vertebrae, or other internal organs. Any penetrating wounds most likely involve some of these structures as well.

Patients suffering from kidney trauma have a history of blunt trauma to the upper lumbar and lower thoracic region. The only outward signs of a kidney contusion or laceration may be bruising or bleeding over the area of contact. The patient may complain of rib pain that increases in intensity during deep inspiration. Cases of severe internal bleeding also produce the signs and symptoms of shock. Palpation of the area generally reveals diffuse tenderness unless a rib is concurrently injured, at which time a more focused pain and crepitus are demonstrated (Fig. 12–18). With severe bleeding, guarding of the abdomen may reflexively occur because of pain (Table 12–6).

Hematuria is a diagnostic sign associated with an injured kidney. Except in the case of severe bleeding within the kidney, the urine may not seem noticeably discolored to the unaided eye, and bleeding can be detected only through laboratory analysis. Urine for further analysis must be collected from a patient suspected of suffering a kidney injury. The absence of blood in the urine immediately after an injury does not rule out the potential of kidney trauma. The use of CT scans or contrast imaging of the urinary tract may be required for a definitive diagnosis.[18] The potential loss of a kidney warrants that individuals demonstrating any of these signs and symptoms be immediately referred to a physician.

Kidney Stones

Kidney stones are the result of a collection of incomplete kidney filtration. Formed by crystals of uric acid, struvite, or calcium, these stones may measure from less than 1 mm to more than 2.5 cm (1 in). A family history of kidney stones,[19] stressful life events,[20] and hypertension[21] may trigger symptomatic kidney stones. The onset of this condition can also be associated with the intake of large amounts of dietary salts[19,22] and other foodstuffs such as apple or grapefruit juice.[23] Ingesting foods and drinks such as caffeinated or decaffeinated coffee, beer, and wine,[23] and increasing the intake of calcium, tea, tomatoes and other potassium-rich

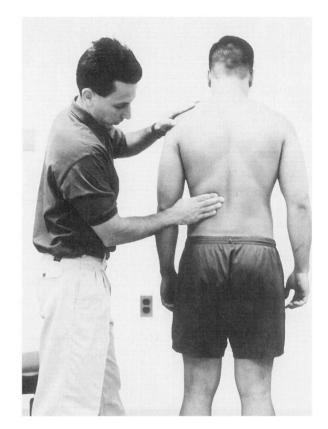

FIGURE 12–18. Palpation of the left kidney. Following an injury, the area overlying the kidneys may become tender to the touch or reveal crepitus secondary to a rib fracture.

foods, and fluids[24] may decrease the possibility of kidney stones.

The first sign of a kidney stone is pain in the left or right side and bladder discomfort may be experienced during urination. Larger stones may be felt as they progress down the ureter to the bladder, producing pain. The most excruciating pain may be experienced as the stone is passed from the urinary bladder through the urethra. When the obstruction occurs in the lower right quadrant, the signs and symptoms of a kidney stone can mimic those of appendicitis.

Patients who are suspected of having kidney stones require a referral to a physician for further evaluation. Mild to moderate kidney stones may be treated through medication and diet modification. Shock-wave lithotripsy can be used to break down small to moderate sized stones; larger stones may require surgical removal.[25]

Urinary Tract Infection

Urinary tract infections (UTIs) are caused by bacterial infections of the bladder or urethra. The ureter and kidney may also be involved. Inflammation of just the bladder, **cystitis**, may also occur. Urinary tract infections may mimic the signs and symptoms of kidney

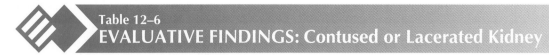

Table 12–6
EVALUATIVE FINDINGS: Contused or Lacerated Kidney

Examination Segment	Clinical Findings	
History	***Onset:***	Acute
	Pain Characteristics:	Posterolateral portion of the upper lumbar and lower thoracic region
	Mechanism:	Blunt trauma or penetrating injury to the kidney (e.g., contusive forces, fractured rib impaling the kidney)
Inspection	Contusion or laceration in the impacted area may be present.	
	Blood is visible on macroscopic or microscopic inspection of the urine.	
	Signs and symptoms of shock may be present.	
Palpation	Tenderness over the impact site	
	Abdominal rigidity may occur	
Functional Tests	Pain possible during urination	
Ligamentous Tests	Not applicable	
Neurologic Tests	Not applicable	
Special Tests	Laboratory findings of hematuria	
Comments	The traumatic forces may also result in a rib fracture or costochondral injury	
	Patients suspected of suffering from a kidney injury should immediately be referred to a physician.	

stones. The patient complains of *dysuria,* the frequent need to urinate, and describes pain in the lower abdominal region. The patient may also describe an abnormal urine color, possibly representing hematuria. Additionally, the urine may have a strong, foul odor. If the infection becomes widespread, fever, nausea, and vomiting may be reported.

Inflammation of the urethra, **urethritis,** may have an onset linked to a specific organism such as gonococcus in the urinary tract; may be attributed to *chlamydia,* gonorrhea, or syphilis; or may have a nonspecific etiology. The onset of urethritis is more frequent in males than females. Urethritis is marked by dysuria, enlarged inguinal lymph nodes, penile discharge, testicular enlargement, and blood in the urine.

Patients suspected of suffering from UTIs or urethritis need to be referred to physicians for antibiotic therapy and tests for associated sexually transmitted diseases (STDs). Likewise, these patients should refrain from sexual activity while the symptoms are present. The patient may also be advised to increase water intake and urinate frequently to flush the infecting agent out of the system.

Appendicitis and Appendix Rupture

Although the onset of appendicitis is rarely attributed to athletic competition, blows to the lower right quadrant may accelerate an existing inflammatory process or cause the inflamed appendix to rupture. Acute appendicitis, commonly occurring in patients who are 15 to 25 years old, is more common in men than in women. The outward symptoms of lower abdominal

tenderness, fever, nausea, and vomiting occur approximately 2 days after the initial inflammation of the appendix. Pain may be referred to the right side of the chest wall as well as the right upper trapezius area. A pus-filled abscess forms 1 to 3 days after the onset of the symptoms. Patients suffering from appendicitis prefer lying supine with the right leg flexed at the hip and knee to lessen the amount of pressure on the lower right quadrant (Table 12–7). Patients suspected of suffering from appendicitis must be immediately referred to a physician. Also, the intake of foods and drinks must be curtailed until permission to resume eating is given by a physician.

Hollow Organ Rupture

Hollow organs are able to absorb the forces from blows to the abdomen, deforming and returning to their initial shape without permanent injury. When a hollow organ is ruptured, the outcome is potentially fatal secondary to hemorrhage, peritoneal contamination, or both.

After a rupture of a hollow organ, the patient describes a history of a blow to the abdomen as well as pain and possible nausea. On further evaluation guarding, abdominal rigidity and tenderness and the signs

---

Dysuria   Painful urination.

Chlamydia   A family of microorganisms that produce infection in the genitals and are sexually transmitted.

Table 12–7
EVALUATIVE FINDINGS: Appendicitis

Examination Segment	Clinical Findings	
History	**Onset:**	Rapid
	Pain Characteristics:	Diffuse in the abdomen; tender and rigid in the lower right quadrant; nausea and possibly vomiting; diarrhea or constipation
	Mechanism:	Infection of the appendix, causing inflammation and eventually possible rupture.
	Predisposing Conditions:	Males between the ages of 15 and 25 years
Inspection	The patient with a sickly appearance; preference to lying supine with the right hip and knee flexed to reduce pressure in the lower right quadrant	
Palpation	Tenderness in the lower right quadrant, especially in the area of **McBurney's point** (see Fig. 12–13) Rebound tenderness	
Functional Tests	As the appendicitis progresses, a fever of at least 99° to 101° F. Rapid pulse Pain with movement Urination and bowel movements increase pressure within the abdominal cavity, thereby increasing pain.	
Ligamentous Tests	Not applicable	
Neurologic Tests	Not applicable	
Special Tests	Not applicable	
Comments	Patients suspected of suffering from appendicitis must immediately be transported to an emergency room. In female athletes, the signs and symptoms of appendicitis are similar to those of pelvic inflammatory disease, ruptured **ectopic pregnancy,** ruptured ovarian cyst, and painful ovulation.	

and symptoms of shock may be noted. Bowel sounds are absent on auscultation.[26]

Because the onset of symptoms associated with hollow organ trauma is gradual, the symptoms may resemble those of a contusion, costal-cartilage sprain, or similar injury. Although the liver is not a hollow organ, its location and relative rigidity predispose it to injury as well. Patients with a seemingly benign abdominal injury must be cautioned to report any increase in symptoms. Patients also need to visually inspect the stool for blood because hemorrhage may leak into the feces.[27] As with all internal organ injuries, patients with suspected ruptures of a hollow organ need to be referred for evaluation at an appropriate medical facility. Because of the possibility of surgery, individuals who have suffered significant trauma to the abdominal organs must refrain from eating or drinking until cleared to do so by a physician.

General Medical Conditions

Gastritis, the inflammation of the stomach lining can result from aspirin or anti-inflammatory medications, alcohol, infection, or bile entering the stomach. When gastric juices backflow into the esophagus **(esophageal reflux),** heartburn, regurgitation of stomach acid, and ulcer-like pain can occur. The symptoms of gastritis can range from simple indigestion and hiccups to nausea, vomiting, and darkened stools.

Irritation of the duodenum can result in the formation of a duodenal (or peptic) **ulcer.** Most duodenal ulcers are caused by the presence of the *Helicobacter pylori* bacteria. However, long-term use of aspirin and other nonsteroidal anti-inflammatory medications can contribute to intestinal ulceration. Ulcers are characterized by abdominal pain, nausea, vomiting, dark stools, fatigue, and weight loss. Esophageal reflux can result in heartburn and indigestion, often mimicking the signs of a heart attack.

Inflammation of the small intestine, **gastroenteritis,** can produce nausea, vomiting, and diarrhea. Bacteria such as *Escherichia coli* and *Salmonella* can trigger the onset of gastroenteritis. Because many of the triggering bacteria are found in foodstuffs, bacterial enteritis is often referred to as "food poisoning." Viral invasion can also cause gastroenteritis, entering the body through drinking water or contaminated food.

Disease, irritation of the bowel, ulceration, ulcers, ischemia, bacteria, stress, or certain antibiotics can lead to the onset of **colitis,** which is inflammation of the large intestine. Colitis may cause frequent bouts of diarrhea, abdominal pain, increased bowel sounds, fever, painful

Ectopic pregnancy   The formation of a fetus outside of the uterine cavity.

defecation, nausea, and vomiting. **Ulcerative colitis** may produce bloody diarrhea in addition to the aforementioned signs and symptoms.

Regional enteritis (Crohn's disease), affects the ileum and produces lower right quadrant pain and cramping. Nausea may be described, but vomiting seldom occurs. A low-grade fever may also be present. Advanced stages of Crohn's disease can produce an abdominal mass, incontinence, and constipation.[28]

The mental and emotional stress associated with athletic competition can give rise to **irritable bowel syndrome,** altering the motility of the muscles of the large intestine. The symptoms of irritable bowel syndrome include alternating bouts of diarrhea and constipation, abdominal pain and tenderness, gas build-up, nausea, vomiting, loss of appetite, and depression. Irritable bowel syndrome is more prevalent in women than in men. Treatment of irritable bowel syndrome includes stress reduction, modifying the diet to include high-fiber foods, and reducing the intake of gastrointestinal stimulants such as caffeine.

PATHOLOGY OF THE REPRODUCTIVE ORGANS

Because of their external location, the male reproductive organs are injured more frequently than the female reproductive organs are. In a direct impact to the genitals, the resulting contusion or lacerations are often embarrassing, especially for younger patients. These conditions must be professionally managed, not only to comfort the patient but also to preserve the integrity of the organs.

Male Reproductive System Pathologies

Trauma to—and disease of—the testicles is potentially a serious medical condition that may lead to infertility and/or hormonal changes.

Testicular Contusion

Direct blows to the testicles result in immediate pain, often at an intensity sufficient to cause vomiting, speech inhibition, and breathing restriction. The priority in managing this condition is to calm the individual. This may be performed by instructing him to inhale deeply and slowly through the nose and exhale through the mouth. Lifting the patient's belt and waistband *may* reduce the feeling of pressure on the testicles and lower abdomen. The efficacy of other anecdotal techniques, such as lifting and dropping the patient on his buttocks, has never been established.

After the pain has been controlled, the patient is instructed to inspect the testicles for normal size and consistency. The trauma may cause the testicle to rupture, giving it a relatively soft, inconsistent texture. Swelling may occur within the testicles, possibly involving the collection of fluids within the scrotum. Either condition warrants immediate follow-up examination by a physician.

Testicular Torsion

Torsion of the spermatic cord occurs as the testicle and spermatic cord is twisted within the scrotal sac. This condition is more common in individuals having an undescended testicle. Unsupported, the testicle and spermatic cord are susceptible to injury from a direct blow or from the simple jarring movements that occur with athletic activity. The use of an athletic supporter decreases the risk of testicular torsion (also referred to as spermatic cord torsion).

An onset caused by acute trauma is associated with intense testicular pain, nausea, and possible vomiting. Symptoms of spermatic cord torsion may have an acute onset of testicular pain caused by the obstruction of the spermatic artery and vein. Inspection reveals a localized swelling of the testicle and, possibly, a mass in the scrotum. Testicular tenderness may be elicited during palpation. The patient requires immediate referral for further evaluation and possible surgery because delayed treatment could lead to loss of the testicle.

Testicular Dysfunction

During fetal development, a channel is formed between the abdomen and scrotum that allows the testicles to fall into the scrotum. As physical maturity develops, the tract normally closes. Incomplete closure can allow fluids from the peritoneum to seep into the scrotum, forming a **hydrocele,** a fluid-filled sac along the spermatic cord. Hydroceles can also be caused by trauma or inflammation of the testicle, epididymis, or secondary to blockage of the spermatic cord's blood supply or the formation of a mass within the serous membrane surrounding the anterior and lateral portion of the testicle (tunica vaginalis). Inguinal hernias may also lead to the onset of a hydrocele.[29] Although the scrotum or testicle (or both) may enlarge, a hydrocele is a painless, benign condition. Other than the outward swelling, the only other symptom is an enlarged testicle that feels like a fluid-filled sack (often described as feeling like a "water balloon"). If the size of the fluid accumulation becomes problematic, the physician may choose to aspirate the hydrocele and close the portal between the scrotum and abdomen. Hydroceles associated with an inguinal hernia require immediate evaluation by a physician.

The formation of *varicose veins* within the scrotum, a **varicocele,** is the result of the obstruction of normal blood flow of the involved veins. In older men, a varicocele can develop secondary to a kidney tumor, altering blood flow from the renal vein through the spermatic vein. The veins within the scrotum may become visible, and the scrotum may appear enlarged. Upon palpation, a painless lump may be felt. The characteristic sign of a varicocele is the scrotum and spermatic cord's feeling like a "bag of worms" during palpation.[30]

Varicose veins   Enlargement of the superficial veins.

Varicoceles are a frequent cause of male infertility. Patients suspected of suffering from a varicocele need a referral to a physician for additional follow-up examination.

The outward signs of a varicocele are similar to those associated with **epididymitis,** or inflammation of the epididymis. Often associated with UTIs, epididymitis is caused by a bacterial infection and may be linked to STDs. Similarly to hydroceles and varicoceles, the scrotum and testicle (or testicles) are enlarged. However, epididymitis is characterized by these structures' being painful to the touch. Pain may also be described during urination, ejaculation, and bowel movements. Bloody discharges and blood in the semen may also be noted. As the infection spreads, the patient may develop a fever and swollen inguinal lymph nodes.

Testicular Cancer

Although unrelated to the acute trauma, testicular cancer is often discovered after testicular injury. Testicular cancer is the most common form of cancer in college-aged male athletes. The risk of onset is greatest between ages 20 to 35 years. A history of undescended testicles (cryptorchidism), *orchitis,* and inguinal hernias increase the risk of developing testicular cancer.[31,32] The patient notices an enlarging and hardening of the involved testicle, and a painless nodule may be noted. Although testicular pain is not always noted, pain may be referred to the low back, inguinal region, and abdomen. Pain may also radiate into the adductor muscle group and appear as an adductor strain. As the disease progresses, blood may be noted in the semen. In the later stages, enlargement of the breasts may occur.

With early detection, the prognosis for most types of testicular cancer is excellent. All men should conduct a testicular self-examination on a monthly basis. Definitive diagnosis of testicular cancer is based on tissue biopsies, ultrasonic imaging, and CT scans. Further information regarding cancer is presented in Chapter 21.

Female Reproductive System Pathologies

The female reproductive organs are well protected within the abdominal cavity. The signs and symptoms tend to duplicate those of appendicitis or trauma to the hollow organs. However, the signs and symptoms may be accompanied by untimely, irregular, or increased menstrual flow. (Injury to the pubic symphysis is discussed in Chapter 8.)

Menstrual Irregularities Associated with Physical Activity

The physical and emotional stresses that accompany many forms of athletics can disrupt or alter female athletes' menstrual cycles. External pressures such as body image, unrealistic target weights, and societal pressures may further disrupt the menstrual cycle.

The absence of the onset of normal **menstruation** by the age of 16 years, **primary amenorrhea,** or the cessation of menstruation for 6 months or more, **secondary**

Table 12–8
FACTORS LEADING TO THE ONSET OF AMENORRHEA

Weight reduction (may be the result of ***anorexia nervosa*** or ***bulimia***)
Obesity
Malnutrition
Hypoglycemia
Cystic fibrosis
Heart disease
Hyperthyroidism
Ovarian disease
Prolonged exercise or overexercising (anorexia athletica)
Pregnancy
Anxiety*
Early menopause*
Pelvic inflammatory disease*

*Secondary amenorrhea only; the remaining factors can be associated with either primary or secondary amenorrhea.

---

amenorrhea, may have a diverse range of causes (Table 12–8). Exercise, weight loss and the resulting decrease in luteinizing hormone, stress, and anxiety may cause irregular menstrual cycles, or **oligomenorrhea.** Because of the association with disease states and nutritional factors, patients experiencing menstrual irregularities need a referral to a gynecologist. Often when the underlying cause of the menstrual irregularity is addressed, regular menstruation resumes. Because of the relationship of amenorrhea to the **female athlete triad,** athletes should be carefully monitored.

Although not normally the result of athletic participation, **dysmenorrhea** can significantly affect an athlete's performance. Dysmenorrhea is characterized by pain or cramping (or both) in the lower abdomen and pelvis starting 1 to 2 days before menstruation. Nausea, vomiting, diarrhea or constipation, and bloating may occur. Patients suffering from dysmenorrhea need referral to a gynecologist because this condition may also be related to *pelvic inflammatory disease (PID),* endometriosis, or

---

Orchitis   Inflammation of the testicle.

Anorexia nervosa   A form of disordered eating characterized by the lack of appetite (or refusal to eat), depression, malaise, and distorted body image most commonly affecting girls and women between the ages of 12 and 21 years.

Bulimia (bulimia nervosa)   A condition marked by periods of insatiable appetite (binge eating) followed by self-induced vomiting (purging).

Hypoglycemia   The state of decreased levels of sugar in the blood, resulting in fatigue, restlessness, and irritability; commonly associated with diabetes.

Pelvic inflammatory disease   An infection of the vagina that spreads to the cervix, uterus, fallopian tubes, and broad ligaments.

other medical conditions. Anti-inflammatory, analgesic, or muscle relaxant medication may be prescribed. Further decrease in symptoms may be accomplished using a moist heat pack placed over the pelvis and abdomen.

The Female Athlete Triad

The female athlete triad syndrome consists of three related components: disordered eating, amenorrhea, and osteoporosis.[33–35] Amenorrhea may also predispose the patient to stress fractures. The American College of Sports Medicine recommends that female athletes who present with one component of the female athlete triad also be screened for the presence of the remaining two components.[34] Table 12–9 presents a list of athletes who are considered as being at risk of acquiring the female athlete triad syndrome.

Individually, any of the components of the female athlete triad poses a significant risk to the health and well being of the athlete. Combined, the components form a potentially fatal condition. Any signs or symptoms of any component of the triad need to be thoroughly evaluated. If left unrecognized or unmanaged, the female athlete triad can lead to a fatal sequence of events.

Currently the best treatment of the female athlete triad is the prevention of the disorder. Athletes should be screened for each of the three components during the pre-participation examination. Athlete, coaches, parents, and health care providers must be educated regarding the predisposing conditions and the signs, symptoms, and potential consequences of the female athlete triad. After a thorough assessment and diagnosis, treatment involves a team approach to address the physical and psychological ramifications of the problem.

Vaginitis

Infection of the vagina, vaginitis, can be classified as bacterial vaginosis, trichomoniasis, or vulvovaginal candidiasis. **Bacterial vaginosis** is caused by a bacterial imbalance within the vagina. **Trichomoniasis** is an STD that involves the infection of the urogenital system in both men and women. In women, trichomoniasis most commonly affects the vagina, but the urethra may also be involved. **Vulvovaginal candidiasis,** commonly referred to as **"yeast infections,"** develops when the yeast cells naturally present in the vagina undergo rapid overgrowth. Vulvovaginal candidiasis has been associated with diabetes mellitus, the use of oral contraceptives or antibiotic medication, and wearing tight-fitting clothing.

The primary sign of bacterial vaginosis is an abnormal, foul-smelling discharge that may be more noticeable after sexual intercourse. Trichomoniasis may be asymptomatic, but a greenish vaginal discharge may be present. Typically, pain is experienced during intercourse and during urination. Vulvovaginal candidiasis is characterized by vaginal redness, burning, and itching. On occasion, a cottage cheese—like discharge from the vagina, may be noted.

Patients suspected of suffering from vaginitis need further evaluation by a gynecologist so that a definitive diagnosis may be made and an appropriate course of treatment determined.

Pelvic Inflammatory Disease

Pelvic inflammatory disease is a general term used to describe inflammation or infection of the uterus, ovaries, or fallopian tubes. The etiology of PID is closely linked to the same bacteria that cause STDs. PID is characterized by vaginal discharge, amenorrhea, dysmenorrhea, or oligomenorrhea, fever, low back and abdominal pain, dysuria, and frequent urination. The inguinal lymph nodes may be enlarged, and the abdomen may be tender to the touch. A referral to a gynecologist is necessary for a definitive diagnosis. The usual course of treatment includes antibiotic medications and, in severe cases, possibly surgery. Prolonged PID can result in infertility.

 ON-FIELD EVALUATION AND MANAGEMENT OF THORACIC AND ABDOMINAL INJURIES

Because trauma to the thorax and abdomen is most often the result of acute, high-velocity impact, the need for on-field evaluation of these conditions is commonplace. At first, injuries to the internal organs may produce only the signs and symptoms of a contusion overlying the impact area. As blood collects within the viscera, outward symptoms of the underlying condition are produced.

RIB FRACTURES

Typically, athletes suffering a rib cage injury leave the area of athletic activity under their own power. In the case of a frank rib fracture or multiple rib fractures,

Table 12–9	
ATHLETES AT RISK OF DEVELOPING ONE OR MORE COMPONENTS OF THE FEMALE ATHLETE TRIAD	
Category	**Example**
Subjectively scored sports	Dance, figure skating, diving, gymnastics
Endurance sports that emphasize a low body weight	Distance running, cycling
Sports that require contour-revealing clothing	Gymnastics, volleyball, swimming, cheerleading
Sports using weight categories	Horse racing, rowing, wrestling
Sports that rely on a prepubertal body type	Figure skating, gymnastics, diving

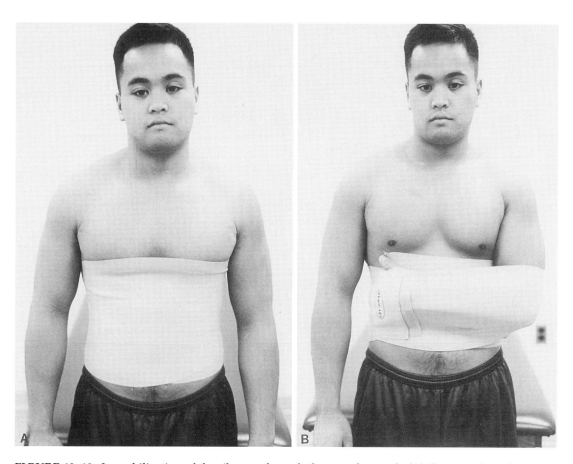

FIGURE 12–19. Immobilization of the rib cage through the use of a swath. **(A)** Compression of the ribs to minimize movement. **(B)** The arm of the involved side may be immobilized to reduce pain that is secondary to movement of the shoulder.

the athlete may not be able to move and must be evaluated on the field. If the presence of a rib fracture is established, further evaluation must be performed to rule out the presence of a pneumothorax or hemothorax. In the absence of these conditions, the athlete is calmed and the area is stabilized before the athlete can be assisted from the field. The area may be stabilized by the use of a rib belt or, more commonly, by wrapping the ipsilateral arm to the side of the athlete with a swathe (Fig. 12–19). The athlete can then be assisted off the field and transported to a medical facility for further evaluation.

FLAIL CHEST

Flail chest must be treated as a medical emergency. Pressure is applied to the flailed ribs by placing a pillow or folded blanket over the area. Treat the athlete for shock, monitor vital signs, and prepare to administer oxygen or assisted respiration. Immediately transport the athlete to a medical facility so that advanced care may be rendered.

PNEUMOTHORAX AND HEMOTHORAX

Patients suspected of having a pneumothorax or hemothorax require continuous vital sign monitoring, treatment for shock, and placement on the affected side in a semi-reclined position, if possible. Oxygen is provided, if available. Prepare to assist with respiration if needed and activate the emergency medical system.

Open Pneumothorax

An open pneumothorax can result from an open rib fracture that also pierces the pleural cavity or from a puncture by an external object (e.g., javelin). An open pneumothorax is characterized by a sucking sound as the athlete attempts to inhale air.

Do not attempt to remove an object that has impaled the athlete. Cover the opening with a sterile dressing and seal it with a nonporous material (e.g., a plastic bag) to prevent the passage of air through the opening (Fig. 12–20). Oxygen may be administered to decrease the amount of respiratory distress.[36]

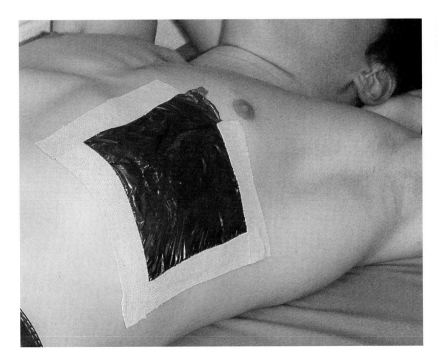

FIGURE 12–20. Management of an open pneumothorax. A one-way valve (upper left-hand corner) is created over the open wound that allows air to escape during exhalation. During inhalation, the valve seals, forcing air to enter the lungs through the trachea

CARDIAC CONTUSIONS

Although the heart is well protected, it may be traumatized by a direct, forceful blow to the sternum or compression of the sternum and anterior rib cage. This force can result in contusions of the pericardial lining, ventricular contusion, or aortic ruptures.[37,38] Within 24 hours after the injury, the subsequent hemorrhage can affect the electrical signals to the heart, causing an irregular heart rhythm.[3]

Symptoms include chest pain, engorgement of the neck vessels, *dyspnea*, and decreased blood pressure. The most severe ramification of cardiac contusions is cardiac arrest. In this event, cardiopulmonary resuscitation (CPR) must be immediately initiated. Patients with suspected cardiac contusions must be immediately referred to a physician.

SOLAR PLEXUS INJURY

The solar plexus (celiac plexus) is injured when an athlete suffers a direct blow to the abdomen or falls on an object, causing transitory paralysis of the diaphragm. The ensuing spasm results in the inability to inhale or, in layman's terms, "have the wind knocked out of you." The athlete is found in apparent respiratory distress, attempting to inspire and unable to communicate. The inability to breathe accompanied by the inability to communicate often leads to panic in the athlete, a condition that warrants treatment equal to that of the injury itself.

Unlike an athlete with an obstruction to the airway who grasps at the throat, this athlete tends to hold the abdomen where the insulting blow was received. Re-

gardless, the examiner must immediately rule out that the airway has been obstructed such as by the athlete's mouthpiece, tooth, or gum.

Although the spasm is a self-limiting condition, the examiner must take actions to hasten the recovery process by reassuring the athlete and using a firm, confident voice. Loosening the athlete's clothes is helpful in lessening the perception of pressure on the abdomen. Instruct the athlete to breathe using long inspirations and short expirations. Also, instructions for the athlete to "pant like a dog" assists in relaxing the diaphragm. Reassuring the athlete further aids in relaxing the spasm. As the athlete's breathing is controlled, obtain a history from the athlete and rule out further internal injury through palpation of the abdomen and monitoring of the athlete's condition, including assessing vital signs as necessary.

BREAST INJURIES

Blunt trauma to the breast can result in hemorrhage or hematoma formation, causing the affected breast to become swollen. Breast trauma may also result in necrosis of the fatty tissue, subsequently with lump formation that could be mistaken for breast cancer during breast examinations.[3] Treat breast contusions with ice to control swelling and pain.

Dyspnea Air hunger marked by labored or difficult breathing; may be a normal occurrence after exertion or an abnormal occurrence indicating cardiac or respiratory distress.

HOLLOW ORGAN INJURIES

Suspected injury to a hollow organ is viewed as a medical emergency. Treat the athlete for shock. For comfort, place the athlete's legs in a hook-lying position and cover him or her with a blanket to maintain body temperature. Continuously monitor and record vital signs, including the time they are taken. These readings should be given to the medical transport team to be delivered with the athlete to the medical facility.

Under no circumstances should the athlete be given anything by mouth. Oral ingestion of solids or liquids may induce vomiting, further injuring the athlete, or may complicate the task of anesthetizing the athlete for any surgical procedure that may be needed.

 REFERENCES

1. Anderson, CR: Case Report: A runner's recurrent abdominal pain. One simple solution. *The Physician and Sportsmedicine*, 20:81, 1992.
2. O'Kane, J, O'Kane, E, and Marquet, J: Delayed complication of a rib fracture. 26:69, 1998.
3. Amaral, JF: Thoracoabdominal injuries in the athlete. *Clin Sports Med*, 16:739, 1997.
4. Proffer, DS, Patton, JJ, and Jackson, DW: Nonunion of a first rib fracture in a gymnast. *Am J Sports Med*, 19:198, 1991.
5. Wasik, M, and McFarland, M: Rib stress fractures: An overview (poster presentation). *J Athletic Training*, 27:156, 1992.
6. Brukner, P, and Khan, K: Stress fracture of the neck of the seventh and eighth ribs: A case report. *Clin J Sport Med*, 6:204, 1996.
7. Taimela, S, Kujala, UM, and Orava, S: Two consecutive rib stress fractures in a female competitive swimmer. 5:254, 1995.
8. Lord, MJ, Ha, KI, and Song, KS: Stress fractures of the ribs in golfers. *Am J Sports Med*, 24:118, 1996.
9. Christiansen, E, and Kanstrup, IL: Increased risk of stress fractures of the ribs in elite rowers. *Scand J Med Sci Sports*, 7:49, 1997.
10. Schramel, FM, Postmus, PE, and Vanderschueren, RG: Current aspects of spontaneous pneumothorax. *Eur Respir J*, 10:1372, 1997.
11. Partridge, RA, et al: Sports-related pneumothorax. *Ann Emerg Med*, 30:539. 1997.
12. Dietzel, DP, and Ciullo, JV: Spontaneous pneumothorax after shoulder arthroscopy: A report of four cases. *Arthroscopy*, 12:99, 1996.
13. Marnejon, T, Sarac, S, and Cropp, AJ: Spontaneous pneumothorax in weightlifters. *J Sports Med Phys Fitness*, 35:124, 1995.
14. Domingo, P, et al: Spontaneous rupture of the spleen associated with pneumonia. *Eur J Clin Microbiol Infect Dis*, 15:733, 1996.
15. Lippstone, MB, et al: Spontaneous splenic rupture and infectious mononucleosis in a forensic setting. *Del Med J*, 70:433, 1998.
16. Fernandes, CM: Splenic rupture manifesting two years after diagnosis of injury. *Acad Emerg Med*, 3:946, 1996.
17. Lawson, DE, et al: Splenic trauma: Value of follow-up CT. *Radiology*, 194:97, 1995.
18. Freitas, JE: Renal imaging following blunt trauma. *The Physician and Sportsmedicine*, 17:59, 1989.
19. Curhan, GC, et al: Family history and risk of kidney stones. *J Am Soc Nephrol*, 8:1568, 1997.
20. Najem, GR, et al: Stressful life events and risk of symptomatic kidney stones. *Int J Epidemiol*, 26:1017, 1997.
21. Cupisti, A, et al: Hypertension in kidney stone patients. *Nephron*, 73:569, 1996.
22. Massey, LK and Whiting, SJ: Dietary salt, urinary calcium, and kidney stone risk. *Nutr Rev*, 53:131, 1995.
23. Curhan, CG, et al: Prospective study of beverage use and the risk of kidney stones. *Am J Epidemiol*, 143:240, 1996.
24. Hirvonen, T, et al: Nutrient intake and use of beverages and the risk of kidney stones among male smokers. *Am J Epidemiol*, 150:187, 1999.
25. Rutz-Danielczak, A; Pupek-Musialik, D and Raszeja-Wanic, B: Effects of extracorporeal shock wave lithotripsy on renal function in patients with kidney stone disease. *Nephron*, 79:162, 1998.
26. Baker, B: Jeunal perforation occurring in contact sports. *Am J Sports Med*, 6:403, 1978.
27. Dauneker, DT, et al: Case report: Intra-abdominal injury to a gymnast. *The Physician and Sportsmedicine*, 7:119, 1979.
28. Morton, PG: *Health Assessment in Nursing* (ed 2). Springhouse, PA, Springhouse Corp, 1993, p. 373.
29. Tanyel, FC, et al: Inguinal hernia revisited through comparative evaluation of peritoneum, processus vaginalis, and sacs obtained from children with hernia, hydrocele, and undescended testis. *J Pediatr Surg*, 34:552, 1999.
30. Comhaire, F, Zalata, A, and Schoonjans, F: Varicocele: Indications for treatment. *Int J Androl*, 18(suppl 2):67, 1995.
31. Pinczowski, D, et al: Occurrence of testicular cancer in patients operated on for cryptorchidism and inguinal hernia. *J Urol*, 146:1291, 1991.
32. Gallagher, RP, et al: Physical activity, medical history, and risk of testicular cancer. *Cancer Causes Control*, 6:398, 1995.
33. West, RV: The female athlete. The triad of disordered eating, amenorrhea, and osteoporosis. *Sports Med*, 26:63, 1998.
34. Otis, CL, et al: American College of Sports Medicine position stand. The female athlete triad. *Med Sci Sports Exerc*, 29:i, 1997.
35. Nattiv, A, et al: The female athlete triad. The inter-relatedness of disordered eating, amenorrhea, and osteoporosis. *Clin Sports Med*, 13:405, 1994.
36. Moore, S: Management of a pneumothorax in a football player. *Athletic Training: Journal of the National Athletic Trainers Association*, 19:129, 1984.
37. Yates, MT, and Aldrete, V: Case report. Blunt trauma causing aortic rupture. *The Physician and Sportsmedicine*, 19:96, 1991.
38. Weiss, RL, et al: The usefulness of transesophageal echocardiography in diagnosing cardiac contusions. *Chest*, 109:73, 1996.

CHAPTER 13

The Shoulder and Upper Arm

The shoulder complex is perhaps the most complicated of the body's articulations because it must provide a large amount of range of motion (ROM) in many anatomical planes. For example, the relationship between the glenohumeral (GH) joint and the scapula allows the humerus to be placed in 16,000 positions that can be differentiated in 1-degree increments.[1]

The shoulder complex lacks the intrinsic bony and ligamentous stabilizers seen in other joints. Relying on its musculature to provide most of its stability, the shoulder complex in general, and specifically the GH joint, is inherently unstable. The GH joint, because of its poor bony stability and weak capsular structures, depends more on the proprioceptive and stabilizing function of its musculature than any other joint in the body.[2] Injury to the shoulder complex may occur from a direct force or secondary to forces transmitted proximally along the upper extremity. The shoulder complex also is predisposed to overuse conditions, especially in individuals participating in sports that require repeated overhead movements.

◆ CLINICAL ANATOMY

The shoulder complex's only attachment to the axial skeleton is at the sternoclavicular (SC) joint. This configuration results in a mechanism whereby the upper extremity is suspended from the torso by muscular attachments. The motions provided by the upper extremity arise from the intricate interactions of the four bones forming the shoulder girdle and the four articulations providing movement. The large ROM provided by the shoulder complex, especially the GH joint, is achieved at the expense of joint stability. Unlike the hip joint, which gains its stability through a deep ball-and-socket joint and strong ligamentous support (at the expense of mobility), the GH joint is characterized by shallow articular surfaces, inconsistent ligamentous support, and an increased reliance on muscular support.

BONY ANATOMY

The shoulder complex, formed by the sternum, clavicle, scapula, and humerus, may be likened to a series of hinges, pulleys, and levers working in unison to choreograph intricate motions in many anatomical planes (Fig. 13–1). A fine degree of ROM, strength, and coordination must be maintained between these bones to ensure that proper biomechanics take place.

The sternum's **manubrium** serves as the site of attachment for each clavicle. Projecting above the body of the sternum, the manubrium's superior surface is indented by the **jugular (suprasternal) notch.** Projecting off each side of the jugular notch is the **clavicular notch,** which accepts the medial head of the clavicle (Fig. 13–2).

Serving as a "strut" between the sternum and scapula, the **clavicle** elevates and rotates to maintain

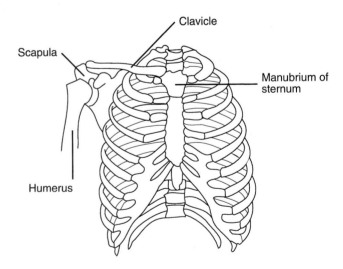

FIGURE 13–1. Bones of the shoulder complex and glenohumeral joint.

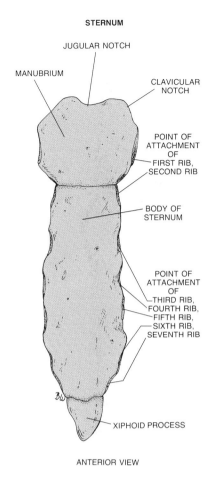

STERNUM

JUGULAR NOTCH

MANUBRIUM

CLAVICULAR
NOTCH

POINT OF
ATTACHMENT
OF
FIRST RIB,
SECOND RIB

BODY OF
STERNUM

POINT OF
ATTACHMENT
OF
THIRD RIB,
FOURTH RIB,
FIFTH RIB,
SIXTH RIB,
SEVENTH RIB

XIPHOID PROCESS

ANTERIOR VIEW

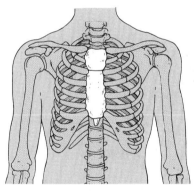

FIGURE 13–2. The sternum, formed by the manubrium, body, and xiphoid process. In preadolescents, the junction between the manubrium and sternal body is pliable, but it fuses with age.

the alignment of the scapula, allowing for additional motion when the arm is raised and preventing excessive anterior displacement of the scapula. The proximal two thirds of the clavicle is characterized by an anteriorly convex bend. The distal one third begins to flatten while curving concavely to meet with the scapula (Fig. 13–3). The point at which the clavicle begins to transi-

tion from a convex to a concave bend, approximately two thirds of the way along its shaft, is relatively weak and is a common site for fractures. The superior surface of the clavicle is not protected by muscle mass, making the bone susceptible to injury. The medial clavicular epiphysis is the last growth plate in the body to ossify and does not fully fuse until approximately age 25 years.[3]

Having no direct bony or ligamentous attachment to the axial skeleton, the **scapula** gains its attachment to the torso by way of the clavicle. Its anterior surface is held against the torso by atmospheric pressure and muscle attachments. The scapula's unique form gives rise to its unique function of serving as both a lever and a pulley.

Thin and triangular, the scapula's anterior costal surface is concave, forming the **subscapular fossa.** The **vertebral (medial) border** is marked by the **inferior** and **superior angles.** The posterior surface is distinguished by the horizontal **scapular spine,** which divides the area into the large **infraspinous fossa** below and the smaller **supraspinous fossa** above. On the lateral end of the scapular spine is the anteriorly projecting **acromion process,** which articulates with the clavicle. Projecting inferiorly and anteriorly to the acromion is the beak-shaped **coracoid process.** The infraspinous, supraspinous, and subscapular fossae merge on the axial border to form the glenoid fossa. Located below the acromion, this fossa articulates with the humeral head (Fig. 13–4).

When the scapula is placed in its anatomical position, the glenoid fossa angles 30 degrees from the frontal plane and its face assumes a downward direction (Fig. 13–5).[4] The angle assumed by the face of the glenoid fossa, the **plane of the scapula,** provides a more functional arc for motion than the cardinal sagittal or frontal planes. This angle also places the rotator cuff muscles in their optimal length-tension relationship. For example, when reaching for an item on an overhead shelf, it is more natural to lift the arm in the plane of the scapula rather than lifting the arm through the sagittal or frontal planes.

The proximal end of the **humerus** is characterized by the medially projecting **humeral head** off of the **anatomical neck** (Fig. 13–6). Bisecting the upper quarter of the anterior surface of the humerus, the **bicipital groove** (intertubercular groove) forms a canal through which the long head of the biceps tendon passes. The lateral edge of the groove is formed by **the greater tuberosity.** The medial border is formed by the **lesser tuberosity.** The inferior borders of the greater and lesser tuberosities mark the **surgical neck,** a name derived because fractures at this location generally require surgical intervention because of the large number of nerves passing through this site. Laterally and slightly above the midshaft is the insertion site for the deltoid muscle group, the **deltoid tuberosity.** The distal structures of the humerus are covered in Chapter 14.

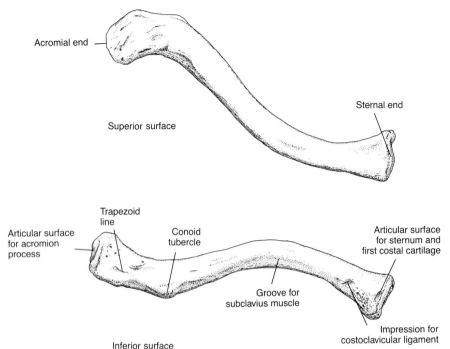

FIGURE 13–3. Clavicle, superior and inferior views.

The **angle of inclination** is the relationship between the shaft of the humerus and the humeral head in the frontal plane, normally 130 to 150 degrees. In the transverse plane, the relationship between the shaft of the humerus and the humeral head is the **angle of torsion,** which varies greatly from individual to individual (Fig. 13–7).[5]

JOINTS OF THE SHOULDER COMPLEX

The motion of the GH joint is augmented by the SC and **acromioclavicular (AC) joints** and the movement between the scapula and the thorax. A change in the mobility or function at any of these associated joints decreases the function at the GH joint.

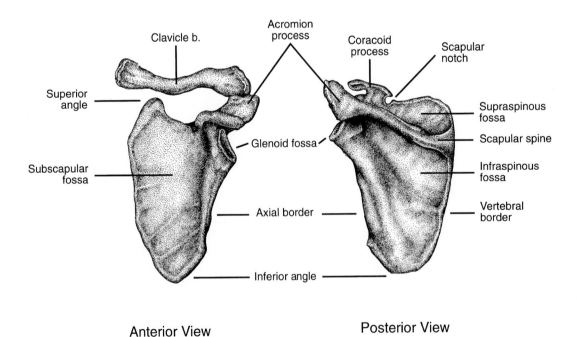

Anterior View

Posterior View

FIGURE 13–4. Bony anatomy of the scapula, anterior (costal), and posterior (dorsal) views, showing the relationship with the clavicle.

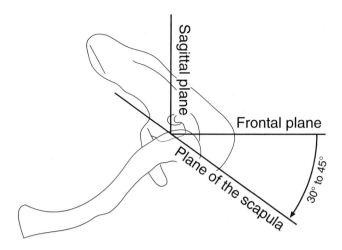

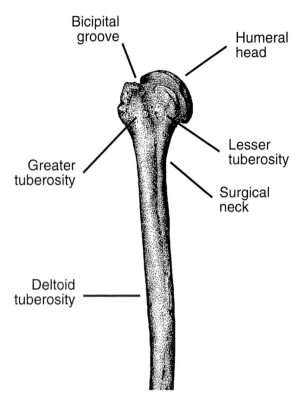

FIGURE 13–5. Plane of the scapula. The face of the glenoid fossa sits at a 30° angle of horizontal adduction in the frontal plane. Movements within the plane of the scapula are more "natural" than movements in the cardinal plane.

FIGURE 13–6. Upper humerus, showing the prominent bony landmarks.

Sternoclavicular Joint

At the SC joint, the proximal portion of the clavicle meets the manubrium of the sternum and a portion of the first costal cartilage to form a gliding joint that allows 3 degrees of freedom of motion: *elevation* and depression, **protraction** and **retraction,** and internal and external rotation.

The articulation between the manubrium and clavicle is inherently incongruent because the proximal end of the clavicle extends one half of its width above the manubrium (Fig. 13–8). The stability of this junction is

enhanced by the presence of a fibrocartilaginous disk. Surrounded by a synovial membrane, the SC joint is supported by the anterior and posterior SC ligaments, the **costoclavicular ligament,** and the **interclavicular ligament.**

The **sternoclavicular disk,** which has qualities similar to the menisci found in the knee, functions as a shock absorber and acts as the axis for clavicular rota-

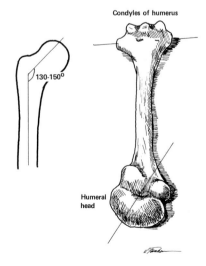

FIGURE 13–7. Angular alignment of the humerus. Angle of inclination representing the angle formed by the long axis of the humeral shaft and the axis of the humeral head. Angle of torsion representing the relationship between the humeral condyles and the humeral head in the transverse plane.

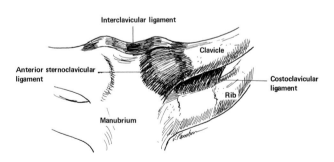

FIGURE 13–8. Ligaments of the SC joint. Although the SC joint does not have inherent bony stability, the ligamentous arrangement provides great strength to the joint.

Elevation   Raising the arm in the scapular plane.

tion. The upper portion of the disk is attached to the clavicle, and its lower portion is attached to the manubrium and first costal cartilage. This disk also serves to divide the joint into two articular cavities, one between the disk and the clavicle and a second between the disk and the manubrium.

The synovial membrane is reinforced by the **anterior** and **posterior sternoclavicular ligaments.** Whereas the anterior fibers resist posterior displacement of the clavicle on the manubrium, the posterior fibers resist anterior displacement. The costoclavicular ligament serves as an axis of clavicular elevation and depression and protraction and retraction. Its anterior fibers limit elevation and lateral clavicular movement. Likewise, the posterior fibers limit elevation and medial movement of the clavicle.

Both of the SC joints are joined by the **interclavicular ligament.** Attaching to the superior proximal ends of the left and right clavicles, the ligament has a common connection on the superior border of the sternum. The interclavicular ligament resists downward movement of the clavicle and assists in dissipating force across the entire upper extremity.

The Acromioclavicular Joint

The distal end of the clavicle meets the scapula's acromion process to form the AC joint. A plane synovial joint, the AC joint allows a gliding articulation between the acromion and the clavicle, capable of 3 degrees of freedom of movement: (1) scapular rotation, (2) scapular winging, and (3) *scapular tipping.* This articulation allows for the motion necessary to maintain the relationship between the scapula and the clavicle in the early and late stages of the GH joint's ROM.

Surrounded by a synovial membrane, the AC joint is supported by the AC ligament and the **coracoclavicular ligament,** which suspend the scapula from the clavicle (Fig. 13–9). A synovial disk is present between the clavicle and the acromion that disappears by the second decade of life and may not be present in the adult's shoulder.

Divided into two separate bands, the superior and inferior portions of the AC ligament function to maintain continuity between the articulating surfaces of the acromion and clavicle. With much of its restraint in the horizontal plane, this ligament maintains stability by preventing the clavicle from riding up and over the acromion process.

Most of the AC joint's intrinsic stability arises from the coracoclavicular ligament. This ligament is divided into two distinct portions: the lateral quadrilateral-shaped **trapezoid ligament** and the medial triangular-shaped **conoid ligament.** Separated by a bursa, the trapezoid ligament limits lateral movement of the clavicle over the acromion. The conoid ligament restricts superior movement of the clavicle. Acting jointly, these ligaments limit rotation of the scapula and provide some degree of horizontal stability. However, a hori-

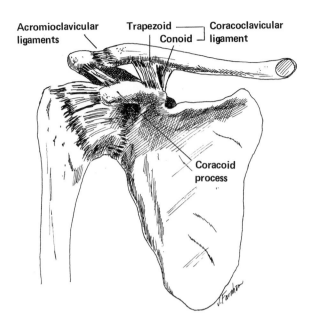

FIGURE 13–9. Ligaments of the acromioclavicular joint. The acromioclavicular ligament provides anterior/posterior stability to the joint. The two portions of the coracoclavicular ligament prevent superior/inferior displacement of the clavicle on the scapula.

zontal dislocation of the AC joint can occur with the coracoclavicular ligament's remaining intact.

The Scapulothoracic Articulation

The articulation between the scapula and the posterior rib cage is not a true anatomical joint because it lacks the typical synovial joint characteristics of connection by fibrous, cartilaginous, or synovial tissues. The movements associated with the scapulothoracic articulation include scapular elevation and depression, protraction and retraction, and upward and downward rotation. The motions rarely occur in an isolated manner. Typically, the motions occur in unison (e.g., protraction and upward rotation). Motion at either the scapulothoracic, AC, or SC joint produces motion of the other two joints.

The Glenohumeral Joint

Formed by the head of the humerus and the scapula's glenoid fossa, the GH articulation is a ball-and-socket joint capable of 3 degrees of freedom of motion: flexion and extension, abduction and adduction, and internal and external rotation. Although not true anatomical motions, horizontal adduction and abduction (or hori-

Scapular tipping The inferior angle of the scapula moving away from the thorax while its superior border moves toward the thorax.

zontal flexion and extension), circumduction, and elevation also occur at the GH joint. Because of its relevance to many athletic movements, elevation is considered as a unique movement throughout this chapter. Most upper extremity motions do not occur in a single isolated plane but, rather, are a combination of movements in two or more planes.

The GH joint is inherently unstable because of the relationship in the sizes of the articular surfaces of the glenoid fossa and the humeral head, a loose joint capsule, and relatively weak ligamentous support. The articulating surface of the glenoid fossa is significantly smaller than that of the humeral head and only vaguely resembles the ball-and-socket joint of the hip. The socket is somewhat deepened by the **glenoid labrum,** which also slightly increases the articular surface. Traditionally thought of as a synovium-lined fibrocartilage, recent findings suggest that the glenoid labrum is actually a fold of dense fibrous connective tissue.[6] Disruption of the glenoid labrum is often associated with recurrent shoulder instability.

Possessing a volume twice the size of the humeral head, the joint capsule arises from the glenoid fossa and glenoid labrum to blend with the muscles of the rotator cuff. Studies on cadavers indicate that the laxity of the capsular arrangement allows the humeral head to be distracted 2 cm or more from the glenoid fossa.[7] The capsule is reinforced by the **glenohumeral ligaments** and the **coracohumeral ligament** (Fig. 13–10).

The three GH ligaments—superior, middle, and inferior—are not distinct joint structures but are actually thickenings in the joint capsule. The specific GH ligament that limits motion depends on the position of the humerus (Table 13–1). The inferior GH ligament possesses an anterior and posterior band with a hammock-like structure, the **inferior pouch,** connecting the two. The area between the superior and middle GH ligaments, the **foramen of Weitbrecht,** is a weak site in the capsule often torn during anterior GH dislocations.

Emanating from the coracoid process, the coracohumeral ligament merges with the superior capsule

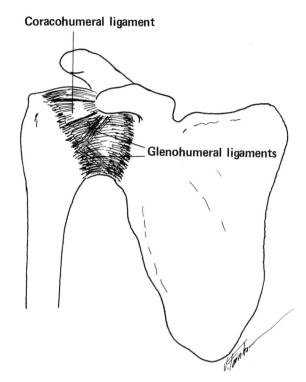

FIGURE 13–10. Ligaments of the GH joint: the coracohumeral and GH ligaments. The GH ligament is divided into superior, middle, and inferior portions. To provide the necessary range of motion to the GH joint, these ligaments must be relatively lax. Much of the stability of this articulation is gained from its muscular arrangement.

and the supraspinatus tendon to insert on the greater tuberosity. The anterior fibers of this ligament limit extension while the posterior fibers limit the amount of GH flexion. The coracohumeral ligament and the superior GH ligament limit external rotation of the humerus when the arm is at the side of the body.

Table 13–1
LIGAMENTS LIMITING HUMERAL MOTION

Position of the Humerus	Ligamentous Structures Limiting Movement
External rotation, 0° abduction	Superior GH ligament Coracohumeral ligament
External rotation, 45° abduction	Middle GH ligament Anterior band of the inferior GH ligament
External rotation, 90° abduction	Inferior GH ligament
Internal rotation, 90° abduction	Posterior band of the inferior GH ligament
Inferior displacement, 0° abduction	Superior GH ligament Coracohumeral ligament
Inferior displacement, 90° abduction	Inferior GH ligament

GH = glenohumeral.

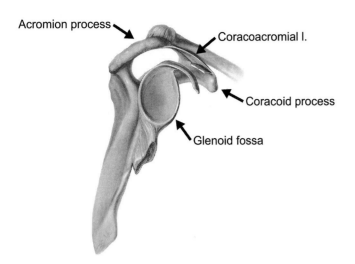

FIGURE 13–11. Coracoacromial arch. The tendons of the rotator cuff, the long head of the biceps brachii tendon, and the subacromial bursa must fit between the arch and the humeral head.

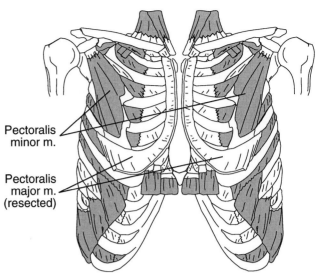

FIGURE 13–12. Pectoralis minor. The pectoralis major has been resected.

When the humerus is hanging at rest in the anatomical position, the articular surfaces of the GH joint have very little contact. Much of the weight of the arm is supported by the superior GH ligament and the inferior portion of the glenoid labrum. When the humerus is abducted to 90 degrees and externally rotated, the entire joint capsule is wound tightly, placing the GH joint in its closed-packed position.

Superior to the humeral head is the **coracoacromial arch,** formed by the **coracoacromial ligament** that traverses from the inferior portion of the acromion process to the posterior portion of the coracoid process (Fig. 13–11). The arch protects the superior portion of the humeral head, the tendons of the rotator cuff muscles, and various bursae from trauma and provides a restraint against superior and anterior GH dislocations. The coracoacromial arch also becomes involved with shoulder impingement syndrome.

MUSCLES OF THE SHOULDER COMPLEX

The function of the shoulder complex and arm is controlled by two groups of muscles: those that act primarily on the scapula and those that function primarily on the humerus. Movements of the shoulder complex involve an intricate series of static and dynamic interactions between these two groups of muscles.

Muscles Acting on the Scapula

The muscles acting on the scapula have two purposes: (1) to move the scapula's glenoid fossa to allow the shoulder complex increased ROM and (2) to fixate the

scapula on the thorax to provide the rotator cuff muscles with a fixed base of support during contractions. The action, origin, insertion, and nerve supply for the muscles acting on the scapula are presented in Table 13–2.

Inserting on the scapula's vertebral border are the **rhomboid minor** and **rhomboid major.** These muscles retract the scapula toward the spine and elevate and downwardly rotate the scapula. The **levator scapulae** acts to elevate and downwardly rotate the scapula. The **serratus anterior,** inserting on the costal surface of the vertebral border, upwardly rotates and protracts the scapula. Working segmentally, the serratus anterior's lower fibers depress the scapula and the upper fibers elevate it. Additionally, this muscle plays a primary function in fixating the scapula's vertebral border to the thorax. A weakness of the serratus anterior or injury to the long thoracic nerve innervating it can result in **scapular winging,** in which the vertebral border lifts away from the thorax. The **pectoralis minor** serves to tilt the scapula forward so that the inferior angle lifts away from the thorax and rotates the inferior angle of the scapula toward the midline of the body (Fig. 13–12).

The **trapezius** muscle is divided into upper, middle, and lower segments (Fig. 13–13). Each of these three segments of the trapezius has a unique action on the scapula. The upper fibers elevate and upwardly rotate, the middle fibers retract, and the lower fibers depress and upwardly rotate the scapula.

Two additional muscles have an indirect force on the scapula. The upper fibers from the **latissimus dorsi** depress the shoulder complex. The clavicular portion of the **pectoralis major** depresses the scapula by its attachment to the clavicle at the AC joint.

Table 13–2
MUSCLES ACTING ON THE SCAPULA

Muscle	Action	Origin	Insertion	Innervation	Root
Latissimus dorsi	Depression of shoulder girdle	• Spinous processes of T6 through T12 and the lumbar vertebrae via the lumbodorsal fascia. • Posterior iliac crest	• Intertubercular groove of the humerus	Thoracodorsal	C6, C7, C8
Levator scapulae	Elevation Downward rotation Extension of cervical spine Rotation of the cervical spine	• Transverse processes of cervical vertebrae C1 through C4	• Superior medial angle of the scapula	Dorsal scapular	C3, C4 C4, C5
Rhomboid major	Scapular retraction Scapular elevation Downward rotation of the scapula	• Spinous processes of T2, T3, T4, and T5	• Vertebral border of scapula (lower two thirds)	Dorsal scapular	C4, C5
Rhomboid minor	Scapular retraction Scapular elevation	• Inferior portion of the ligamentum nuchae • Spinous processes C7 and T1	• Vertebral border of scapula (near the medial border of the scapular spine)	Dorsal scapular	C4, C5
Serratus anterior	Upward rotation Protraction Depression (lower fibers) Elevation (upper fibers) Fixation of the scapula to the thorax	• Anterior portion of 1st through 8th or 9th ribs • Aponeuroses of the intercostal muscles	Costal surfaces of the: • Superior angle of scapula • Vertebral border of scapula • Inferior angle of scapula	Long thoracic	C5, C6, C7
Trapezius (upper one third)	Elevation of scapula Upward rotation of scapula Rotation of C-spine to the opposite side Extension of C-spine	• Occipital protuberance • Superior nuchal line of the occipital bone • Upper portion of the ligamentum nuchae • Spinous process of C7	• Distal/lateral one third of clavicle • Acromion process • Scapular spine	Accessory	CN XI
Trapezius (middle one third)	Retraction of scapula Fixation of thoracic spine	• Lower portion of the ligamentum nuchae • Spinous processes of the 7th cervical vertebra and T1 through T5	• Acromion process • Spine of the scapula (superior, lateral border)	Accessory	CN XI
Trapezius (lower one third)	Depression of scapula Retraction of scapula Fixation of thoracic spine	• Spinous processes and supraspinal ligaments of T8 through T12	• Spine of the scapula (medial portion)	Accessory	CN XI
Pectoralis major	Depression of the shoulder girdle (clavicular fibers)	• Medial one-half of the clavicle • Anterolateral portion of the sternum	• Greater tuberosity of the humerus—lateral lip of the bicipital groove.	Lateral and medial pectoral	C6, C7, C8, T1
Pectoralis minor	Forward (anterior) tilting	• Costalcartilages of ribs 6 through 7 • Anterior portion of 3rd through 5th ribs	• Coracoid process of scapula	Lateral pectoral	C7, C8, T1

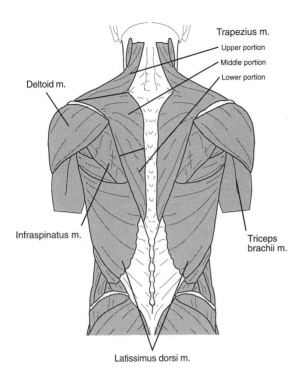

FIGURE 13–13. Superficial posterior muscles acting on the scapula and GH joint. The trapezius (upper, middle, and lower portions), latissimus dorsi, infraspinatus, posterior portion of the deltoid, and the triceps brachii.

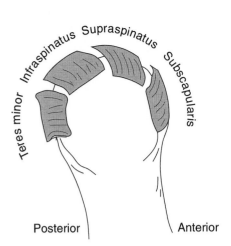

FIGURE 13–14. Muscles of the rotator cuff as they attach to the humeral head.

Muscles Acting on the Humerus

Motion at the shoulder joint can occur as GH motion. However, as is the case of sport-specific motions, motion at the shoulder joint can be the result of the motion provided by the entire shoulder complex. The action, origin, insertion, and nerve supply for the muscles acting primarily on the humerus are presented in Table 13–3.

Four muscles arising off the scapula form the **rotator cuff muscle group** (Fig. 13–14). As a group, the rotator cuff internally and externally rotates the humerus and stabilizes the humeral head in the glenoid fossa. During the later stages of abduction, the rotator cuff muscle group also provides a downward pull on the humeral head, allowing for its unimpeded passage under the acromion. The **subscapularis muscle** is the only member of the rotator cuff group that internally rotates the humerus. The **supraspinatus** assists in abducting and externally rotating the humerus. The remaining two members of the rotator cuff, the **infraspinatus** and **teres minor**, externally rotate the humerus and provide a degree of assistance during horizontal abduction. Additionally, the teres minor is an assistive mover during extension of the GH joint. The eccentric contractions of the infraspinatus and teres minor muscles decelerate the humerus at the end of overhead throwing motions. Closely associated with the muscles of the rotator cuff

is the teres major, which assists with internal rotation, adduction, and extension of the humerus.

Although having a common insertion on the deltoid tuberosity of the humerus, each section of the **deltoid muscle group** should be considered independently. As a whole, the deltoid muscle group is the prime mover during abduction. Considered as individual units, the **anterior fibers** flex the GH joint, horizontally adduct, and internally rotate the humerus. The **middle fibers** serve to abduct the humerus. The **posterior fibers** act to extend, horizontally abduct, and externally rotate the humerus. The deltoid group and the upper fibers of the trapezius merge at the AC joint and assume the role of secondary stabilizers of this articulation.

During abduction, a *force couple* exists between the line of pull between the supraspinatus and the deltoid muscle group. The line of force created by the deltoid's contraction tends to pull the head of the humerus upward against the inferior portion of the acromion process and the coracoacromial ligament. In the early stages of abduction, the rotator cuff's angle of pull must be sufficient to hold the head of the humerus close against the glenoid fossa. After the humerus moves past 90 degrees, the rotator cuff's angle of pull changes so that its force rolls the humeral head inferiorly on the glenoid fossa, creating clearance to pass under the acromion process and the coracoacromial ligament (Fig. 13–15). A damaged or weak rotator cuff group changes the dynamics of the force couple, resulting in the impingement of the rotator cuff and long head of the biceps brachii tendon between the humeral head, subacromial bursa, and acromion process.

Force couple Coordination between dynamic and isometric contractions of opposing muscle groups to perform a movement of a joint.

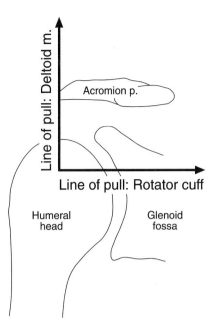

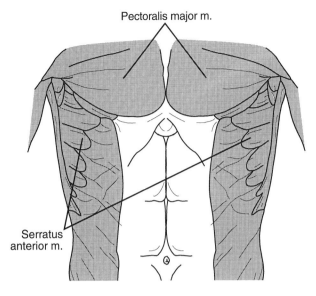

FIGURE 13–16. Pectoralis major and serratus anterior.

FIGURE 13–15. Scapulohumeral force couple. Contraction of the deltoid muscle pulls the humeral head upward. To prevent contact between the humeral head and the acromion process during abduction, the rotator cuff must hold the humeral head close to the glenoid fossa and, when the humerus approaches 90° of abduction, must serve to glide the humerus inferiorly.

The **pectoralis major** is divided into two portions, the clavicular portion and the sternal portion, each having a common insertion on the greater tuberosity (Fig. 13–16). As a whole, the pectoralis major adducts, horizontally adducts, and internally rotates the humerus. The clavicular portion flexes, internally rotates, and horizontally adducts the humerus. The sternal portion depresses the shoulder girdle and assists in horizontal adduction.

The **latissimus dorsi** has a broad origin on the lumbar spine, thoracodorsal fascia, and iliac crest. Inserting on the intertubercular groove of the humerus, the latissimus dorsi adducts, internally rotates, and extends the humerus. Attaching to the infraglenoid tuberosity of the scapula, the **long head of the triceps brachii** is an adductor and extensor of the humerus, especially when the elbow is flexed.

The **coracobrachialis** acts on the humerus as a flexor and adductor. Both heads of the **biceps brachii** have an attachment on the scapula (Fig. 13–17). The short head attaches to the coracoid process, and the long head passes through the bicipital groove to attach on the supraglenoid tuberosity. Stability within the bicipital groove is maintained by the **transverse humeral ligament,** lined by a capsular sheath emanating from the GH capsule. Both heads assist in GH flexion and, when the humerus is externally rotated, the long head assists in GH abduction.

The long head of the biceps enters the joint capsule through an invagination between the supraspinatus and subscapularis muscles. Whereas the capsule is penetrated, the tendon does not enter the synovial membrane of the articulation. During the motions of humeral flexion and abduction, the tendon must slide within the bicipital groove. Although the biceps produces little force during these motions, an inflammatory response or damage to the transverse humeral ligament results in pain and disrupts the normal mechanics of the GH joint.

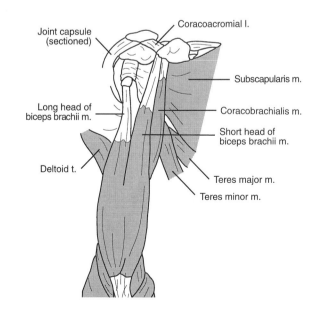

FIGURE 13–17. Coracobrachialis and attachment of the long and short heads of the biceps brachii muscle.

Table 13–3
MUSCLES ACTING ON THE HUMERUS

Muscle	Action	Origin	Insertion	Innervation	Root
Biceps brachii	Flexion Abduction	Long head: Supraglenoid tuberosity of scapula Short head: Coracoid process of scapula	Radial tuberosity and aponeurosis	Musculocutaneous	C5, C6
Coracobrachialis	Flexion Adduction	Coracoid process	Medial shaft of the humerus, adjacent to the deltoid tuberosity	Musculocutaneous	C6, C7
Deltoid (anterior one third)	Flexion Abduction Horizontal adduction Internal rotation	Lateral one third of the clavicle	Deltoid tuberosity	Axillary	C5, C6
Deltoid (middle one third)	Abduction Flexion	Acromion process	Deltoid tuberosity	Axillary	C5, C6
Deltoid (posterior one third)	Extension Horizontal abduction Abduction External rotation	Spine of the scapula	Deltoid tuberosity	Axillary	C5, C6
Infraspinatus	External rotation Horizontal abduction Humeral head stabilization	Infraspinous fossa of the scapula	• Lateral portion of the greater tuberosity of the humerus • GH joint capsule	Suprascapular	C5, C6
Latissimus dorsi	Extension Internal rotation Adduction	• Spinous processes of T6 through T12 and the lumbar vertebrae via the lumbodorsal fascia. • Posterior iliac crest	Floor of the bicipital groove of the humerus	Thoracodorsal	C6, C7, C8

Muscle	Action	Origin	Insertion	Nerve	Roots
Pectoralis major	Adduction Horizontal adduction Flexion (clavicular segment) Internal rotation	• Medial one-half of the clavicle • Anterolateral portion of the sternum • Costalcartilages of ribs 6 through 7	Greater tuberosity of the humerus	Lateral and medial pectoral	C6, C7, C8, T1
Subscapularis	Internal rotation Humeral head stabilization	Anterior surface (subscapular fossa) and axillary border of the scapula	• Lesser tuberosity of the humerus • Ventral portion of the GH capsule	Upper and lower subscapular	C5, C6, C7
Supraspinatus	Abduction External rotation Humeral head stabilization	Supraspinous fossa (medial two thirds) of the scapula	• Medial aspect of the greater tuberosity • GH joint capsule	Suprascapular	C4, C5, C6
Teres major	Extension Internal rotation Adduction	Inferior angle of scapula Lower one third of the axillary border of the scapula	Medial lip of the bicipital groove	Lower subscapular	C5, C6, C7
Teres minor	External rotation Horizontal abduction	Lateral upper two thirds of axillary border of the scapula	Lateral aspect of the greater tuberosity	Axillary	C5, C6
Triceps brachii	Extension (long head) Adduction	Long head: Infraglenoid tuberosity of scapula Lateral head: Lateral and posterior surface of the proximal 1/2 of the humerus Medial head: Distal 2/3 of medial and posterior humerus	Olecranon process of ulna	Radial	C6, C7, C8, T1

GH = glenohumeral.

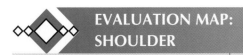

EVALUATION MAP: SHOULDER

1. HISTORY

Location of the pain
Onset
Activity
Injury mechanism
Symptoms
Prior injury

2. INSPECTION

General
The position of the head
The position of the arm

Anterior Structures
Level of the shoulders
Contour of the clavicles
Symmetry of the deltoid muscle
    groups
Anterior humerus
Biceps brachii

Lateral Structures
Deltoid muscle group
Acromion process
    Step deformity
Position of the humerus

Posterior Structures
Alignment of the spinal vertebrae
Position of the scapula
Muscle tone
Position of the humerus

3. PALPATION

Anterior Structures
Jugular notch
SC ligament
Clavicular shaft
Acromion process
    Piano key sign
Coracoid process
Pectoralis major
Pectoralis minor
Deltoid muscle group

Humerus
Humeral head
Greater/lesser tuberosities
Bicipital groove
Humeral shaft
Coracobrachialis
Biceps brachii
    Long head tendon
    Short head tendon

Scapula
Spine of the scapula
Superior angle
Inferior angle
Rotator cuff
Teres major
Rhomboids
Levator scapulae
Trapezius
Latissimus dorsi
Triceps brachii

4. RANGE OF MOTION TESTS

Active Range of Motion
Flexion
Extension
    Gerber lift-off test
Abduction
Adduction
Internal rotation
External rotation
Horizontal adduction
Horizontal abduction

Passive Range of Motion
Flexion
Extension
Abduction
Adduction
Internal rotation
External rotation
Horizontal adduction
Horizontal abduction

Resisted Range of Motion
Flexion
Extension
Abduction
Adduction
Internal rotation
External rotation
Horizontal adduction
Horizontal abduction

Scapular Movements
Elevation
Depression
Retraction
Protraction
Rotation

5. LIGAMENTOUS TESTS

SC glide
AC glide
GH joint
    Apprehension test
    GH glide

6. NEUROLOGIC TESTS

Brachial plexus
Cervical nerve root

Thoracic outlet syndrome
Adson's test
Allen test
Military brace position

7. SPECIAL TESTS

Acromioclavicular joint sprain
AC traction test
AC compression test

Glenohumeral pathology
Relocation test
Posterior apprehension test
Posterior apprehension test in the
    plane of the scapula
Sulcus sign
Active compression test

Rotator cuff pathology
Drop arm test
Neer impingement test
Hawkins shoulder impingement test
Empty can test

Biceps tendon pathology
Yergason's test
Speed's test
Ludington's test

AC = acromioclavicular; GH = glenohumeral; SC = sternoclavicular.

SCAPULOTHORACIC RHYTHM

For the hand to obtain its maximal arc of motion, the GH and scapulothoracic articulation must combine their ROMs. If the humeral head were rigidly fixated in the glenoid fossa in a manner eliminating GH movement, the humerus could still be elevated to 60 degrees through upward rotation of the scapula. For the humerus to be elevated to its maximum ROM of 180 degrees, the GH and scapulothoracic articulation must function together. An approximate two-to-one ratio is found between GH elevation and upward scapular rotation. For 180 degrees of humeral elevation to occur, 120 degrees is from GH movement and 60 degrees is through upward rotation of the scapula.

This ratio is not smooth or consistent. Early in the ROM, elevation occurs primarily at the GH joint, with the scapula fixating to provide stability for the contracting muscles. During the intermediate stages of humeral elevation, the ratio between the GH joint and the scapula is approximately one to one.[8] At the extremes of these movements, these motions again occur primarily at the GH joint. Maintenance of this rhythm is based on the coordination of the prime movers of the humerus and the synergistic contractions of the scapular stabilizers.

BURSA OF THE SHOULDER COMPLEX

Although commonly fused into a single unit commonly referred to as the subacromial bursa, two bursae are actually located at the GH joint: the **subacromial bursa** and the **subdeltoid bursa.** The subacromial bursa is located above the superior surface of the supraspinatus tendon and serves to lubricate the movement of the overlying fibers of the deltoid muscle, acting as a secondary joint cavity.[9] When the humerus is elevated, the bursa buffers the supraspinatus tendon against its contact with the acromion process and the coracoacromial ligament. When the bursa becomes inflamed, the structures within the subacromial space become compressed, potentially leading to rotator cuff impingement.

 ## CLINICAL EVALUATION OF SHOULDER INJURIES

Because of the interrelationship of the shoulder complex to the cervical and thoracic spine, torso, abdomen, and elbow, clinicians must be prepared to undertake thorough evaluations of these areas. Chapter 11 discusses pain that may be referred from the cervical spine, and Chapter 12 describes visceral pain that is referred into the shoulder and upper arm.

HISTORY

During the history-taking phase of the examination, the onset and duration of the condition must be ascertained and the location of the pain identified. Because the shoulder and upper arm are common sites for referred pain from orthopedic or visceral origins, a complete examination of the cervical spine, thorax, and abdomen may be indicated, particularly when a patient presents with a vague history of injury to the shoulder complex (see Fig. 12–15).

The following information should be obtained during the history-taking process so that the mechanism of injury, prior injuries, structures involved in the injury, and nature of the pain can be determined:

- **Location of the pain:** The examination begins by localizing the area of pain, the type of pain, and any dysfunction reported by the patient. Shoulder pathology typically produces pain within the GH joint that may project laterally into the upper arm or medially into the trapezius. Pain that begins in the trapezius and radiates into the upper arm, forearm, or hand implicates cervical nerve root involvement.

- **Onset:** The onset of pain often indicates the underlying pathology. Pain with an acute onset may indicate a fracture, GH joint dislocation and subluxation, or an AC sprain. Inflammatory conditions of the shoulder complex, such as tendinitis, bursitis, or osteoarthritis, usually have an insidious onset. In these cases, pain may first be noticed after activity. This then progresses to pain during activity and, eventually, constant pain.

- **Activity and injury mechanism:** An external force applied to the shoulder complex, such as a direct blow or joint force beyond normal limits, results in acute soft tissue or bony injury. A history of repetitive overhead motion activities such as throwing, swimming, or tennis may indicate an overuse injury such as rotator cuff inflammation.

- **Symptoms:** The symptoms to be noted include resting pain, pain with movement, and dysfunction of the shoulder complex. The patient may describe the shoulder as "going out of place," indicating GH instability; decreased velocity or poor accuracy when throwing; or discomfort when performing overhand motions, indicating inflammatory conditions. Question the patient about radiating pain and numbness possibly indicating nerve pathology. Box 13–1 presents the phases of the pitching motion and relates the structures involved with each.

- **Prior injury:** A history of previous injury to the AC or GH joints can alter the biomechanics of the shoulder complex. Because cervical spine pathology can result in referred pain to the upper extremity, the previous injury history of the cervical spine must be ascertained. If a history of injury to the cervical spine or thorax has been described, the cervical spine and peripheral nerves are further evaluated so that the possible relationship to the existing condition can be determined.

Box 13–1
PHASES OF THE PITCHING MOTION

	Wind-up	Cocking	Acceleration	Deceleration	Follow Through
Glenohumeral Joint Position	Neutral	90° abduction Maximum external rotation	90° abduction Moving to internal rotation	90° abduction Internal rotation	Horizontal abduction Internal rotation Decreasing abduction
Glenohumeral Joint Stresses	Low joint stresses	Anterior joint capsule Inferior joint capsule	Anterior joint capsule	Posterior joint capsule Distraction of GH joint	Posterior joint capsule Distraction of GH joint
Elbow Position	Some degrees of flexion	Approximately 90° flexion Increased valgus forces on the elbow	90° flexion moving into extension	20° to 30° flexion moving into extension	Extension
Concentric Muscle Contraction	Muscular forces mostly generated by the lower extremity	External rotators	Internal rotators Serratus anterior Upper trapezius Trunk and lower extremity	Internal rotators Triceps brachii	Internal rotators
Eccentric Muscle Contraction		Internal rotators	External rotators Rhomboids Middle and lower trapezius	External rotators Biceps brachii Brachialis	External rotators
Center of Gravity	Elevated over pivot foot	Over pivot foot	Between pivot foot and plant foot	Over plant foot	Forward of plant foot

GH = glenohumeral.

The preceding list is not all inclusive for the questions to be asked during the history-taking process. The scope of the questions expands for cases involving an insidious onset. When an acute traumatic injury is being assessed, the history-taking process should become more focused based on the mechanism of injury.

INSPECTION

The patient should wear clothing that allows full inspection of both shoulders and the cervical, thoracic, and lumbar spine.

- **Position of the head:** Observe the position of the head, which normally assumes an upright position. A head that is side bent or rotated may indicate muscle spasm, pressure on a cervical nerve root, or stretching of the cervical nerves. Conditions relating to the cervical spine and its nerve network are discussed in Chapter 11.
- **Position of the arm and willingness to move the involved limb:** Note whether the arm is splinted alongside the body or if it simply hangs limp at the side. Traumatic shoulder injuries are often voluntarily splinted with the humerus along the lateral portion of the rib cage and the forearm supported across the chest. Brachial plexus injuries are characterized by the arm's hanging limply at the side (see Chapter 11). With GH dislocations, the humerus is locked into a fixed position (e.g., anterior dislocations result in the humerus' being abducted and externally rotated).

  Does the patient gesture with the involved arm or duplicate the motion or position causing pain? Observe his or her willingness to move the involved limb throughout the examination. For instance, does the patient raise the involved arm when removing his or her shirt or jacket or does the arm remain at the side with the clothing dropped down over it? Unwillingness to move the arm may indicate apprehension or an increased severity of the condition.

Inspection of the Anterior Structures

- **Level of the shoulders:** Observe the height of the AC joints, the clavicle, and the SC joints. These should align bilaterally, but the dominant shoulder may appear slightly lower than the nondominant one (Fig. 13–18).

  A painful shoulder is often held in an elevated position.[10] Unilateral elevation may also indicate upper trapezius hypertrophy on the raised side or atrophy on the depressed side. Another cause is the presence of scoliosis (see the "Inspection of the Posterior Structures" section). Bilaterally raised shoulders may result from well-developed upper trapezius muscles or unwanted spasm in these muscle groups. Shoulders that are abnormally depressed bilaterally may occur as a result of decreased upper trapezius muscle tone. Bilaterally or unilaterally depressed shoulder complexes can place pressure on the arterial, venous, and nervous supply of the arm, predisposing the patient to **thoracic outlet syndrome** (see the "Pathologies and Related Special Tests" section of this chapter). Rounded shoulders can indicate tightness of the pectoralis major and minor muscles.
- **Contour of the clavicles:** Inspect the clavicle, easily visible in thin patients or those with well-defined upper body musculature. Observe the SC joint, the shaft of the clavicle, and the clavicle's termination at the AC joint for symmetry and compare them bilaterally.

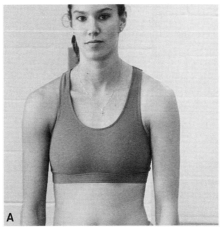
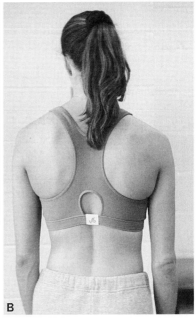

FIGURE 13–18. (A) Anterior and **(B)** posterior view of the shoulders. Note that the shoulder of the dominant right arm hangs lower than the shoulder of the nondominant arm.

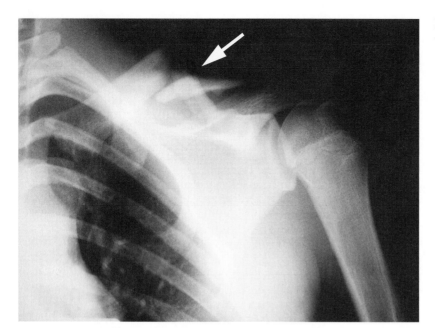

FIGURE 13–19. Radiograph of a fractured clavicle.

Acute traumatic conditions involving the clavicle are typically identifiable during the inspection process. SC or AC joint sprains may be marked by a gross deformity at the articulation, with one side having a more predominant protrusion than the other side. Any previous history involving these joints must be established because deformity may be residual from past trauma.

Complete clavicular fractures are indicated by a clear deformity of the shaft (Fig. 13–19). Although these fractures usually occur at the juncture between the concave and convex bends (the distal third of the shaft), they can occur anywhere along the clavicle. Patients suffering from a fractured clavicle tend to support the involved arm next to the body and rotate the head to the opposite side. If a fractured clavicle is suspected, terminate the evaluation, immobilize the arm with a sling, and refer the patient to a physician.

- **Symmetry of the deltoid muscle groups:** Note the bilateral symmetry of the deltoid muscle tone. Normally, this muscle group has a rounded contour. The deltoid of the dominant arm may be hypertrophied compared with the deltoid of the nondominant side. Atrophy of this muscle group may indicate a lack of use of the involved arm or may reflect pathology to the C5 and C6 nerve roots (axillary nerve involvement).

A dislocated GH joint disrupts the contour of the deltoid group by flattening the area passing over the head of the humerus (Fig. 13–20). In some instances, the humeral head may protrude anteriorly; distal pulses should always be checked. The absence of a distal pulse indicates potentially catastrophic impingement of the neurovascular bundle supplying the arm, wrist, and hand and requires immediate referral for further medical attention.

- **Anterior humerus and biceps brachii muscle group:** Note the shape and contour of the biceps brachii and any unilateral bulges within the muscle. A tendon rupture is characterized by the muscle's shortening

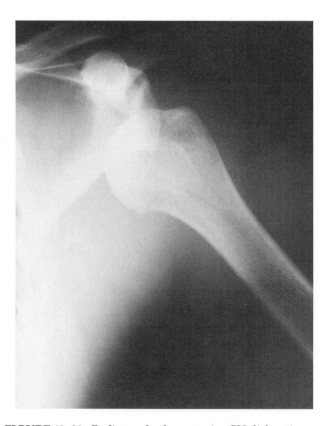

FIGURE 13–20. Radiograph of an anterior GH dislocation.

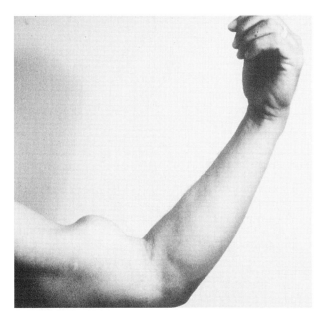

FIGURE 13–21. Rupture of the long head of the biceps brachii tendon.

away from the involved structure (Fig. 13–21). A careful inspection of the entire muscle is necessary because the distal tendon can rupture from its insertion at the elbow, causing a unilateral deformity.

Inspection of the Lateral Structures

- **Deltoid muscle group:** This portion of the inspection process is a continuation of the observation of the anterior portion of the deltoid. The contour of this

group is noted and compared with the contralateral side, giving special attention to the roundness of the muscle as it passes over the humeral head.

- **Acromion process:** The junction between the clavicle and the acromion process usually appears smooth and even. Note for the presence of a **step deformity.** This condition involves the clavicle's riding above the acromion process, indicating an AC sprain (Fig. 13–22). This finding is confirmed during the palpation phase **(piano key sign)** and during the special tests portion **(AC traction test).**
- **Position of the humerus:** Normally, the humerus hangs in the anatomical position. Adhesions within the GH joint, muscle spasm, or pain associated with bursitis and tendinitis may cause the patient to splint the humerus to guard against motion.

Inspection of the Posterior Structures

- **Alignment of the vertebral column:** Inspect the alignment of the cervical, thoracic, and lumbar spine to evaluate for scoliosis. This malady can cause altered biomechanics of the shoulder complex.
- **Position of the scapulae:** Observe the vertebral borders of both scapulae, which usually rest an equal distance from the spinous processes of the thoracic vertebrae. The superior angle normally sits at the level of the T2 spinous process and the inferior angle at the T7 spinous process. The most medial aspect of the scapular spine is located at the level of the third thoracic vertebra. In the anatomical position, the scapula is in full contact with the thorax. Note the presence of the inferior angle lifting away from the thorax (winging scapula). Also observe for any unilateral scapular protraction, retraction, or tilting.

FIGURE 13–22. Radiograph of a third-degree AC sprain. The superior displacement of the clavicle's distal aspect creates a characteristic "step deformity."

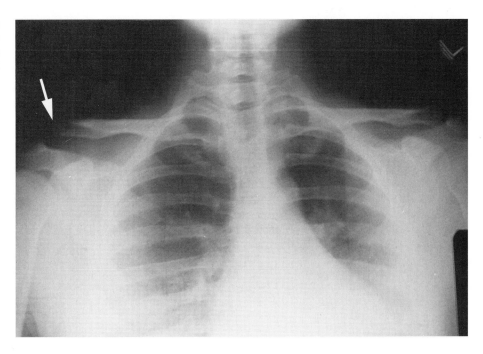

Sprengel's deformity, a congenitally undescended scapula, may occur on one scapula or both. A high-riding scapula may indicate poorly developed or malformed scapular elevators. The clinical ramifications of this condition vary from little or no dysfunction to extreme disability. Clinicians may expect to find a decreased ROM in the involved extremity in athletes.

- **Muscle tone:** Inspect the posterior musculature for symmetry on each side. The superficial muscles of well-developed individuals are usually easily identifiable, as are the prominent bony landmarks. Any spasm, deformity, or discoloration of the musculature or skin should be noted as well.

  Observe the prominence of the scapular spine. Atrophy of the supraspinatus or infraspinatus muscles leads the spine of the scapula to become more visible and palpable. Chronic rotator cuff tears are classically marked by the wasting of the infraspinatus muscle.[10] The scapular stabilizers should also be observed for tone and symmetry.

- **Position of the humerus:** Check patients with acute shoulder injuries for possible posterior GH dislocation, although it is rare. The head of the humerus, when posteriorly dislocated, usually rests on the infraspinous fossa. This injury is associated with possible bony and articular surface injury and neurovascular damage. This condition may be masked by patients with well-developed shoulder muscles.

PALPATION

To rule out fractures, dislocations, and gross joint injury, the bony structures are palpated prior to the soft tissue structures. If palpation reveals any gross deformity, the examination should be terminated, the shoulder immobilized, and the patient referred to a physician for a definitive diagnosis.

Palpation of Anterior Shoulder

1. **Jugular notch:** Begin the palpation process by locating the jugular notch on the manubrium. Palpate the common junction provided by the interclavicular ligament between the SC joints.
2. **Sternoclavicular joint:** Proceed laterally to identify the SC joint, checking for point tenderness over the articulation. Dislocations of the SC joint tend to displace the clavicular head medial and superior to the clavicular notch. **Posterior SC dislocations are a medical emergency** because posterior displacement of the clavicle may jeopardize the integrity of the neurovascular structures directly posterior to the joint or may place pressure on the trachea, lung, or both.
3. **Clavicular shaft:** From the SC joint, continue to palpate laterally along the shaft of the clavicle, noting any crepitus or pain. The superior surface is easily palpable because of the absence of muscle attachments. Prior clavicular fractures may be marked by

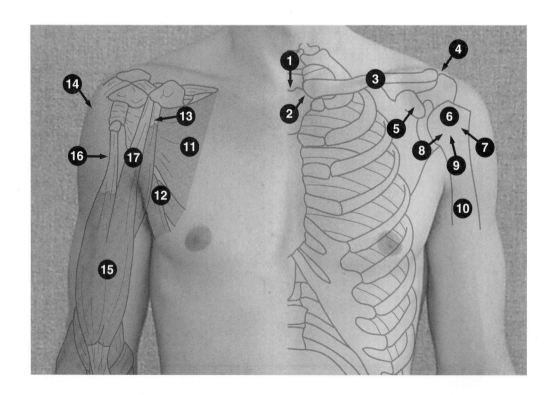

palpable bony callus formation over the healed fracture site.

4. **Acromion process and AC joint:** As the clavicle extends laterally, expect that it may become less palpable in patients who have well-developed pectoralis major and deltoid musculature. The acromion process may be more easily located by palpating to the lateral end of the scapular spine.

   If a step deformity is observed during the observation phase of the examination, note for bobbing of the clavicle when downward pressure is applied. Known as the **piano key sign,** this test checks the integrity of the coracoclavicular ligaments.

5. **Coracoid process:** From the acromion process, move two fingers' breadths medially. From this point, move approximately 1 inch below the clavicle, applying gentle pressure laterally. Feel for the coracoid process just above and behind the tendon of the pectoralis major. To confirm that the coracoid process has been located, passively move the GH joint through 15 to 30 degrees of flexion and extension and abduction and adduction. No movement of the coracoid process should be felt within this ROM. If movement is felt beneath the fingers, the humeral head is most probably being palpated. In this case, move the fingers medially and attempt this procedure again.

   The coracoid process serves as the point of insertion for the pectoralis minor and is the origin of the short head of the biceps brachii tendon and the coracobrachialis muscle. In addition, it provides a source of attachment for several ligaments. Apply pressure carefully when palpating this area because it is easily irritated.

6. **Humeral head:** Moving laterally from the acromion process, palpate the anteromedial portion of the humeral head in the axilla posterior to the tendon of pectoralis major. The relationship of the humeral head to the glenoid fossa must be determined. Direct palpation of the humeral head may not be possible in patients with well-developed shoulder musculature. However, an anteriorly or inferiorly displaced humeral head is easily palpable.

7. **Greater tuberosity:** Locate the greater tuberosity in the anatomical position approximately one finger's breadth below the lateral edge of the anterior portion of the acromion process. This structure is more easily palpated by passively extending the humerus, causing the greater tuberosity to move from beneath the acromion process.

8. **Lesser tuberosity:** With the humerus externally rotated to ease palpation, locate the medial border of the bicipital groove formed by the lesser tuberosity.

9. **Bicipital groove:** Externally rotate the humerus to make the bicipital groove more palpable. The groove is felt as an indentation in the bone just medial to the greater tuberosity. Gently palpate this area along its length to elicit any tenderness caused by bicipital tendinitis or damage to the transverse humeral ligament. Note that this area is typically tender and should be compared with the opposite side to determine a relative difference in pain.

10. **Humeral shaft:** Palpate the shaft of the humerus, more easily palpated along its medial and lateral borders under the belly of the biceps brachii and brachioradialis muscles.

11. **Pectoralis major:** Locate the pectoralis major on the anterior thoracic cavity. Palpate this muscle as it flares into its tendon, noting the integrity and any point tenderness as it crosses the GH capsule and attaches on the greater tuberosity of the humerus.

12. **Pectoralis minor:** Attempt to palpate the tendon insertion on the coracoid process of the pectoralis minor. Located beneath the pectoralis major, the bulk of the pectoralis minor is not palpable.

13. **Coracobrachialis:** Locate the coracobrachialis muscle as it originates off the coracoid process. It may be palpable at this point. Its body and insertion lie deep in the superficial musculature of the humerus and are therefore difficult to palpate.

14. **Deltoid group:** Palpate each of the three portions of the deltoid from its unique origin to the common insertion on the humerus.

15–17. **Biceps brachii:** From the belly of the biceps brachii, palpate each of the two heads. Feel for the long head of the biceps (16) as it travels through its passage in the bicipital groove under the transverse humeral ligament until it passes beneath the anterior deltoid. Palpate the biceps' short head (17) along its length as it passes beneath the pectoralis major tendon and attaches on the coracoid process.

Palpation of Posterior Shoulder

1. **Spine of the scapula:** Locate the spine of the scapula by finding the acromion process. Palpate posteriorly along the bony surface of the acromion to meet with the scapular spine. Continue palpation medially along the length of the spine to its termination along the scapula's vertebral border.

2. **Superior angle:** From the vertebral border, palpate upward to find the superior angle of the scapula. This landmark may be obstructed by muscle mass of the upper portion of the trapezius and levator scapulae.

3. **Inferior angle:** Moving inferiorly along the vertebral border, feel for the apex of the inferior angle of the scapula. Ask the patient to touch the inferior angle of the opposite scapula from below, causing the scapula undergoing examination to wing and making the inferior angle and the lower portions of the vertebral and axial borders more easily palpable.

4–6. **Rotator cuff:** Palpate the mass of three of the four rotator cuff muscles on the scapula. Palpate the infraspinatus (4), teres minor (5), and supraspinatus (6) along their lengths until they disappear beneath the mass of the deltoid. By passively extending the GH joint from the anatomical position, the greater

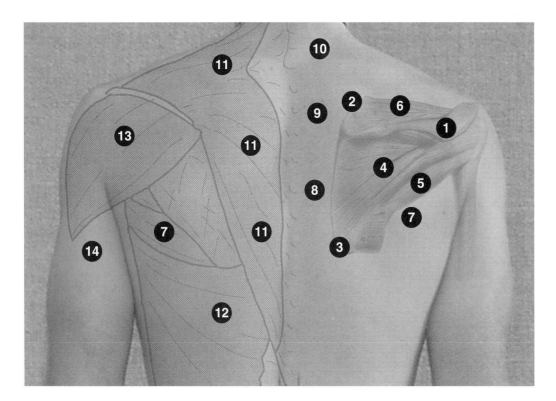

tuberosity becomes prominent, allowing for the palpation of these muscles' insertions on the humerus. Although the individual tendons are not distinguishable from each other, any pain or tenderness elicited during palpation should be noted because it may indicate rotator cuff pathology. The origin, mass, and tendinous insertion of the subscapularis muscle are not directly palpable.

7. **Teres major:** Locate the origin and body of the teres major muscle immediately inferior to the teres minor. The insertion of this muscle cannot be directly palpated. This muscle is a common site for trigger points in swimmers and in athletes who participate in sports with overhead movements. Note any hypersensitive areas.

8–9. **Rhomboid:** The rhomboid major (8) and rhomboid minor (9) cannot be directly palpated and are indistinguishable from each other except for their relative locations.

10. **Levator scapulae:** Although largely covered by the upper portion of the trapezius muscle, palpate the origin of the levator scapulae on the transverse processes of the first through the fourth cervical vertebrae to its insertion on the medial border of the scapula, just inferior to the superior angle.

11. **Trapezius:** Palpate the trapezius muscle relative to its upper, middle, and lower portions. This muscle is the most superficial of the muscles acting on the scapula and therefore overlies the levator scapulae and the rhomboid muscle group.

12. **Latissimus dorsi:** Locate the latissimus dorsi tendon inferior to the teres major. Follow this tendon through the axilla to its attachment on the floor of the bicipital groove.

13. **Posterior deltoid:** Palpate the posterior portion of the deltoid muscle group noting for atrophy, spasm, or localized areas of pain.

14. **Triceps brachii:** Palpate the long head of the triceps brachii tendon superiorly until the insertion disappears under the posterior deltoid.

RANGE OF MOTION TESTING

The motion occurring at the GH, AC, and SC joints, as well as the motion of the scapula, is evaluated during functional testing, keeping in mind the interrelationship among these articulations. A deficit at one joint affects the motion of the others. These functional tests must not be performed when severe traumatic injuries such as fractures, joint dislocation, or complete muscle tears are suspected.

The amount of motion that the GH joint is capable of producing depends on the position of the greater and the lesser tuberosities relative to the scapula's bony structures. To achieve complete abduction, the humerus must be externally rotated to allow the greater tuberosity to clear under the acromion process. The motion of flexion does not depend on relative internal or external rotation of the humerus because the greater tuberosity depresses inferiorly and passes beneath the acromion process.[11] Goniometric evaluation of shoulder ROM is presented in Box 13–2.

Box 13–2
SHOULDER GONIOMETRY

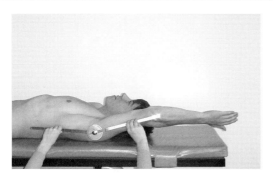

Flexion

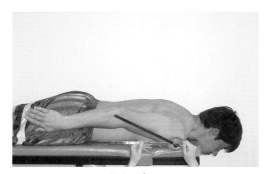

Extension

PATIENT POSITION	Supine	Prone
GONIOMETER PLACEMENT		
FULCRUM	Aligned lateral to the acromion process	Aligned lateral to the acromion process
STATIONARY ARM	Aligned parallel to the table top	Aligned parallel to the table top
MOVEMENT ARM	Centered over the midline of the lateral humerus	Centered over the midline of the lateral humerus

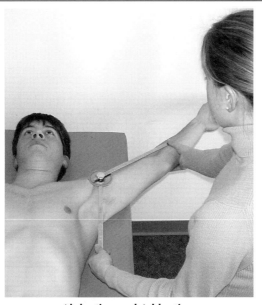

Abduction and Adduction

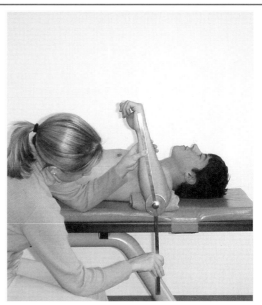

Internal and External Rotation

PATIENT POSITION	Supine or sitting	Supine with the elbow flexed to 90°
GONIOMETER PLACEMENT		
FULCRUM	Anterior to the acromion process	Centered lateral to the olecranon process
STATIONARY ARM	Parallel to the long axis of the torso	Perpendicular to the floor or parallel to the tabletop
MOVEMENT ARM	Centered over the midline of the anterior humerus	Centered over the long axis of the ulna

Table 13–4
MUSCLES CONTRIBUTING TO SCAPULAR MOVEMENTS

Elevation	Protraction	Upward Rotation
Levator scapulae Rhomboid major Rhomboid minor Serratus anterior (upper portion) Trapezius (upper portion)	Serratus anterior	Serratus anterior Trapezius (upper and lower portion)
Depression	**Retraction**	**Downward Rotation**
Serratus anterior (lower portion) Trapezius (lower portion) Pectoralis major (clavicular portion)	Rhomboid major Rhomboid minor Trapezius (middle fibers) Trapezius (lower fibers)	Rhomboid major Rhomboid minor Levator scapulae

In healthy individuals, strength is equal in both extremities.[12] This strength relationship may vary among athletes involved in throwing and racquet sports. The dominant shoulder of collegiate tennis players produce a significantly greater amount of torque and power during internal rotation than the nondominant shoulder does.[13] Professional baseball pitchers do not display a significant difference in the amount of peak torque produced during internal rotation when compared bilaterally, but a significant difference does arise at high speeds (greater than or equal to 300° per second) during external rotation, with the dominant arm producing more torque.[14] The strength ratio of internal to external rotators is 3:2 for concentric contractions and 3:4 for eccentric contractions.[15]

Active Range of Motion

The muscles contributing to the scapula are presented in Table 13–5 and those contributing to the humerus in Table 13–5. An evaluation of the aggregate motion available to the shoulder complex can be quickly determined through the Apley's scratch test (Box 13–3). Each of the three components of this test should be compared bilaterally to determine a decrease in the ROM, pain, and the willingness to move.

• **Flexion and extension:** The shoulder complex is capable of producing 220 to 240 degrees of movement in the sagittal plane (Fig. 13–23). The majority of this ROM, accounting for 170 to 180 degrees of motion from the anatomical position, is provided by flexion. The remaining 50 to 60 degrees occur from the limb's moving from the anatomical position to extension.

• **Abduction and adduction:** Occurring in the frontal plane, the normal ROM for abduction is 170 to 180 degrees (Fig. 13–24). The motion of adduction is blocked in the anatomical position and any further movement requires that the GH joint be flexed or extended so that the humerus can pass in front of or behind the torso. The patient's ability to control adduction should be noticed. An arm that falls uncontrollably

Table 13–5
MUSCLES CONTRIBUTING TO HUMERAL MOVEMENTS

Flexion	Adduction	Horizontal Adduction	Internal Rotation
Biceps brachii Coracobrachialis Deltoid (anterior one third) Deltoid (middle one third) Pectoralis major (clavicular fibers)	Coracobrachialis Latissimus dorsi Pectoralis major Teres major Triceps brachii	Deltoid (anterior one third) Pectoralis major	Deltoid (anterior one third) Latissimus dorsi Pectoralis major Subscapularis Teres major
Extension	**Abduction**	**Horizontal Abduction**	**External rotation**
Deltoid (posterior one third) Latissimus dorsi Teres major Triceps brachii (long head)	Biceps brachii Deltoid (anterior one third) Deltoid (middle one third) Deltoid (posterior one third) Supraspinatus	Deltoid (posterior one third) Infraspinatus Teres minor	Deltoid (posterior one third) Infraspinatus Teres minor Supraspinatus

Box 13–3
APLEY'S SCRATCH TESTS

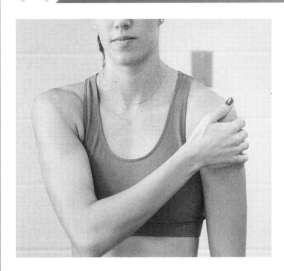

The patient touches the shoulder opposite the front
Motions produced: GH adduction, horizontal adduction, and internal rotation; scapular protraction

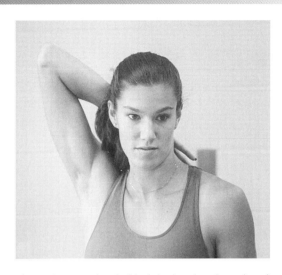

The patient reaches behind the head and touches the opposite shoulder from behind
Motions produced: GH abduction and external rotation; scapular protracton, elevation, and upward rotation

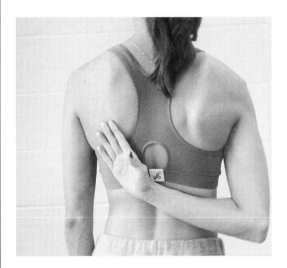

The patient reaches behind the back and touches the opposite scapula
Motions produced: GH adduction and internal rotation; scapular retraction and downward rotation

GH = glenohumeral.

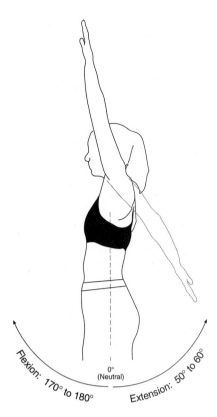

FIGURE 13–23. Range of motion for shoulder flexion and extension.

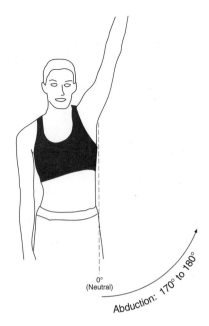

FIGURE 13–24. Range of motion for shoulder abduction and adduction.

from 90 degrees of abduction indicates a positive **drop arm test** for rotator cuff pathology (Box 13–4). The inability to control the descent of the arm may indicate a rotator cuff tear or poor eccentric control of the scapula.

The patient may describe an area within the ROM that elicits pain. This painful arc, usually occurring between 60 and 120 degrees of abduction, is often associated with impingement of the rotator cuff musculature between the humeral head and the coracoacromial arch.

● **Internal and external rotation:** Internal and external rotation is tested in both the neutral position and in 90 degrees of abduction. In the neutral position, the humeral head and the greater tuberosity are allowed to rotate beneath the acromion without interference. During internal rotation, the torso blocks the motion. External rotation in this position, usually 40 to 50 degrees, is less than when the humerus is abducted 90 degrees. This motion is limited by the superior GH and coracohumeral ligaments.

When abducted to 90 degrees so that the greater and lesser tuberosities can clear the structures of the scapula, the GH joint can obtain an increased amount of internal and external rotation (Fig. 13–25). With the humerus in 90 degrees of abduction with the elbow flexed to 90 degrees, the normal ROM in

this position is 80 to 90 degrees of external rotation and 70 to 80 degrees of internal rotation. These motions are restricted by the inferior GH ligament.

Another method of measuring internal rotation is to have the patient reach behind and up the back (Fig. 13–26). This measurement is more representative of functional motion than standard goniometry. The measurement is taken from the spinal level where the thumb rests at maximal motion. With the dominant hand, the patient should generally be capable of obtaining a spinal level that is equal to or greater than that obtainable on the nondominant side.

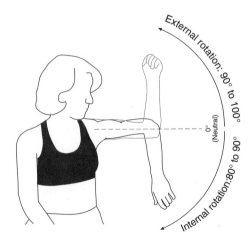

FIGURE 13–25. Range of motion for shoulder internal rotation and external rotation.

Box 13–4
DROP ARM TEST FOR ROTATOR CUFF TEARS

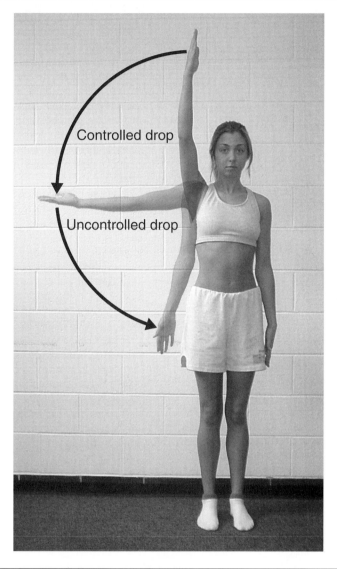

Controlled drop

Uncontrolled drop

PATIENT POSITION	Standing or sitting The humerus fully abducted and externally rotated and the forearm supinated
POSITION OF EXAMINER	Standing lateral to, or behind, the involved extremity
EVALUATIVE PROCEDURE	The patient slowly lowers the arm to the side
POSITIVE TEST	The arm falls uncontrollably from a position of approximately 90° abduction to the side
IMPLICATIONS	The inability to lower the arm in a controlled manner is indicative of lesions to the rotator cuff, especially the supraspinatus.
MODIFICATION	If the patient is able to lower the arm in a controlled manner through the ROM, a derivative of the drop arm test may be implemented: • The patient holds the humerus in 90° abduction. • The examiner applies gentle pressure on the distal forearm. • A positive test result causes the arm to fall against the side of the body, indicating lesions to the rotator cuff

ROM = range of motion.

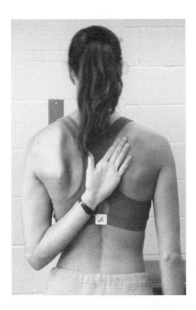

FIGURE 13–26. Method of checking for shoulder internal rotation as recommended by the American Academy of Orthopaedic Surgeons. The amount of internal GH rotation is determined by measuring the distance up the spinal column the patient can reach and comparing this result to that of the opposite shoulder.

- **Horizontal adduction and abduction:** The neutral position for horizontal adduction and abduction is 90 degrees of abduction with the arm flexed at a 30 degree angle from the torso in the plane of the scapula (see Fig. 13–5). Occurring in the horizontal plane, the expected ROM is 120 degrees of horizontal

adduction and 45 degrees of horizontal abduction relative to the plane of the scapula.

Passive Range of Motion

- **Flexion and extension:** Passive ROM (PROM) may be isolated to the GH joint or may encompass the entire motion allowed by the shoulder complex. To isolate the GH joint, the scapula must be stabilized to prevent its contribution to shoulder motion. When the entire motion provided by the shoulder complex is evaluated, the thorax must be stabilized. Each of these two methods of stabilization is more easily accomplished with the patient sitting or lying supine during flexion and prone during extension (Fig. 13–27).

Flexion should have a firm end-feel for both GH and shoulder complex motions. During GH flexion, the terminal motion is checked by the tightening of the GH capsule (especially the coracohumeral ligament and the posterior capsular fibers) and the teres minor, teres major, and infraspinatus muscles. The muscles attaching to the anterior portion of the humerus, especially the pectoralis major and the latissimus dorsi, normally terminate flexion accomplished by the entire shoulder complex.

The two types of passive extension result in a firm end-feel. During isolated GH extension, the coracohumeral ligament and the anterior joint capsule become taut. During extension of the shoulder complex, the pectoralis major (clavicular fibers) and serratus anterior muscles contribute to the end-feel.

Pain occurring at the end range of passive flexion may indicate impingement of the supraspinatus ten-

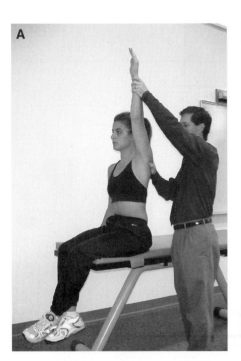

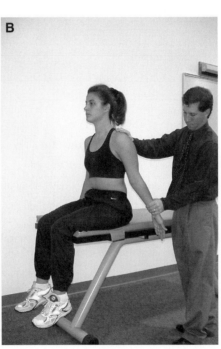

FIGURE 13–27. Passive range of motion testing for **(A)** shoulder flexion and **(B)** shoulder extension.

FIGURE 13–28. Passive range of motion testing for shoulder abduction **(A)** and adduction **(B).**

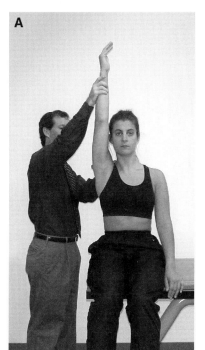

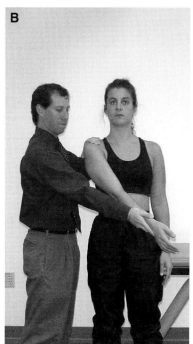

don, long head of the biceps brachii, or the subacromial bursa between the inferior portion of the acromion process and the humeral head. Pain during passive extension may result from damage to the anterior portion of the GH capsule or the coracohumeral ligament.

- **Abduction and adduction:** As in the case of flexion and extension, abduction is the result of motion's arising from the shoulder complex or isolated to its pure GH movement. When attempting to isolate GH abduction, the scapula is stabilized to prevent its upward rotation and elevation. To restrict motion to the shoulder complex, the thorax is stabilized to eliminate lateral bending of the spine. Passive abduction may be examined with the patient sitting or supine (Fig. 13–28).

The normal ROM resulting from purely GH movement has a firm end-feel because of the stress placed on the inferior GH ligament, the inferior capsule, and the pectoralis major and latissimus dorsi muscles. During abduction arising from the entire shoulder complex, the rhomboids and the middle and lower fibers of the trapezius muscle contribute to the end-feel.

Passive ROM measurements and end-feels are not normally taken for adduction because of the humerus striking the body. However, hyperadduction may be measured by moving the arm in front of the torso. Note for the presence of a painful arc, indicating rotator cuff impingement, when passively moving the arm from abduction to adduction. Pain experienced during both passive abduction and pas-

sive adduction may indicate inflammation of the subacromial structures.

- **Internal and external rotation:** PROM for rotation of the humerus is measured with the GH joint abducted to 90 degrees and the elbow flexed to 90 degrees. These motions can be tested with the patient in the seated or supine positions. To isolate rotation at the GH joint, the scapula is stabilized to prevent elevation, depression, and tilting. When measuring motion produced by the shoulder complex, the thorax is stabilized to prevent flexion or extension of the spine (Fig. 13–29).

The firm end-feel associated with normal internal rotation is caused by tightening of the posterior fibers of the GH capsule and the infraspinatus and teres minor muscles. During internal rotation with the scapula unstabilized, the rhomboid muscle group and the middle and lower fibers of the trapezius contribute to the end-feel.

During external rotation, the GH ligaments, the coracohumeral ligament, and the joint capsule wind tight, resulting in a firm end-feel for both isolated GH movements and the shoulder complex as a whole. Muscular contributions lending to the end-feel for GH motion include the subscapularis, pectoralis major, latissimus dorsi, and the teres major muscles.

Athletes who throw overhand, such as baseball players, javelin throwers, tennis players, and quarterbacks, often have an increased range of external rotation and decreased internal rotation. However, the combined amount of internal and external rotation is usually equal bilaterally.

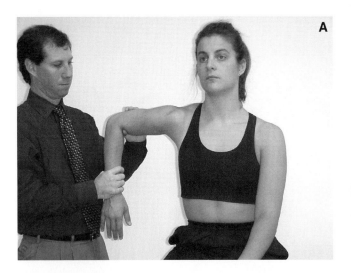

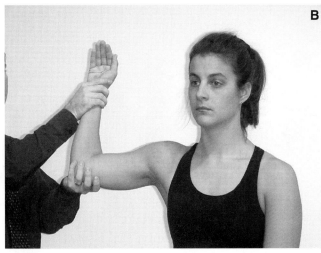

FIGURE 13–29. Passive range of motion testing for shoulder internal rotation **(A)** and external rotation **(B).**

Examination of passive external rotation must be delayed until the end of the assessment procedure when a GH dislocation, subluxation, or chronic instability is suspected. In such instances, the examination proceeds with great care. Passive external rotation of the GH joint is the same procedure as the **apprehension test** (Box 13–5).

The GH joint is palpated during passive internal and external rotation to determine the presence of crepitus, which may indicate rotator cuff or bicipital tendinitis and subacromial bursitis, or "clicks," which may indicate a labral tear.

• **Horizontal adduction and abduction:** To isolate GH motion, the scapula must be stabilized to prevent protraction and retraction. During evaluation of the entire shoulder complex, the torso is stabilized so that spinal motion does not contribute to motion of the shoulder (Fig. 13–30).

Horizontal adduction may have a soft end-feel because of soft tissue approximation when the pectoralis major, biceps, and anterior deltoid muscles are well developed. Soft end-feel also may be found in obese individuals. If this is not the case, a firm end-feel is associated with stretching of the posterior GH capsule and tension developed by the posterior deltoid muscle.

A firm end-feel is expected during horizontal abduction because of the tightening of the anterior GH capsule and the middle and inferior GH ligaments. Some tension may also be developed by the anterior deltoid and pectoralis major. During horizontal abduction obtained through motions of the entire shoulder complex, additional tension is developed by the pectoralis major.

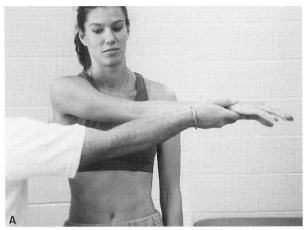

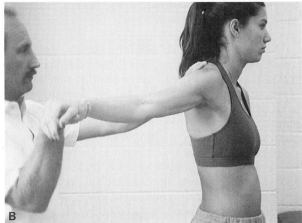

FIGURE 13–30. Passive range of motion testing for **(A)** shoulder horizontal adduction and **(B)** shoulder horizontal abduction.

Box 13–5
APPREHENSION TEST FOR ANTERIOR GLENOHUMERAL LAXITY

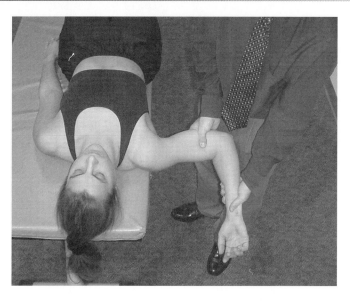

PATIENT POSITION	Supine, standing, or sitting The GH joint abducted to 90° and the elbow flexed to 90°
POSITION OF EXAMINER	Positioned in front of or beside the patient on the involved side The examiner supporting the humerus at midshaft while the forearm is grasped proximal to the wrist
EVALUATIVE PROCEDURE	While supporting the humerus at 90° abduction, the examiner passively externally rotates the GH joint by slowly applying pressure to the anterior forearm.
POSITIVE TEST	The patient displays apprehension that the shoulder may dislocate and resists further movement. Pain is centered in the anterior capsule of the GH joint.
IMPLICATIONS	The anterior capsule, inferior GH ligament, or glenoid labrum have been compromised, allowing the humeral head to dislocate or subluxate anteriorly on the glenoid fossa.
CAUTION	Pressure should be applied gradually and the test terminated at the first sign of apprehension. Do not perform this test when there is obvious dislocation or subluxation of the GH joint

GH = glenohumeral.

Resisted Range of Motion

Box 13–6 describes the resisted ROM (RROM) for the shoulder complex. The Gerber lift-off test is a sensitive method of isolating the subscapularis (Box 13–7).[16,17,18]

Scapular Movements

Observe the motion of the scapula during active humeral movements, noting any winging of the scapula and comparing the scapulothoracic rhythm on one side with that of the opposite side. A greater than normal contribution to humeral elevation is usually observed in patients suffering from GH instability, rotator cuff pathology, or impingement syndromes.[10]

Winging of the vertebral border may occur during elevation of the humerus and during the eccentric return to the neutral position.[10] Scapular winging may occur secondary to weakness of the serratus anterior muscle or inhibition of the long thoracic nerve. The most common clinical approach to determining the presence of a winging scapula is to have the patient push against the wall while observing the relative scapular alignment (Fig. 13–31). Winging of the scapula is immediately apparent when the cause is inhibition of the long thoracic nerve.

Winging caused by weakness of the serratus anterior may not become apparent until the muscle is fatigued. For this reason, the patient should perform this maneuver a minimum of 10 times.

Box 13–6

RESISTED RANGE OF MOTION FOR THE SHOULDER

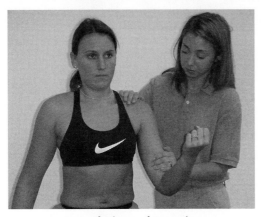

Flexion and Extension

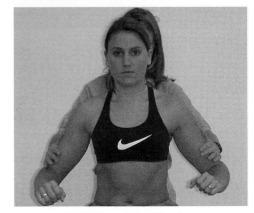

Abduction and Adduction

STARTING POSITION	Seated The humerus in the neutral position	Seated The humerus abducted to approximately 30°
STABILIZATION	Superior aspect of the shoulder	The torso, possibly although the patient's body weight may be sufficient
RESISTANCE	Distal humerus, just proximal to the elbow on the side toward the motion being tested	Distal humerus, just proximal to the elbow on the side toward the motion being tested
MUSCLES TESTED	**Flexion:** anterior deltoid, pectoralis major (clavicular portion), coracobrachialis, middle deltoid, biceps brachii **Extension:** posterior deltoid, latissimus dorsi, teres major, triceps brachii (long head)	**Abduction:** deltoid muscle group, supraspinatus, biceps brachii **Adduction:** pectoralis major, coracobrachialis, latissimus dorsi, teres major, triceps brachii

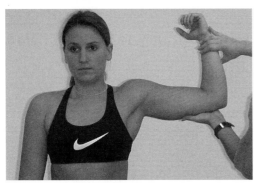

Internal and External Rotation

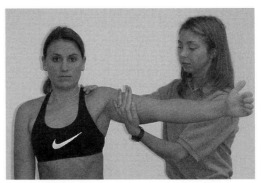

Horizontal Abduction and Adduction

STARTING POSITION	Seated The humerus in neutral position or abducted to 90° The elbow flexed to 90°	Seated or supine The elbow extended
STABILIZATION	The distal humerus is stabilized just proximal to the elbow.	Superior aspect of the shoulder (if needed)
RESISTANCE	Distal forearm on the side toward the motion being tested	Mid-humerus on the side toward the motion being tested
MUSCLES TESTED	**Internal rotation:** anterior deltoid, latissimus dorsi, pectoralis major, subscapularis, teres major **External rotation:** posterior deltoid, infraspinatus, supraspinatus, teres minor	**Horizontal abduction:** posterior deltoid, infraspinatus, teres minor **Horizontal adduction:** anterior deltoid, pectoralis major

Box 13–7

GERBER LIFT-OFF TEST FOR SUBSCAPULARIS WEAKNESS

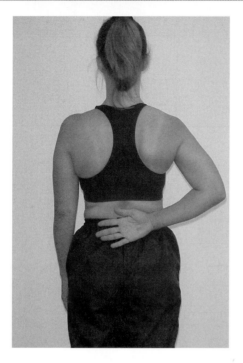
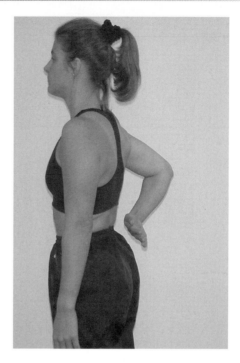

PATIENT POSITION	Standing with the humerus internally rotated The dorsal surface of the hand placed against the mid-lumbar spine
POSITION OF EXAMINER	Standing behind the patient
EVALUATIVE PROCEDURE	The patient attempts to actively lift the hand off the spine while the humerus stays in extension.
POSITIVE TEST	The inability to lift the hand off the spine
IMPLICATIONS	Positive test findings are associated with tears and weakness of the subscapularis muscle.
MODIFICATION	Resistance can be applied to the patient's palm.

FIGURE 13–31. Test for scapular winging. In the presence of a weakened serratus anterior muscle, or long thoracic nerve injury, performing a "push-up" against a wall causes the vertebral border of the scapula to lift off the thorax.

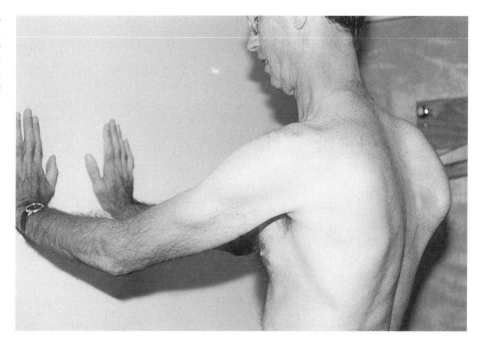

Box 13–8
MANUAL MUSCLE TESTING OF THE SCAPULAR MUSCLES

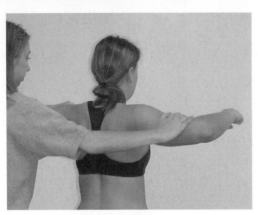

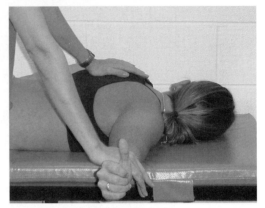

	Rhomboids	Middle Trapezius
STARTING POSITION	While in the seated position, the elbow is flexed; the humerus is adducted and slightly extended.	In the prone position, the elbow is extended and the humerus is abducted to 90° and externally rotated so that the thumb points upwards.
STABILIZATION	Not applicable	Not applicable
RESISTANCE	The examiner attempts to horizontally abduct the humerus while noting for scapular protraction indicating weakness.	A downward pressure is applied to the distal humerus.

Active ROM (AROM) and RROM shoulder elevation is used to determine the integrity of the levator scapulae and upper fibers of the trapezius (Fig. 13–32). Active protraction and retraction may also be assessed by hav-

ing the patient roll the shoulders forward and bring the shoulders back into the military "attention" position. Manual muscle testing of the scapular muscles is presented in Box 13–8.

LIGAMENTOUS AND CAPSULAR TESTING

The integrity of the ligaments and capsules of the shoulder complex are determined through joint glide. Because of the relative difficulty in manipulating the clavicle, the findings for tests for SC and AC joint instability are more subtle than the findings for the other joints in the body. Generally, the findings are positive only in the more severe cases. These tests are contraindicated when a fracture or joint dislocation is suspected.

Test for Sternoclavicular Joint Laxity

To determine the stability of the SC joint, position the patient supine and while sitting at the head of the patient, grasp the clavicle just distal to the medial clavicular head. Apply gliding pressures that force the medial clavicle downward, upward, anteriorly, and posteriorly while noting any pain or bilateral laxity that is elicited:

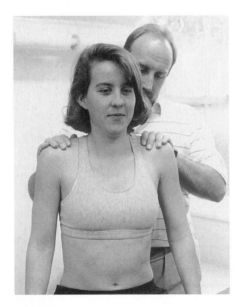

FIGURE 13–32. Resistive testing of shoulder elevation (shoulder shrug).

Clavicular Motion	Structures Involved
Inferior	Interclavicular L.
Superior	Costoclavicular L. (anterior and posterior fibers)
Anterior	SC L. (posterior fibers)
Posterior	SC L. (anterior fibers)

Pain that is evoked during all movements may result from either damage to the SC joint disk or a complete disruption of the joint capsule, indicating a possible dislocation or subluxation of the joint.

Test for Acromioclavicular Joint Laxity

With the patient supine, the AC joint is manipulated by grasping the clavicle along its distal one third and gliding the joint in the following directions, noting any pain or laxity:

Clavicular Motion	Structures Involved
Inferior	AC L. (superior fibers)
Superior	Conoid L* Trapezoid L* AC L (inferior fibers)
Anterior	AC L Coracoclavicular L (in the absence of the AC ligament)
Posterior	Clavicle contacting acromion (posterior block) Stress on the AC L

*Portions of the coracoclavicular L.

Test for Glenohumeral Joint Laxity

Assessment of true GH glide involves the sliding of the humeral head relative to the glenoid fossa. The ligaments tested during this procedure are also stressed during many of the special tests used to determine GH laxity. Laxity and instability are not synonymous. A lax shoulder can still be functionally stable. Also, an unstable shoulder may not demonstrate laxity during glide, especially when the patient is awake, not anesthetized, because of reflex muscle guarding.

The glide tests are performed in three directions (i.e., anterior, posterior, and inferior), with the humerus in the neutral (open pack) position and the scapula stabilized (Box 13–9). All motions occur relative to the plane of the scapula. Therefore, anterior glide is not tested by drawing the humerus forward relative to the sagittal plane but, rather, forward relative to the face of the glenoid fossa perpendicular to the plane of the scapula.[19] The degree of laxity is based on the amount of translation relative to the opposite limb. Any situation in which the humeral head can be displaced past the labral rim warrants further examination by a physician.

Superior glide is not tested because of the bony block formed between the humeral head and the coracoacromial arch. The Pathology and Related Special Tests section of this chapter discusses multidirectional instabilities.

GH glide tests can be modified using the **load and shift technique.** During standard GH glide testing, the humerus is distracted from the glenoid fossa. During load and shift testing, an axial load is placed upon the humerus, compressing the humeral head into the glenoid fossa, centering the joint in its anatomical position. The following scale is used during load and shift testing:[20]

Grade	Amount of humeral head translation
Trace (0)	No translation of the humeral head
Grade I	Translation of the humeral head to the glenoid rim, but not over it
Grade II	Translation of the humeral head over the glenoid rim, but without the head spontaneously reduces
Grade III	Dislocation of the humeral head without spontaneous reduction

When a three-point grading scale is used, poor intra- and inter-tester reliability occurs.[21] If the grading scale is modified to a two-point scale (the humerus does not subluxate or the humerus does subluxate), the reliability of the test greatly improves.[22]

NEUROLOGIC TESTING

Cervical nerve root trauma, brachial plexus injury, thoracic outlet syndrome, and other nerve pathologies can produce neurologic symptoms in the shoulder and upper extremity (Fig 13–33). An upper quarter neurologic screen can be used to identify the involved

FIGURE 13–33. Neuropathies of the shoulder and upper arm. Pain may also be referred to this area from the thorax (see Figure 12–15) and the brachial plexus (see Chapter 11 and Box 1–6).

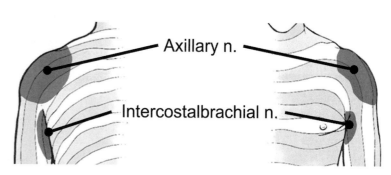

Box 13–9
GLENOHUMERAL GLIDE TESTS

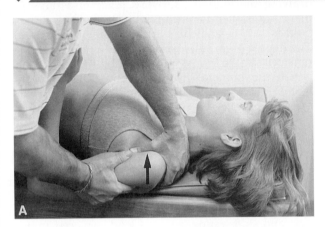

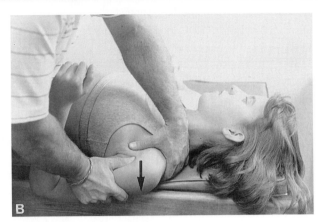

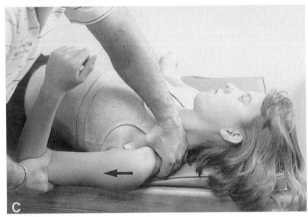

PATIENT POSITION	Lying supine with the GH joint over the edge of the table
POSITION OF EXAMINER	Standing lateral to the side being tested with one hand stabilizing the shoulder complex by grasping the scapula and the other grasping the humerus just below the surgical neck.
EVALUATIVE PROCEDURE	The examiner applies a gentle, yet firm force that moves the humeral head anteriorly relative to the glenoid fossa while applying a slight distraction to the joint to separate the humeral head from the fossa. This procedure is then repeated in the posterior and inferior direction.
POSITIVE TEST	Pain or increased motion compared with the same direction on the opposite shoulder.
IMPLICATIONS	Laxity of the static stabilizers of the GH joint: **(A) Anterior:** coracohumeral ligament, superior and middle GH ligaments, anterior joint capsule, labral tear **(B) Posterior:** posterior joint capsule, labral tear. **(C) Inferior-anterior:** inferior joint capsule, superior GH ligament, coracohumeral ligament (see the description in the "Glenohumeral Instability" section of this chapter)
MODIFICATION	In the case of large patients, a second examiner can be used to assist in stabilizing the scapula.

GH = glenohumeral.

Table 13–6
EVALUATIVE FINDINGS: Sternoclavicular Joint Injury

Examination Segment	Clinical Findings	
History	***Onset:***	Acute
	Pain Characteristics:	Limited to the SC joint area; pressure on the underlying neurovascular network can cause paresthesia in the upper extremity; pressure on the esophagus and trachea may impede swallowing and breathing
	Mechanism:	Force applied longitudinally to the clavicle, such as falling on an outstretched arm, or forceful distraction of the arm and distal shoulder complex
Inspection	Dislocations are marked by displacement of the clavicular head anteriorly, superiorly, or posteriorly. Sprains may present with localized swelling over the joint; discoloration may or may not be present. The patient's neck may be tilted toward the involved joint.	
Palpation	Obvious joint displacement is often felt. Pain may be reported over the SC joint. Crepitus is present over the articulation.	
Range of Motion	For joint sprains, pain is elicited at the extreme range of abduction, flexion, or horizontal abduction because of the rotation and elevation that occurs at the SC joint. Pain may be elicited during scapular protraction and retraction.	
Ligamentous Tests	SC glide tests. Joint play movements elicit pain for 1st-degree sprains; 2nd- and 3rd-degree sprains are marked by hypermobility. Ligamentous tests should not be performed on obvious dislocations.	
Neurologic Tests	Not applicable	
Special Tests	None	
Comments	Posterior SC dislocations are considered medical emergencies because of the potential threat to the underlying neurovascular structures, the esophagus, and trachea. Fractures of the medial 1/3 of the clavicle can produce a pseudo-dislocation.	

SC = sternoclavicular.

nerve root (or roots) (see Box 1–6). Chapter 11 describes the brachial plexus and the actual mechanisms and tests for cervical nerve root impingement, and Chapter 12 discusses visceral origins of referred pain into this area.

◆ PATHOLOGIES OF THE SHOULDER COMPLEX AND RELATED SPECIAL TESTS

Because of the number of bones, muscles, articulations, ligaments, and other supporting structures associated with the shoulder complex, this complex is susceptible to a wide range of injuries. This section presents major orthopedic and athletic injuries to each segment and describes the signs, symptoms, and special evaluative procedures used to reach the appropriate conclusions. The clinician should structure the examination approach to include only those special tests that are relevant to confirm or deny the suspected pathology.

STERNOCLAVICULAR JOINT SPRAINS

Injuries to the SC joint usually occur from a longitudinal force being placed on the clavicle. This mechanism commonly occurs by falling on an outstretched arm or from a force being placed on the lateral portion of the shoulder. Less frequently, traction forces, such as those experienced by gymnasts performing on the rings, high bar, or uneven bars in which the athlete is suspended by the arms, may disrupt the integrity of the joint capsule.

SC sprains are marked by pain during joint play movements. Protraction and retraction of the scapula can reproduce pain associated with ligamentous or disk damage. Dislocations of this joint commonly occur anteriorly, superiorly, or posteriorly relative to the sternum.[23] Anterior dislocations are more common than posterior (retrosternal) dislocations because the anterior SC ligament is relatively weak.

Because of the potential threat to the subclavian artery, subclavian vein, trachea, and esophagus, posterior SC dislocations are a medical emergency.[3] Pressure can be placed on the superior mediastinum, blocking the cranial vessels, trachea, and esophagus, producing dizziness, nausea, neurovascular symptoms in the upper extremity, dyspnea, and *dysphagia* (Table 13–6).[3,24]

Dysphagia   Difficulty with swallowing or the inability to swallow.

The clavicle's medial epiphysis does not completely fuse until approximately age 25 years. The similarities in the signs and symptoms of a SC joint sprain or dislocation and those associated with an epiphyseal injury, a **pseudo-dislocation,** are similar, injuries to the growth plate must be ruled out in patients younger than age 25 years.[3,25] A definitive evaluation of the integrity of the SC joint can be made using magnetic resonance imaging (MRI).

Unstable or irreducible posterior SC dislocations often require surgical repair and internal fixation of the joint.[26] Anterior or superior SC dislocations may be managed through closed reduction and immobilization of the involved arm.

Treatment of a SC joint sprain typically involves palliative measures to decrease the signs and symptoms of inflammation and allow the injury to heal. The use of ice and sling immobilization as necessary to decrease the traction on the joint and ROM to the cervical spine and upper extremity are used initially. As the pain and swelling at the joint decrease, strengthening of the surrounding musculature is initiated with a progressive return to functional activities.

ACROMIOCLAVICULAR JOINT SPRAINS

Horizontal (anterior and posterior) stability of the AC joint is maintained by the AC ligament. Superior stability is maintained by the conoid and trapezoid segments of the coracoclavicular ligament. Commonly referred to as a "separated shoulder," rupture of these ligaments results in instability or dislocation of the joint. There-fore, these ruptures are more correctly referred to as sprains. The most common mechanisms for acute injury of the AC joint are characterized by the acromion's being driven away from the clavicle or vice versa. Examples of these mechanisms include:

- Landing on a forward-flexed outstretched arm or the point of the elbow, which drives the scapula posterior to the clavicle
- A blow to the acromion process, which drives the scapula inferior to the clavicle
- A force that drives the clavicle away from the scapula when the scapula is fixated

The AC joint may also be traumatized by overuse, repetitive stress mechanisms. Classification of AC sprains is based on the structures involved, the degree of instability, and the direction in which the clavicle has been displaced relative to the acromion and coracoid process (Table 13–7).

Evaluations of patients with acute AC injuries reveal a history describing one of the aforementioned mechanisms (Table 13–8). Pain is located over the distal clavicle, AC joint, anterolateral neck, superior scapula, and the lateral deltoid.[27] On inspection, advanced sprains (type II and above) normally result in noticeable displacement of the clavicle from the acromion process, creating a **step deformity** (see Fig. 13–22). Palpation of the involved area may produce hypermobility of the distal clavicle. The **piano key sign** represents a bob of the clavicle vertically, with the distal clavicle depressing and elevating with manual palpation, indicating trauma to the coracoclavicular ligament.

Table 13–7
CLASSIFICATION SYSTEM FOR ACROMIOCLAVICULAR JOINT SPRAINS

Grade	Structures Involved	Signs and Symptoms
Type I	Slight to partial damage of the AC ligament and capsule	Point tenderness over the AC joint; no laxity or deformity noted
Type II	Rupture of the AC ligament and partial damage to the coracoclavicular ligament	Slight laxity and deformity of the AC joint Slight step deformity
Type III	Complete tearing of the AC and coracoclavicular ligaments; possible involvement of the deltoid and trapezius fascia	Obvious dislocation of the distal end of the clavicle from the acromion process
Type IV	Complete tearing of the AC and coracoclavicular ligaments and tearing of the deltoid and trapezius fascia	Posterior clavicular displacement into the insertion of the upper fibers of the trapezius.
Type V	Same as type IV	Displacement of the involved clavicle from the acromion 100% to 300%, as compared with the opposite limb; clavicle posteriorly displaced with stripping away of the deltoid-trapezius aponeurosis
Type VI	Same as type IV	Displacement of the clavicle inferiorly under the coracoid (possible involvement of the brachial plexus)

AC = acromioclavicular.

Table 13–8
EVALUATIVE FINDINGS: Acromioclavicular Joint Sprains

Examination Segment	Clinical Findings	
History	**Onset:**	Acute
	Pain Characteristics:	Primarily localized at the AC joint; also possibly including the upper trapezius, and upper scapula (secondary to trapezius spasm)
	Mechanism:	Falling on the point of the shoulder, landing on the AC joint
		Force applied longitudinally to the clavicle, such as falling on an outstretched arm
Inspection	Displacement of the clavicle may be present.	
	Step deformities indicate damage to the coracoclavicular ligament.	
Palpation	Superior displacement of the clavicle that is reduced with manual pressure (**piano key sign**).	
Range of Motion	**AROM:**	Pain with elevation of the humerus and during protraction and retraction of the scapula
	PROM:	Pain produced during elevation of the humerus owing to movement at the AC joint
	RROM:	Decreased strength possibly noted for all movements due to pain, especially with those muscles having an attachment on the acromion or clavicle
		Pain is produced during resisted horizontal adduction.
Ligamentous Tests	Joint play movements reveal hypermobility of the AC joint.	
Neurological Tests	Not applicable	
Special Tests	AC traction test, AC compression test	
Comments	Fractures of the distal clavicle may present with the clinical signs and symptoms of an acromioclavicular joint sprain.	
	Radiographs should be obtained to rule out clavicular fracture and determine the severity of the sprain.	

AC = acromioclavicular; AROM = active range of motion; PROM = passive range of motion; RROM = resisted range of motion.

Tests for AROM and PROM produce pain on most movements, especially those occurring above 90 degrees and during the **Apley's scratch tests** (see Box 13–3). RROM tests are diminished in all planes. Active and resisted horizontal adduction also elicit pain from the AC joint. The **AC traction test** (Box 13–10) reveals trauma to the coracoclavicular ligament, and the **AC compression test** (Box 13–11) reproduces horizontal AC instability.

Patients displaying a hypermobile AC articulation should be referred to a physician for evaluation because, in some instances, fractures of the distal clavicle may clinically mimic a dislocation of the AC joint.[28] Radiographically, stress radiographs can be used to differentiate between injuries that are isolated to the AC ligament and those that include the coracoclavicular ligament.

Chronic AC joint pain may be the result of a degenerative process within the articulation, previous injury, or aging. Its symptoms may be easily confused with rotator cuff symptoms and may result in, or be caused by, rotator cuff injuries.[29,30] Pain is produced when the arm is internally rotated or abducted, the AC joint is stressed, or when the GH joint is placed in the classic impingement position of forward flexion and abduction.[29,31] Pain arising from the AC joint can be differentiated from that arising from the subacromial bursa and rotator cuff by its location. AC joint pain radiates into the scapula and neck. Subacromial joint pathology tends to only radiate pain laterally.[27] During chronic AC joint degeneration, many of the signs and symptoms of an acute AC joint injury are present, but there is no history of trauma to the AC joint. Although the joint may be painful on palpation, instability is not generally demonstrated. Radiographic examination may show degenerative changes within the joint's articulating space.

For patients suffering with grade I or II AC sprains and those with chronic joint degeneration, conservative management is usually recommended. Local corticosteroid injections can provide short-term relief of symptoms, but they do not alter the long-term progression of the condition.[32]

For patients with AC sprains that are grade II and higher, surgical or conservative management is used. However, there is little difference in the long-term outcome between the two approaches.[33] Conservative management requires a decreased period of immobilization and yields a reduced amount of time lost from activity. Patients being treated conservatively demonstrate strength and ROM that is at least equal to patients undergoing surgery.[33,34] Although the level of function between the two groups is equal, the amount of long-term deformity is higher in patients managed conservatively. For patients being managed surgically, the patient's subjective pain scores commonly are lower after surgery.[33–35]

Box 13–10
ACROMIOCLAVICULAR TRACTION TEST

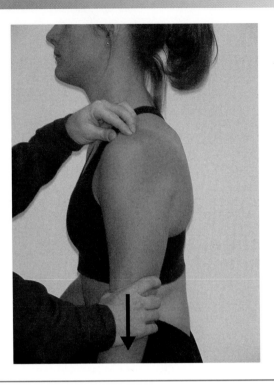

The principle behind the AC traction test is similar to a stress radiograph used to diagnose AC instability.

PATIENT POSITION	Sitting or standing The arm hanging naturally from the side
POSITION OF EXAMINER	Standing lateral to the involved side The clinician grasps the patient's humerus proximal to the elbow. The opposite hand gently palpates the AC joint.
EVALUATIVE PROCEDURE	The examiner applies a downward traction on the humerus.
POSITIVE TEST	The humerus and scapula move inferior to the clavicle, causing a step deformity, pain, or both.
IMPLICATIONS	Sprain of the AC or costoclavicular ligaments (see Table 13–7 for grades).
COMMENT	Patients displaying positive AC traction test results should be referred to a physician for follow-up radiographic stress testing and to rule out a clavicular fracture.

AC = acromioclavicular.

Conservative management focuses on sling immobilization only for as long as is needed for pain relief. Extended use of a sling or the use of special slings that place pressure on the distal clavicle does not make a difference in long-term results. Local modalities and treatment of subsequent trapezius muscle spasm highlight early treatment. The patient can progress through ROM and shoulder strengthening exercises as tolerated. With grade I AC joint sprains, this may occur within the first week. With more severe injuries, 3 to 4 weeks may be necessary. Because of the increased stress on the AC and GH joints in the terminal ranges of overhead movement, motion and strengthening in these extreme ranges may be limited early on.

Surgical intervention is associated with several potential long-term detriments. Resection of the distal clavicle or disruption of the AC joint capsule can result in dysfunction of both the AC and GH joints.[36]

Box 13–11
ACROMIOCLAVICULAR COMPRESSION TEST

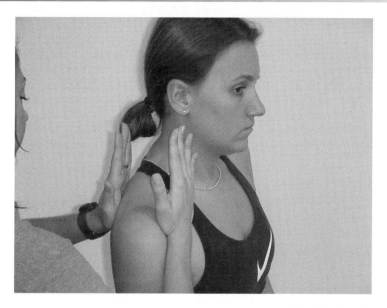

PATIENT POSITION	Sitting or standing with the arm hanging naturally at the side
POSITION OF EXAMINER	Standing on the involved side with the hands cupped over the anterior and posterior joint structures
EVALUATIVE PROCEDURE	The examiner squeezes the hands together, compressing the AC joint.
POSITIVE TEST	Pain at the AC joint or excursion of the clavicle over the acromion process
IMPLICATIONS	Damage to the AC ligament and possibly the coracoclavicular ligament.

AC = acromioclavicular.

GLENOHUMERAL INSTABILITY

The GH joint may present with instability anteriorly, posteriorly, inferiorly, or in multiple planes. It is the result of ligamentous or labral pathology, capsular instability, or muscular weakness. The severity of the instability is graded based on **joint glide movements,** the relative displacement of the humeral head on the glenoid fossa.

The primary passive supports of the GH joint have been described as being the GH ligaments, the joint capsule, and the coracohumeral ligament, which provide stability, limit the extremes of motion, and align the humeral head during movement.[37] These passive restraints are augmented by the rotator cuff and other GH musculature to provide coordinated motion of the shoulder complex. This close relationship between the passive and dynamic stabilizers indicates that pathological changes in the rotator cuff may result in GH instability (Table 13–9).[38]

Anterior Instability

Anterior instability is the result of laxity of the anterior stabilizing structures such as the middle GH ligament and, more specifically, the anterior band of the inferior GH ligament.[39] The superior and middle GH ligaments [40] and large tears or weakness of the rotator cuff musculature may also contribute to anterior GH instability.[41] The inferior GH ligament may be avulsed from the labrum or may be avulsed along with a portion of the labrum, forming a **Bankart lesion.** Bankart lesions are difficult to identify clinically, with the primary complaints being pain and crepitus as the humeral head moves against the anterior labrum during GH glide testing, load and shift testing, or external rotation of the humerus.

The primary mechanism for anterior dislocations of the humeral head is excessive external rotation and abduction of the humerus. In this position, the anterior capsule is reinforced by the anterior fibers of the deltoid

Table 13–9
DIFFERENTIAL FINDINGS OF CHRONIC GLENOHUMERAL INSTABILITY

	Anterior Instability	Posterior Instability	Multidirectional Instability
Onset	Chronic	Chronic	Insidious or chronic
Pain	Diffuse ache during ADLs along with the sensation that the shoulder is "loose" when brought into abduction with external rotation	Diffuse ache during ADLs; the patient reports that the shoulder feels unstable when it is brought across the body	Pain in the shoulder that increases with ADLs; the patient reports that the shoulder is "loose" with positions in the extremes of rotation motions
Mechanism	A specific mechanism of injury may be described, but chronic anterior instability is often caused by repetitive microtrauma involving external rotation when the GH joint is abducted to 90°.	Patient may describe a specific mechanism of injury but chronic posterior instability is generally caused by repetitive microtrauma involving longitudinal force on the length of the humerus while internally rotated and the GH joint flexed to 90° and horizontally adducted.	Although the instability is multidirectional, the chief complaint is typically pain during external rotation with the shoulder abducted to 90°. A sensation of instability may be described during the midrange of motion.
Predisposition	Joint hypermobility	Joint hypermobility	Joint hypermobility
Inspection	A flattened deltoid is possible as chronic cases can cause atrophy of the deltoid muscle group and the scapular muscles. Possible atrophy of the rotator cuff muscles	Chronic cases can cause atrophy of the deltoid muscle group, rotator cuff muscles, and scapular muscles.	Chronic cases can cause atrophy of the deltoid muscle group and the scapular muscles.
Palpation	Tenderness of the anterior GH joint	Tenderness of the posterior GH joint	Tenderness in the anterior GH joint
Range of Motion			
AROM	Decreased external rotation secondary to sensation of instability and/or pain	Decreased internal rotation	Possible limitation at the end ranges of motion secondary to a sensation of instability
PROM	Decreased external rotation secondary to sensation of instability and/or pain	Decreased internal rotation	Limited end range due to pain and instability
RROM	Pain and weakness during external rotation in advanced cases and/or pain	Pain and weakness during internal rotation in advanced cases	Pain and weakness during internal and external rotation
Ligamentous Tests	Increased anterior glide, although it may not appear increased to the contralateral side due to the bilateral nature of instability in chronic cases	Increased posterior glide, although it may not appear increased to the contralateral side due to the bilateral nature of instability in chronic cases	Increased glide in all directions
Special Tests	Apprehension test, relocation test	Posterior apprehension test; test for posterior instability in the plane of the scapula	Apprehension test; Relocation test; Posterior apprehension test; Test for posterior instability in the plane of the scapula.
Comments	Chronic cases may have a predisposition to bilateral involvement. Chronic atraumatic instability usually occurs in patients less than 30 years old.	Chronic cases may have a predisposition to bilateral involvement. Chronic atraumatic instability usually occurs in patients less than 30 years old.	Chronic cases may have a predisposition to bilateral involvement. Multidirectional instability usually occurs in patients less than 30 years old.

AROM = active range of motion; PROM = passive range of motion; RROM = resisted range of motion.

Box 13–12
RELOCATION TEST FOR ANTERIOR GLENOHUMERAL LAXITY

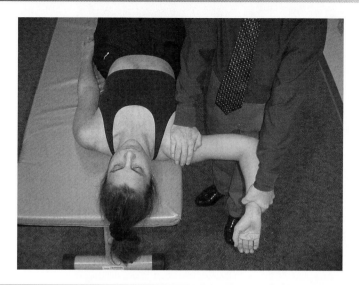

PATIENT POSITION	Supine The GH joint abducted to 90° The elbow flexed to 90°
POSITION OF EXAMINER	Standing beside the patient, inferior to the humerus on the involved side The forearm grasped proximal to the wrist to provide leverage during external rotation of the humerus The opposite hand held over the humeral head
EVALUATIVE PROCEDURE	The examiner externally rotates the humerus until pain, discomfort, or apprehension of a dislocation is experienced by the patient or the normal ROM is met. Posterior pressure is then applied to relocate the subluxated joint.
POSITIVE TEST	Decreased pain or increased ROM (or both) compared with the anterior apprehension test
IMPLICATIONS	Anterior pain may be the result of increased laxity in the anterior ligamentous and capsular structures. Posterior pain may be from the impingement of the posterior capsule or labrum. A positive test result supports the conclusion of increased laxity in the anterior capsule owing to capsular damage or labrum tears. The manual pressure applied by the examiner increases the stability of the anterior portion of the GH capsule, allowing more external rotation to occur.
COMMENT	The relocation test is usually performed after the anterior apprehension test.

GH = glenohumeral; ROM = range of motion.

muscle group and the anterior rotator cuff tendons, reducing the anterior shear forces across the glenoid fossa and forcing the humeral head inferiorly.[42] Passive external rotation of the humerus must be performed with caution, especially when the shoulder is in 90 degrees of flexion as this is similar to the **apprehension test ("crank test") for anterior instability** (see Box 13–5). Positive apprehension test results are followed up with the **relocation test for anterior instability,** in which manual pressure is applied on the anterior humeral head to keep the joint from dislocating (Box 13–12).

A common finding associated with an anterior GH dislocation is a **Hill-Sachs lesion,** a small defect in the posterior humeral head's articular cartilage caused by the impact of the humeral head on the glenoid fossa as the humerus attempts to relocate (Fig. 13–34). The lesion is used as a diagnostic tool in determining the severity of the dislocation. In patients who report that the shoulder dislocated but spontaneously relocated, the lesion may be present on radiographic examination. The lesion itself is rarely symptomatic but may lead to early degeneration of the GH joint.

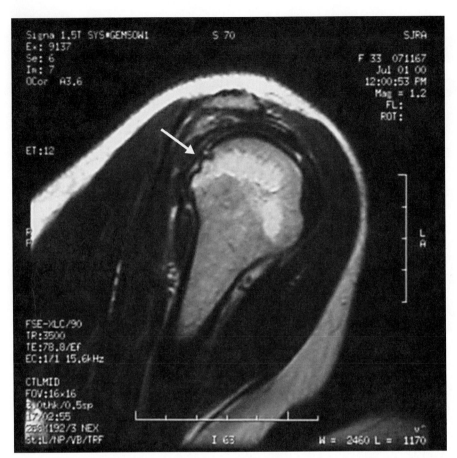

FIGURE 13–34. An MRI of a Hill-Sachs lesion.

Posterior Instability

Posterior GH instability is relatively rare, accounting for approximately 3 percent of all shoulder instabilities.[43] This type of instability most often occurs when the humerus is flexed and internally rotated while a longitudinal posterior force is placed on the humerus. Although posterior instability may be the result of a single traumatic event, it often appears to be the result of accumulated microtrauma secondary to repeated blows on a forward-flexed arm, such as during blocking in football, the follow-through phase of throwing or overhand tennis volleys, or overhead swimming strokes.[43,44]

Posterior instability results from weakness of the subscapularis muscle, the primary dynamic restraint against posterior humeral displacement. The coracohumeral and posterior band of the inferior GH ligaments also provide restraint when the humerus is in its neutral position or internally rotated, respectively. The long head of the biceps brachii tendon also provides posterior stability.[45] The **posterior apprehension test** (Box 13–13) and the **test for posterior instability in the plane of the scapula** (Box 13–14) are used to evaluate posterior GH instability. Lesions found on the anterior portion of the humeral head after a posterior dislocation are termed **reverse Hill-Sachs lesions.**

Inferior Instability

The primary restraint against inferior translation of the GH joint depends on the position of the humerus. In the neutral position, the primary restraint against inferior translation is the superior GH ligament, with little or no assistance provided by the coracohumeral ligament. When the humerus is abducted to 45 degrees in neutral rotation, the anterior portion of the inferior GH ligament is the primary restraint; this position also shows the greatest amount of translation. After further abducting the humerus to 90 degrees, the entire inferior GH ligament is responsible for restricting inferior displacement, but the posterior band is perhaps the most important restraint.[46] The presence of rotator cuff tears or weakness also increases inferior GH laxity.[41] Superior translation of the humeral head is limited by the presence of the coracoacromial arch and the acromion process.

The **sulcus sign** is used to identify the presence of multidirectional instability (Box 13–15). If the shoulder demonstrates laxity in the neutral position, it can be assumed to be lax in all positions. A positive sulcus sign with the humerus flexed to 90 degrees may indicate inferior instability.

Box 13–13
POSTERIOR APPREHENSION TEST FOR GLENOHUMERAL LAXITY

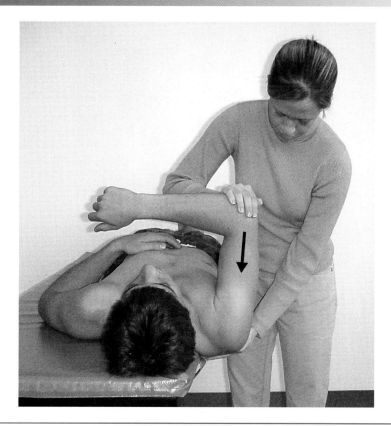

PATIENT POSITION	Sitting or supine The shoulder flexed to 90° and the elbow flexed to 90° The GH joint being tested off to the side of the table
POSITION OF EXAMINER	Standing on the involved side One hand grasping the forearm The opposite hand stabilizing the posterior scapula
EVALUATIVE PROCEDURE	The examiner applies a longitudinal force to the humeral shaft, encouraging the humeral head to move posteriorly on the glenoid fossa. The examiner may choose to alter the amount of flexion and rotation of the humerus.
POSITIVE TEST	The patient displays apprehension and produces muscle guarding to prevent the shoulder from subluxating posteriorly.
IMPLICATIONS	Laxity in the posterior GH capsule, torn posterior labrum

GH = glenohumeral.

Box 13–14
TEST FOR POSTERIOR INSTABILITY IN THE PLANE OF THE SCAPULA

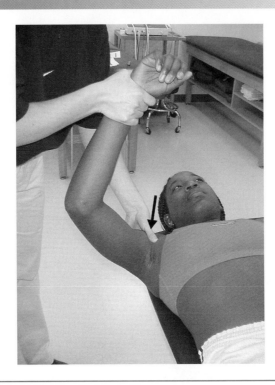

PATIENT POSITION	Lying supine The shoulder in 90° of abduction and horizontally adducted to approximately 30° to place the humerus in the plane of the scapula The elbow flexed to a comfortable position The GH joint being tested off to the side of the table
POSITION OF EXAMINER	One hand supports the weight of the arm at the elbow The opposite palm or thumb is placed over the anterior portion of the GH capsule.
EVALUATIVE PROCEDURE	Using the thumb or palm, a pressure is applied to the humeral head, attempting to drive it posteriorly on the glenoid fossa. Additional force may be used by applying a longitudinal force on the humerus by applying pressure from the elbow.
POSITIVE TEST	Pain or laxity in the posterior GH capsule or the patient displaying apprehension of a posterior subluxation
IMPLICATIONS	Laxity in the posterior GH capsule, coracohumeral ligament

GH = glenohumeral.

SULCUS SIGN FOR INFERIOR GLENOHUMERAL LAXITY

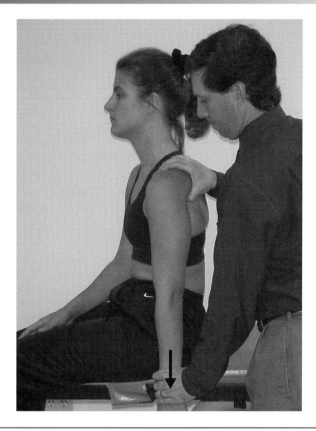

PATIENT POSITION	Sitting Arm hanging at the side
POSITION OF EXAMINER	Standing lateral to the involved side The patient's arm gripped distal to the elbow
EVALUATIVE PROCEDURE	A downward (inferior) traction force is applied to the humerus
POSITIVE TEST	An indentation (sulcus) appears beneath the acromion process To differentiate the results of this test from those of the AC traction test for AC joint instability, the movement of the humeral head is away from the scapula and clavicle in this test. In the AC traction test, the humerus and scapula move away from the clavicle.
IMPLICATIONS	The humeral head slides inferiorly on the glenoid fossa, indicating laxity in the superior GH ligament.

AC = acromioclavicular; GH = glenohumeral.

Multidirectional Instability

Multidirectional instabilities are a combination of two or more unidirectional instabilities. Evaluation of shoulder instability must be performed carefully to differentiate between unidirectional and multidirectional instabilities. Treatment of only one of the unidirectional instabilities in the presence of a multidirectional instability can worsen the condition because only one aspect of the joint is strengthened, potentially increasing the chance of instability in the other involved plane.

ROTATOR CUFF PATHOLOGY

A cause-and-effect relationship exists between rotator cuff inflammation and rotator cuff impingement syndrome. Impingement of the rotator cuff muscles occurs when there is decreased space through which the rotator cuff tendons pass under the coracoacromial arch. In its initial stages, the impingement often results in the inflammation of the rotator cuff tendons. Likewise, inflammation of the rotator cuff tendons results in the enlargement of the tendons, decreasing the subacromial space and increasing the likelihood of impinging the tendons. The source of rotator cuff impingement is classified as being compressive or tensile and ranked into primary and secondary sources (Table 13–10).

This sequence of events creates a closed cycle in which one condition exacerbates the other. When allowed to proceed unchecked, the ultimate outcome is a shoulder with greatly diminished function. To athletes participating in overhead sports or workers who perform repetitive overhead movements, impingement syndrome or rotator cuff pathology can be career threatening.

Rotator Cuff Impingement Syndrome

Caused by a reduction in the space below the coracoacromial arch, the structures that lie beneath this

Table 13–10
CAUSES OF ROTATOR CUFF IMPINGEMENT

Force	Source
Primary compression	Irregularly shaped acromion Coracoacromial ligament Enlarged bursa Thickened rotator cuff tendons
Secondary compression	Loss of humeral head depression/stabilization Poor posture Repetitive overhead movement
Primary tensile	Repetitive overload Eccentric forces
Secondary tensile	*Scapular dyskinesis* Rotator cuff muscle weakness GH instability

area, the rotator cuff tendons (primarily the supraspinatus tendon), the long head of the biceps brachii tendon, the subacromial bursa, the GH joint capsule, and the head of the humerus are compressed between the acromion process and the humeral head (Fig. 13–35). The most common cause of impingement is anatomical variation in the coracoacromial arch that produces a mechanical wear on the rotator cuff, subacromial bursa, and the long head of the biceps tendon.[47] Fatigue from overuse or decreased strength of the rotator cuff can also contribute to impingement syndrome. Decreased strength or fatigue leads to decreased humeral head depression as the humerus is

Scapular dyskinesis An improperly moving scapula (term is discussed in Table 13–10).

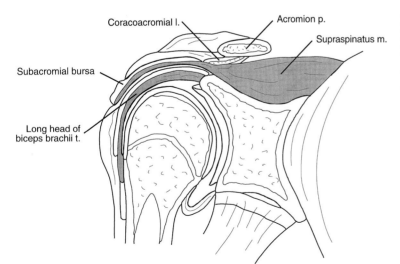

Coracoacromial l.
Acromion p.
Supraspinatus m.
Subacromial bursa
Long head of biceps brachii t.

FIGURE 13–35. Structures involved in shoulder impingement syndrome. If the humeral head does not depress during abduction, the long head of the biceps brachii, the subacromial bursa, and the supraspinatus tendon are impinged between the coracoacromial arch and the head of the humerus.

brought into overhead positions, causing impingement of the structures. Impingement can occur anywhere along the coracoacromial arch and under the AC joint.

A relationship between poor scapular biomechanics and impingement syndromes has been suggested.[48,49] In this case, the scapula does not upwardly rotate appropriately to allow the rotator cuff muscles and the long head of the biceps tendon to pass beneath the coracoacromial arch.

The chief complaint associated with rotator cuff impingement is pain during overhead movements and an associated painful arc (Table 13–11). The patient may describe a relief of symptoms when the GH joint is maintained in slight abduction. The physical impingement of supraspinatus tendon between the acromion process and the greater tuberosity begins with GH joint is forward flexed and the humerus abducted to 30 degrees and reaches its peak at 90 degrees of abduction with the humerus internally rotated.[50] The **Neer impingement test** (Box 13–16) and the **Hawkins (Kennedy-Hawkins) impingement test** (Box 13–17) are the most commonly used clinical evaluation techniques for patients suspected of having this condition.

Rotator Cuff Tendinitis

Rotator cuff tendinitis typically presents with a slow onset of the symptoms. In the early stages, the chief complaint is pain deep within the shoulder in the subacromial area after activity. The symptoms then progress to pain during activity and, finally, to constant pain with most activities of daily living. Factors contributing to the onset of rotator cuff pathology include a decreased muscle balance between the internal and external rotators, capsular laxity, poor scapular control, and impingement syndromes.

The shoulder is predisposed to rotator cuff tendinitis by the relatively poor vascularization of the tendons, a fact that also hinders the healing process. The supraspinatus tendon is the most susceptible of the rotator cuff group to inflammatory conditions, especially at the convergence zone of the anterior and posterior circumflex arteries, just proximal to the greater tuberosity.[51] In addition to its poor blood supply, pressure is placed on this tendon by the humeral head "wringing" it dry of blood and other vital nutrients.

Table 13–11
EVALUATIVE FINDINGS: Rotator Cuff Impingement

Examination Segment	Clinical Findings	
History	*Onset:*	Insidious
	Pain Characteristics:	Beneath the acromion process and radiating to the lateral arm
	Mechanism:	Repetitive overhead motion impinging the rotator cuff muscles (especially the supraspinatus) and long head of the biceps tendon between the humeral head and coracoacromial arch
	Predisposing conditions:	Tight posterior capsule and ligamentous tissues, irregularly shaped acromion (curved or hooked), subacromial spurs, scapular dyskinesis, rotator cuff weakness
Inspection	The shoulder may be postured for comfort by holding the arm close to the body and avoiding overhead arm motions.	
Palpation	Tenderness exists beneath the acromion process, over the supraspinatus insertion at the greater tuberosity, and over the bicipital groove.	
Range of Motion	Active, passive, and resisted movements of GH internal and external rotation and flexion result in pain and/or weakness, especially when the arm is abducted above 90°. Active abduction in an arc of motion from about 70° to 120° results in pain. Activities of daily living and athletic events requiring overhead movement result in pain.	
Ligamentous Tests	A complete ligamentous and capsular screen is necessary to rule out GH and AC laxity.	
Neurologic Tests	Not applicable	
Special Tests	The Neer and Hawkins impingement tests and the empty can test are usually painful.	
Comments	Impingement may occur secondary to GH instability in younger patients. The inflammatory response caused by rotator cuff impingement, if untreated, can lead to rotator cuff tears.	

AC = acromioclavicular; GH = glenohumeral.

Box 13–16
THE NEER SHOULDER IMPINGEMENT TEST

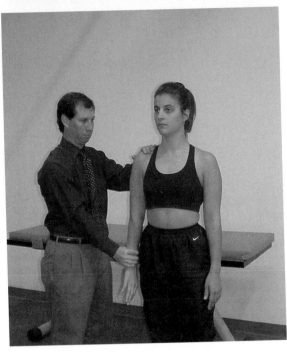
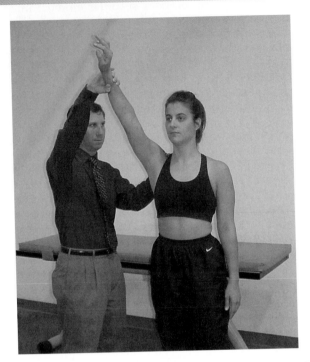

PATIENT POSITION	Standing or sitting The shoulder, elbow, and wrist in the anatomical position
POSITION OF EXAMINER	Standing lateral or forward of the involved side The patient's shoulder stabilized on the posterior aspect The examiner's other hand gripping the patient's arm distal to the elbow joint
EVALUATIVE PROCEDURE	With the elbow extended, the humerus is placed in internal rotation and the forearm is pronated. The GH joint is then forcefully moved through forward flexion as the scapula is stabilized.
POSITIVE TEST	Pain with motion, especially near the end of the ROM.
IMPLICATIONS	Pathology is present in the rotator cuff group (especially the supraspinatus) or the long head of the biceps brachii tendon. The motion of the test impinges these structures between the greater tuberosity and the inferior side of the acromion process and AC joint.

AC = acromioclavicular; GH = glenohumeral; ROM = range of motion.

⟫⟫⟫ **Box 13–17**
THE HAWKINS SHOULDER IMPINGEMENT TEST

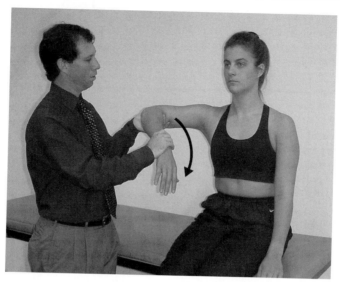

PATIENT POSITION	Sitting or standing The shoulder, elbow, and wrist in the anatomical position
POSITION OF EXAMINER	Standing lateral or forward of the involved side The examiner's other hand gripping the patient's arm at the elbow joint
EVALUATIVE PROCEDURE	With the elbow flexed, the GH joint elevated to 90° in the scapular plane. At this point, the humerus is passively internally rotated.
POSITIVE TEST	Pain with motion, especially near the end of the ROM
IMPLICATIONS	Pathology is present in the rotator cuff group (especially the supraspinatus) or the long head of the biceps brachii tendon. The motion of the test impinges these structures between the greater tuberosity and the inferior side of the acromion process.
COMMENT	If the humerus is brought in toward the sagittal plane, the chance of eliciting a false-positive result secondary to AC joint pathology increases.

AC = acromioclavicular; GH = glenohumeral; ROM = range of motion.

Box 13–18
CLASSIFICATION OF ACROMION SHAPES

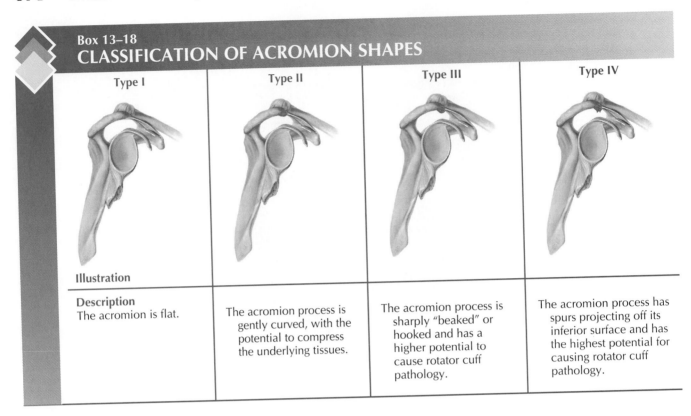

	Type I	Type II	Type III	Type IV
Illustration				
Description	The acromion is flat.	The acromion process is gently curved, with the potential to compress the underlying tissues.	The acromion process is sharply "beaked" or hooked and has a higher potential to cause rotator cuff pathology.	The acromion process has spurs projecting off its inferior surface and has the highest potential for causing rotator cuff pathology.

Table 13–12
EVALUATIVE FINDINGS: Rotator Cuff Tears

Examination Segment	Clinical Findings	
History	**Onset:**	Insidious or acute
	Pain Characteristics:	Deep within the shoulder beneath the acromion process. Pain usually radiating into the lateral arm.
	Mechanism:	Insidious: Chronic impingement or weakening of the rotator cuff tendons over time due to aging; a single traumatic episode may cause the final rupture of a weakened tendon.
		Acute: Dynamic overloading of the tendon.
	Predisposing conditions:	Rotator cuff impingement, chronic rotator cuff tendinitis, acromion changes, repetitive overhead motion, repetitive eccentric loading
Inspection	In chronic cases, inspection of the scapula possibly revealing atrophy of the infraspinatus and/or supraspinatus	
Palpation	Tenderness in the subacromial space and at the insertion of the supraspinatus tendon into the greater tuberosity	
Range of Motion Tests	Pain with isolation of the supraspinatus muscle	
	Pain during overhead motions	
	Pain possible with resisted range of motion tests, especially abduction, internal rotation, and external rotation	
Ligamentous Tests	Tests to rule out GH and AC laxity and impingement	
Neurologic Tests	Not applicable	
Special Tests	Drop arm test; empty can test	
	Impingement tests may be positive.	
Comments	Rotator cuff impingement tests are often positive.	
	A history of rotator cuff tendinitis often precedes rotator cuff tears.	

AC = acromioclavicular; GH = glenohumeral.

The shape and location of the acromion process may also precipitate the onset of rotator cuff inflammation. The rate of rotator cuff pathology is markedly increased when the lateral acromion angle is less than 70 degrees, forming an acromial spur.[52] Shoulders that are affected by chronic rotator cuff pathology are also characterized by an increased number of acromial osteophytes (Box 13–18).[53]

The posterior rotator cuff muscles, the infraspinatus and teres minor, play an important role in the throwing motion. In addition to externally rotating the humerus during the cocking phase of the throw, these muscles eccentrically contract to decelerate the arm during the follow-through phase. The eccentric contraction can lead to microtearing or inflammation of these muscles, eventually giving way to larger tears.

The relative severity of rotator cuff pathology is based on the presence of tearing within the tendons (Table 13–12). Tears to the tendons may result from a single traumatic force or, more commonly and especially in the older population, from the accumulation of microtrauma (overuse injuries). **Partial-thickness tears** are short, longitudinal lesions in the tendon, initially involving the superficial or midsubstance fibers. When partial-thickness tears go untreated, a **full-thickness tear** may develop (full-thickness tears may also develop secondary to a single traumatic force). Severe dysfunction of the supraspinatus or infraspinatus muscles may lead to atrophy that is visible during inspection of the scapula.

During the controlled motion from full abduction to adduction, individuals suffering from tears in the rotator cuff tendons are unable to control the rate of fall after the humerus reaches 90 degrees of abduction as demonstrated by the **drop arm test** (see Box 13–4). The **empty can test** isolates the supraspinatus tendon for weakness or pain (Box 13–19).

Box 13–19
EMPTY CAN TEST FOR SUPRASPINATUS PATHOLOGY

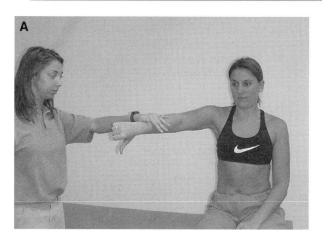
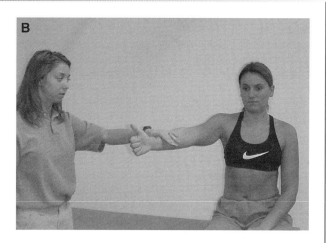

PATIENT POSITION	Sitting or standing The GH abducted to 90° in the scapular plane, the elbow extended, and the humerus internally rotated and the forearm pronated so that the thumb points downward (internally rotated) **(A).**
POSITION OF EXAMINER	Standing facing the patient One hand placed on the superior portion of the midforearm to resist the motion of abduction in the scapular plane
EVALUATIVE PROCEDURE	The evaluator resists abduction (applies a downward pressure).
POSITIVE TEST	Weakness or pain accompanying the movement
IMPLICATIONS	The supraspinatus tendon (1) is being impinged between the humeral head and the coracoacromial arch, (2) is inflamed, or (3) contains a lesion.
MODIFICATION	This test can be performed with the humerus externally rated and the forearm supinated so that the thumb is facing upward, the **full can test (B).**

GH = glenohumeral.

Subacromial Bursitis

Chronic rotator cuff impingement or rotator cuff tears, if untreated, ultimately lead to inflammation of the subacromial bursa. Often occurring concurrently, it is difficult to differentiate between rotator cuff pathology and subacromial bursitis. Subacromial bursitis causes positive results from impingement tests and tests for supraspinatus tendinitis as the three conditions are often related.

Management of Rotator Cuff Pathologies and Impingement Syndromes

Nonsurgical approaches to managing patients with rotator cuff pathology and impingement syndromes emphasize modification of activity, control of inflammation through the use of medications and therapeutic modalities, and rotator cuff flexibility and strengthening programs.[54] The restoration of capsular flexibility for rotator cuff pathology focuses on decreasing the tightness of the posterior shoulder structures. Tightness of the posterior structures restricts internal rotation (internal rotation deficiency) and increases forces causing elevation of the humeral head under the coracoacromial arch. These structures are isolated during stretching routines by stabilizing the scapula while taking the arm into internal rotation and during joint mobilization.

Strengthening must focus on the scapular musculature, the rotator cuff, and other shoulder muscles. The strength and use of the legs and trunk also must be analyzed. Much of the forces derived in an activity, such as throwing a baseball, originate in the legs, pelvis, and trunk. Decreased contributions from these areas call for increased activity of the rotator cuff muscles, exposing it to potentially injurious force and overuse injuries.

The patient should be able to control the scapula throughout the ROM. Strengthening of the rotator cuff must occur in conjunction with scapular stabilization. Initially, the rotator cuff can be strengthened in the scapular plane with the humerus in slight abduction to prevent overstressing the rotator cuff. As the patient progresses, the humerus can be elevated to overhead positions that place more functional stresses on the tendons. A well-rounded rehabilitation program also includes strengthening of the distal arm.

Surgery may be required to debride the subacromial space, resect the lateral portion of the clavicle (thus increasing the subacromial space), or repair the tear.[54] Based on the pathology, especially the size of any rotator cuff tear, the physician determines if surgery is done arthroscopically, with a mini-open technique (small scar over the superior aspect of the shoulder), or full open repair. Most small to medium sized tears can be repaired with arthroscopy or the mini-open technique.

Postoperatively, rehabilitation is dictated by the type of surgery required. Although debridements of the sub-acromial space and rotator cuff can progress based on the patient's tolerance, rotator cuff repairs require careful use of active and resisted motions in the repaired tissues for a period of 6 to 8 weeks to allow healing to occur.

BICEPS TENDON PATHOLOGY

The long head of the biceps tendon provides very little force in moving the GH joint, but pathology of this structure can decrease the strength, ROM, and stability of the GH joint.[55] During overhead movements, the tendon slides within its sheath that is located in the bicipital groove. When the tendon is inflamed, these movements produce pain and decrease the GH joint's functional ability.

Bicipital Tendinitis

Bicipital tendinitis may result from rotator cuff dysfunction, from overuse of the biceps brachii muscle, or from impingement. The transverse humeral ligament, which holds the tendon in the bicipital groove, may become stretched or torn as the result of sudden forceful extension or external rotation of the shoulder accompanied by elbow flexion. Disruption of the transverse humeral ligament can cause the long head of the biceps tendon to sublux from the bicipital groove, especially when the elbow is flexed and the humerus is externally rotated. Tears of the supraspinatus or infraspinatus tendons are often associated with dislocation or subluxation of the long head of the biceps brachii tendon.[56]

The **Yergason's test** can reproduce subluxation of the long head of the biceps tendon or cause pain in the presence of bicipital tendinitis (Box 13–20). Pain caused by a subluxating tendon can be differentiated by **Speed's test,** which only has positive test results in the presence of bicipital tendinitis (Box 13–21). MRI can also be used to differentiate between the two conditions.[57] **Ludington's test** can be used to identify a rupture of the biceps tendon or the muscle itself (Box 13–22).[58]

Bicipital tendinitis and rotator cuff tendinitis often occur simultaneously. Conservative rehabilitation includes decreasing inflammation with the use of oral medications, *phonophoresis,* or *iontophoresis.* Stretching and strengthening of the shoulder complex muscles should progress in a manner similar to that used for rotator cuff tendinitis.

Phonophoresis   The use of therapeutic ultrasound to introduce medication into the body.

Iontophoresis   The use of a direct current to introduce medication into the body.

Box 13–20
YERGASON'S TEST FOR SUBLUXATION OF THE BICEPS TENDON

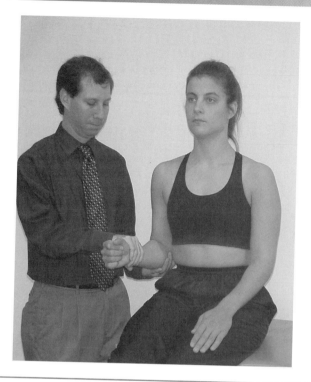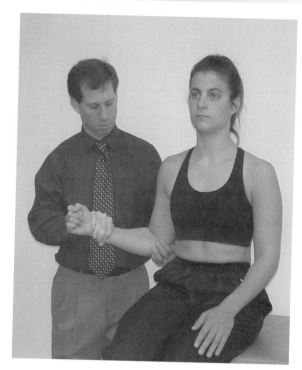

PATIENT POSITION	Sitting or standing GH joint in the anatomical position The elbow flexed to 90° The forearm positioned so that the lateral border of the radius faces upward (neutral position).
POSITION OF EXAMINER	Positioned lateral to the patient on the involved side The olecranon stabilized inferiorly and maintained close to the thorax The forearm stabilized proximal to the wrist
EVALUATIVE PROCEDURE	The patient provides resistance while the examiner concurrently moves the GH joint into external rotation and the proximal radioulnar joint into supination.
POSITIVE TEST	Pain or snapping (or both) in the bicipital groove
IMPLICATIONS	**Primary:** snapping or popping in the bicipital groove indicates a tear or laxity of the transverse humeral ligament. This pathology prevents the ligament from securing the long head of the tendon in its groove. **Secondary:** pain with no associated popping in the bicipital groove may indicate bicipital tendinitis.

GH = glenohumeral.

Box 13–21
SPEED'S TEST FOR LONG HEAD OF THE BICEPS BRACHII TENDINITIS

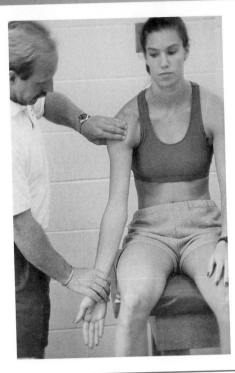

PATIENT POSITION	Sitting or standing The elbow extended The GH joint in neutral position or slightly extended to stretch the biceps brachii
POSITION OF EXAMINER	Standing lateral to and in front of the involved limb The fingers of one hand positioned over the bicipital groove while stabilizing the shoulder The forearm stabilized proximal to the wrist
EVALUATIVE PROCEDURE	The clinician resists flexion of the GH joint and elbow while palpating for tenderness over the bicipital groove.
POSITIVE TEST	Pain along the long head of the biceps brachii tendon, especially in the bicipital groove
IMPLICATIONS	Inflammation of the long head of the biceps tendon as it passes through the bicipital groove Possible tear of the transverse humeral ligament with concurrent instability of the long head of the biceps tendon as it passes through the bicipital groove

GH = glenohumeral.

Box 13–22
LUDINGTON'S TEST FOR BICEPS BRACHII PATHOLOGY

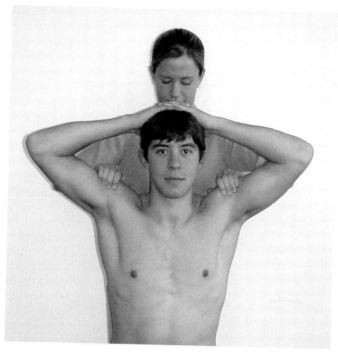

PATIENT POSITION	Standing or sitting The hands on top of the head with the fingers interlocked, supporting the weight of the arms
POSITION OF EXAMINER	Standing behind the patient, palpating the long head of the biceps brachii
EVALUATIVE PROCEDURE	The patient contracts the biceps brachii by applying force to the top of the head. The examiner palpates the long head of the biceps tendon, noting tension within the tendon.
POSITIVE TEST	Decreased or no tension is felt under the involved tendon; the tendon should be felt developing tension in the uninvolved muscle. Pain is increased
IMPLICATIONS	Rupture of the long head of the biceps brachii tendon

Table 13–13
CLASSIFICATION OF SLAP LESIONS

Type	Pathology
I	Fraying of the labrum near the insertion of the LHB tendon.
II	Avulsion of the glenoid labrum with an associated tear of the LHB.
III	A bucket-handle tear of the labrum with displacement of the fragment. No involvement of the LHB tendon.
IV	Bucket-handle tear of the labrum with associated tearing of the LHB tendon.

LHB = long head of the biceps.

Superior Labrum Anteroposterior Lesions

Superior labrum anteroposterior (SLAP) lesions are tears in the superior glenoid labrum located near the attachment of the long head of the biceps brachii tendon. Tension of the long head of the biceps tendon, such as that experienced during the follow-through phase of pitching when the biceps works to decelerate the elbow, pulls the labrum away from the glenoid fossa. Other compression and inferior traction mechanisms can also produce SLAP lesions.[59,60] Although usually having an acute onset, SLAP lesions present with clinically inconsistent symptoms. SLAP lesions can sometimes be seen on MRI or computed tomography (CT) scans, but are most commonly found during surgery. Table 13–13 presents four classifications of SLAP lesions. Clinically, SLAP lesions can be identified using the **active compression test (O'Brien test)** (Box 13–23).[61]

Postoperative management of a patient with a SLAP lesion depends on whether the tear was debrided or repaired. Although cases of debridement can usually progress as tolerated, repairs of SLAP lesions progress more slowly. Most importantly after a surgical SLAP repair, contraction of the biceps tendon and other traction forces from the tendon placed on the repair must be controlled for 6 to 8 weeks.

THORACIC OUTLET SYNDROME

Thoracic outlet syndrome is caused by pressure on the trunks and medial cord of the brachial plexus, the subclavian artery, or the subclavian vein (collectively known as the neurovascular bundle). Its etiology may be linked to the presence of a cervical rib, pressure placed on the neurovascular bundle as it is impinged between the clavicle and the first rib, compression between the pectoralis minor and rib cage, or tightness of the anterior and middle scalene muscles.

Present in a small percentage of the population, the cervical rib is a congenital outgrowth of the seventh cervical vertebra. This structure places pressure on the neurovascular bundle, especially when the shoulder complex is pulled inferiorly. The presence of a cervical rib is not necessarily a predisposition to thoracic outlet syndrome. Of all individuals possessing cervical ribs, fewer than 10 percent display the clinical signs and symptoms of thoracic outlet syndrome.[62]

The neurovascular bundle passes between the clavicle and the first thoracic rib and is therefore susceptible to pressure on its anterior surface. Poor posture, drooping shoulders that depress the clavicles, forward shoulder posture, prolonged pressure on the upper surfaces of the first rib such as wearing a backpack, or acute trauma may lead to the onset of thoracic outlet syndrome. The incidence of thoracic outlet syndrome is increased in athletes who perform repetitive overhead movements such as throwing or swimming.

The signs and symptoms of thoracic outlet syndrome may be neurologic or vascular in nature (Table 13–14).

Pallor   Lack of color in the skin.

Table 13–14
NEUROVASCULAR FINDINGS: Thoracic Outlet Syndrome

Onset	Signs and Symptoms
Neurological onset*	Numbness Pain Paresthesia
Arterial onset	Coldness of the skin *Pallor* Cyanosis in the fingers Muscular weakness
Venous onset	Muscular and joint stiffness Edema Venous engorgement Thrombophlebitis

*Note: These symptoms normally occur over the ulnar nerve distribution.

> **Box 13–23**
> ## ACTIVE COMPRESSION TEST (O'BRIEN TEST)

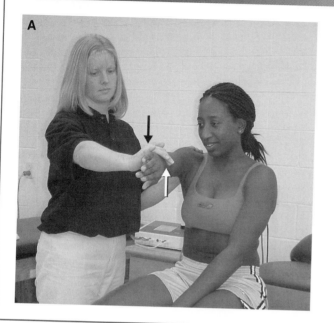

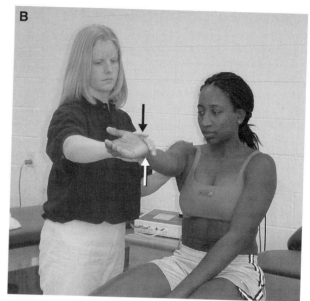

PATIENT POSITION	Standing The GH joint is flexed to 90° and horizontally adducted 15° from the sagittal plane. The humerus in full internal rotation and the forearm pronated **(A)**.
POSITION OF EXAMINER	In front of the patient One hand placed over the superior aspect of the patient's distal forearm
EVALUATIVE PROCEDURE	The patient resists the examiner's downward force. The test is repeated with the humerus externally rotated and the forearm supinated **(B)**.
POSITIVE TEST	Pain that is experienced with the arm internally rotated but is decreased during external rotation: **1.** Pain or clicking within the GH joint may indicate a labral tear. **2.** Pain at the AC joint may indicate AC joint pathology.
IMPLICATIONS	SLAP lesion
COMMENTS	The presence of rotator cuff pathology may produce false-positive results.

AC = acromioclavicular; GH = glenohumeral; SLAP = superior labrum; anterior to posterior tear.

Neurologic symptoms commonly are found along the distribution of the medial cord of the brachial plexus (C8 and T1) because of its proximity to the first thoracic rib. Generally, clinical symptoms are produced along the distribution of the ulnar nerve; decreased function along the median nerve may also be noted.

Vascular signs and symptoms reflect the specific structure being obstructed. Occlusion of the subclavian artery presents signs and symptoms typical of decreased blood flow. Blockage of the subclavian vein is characterized by edema in the distal upper extremity and, if untreated, may result in thrombophlebitis.

The underlying principle for thoracic outlet syndrome tests is related to the placement of pressure on the neurovascular bundle. **Adson's test** attempts to depress the shoulder complex and place the medial cord of the brachial plexus, the subclavian artery, and the subclavian vein on stretch while simultaneously placing pressure on the bundle from the anterior scalene muscle (Box 13–24). Thoracic outlet syndrome caused by the pectoralis minor muscle can be detected via the **Allen test** (Box 13–25). Costoclavicular etiology is tested via the **costoclavicular syndrome test** (military brace position) (Box 13–26).

Positive test results for thoracic outlet syndromes are not necessarily definitive of any underlying pathology. Patients who test positive for thoracic outlet syndrome need to be referred to a physician for further evaluation.

Box 13–24
ADSON'S TEST FOR THORACIC OUTLET SYNDROME

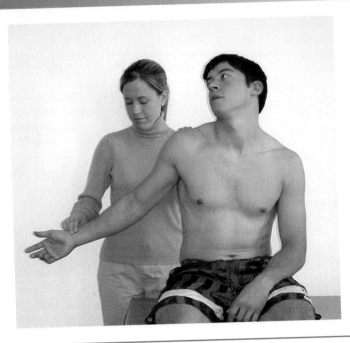

PATIENT POSITION	Sitting The shoulder abducted to 30° The elbow extended with the thumb pointing upward The humerus externally rotated
POSITION OF EXAMINER	Standing behind the patient One hand positioned so that the radial pulse is palpable
EVALUATIVE PROCEDURE	While still maintaining a feel for the radial pulse, the examiner externally rotates and extends the patient's shoulder while the face is rotated toward the involved side and extends the neck. The patient is instructed to inhale deeply and hold the breath.
POSITIVE TEST	The radial pulse disappears or markedly diminishes.
IMPLICATIONS	The subclavian artery is being occluded between the anterior and middle scalene muscles and the pectoralis minor.
COMMENT	This test often produces false-positive results.

Box 13–25
ALLEN TEST FOR THORACIC OUTLET SYNDROME

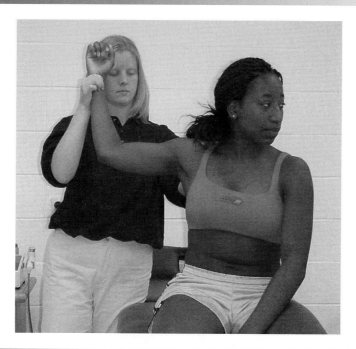

PATIENT POSITION	Sitting The head facing forward
POSITION OF EXAMINER	Standing behind the patient One hand positioned so that radial pulse is felt
EVALUATIVE PROCEDURE	The elbow is flexed to 90° while the clinician abducts the shoulder to 90°. The shoulder is then passively horizontally abducted and placed into external rotation. The patient then rotates the head towards the opposite shoulder.
POSITIVE TEST	The radial pulse disappears.
IMPLICATIONS	The pectoralis minor muscle is compressing the neurovascular bundle.
COMMENT	This test often produces false-positive results.

Box 13–26
MILITARY BRACE POSITION FOR THORACIC OUTLET SYNDROME

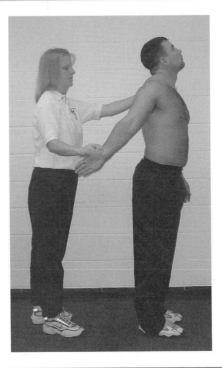

PATIENT POSITION	Standing The shoulders in a relaxed posture The head looking forward
POSITION OF EXAMINER	Standing behind the patient One hand positioned to locate the radial pulse on the involved extremity
EVALUATIVE PROCEDURE	The patient retracts and depresses the shoulders as if coming to military attention. The humerus is extended and abducted to 30°. The neck and head are hyperextended.
POSITIVE TEST	The radial pulse disappears.
IMPLICATIONS	The subclavian artery is being blocked by the costoclavicular structures of the shoulder.

Management of thoracic outlet syndrome focuses on correcting postural causes and muscle tightness that are compressing the neurovascular bundle. Postural awareness training and the use of ergonomically correct positioning, especially while driving, using a computer, or any repetitive activity, is indicated. The use of *nerve gliding* is also proposed to maintain the brachial plexus' moving freely from compression throughout its course.

 ON-FIELD EVALUATION OF SHOULDER INJURIES

The most important findings to be ruled out during the on-field evaluation of injuries to the shoulder complex are fractures and dislocations, which may often be con-

firmed through visual inspection or palpation of the area. When a humeral fracture or GH joint dislocation is suspected, the presence of a distal pulse must be determined. The absence of this pulse warrants the athlete's immediate transportation to a hospital.

Pain radiating through the shoulder and into the arms may indicate damage to one or more cervical nerve roots. A complete evaluation of the cervical or thoracic spine must be performed first when the mech-

Nerve gliding Movement of the nerve through surrounding tissues by placing the limb in various positions. The ability of the nerve to move freely during functional activity is assessed.

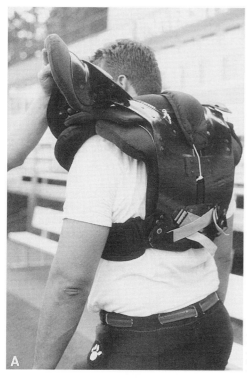
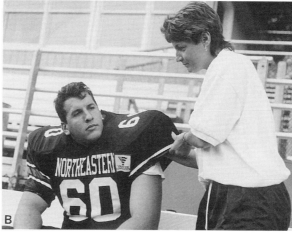

FIGURE 13–36. (A) The cantilever of football shoulder pads. **(B)** By reaching under the cantilever, the humeral head, AC joint, and distal clavicle can be palpated.

anism of injury or description of the symptoms implicates possible cervical spine trauma (see Chapter 11). The athlete is not moved until the possibility of spinal injury has been eliminated. Trauma to the spleen or myocardial dysfunction may also refer pain into the shoulder.

The on-field evaluation of patients with shoulder injuries is complicated by the presence of shoulder pads in sports such as football, ice hockey, and lacrosse. The examiner must become familiar with how to work around these pads and, if necessary, how to remove them without further aggravating the injury.

EQUIPMENT CONSIDERATIONS

Palpation Under the Shoulder Pads

Shoulder pads have at least one cantilever that arches over the acromion process and the deltoid muscle group (Fig. 13–36). The space provided by the cantilever provides enough room to reach under the jersey and palpate the humeral head, AC joint, and distal clavicle. By unfastening the strap that passes beneath the axilla and loosening the sternal fasteners, more room may be provided. It is also possible to palpate the proximal structures of the shoulder complex by entering the shoulder pads from the neck opening.

Because the clinician is palpating these structures without actually being able to see them, care must be used when applying pressure. The initial palpation must be performed gently, following the contours of the shoulder complex while checking for gross deformity.

Removal of the Shoulder Pads

Certain injuries such as AC or SC joint sprains, GH dislocations, or clavicular fractures require the removal of the shoulder pads to further evaluate the condition, begin treatment of the area, or transport the athlete. This must be done with as little movement of the injured extremity as possible to prevent further insult to the injured structures.

If the athlete's jersey is loose fitting, the examiner first removes the uninjured arm. After this is completed, the examiner slides the shirt up and over the head, then drops it down over the injured arm. In many cases, it is easier to remove the shirt and shoulder pads as a single unit (Fig. 13–37). If the shirt is extraordinarily tight fitting or is a practice jersey or in the case of a medical emergency, it may be cut off the athlete.

ON-FIELD HISTORY

- **Location of pain:** Trauma to the AC joint is described as pain localized to the upper shoulder, possibly projecting into the deltoid. Pain that involves the upper trapezius and radiates into the shoulder and arm that also is accompanied by weakness may indicate brachial plexus involvement.
- **Mechanism of injury:** A force that internally or externally rotates the GH joint can result in a GH subluxation or dislocation, especially if the humerus was abducted at the time of the injury. Falling on the tip of the shoulder or landing on an outstretched arm can result in a clavicular fracture, AC sprain, or SC sprain.

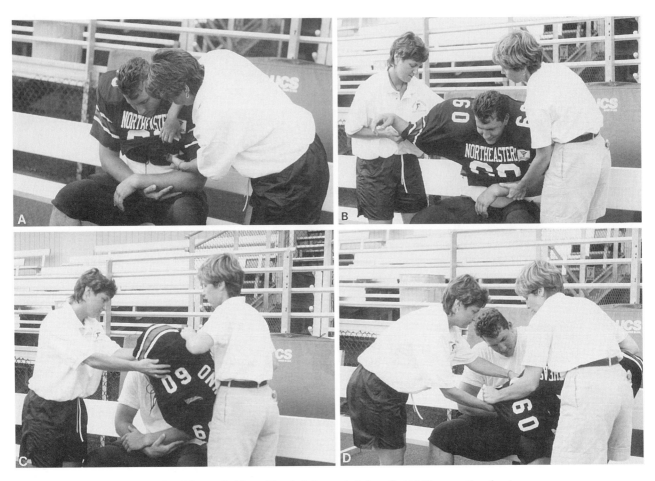

FIGURE 13–37. Removing shoulder pads (the athlete's left arm is injured). **(A)** Unsnap the chest straps. **(B)** Pull the shirt off the uninjured arm. **(C)** Lift the shoulder pads and shirt over the athlete's head. **(D)** Slide the shoulder pads from around the injured arm.

ON-FIELD INSPECTION

- **Arm posture:** The position of the shoulder, humerus, and arm can provide useful clues to the possible pathology.

  ○ **Arm splinted against the torso:** The humerus' being splinted against the ribs with the forearm supported across the body and the athlete's head looking away from the involved side can indicate a clavicular fracture or AC joint pathology.

  ○ **Arm hanging limply at the side:** The arm's dangling limply to the side often indicates **brachial plexus pathology** (see Chapter 11).

  ○ **Arm "locked":** The humerus' being locked in various positions can indicate a GH dislocation, with the position of the arm providing evidence of the direction of the dislocation. If it is **adducted and externally rotated,** suspect anterior or inferior GH dislocation; inferior dislocations are marked by a limited amount of abduction. If it is **abducted and internally rotated,** suspect posterior GH dislocation.

- **Gross deformity:** Initial inspection of the shoulder complex may be hindered by shoulder pads and jerseys. Gross deformity may be identified during palpation or visually after the equipment has been removed.

ON-FIELD PALPATION

- **Position of the humeral head:** If the GH joint is dislocated, the humeral head can be palpated sitting anterior, posterior, or inferior relative to the glenoid fossa.
- **AC joint alignment:** The AC joint is palpated for any abnormal play, including the **piano key sign.**
- **Clavicle:** Fractures of the clavicle are often readily apparent. If no visible sign of a fracture is present, palpate the length of the clavicle to identify subcutaneous discontinuity or areas of point tenderness.
- **Sternoclavicular joint:** The SC joint is palpated for bilateral symmetry and continuity.
- **Humerus:** The length of the humerus is palpated for signs of a fracture, especially in the area of the surgical neck.

ON-FIELD FUNCTIONAL TESTS

If the signs of a joint dislocation or bony fracture have been ruled out, the Apley's scratch test (see Box 13–3) can be used as a gross assessment of the athlete's willingness to move the involved extremity and the amount of motion available. The remaining ROM tests can be conducted on the sideline in the manner described in the ROM section of this chapter.

ON-FIELD NEUROLOGIC TESTS

Brachial plexus injuries cause pain, numbness, and paresthesia in the upper extremity, but the trauma actually involves the cervical nerve roots (see Chapter 12).

INITIAL MANAGEMENT OF ON-FIELD SHOULDER INJURIES

The following is suggested protocol for the initial management of major injuries to the shoulder complex and upper arm. In emergencies or when proper splinting materials are not available, the athlete's jersey may be used as a sling or the hand can be tucked into the belt of the pants (Fig. 13–38).

SCAPULAR FRACTURES

Although rare, reports of scapular fractures in football players have been reported.[63,64] Incidence of scapular fractures is highest among players who wear relatively small shoulder pads. Fractures may occur to the body

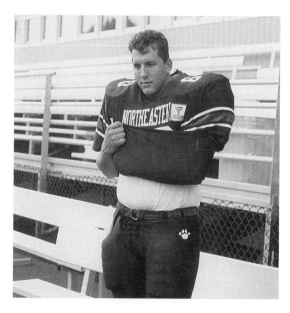

FIGURE 13–38. A temporary sling can be made by pulling the shirt up and over the involved arm.

of the scapula, but most often in the glenoid fossa, glenoid neck, or coracoid process secondary to a GH dislocation.

Patients with fractures of the glenoid fossa may present with many of the signs and symptoms of rotator cuff inflammation through decreased strength during abduction and external rotation. Any athlete suffering from a GH dislocation also needs a radiographic evaluation to rule out a secondary fracture to the glenoid or coracoid process.

To prevent motion, suspected scapular fractures are managed by immobilizing the arm on the affected side in a comfortable position. The athlete then is transported for further medical evaluation.

CLAVICULAR INJURIES

Clavicular Fractures

When fractures of the clavicle are suspected, the arm must be immobilized to prevent movement of the fractured segments. The athlete also is transported to a physician for a definitive diagnosis. Although rare, secondary damage to nerves and blood vessels may result from clavicular fractures.[65]

The shoulder may be immobilized using a sling or triangular bandage. A sling and swath approach may be more comfortable for the athlete by taking the weight of the arm off the involved clavicle.

Sternoclavicular Joint Injuries

The immediate concern with SC dislocations is the potential compromise to the underlying structures from a posterior dislocation. A neurologic and vascular examination of the extremity and carotid artery on the involved side must be performed immediately. Any absent or diminished findings are considered a medical emergency. The involved arm is immobilized using the procedure described for clavicular fractures and the athlete is immediately transported to an emergency medical facility. To avoid placing pressure on the structures posterior to the SC joint, the athlete must not be transported in the supine position.

Acromioclavicular Joint Injuries

Athletes displaying the signs and symptoms of an AC joint sprain require immobilization in a position that lessens the displacement between the clavicle and the acromial process. Initially, this may be achieved through the use of a foam pad with a hard shell held in place over the acromial process by a spica wrap and a sling supporting the weight of the arm (Fig. 13–39).

Most commonly, physicians choose to treat all but the most severe AC sprains nonsurgically.[12,29,66] Comparative follow-up studies of surgical and nonsurgical management of AC dislocations indicate that shoulders treated nonsurgically display little residual decrease in ROM or in strength deficits.[12]

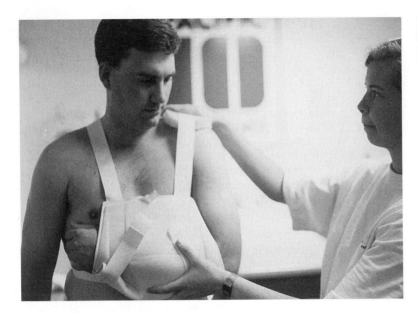

FIGURE 13–39. Management of an acromioclavicular joint sprain. A commercially available device (shown) or a sling and swath can be used to immobilize the shoulder and apply pressure to the AC joint.

Athletes suffering from AC joint contusions, in addition to the standard modality protocol, need to have the joint protected with additional padding during activity. Such protection may be obtained through the use of a foam doughnut pad with a hard shell held in place by an elastic spica wrap or elastic tape.

GLENOHUMERAL DISLOCATIONS

Because of the possibility of a dislocated humeral head causing additional trauma to the blood and nerve supply to the arm, it is important to monitor the distal pulses, check for circulation in the fingertips, and perform a sensory screen of the involved arm. Absence of a pulse indicates a medical emergency.

To transport the athlete, the arm is fixed in the position it has assumed through the use of a moldable splint (metal or vacuum) or towels placed between the humerus and torso. A sling or elastic wrap may be used to support the weight of the arm. It is important to keep the wrist and hand exposed so that the pulses may be rechecked.

Because of the threat of causing additional trauma to the GH structures, on-field reductions of GH dislocations should not be performed by anyone other than a physician. Forced reduction of the humeral head may damage the glenoid fossa, the coracoid process, or the neurovascular structures in the area. The athlete must be immediately transported to a physician as soon as the shoulder has been immobilized.

HUMERAL FRACTURES

Fractures of the humeral shaft and neck are often marked by extreme pain, dysfunction, and obvious deformity. Most humeral fractures occur as the result of a high-impact force. Spontaneous fractures occurring during pitching also have been reported.[67] Fractures in the region of the surgical neck can threaten the radial nerve. Fractures of the humeral head may occur secondary to GH dislocations and therefore initially go unnoticed because of the attention placed on the joint.

Fractures of the humeral shaft are splinted in the position they are found, using a moldable aluminum splint or a vacuum splint. The wrist and fingers remain exposed so that the radial pulse, circulation to the fingers, and sensation of the fingers can be monitored. The athlete is transported supine or on a stretcher. An immediate physician referral is indicated.

◆ REFERENCES

1. Perry, J: Normal upper extremity kinesiology. *Phys Ther*, 58:265, 1978.
2. Nyland, JA, Caborn, DN, and Johnson, DL: The human glenohumeral joint. A proprioceptive and stability alliance. *Knee Surg Sports Traumatol Arthrosc*, 6:50, 1998.
3. Wroble, RR: Sternoclavicular injuries. Managing damage to an overlooked joint. *The Physician and Sportsmedicine*, 23:19, 1995.
4. Culham, E, and Peat, M: Functional anatomy of the shoulder complex. *J Orthop Sports Phys Ther*, 18:342, 1993.
5. Norkin, CC, and Levangie, PK: The shoulder complex. In Norkin, CC, and Levangie, PK (eds): *Joint Structure and Function: A Comprehensive Analysis* (ed 2). Philadelphia, FA Davis, 1992, p 219.
6. Norkin, CC, and Levangie, PK: The shoulder complex. In Norkin, CC, and Levangie, PK (eds): *Joint Structure and Function: A Comprehensive Analysis* (ed 2). Philadelphia, FA Davis, 1992, p 220.
7. Kessler, RM, and Hertling, D: The shoulder and shoulder girdle. In Hertling, D, and Kessler, RM (eds): *Management of Common Musculoskeletal Disorders. Physical Therapy Principles and Procedures* (ed 2). Philadelphia, JB Lippincott, 1990, p 171.
8. Doody, SG, and Waterland, JC: Shoulder movements during abduction in the scapular plane. *Arch Phys Med Rehabil*, 51:595, 1970.
9. Hollinshead, WH, and Jenkins, DB: The shoulder. In Hollinshead, WH, and Jenkins, DB (eds): *Functional Anatomy of the Limbs and Back* (ed 5). Philadelphia, WB Saunders, 1981.
10. Boublik, M, and Hawkins, RJ: Clinical examination of the shoulder complex. *J Orthop Sports Phys Ther*, 18:379, 1993.
11. Norkin, CC, and Levangie, PK: The shoulder complex. In Norkin, CC, and Levangie, PK (eds): *Joint Structure and Func-*

tion: *A Comprehensive Analysis* (ed 2). Philadelphia, FA Davis, 1992, p 223.

12. Tibone, J, Sellers, R, and Tonino, P: Strength testing after third degree acromioclavicular dislocations. *Am J Sports Med*, 20:328, 1992.

13. Chandler, TJ, et al: Shoulder strength, power, and endurance in college tennis players. *Am J Sports Med*, 20:445, 1992.

14. Wilk, KE, et al: The strength characteristics of internal and external rotator muscles in professional baseball pitchers. *Am J Sports Med*, 21:61, 1993.

15. Reynolds, RS, and Hirschman, LD: An examination of the concentric and eccentric strength of the shoulder rotators (abstr). *Athletic Training: Journal of the National Athletic Trainers Association*, 26:154, 1991.

16. Gerber, C, and Krushell, RJ: Isolated rupture of the tendon of the subscapularis muscle. Clinical features in 16 cases. *J Bone Joint Surg*, 73(B):389, 1991.

17. Kelly, BT, Kadrmas, WR and Speer, KP: The manual muscle examination for rotator cuff strength. An electromyographic investigation. *Am J Sports Med*, 24:581, 1996.

18. Greis, PE, et al: Validation of the Lift-off test and analysis of subscapularis activity during maximal internal rotation. *Am J Sports Med*, 24:589, 1996.

19. Speer, KP: Anatomy and pathomechanics of shoulder instability. *Operative Techniques in Sports Medicine*, 1:252, 1993.

20. Hawkins, RJ, and Bokor, DJ: Clinical evaluation of shoulder problems. In Rockwood, CA, and Masten, FA (eds): *The Shoulder* (vol 1). Philadelphia, WB Saunders, 1990, pp 149–177.

21. Levy, AS, et al: Intra- and interobserver reliability of the shoulder laxity examination. *Am J Sports Med*, 27:460, 1999.

22. McFarland, EG, Campbell, G, and McDowell, J: Posterior shoulder laxity in asymptomatic athletes. *Am J Sports Med*, 24:468, 1996.

23. Prime, HT, Doig, SG, and Hooper, JC: Retrosternal dislocation of the clavicle: A case report. *Am J Sports Med*, 19:92, 1991.

24. Jougon, JB, Lepront, DJ, and Dromer, CE: Posterior dislocation of the sternoclavicular joint leading to mediastinal compression. *Ann Thorac Surg*, 61:711, 1996.

25. Brinker, MR, and Simon, RG: Pseudo-dislocation of the sternoclavicular joint. *J Orthop Trauma*, 13:222, 1999.

26. Brinker, MR, et al: A method for open reduction and internal fixation of the unstable posterior sternoclavicular joint dislocation. *J Orthop Trauma*, 11:378, 1997.

27. Gerber, C, Galantay, RV, and Hersche, O: The pattern of pain produced by irritation of the acromioclavicular joint and the subacromial space. *J Shoulder Elbow Surg*, 7:352, 1998.

28. Bach, BR, VanFleet, TA, and Novak, PJ: Acromioclavicular injuries: Controversies in treatment. *The Physician and Sports Medicine*, 20:87, 1992.

29. Bach, BR, and Novack, PJ: Chronic acromioclavicular joint pain: An overlooked problem. *The Physician and Sports Medicine*, 21:63, 1993.

30. Gartsman, GM: Arthroscopic resection of the acromioclavicular joint. *Am J Sports Med*, 21:71, 1993.

31. Gartsman, GM, et al: Arthroscopic acromioclavicular joint resection: An anatomical study. *Am J Sports Med*, 19:2, 1991.

32. Jacob, AK, and Sallay, PI: Theraputic efficacy of corticosteroid injections in the acromioclavicular joint. *Biomed Sci Instrum*, 34:380, 1997.

33. Phillips, AM, Smart, C, and Groom, AF: Acromioclavicular dislocation. Conservative or surgical therapy. *Clin Orthop*, Aug:10, 1998.

34. Press, J, et al: Treatment of grade III acromioclavicular separations. Operative versus nonoperative management. *Bull Hosp Jt Dis*, 56:77, 1997.

35. Rawes, ML and Dias, JJ: Long-term results of conservative treatment for acromioclavicular dislocation. *J Bone Joint Surg*, 78(B):410, 1996.

36. Shaffer, BS: Painful conditions of the acromioclavicular joint. *J Am Acad Orthop Surg*, 7:176, 1999.

37. Terry, GC, et al: The stabilizing function of passive shoulder restraints. *Am J Sports Med*, 19:26, 1991.

38. Jobe, FW, et al: Anterior capsulolabral reconstruction of the shoulder in athletes in overhand sports. *Am J Sports Med*, 19:428, 1991.

39. Stefko, JM, et al: Strain of the anterior band of the inferior glenohumeral ligament during capsule failure. *J Shoulder Elbow Surg*, 6:473, 1997.

40. Steinbeck, J, Liljenqvist, U, and Jerosch, J: The anatomy of the glenohumeral ligamentous complex and its contribution to anterior shoulder stability. *J Shoulder Elbow Surg*, 7:122, 1998.

41. Hsu, HC, et al: Influence of rotator cuff tearing on glenohumeral stability. *J Shoulder Elbow Surg*, 6:413, 1997.

42. Tsia, L, et al: Shoulder function in patients with unoperated anterior shoulder instability. *Am J Sports Med*, 19:469, 1991.

43. Hurley, JA, et al: Posterior shoulder instability: Surgical versus conservative results with evaluation of glenoid version. *Am J Sports Med*, 20:396, 1992.

44. Greenan, TJ, et al: Posttraumatic changes in the posterior glenoid and labrum in a handball player. *Am J Sports Med*, 21:153, 1993.

45. Blasier, RB, et al: Posterior glenohumeral subluxation: active and passive stabilization in a biomechanical model. *J Bone Joint Surg*, 79(A):433, 1997.

46. Warner, JJP, et al: Static capsuloligamentous restraints to superior-inferior translation of the glenohumeral joint. *Am J Sports Med*, 20:675, 1992.

47. Burns, TP, and Turba, JE: Arthroscopic treatment of shoulder impingement in athletes. *Am J Sports Med*, 20:13, 1992.

48. Kamkar, A, Irrgang, JJ, and Whitney, SL: Nonoperative management of secondary shoulder impingement syndrome. *Am J Sports Med*, 17:212, 1993.

49. Shankwiler, JA, and Burkhead, WZ: Diagnosis, evaluation, and conservative treatment of impingement syndrome. *Operative Techniques in Sports Medicine*, 1:89, 1994.

50. Brossmann, J, et al: Shoulder impingement syndrome: Influence of shoulder position on rotator cuff impingement: An anatomic study. *AJR Am J Roetgenol*, 167:1511, 1996.

51. Determe, D, et al: Anatomic study of the tendinous rotator cuff of the shoulder. *Surg Radiol Anat*, 18:195, 1996.

52. Banas, MP, Miller, RJ, and Totterman, S: Relationship between the lateral acromion angle and rotator cuff disease. *J Shoulder Elbow Surg*, 4:454, 1995.

53. Cuomo, F, et al: The influence of acromioclavicular joint morphology on rotator cuff tears. *J Shoulder Elbow Surg*, 7:555, 1998.

54. McConville, ORu and Iannotti, JP: Partial-thickness tears of the rotator cuff: Evaluation and management. *J Am Acad Orthop Surg*, 7:32, 1999.

55. Norkin, CC, and Levangie, PK: The shoulder complex. In Norkin, CC, and Levangie, PK (eds): *Joint Structure and Function: A Comprehensive Analysis* (ed 2). Philadelphia, FA Davis, 1992, p. 228.

56. Walch, G, et al: Subluxations and dislocations of the tendon of the long head of the biceps. *J Shoulder Elbow Surg*, 7:100, 1998.

57. Zanetti, M, et al: Tendinopathy and rupture of the tendon of the long head of the biceps brachii muscle: Evaluation with MR arthography. *AJR Am J Rotentgenol*, 170:1557, 1998.

58. Ludington, NA: Rupture of the long head of the biceps cubiti muscle. *Ann Surg*, 77:358, 1923.

59. Handelberg, F, et al: SLAP Lesions: A retrospective multicenter study. *Arthroscopy*, 14:856, 1998.

60. Morgan, CD, et al: Type II SLAP lesions: Three subtypes and their relationships to superior instability and rotator cuff tears. *Arthroscopy*, 14:553, 1998.

61. O'Brien, SJ, et al: The active compression test: A new and effective test for diagnosing labral tears and acromioclavicular joint abnormalities. *Am J Sports Med*, 26:610, 1998.

62. Baker, CL, and Liu, SH: Neurovascular injuries to the shoulder. *J Orthop Sports Phys Ther*, 18:360, 1993.

63. Culpepper, MI, and Roberts, JM: Case report: Fracture of the scapula in a professional football player. *Athletic Training: Journal of the National Athletic Trainers Association*, 20:35, 1985.

64. Cain, TE, and Hamilton, WP: Scapular fractures in professional football players. *Am J Sports Med*, 20:363, 1992.

65. Bartosh, RA, Dugdale, TW, and Nelson, R: Isolated musculocutaneous nerve injury complicating closed fracture of the clavicle: A case report. *Am J Sports Med*, 20:356, 1992.

66. Martel, JR: Clavicular nonunion: Complications with the use of mersilene tape. *Am J Sports Med*, 20:360, 1992.

67. Branch, T, et al: Spontaneous fractures of the humerus during pitching: A series of 12 cases. *Am J Sports Med*, 20:468, 1992.

14

The Elbow and Forearm

Serving as the link between the powerful movements of the shoulder and the *fine motor control* of the hand, the elbow is often overlooked as an area of potentially disabling injury. Even minor injuries to the elbow can severely hamper the ability to perform the most rudimentary movements. Fractures or other trauma involving the elbow or forearm can result in impairment of the neurovascular structures supplying the wrist, hand, and fingers. Therefore, examination of the elbow and forearm is often expanded to include the hand and shoulder.

 CLINICAL ANATOMY

The humerus, radius, and ulna form the elbow joint. The radius and ulna continue on to form the proximal and distal radioulnar joints of the forearm. The distal end of the humerus flares to form the medial and lateral epicondyles. The larger of these epicondyles, the **medial epicondyle,** is demarcated on its distal anteromedial border by the **trochlea.** Covered by articular cartilage, this epicondyle serves as the axis for rotation of the ulna on the humerus. Separated from the trochlea by the trochlear groove, the **capitellum** forms the lateral humeral articulating surface on the distal border of the **lateral epicondyle.** Unlike the trochlea, the dome-shaped capitellum does not extend to the posterior aspect of the humerus. Located immediately above the capitellum, the **radial fossa** is an indentation in the lateral epicondyle that accepts the radial head during elbow flexion (Fig. 14–1). The distal end of the humerus is anteriorly rotated 30 degrees relative to the humeral shaft.[1]

The **ulna** forms the medial border of the forearm. Proximally, the ulna articulates with the humerus and radius. The **semilunar notch,** an indentation lined with articular cartilage, fits snugly around the humeral trochlea. The proximal border of the ulna is formed by the **olecranon process,** a projection that fits into the humeral **olecranon fossa** during complete extension of the elbow. The distal border of the semilunar notch is

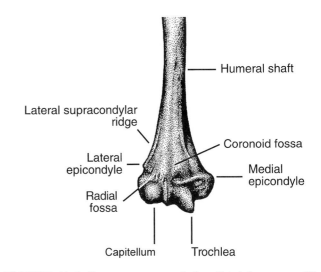

FIGURE 14–1. Bony anatomy of the distal humerus. The trochlea articulates with the ulna; the capitellum, with the radial head.

formed by the **coronoid process.** The ulnar coronoid process is received by the **coronoid fossa** of the humerus during elbow flexion. Lateral and slightly distal to the coronoid process, the **radial notch** is an indentation that accepts the radial head to form the **proximal radioulnar joint** (Fig. 14–2).

Located on the thumb-side of the forearm, the **radius** is lateral to the ulna when the body is in its anatomical position. The proximal articulating surface, the **radial head,** is disk shaped and concave to allow gliding and rotation on the capitellum. The border of the proximal radius is also covered with articular cartilage to allow it to rotate on the ulna. Distal to the radial head is the **bicipital tuberosity** (radial tuberosity), the insertion

---

Fine motor control   Specific control of the muscles allowing for completion of small, delicate tasks.

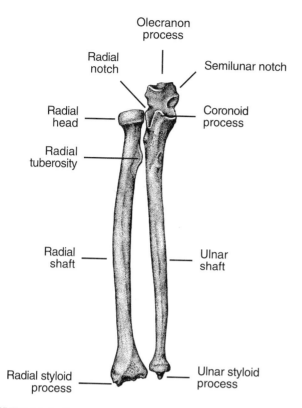

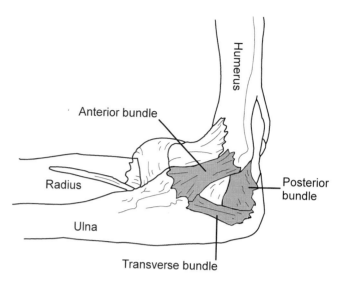

FIGURE 14–2. Bony anatomy of the radius and ulna.

FIGURE 14–3. Ulnar collateral ligament complex. This ligament is formed by the anterior oblique ligament, the posterior oblique ligament, and the transverse oblique ligament.

site for the biceps brachii. The **radial shaft** is triangular in shape and broadens medially and laterally at its distal end. The **radial styloid process** projects off the lateral border of the distal radius. **Lister's tubercle** projects off the posterior portion of the distal radius.

ARTICULATIONS AND LIGAMENTOUS ANATOMY

To function properly, the elbow must rely on the integrity of four individual articulations: the humeroulnar joint, humeroradial joint, proximal radioulnar joint, and distal radioulnar joint. The motion of elbow flexion and extension occurs at the humeroulnar and humeroradial joint. The motion of forearm *supination* and *pronation* occurs at the humeroradial, superior radioulnar, and inferior radioulnar joints.

Humeroulnar and Humeroradial Joints

A modified hinge joint, the **humeroulnar articulation,** allows for 1 degree of freedom of movement: flexion and extension. The design of this joint may allow up to 5 degrees of internal rotation of the ulna on the humerus, but this motion is an accessory one.

Also a modified hinge joint, the **humeroradial joint** permits 2 degrees of freedom of movement: (1) flexion and extension as the radial head glides around the capitellum and (2) rotation of the radius on the capitellum during the movements of pronation and supination.

Proximal and Distal Radioulnar Joints

The **proximal radioulnar joint** is formed by the convex radial head and the concave radial notch of the ulna. The **distal radioulnar joint** is formed by an articular disk between the radius and ulna where the concave ulnar notch of the radius articulates with the convex region of the ulna. The radioulnar joints have 1 degree of freedom of movement, pronation and supination. Their alignment is maintained by an interosseous membrane spanning the median (facing) borders of the bones, classifying it as a syndesmotic joint. During pronation, proximal joint motion occurs as the radius rotates within the radial notch of the ulna, causing the radius to cross over the ulna. At the distal joint, the disk and ulnar notch of the radius sweep across the ulna. The reverse occurs during supination.

Ligamentous Support

Support of the medial elbow against valgus forces is obtained from the **ulnar collateral ligament** (UCL), which is divisible into three unique sections, the anterior, transverse, and posterior bundles (Fig. 14–3). The **anterior bundle** originates from the inferior surface of the medial epicondyle and passes anterior to the axis of

---

Supination (forearm)   Movement at the radioulnar joints allowing for the palm to turn upward, as if holding a bowl of soup.

Pronation (forearm)   Movement at the radioulnar joints allowing for the palm to be turned downward.

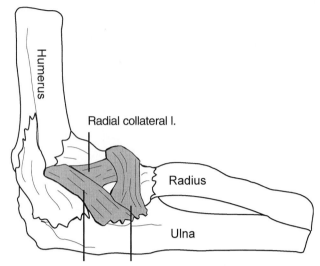

FIGURE 14–4. Lateral ligaments of the elbow. This group is formed by the radial collateral ligament, the lateral ulnar collateral ligament, and the annular ligament. The annular ligament is responsible for maintaining the relationship between the proximal radius and ulna.

rotation to insert on the medial aspect of the coronoid process. Unlike the other elbow ligaments, the anterior bundle is easily distinguishable from the joint capsule. Taut throughout the elbow's range of motion (ROM), this band is the primary restraint against valgus force. The **transverse bundle,** originating from the medial epicondyle and inserting on the coronoid process, provides little, if any, support to the medial elbow.[1] Inserting on the olecranon process, the **posterior bundle** is taut in flexion beyond 60 degrees.

Lateral support of the elbow is derived from the radial collateral, annular, lateral ulnar collateral, and the accessory lateral collateral ligaments (Fig. 14–4). The most important lateral stabilizing structure is the **lateral ulnar collateral ligament** (LUCL). Arising from the middle of the lateral epicondyle and inserting on the tubercle of the ulna, the LUCL provides lateral support of the ulna that is independent of the other lateral ligaments. Disruption of this ligament results in rotatory instability of the elbow joint.

The **radial collateral ligament** (RCL) is a thickened area in the lateral joint capsule between the lateral epicondyle and the annular ligament. In addition to resisting varus stresses, the RCL assists in maintaining the close relationship between the humeral and radial articulating surfaces.

Encircling the radial head, the **annular ligament** is a fibro-osseous structure that permits internal and ex-

ternal rotation of the radial head on the capitellum of the humerus. Both ends of the annular ligament attach to the coronoid process and form four fifths of a circle. The remaining one fifth of the circle is formed by the radial notch. This articulation receives additional support from the attachment of the RCL and the fibrous attachment of the supinator muscle. The distal end of the annular ligament narrows to conform to the shape of the radial head, preventing the radius from sliding distally.

During excessive supination, the anterior fibers of the annular ligament become taut; at the end of pronation, the posterior fibers are taut. When a varus stress is applied to the elbow, the **accessory lateral collateral ligament** (ALCL) assists the annular ligament and the RCL in preventing the radius from separating from the ulna.

Interosseous Membrane

A dense band of fibrous connective tissue, the fibers of the interosseous membrane run obliquely from the radius to the ulna and span the distance between the proximal and distal radioulnar joints (Fig. 14–5). This fibrous arrangement serves as a stabilizer against axial forces applied to the wrist, transmitting force from the radius to the ulna. This force is then transmitted to the humerus. The interosseous membrane also serves as the origin for many of the muscles acting on the wrist and hand.

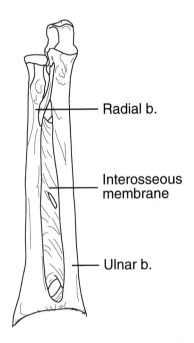

FIGURE 14–5. Interosseous membrane. The fibrous arrangement of this structure transmits force absorbed by the radius at the wrist to the ulna.

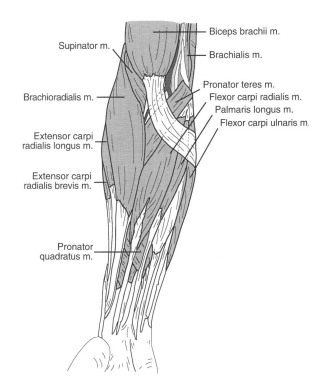

FIGURE 14–6. Anterior muscles of the forearm. These muscles serve primarily to flex the wrist and fingers and rotate the forearm.

MUSCULAR ANATOMY

The muscles inserting on the proximal radius and ulna act to flex or extend the elbow and pronate or supinate the forearm. Many of the prime movers of the wrist and hand originate from the humeral epicondyles and the proximal radius and ulna. The actions, origins, insertions, and innervation of the muscles producing elbow and forearm motion are presented in Table 14–1. Chapter 15 discusses the forearm muscles acting on the wrist and hand.

Elbow Flexor and Supinator Group

The **biceps brachii, brachialis,** and **brachioradialis** are the prime flexors of the elbow. The relative position (i.e., pronated, supinated, or neutral) of the forearm determines which of the muscles provides the primary contribution to the movement. When the forearm is supinated, the biceps brachii is the prime elbow flexor; when the forearm is pronated, the brachialis is the primary contributor to elbow flexion. When the forearm is in its neutral position (radial side upward), the brachioradialis is the primary elbow flexor. The **supinator** is assisted by the biceps brachii during forceful supina-

tion. The brachioradialis contributes to both pronation and supination when the forearm is at the end of the opposite motion (i.e., the brachioradialis contributes to pronation when the forearm is fully supinated). The lateral bulk of the forearm muscles is formed by the extensor carpi radialis longus, extensor carpi radialis brevis, extensor carpi ulnaris, and extensor digitorum communis muscles (Fig. 14–6).

Elbow Extensor and Pronator Group

The muscles acting to extend the elbow, the **triceps brachii** and **anconeus,** do not influence pronation or supination of the forearm. However, the anconeus does stabilize the ulna during these movements (Fig. 14–7). The primary pronators of the forearm are the **pronator teres,** arising from just above the medial epicondyle of the humerus and inserting on the anterolateral aspect of the radius, and the **pronator quadratus,** located on the distal forearm running obliquely from the medial aspect of the ulna to the radius. The remaining medial bulk of the proximal forearm is formed by the flexor carpi radialis, palmaris longus, flexor digitorum superficialis, and flexor carpi ulnaris muscles, which are discussed in Chapter 15.

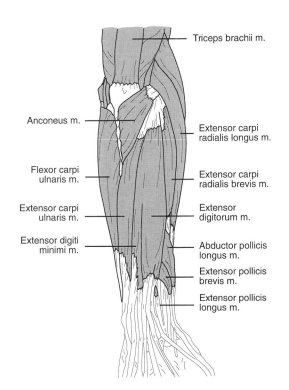

FIGURE 14–7. Posterior muscles of the forearm. These muscles serve to extend the wrist and fingers.

Table 14–1
MUSCLES ACTING ON THE ELBOW AND FOREARM

Muscle	Origin	Insertion	Action	Innervation	Root
Anconeus	• Posterior surface of the lateral epicondyle	• Lateral border of the olecranon process	Elbow extension Stabilization of ulna during pronation and supination	Radial	C7, C8
Biceps brachii	• Long head: Supraglenoid tuberosity of scapula • Short head: Coracoid process of scapula	• Radial tuberosity	Elbow flexion Forearm supination Shoulder flexion	Musculocutaneous	C5, C6
Brachialis	• Distal one-half of anterior humerus	• Coronoid process of ulna • Ulnar tuberosity	Elbow flexion	Musculocutaneous	C5, C6
Brachioradialis	• Lateral supracondylar ridge of humerus	• Styloid process of radius	Elbow flexion Forearm pronation May assist with forearm supination	Radial	C5, C6
Extensor carpi radialis brevis	• Lateral epicondyle via the common extensor tendon • Radial collateral ligament	• Base of the 3rd metacarpal	Wrist extension Radial deviation	Radial	C6, C7
Extensor carpi radialis longus	• Supracondylar ridge of humerus	• Radial side of the 2nd metacarpal	Wrist extension Radial deviation Elbow flexion	Radial	C6, C7
Extensor carpi ulnaris	• Lateral epicondyle via the common extensor tendon	• Ulnar side of the base of the 5th metacarpal	Wrist extension Ulnar deviation	Deep radial	C6, C7, C8
Extensor digitorum communis	• Lateral epicondyle via the common extensor tendon	• Into the dorsal surface of the base of the middle and distal phalanges of each of the four fingers	Wrist extension MCP extension PIP extension	Deep radial	C6, C7, C8
Flexor carpi radialis	• Medial epicondyle via the common flexor tendon	• Palmar aspect of the bases of the 2nd and 3rd metacarpal bones	Forearm pronation Wrist flexion Radial deviation Elbow flexion	Median	C6, C7
Flexor carpi ulnaris	• Humeral head: Medial epicondyle via the common flexor tendon • Ulnar head: Medial border of the olecranon; proximal two-thirds of the posterior ulna	• Pisiform • Hamate • Palmar aspect of the base of the 5th metacarpal	Wrist flexion Ulnar deviation Elbow flexion	Ulnar	C8, T1

Muscle	Action	Proximal attachment	Distal attachment	Nerve	Root
Flexor digitorum profundus	DIP flexion PIP flexion Wrist flexion	• Anteromedial proximal three fourths of the ulna and associated interosseous membrane	• Bases of the distal phalanges of the second through fifth digits	Lateral: Median nerve Medial: Ulnar nerve	C8, T1

Flexor digitorum superficialis	PIP flexion
	MCP flexion
	Wrist flexion
		• Humeral head:
		  Medial epicondyle via the common flexor tendon; ulnar collateral ligament
		• Ulnar head:
		  Coronoid process
		• Radial head:
		  Oblique line of radius
			• Middle phalanges of the second through fifth digits	Median	C7, C8, T1

Palmaris longus	Wrist flexion	• Medial epicondyle via the common flexor tendon	• Flexor retinaculum • Palmar aponeurosis	Median	C6, C7
Pronator quadratus	Forearm pronation	• Anterior surface of the distal one fourth of ulna	• Lateral portion of the distal one fourth of the radius	Anterior interosseous nerve	C8, T1

Pronator teres	Forearm pronation
	Elbow flexion
		• Humeral head:
		  Proximal to the medial epicondyle of humerus
		• Ulnar head:
		  Coronoid process
			• Middle one third of the lateral radius	Median	C6, C7

Supinator	Forearm supination	• Lateral epicondyle • Radial collateral ligament • Annular ligament • Supinator crest of ulna	• Proximal one third of radius	Deep radial	C6, C7, C8

Triceps brachii	Elbow extension
	Shoulder extension
		• Long head:
		  Infraglenoid tuberosity of scapula
		• Lateral head:
		  Posterolateral surface of the proximal one-half of the humeral shaft
		• Medial head:
		  Posteromedial surface of the humerus
			• Olecranon process of the ulna	Radial	C7, C8

DIP = distal interphalangeal; MCP = metacarpophalangeal; PIP = proximal interphalangeal.

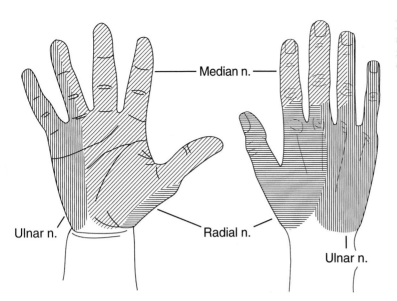

FIGURE 14–8. The median, ulnar, and radial nerve sensory distribution in the hand. Note that texts differ on the exact delineation between the cutaneous distribution of the individual nerves.

NERVES

Three primary nerves cross the elbow: the median nerve, ulnar nerve, and radial nerve. Their relatively superficial course across the elbow and in the distal portion of the forearm predispose them to acute traumatic injury. Figure 14–8 presents the sensory distribution of these nerves in the hand.

Median Nerve

Crossing the anterior elbow in the same path as the brachial artery, the median nerve travels deep within the forearm muscles to follow the flexor digitorum superficialis down the middle of the anterior forearm. As it approaches the wrist, the median nerve becomes superficial once again as it passes between the flexor digitorum superficialis and flexor carpi radialis tendons (beneath the palmaris longus) to pass through the carpal tunnel and enter the hand. With the exception of the flexor carpi ulnaris and the medial portion of the flexor digitorum profundus, the median nerve supplies all of the wrist flexor muscles and the pronator teres and pronator quadratus. Shortly after crossing the elbow joint, the **anterior interosseous nerve** projects off the median nerve to pass under the two heads of the pronator teres.

Ulnar Nerve

The ulnar nerve enters the elbow by traveling between the olecranon process and the medial epicondyle. After superficially crossing the joint line, it courses deep to follow the ulnar artery to the middle of the forearm. At this point, it moves medial to the flexor carpi ulnaris tendon and crosses the wrist joint superficial to the flexor retinaculum, traveling between the pisiform and the hook of the hamate **(tunnel of Guyon)** to provide sensory and motor innervation to the hand. The ulnar nerve innervates the flexor carpi ulnaris muscle and the medial portion of the flexor digitorum profundus in the forearm.

Radial Nerve

The radial nerve courses distally on the posterior aspect of the humerus and then crosses the lateral aspect of the elbow's joint line between the brachioradialis and brachialis muscles. Then it diverges into two branches, the superficial and deep branches. The **superficial branch,** the direct continuation of the radial nerve, provides sensation to the dorsum of the wrist, hand, and thumb (see Fig. 14–8). The **deep branch** provides motor innervation exclusively to the extensor carpi radialis longus and brevis, supinator, brachioradialis, extensor pollicis longus, abductor pollicis longus, extensor pollicis brevis, and extensor digitorum muscles. Therefore, it is possible to injure the deep branch of the radial nerve without experiencing any sensory loss. However, critical motor loss does occur.

BURSAE

Several bursae are found in the elbow region, but few have clinical significance. The **subcutaneous olecranon bursa,** located between the olecranon process and the skin, is susceptible to trauma. This bursa is usually injured after a direct blow to the olecranon process. The other significant bursa is the **subtendinous olecranon bursa.** This structure is located between the tendon of triceps brachii and the olecranon process. This bursa may become inflamed secondary to repetitive stresses applied to the joint.

CLINICAL EVALUATION OF THE ELBOW AND FOREARM

The elbow may be traumatized by valgus or varus forces, forced hyperextension, direct blows to the olecranon process or the epicondyles, or most commonly, secondary to overuse from the inherently unnatural motion of throwing. The stresses placed on the elbow are increased when improper technique is used or when an individual compensates for shoulder pain or decreased ROM by altering elbow motion.

HISTORY

The onset and location of the symptoms are among the most important history findings surrounding elbow trauma. Determining the cause-and-effect relationship between the mechanism and the onset of the symptoms is helpful in developing a successful treatment plan. In addition, because the elbow may be the site of referred pain from the cervical spine, all other possible sources of pain must be ruled out.

EVALUATION MAP: ELBOW AND FOREARM

1. HISTORY

Location of the pain
Onset of the symptoms
Mechanism of injury
Technique
Associated sounds
Associated sensations
Previous history
General medical health

2. INSPECTION

Anterior Structures
Carrying angle
Cubital fossa

Medial Structures
Medial epicondyle
Flexor muscle mass

Lateral Structures
Alignment
Cubital recurvatum
Extensor muscle mass

Posterior Structures
Bony alignment
Olecranon process and bursa

3. PALPATION

Anterior Structures
Biceps brachii
Cubital fossa
Brachioradialis
Wrist flexor group
Pronator quadratus

Medial Structures
Medial epicondyle
Ulna
Ulnar collateral ligament

Lateral Structures
Lateral epicondyle
Radial head
Lateral ulnar collateral ligament
Capitellum
Annular ligament
Radial collateral ligament

Posterior Structures
Olecranon process
Olecranon fossa
Triceps brachii
Anconeus
Ulnar nerve
Wrist extensors
Finger extensors
Thumb musculature

4. RANGE OF MOTION TESTS

Active Range of Motion
Flexion
Extension
Pronation
Supination

Passive Range of Motion
Flexion
Extension
Pronation
Supination

Resisted Range of Motion
Flexion
Extension
Pronation
Supination

5. LIGAMENTOUS TESTS

Valgus stress test
Varus stress test

6. NEUROLOGIC TESTS

Radial nerve
Medial nerve
Ulnar nerve

7. SPECIAL TESTS

Elbow Sprains
Posterolateral rotatory instability test

Epicondylitis
Tennis elbow test

Nerve trauma
Tinel's sign

- **Location of the symptoms:** The examination begins by localizing the area of pain, the type of pain, and any dysfunction that is reported, remembering the possibility of these symptoms being referred by pathology that is proximal or distal to the elbow (Table 14–2). Referred pain usually presents with symptoms localized within the distribution of a specific nerve or nerve root.
- **Onset of the symptoms:** Elbow pain may have an acute or chronic onset. Traumatic injury is traced to a specific onset of pain and symptoms. Chronic conditions of the elbow may initially produce minor symptoms related to activity but can rapidly progress to constant pain during all activities of daily living (ADLs).
- **Mechanism of injury:** The elbow is well protected at the side of the body and is not subjected to an overburden of harmful stress. The elbow can be acutely injured by the high amount of stress generated while throwing or during weight lifting. The elbow can also be acutely injured if the hand is planted on the ground so that it is away from the side of the body and forces are transmitted across the joint.

    Most elbow injuries tend to be caused by repetitive low-load stresses. Throwing a ball or using a racquet can cause stresses capable of resulting in tendinitis or neuritis in the elbow. Adolescents are vulnerable to repetitive stress injuries at open growth plates as stresses are transmitted across these areas. Question athletes who are involved in throwing activities about the level of activity, including the number of throws, time span in which the throws occurred, and any changes in the throwing technique. The use of computers, musical instruments, or machinery that requires repetitive wrist and finger mo-

tions may also produce symptoms or exacerbate the current symptoms.

- **Technique:** Overuse injuries commonly lead to suspicion of improper technique or poor elbow biomechanics or weak muscles. Ask the patient about changes in technique or equipment or increases in the intensity or duration of play. Questions raised during the history-taking process regarding biomechanics may necessitate that the examiner work with the athlete and coach in further evaluating technique and making corrections as needed.
- **Associated sound and sensations:** An elbow that chronically locks, clicks, or pops during movement may indicate osteochondritis dessicans or an unstable joint. The presence of these structures may be confirmed through diagnostic imaging.
- **Previous history:** Pain that is associated with seasonal activity may be related to poor conditioning. Because of the possibility of referred pain, patients with nontraumatic origin of pain or suspected of having referred pain from the cervical spine require investigation about a history of previous trauma, paresthesia, strength loss, or other dysfunction in this area.
- **General medical health:** A history of other medical conditions needs to be ascertained. Certain vascular problems, neurologic involvement, or systemic diseases may predispose the elbow to inflammatory or degenerative injuries or illnesses.

INSPECTION

The upper arm, elbow, and forearm are inspected for the evidence of contusions, ecchymosis, scars, and swelling. These conditions can place pressure on the ra-

Table 14–2
POSSIBLE TRAUMA BASED ON THE LOCATION OF PAIN

	Location of Pain			
	Lateral	**Anterior**	**Medial**	**Posterior**
Soft tissue injury	Annular ligament sprain Radial collateral ligament sprain Radiocapitellar chondromalacia Lateral epicondylitis (tennis elbow) Radial nerve trauma	Biceps brachii tendinitis Rupture of the biceps brachii tendon Median nerve trauma Anterior capsule sprain	Ulnar collateral ligament sprain Medial epicondylitis Ulnar nerve trauma	Olecranon bursitis Triceps brachii tendinitis Triceps tendon rupture
Bony injury	Avulsion of the common extensor tendon Lateral epicondyle fracture Radius fracture Radial head fracture Radial head dislocation	Osteochondral fracture Avulsion of the biceps brachii tendon	Avulsion of the common flexor tendon Medial epicondyle fracture Ulna fracture Osteophyte formation	Fracture of the olecranon process

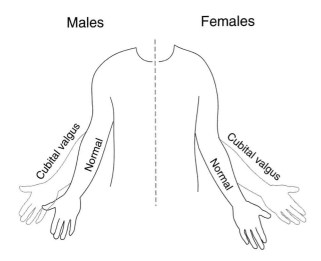

FIGURE 14–9. Angular relationships at the elbow. On average, women have an increased angle between the midline of the forearm and the humerus (the "carrying angle") relative to men. Long term participation in overhand throwing sports increases this angle.[2]

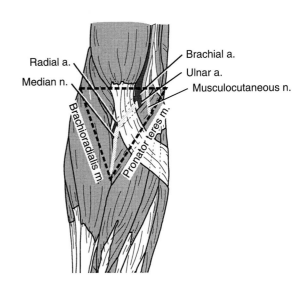

FIGURE 14–10. The cubital fossa is a triangular area demarcated by the brachioradialis muscle laterally and the pronator teres medially. The brachial artery and its two subdivisions (the radial and ulnar arteries), the median nerve, and the musculocutaneous nerve pass through this fossa.

dial, median, and ulnar nerves, causing symptoms to radiate to the forearm and hand.

Inspection of the Anterior Structures

- **Carrying angle:** The angle formed by the long axis of the humerus and ulna, the carrying angle, ranges from 10 to 15 degrees of valgus in women and 5 to 10 degrees in men. Normally this angle is reduced or entirely eliminated during flexion.[1] With the elbow fully extended and the forearm supinated, note the presence of an increased carrying angle, **cubitus valgus,** or a decreased angle, **cubitus varus** (Fig. 14–9). Baseball pitchers may exhibit cubitus valgus in the throwing arm, an adaptation to repeated valgus loading during the throwing motion.[2] Other deviations of this angle may reflect a fracture of one or more bones or their epiphyseal plates.
- **Cubital fossa:** Swelling within the cubital fossa can place pressure on the local neurovascular structures, raising the suspicion of injury to the nearby soft tissues, including the distal biceps tendon (Fig. 14–10).

Inspection of the Medial Structures

- **Medial epicondyle:** The medial epicondyle is the most prominent structure on the medial aspect of the elbow, but it may become masked by excessive swelling.
- **Flexor muscle mass:** The wrist flexor muscle mass is observable along the medial aspect of the elbow and forearm. The mass widens approximately 2 to 3 inches below the elbow. Loss of girth along the medial forearm may occur secondary to prolonged immobilization or disuse associated with long-term tendinitis.

Inspection of the Lateral Structures

- **Alignment of the wrist and forearm:** The wrist should be centered on the forearm. Compression of the radial nerve as it crosses the elbow joint can inhibit the wrist extensors, resulting in drop wrist syndrome (see Chapter 15).[3]
- **Cubital recurvatum:** The alignment of the forearm and humerus when the elbow is fully extended is noted. Although normally a straight line, extension beyond 0 degrees (cubital recurvatum) is common, especially in women (Fig. 14–11).
- **Extensor muscle mass:** The wrist extensor muscle mass is observable along the lateral aspect of the elbow and forearm. The mass widens approximately 1 to 2 inches below the elbow. Loss of girth along the lateral forearm can occur secondary to prolonged immobilization or disuse after long-term tendinitis or radial nerve involvement.

Inspection of the Posterior Structures

- **Bony alignment:** When the elbow is flexed to 90 degrees, the medial epicondyle, lateral epicondyle, and olecranon process form an isosceles triangle. When the elbow is extended, these structures typically lie within a straight line. Deviation from this alignment may reflect bony pathology.
- **Olecranon process and bursa:** Flexion of the elbow makes the bony contour of the olecranon process visible. Acute injury or overuse conditions may cause the olecranon bursa to rupture, swell, or inflame, masking the outline of the olecranon (Fig. 14–12).

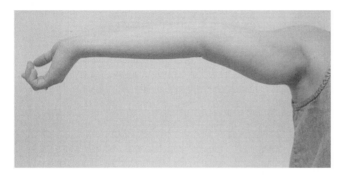

FIGURE 14–11. Cubital recurvatum. A normal hyperextension of the elbow.

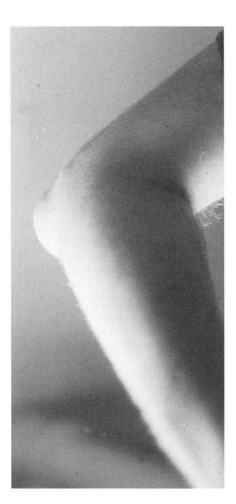

FIGURE 14–12. Inflammation of the subcutaneous olecranon bursa. This structure is often traumatized by a direct blow to the olecranon process.

PALPATION

Many of the structures of the upper extremity insert or originate at the elbow, making careful, precise palpation a must for the examiner. Tenderness elicited with palpation must be correlated with other subjective and physical objective findings. Some areas, such as the humeral condyles, may be tender in the uninjured elbow.

Palpation of the Anterior Structures

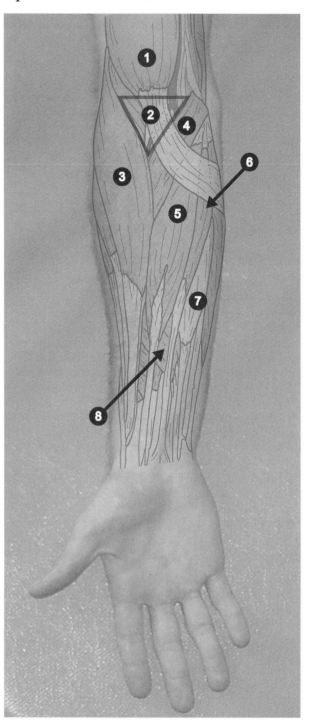

FIGURE 14–13. Making the brachioradialis more prominent. An isometric contraction with the forearm in the neutral position and the elbow flexed to 90° causes the brachioradialis to become prominent.

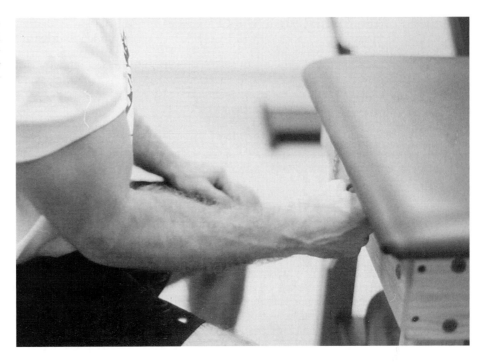

1. **Biceps brachii:** Palpate the muscle belly of the biceps brachii along the anterior aspect of the humerus until its tendon inserts onto the radius. The tendon is more easily recognized if the elbow is held in 90 degrees of flexion. The distal biceps brachii tendon can be ruptured with a forceful eccentric contraction, resulting in deformity of the muscle.

2. **Cubital fossa:** Passing within the cubital fossa, palpate the brachial artery medial to the biceps brachii tendon. In some individuals, the median nerve can be palpated within the fossa. The musculocutaneous nerve also passes through this area but cannot be palpated because it runs underneath the pronator teres muscle (see Fig. 14–10).

3. **Brachioradialis:** To palpate the brachioradialis, place the forearm in the neutral position. The most lateral of the elbow flexor muscles, the brachioradialis is made prominent by resisting elbow flexion while the forearm is held in this position (Fig. 14–13). Palpate the length of the brachioradialis muscle from its attachment on the lateral supracondylar ridge to the distal attachment on the radial styloid process.

4–7. **Wrist flexor group:** Near their origin on the medial epicondyle, the bellies of the wrist flexors cannot be distinguished from one another. As they progress distally, the individual tendons of the pronator teres (4), flexor carpi radialis (5), palmaris longus (absent in some individuals) (6), and the flexor carpi ulnaris (7), become identifiable as they near the wrist. Figure 14–14 presents a memory aid to assist in identifying these muscles.

8. **Pronator quadratus:** Laying deep to the wrist and finger flexors, palpate the area over the pronator quadratus muscle on the distal aspect of the anterior forearm.

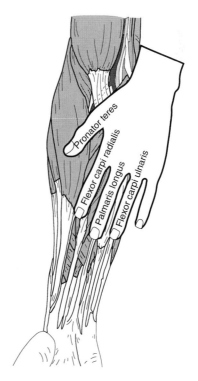

FIGURE 14–14. Method of approximating the superficial muscles of the flexor forearm.

Palpation of the Medial Structures

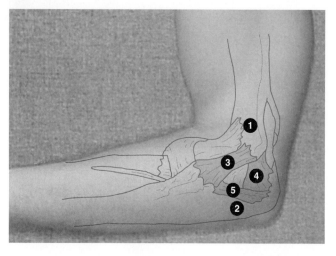

1. **Medial epicondyle:** Locate the medial epicondyle, prominent along the distal aspect of the humerus as it flares away from the shaft of the bone. The common wrist flexor tendon attaches at the epicondyle; palpation of the epicondyle elicits exquisite tenderness in the presence of medial epicondylitis.
2. **Ulna:** Identify the base of the ulna, located distal to the elbow's medial joint space. The shaft is prominent throughout its length, especially along its medial and posterior (dorsal) surfaces. The anterior aspect of the shaft can be palpated along the distal two thirds of its length as it arises from beneath the mass of the wrist flexors to its point of articulation with the wrist.
3–5. **Ulnar collateral ligament:** To better identify the UCL, have the patient flex the elbow to between 20 and 30 degrees. The anterior band (3) of this ligament can be directly palpated as it crosses the angle formed by the humerus and ulna. Continue around the medial aspect of the elbow to palpate the area over the posterior (4) and transverse bundles (5) of the UCL.

Palpation of the Lateral Structures

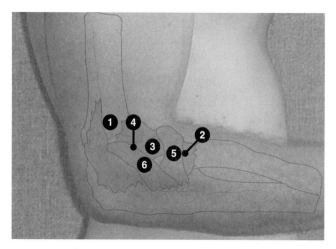

1. **Lateral epicondyle:** Smaller than the medial epicondyle, identify the lateral epicondyle, prominent as it projects from the distal end of the humerus. Palpate this structure for tenderness caused by inflammation of the common origin of the wrist extensors.
2. **Radial head:** Moving slightly distal from the lateral joint line, locate and palpate the head of the radius underneath the posterior aspect of the wrist extensor muscles. It becomes more identifiable as it rolls beneath the examiner's finger as the forearm is pronated and supinated. During flexion and extension of the elbow, the radial head moves with the forearm.
3. **Radial collateral ligament:** Locate the RCL between the radial head and the lateral epicondyle. Although the RCL is not normally identifiable, its length is palpated for signs of tenderness.
4. **Capitellum:** Moving proximally from the radial head across the joint line, find the rounded capitellum. While passively pronating and supinating the forearm with the elbow bent to various degrees of flexion, palpate the capitellum and radial head for the presence of crepitus, which indicates radiocapitular chondromalacia.[4]
5. **Annular ligament:** Although this structure cannot be identified directly during palpation, palpate the area overlying the radial head for evidence of tenderness, crepitus, or swelling.
6. **Lateral ulnar collateral ligament:** Move superiorly and anteriorly from the radial head to locate the LUCL as it crosses the lateral joint line. Passively extending the forearm may make this structure more palpable.

Palpation of the Posterior Structures

1. **Olecranon process:** Locate the ulna's olecranon process, the prominent rounded bone on the posterior aspect of the elbow. Palpate this structure for tenderness and mobility. A forced hyperextension of the elbow or a direct backward fall on the elbow may cause a fracture. The **olecranon bursa** is not palpable unless it is inflamed, in which case it can potentially result in a large amount of swelling and tenderness and mask the underlying bone.
2. **Olecranon fossa:** With the elbow partially flexed and the triceps muscle relaxed, palpate the olecranon fossa on the posterior humerus, located just superior to the olecranon process.
3. **Triceps brachii:** Slightly flex the elbow to make the fibers of the triceps brachii tendon stand out from its attachment on the olecranon. The posterolateral portion of this muscle is formed by the lateral head of the triceps and the posteromedial portion by the long head. The medial head runs deep to the long head but becomes palpable over the medial aspect of the distal humerus. The length of the triceps brachii is palpated for tenderness or deformity.
4. **Anconeus:** Palpate the anconeus between the lateral epicondyle and the olecranon process.

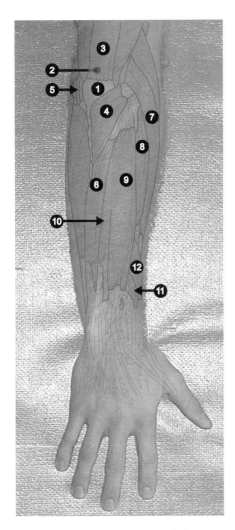

5. **Ulnar nerve:** With the elbow in full extension, palpate the sulcus formed by the medial epicondyle
and the medial border of the olecranon process for
the ulnar nerve, identifiable as a thin, cordlike
structure. Determine if the ulnar nerve can be displaced from the sulcus by gently moving it medi-

ally and laterally. Inflammation of the nerve may
result in a positive Tinel's sign, burning, pain, or
paresthesia along the medial border of the forearm
and little finger-during palpation. Also palpate the
ulnar nerve as the elbow is flexed and extended to
determine if the nerve subluxates out of its groove.

6–8. **Wrist extensors:** Resist wrist extension to make
the extensor carpi ulnaris (6), extensor carpi radialis
brevis (7), and extensor carpi radialis longus (8),
muscles become prominent. With the forearm
pronated, the wrist extensors can be palpated distal
to the lateral epicondyle. The superficial muscle is
the extensor carpi radialis longus; the inferior, the
extensor carpi radialis brevis.

9–10. **Finger extensors:** Resist finger extension to make
the extensor digitorum (9) and extensor digiti minimi muscles (10) prominent.

11–12. **Thumb musculature:** Ask the patient to extend
and abduct the thumb to more easily identify the
extensor pollicis brevis (11) and abductor pollicis
longus muscles (12).

RANGE OF MOTION TESTING

The motions at the elbow joint are limited to flexion
and extension and pronation and supination. If epicondylitis or trauma to the ulnar, median, or radial
nerve is suspected, ROM testing of the wrist and fingers must be incorporated. Box 14–1 presents goniometric measurement of elbow flexion and extension.

Active Range of Motion

• **Flexion and extension:** Most of the elbow's ROM is
composed of flexion, ranging between 145 and 155
degrees from the neutral position and occurs in the
sagittal plane around a coronal axis (Fig. 14–15). Extension is usually limited at 0 degrees by the olecranon process, but hyperextension is common (see Fig.
14–11).

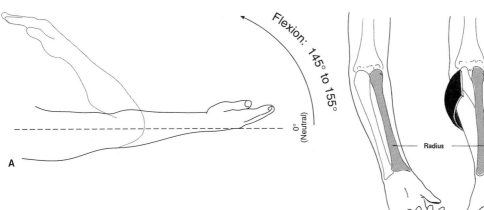

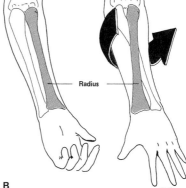

FIGURE 14–15. Active range of motion at the elbow.
(A) Elbow flexion and extension; **(B)** forearm pronation and supination.

Box 14–1
ELBOW GONIOMETRY

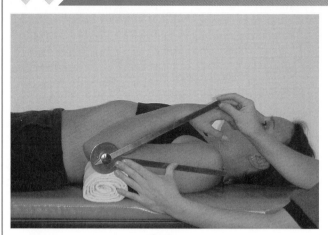

Flexion

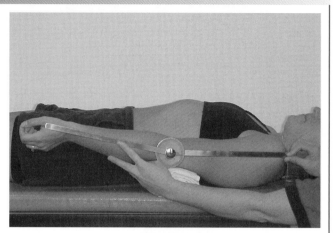

Extension

PATIENT POSITION	Supine with the humerus close to the body, the shoulder in the neutral position, and the forearm supinated A bolster placed under the distal humerus
GONIOMETER ALIGNMENT	
FULCRUM	Centered over the lateral epicondyle
STATIONARY ARM	Aligned with the long axis of the humerus, using the acromion process as the proximal landmark
MOVEMENT ARM	Aligned with the long axis of the radius, using the styloid process as the distal landmark.

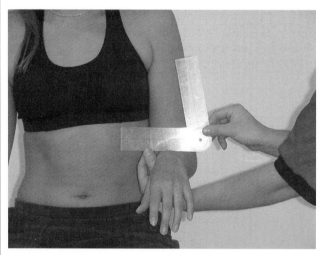

Pronation

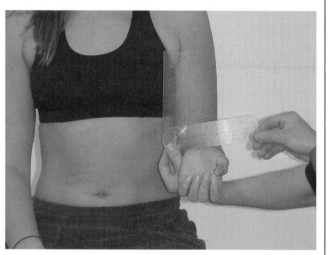

Supination

PATIENT POSITION	Sitting with the humerus held against the torso The elbow flexed to 90°	
GONIOMETER ALIGNMENT		
FULCRUM	Centered lateral to the ulnar styloid process	
STATIONARY ARM	Aligned parallel to the midline of the humerus	
MOVEMENT ARM	Across the dorsal portion of the forearm	Across the ventral portion of the forearm

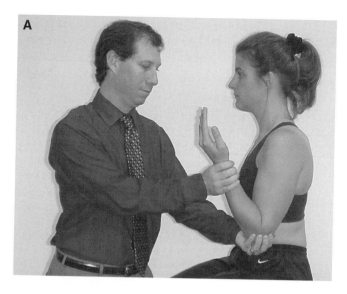

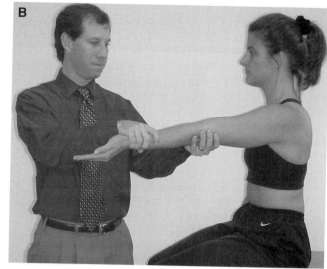

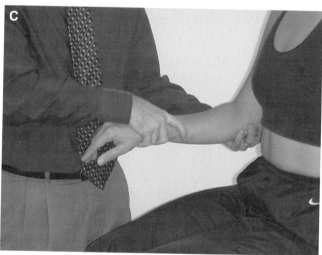

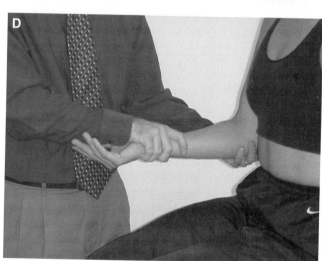

FIGURE 14–16. Passive range of motion for **(A)** and **(B)** flexion and extension and **(C)** and **(D)** pronation and supination.

- **Pronation and supination:** The neutral position for forearm pronation and supination is the thumb and radius pointing upward. The total ROM is 170 to 180 degrees, with approximately 90 degrees of motion in each direction. This movement occurs in the transverse plane around the longitudinal axis relative to the anatomical position.

Passive Range of Motion

- **Flexion and extension:** Position the elbow in extension with the forearm supinated and the shoulder joint stabilized to prevent compensatory motion (Fig. 14–16). Flex the elbow until soft tissue approximation between the bulk of the biceps brachii muscle and the muscles of the anterior forearm limits the motion, creating a soft end-feel. Extension produces a hard end feel by the bony contact between the olecranon process and the olecranon fossa.

- **Pronation and supination:** Position the shoulder in the neutral position and flex the elbow to 90 degrees. Support the forearm so that the radius and thumb are pointing upward and the elbow is stabilized against the torso to prevent shoulder motion. During pronation, the end-feel may be hard as the radius and ulna contact each other or firm secondary to stretching of the proximal and distal radioulnar ligaments and the interosseous membrane. Supination normally meets with a firm end-feel caused by the stretching of the proximal and distal radioulnar ligaments and the interosseous membrane.

Resisted Range of Motion

Resisted ROM is illustrated in Box 14–2. However, even injured patients are capable of overpowering the clinician during pronation and supination testing. An alternative method of resisting pronation and supination is

Box 14–2
RESISTED RANGE OF MOTION FOR THE ELBOW

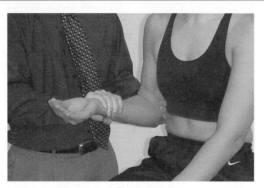

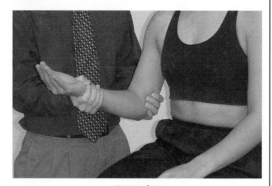

	Flexion	**Extension**

STARTING POSITION	Sitting or standing
	The shoulder in the neutral position
	To isolate a specific muscle during the test:
	  Biceps brachii: forearm supinated
	  Brachialis: forearm pronated
	  Brachioradialis: forearm neutral
		Sitting or standing
		The shoulder in the neutral position
		The forearm supinated

STABILIZATION	Anterior humerus, being careful not to compress the involved muscles	Posterior humerus, being careful not to compress the involved muscles
RESISTANCE	Over the distal forearm	Over the posterior aspect of the distal forearm
MUSCLES TESTED	See forearm position	Triceps brachii, anconeus

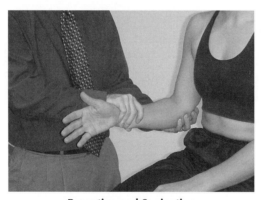

Pronation and Supination

STARTING POSITION	Seated The shoulder in the neutral position and the elbow flexed to 90° The radius facing upwards
STABILIZATION	Proximal to the elbow to prevent abduction or adduction of the glenohumeral joint
RESISTANCE	**Pronation:** resistance applied to the palmar aspect of the forearm **Supination:** resistance applied to the dorsal surface of the forearm
MUSCLES TESTED	**Pronation:** pronator quadratus, pronator teres, brachioradialis **Supination:** biceps brachii, supinator

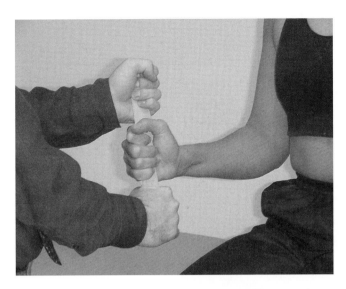

FIGURE 14–17. Alternate method for resisted range of motion testing during pronation and supination.

through the use of a 1-inch diameter dowel. The patient grasps the middle of the dowel as if holding a hammer. The examiner then applies resistance to both ends of the dowel as the patient pronates and supinates the forearm (Fig. 14–17). This test for pronation and supination is more functionally oriented than the clinical test, but the patient is more likely to compensate using humeral movements.

LIGAMENTOUS TESTING

Single-plane instability of the elbow joint can be tested only in the frontal plane when the joint is not fully extended. Valgus and varus stress ligamentous testing of

the fully extended elbow is meaningless because the olecranon process is securely locked within its humeral fossa. However, laxity demonstrated in this position may indicate an epiphyseal fracture.

Test for Medial Ligament Laxity

The anterior oblique portion of the UCL is the primary restraint of the medial elbow against valgus stress. Trauma to this structure displays valgus laxity throughout the ROM, and injury to the other medial ligaments is unlikely without first damaging the anterior oblique portion of the UCL (Box 14–3).

Test for Lateral Ligament Laxity

Less common than medial ligament laxity, straight-plane varus laxity of the elbow occurs when the RCL is damaged. Involvement of the annular ligament, ALCL, or LUCL increases the laxity by allowing the radial head to separate from the ulna. The integrity of these structures is determined through varus stress tests (Box 14–4).

NEUROLOGIC TESTING

The muscles innervated by the brachial plexus range from the shoulder into the elbow, forearm, and hand. Nerve impingement occurring in the cervical or shoulder region can result in disruption of the sensory or motor function (or both) in the elbow, forearm, and hand. Likewise, nerve trauma in the elbow refers its symptoms into the wrist, hand, and fingers (Fig. 14–18). Neurologic testing may also require that an upper quarter screen be performed (see Box 1–6).

FIGURE 14–18. Local neuropathies of the elbow, forearm, and hand. Correlate these findings with those of an upper quarter neurological screen (see Box 1–6).

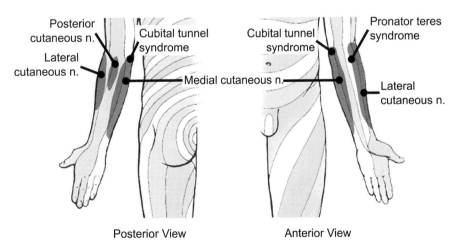

Box 14–3
VALGUS STRESS TEST

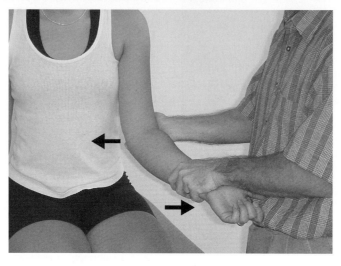

PATIENT POSITION	Standing or sitting The elbow flexed to 25°
POSITION OF EXAMINER	Standing lateral to the joint being tested One hand supporting the lateral elbow with the fingers reaching behind the joint to palpate the medial joint line with the opposite hand grasping the distal forearm
EVALUATIVE PROCEDURE	A valgus force is applied to the joint. The procedure is repeated with the elbow in various degrees of flexion.
POSITIVE TEST	Increased laxity compared with the opposite side, or pain, or both
IMPLICATIONS	Sprain of the ulnar collateral ligament, especially the anterior oblique portion. Laxity beyond 60° of flexion also implicates involvement of the posterior oblique fibers.
COMMENT	Laxity may also indicate epiphyseal injury.

 ## PATHOLOGIES AND RELATED SPECIAL TESTS

This section discusses the evaluation of patients with acute and chronic elbow injuries. The number of special tests for the elbow is relatively limited compared with those associated with the other joints described in this text. The conclusion of specific injuries is largely based on the correlation between the history of injury and examination findings.

ELBOW SPRAINS

Because the elbow is stabilized by the locking of the olecranon process in its fossa when the joint is extended, strain is placed on the ligaments when the elbow is flexed. A valgus or varus stress from a blow or forceful motion delivered to a flexed elbow is dissi-pated by the collateral ligaments. The trauma becomes more complex when a rotational component is added to the elbow. When a valgus or varus force is placed on an extended elbow, the olecranon process, in addition to the collateral ligament, must be evaluated for injury. A hyperextension mechanism can stress the elbow's anterior capsule or compress the posterior structures.

Ulnar Collateral Ligament

The UCL is stressed secondary to a valgus loading of the humeroulnar joint. Acutely, this stress results from a force delivered to the lateral elbow. Valgus loading of the UCL also occurs during normal athletic movements but is especially great during the overhand pitching motion. The force load generated during this motion is so great that the UCL cannot tolerate the tension on its own. As a result, the UCL must rely on the triceps brachii, the wrist flexor-pronator muscles, and the an-

Box 14–4
VARUS STRESS TEST

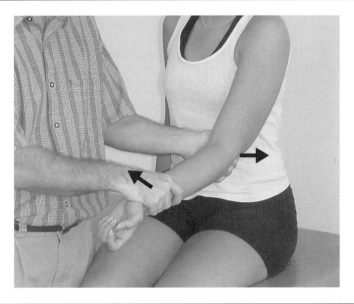

PATIENT POSITION	Standing or sitting The elbow flexed to 25°
POSITION OF EXAMINER	Standing medial to the joint being tested One hand supporting the medial elbow with the fingers reaching behind the joint to palpate the lateral joint line with the opposite hand grasping the distal forearm
EVALUATIVE PROCEDURE	A varus force is applied to the elbow. This process is repeated with the joint in various degrees of flexion.
POSITIVE TEST	Increased laxity compared with the opposite side, and/or pain is produced.
IMPLICATIONS	Moderate laxity reflects trauma to the radial collateral ligament. Gross laxity may also indicate damage to the annular or accessory lateral collateral ligament, causing the radius to displace from the ulna.
COMMENT	Laxity may also indicate epiphyseal injury.

coneus to provide dynamic stabilization to counteract the valgus force placed on this joint.[5] The LUCL can also be injured if the force is sufficient.

The chief complaint is pain on the medial aspect of the elbow that intensifies with motion. Compression of the radial nerve may produce radicular pain in the forearm and fingers. Tensile forces placed on the ulnar nerve can cause paresthesia in the distal ulnar nerve distribution. Swelling may be present on the anterior, medial, and posterior borders of the joint. In most medial sprains, the anterior oblique section of the UCL is traumatized. Tenderness is noted along its length from the medial epicondyle to the coronoid process. If the elbow is flexed past 60 degrees, the posterior oblique band may also be painful. ROM testing may reveal pain secondary to stretching of the ligaments or from joint instability. Valgus stress testing demonstrates pain and laxity at various degrees of flexion (Table 14–3). Be-

cause of the relationship of the ulnar nerve to the medial elbow, a neurologic examination of the forearm, wrist, hand, and fingers may also be required.

Tears of the LUCL permit a transient rotatory subluxation of the humeroulnar joint and an associated subluxation of the radiohumeral joint.[6] This results in the radius and ulna acting as a single unit as they rock away from the articulating surfaces of the humerus. Clinically, patients with this condition may be evaluated through the **posterolateral rotatory-instability test** (Box 14–5).

In cases of chronic overload to the medial side of the elbow, the initial treatment is to alleviate any repetitive forces on the elbow. Local modalities are helpful to decrease pain and inflammation. ROM is progressed in a pain-free manner. Strengthening of the muscles surrounding the joint is performed to assist in stabilizing the elbow against valgus forces. In athletes who perform

Table 14–3
EVALUATIVE FINDINGS: Ulnar Collateral Ligament Sprain

Examination Segment	Clinical Findings	
History	***Onset:***	Acute or insidious
	Pain characteristics:	Medial aspect of elbow
	Mechanism:	Acute: valgus stress placed on the ulnar collateral ligament
		Insidious: repeated valgus loading of the elbow.
	Predisposing conditions:	Repeated activities that exert tensile stresses on the medial aspect of the elbow (e.g., throwing); internal rotation deficits in the throwing athlete
Inspection	Swelling may be present in the anterior medial, and posterior aspects of the elbow.	
Palpation	Palpation of the medial elbow from the medial epicondyle to the coronoid process may elicit tenderness and crepitus.	
Functional Tests	***AROM:***	Limited secondary to pain because of stretching of the ligaments or joint instability
	PROM:	Pain elicited by stretching of the ligaments
	RROM:	Strength decreased secondary to pain and joint instability
Ligamentous Tests	Valgus testing at 25° of flexion demonstrates increased laxity and pain at the medial elbow and may elicit paresthesia in the ulnar nerve distribution.	
	Testing at other degrees of flexion (e.g. 45°, 60°, and 90°) may elicit symptoms	
Neurologic Tests	Sensory and motor testing of the ulnar nerve distribution may be affected.	
	Tinel sign at the ulnar nerve may be positive if the nerve has been traumatized.	
Special Tests	Posterolateral rotatory instability test of the elbow	

AROM = active range of motion; PROM = passive range of motion; RROM = resisted range of motion.

Box 14–5
POSTEROLATERAL ROTATORY INSTABILITY TEST

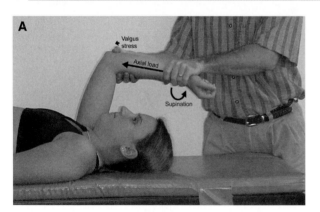 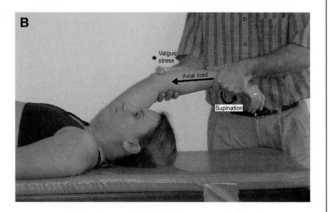

Test for posterolateral rotatory instability of the elbow consists of extending the elbow with a axial load, valgus stress, and forearm supination. The elbow subluxates as it nears full extension. A palpable reduction may be felt as the elbow is moved back into flexion.

PATIENT POSITION	Supine
	The shoulder and elbow flexed to 90° and the forearm is fully supinated.
POSITION OF EXAMINER	Standing at the head of the patient
	One hand grasping the proximal forearm with the other hand grasping the distal forearm at the wrist (**A**).
EVALUATIVE PROCEDURE	While applying a valgus stress and axial compression, the elbow is extended and the forearm is maintained in full supination (**B**).
	The elbow then can be taken back into flexion (not shown).
POSITIVE TEST	The elbow subluxates as it is extended and can be felt to relocate as it is flexed.
IMPLICATIONS	Chronic instability of the elbow

throwing motions, the ROM at the shoulder also requires assessment. Over time, throwers lose shoulder internal rotation and gain excessive amounts of external rotation. A tremendous amount of valgus force is placed on the medial elbow during the cocking and acceleration phases of overhead pitching. Inclusion of ROM exercises for increasing internal rotation of the shoulder is often needed to balance the stresses at the medial elbow.

Radial Collateral Ligament

Injury to the RCL complex is rare because in most positions, the body shields the elbow from varus forces. Additionally, the stresses placed on the elbow joint during throwing and racquet sports are absorbed by the UCL and the wrist extensor muscles.

Varus forces placed on the lateral elbow ligaments can result in trauma to the RCL and, possibly, the annular ligament. Trauma to the RCL or its component parts (see Fig. 14–4) not only results in varus laxity but also may disrupt the articulation between the radial head and the capitellum. The signs and symptoms of RCL sprains are similar to those of UCL trauma but may be compounded by pain, laxity, or weakness during pronation and supination.

The treatment for patients with radial collateral ligament sprains is similar to that for those with medial elbow sprains. With radial collateral sprains, strengthening focuses on strengthening the wrist extensors, supinators, brachioradialis, and the surrounding elbow muscles to provide dynamic stabilization against varus stresses.

EPICONDYLITIS

Both the lateral and medial epicondyles serve as the origin for many of the muscles acting on the wrist and fingers. The most common ailment afflicting the epicondyles is inflammation of the periosteum and the associated tendons. Prolonged stressful loads may result in stress- or avulsion fractures.

Lateral Epicondylitis

Inflammation of the lateral epicondyle irritates the common attachment of the wrist extensor group (extensor carpi ulnaris, extensor carpi radialis longus, extensor carpi radialis brevis, extensor digitorum communis, and supinator). Although any or all of these muscles' functions may be inhibited, the extensor carpi radialis brevis is the muscle most commonly affected. Repeated, forceful eccentric contractions of the wrist extensor muscles result in the accumulation of degenerative forces at their attachment site.[7] The relatively small area of attachment for these muscles causes a great force load to be applied to the bone as these muscles contract.

Lateral epicondylitis is prevalent in racquet sports, affecting more than half of all regular tennis players,[8] leading to its colloquial name, **"tennis elbow."** Most common in individuals older than age 40 years, the chief complaint is pain over the lateral epicondyle, decreased grip strength, and pain with gripping. In patients who play racquet sports, the symptoms are increased during backhand strokes.

Inspection of the painful area may reveal swelling, and palpation of the area may produce pain. Active wrist extension results in pain that worsens with resisted motion. Pain elicited during passive stretching of the extensor muscles and resisted finger extension has also been demonstrated to be a reliable indicator of this condition.[9] The **tennis elbow test** is sensitive to even mild cases of lateral epicondylitis (Box 14–6). Entrapment of the radial nerve may produce symptoms that are similar to lateral epicondylitis (Table 14–4).

Treatment of lateral epicondylitis involves avoiding the activities that aggravate the condition. Oral anti-inflammatory medications and local anti-inflammatory modalities also are used. Local corticosteroid injections may be beneficial, allowing the patient to progress through the rehabilitation program of flexibility and strengthening.[10] Therapeutic exercises involve stretching and strengthening around the elbow with the main focus on the wrist extensor group. Although many advocate the use of "tennis elbow" straps, the full benefits of these devices are inconclusive.[1]

As the patient recovers, a return to the initial activities creating the inflammation may require an assessment of the equipment being used (i.e., racquet size and stiffness, ergonomic assessment of computer work station) and the technique being used. Many patients who develop this condition from athletic participation may benefit from a coach's lesson to improve their techniques. Sometimes activity modifications that reduce or eliminate repetitive contraction of the wrist extensors may be beneficial.

Medial Epicondylitis

Activities involving the swift, powerful snapping of the wrist and pronation of the forearm load the medial epicondyle. As with its lateral counterpart, medial epicondylitis involves point tenderness at the origin of the pronators teres, flexor carpi radialis, palmaris longus, and flexor carpi ulnaris tendon on the medial epicondyle. The length of the pronator teres muscle also may be tender (Table 14–5). In young baseball pitchers, the tension build-up in the medial epicondyle may result in avulsion of the common tendon from its attachment site, **"little leaguer's elbow"** (Fig. 14–19). Medial epicondylitis may cause neuropathy of the ulnar nerve, causing symptoms to radiate into the medial forearm and fingers.[11]

The treatment of patients with medial epicondylitis follows the protocol described for those with lateral epicondylitis.

Box 14–6
TEST FOR LATERAL EPICONDYLITIS ("TENNIS ELBOW" TEST)

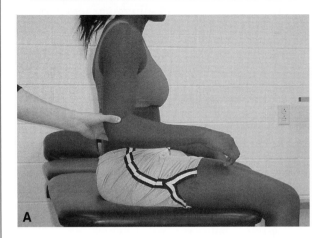

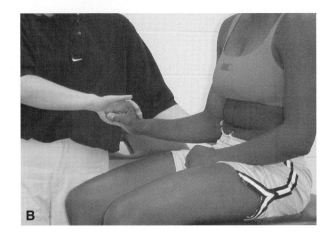

(A) The location of the thumb on the lateral epicondyle. **(B)** Resisted wrist extension.

PATIENT POSITION	Seated with the tested elbow flexed to 90°, the forearm pronated, and the fingers flexed.
POSITION OF EXAMINER	Standing lateral to the patient with one hand positioned over the dorsal aspect of the wrist and hand
EVALUATIVE PROCEDURE	The examiner resists wrist extension while palpating the lateral epicondyle and common attachment of the wrist extensors.
POSITIVE TEST	Pain in the lateral epicondyle
IMPLICATIONS	Lateral epicondylitis (tennis elbow)
MODIFICATION	This test may also be performed with the elbow in extension.

Table 14–4
EVALUATIVE FINDINGS: Lateral Epicondylitis

Examination Segment	Clinical Findings	
History	***Onset:***	Insidious
	Pain characteristics:	Lateral epicondyle and proximal portion of the common tendons of the wrist extensors; radicular pain into the wrist extensor muscles is possible with advanced cases
	Mechanism:	Overuse syndrome involving repeated, forceful wrist extension; radial deviation, supination, or grasping in an overhand position
	Predisposing conditions:	Repeated eccentric loading of the wrist extensor muscles
Inspection	Swelling possibly present over the lateral epicondyle	
Palpation	Pain and possible crepitus over the lateral epicondyle and proximal portion of the common wrist extensor tendon	
Functional Tests	***AROM:***	Pain with combined wrist extension and elbow flexion; radial deviation also possibly painful
	PROM:	Pain during passive wrist flexion, especially with elbow extension
	RROM:	Pain with resisted wrist extension and resisted finger extension when elbow extended
Ligamentous Tests	Not applicable	
Neurologic Tests	Not applicable	
Special Tests	Test for lateral epicondylitis ("tennis elbow" test)	
Comments	In racquet sports, pain is worsened with the backhand stroke and may be related to improper size of the racquet handle grip or a racquet that is too tightly strung.	

AROM = active range of motion; PROM = passive range of motion; RROM = resisted range of motion.

Table 14–5
EVALUATIVE FINDINGS: Medial Epicondylitis

Examination Segment	Clinical Findings	
History	*Onset:*	Insidious
	Pain characteristics:	Medial epicondyle and the proximal portion of the adjacent wrist flexor and pronator muscles.
	Mechanism:	Repeated, forceful flexion or pronation of the wrist (or both)
	Predisposing conditions:	Repeated activities that eccentrically load the medial elbow muscles (e.g., throwing, golfing)
Inspection	Swelling in the area over the medial epicondyle	
Palpation	Point tenderness and crepitus over the medial epicondyle; tenderness in the proximal portion of the wrist flexor group, especially the pronator teres	
Functional Tests	*AROM:*	Pain during wrist flexion; wrist extension possibly resulting in pain secondary to stretching the involved muscles
	PROM:	Pain during wrist extension, especially with elbow extension
	RROM:	Decreased strength and pain during wrist flexion, pronation, or ulnar deviation
Ligamentous Tests	Not applicable	
Neurologic Tests	Sensory and motor tests to identify potential ulnar nerve neuropathy	
Special Tests	None	

AROM = active range of motion; PROM = passive range of motion; RROM = resisted range of motion.

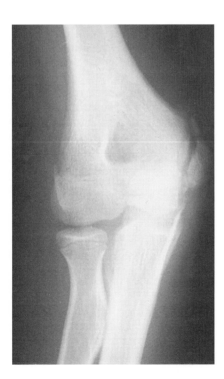

FIGURE 14–19. Avulsion of the origin of the wrist flexor muscles, "little leaguer's elbow." This condition can mimic medial epicondylitis.

DISTAL BICEPS TENDON RUPTURE

Rupture of the distal biceps tendon is debilitating because of the loss of strength during elbow flexion and supination. The mechanism of injury involves the eccentric loading of the biceps brachii when the elbow is extended.[12–14] The patient reports immediate pain and the sensation of a "pop" within the elbow. A loss of arm strength during elbow flexion and forearm supination is also apparent.

Inspection of the cubital fossa reveals swelling and ecchymosis. A palpable defect in the distal biceps tendon may also be noted. Active ROM (AROM) and passive ROM (PROM) may remain within normal limits, but a definitive decrease in strength during resisted ROM (RROM) testing for elbow flexion and supination is present. (Table 14–6). Routine radiographs can be used to rule out avulsion of the bicipital (radial) tuberosity.

Conservative treatment of distal biceps tendon rupture has usually resulted in less than desirable outcomes. Thus surgical repair is the preferred method of treatment.[15–17] Postsurgical rehabilitation consists of a progressive return of ROM after a 1-week period of total immobilization. Submaximal strengthening is begun at 4 weeks and progressed as tendon healing in the bone solidifies by week 8.[14]

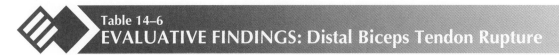

Table 14–6
EVALUATIVE FINDINGS: Distal Biceps Tendon Rupture

Examination Segment	Clinical Findings	
History	*Onset:*	Acute
	Pain characteristics:	Pain in the cubital fossa that decreases over time
	Mechanism:	Eccentric loading of the biceps brachii while the elbow is extended
	Predisposing conditions:	More commonly seen after the third decade of life as the tensile strength of the tendon decreases
Inspection	Swelling and ecchymosis in the cubital fossa	
Palpation	Palpable defect in the distal biceps tendon; the lesion may be more easily recognized if the patient attempts to hold the elbow in 90° of flexion	
Functional Tests	*AROM:*	Possibly within normal limits or slightly decreased during elbow flexion and extension and forearm pronation and supination secondary to pain
	PROM:	Within normal limits; a partial tearing of the tendon may produce pain during elbow extension and pronation as the remaining fibers are stretched
	RROM:	Decreased strength for elbow flexion and supination
Ligamentous Tests	None	
Neurologic Tests	None	
Special Tests	None	
Comments	The radial tuberosity (the distal attachment site for the biceps brachii) may be avulsed.	

AROM = active range of motion; PROM = passive range of motion; RROM = resisted range of motion.

OSTEOCHONDRITIS DESSICANS OF THE CAPITULUM

Osteochondritis dessicans of the capitellum develops gradually because of increased valgus loading compressing the radial head and capitellum with overhead throwing. Although the exact etiology is not known, osteochondritis dessicans is thought to be the result of disrupted blood flow to the area creating an osteochondral defect over time.

The patient complains of lateral elbow pain that increases with activity. A flexion contracture is usually present. Radiographic examination reveals either a nondisplaced fragmented defect or a loose body within the joint (Table 14–7). If the fragment has not separated, rest along with a progressive program of ROM and strengthening is used. A loose body warrants surgical intervention to remove the fragment and curettage the defect. In either case, the return to previous athletic endeavors is guarded, especially in the throwing athlete.

NERVE TRAUMA

The superficial location of the ulnar nerve and the anatomical tunnels through which the radial and median nerves pass can result in traumatic or insidious impairment of their functions. Inhibition of these nerves in the area of the elbow causes the symptoms to radiate distally, resulting in dysfunction in the wrist, hand, and fingers. This dysfunction is characterized by paresthesia, decreased grip strength, and the inability to actively extend the wrist depending on the nerve involved.

As the **ulnar nerve** crosses the medial aspect of the elbow's joint line, it is relatively superficial, predisposing it to concussive forces. If the nerve's supporting structures are unstable, the nerve may chronically subluxate as the forearm is flexed, resulting in a progressive inflammation. The increased size of the inflamed structures causes a decrease in the cross-sectional size of the cubital tunnel leading to compression of the ulnar nerve.[18]

Impairment of the ulnar nerve manifests its symptoms through decreased sensory and motor function in the hand and fingers. Acute trauma of the ulnar nerve causes a burning sensation in the medial forearm, little finger, and ring finger and decreased strength of the finger flexor muscles, lumbricals, interossei, thumb abductors, and flexor carpi ulnaris. Chronic neurologic deficit to these muscles causes the hand to deviate radially during flexion. This deficit also inhibits the individual's ability to make a fist because of a lack of flexion in the fourth and fifth distal interphalangeal (DIP) joints, characterized by a *clawhand* position (see Chapter 15).

Clawhand Hand positioning characterized by hyperextension of the metacarpophalangeal joints and flexion of the middle and distal phalanges resulting from trauma to the median and ulnar nerves.

Table 14–7
EVALUATIVE FINDINGS: Osteochondritis Dessicans of the Capitulum

Examination Segment	Clinical Findings	
History	**Onset:**	Insidious
	Pain characteristics:	Dull, lateral elbow pain that is increased with activity
	Mechanism:	Repetitive valgus loading of the elbow joint; compressive loading of the humeroulnar joint
	Predisposing conditions:	Improper biomechanics
Inspection	Arm possibly postured with the elbow in flexion	
Palpation	Tenderness over the lateral epicondyle and lateral joint line	
Functional Tests	**AROM:**	Decreased extension; flexion contracture possible
	PROM:	Decreased extension; flexion contracture possible
	RROM:	Pain secondary to compression placed through the joint
Ligamentous Tests	None	
Neurologic Tests	None	
Special Tests	None	
Comments	Typically seen in adolescents participating in throwing athletics. The prognosis for a full return to activity is guarded.	

AROM = active range of motion; PROM = passive range of motion; RROM = resisted range of motion.

The **radial nerve** is most often injured by deep lacerations of the elbow or secondary to fractures of the humerus or radius. The deep branch of the radial nerve is dedicated to motor function of the thumb's extensors, wrist extensors, finger extensors, and supinators. Thus, there is no sensory loss associated with trauma to this nerve segment. If the superficial branch is lacerated, sensory loss results on the posterior forearm and hand. Inflammation or irritation of the ulnar and radial nerves as they cross the elbow joint can be detected through Tinel's sign (Fig. 14–20).

Entrapment of the radial nerve, **radial tunnel syndrome** (RTS), clinically resembles lateral epicondylitis. Radial tunnel syndrome differs from epicondylitis in that the symptoms of RTS persist for more than 6 months with tenderness over the radial tunnel. Also, the symptoms may reproduced with resisted supination and during resisted extension of the middle finger, possibly resembling the findings of lateral epicondylitis.[19]

The **median nerve** is typically injured or compressed on the distal portion of the forearm. However, pressure in the cubital fossa may compress the nerve as it crosses the joint line. The most common clinical manifestation of median nerve trauma, **carpal tunnel syndrome,** is discussed in Chapter 15. A branch of the median nerve, the anterior interosseous nerve, can become compressed by the pronator teres, causing **pronator teres syndrome.** This syndrome is characterized by the patient's ability to pinch the tips of the thumb and index fingers together.

Forearm Compartment Syndrome

The forearm contains three identifiable compartments: the volar, dorsal, and mobile wads.[20] Increased pressures within these compartments, possibly the result of hypertrophic muscles, hemorrhage, or fractures of the mid forearm, distal radius, or supracondylar area, increases the risk for compromising circulation and neurologic function of the hand.[20,21]

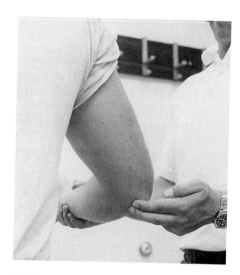

FIGURE 14–20. Tinel's sign for neuropathy. In the presence of neuropathy, tapping on the ulnar (shown) or radial nerve results in a burning sensation in the hand.

In its early stages, forearm compartment syndrome is marked by complaints of pressure in the forearm, sensory disruption in the hand and fingers, decreased muscular strength, and pain during passive elongation of the involved muscles. Because of their deep location, the flexor digitorum profundus and the flexor pollicis longus are the most commonly affected muscles.[20] As the condition becomes more chronic or increases in severity, a decrease or absence of the radial or ulnar pulses are noted and **Volkmann's ischemic contracture** may develop (see Chapter 15). Surgery is often required to relieve the increased intracompartmental pressure.

 ## ON-FIELD EVALUATION OF ELBOW AND FOREARM INJURIES

In most instances, acute injuries of the elbow do not require an on-field evaluation and subsequent management of the condition. The exceptions to this are elbow dislocations and fractures of the forearm or humerus. In these cases, the athlete remains down on the playing surface.

ON-FIELD HISTORY

After the possibility of a fracture or dislocation has been ruled out, the circumstances surrounding the injury must be established:

- **Position of the arm:** When the hand is supporting the body weight, the arm is in a closed kinetic chain. Blows to the forearm, elbow, or humerus must be absorbed by the elbow's supportive structures, increasing the suspicion of acute ligamentous injuries.
- **Type of force involved:** The nature of the force delivered to the elbow must be determined. Landing on the palm of the hand delivers a longitudinal force up the radius that is transferred to the ulna by the interosseous membrane. A force to the lateral side of the elbow places stress on the UCL, and a medial force stresses the RCL. A force from the posterior aspect of the elbow results in hyperextension of the joint and places shear forces on the olecranon process. A blunt force places compressive forces on the tissues beneath the location of the impact.

ON-FIELD INSPECTION

The primary tool in the evaluation of these conditions is inspection of the injured area. Elbow dislocation and forearm or humeral fractures tend to result in gross deformity, but radial and ulnar fractures are inherently more noticeable.

- **Alignment of forearm and wrist:** Observe the length of the radius and ulna for gross deformity and note the relationship between the forearm and wrist. A

complete fracture of either of the long bones may alter the wrist's position relative to the forearm.
- **Posterior triangle of the elbow:** Note the alignment of the medial epicondyle, lateral epicondyle, and the olecranon process. These structures should form an isosceles triangle when the elbow is flexed to 90 degrees. Any deviation of this relationship may indicate a dislocation. In the event of a posterior dislocation, the olecranon process becomes overly prominent. If either condition exists, the evaluation must be terminated immediately and the athlete must be referred to a physician after appropriate immobilization.

ON-FIELD PALPATION

Palpation is performed to confirm the suspicion of injury established during the history-taking process while also ruling out any other gross trauma.

- **Alignment of the elbow:** Palpate the medial epicondyle, lateral epicondyle, and olecranon for tenderness, crepitus, and improper alignment.
- **Collateral ligaments:** Palpate the RCL and UCL along their lengths to identify any pain or crepitus along these structures. Crepitus at the ligament's origin or insertion may indicate an avulsion.
- **Radius and ulna:** Palpate the length of the radius and ulna for tenderness, deformity, or false joints indicative of a fracture.

ON-FIELD RANGE OF MOTION TESTS

Before deciding whether to splint the arm, the athlete's willingness and ability to move the elbow must be established:

- **AROM:** Ask the athlete to wiggle the fingers, move the wrist through flexion and extension and radial and ulnar deviation, and then through forearm pronation and supination and elbow flexion and extension. The inability to perform any one of these steps or significant pain with these motions warrants the immobilization of the elbow, forearm, and wrist before the athlete is removed from the field.
- **PROM:** After the athlete has displayed the ability to actively and willingly move the elbow, passively move the joint through its ROMs. Osteochondral fractures cause a premature end-point in the ROM. Fractures of the olecranon process cause pain at the terminal range of extension.
- **RROM:** Although this portion of the examination can be delayed until the athlete is removed to the sideline, establish a baseline of strength for future comparison. Nerve root compression may result in a short-term loss of strength that rapidly returns to normal.

FIGURE 14–21. Posterior dislocation of the elbow. This condition results in obvious deformity of the joint. Note that the humeroulnar and humeroradial joints are involved.

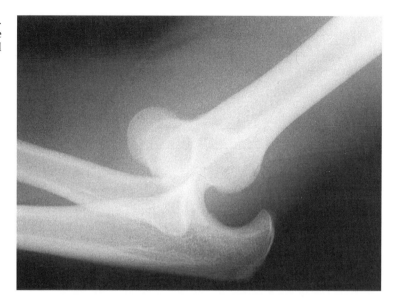

ON-FIELD NEUROLOGIC TESTS

The immediate evaluation of elbow injuries may necessitate the neurologic assessment of the forearm and hand. Refer to the section of this chapter on neurologic testing and see Figure 14–8.

 ## ON-FIELD MANAGEMENT OF ELBOW AND FOREARM INJURIES

The most significant injuries facing athletic trainers during the on-field evaluation are dislocations of the elbow joint and fractures of the forearm (Fig. 14–21). These conditions require careful management to prevent further trauma to the involved structures and protect the neurovascular network supplying the hand. Fractures of the forearm or dislocations of the elbow may lead to the onset of **Volkmann's ischemic contracture** (see Chapter 15).

ELBOW DISLOCATIONS

The forces needed to dislocate the elbow are very high, typically requiring an axial force through the forearm while the elbow is slightly flexed. Injuries of this magnitude cause extreme pain and perhaps hysteria in the athlete. The involved elbow is obviously deformed and the ability to actively move the elbow is lost. The onset of swelling can be rapid, possibly masking the underlying deformity if there is a delay in evaluating the condition. Because of the potential compromise of the blood vessels and nerves crossing the joint, the patient's distal neurovascular function must be assessed.

The elbow is immobilized in the position in which it is found, while still allowing the distal pulse to be monitored. The athlete must be immediately transported for further medical treatment by a physician.

FRACTURE ABOUT THE ELBOW

Supracondylar fractures are almost exclusively found in adolescent athletes, resulting from a fall directly onto a flexed elbow or a hyperextension mechanism. Pain occurs over the supracondylar region. Angular deformity of the humerus may be noted, except in the case of nondisplaced fractures.

Fractures of the olecranon process are more common in skeletally mature athletes. Being relatively unprotected by overlying muscle, the olecranon is most predisposed to direct blows such as falling on a flexed elbow. Pain, crepitus, and deformity are noted on palpation. Acute swelling may arise directly from the trauma to the olecranon or arise secondary to injury of the olecranon bursa. Pain is also described during active extension of the elbow and with passive overpressure during extension.

Fractures of the radius and ulna may compromise the neurovascular supply to the wrist and hand. Because of this, distal pulses must be monitored constantly after the injury. At that time, the elbow, forearm, and wrist must be immobilized to minimize movement of the fractured bones. After the area has been stabilized, the athlete must be immediately transported and treated for shock.

REFERENCES

1. Stroyan, M, and Wilk, KE: The functional anatomy of the elbow complex. *J Orthop Sports Phys Ther*, 17:279, 1993.
2. King, JW, Brelsford, HJ, and Tullos, HS: Analysis of the pitching arm of the professional baseball pitcher. *Clin Orthop*, 67:116, 1969.
3. Doughty, MP: Drop wrist: Complications following a comminuted fracture of the radius. Orthotic glove designed to permit participation. *Athletic Training: Journal of the National Athletic Trainers Association*, 22:221, 1987.
4. Andrews, JR, et al: Physical examination of the thrower's elbow. *J Orthop Sports Phys Ther*, 17:269, 1993.

5. Werner, SL, et al: Biomechanics of the elbow during baseball pitching. *J Orthop Sports Phys Ther*, 17:274, 1993.
6. Nestor, BJ, O'Driscoll, SW, and Morrey, BF: Ligamentous reconstruction for posterolateral rotatory instability of the elbow. *J Bone Joint Surg Am*, 74:1235, 1992.
7. Lieber, RL, Ljung, BO, and Friden, J: Sarcomere length in wrist extensor muscles. Changes may provide insights into the etiology of chronic lateral epicondylitis. *Acta Orthop Scand*, 68:249, 1997.
8. Sterling, JC, et al: Tennis elbow: A brief review of treatment. *Athletic Training: Journal of the National Athletic Trainers Association*, 23:316, 1988.
9. Haker, E: Lateral epicondylalgia: Diagnosis, treatment, and evaluation. *Crit Rev Phys Rehabil Med*, 5:129, 1993.
10. Assendelft, WJ, et al: Corticosteroid injections for lateral epicondylitis: a systematic overview. *Br J Gen Pract*, 46:209, 1996.
11. Gabel, GT, and Morrey, BF: Operative treatment of medial epicondylitis. Influence of concomitant ulnar neuropathy at the elbow. *J Bone Joint Surg*, 77(A):1065, 1995.
12. Agins, HJ, et al: Rupture of the distal insertion of the biceps tendon. *Clin Orthop*, 234:34, 1988.
13. D'Allesandro, DF, et al: Repair of distal biceps tendon ruptures in athletes. *Am J Sports Med*, 21:114, 1993.
14. D'Arco, P, et al: Clinical, functional, and radiographic assessments of the conventional and modified Boyd-Anderson surgical procedures for repair of distal biceps tendon ruptures. *Am J Sports Med*, 26:254, 1998.
15. Baker, BE, and Bierwagen, D: Rupture of the distal tendon of the biceps brachii: Operative versus non-operative treatment. *J Bone Joint Surg*, 67(A):414, 1985.
16. Friedmann, E: Rupture of the distal biceps brachii tendon: Report on 13 cases. *J Am Med Assoc*, 184:60, 1963.
17. Morrey BF, Askew LJ, An, KN, at al: Rupture of the distal tendon of the biceps brachii: A biomechanical study. *J Bone Joint Surg*, 67(A):418, 1985.
18. Barker, C: Evaluation, treatment, and rehabilitation involving a submuscular transposition of the ulnar nerve at the elbow. *Athletic Training: Journal of the National Athletic Trainers Association*, 23:10, 1988.
19. Lutz, FR: Radial tunnel syndrome: An etiology of chronic lateral elbow pain. *J Orthop Sports Phys Ther*, 14:14, 1991.
20. Botte, MJ, and Gelberman, RH: Acute compartment syndrome of the forearm. *Hand Clin*, 14:391, 1998.
21. Peters, CL, and Scott, SM: Compartment syndrome in the forearm following fractures of the radial head or neck in children. *J Bone Joint Surg*, 77(A):1070, 1995.

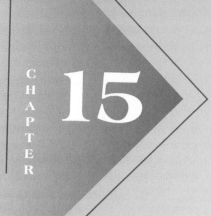

C H A P T E R

15 > The Wrist, Hand, and Fingers

Unrestricted use of the wrist, hand, and fingers is necessary, thus limiting the amount of protective equipment that can reasonably be worn during work or sports activities.[1] Injury to this area include impairment of gross and fine motor movements. An athlete's disability after injury to these body areas depends on the sport, position, and the dominance of the injured hand. In football, a hand injury that has little consequence to a lineman could be disabling to a quarterback or wide receiver. In a sport such as basketball, injuries to the non-shooting hand impact the athlete's ability less than those involving the shooting hand.

◆ **CLINICAL ANATOMY**

The distal portions of the radius and ulna, eight carpal bones, five metacarpals, and 14 phalanges, form the skeleton of the wrist, hand, and fingers (Fig. 15–1). The **distal radius** broadens to form a small **ulnar notch** on its medial surface to accept the ulnar head, and the **radial styloid process** projects off its anterolateral border. The **ulnar head** is more circular, with the **ulnar styloid process** arising from its medial surface.

Having unusual shapes and irregular surfaces, the **carpal bones** are aligned in two rows (Fig. 15–2). From the radial to ulnar sides, the proximal row consists of the scaphoid (navicular), lunate, triquetrum, and the pisiform bones. The distal row is formed by the trapezium, trapezoid, capitate, and hamate bones. In the

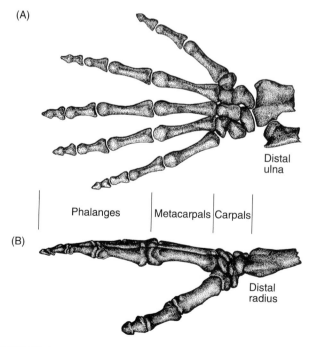

(A)

(B)

Phalanges | Metacarpals | Carpals

Distal ulna

Distal radius

FIGURE 15–1. Bones of the wrist and hand, formed by the radius and ulna, 8 carpal bones, 5 metacarpals, and 14 phalanges.

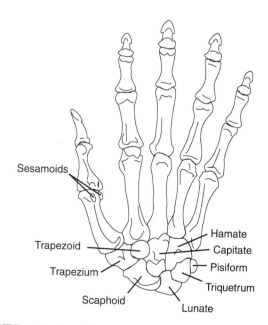

Sesamoids

Trapezoid

Trapezium

Scaphoid

Hamate

Capitate

Pisiform

Triquetrum

Lunate

FIGURE 15–2. Carpal bones of the hand.

distal carpal row, the trapezium aligns with the first **metacarpal,** the trapezoid with the second metacarpal, the capitate with the third metacarpal, and the fourth and fifth metacarpals to the hamate. The pisiform "floats" on the triquetrum, acting as a sesamoid bone for the flexor carpi ulnaris muscle, modifying its angle of pull. The scaphoid is the most commonly fractured of the carpals, and the lunate is the most commonly dislocated.

Much of the length of the hand is formed by the metacarpals, numbered from I (thumb) to V (little finger). Shaped similarly to long bones, the proximal articulating surfaces are concave to accept the convex surface of the carpals. The distal surfaces are convex to accept the concave surface of the proximal phalanx of each of the fingers. Each finger (except the thumb, which has only a proximal and distal phalanx) has a **proximal, middle,** and **distal phalanx.** The proximal aspect of these bones is referred to as the base, and the distal aspect is referred to as the head.

Two small sesamoid bones are located over the palmar aspect of the distal end of the first metacarpal (see Fig. 15–2). These mobile bones improve the mechanical line of pull of the flexor pollicis brevis, abductor pollicis brevis, and adductor pollicis muscles.

ARTICULATIONS AND LIGAMENTOUS SUPPORT

The motion produced by the wrist, hand, and fingers occurs through the interaction of several joints, which form numerous force couples with their associated muscles. An overview of the interactions involving specific joints is described in this section.

Distal Radioulnar Joint

The distal radioulnar articulation, formed by the ulnar head and the ulnar notch of the radius, allows 1 degree of freedom of movement: pronation and supination. The distal and proximal radioulnar joints work together to produce those motions. Restriction of motion at either of these joints limits pronation and supination of the entire forearm. At the distal radioulnar joint, pronation and supination is produced by the radius' gliding around the ulna. However, the ulna moves slightly anteriorly and medially during supination and posteriorly and laterally during pronation.

Radiocarpal Joint

The radiocarpal articulation is an ellipsoid joint that provides 2 degrees of freedom of movement: flexion and extension and radial and ulnar deviation. The joint is formed by the distal end of the radius' articulation with the scaphoid and lunate. Another joint is formed by the triangular fibrocartilaginous disk's articulation with the lunate and triquetrum.

The joint is covered by a fibrous capsule reinforced by ligamentous thickenings (Fig. 15–3). The **radial collateral ligament** (RCL), originating off the styloid process and inserting on the scaphoid and trapezium, limits *ulnar deviation* and becomes taut when the wrist is at the extreme ranges of flexion and extension.

The most important ligament for controlling motion and wrist stability is the **palmar (volar) radiocarpal ligament.**[2] This structure originates from the anterior surface of the distal radius and courses obliquely and medially to split into three individual segments, each named for the bone to which it attaches: the **radiocapitate ligament, radiotriquetral ligament,** and **radioscaphoid ligament.** As a unit, these ligaments maintain the alignment of the associated joint structures and limit hyperextension of the wrist.

The **dorsal radiocarpal ligament** is the only major ligament on the *dorsal* surface of the wrist (Fig. 15–4). Arising from the posterior surface of the distal radius and styloid process, this ligament attaches to the lunate and triquetrum to limit wrist flexion.

The ulna is buffered from the proximal row of carpals by the triangular fibrocartilaginous disk. The **ulnar collateral ligament** (UCL) arises from the ulna's styloid process and attaches on the medial aspect of the triquetrum dorsally and the pisiform palmarly. This ligament checks *radial deviation* and becomes taut at the end-ranges of flexion and extension. Medially, the small palmar (volar) ulnocarpal ligament originates from the distal ulna, blends in with the UCL and attaches to the lunate and triquetrum.

Intercarpal Joints

Each carpal bone is fixated to its contiguous carpal in the same row by small palmar, dorsal, and interosseous ligaments. This ligamentous arrangement allows for very little gliding movement between the bones adjacent to one another within a row.

Intermetacarpal Joints

The proximal and distal carpal rows are separated by a single joint cavity with small fibrous projections connecting the rows. This structure allows limited gliding movements of flexion and extension and radial and ulnar deviation that are needed to obtain the normal amount of wrist flexion and extension.

Ulnar deviation Movement of the hand toward the ulnar side of the forearm.

Dorsal (upper extremity) The posterior aspect of the hand and forearm relative to the anatomical position.

Radial deviation Movement of the hand toward the radial (thumb) side.

FIGURE 15–3. Palmar (volar) ligaments of the wrist and hand.

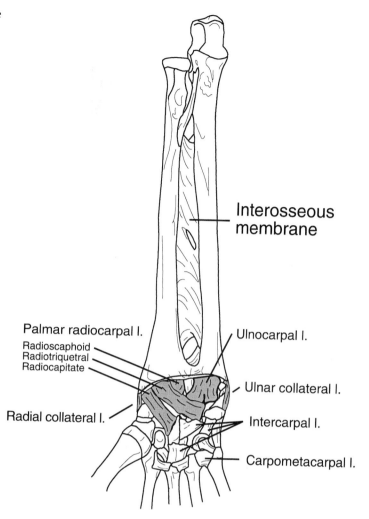

Interosseous membrane

Palmar radiocarpal l.
Radioscaphoid
Radiotriquetral
Radiocapitate

Ulnocarpal l.

Ulnar collateral l.

Radial collateral l.

Intercarpal l.

Carpometacarpal l.

FIGURE 15–4. Ligaments of the wrist and hand: dorsal **(A)**; palmar **(B)**.

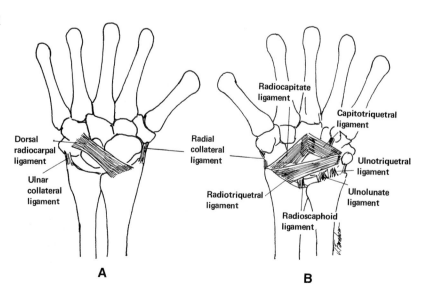

Dorsal radiocarpal ligament

Ulnar collateral ligament

Radial collateral ligament

Radiocapitate ligament

Capitotriquetral ligament

Ulnotriquetral ligament

Ulnolunate ligament

Radiotriquetral ligament

Radioscaphoid ligament

A

B

Carpometacarpal Joints

The first three metacarpals articulate with a single carpal: metacarpal I with the trapezium; metacarpal II with the trapezoid; and metacarpal III with the capitate. The fourth and fifth metacarpals articulate with the hamate to form one of the **carpometacarpal (CMC) joints** (see Fig. 15–2).

The first CMC joint, that of the thumb, has a synovial cavity separate from the lateral four joints. Classified as a saddle joint, the first CMC joint is capable of 2 degrees of freedom of movement: flexion and extension and abduction and adduction. An accessory rotational component occurs concurrently with these motions, allowing for **opposition,** a combined movement that allows the thumb to touch each of the four fingers (the return motion from opposition is **reposition**).

The CMC joints II through IV are *plane synovial joints* that have 1 degree of freedom of movement, flexion and extension. The fifth CMC joint has 2 degrees of movement, flexion and extension and abduction and adduction. Several small ligaments support these joints and allow progressively more motion with each medial joint. The second and third CMC joints are practically immobile, but the fourth and fifth have greater mobility, allowing the hand to strongly grip small objects.

Metacarpophalangeal Joints

Condyloid joints capable of 2 degrees of freedom of movement, flexion and extension and abduction and adduction. The five metacarpophalangeal (MCP) articulations represent the union between the concave articular surface of the proximal phalanx of each finger and the convex articular surface of the associated metacarpal. Although the thumb is capable of abducting and adducting at any point in the range of motion (ROM), the maximum amount of this abduction and adduction in the lateral four fingers is possible only when they are fully extended.

Support against valgus and varus forces is provided by pairs of collateral ligaments running obliquely from the dorsal aspect of the side of the metacarpal to the palmar aspect of the phalanx. As the fingers are flexed, these ligaments tighten, limiting the amount of abduction and adduction available to the joint in this position.

The palmar aspect of the MCP joints is reinforced by a thick fibrocartilaginous **palmar (volar) ligament.** The dorsal aspects of the lateral four MCP joints are reinforced by the expansion of the extensor hood. Reinforcement is also provided by the deep transverse metacarpal ligament. These strong bands limit abduction and adduction and reinforce the palmar ligaments.

MUSCULAR ANATOMY

The muscles of the wrist and hand function under a broad spectrum of circumstances and demands. The

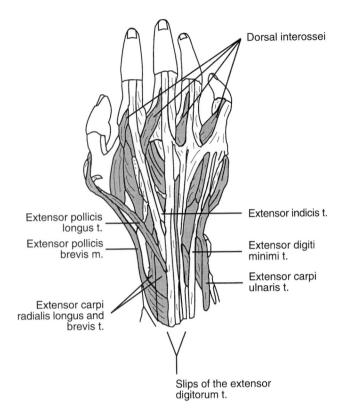

FIGURE 15–5. Intrinsic muscles of the dorsal hand and attachments of the long finger extensors.

same muscles that are used to grip strongly are also called on to perform the most delicate of fine motor skills. The extrinsic muscles acting on the wrist, including the long muscles of the fingers, are described in Table 15–1. The intrinsic muscles of the hand are presented in Table 15–2.

The natural, relaxed position of the hand and fingers is one of slight flexion. This positioning is caused by the relative shortness of the finger flexors. This concept can be demonstrated by noting how the fingers flex as the wrist is passively extended.

Extensor Muscles

Located on the posterolateral portion of the forearm, the wrist's extensor muscles are divided into two groups, both innervated by the **radial nerve.** Figures 14–6 and 14–7 show the locations of these muscles relative to the forearm, and Figures 15–5 and 15–6 show the locations of their insertions on the wrist and hand.

The superficial muscles, **extensor carpi radialis longus and brevis** and **extensor carpi ulnaris,** are the primary wrist extensors. The **extensor digitorum com-**

Plane synovial joint   A synovial joint formed by the gliding between two or more bones.

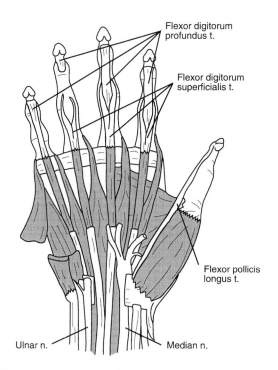

FIGURE 15–6. Intrinsic palmar muscles and long finger flexors. Note the location of the ulnar and median nerves.

munis, the primary extensor of the lateral four fingers' interphalangeal (IP) joints, serves to assist in wrist extension. The brachioradialis is also located in the superficial compartment, but it does not directly influence wrist movement.

The deep compartment contains the thumb's extensors, the **extensor pollicis longus** and the **extensor pollicis brevis,** and its primary abductor, the **abductor pollicis longus.** The long extensor of the second finger, the **extensor indicus,** is also located in this compartment. The remaining deep muscle, the **supinator,** is capable of supinating the forearm at all angles of elbow flexion but has no action on the hand or fingers.

The extensor muscles are secured to the posterior portion of the distal radius and ulna by the **extensor retinaculum.** This strong, transverse band increases the efficiency of the muscles' pull and prevents "bow stringing" when the wrist is extended.

Flexor Muscles

The anteromedial forearm is also divided into two compartments, superficial and deep. The superficial compartment houses the wrist's flexor muscles, the **flexor carpi radialis, palmaris longus** (absent in approximately 10% of the population), and **flexor carpi ulnaris.** The **flexor digitorum superficialis,** responsible for flexion of the four proximal interphalangeal (PIP) joints, and the **pronator teres** are also located in this compartment. The location of these muscles is presented in Figure 14–6, and their insertion on the wrist and hand is given in Figure 15–6. The deep compartment is formed

by the **flexor digitorum profundus,** flexing both the PIP and distal interphalangeal (DIP) joints; the **flexor pollicis longus;** and the **pronator quadratus.**

The flexor muscles are innervated by the **median nerve.** The exception is the flexor carpi ulnaris and the fourth and fifth portions of the flexor digitorum profundus. These are supplied by the **ulnar nerve.**

Palmar Muscles

The hand's intrinsic muscles are grouped into the thenar, central, hypothenar, and adductor interosseous compartments. The **thenar eminence,** the mass found over the thumb's palmar surface, is formed by the **abductor pollicis brevis, flexor pollicis brevis,** and **opponens pollicis muscles** and the tendon of the **flexor pollicis longus muscle** (Fig. 15–7). On the ulnar aspect, the fleshy mound at the base of the little finger, the **hypothenar eminence,** contains the **abductor digiti minimi, flexor digiti minimi brevis,** and the **opponens digiti minimi muscles.**

The tendons of **flexor digitorum superficialis** and **flexor digitorum profundus** pass through the central compartment. Four **lumbrical** muscles originate off the radial side of each slip of the flexor digitorum profundus tendon. Crossing the MCP joint on the palmar side, the lumbrical muscle continues around the phalanx to insert into the extensor hood. Because of their attachment on the extensor hood, the lumbrical muscles serve to flex the MCP joints and extend the PIP and DIP joints (forming the "table top" position). The entire central compartment is covered by the **palmar aponeurosis** (volar plate).

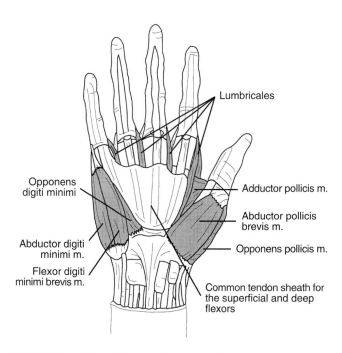

FIGURE 15–7. Intrinsic muscles of the thumb and little finger.

Table 15–1
EXTRINSIC MUSCLES ACTING ON THE WRIST AND HAND

Muscle	Action	Origin	Insertion	Innervation	Root
Abductor pollicis longus	1st CMC joint abduction 1st CMC joint extension Assists in radial deviation of the wrist	• Posterior surface of the distal ulna • Posterior surface of the distal radius • Adjoining interosseous membrane	• Radial side of the base of the 1st metacarpal	Median	C6, C7
Extensor carpi radialis brevis	Wrist extension Radial deviation	• Lateral epicondyle via the common extensor tendon • Radial collateral ligament	• Base of the 3rd metacarpal	Radial	C6, C7
Extensor carpi radialis longus	Wrist extension Radial deviation	• Supracondylar ridge of humerus	• Radial side of the 2nd metacarpal	Radial	C6, C7
Extensor carpi ulnaris	Wrist extension Ulnar deviation	• Lateral epicondyle via the common extensor tendon	• Ulnar side of the base of the 5th metacarpal	Deep radial	C6, C7, C8
Extensor digitorum communis	Wrist extension MCP extension IP extension Radial deviation of the wrist	• Lateral epicondyle via the common extensor tendon	• The dorsal surface of the proximal base of the middle and distal phalanges of each of the four fingers	Deep radial	C6, C7, C8
Extensor pollicis brevis	1st MCP joint extension 1st CMC joint extension 1st CMC joint abduction Assists in wrist radial deviation	• Posterior surface of the distal radius • Adjoining interosseous membrane	• Dorsal surface of the base of the proximal phalanx of the thumb	Deep radial	C6, C7
Extensor pollicis longus	1st IP joint extension 1st MCP joint extension 1st CMC joint extension Assists in wrist extension Assists in wrist radial deviation	• Posterior surface of the middle one-third of the ulna • Adjoining interosseous membrane	• Dorsal surface of the base of the distal phalanx of the thumb	Deep radial	C6, C7, C8
Flexor carpi radialis	Wrist flexion Forearm pronation Radial deviation	• Medial epicondyle via the common flexor tendon	• Bases of the 2nd and 3rd metacarpal bones	Median	C6, C7

524

Muscle	Action	Attachments	Innervation	Nerve roots
Flexor carpi ulnaris	Wrist flexion Ulnar deviation	**Humeral head** • Medial epicondyle via the common flexor tendon **Ulnar head** • Medial border of the olecranon • Proximal two thirds of the posterior ulna • Pisiform • Hamate • 5th metacarpal	Ulnar	C8, T1
Flexor digitorum profundus	DIP flexion PIP flexion Wrist flexion	• Anteromedial proximal three fourths of ulna and associated interosseous membrane • Bases of the medial phalanges of digits II through V	Palmar interosseous	C8, T1
Flexor digitorum superficialis	PIP flexion MCP flexion Wrist flexion	**Humeral head** • Medial epicondyle via the common flexor tendon • Ulnar collateral ligament **Ulnar head** • Coronoid process **Radial head** • Oblique line of radius • Sides of the middle phalanges of digits II through V	Median	C7, C8, T1
Flexor pollicis longus	1st IP joint flexion 1st MCP joint flexion Assists in wrist flexion	• Anterior surface of the radius • Adjoining interosseous membrane • Coronoid process of ulna • Palmar surface of the base of the distal phalanx of the thumb	Palmar interosseous	C8, T1
Palmaris longus	Wrist flexion	• Medial epicondyle via the common flexor tendon • Flexor retinaculum • Palmar aponeurosis	Median	C6, C7

CMC = carpometacarpal; DIP = distal interphalangeal; IP = interphalangeal; MCP = metacarpophalangeal; PIP = proximal interphalangeal.

Table 15–2
INTRINSIC MUSCLES ACTING ON THE HAND

Muscle	Action	Origin	Insertion	Innervation	Root
Abductor digiti minimi	Abduction of the 5th finger Assists in opposition	• Tendon of flexor carpi ulnaris • Pisiform	By two slips into the 5th finger • Ulnar side of the base of the proximal phalanx • Ulnar border of the extensor expansion	Ulnar	C8, T1
Abductor pollicis brevis	1st CMC joint abduction 1st MCP joint abduction Assists in opposition	• Flexor retinaculum • Trapezium • Scaphoid	• Radial surface of the base of the proximal phalanx of the thumb • Via a slip into the extensor expansion	Median	C6, C7
Adductor pollicis	1st CMC joint adduction 1st MCP joint adduction 1st MCP joint flexion Assists in opposition	• Capitate bone • Bases of 2nd and 3rd metacarpals • Palmar surface of 3rd metacarpal	• Ulnar surface of the base of the proximal phalanx of the thumb • Via a slip into the extensor expansion	Deep palmar branch	C8, T1
Dorsal interossei	Abduction of the 3rd, 4th and 5th fingers Assists in MCP flexion Assists in extension of the IP joints	**Thumb** • Ulnar border of 1st metacarpal • Radial border of 2nd metacarpal **2nd, 3rd, and 4th fingers** • Adjacent sides of metacarpals	**Thumb** • Radial border of the 2nd finger **2nd** • Radial side of the 3rd finger **3rd** • Ulnar side of 3rd finger **4th** • Ulnar side of 4th finger	Deep palmar branch	C8, T1
Flexor digiti minimi	5th MCP joint flexion Assists in opposition	• Hook of the hamate bone • Flexor retinaculum	• Ulnar border of the proximal phalanx of the 5th finger	Ulnar	C8, T1
Flexor pollicis brevis	1st MCP joint flexion 1st CMC joint flexion Assists in opposition	• Flexor retinaculum • Trapezoid • Capitate	• Radial surface of the base of the proximal phalanx • Via a slip into the extensor expansion	Median Deep palmar branch	C6, C7 C8, T1

Muscle	Action	Proximal attachment	Distal attachment	Innervation	Root
Lumbricales	Flexion of the 2nd through 5th MCP joints Extension of the PIP and DIP joints	**1st and 2nd** • Radial surface of flexor profundus tendons **3rd** • Adjacent sides of flexor profundus tendons of 3rd and 4th fingers **4th** • Adjacent sides of flexor profundus tendons of the 4th and 5th fingers	• Radial border of the extensor tendons of the respective digits	1st and 2nd: median 3rd and 4th: deep palmar branch	C6, C7 C8, T1
Opponens digiti minimi	Opposition of the 5th finger	• Hook of the hamate bone • Flexor retinaculum	• Ulnar border of the length of the 5th metacarpal	Ulnar	C8, T1
Opponens pollicis	Thumb opposition	• Flexor retinaculum • Trapezium	• Length of the 1st metacarpal	Median	C6, C7
Palmar interossei	Adducts 1st, 2nd, 4th and 5th fingers Assists in flexion of the MCP joints	**Thumb** • Ulnar border of the 1st metacarpal **2nd** • Ulnar border of the 2nd metacarpal **3rd** • Radial border of the 4th metacarpal **4th** • Radial border of the 5th metacarpal	**Thumb** • Ulnar border of thumb **2nd** • Ulnar side of 2nd finger **3rd** • Radial side of ring finger • Radial side of little finger	Deep palmar branch	C8, T1

CMC = carpometacarpal; DIP = distal interphalangeal; IP = interphalangeal; MCP = metacarpophalangeal; PIP = proximal interphalangeal.

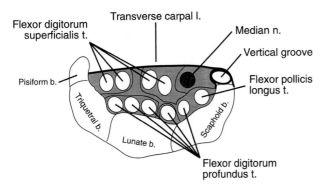

FIGURE 15–8. The carpal tunnel. Inflammation of the tendons passing through the carpal tunnel increases the volume within this fixed space. If the volume continues to increase, the median nerve is compressed, resulting in neurologic symptoms in the hand.

The palmar adductor interosseous compartment fills the void between metacarpals. The webspace between the thumb and index finger is filled by the **adductor pollicis muscle.** Three spaces between the remaining metacarpals are filled by four palmar and four dorsal interosseous muscles. Using the third metacarpal as the midline reference, the palmar interossei adduct the fingers, and the dorsal interossei abduct them.

THE CARPAL TUNNEL

Many of the anterior muscles acting on the wrist and fingers cross the radiocarpal joint through the carpal tunnel (Fig. 15–8). A fibro-osseous structure, the tunnel's floor is formed by the proximal carpal bones. Its roof is formed by the transverse carpal ligament. Ten structures pass through the tunnel: the median nerve, the flexor pollicis longus tendon, the four slips of the flexor digitorum superficialis, and the flexor digitorum

profundus tendons. Inflammation of these structures compresses the median nerve, resulting in paresthesia in the median nerve distribution in the palmar aspect of the second, third, and fourth fingers. Grip strength is decreased because of inhibition of the motor nerves supplying the thumb's flexors and opposition muscles.

CLINICAL EVALUATION OF INJURIES TO THE WRIST, HAND, AND FINGERS

An evaluation of the elbow, shoulder, and cervical spine may also be indicated when a patient's history, mechanism, or symptoms suggest involvement of these structures. Impairment of the nerves in these proximal areas may manifest their symptoms through decreased sensation and strength in the hand.

HISTORY

- **Location of pain:** Because the structures of the wrist and hand are so close to one another, enough details should be gained during the history-taking process to localize the symptoms as specifically as possible. Trauma to the cervical spine, shoulder, elbow, and forearm can radiate symptoms into the wrist and hand. Injury to the median, ulnar, and radial nerves can radiate symptoms into their specific sensory or motor distributions in the hand (Fig. 15–9).
- **Mechanism of injury:** In the case of acute trauma, identify the mechanism of injury to localize the injured structure or structures. Ask patients describing an injury of insidious onset about activities that increase or decrease the symptoms. When evaluating patients with hand injuries that have an insidious onset, pay particular attention to specific postures that may be assumed.

FIGURE 15–9. Nerve distribution in the hand.

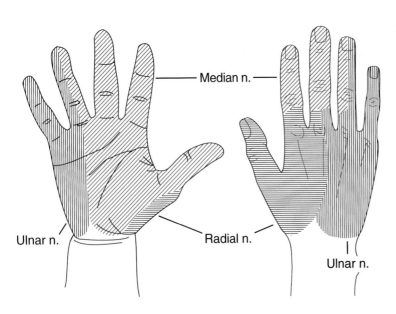

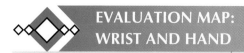

EVALUATION MAP: WRIST AND HAND

1. HISTORY

Location of pain
Mechanism of injury
Relevant sounds
Relevant sensation
Duration of symptoms
Description of symptoms
Previous history
General medical health

2. INSPECTION

General
Posture of the hand
Gross deformity
Palmar creases
Areas of cuts or scars

Wrist and Hand
Continuity of the distal radius and
   ulna
Continuity of the carpals and
   metacarpals
Alignment of the MCP joints
Posture of the wrist and hands
Ganglion cyst

Thumb and Fingers
Skin and fingernails
   Subungual hematoma
   Felon
   Paronychia
Alignment of fingernails
Finger deformities

3. PALPATION

Palpation of the Hand
Metacarpals
MCP collateral ligaments

Phalanges
IP collateral ligaments
Thenar compartment
Thenar webspace
Central compartment
Hypothenar compartment
Ulna
   Ulnar styloid process
   Ulnar collateral ligament
Radius
   Radial styloid process
   Lister's tubercle
   Radial collateral ligament

Palpation of the Carpals
Scaphoid
Trapezium
Lunate
Pisiform
Hamate
Capitate
Trapezoid

4. RANGE OF MOTION TESTS

Wrist
AROM
PROM
RROM
   Flexion
   Extension
   Radial deviation
   Ulnar deviation

Thumb–CMC
AROM
PROM
RROM
   Flexion
   Extension
   Abduction
   Adduction
   Opposition

Fingers
AROM
PROM
RROM
   Flexion—MCP
   Extension—MCP
   Abduction—MCP
   Adduction—MCP
   Flexion—IP joints
   Extension—IP joints
   Grip dynamometry

5. LIGAMENTOUS TESTS

Valgus stress testing—radiocarpal
   joint
Varus stress testing—radiocarpal
   joint
Glide testing of the wrist
Valgus stress testing—IP joints
Varus stress testing—IP joints
Ulnar collateral ligament— thumb

6. NEUROLOGIC TESTS

Radial nerve
Median nerve
Ulnar nerve

7. SPECIAL TESTS

Carpal Tunnel Syndrome
Phalen's test

DeQuervain's Syndrome
Finkelstein test

AROM = active range of motion: IP = interphalangeal; PROM = passive range of motion; RROM = resisted range of motion.

- **Relevant sounds or sensations:** Question the patient about any sounds or sensations experienced by the patient. Fractures, dislocations, and tendon injuries such as a **trigger finger** may have an associated popping sound that is accompanied by a sensation of snapping.
- **Duration of symptoms:** Correlate the injury mechanism with the duration of symptoms. Nagging wrist pain that does not decrease in severity may indicate a **scaphoid fracture** or a **tear of the triangular fibrocartilaginous complex** (TFCC).
- **Description of symptoms:** Ask the patient to describe the symptoms felt. Pain that is described as "aching" or "throbbing" is often associated with trauma to the involved bony or soft tissues. "Burning" or "tingling" sensations suggest neurologic or vascular involvement.
- **Previous history:** Determine the previous history of injury and any resulting loss of function.
- **General medical health:** Question the patient about a history of other disorders. Systemic diseases such as rheumatoid arthritis often affect the fingers before the other joints in the body. This area is often the first to be affected by *peripheral vascular disease (PVD)* or **Raynaud's phenomenon.**

INSPECTION

General Inspection

- **Posturing of the hand:** The natural, relaxed posture of the hand is that of slight flexion, with a slight arch in the palm. The absence of this arch may indicate an avulsion of one or more finger flexors or atrophy of the hand's intrinsic muscles in the case of chronic injuries (Box 15–1).
- **Gross deformity:** Note areas of swelling, discoloration, or gross deformity. Dislocation of the MCP or IP joints results in obvious deformity of the joint's articulating surfaces (Fig. 15–10). A fracture of the metacarpals shows as a protrusion or depression along the usually flat dorsal surface of the hand.
- **Palmar creases:** Swelling in one or more of the hand compartments can obliterate the normal palmar creases.
- **Areas of cuts or scars:** The tendons and nerves of the wrist and hand are superficial, causing them to be vulnerable to even minor cuts. Acute or prior lacerations and previous surgeries may have permanently injured the underlying structures, resulting in paresthesia or the loss of function in one or more fingers.

  In female athletes, abrasions, small cuts, or callosities over the dorsal surface of the MCP or IP joints, **Russell's sign,** can be one of the few outward signs of bulimia. These lesions are caused by repeated contact with the teeth during self-induced vomiting.[3]

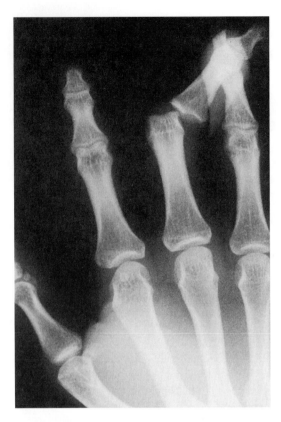

FIGURE 15–10. Dislocation of the proximal interphalangeal joint of the third finger. This type of injury results in obvious visible deformity.

Inspection of the Wrist and Hand

- **Continuity of the distal radius and ulna:** Observe the symmetry of the distal radius and ulna. A loss of continuity in one bone relative to the other may indicate a fracture.
- **Continuity of the carpals and metacarpals:** Although the carpal bones are normally indistinguishable from one another during inspection of the hand, observe the metacarpal shafts for gross discontinuity. Also observe the area overlying the lunate for an abnormal contour that may indicate a dislocation.
- **Alignment of the MCP joints:** Look for the MCP joints to be normally aligned relative to the noninvolved side. A depressed or shortened knuckle may indicate a metacarpal fracture.
- **Posture of the wrist and hand:** Note the posture of the wrist and hand. Trauma to the structures that lie between the cervical spine and wrist may cause the wrist and hand to assume an abnormal posture such

Peripheral vascular disease (PVD) A syndrome involving an insufficiency of arteries or veins in maintaining proper circulation.

Box 15–1
PATHOLOGICAL HAND AND FINGER POSTURES

Ape Hand

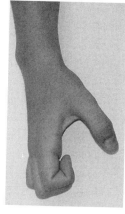

Pathology

Inhibition of the median nerve results in atrophy of the muscles within the thenar eminence. The extensor muscles draw the thumb parallel with the fingers and the patient's ability to flex or oppose the thumb is lost.

Bishop's Deformity

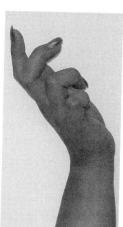

Inhibition of the ulnar nerve results in atrophy of the hypothenar, interossei, and the medial two lumbrical muscles. The finger assumes a posture of flexion in the PIP and DIP joints that is more pronounced in the 4th and 5th fingers; also known as **"Benediction deformity."**

Claw Hand

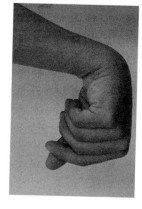

Extension of the MCP joint and flexion of the PIP and DIP joints as the result of pathology of the ulnar and median nerve.

Dupuytern's Contracture

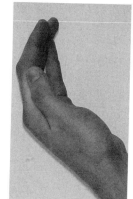

Pathology

Flexion contracture of the MCP and PIP joints is caused by a shortening or adhesion (or both) of the palmar fascia. This condition most commonly affects the 4th and 5th fingers.

Swan-Neck Deformity

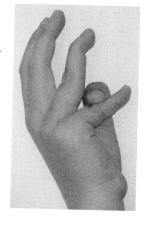
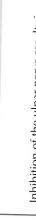

Pathology

Characterized by flexion of the MCP and DIP joints and hyperextension of the PIP joint, swan-neck deformity can be caused by a wide range of pathologies, including volar plate injuries, malunion fractures of the middle phalanx, trauma to the finger flexor or extensor muscles, or rheumatoid arthritis.

Volkmann's Ischemic Contracure

A decrease in the blood supply to the forearm muscles can result in a flexion contracture of the wrist and fingers **(claw fingers)**. Volkmann's contracture can occur after a forearm fracture, fracture or dislocation of the elbow, or forearm compartment syndrome.

DIP = distal interphalangeal; MCP = metacarpophalangeal; PIP = proximal interphalangeal.

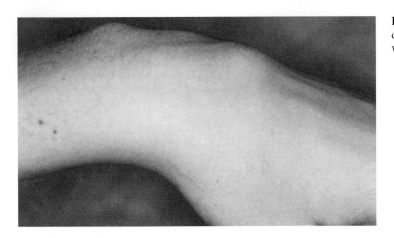

FIGURE 15–11. Ganglion cyst of the wrist extensor tendon. These deformities, caused by a build-up of fluid within the tendon's sheath, are often asymptomatic.

as **Volkmann's ischemic contracture** (see Box 15–1). Inhibition of the radial nerve may result in paralysis of the wrist and finger extensors and cause **drop-wrist deformity,** indicating the inability to extend the wrist.

• **Ganglion cyst:** Note any collection of fluid or the formation of a mass. A benign collection of thick fluid within a tendinous sheath or joint capsule, ganglion cysts are commonly found in the wrist and hand complex (Fig. 15–11). When the cyst becomes symptomatic, pain is caused by motion and the ganglion is tender to the touch and hardens with time. Patients with symptomatic cysts should be referred to a physician for further evaluation and treatment.

Inspection of the Thumb and Fingers

• **Inspection of the skin and fingernails:** Trophic changes such as discoloration and changes in hair patterns or skin and nail texture may indicate peripheral vascular disease, reflex sympathetic dystrophy, or Raynaud's phenomenon. Clubbing or cyanosis of the nail sometimes indicates pulmonary disease, Marfan syndrome, cardiovascular disorder, or other disease states.

○ **Subungual hematoma:** The formation of a hematoma is characterized by discoloration beneath the fingernail. Observe for the presence of the crescent-shaped *lumina.* If the lumina is absent, the fingernail will eventually be lost.

○ **Felon:** An infection or abscess at or distal to the DIP joints, felons arise secondary to contusions or lacerations. The distal end of the finger is red, enlarged, tender to the touch, and warm. Felons must be treated with antibiotics to prevent them from spreading proximally in the finger and hand.

○ **Paronychia:** An infection around the periphery of the fingernail, a paronychia results in redness, swelling, and possible drainage around the nailbed (Fig. 15–12). A paronychia should be treated with

---

Lumina   The growth plate of a fingernail or toenail.

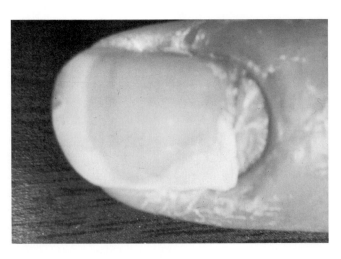

FIGURE 15–12. A paronychina.

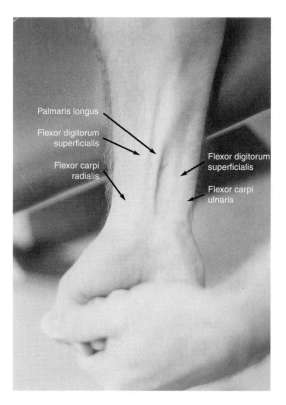

FIGURE 15–13. Surface anatomy of the muscles crossing the anterior wrist.

warm soaks. A physician may prescribe oral antibiotics or drain the affected area.

- **Alignment of fingernails:** During finger flexion, the lateral four fingernails usually assume approximately the same alignment. A finger that deviates from the rest may indicate a spiral fracture of a phalanx or metacarpal.

- **Individual finger deformities:** Irregular posture of one finger may indicate an acute injury or previous trauma (Box 15–2). Deformities along the shaft of the bone may indicate a fracture; deformities at the joint indicate a dislocation.

PALPATION

Detailed palpation of the muscles acting on the wrist and hand is described in Chapter 14.

Palpation of Wrist and Finger Flexor Muscle Group

Starting at their origin on the medial humeral epicondyle, palpate the wrist flexor group through its mass to the point where the individual tendons become distinguishable (Fig. 15–13). Palpate the flexor carpi ulnaris, flexor digitorum profundus, flexor digitorum radialis, and flexor carpi radialis from their origin on the anterior arm to their respective attachment on the hand and wrist. Locate the palmaris longus as it travels up the middle of the forearm by moving medially from the flexor carpi radialis. Absent in 12 to 15 percent of the population, the palmaris longus is more easily identified when the thumb and fifth finger are opposed and the wrist is flexed (Fig. 15–14).

On the anterior portion of the wrist, palpate the area of the carpal tunnel for warmth, swelling, and tenderness that may radiate distally into the hand (see Fig. 15–8).

Palpation of the Wrist and Finger Extensor Muscle Group

Starting at their common origin on the lateral epicondyle of the humerus, palpate the wrist and finger extensor group. The extensor digitorum communis is palpated along its distal length, where it becomes tendinous and splits into the four tendons leading to the fingers (Fig. 15–15). The thumb extensors, extensor pollicis longus, and extensor pollicis brevis (radial side) are identifiable by their location around the anatomical snuffbox. The extensor pollicis longus tendon forms the medial (ulnar) border; the abductor pollicis longus and extensor pollicis brevis tendons form the lateral (radial) border. Palpate the length of these tendons to their insertion on the thumb (Fig 15–16). A portion of the abductor pollicis longus may also be palpable.

FIGURE 15–14. The palmaris longus tendon becomes prominent during wrist flexion and opposition of the thumb and little finger.

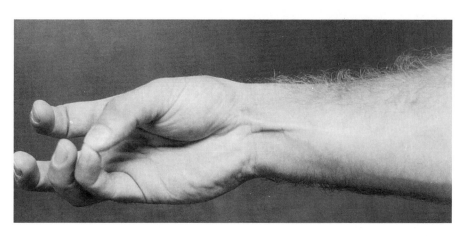

Box 15–2
ACUTE FINGER PATHOLOGIES

	Jersey Finger	Mallet Finger	Boutonnière Deformity
Observation			
Illustration	FDP FDS		**Boutonnière Deformity** Volar plate **Pseudo Boutonnière Deformity**
Pathology	Avulsion of the flexor digitorum profundus tendon	Avulsion of the extensor digitorum longus tendon	**Boutonnière deformity:** a rupture of the central extensor tendon **Pseudo-boutonnière deformity:** a rupture of the volar plate
Posture	Inability to actively flex the DIP joint.	Inability to actively extend the distal phalanx, which assumes the posture of 25° to 35° of flexion	Extension of the MCP and DIP joints and flexion of the PIP joint; acutely, the PIP joint can be actively extended in those with boutonnière deformities but cannot be actively extended in those with pseudo-boutonnière deformities

DIP = distal interphalangeal; MCP = metacarpophalangeal; PIP = proximal interphalangeal.

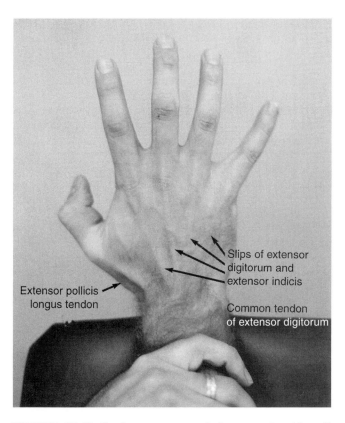

FIGURE 15–15. Surface anatomy of the posterior (dorsal) wrist and forearm, showing the four slips of the extensor digitorum communis (longus) tendon.

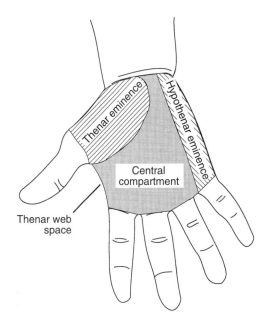

FIGURE 15–17. Zones of the hand.

Palpation of the Hand

The intrinsic muscles of the hand cannot be individually identified during palpation. The palpation of these structures is broken down into compartmental zones: thenar eminence, central compartment, and hypothenar eminence. (Fig. 15–17).

FIGURE 15–16. Borders of the anatomical snuffbox.

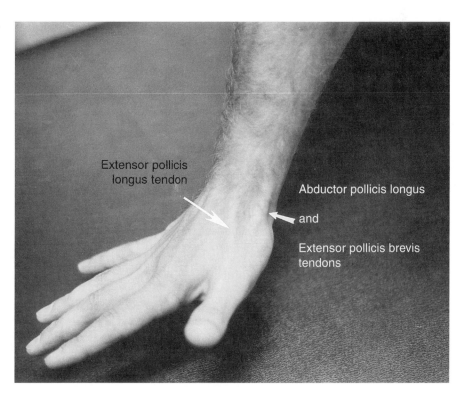

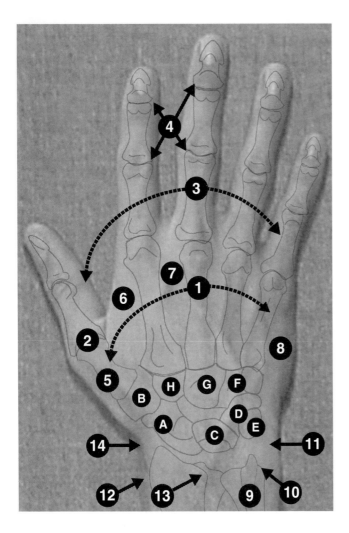

1. **Metacarpals:** All five metacarpals are palpable along their entire length. Begin the palpation of each metacarpal at the MCP joint and proceed proximally to the CMC joint, noting for areas that elicit pain, deformity, or crepitation.
2. **Collateral ligaments of the metacarpophalangeal joints:** The thumb's UCL and RCL are relatively subcutaneous as they cross the first MCP joint. The RCL of the second MCP joint and the UCL of the fifth MCP joint are the only other collateral ligaments directly palpable.
3. **Phalanges:** Each phalanx of the fingers is palpated for the presence of pain, crepitus, or deformity. Pay extra attention to the flares adjoining the bases and heads with the shafts. Abduction, adduction, or other injury to the IP joints may result in a fracture through these areas.
4. **Collateral ligaments of the IP joints:** The collateral ligaments of each of the nine IP joints are easily palpated as they cross the joint line. Palpate these ligaments from their origin on the proximal bone to their insertion on the distal bone.
5. **Thenar compartment:** The small but prominent thenar muscle mass is palpated on the palmar sur-

face of the hand near the base of the thumb. The opponens pollicis sits deep within the compartment, covered by the abductor pollicis brevis and the flexor pollicis brevis muscles and the tendon of the flexor pollicis longus tendon.
6. **Thenar webspace:** The adductor pollicis is palpated within the webspace between the thumb and index finger and is more easily identified if the thumb is actively abducted.
7. **Central compartment:** Lying between the thenar and hypothenar compartments, the palmar aponeurosis is the most superficial structure within the central compartment. Palpation along the metacarpals may reveal the fingers' flexor tendons.
8. **Hypothenar compartment:** The hypothenar mass is palpated along the ulnar border of the palm. The muscles within this area (i.e., the abductor digiti minimi, flexor digiti mini brevis, and opponens digiti minimi muscles) cannot be identified specifically.
9. **Ulna:** The distal two thirds of the ulna is palpated starting at the point where it emerges from the bulk of the wrist flexors on the dorsal aspect of the forearm. As the ulna approaches the wrist articulation, its head becomes prominent and palpable on its anterior, medial, and posterior borders.
10. **Ulnar styloid process:** The ulnar styloid process is palpated on the distal posteromedial border for tenderness or crepitus.
11. **Ulnar collateral ligament:** The wrist's UCL is palpated as it arises from the styloid process and crosses the joint space to attach to the triquetrum dorsally and the pisiform palmarly.
12. **Distal radius and styloid process:** The distal radius is palpated on the anterior, lateral, and posterior sides of the forearm. The small styloid process can be located on the most distal aspect of the lateral radius.
13. **Lister's tubercle** is palpable on the dorsal surface of the distal radius.
14. **Radial collateral ligament:** After locating the RCL from its attachment on the radial styloid process, this structure is palpated as it crosses the joint line to its attachment on the scaphoid.

Palpation of the Carpals

The individual carpals are not always identifiable from one another, but the area overlying these bones can be palpated on the dorsal side of the hand.

A. **Scaphoid:** Locate the scaphoid bone, which serves as the floor of the **"anatomical snuffbox,"** making it easily identifiable and a good starting point for palpating the carpals. Actively extending the thumb and first metacarpal makes the abductor pollicis longus, extensor pollicis brevis, and extensor pollicis longus more distinct. The scaphoid is located within these two boundaries (see Fig. 15–16). To differentiate between the scaphoid and trapezium bones, palpate the wrist just distal from the radius while the wrist is ulnarly deviated. The scaphoid bone will be felt to "pop" into position under the finger.

B. **Trapezium:** Locate and palpate the trapezium between the scaphoid bone and the thumb's metacarpal.

C. **Lunate:** Return to the scaphoid bone and then move toward the ulna. The lunate is prominent across the joint line from the medial radial head, approximately in line with the third metacarpal. A technique for locating the lunate is to find Lister's tubercle on the dorsal aspect of the distal radius first, then palpate distally to locate a depression in the joint line. The lunate will fill this void as the patient's wrist is passively flexed.

D. **Triquetrum:** Palpate the triquetrum along the most proximal aspect of the hand approximately one finger's breadth distal to the ulnar styloid process.

E. **Pisiform:** Palpate directly anterior to the triquetrum for the pisiform, prominent as a small, rounded protuberance on the palmar side of the most proximal aspect of the hypothenar group. This bone is mobile as it lies in the tendon of the flexor carpi ulnaris muscle when the muscle is relaxed by passive wrist flexion.

F. **Hamate:** Identify the hamate by its palmarly projecting hook. Locate the center of the ulna and palpate immediately across the joint line, distal to the pisiform. The hook of the hamate feels like a hard palmar projection that moves with the hand as the wrist is flexed and is palpated on the palmar side.

G. **Capitate:** From the hamate, move toward the thumb side of the hand to locate the capitate, just proximal to the base of the third metacarpal on the palmar aspect of the hand.

H. **Trapezoid:** Locate the trapezoid lying at the base of the second metacarpal. This structure is more easily palpated from the dorsal aspect of the hand.

RANGE OF MOTION TESTING

A summary of the end-feels obtained from passive ROM (PROM) testing for the wrist, hand, fingers, and thumb is presented in Table 15–3. Refer to Tables 15–1 and 15–2 for the innervations of these muscles. Goniometric evaluation of the wrist and fingers is presented in Boxes 15–3 and 15–4.

Wrist Range of Motion Testing

The motions of pronation and supination are described in Chapter 14.

Table 15–3
NORMAL END-FEELS OBTAINED DURING PASSIVE RANGE OF MOTION TESTING

Area	Motion	End-Feel	Tissues
Wrist	Flexion	Firm	Dorsal radiocarpal ligament and joint capsule
	Extension	Firm	Palmar radiocarpal ligament and joint capsule
	Radial deviation	Hard	Scaphoid striking styloid process of radius
	Ulnar deviation	Firm	Radiocarpal ligaments and tendons
Thumb	Flexion	Soft	Approximation of thenar eminence and the palm
(CMC)	Extension	Firm	Anterior joint capsule, flexor pollicis brevis, opponens pollicis, first interossei
	Abduction	Firm	Stretching of the webspace
	Adduction	Soft	Approximation of thenar eminence and palm
	Opposition	Firm	Thumb and 5th finger touching
Fingers and	Flexion	Hard	Proximal phalanx contacts the metacarpal
thumb	Extension	Firm	Tension in the volar plate
(MCP)	Abduction	Firm	Stretching of the collateral ligaments and webspace
	Adduction	Firm	Stretching of the collateral ligaments and webspace
Fingers	Flexion	Hard	Proximal and middle phalanges contact
(PIP)	Extension	Firm	Stretching of the volar plate
Fingers	Flexion	Firm	Tension in dorsal joint capsule and collateral ligaments
(DIP) and thumb (IP)	Extension	Firm	Stretching of palmar joint capsule and volar plate

CMC = carpometacarpal; DIP = distal interphalangeal; IP = interphalangeal;
MCP = metacarpophalangeal; PIP = proximal interphalangeal.

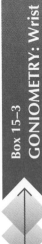

Box 15–3
GONIOMETRY: Wrist

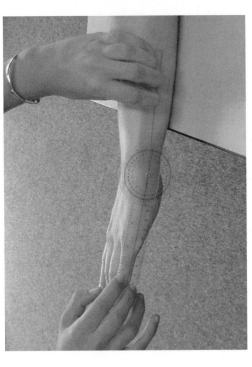

Flexion and Extension

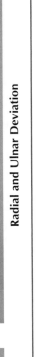

Radial and Ulnar Deviation

	Flexion and Extension	Radial and Ulnar Deviation
PATIENT POSITION	Forearm is pronated with the hand off the edge of the table. During wrist flexion, the fingers are allowed to extend. During wrist extension, the fingers are allowed to flex.	Forearm is pronated with the hand resting on the table
GONIOMETER PLACEMENT		
FULCRUM	Over the lateral joint line of the wrist	Aligned with the center of the distal radioulnar joint, just proximal to the capitate
STATIONARY ARM	Centered on the midline of the ulnar shaft	Centered over the midline of the forearm
MOVEMENT ARM	Centered on the midline of the fifth metacarpal	Centered over the third metacarpal

Box 15–4

GONIOMETRY: Finger

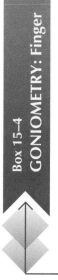

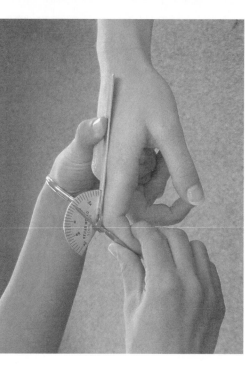

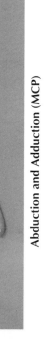

	Flexion and Extension (MCP, PIP, and DIP)	**Abduction and Adduction (MCP)**
PATIENT POSITION	The hand is placed in its neutral position.	The hand is placed in its neutral position.
GONIOMETER PLACEMENT		The hand is in its neutral position with the fingers slightly spread
FULCRUM	Positioned over the dorsal aspect of the joint being tested	
STATIONARY ARM	Centered on the midline of the bone proximal to the joint being tested	Centered over the MCP joint being tested
MOVEMENT ARM	Centered on the midline of the bone distal to the joint being tested	Centered over the proximal phalange of the joint being tested

DIP = distal interphalangeal; MCP = metacarpophalangeal; PIP = proximal interphalangeal.

(A)

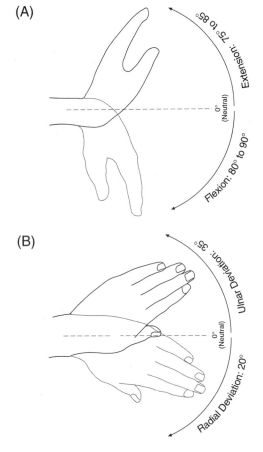

Extension: 75° to 85°

0° (Neutral)

Flexion: 80° to 90°

(B)

Ulnar Deviation: 35°

0° (Neutral)

Radial Deviation: 20°

Active Range of Motion

- **Flexion and extension:** A total of 155 to 175 degrees of motion occurs in the sagittal plane around a coronal (medial-lateral) axis. Flexion accounts for 80 to 90 degrees and extension ranges from 75 to 85 degrees. The fingers should be relaxed to ensure the maximum amount of motion (Fig. 15–18A).
- **Radial and ulnar deviation:** Approximately 55 degrees of motion is permitted through the range of radial and ulnar deviation. This motion occurs in the frontal plane around an anteroposterior axis. From the neutral position, 35 degrees of ulnar deviation and 20 degrees of radial deviation are permitted by the joint structure (Fig. 15–18B).

Passive Range of Motion

- **Flexion and extension:** Position the wrist over the edge of the table with the elbow flexed to 90 degrees and the hand facing downward. Stabilize the forearm to prevent pronation and supination. The fingers should be relaxed (Fig. 15–19A and B).
- **Radial and ulnar deviation:** Position the wrist and forearm in the same manner as for passive flexion and extension (Fig. 15–19C and D).

Resisted Range of Motion

Resisted ROM (RROM) of the wrist is highlighted in Box 15–5.

FIGURE 15–18. (A) Active range of motion for wrist flexion and extension. **(B)** Active range of motion for radial and ulnar deviation of the wrist.

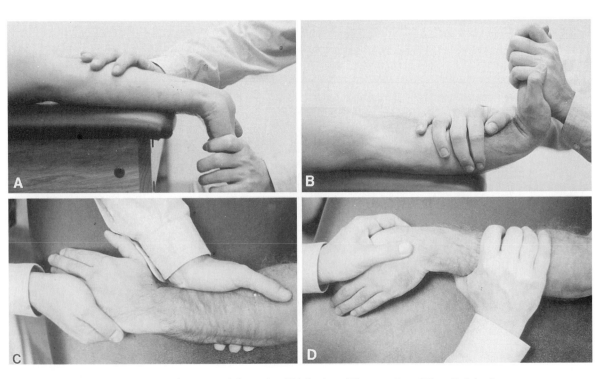

FIGURE 15–19. Passive range of motion of the wrist: **(A)** flexion; **(B)** extension; **(C)** radial deviation; **(D)** ulnar deviation.

Box 15–5
RESISTED RANGE OF MOTION FOR THE WRIST

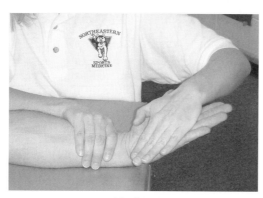

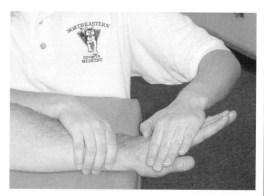

	Flexion	**Extension**
STARTING POSITION	The forearm is supinated and the wrist is extended	The forearm is pronated and the wrist is flexed
STABILIZATION	Posterior portion of the mid-forearm	Anterior portion of the mid-forearm
RESISTANCE	Palmar surface of the hand	Dorsal surface of the hand
MUSCLES TESTED	Flexor carpi radialis, flexor carpi ulnaris, flexor digitorum profundus, flexor digitorum superficialis, palmaris longus, flexor pollicis longus	Extensor carpi radialis longus, extensor carpi radialis brevis, extensor carpi ulnaris, extensor digitorum communis, extensor pollicis longus

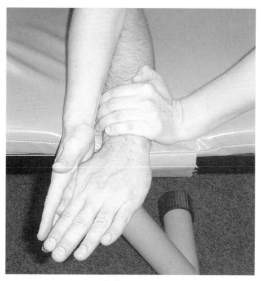

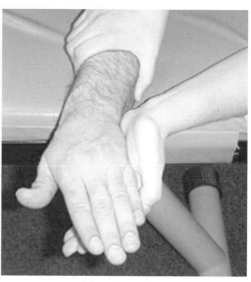

	Radial Deviation	**Ulnar Deviation**
STARTING POSITION	The forearm is supinated with the wrist in a neutral position.	The forearm is supinated with the wrist in a neutral position.
STABILIZATION	Distal forearm	Distal forearm
RESISTANCE	Radial side of the hand	Ulnar side of the hand
MUSCLES TESTED	Extensor carpi radialis longus, extensor carpi radialis brevis, abductor pollicis longus, extensor pollicis longus, extensor pollicis brevis	Extensor carpi ulnaris, flexor carpi ulnaris

Thumb Range of Motion Testing: Carpometacarpal Joint

The thumb is discussed as an individual unit as it pertains to the CMC joint. Its MCP and IP joints are described in the section on finger ROM. The motions of the thumb's CMC joint tend to be confusing, especially when compared with those of the remaining four fingers. Although abduction and adduction of the fingers occur in the frontal plane, abduction and adduction of the thumb (palmar abduction and adduction) occurs in the sagittal plane. Likewise, flexion and extension of the fingers occur in the sagittal plane. In the thumb, these motions occur in the frontal plane.

Active Range of Motion

- **Flexion and extension:** Thumb flexion and extension occur in the frontal plane around an anteroposterior axis. The majority of this motion, 60 to 70 degrees, is flexion (Fig. 15–20A). Only a trace amount of true CMC extension is permitted.
- **Abduction and adduction:** In the anatomical position, this motion occurs in the sagittal plane around a coronal axis. Abduction, best exemplified by the position the thumb assumes when holding a can, accounts for the total motion of 70 to 80 degrees (Fig. 15–20B). True adduction is limited by the phalanx striking the second metacarpal.

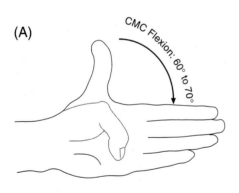

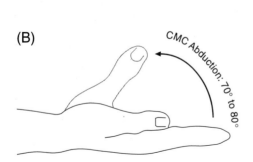

FIGURE 15–20. Active range of motion of the first carpometacarpal joint: **(A)** flexion; **(B)** abduction.

- **Opposition:** Opposition is the combined motion of flexion, abduction, and rotation of the thumb and is demonstrated by touching the thumb to the little finger (see Fig. 15–14).

Passive Range of Motion

- **Flexion and extension:** Flexion and extension are measured with the forearm supinated and resting on a table with the wrist and IP joint in the neutral position. The carpal bones are stabilized to prevent motion from occurring at the wrist (Fig. 15–21A and B).
- **Abduction and adduction:** The medial forearm is rested on the table in the neutral position. The wrist, CMC, MCP, and IP joints are placed in 0 degrees of extension. Stabilization is provided to the carpal bones and second metacarpal (Fig. 15–21C and D).
- **Opposition:** The forearm is fully supinated and the wrist is placed in its neutral position. The examiner brings the thumb and fifth finger toward each other. Normally, the two fingers should touch each other.

Resisted Range of Motion

Resisted ROM for the thumb is presented in Box 15–6.

Finger Range of Motion Testing

Active Range of Motion

- **Flexion and extension of the MCP joints:** Flexion and extension of the MCP joints occur in the sagittal plane around a coronal axis. A maximum of 105 to 135 degrees of motion is allowed at the MCP joint, with 20 to 30 degrees occurring during extension and the remaining 85 to 105 degrees accounted for during flexion (Fig. 15–22A).

  Locking that occurs during finger flexion can indicate **"trigger finger,"** adhesions in the flexor tendon sheath. During active flexion, the sheath adheres to the surrounding tissues and requires additional effort to gain flexion. As the tendon releases, an audible snap is heard and the finger snaps into flexion. During the latter stages of this condition, full flexion may be restricted.
- **Abduction and adduction of the MCP joints:** Twenty to 25 degrees of motion are allowed during abduction and the return motion of adduction. The movement occurs in the frontal plane around an anteroposterior axis with the third metacarpal serving as the reference point (Fig. 15–22B).
- **Flexion and extension of the IP joints:** Flexion and extension of the IP joints range from 80 to 90 degrees at the thumb, 110 to 120 degrees at the PIP, and 80 to 90 degrees at the DIP joints of the fingers (Fig. 15–22C and D).

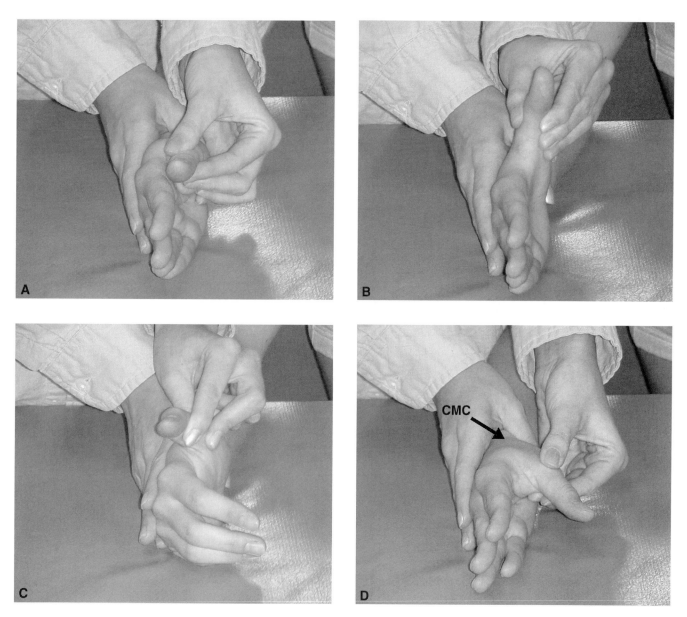

FIGURE 15–21. Passive range of motion of the first carpometacarpal joint: **(A)** flexion, **(B)** extension, **(C)** adduction, **(D)** abduction. Do not confuse CMC motion with motion produced by the MP joint (refer to Figure 15–21D for the location of the CMC joint).

FIGURE 15–22. Illustration of finger range of motion: **(A)** metacarpophalangeal flexion and extension; **(B)** metacarpophalangeal abduction; **(C)** flexion of the proximal interphalangeal joint; **(D)** flexion of the proximal and distal interphalangeal joints.

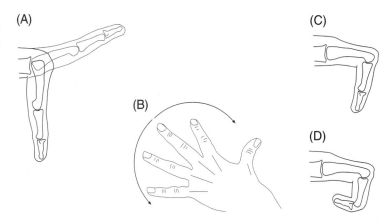

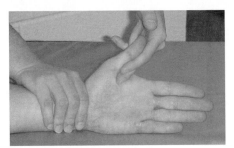

Flexion

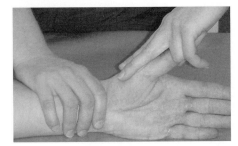

Extension

STARTING POSITION	Neutral position	Neutral position
STABILIZATION	Carpal bones	Carpal bones
RESISTANCE	Palmar aspect of the first phalanx	Dorsal aspect of the first phalanx
MUSCLES TESTED	Flexor pollicis longus, flexor pollicis brevis	Extensor pollicis longus, extensor pollicis brevis, abductor pollicis longus
	IP joint: flexor pollicis longus	**IP joint:** extensor pollicis longus extensor pollicis brevis

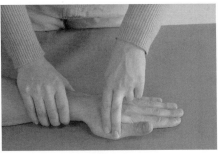

Abduction

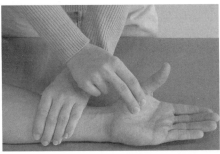

Adduction

STARTING POSITION	Neutral position	Neutral position
STABILIZATION	Wrist and lateral four metacarpals	Wrist and lateral four metacarpals
RESISTANCE	Lateral border of the first metacarpal	Medial border of the first metacarpal
MUSCLES TESTED	Abductor pollicis longus, abductor pollicis brevis, extensor pollicis brevis	Adductor pollicis

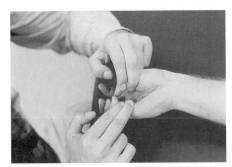

Opposition

STARTING POSITION	The thumb and fifth fingers opposed
STABILIZATION	Not applicable
RESISTANCE	The examiner attempts to separate the fingers
MUSCLES TESTED	Opponens pollicis, opponens digiti minimi

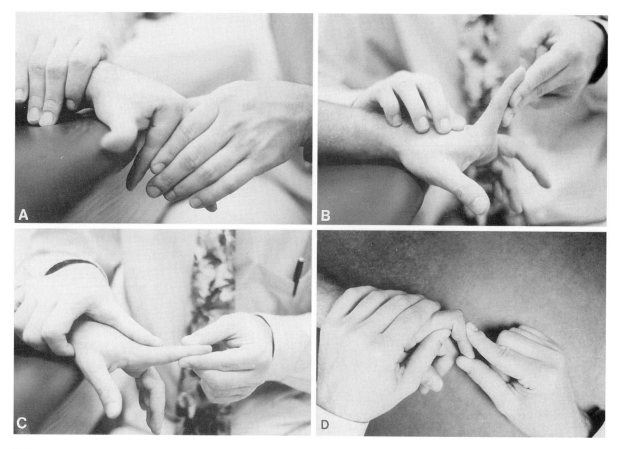

FIGURE 15–23. Passive finger range of motion: **(A)** flexion and **(B)** extension of the metacarpophalangeal joint; **(C)** extension of the proximal interphalangeal joint; **(D)** flexion of the proximal interphalangeal joint.

Passive Range of Motion

- **Flexion and extension of the MCP joints:** While stabilizing the metacarpal, grasp the proximal phalanx of the finger being tested (Fig. 15–23A and B).

- **Abduction and adduction of the MCP joints:** Grasp the finger over the PIP joint. The patient's arm is positioned so that the palm is resting flat against the table with the metacarpals stabilized to prevent wrist motion.

- **Flexion and extension of the interphalangeal joints:** Stabilize the phalanx proximal to the joint being tested while applying force to the phalanx of the distal bone. The normal end-feel for the PIP joint is hard during flexion as the two phalanges contact each other, but a soft end-feel can occur by soft tissue approximation (Fig. 15–23 C and D).

Resisted Range of Motion

Resisted ROM for the finger is presented in Box 15–7. A manual dynamometer can be used to quantitatively measure grip strength (Box 15–8).

LIGAMENTOUS AND CAPSULAR TESTING

The ligaments of the wrist are stressed with overpressure during the evaluation of PROM (Table 15–4). Avulsion fractures of a ligament's attachment may

Table 15–4
LIGAMENTS STRESSED DURING WRIST PASSIVE RANGE OF MOTION

	Ligaments Stressed	
Passive movement	**Primary**	**Secondary**
Extension	Palmar ulnocarpal Palmar radiocarpal	Radial collateral Ulnar collateral
Flexion	Dorsal radiocarpal	Radial collateral Ulnar collateral
Radial deviation	Ulnar collateral	Palmar ulnocarpal
Ulnar deviation	Radial collateral	Palmar radiocarpal

Box 15–7
RESISTED RANGE OF MOTION FOR THE FINGERS

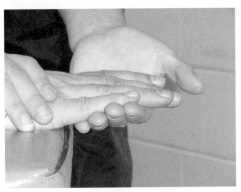

Flexion

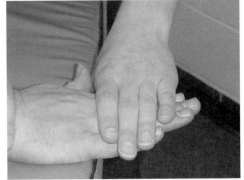

Extension

STARTING POSITION	The joint being tested is placed in the neutral position	The joint being tested is placed in the neutral position
STABILIZATION	At the joint (or joints) proximal to the joint being tested	At the joint (or joints) proximal to the joint being tested
RESISTANCE	On the palmar aspect of the phalanx distal to the joint being tested	On the dorsal aspect of the phalanx distal to the joint being tested
MUSCLES TESTED	**MCP joint:** interossei, lumbricales, flexor digitorum profundus, flexor digitorum superficialis, flexor digiti minimi (5th finger) **PIP joint:** flexor digitorum profundus, flexor digitorum superficialis **DIP joint:** flexor digitorum profundus	**MCP joint:** extensor digitorum communis **PIP and DIP joints:** extensor digitorum communis, interossei, lumbricales

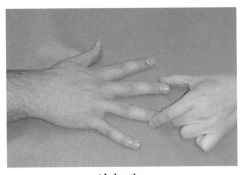

Abduction

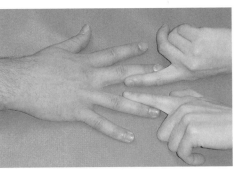

Adduction

STARTING POSITION	The joint being tested is placed in the neutral position	The joint being tested is placed in the neutral position
STABILIZATION	Not applicable	Not applicable
RESISTANCE	As above	As above
MUSCLES TESTED	Dorsal interossei, abductor digiti minimi (5th finger)	Palmar interossei

DIP = distal interphalangeal; MCP = metacarpophalangeal; PIP = proximal interphalangeal.

Box 15–8
GRIP DYNAMOMETRY

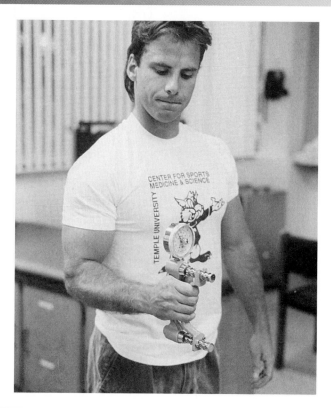

PATIENT POSITION	Holding the grip dynamometer with the elbow flexed to 90° and the radioulnar joint in its neutral position
POSITION OF EXAMINER	Standing in front of the patient, viewing the dynamometer's gauge
EVALUATIVE PROCEDURE	The dynamometer is set at one of five specified settings (1, 1.5, 2, 2.5, and 3 inches). The patient squeezes the dynamometer's handle with maximum force at every setting, with adequate recovery time allowed between bouts. The values are recorded and the test is repeated on the opposite hand.
POSITIVE TEST	Injured nondominant hand: more than 10% bilateral strength deficit compared with the dominant hand Injured dominant hand: more than 5% bilateral strength deficit compared with the nondominant hand
IMPLICATIONS	Pathology that inhibits grip strength, the underlying cause of the weakness must be determined.
COMMENT	Because of the wide range of variation in grip strength, the outcome of each of these tests is most meaningful when compared with a baseline measure. This test can be repeated 3 times at any one setting and the results averaged.

produce positive results during stress testing. Because the fracture can involve the joint's articular surface, sprains should be radiographed to rule out joint pathology.

Tests for Collateral Support of the Wrist Ligaments

The UCL provides lateral support against valgus forces (radial deviation), and the RCL checks varus forces (ulnar deviation). These two ligaments also function cooperatively to limit wrist flexion and extension. Their integrity may be partially established through valgus and varus stress testing (Box 15–9) and by assessing glide between the proximal carpal row and the radius (Box 15–10). These tests not only check the integrity of the collateral ligaments but may also elicit signs of trauma to the triangular fibrocartilage.

Tests for Collateral Support of the Interphalangeal Joints

The integrity of the IP joints' collateral ligaments can be determined through valgus and varus stress testing. Although these tests demonstrate laxity in cases of a complete rupture of the ligament, pain may also be

used as a measure of the relative severity of the injury (Box 15–11).

Test for Support of the Ulnar Collateral Ligament

The only MCP joint that is routinely stress tested is the thumb's UCL (Box 15–12). Because of the alignment of the fingers, the only other MCP collateral ligaments frequently injured are the UCL of the MCP joint of the index finger and the RCL of the little finger.

NEUROLOGIC TESTING

Most commonly, nerves of the hand, wrist, and fingers are affected by pathology proximal to the forearm, but trauma in this region can lead to localized symptoms. **Carpal tunnel syndrome** (CTS), discussed later in this chapter, causes dysfunction in the distal median nerve distribution (Fig. 15–24). The ulnar nerve can become compressed as it passes through the tunnel of Guyon, located between the hook of the hamate and the pisiform. Radial nerve pathology in the elbow can result in **drop wrist syndrome,** which is the inability to actively extend the wrist and fingers. A complete upper quarter screen may be indicated (see Box 1–6).

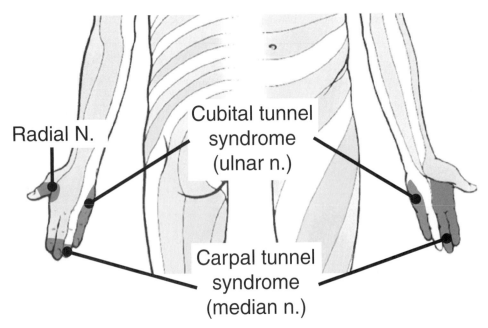

FIGURE 15–24. Local neuropathies of the hand. Correlate these findings with those of an upper quarter neurological screen (see Box 1–6).

Box 15–9
VALGUS AND VARUS STRESS TESTING OF THE WRIST

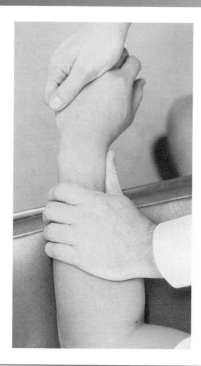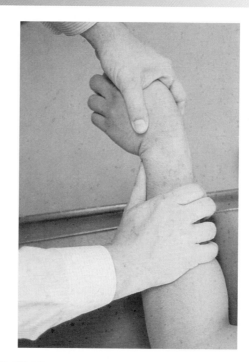

PATIENT POSITION	Sitting The elbow flexed to 90°, the forearm pronated, and the fingers assuming the relaxed position of flexion
POSITION OF EXAMINER	Sitting or standing lateral to the wrist being tested One hand grips the distal forearm and the other grasps the hand across the metacarpals
EVALUATIVE PROCEDURE	UCL: a valgus stress is applied, radially deviating the wrist RCL: a varus stress is applied, ulnarly deviating the wrist
POSITIVE TEST	Pain or laxity (or both) compared with the same ligament on the opposite wrist
IMPLICATIONS	Stretching or tearing of the UCL or RCL
COMMENT	Pain may be elicited in the presence of trauma to the triangular fibrocartilage, scaphoid fractures, or the palmar or dorsal radiocarpal or ulnocarpal ligaments.

RCL = radial collateral ligament; UCL = ulnar collateral ligament.

Box 15–10
WRIST GLIDE TESTS

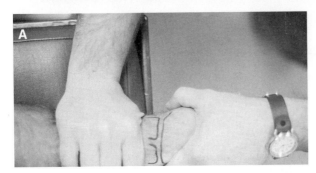

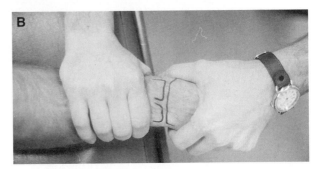

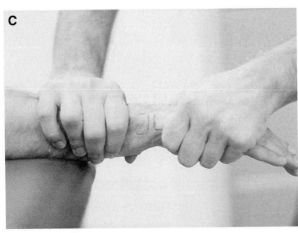

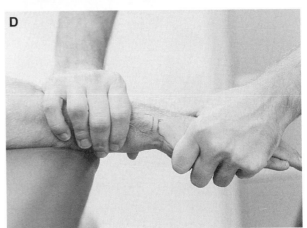

Glide testing of the wrist: radial glide (**A**); ulnar glide (**B**); superior glide (**C**); and inferior glide (**D**).

PATIENT POSITION	Sitting The elbow flexed to 90°, the forearm pronated, and the fingers assuming the relaxed position of flexion
POSITION OF EXAMINER	Sitting or standing lateral to the wrist being tested One hand grips the distal radius and the other hand grasps the proximal carpal row
EVALUATIVE PROCEDURE	A shear force is applied to the wrist by gliding the distal segment in a radial and ulnar direction and then in a volar and dorsal direction.
POSITIVE TEST	Pain or significant change in glide compared with the opposite side
IMPLICATIONS	Tear or stretching of the collateral or intercarpal ligaments or trauma to the triangular fibrocartilage. Decreased glide may indicate adhesions and capsular stiffness after injury or surgery.
COMMENT	This motion stresses both collateral ligaments; the determination of which ligament is involved is based on the location of pain.

Box 15–11
VALGUS AND VARUS TESTING OF THE INTERPHALANGEAL JOINTS

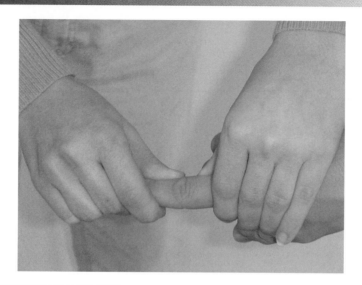

Stress testing the ulnar collateral ligament of the PIP joint. This test should be repeated using varus stress for the radial collateral ligament.

PATIENT POSITION	Sitting or standing The joint being tested is in extension.
POSITION OF EXAMINER	Standing if front of the patient, stabilizing the phalanx proximal to the joint being tested
EVALUATIVE PROCEDURE	The examiner grasps the phalanx distal to the joint being tested and applies a valgus stress to the joint. A varus stress is then applied to the joint.
POSITIVE TEST	Increased gapping, compared with the same motion on the same finger of the opposite hand Pain
IMPLICATIONS	Collateral ligament sprain
COMMENT	Except in the case of a complete disruption of the ligament, the degree of injury to the ligament cannot be established.

PIP = proximal interphalangeal.

Box 15–12
TEST FOR LAXITY OF THE COLLATERAL LIGAMENTS

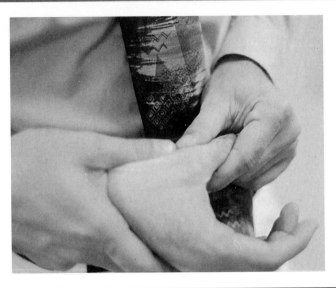

PATIENT POSITION	Sitting or standing
POSITION OF EXAMINER	Standing in front of the patient
EVALUATIVE PROCEDURE	The examiner stabilizes the first metacarpal with one hand and its proximal phalanx with the other. While stabilizing the first metacarpal with the thumb slightly abducted and extended, the examiner applies a valgus stress to the ulnar collateral ligament. The test is repeated with the joint in varying degrees of flexion to evaluate the dorsal capsule of the joint.
POSITIVE TEST	The ulnar side of the first metacarpophalangeal joint gaps farther than the uninjured side or the patient describes pain (or both).
IMPLICATIONS	Stretching or tearing of the ulnar collateral ligament

 PATHOLOGIES OF THE WRIST, HAND, AND FINGERS AND RELATED SPECIAL TESTS

Any injury to this area involves the possible ramification of significant disability in both athletic competition and activities of daily living (ADLs). Although similar in nature, trauma to the thumb and trauma to the fingers are discussed in separate sections because of the potential differences in the functional outcomes.

WRIST PATHOLOGY

Trauma to the wrist can affect the distal portion of the radius and ulna; the collateral, volar, and dorsal ligaments; the triangular fibrocartilage; or the neurovascular structures. The mechanisms of injury for most of these conditions are similar, calling for careful inspection, palpation, and functional testing of the involved structures.

Wrist Sprains

Because wrist ligament sprains are caused by many of the same mechanisms as for other pathologies of the wrist and hand, the conclusion of a wrist sprain is often based on the exclusion of other injuries.[4] The possibilities of carpal fractures (especially the scaphoid), triangular fibrocartilage tears, and CTS must first be eliminated before making the determination of a wrist sprain. Sprains of the distal radioulnar ligaments can lead to a dislocation of the distal ends of these two bones, especially in the presence of an associated fracture.[5]

AROM is limited in all directions secondary to pain, with the restriction occurring equally during flexion and extension. Although pain may be duplicated by the ligaments' being pinched between two bones, pain typically occurs during PROM or during valgus and varus stress testing as the involved ligaments are stretched with overpressure (Table 15–5).

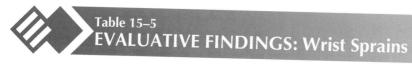

Table 15–5
EVALUATIVE FINDINGS: Wrist Sprains

Examination Segment	Clinical Findings	
History	*Onset:*	Acute
	Pain characteristics:	Pain emanating from the palmar and dorsal aspects of the wrist near the joint line
	Mechanism:	Tensile forces placed on the ligaments as the joint is forced past its normal ROM
Inspection	Swelling localized to the joint line	
Palpation	Tenderness usually more diffuse over the wrist joint than with other wrist injuries such as scaphoid fractures or tears of the triangular fibrocartilage	
Functional Tests	*AROM:*	Limited as the sprained tissues are placed on stretch; motion in the opposite direction also possibly limited as the capsule and ligamentous tissues become pinched as the movement is performed
	PROM:	Limited as the sprained tissues are placed on stretch
	RROM:	Pain possibly absent with isometric testing in a neutral position; providing resistance through the ROM exhibiting weakness secondary to pain
Ligamentous Tests	Wrist glide tests	
Neurologic Tests	Not applicable	
Special Tests	None	
Comments	The diagnosis of a wrist sprain is made after the possibility of carpal fractures, triangular fibrocartilage tears, and other traumatic injury has been ruled out.	

AROM = active range of motion; PROM = passive range of motion; ROM = range of motion; RROM = resisted range of motion.

Triangular Fibrocartilage Complex Injury

Trauma to the TFCC and the UCL can result in permanent disability of the wrist if left unrecognized and untreated.[6] Athletes who compete in sports that place the upper extremity in a closed kinetic chain are at an increased risk of TFCC injury.

Forced hyperextension results in pain along the ulnar side of the wrist and is accompanied by decreased wrist motion secondary to pain. During palpation, close attention must be devoted to the ulnar styloid process because it can be avulsed by the UCL concurrently with injury to the TFCC (Table 15–6). Any suspicion of injury to the TFCC should warrant referral to a physician for further evaluation.

Carpal Tunnel Syndrome

Carpal tunnel syndrome refers to the signs and symptoms caused by the compression of the median nerve as it passes through the carpal tunnel (see Fig. 15–8). The most frequently cited cause of CTS is fibrosis of the synovium of the flexor tendons secondary to tenosynovitis.[7,8] CTS may occur with repetitive microtrauma, with acute trauma to the carpal tunnel, or as the result of progressive degeneration of the carpal tunnel's structures. The resulting symptoms of CTS can have detrimental effects on both athletic ability and ADLs.

Paresthesia and pain are described along the median nerve distribution (thumb, index, middle, and lateral half of the ring finger), with the symptoms often occurring at night because of impeded venous return.[9] Inspection of the hand may reveal atrophy of the thenar muscles, and grip strength is often decreased.[10] Manual muscle testing of the abductor pollicis brevis and the opponens pollicis reveals weakness on the involved side (Table 15–7).[11] A positive **Tinel's sign** is elicited over the carpal tunnel (Fig. 15–25), and results of **Phalen's test** are positive (Box 15–13). An achy pain may be described in the volar aspect of the forearm.

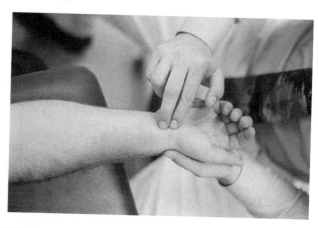

FIGURE 15–25. Tinel's test performed over the median nerve. In the presence of carpal tunnel syndrome, this test results in pain and paresthesia radiating into the middle finger.

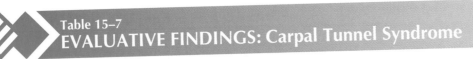

Table 15–6
EVALUATIVE FINDINGS: Injury to the TFCC

Examination Segment	Clinical Findings	
History	**Onset:**	Acute; the patient may not report the injury for some time after its onset
	Pain characteristics:	Distal to the ulna along the medial one half of the wrist; the UCL of the wrist may also be tender
	Mechanism:	Forced hyperextension of the wrist, compressing the triangular fibrocartilage
Inspection	Diffuse swelling around the wrist is possible, although acutely, no swelling may be visible.	
Palpation	Point tenderness distal to the ulna along the medial one half of the wrist's joint line; the UCL may also display tenderness.	
Functional Tests	**AROM:**	Motion is limited, especially into extension and ulnar deviation.
	PROM:	Motion is limited, especially into extension and ulnar deviation.
	RROM:	Isometric testing may be normal; resistance through the ROM is limited, especially as the wrist is brought into extension and ulnar deviation.
Ligamentous Tests	Stressing the UCL elicits pain, although laxity may not be present. Ulnar deviation produces pain.	
Neurologic Tests	Not applicable	
Special Tests	None	
Comments	Triangular fibrocartilage complex tears may be easily confused with a sprain of the wrist's UCL; persistence of symptoms should alert the examiner to injury beyond a simple wrist sprain. Patients suspected of suffering from triangular fibrocartilage complex tears should be referred to a physician for further evaluation.	

AROM = active range of motion; PROM = passive range of motion; ROM = range of motion; RROM = resisted range of motion; UCL = ulnar collateral ligament.

Table 15–7
EVALUATIVE FINDINGS: Carpal Tunnel Syndrome

Examination Segment	Clinical Findings	
History	**Onset:**	Insidious
	Pain characteristics:	Paresthesia or pain in the hand, wrist, and fingers (median nerve distribution), possibly radiating up the length of the arm and worsening during sleep secondary to a flexed posture of the elbow, wrist, and fingers
	Mechanism:	Repetitive wrist movement involving flexion and extension or finger flexion and extension
	Predisposing conditions:	Poor posture or biomechanics
Inspection	Palmar aspect of the wrist possibly appearing thickened	
Palpation	Possible tenderness on palpation directly over the palmar aspect of the wrist	
Functional Tests	**AROM:**	The wrist motion may be slightly limited owing to stiffness, although AROM may be normal.
	PROM:	Median nerve symptoms may increase as the wrist is fully extended or fully flexed.
	RROM:	In chronic cases, the strength of the abductor pollicis brevis, flexor pollicis brevis, or opponens pollicis may be decreased.
Ligamentous Tests	Not applicable	
Neurologic Tests	Possible decreased sensation along the median nerve distribution of the hand (palmar aspect of the thumb, fingers II and III, and the lateral aspect of IV)	
Special Tests	Tinel's sign; Phalen's test	
Comments	This condition is typically found in individuals who perform repetitive wrist and hand movements such as typing and may become more pronounced in a student–athlete population with the increase in computer use in academic work.	

AROM = active range of motion; PROM = passive range of motion; ROM = range of motion; RROM = resisted range of motion.

Box 15–13
PHALEN'S TEST FOR CARPAL TUNNEL SYNDROME

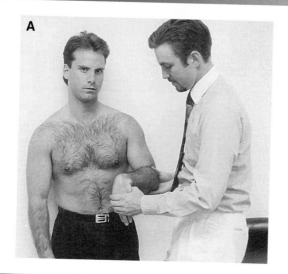

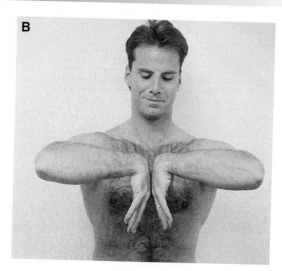

(A) Modification of Phalen's test (described below), **(B)** Original test as described by Phalen.

PATIENT POSITION	Standing or seated
POSITION OF EXAMINER	Standing in front of the patient
EVALUATIVE PROCEDURE	The examiner applies overpressure during passive wrist flexion and holds the position for 1 min. This procedure is then repeated for the opposite extremity.
POSITIVE TEST	Tingling in the distribution of the median nerve distal to the carpal tunnel.
IMPLICATIONS	Median nerve compression
MODIFICATION	The traditional version of this test, in which the patient maximally flexes the wrists by pushing the dorsal aspects of the hands together, is not recommended because the patient may shrug the shoulders, causing compression of the median branch of the brachial plexus as it passes through the thoracic outlet.

The signs and symptoms of CTS closely resemble the peripheral symptoms associated with impingement of the C7 nerve root and proximal neuropathy of the median nerve. A careful differential evaluation must be made to identify the cause of the symptoms.

Initially, patients with CTS are managed conservatively. The basic treatment plan focuses on rest from aggravating activities and activity modification and ergonomic changes in posture, work stations, and computer usage. Initial treatments also include the use of nonsteroidal anti-inflammatory drugs (NSAIDs) to decrease inflammation and splinting to remove harmful physical stresses. Initially splinting may be used only at night. Severe or nonresponsive cases may require splint use throughout the day. Attempts at stretching and strengthening usually do not affect the course of the treatment.

Surgery may be required to relieve the compression on the median nerve. After an initial period of taking NSAIDs and immobilization to allow for healing, AROM and strengthening exercises are begun.

Wrist Fractures

Fractures of the distal radius or ulna frequently occur secondary to landing on an outstretched arm. The term **"Colles' fracture"** is often used to describe any fracture of the distal radius. However, a true Colles' fracture is a nonarticular fracture of the radius approximately 1.5 inches proximal to the radiocarpal joint, where the distal radius is displaced dorsally.[12] On a lateral radiographic view, the wrist appears as an upside-down fork (Fig. 15–26). The terms **"Smith's fracture"** and **"reverse Colles' fracture"** are used to describe a fracture in which the distal radius is displaced palmarly.[13] Fractures of the wrist involve the immediate loss of function and possible deformity (Table 15–8).

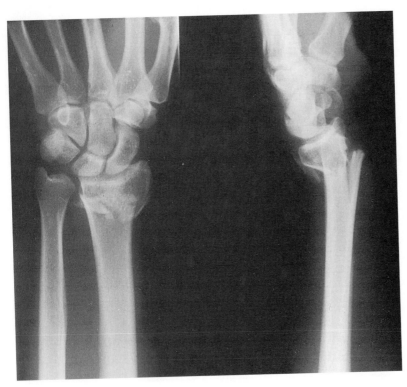

FIGURE 15–26. Radiograph of a Colles' fracture. Note the dorsal displacement of the radius.

HAND PATHOLOGY

The majority of injuries to the hand, the carpals and metacarpals, have an acute onset. The carpals are most commonly injured after hyperflexion or hyperextension of the wrist. Injury to the metacarpals typically follows axial loading of the bone. Both groups of bones are also susceptible to crushing forces.

Scaphoid Fractures

The majority of all carpal fractures involve the scaphoid bone because of its function as a bony block limiting wrist extension.[14] Receiving its blood supply from the distal end, a fracture compromises nutrition to the proximal portion, causing a high incidence of nonunion fractures and malunion fractures secondary to avascu-

◢◢◢ **Table 15–8**
EVALUATIVE FINDINGS: Wrist and Distal Forearm Fractures

Examination Segment	Clinical Findings	
History	**Onset:**	Acute
	Pain characteristics:	Distal forearm, proximal wrist; the patient may describe hearing and feeling a cracking sensation
	Mechanism:	A hyperextension mechanism, possibly combined with a rotatory component, placing tensile, compressive, or shear forces on the radius, ulna, or both (e.g., landing on an outstretched arm)
Inspection	Gross deformity of the long bones possible; rapid onset of swelling	
Palpation	Discontinuity of the long bones may be felt and the area is tender to the touch. The bony palpation phase may be omitted if gross deformity is present. The examiner must locate the radial and ulnar pulses to ensure an adequate blood supply to the hand and fingers.	
Functional Tests	In the event of obvious gross deformity of the long bones, ROM testing is not conducted.	
Ligamentous Tests	Not applicable	
Neurologic Tests	Establish the presence of the distal pulses and innervation, including capillary refill.	
Special Tests	Not applicable	
Comments	Suspected fractures should be appropriately splinted and the patient immediately referred to a physician.	

ROM = range of motion.

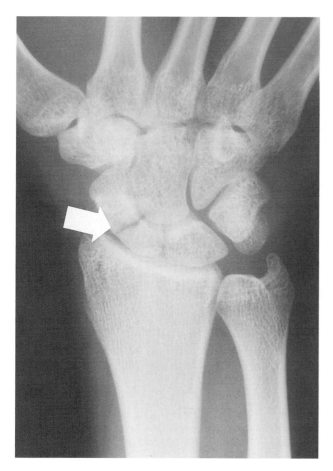

FIGURE 15–27. Radiograph of a scaphoid fracture.

lar necrosis (Fig. 15–27).[15] Unresolved fractures or chronically impaired circulation to the scaphoid may result in the development of *Preiser's disease.*

The chief complaint is of an ache in the area of the anatomical snuffbox that is worsened with palpation on its palmar and dorsal aspects (see Fig. 15–12). Pain occurs with active and resisted wrist extension near the end of the ROM, where the scaphoid contacts the radius. Severe pain is produced with overpressure during passive flexion, extension, and radial deviation. Grip strength may be decreased on the involved side. Compression of the first metacarpal toward the scaphoid may also produce pain.

Patients with an injury that produces pain in the area of the anatomical snuffbox after a hyperextension mechanism, such as falling on an outstretched arm, must be treated as having a fracture of the scaphoid (Table 15–9). The wrist and thumb require immobilization and the patient is referred to a physician. Fracture lines are not always visible on the initial radiographic examination, and follow-up radiographs may be ordered as indicated.[16] Bone scans, computed tomography (CT) scans, and magnetic resonance imaging (MRI) scans can identify the presence of a scaphoid fracture earlier than can standard radiographs.

No one course of treatment for patients with scaphoid fractures is universally accepted. Some orthopedists choose to treat these fractures in a short arm cast. Other physicians elect to use a long arm thumb spica cast for 6 weeks followed by a short arm thumb spica cast for 6 weeks. The long arm cast eliminates movement at the fracture site caused by forearm pronation and supination. This treatment course may decrease the number of non- and malunions with these fractures. After adequate healing has taken place and the cast has been removed, the initial treatment focuses on restoration of ROM followed by strengthening. Displaced fractures that cannot be adequately reduced require open reduction and internal fixation. In some athletes, the treatment of choice may also be to immediately surgically fixate the fracture. This allows for an increased chance of healing as well as earlier motion with less chance of motion loss.

Perilunate and Lunate Dislocation

Forced hyperextension of the wrist and hand may disassociate the lunate from the rest of the carpals, resulting in its displacement either dorsally or palmarly. As the limits of the wrist and hand extension are exceeded, the scaphoid bone strikes the radius, rupturing the volar ligaments connecting the scaphoid to the lunate. As the force continues, the distal carpal row is stripped away from the lunate, resulting in the lunate's resting dorsally relative to the other carpals, a **perilunate dislocation.** Further extension leads to rupture of the dorsal ligaments, relocating the carpals and rotating the lunate. The lunate then rests volarly relative to the carpals, a **lunate dislocation.** Each of these types of dislocations may spontaneously reduce.

The chief complaint is pain along the radial side of the palmar or dorsal aspect of the wrist that limits ROM. A bulge may be visible on the palmar or dorsal aspect of the hand proximal to the third metacarpal (Table 15–10). The displacement of the lunate or swelling can cause paresthesia in the middle finger. With a lunate dislocation, the third knuckle is level with the other knuckles (it normally assumes a superior position).[17] A fracture of the scaphoid bone should be suspected with any lunate dislocation because of the similarity in their mechanisms of injury. However, patients with these injuries may present with no significant physical findings other than pain, so a definitive diagnosis is made using radiographs.

Repeated trauma to the lunate may compromise its vascular supply, resulting in *Kienböck's disease.* Untreated, Kienböck's disease may result in a loss of ulnar deviation; tenderness, pain, and swelling over the

Preiser's disease Osteoporosis of the scaphoid, resulting from a fracture or repeated trauma.

Kienböck's disease Osteochondritis or slow degeneration of the lunate bone.

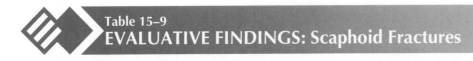

Table 15–9
EVALUATIVE FINDINGS: Scaphoid Fractures

Examination Segment	Clinical Findings	
History	*Onset:*	Acute, although the patient may delay seeking assistance because of the initial "minor" nature of the injury
	Pain characteristics:	Proximal portion of the lateral wrist in the anatomical snuffbox
	Mechanism:	Forceful hyperextension of the wrist that compresses the scaphoid
Inspection	Swelling possible in the anatomical snuffbox	
Palpation	Palpation of the scaphoid as it sits in the anatomical snuffbox elicits pain and tenderness; crepitus may be present. Pain may also be produced during palpation of the scaphoid's palmar aspect. Compression of the first metacarpal toward the scaphoid may elicit pain.	
Functional Tests	*AROM:*	Pain is produced at the terminal ROM, especially during extension. Radial deviation increases pain as the scaphoid is impinged between the radius, lunate, and trapezium.
	PROM:	Overpressure produces exquisite pain during extension. Pressure during flexion may also produce pain. Radial deviation increases pain.
	RROM:	Grip strength may be reduced.
Ligamentous Tests	Not applicable	
Neurologic Tests	Not applicable	
Special Tests	Not applicable	
Comments	Patients describing pain in the anatomical snuffbox after a mechanism involving forced hyperextension of the wrist should be managed as if they have a scaphoid fracture until it is ruled out by a physician. Scaphoid fractures may not appear on standard radiographs until several weeks after the injury but may be recognized on a bone scan within 72 hours after injury.	

AROM = active range of motion; PROM = passive range of motion; ROM = range of motion; RROM = resisted range of motion.

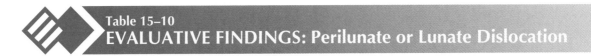

Table 15–10
EVALUATIVE FINDINGS: Perilunate or Lunate Dislocation

Examination Segment	Clinical Findings	
History	*Onset:*	Acute
	Pain characteristics:	Lateral wrist and hand
		Paresthesia along the median nerve distribution
	Mechanism:	Forced hyperextension of the wrist and hand
Inspection	A bulge caused by the displacement of the lunate may be seen on the palmar or dorsal aspect of the hand.	
Palpation	The lunate can be prominent during palpation, especially when it is displaced dorsally. Point tenderness and crepitus are present over the lunate.	
Functional Tests	ROM in all planes is limited secondary to pain.	
Ligamentous Tests	Not applicable	
Neurologic Tests	The sensory distribution of the median nerve requires evaluation for paresthesia.	
Special Tests	None	
Comments	An associated scaphoid fracture must be suspected with both perilunate and lunate dislocations.	

ROM = range of motion.

lunate; decreased grip strength; and weakness during wrist extension. A characteristic finding of Kienböck's disease is pain during passive extension of the third finger.

Lunate dislocations that are seen early after the injury may be amenable to closed reduction. If reduction is successful, the wrist is then immobilized in flexion for 6 to 8 weeks. The site of reduction requires frequent follow-up evaluations with radiographic examination. If the reduction is lost, percutaneous pinning of the lunate in the reduced position or open reduction may be needed.

If the patient is seen within 3 weeks of the initial injury, perilunate dislocations may be treated with closed reduction. If good anatomic reduction is demonstrated on radiographic examination, the wrist is then immobilized with slight flexion for 6 to 8 weeks. Loss of the reduction, even with casting, is common. Percutaneous pinning or open reduction are generally needed to maintain stable reduction.

Metacarpal Fractures

The metacarpals are typically fractured secondary to a compressive force along the bone's shaft, such as improperly punching with a fist. In football players, the incidence of fractures involving metacarpals is evenly divided among the five digits. In basketball players, most fractures involve the fourth and fifth metacarpals.[18] It is common for the patient to hear the bone snapping as it fractures and describe immediate pain along one or more metacarpals. Gross deformity at the fracture site may be observed as one end of the bone rides over the other end, or the fracture site may be obscured by localized swelling along the dorsum of the hand (Fig. 15–28). Palpation reveals local tenderness over the fracture site. The actual bony fragments or crepitus may be palpated and the presence of a false joint established. The presence of a nondisplaced fracture may be confirmed through a variation of the long bone compression test (Fig. 15–29). The ROM of the involved finger, and possibly the hand, is limited by pain. The patient is unable to make a fist (Table 15–11). As the patient attempts to flex the hand, the fingers should remain parallel to one another. With metacarpal fractures, the involved segment may rotate so that the finger flexes under or on top of the finger next to it.

Fractures of the fifth metacarpal are termed **"boxer's fractures"** because of their common incidence after an improperly thrown punch. This type of fracture is characterized by a depressed fifth MCP joint that, on radiographic examination, reveals an overlapping of the bone.

Treatment for metacarpal fractures depends on the presence of rotation at the fracture site. In the absence of rotation, a conservative approach of casting may be used. The presence of rotation at the fracture site necessitates open reduction with internal fixation to ensure favorable functional outcomes.[19] After adequate heal-

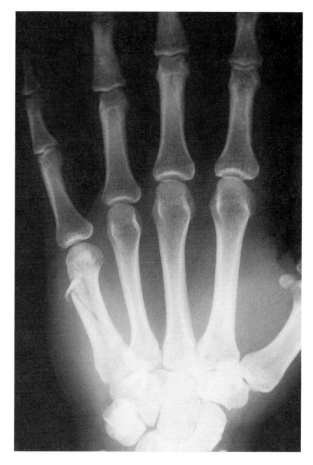

FIGURE 15–28. Radiograph of a metacarpal fracture, the so-called "boxer's fracture."

ing has taken place, AROM can be started and progressed to PROM, if needed, at about 8 weeks after the fracture. Strengthening of the wrist and hand is incorporated to counteract the effects of immobilization on the skeletal muscle.

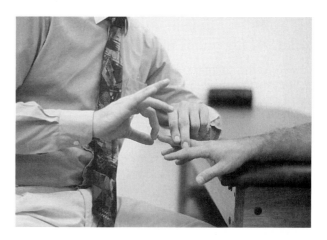

FIGURE 15–29. Long bone compression test for phalanx fracture. The examiner flicks the tip of the finger. Pain arising from a phalanx is a positive result.

Table 15–11
EVALUATIVE FINDINGS: Metacarpal Fractures

Examination Segment	Clinical Findings	
History	***Onset:***	Acute
	Pain characteristics:	Along the shaft of one or more metacarpals
	Mechanism:	Longitudinal compression of the bone (direct contact), a crushing force (being stepped on), or a shear force (hyperextension of the finger)
Inspection	Gross deformity of the bone may be visible. There is localized swelling over the involved metacarpal(s), and MCP joint(s), which may spread to the entire dorsum of the hand. Fractures of the 5th, and possibly 4th, metacarpals may result in a depression or shortening of the knuckles. The fingernail may be abnormally rotated when a fist is made.	
Palpation	Severe tenderness is present over the fracture site. Bony fragments or crepitus may be present. A false joint may be displayed. Palpation should not be performed if a fracture is evident.	
Functional Tests	***AROM:***	Limited secondary to pain; in some instances, the patient is unable to make a fist
	PROM:	Limited secondary to pain
	RROM:	Limited secondary to pain ROM testing should not be performed if a fracture is evident.
Ligamentous Tests	Not applicable	
Neurologic Tests	Not applicable	
Special Tests	Long bone compression test.	
Comments	If a fracture is evident during inspection, the evaluation should be immediately terminated, the hand appropriately splinted, and the patient immediately referred to a physician.	

AROM = active range of motion; PROM = passive range of motion; ROM = range of motion; RROM = resisted range of motion.

FINGER PATHOLOGY

Frequently finger injuries go unreported or there is a significant lapse between the onset of the injury and its report. Often gross deformity is associated with these conditions, especially with joint dislocations. However, the patient may self-reduce a dislocation before seeking medical attention.

Collateral Ligament Injuries

Trauma to the collateral ligaments can range from simple sprains to complete dislocations caused from a unilateral stress being applied to an extended finger. Pain is experienced at the affected joint and the person may report self-reducing the joint after a dislocation. Active motion and passive motion are limited secondary to pain and swelling. With the exception of a complete disruption of the ligament, valgus and varus stress testing does not accurately distinguish the severity of the injury.

Boutonnière Deformity

A rupture of the central extensor tendon causes it to slip palmarly on each side of the PIP joint, changing its

line of pull on this joint from that of an extensor to one of a flexor. The resulting position of the finger is extension of the DIP and MCP joints and flexion of the PIP joint, a boutonnière deformity (see Box 15–2). The patient describes a longitudinal force on the finger, such as being struck with a ball. Pain occurs on the dorsal aspect of the PIP joint, and the boutonnière deformity is visible. In acute cases, the PIP joint cannot be actively extended, but the examiner can passively return the joint to its normal position. The signs and symptoms of a tendon rupture may not be recognized for some time after the injury.[1] In chronic cases, the tendon becomes fibrotic, forming a mechanical block against even passive extension of the joint.

An injury to the volar plate can cause a flexion deformity of the PIP joint that resembles a boutonnière deformity, a **pseudo-boutonnière deformity** (see Box 15–2). Hyperextension of the finger causes the volar plate to split along the finger's long axis and slide dorsally past the joint's axis. The PIP joint cannot be extended either actively or passively.

Finger Fractures

Fractures of the **distal phalanx,** the most common fractures of the hand, occur most frequently in the thumb and middle finger. One reason for this high incidence of injury is the attachments of the flexor and extensor tendons. Avulsions of these tendons result in the inability to completely flex or extend the distal phalanx. The distal phalanx is also vulnerable to crushing mechanism (e.g., being stepped on) and longitudinal compression and rotation (e.g., a blow to the tip of the finger). The **middle phalanx** is the least frequently fractured phalanx and tends to fracture at the distal portion of the shaft. Injuries to the **proximal phalanx** usually have concurrent tendon and skin trauma. A direct blow to the finger often results in a transverse or comminuted fracture; a twisting or rotational force causes a spiral fracture (Fig. 15–30).

The signs and symptoms of phalanx fractures are similar to those of metacarpal fractures (see Table 15–11). An audible "snap" at the time of injury may be reported, especially when the proximal or middle phalanges are injured. Pain is centered over the fracture site, and gross deformity may be present in the finger's alignment. Soft tissue swelling and hematoma formation increase the amount of pain associated with the fracture and impair the ability to palpate the injured area. AROM is limited by pain or bony derangement. During finger flexion, a spiral or oblique fracture causes

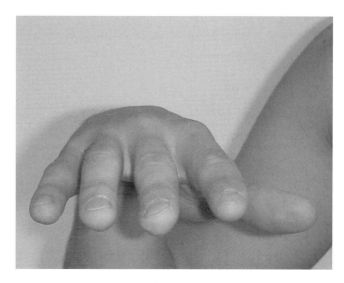

FIGURE 15–31. Rotational malalignment associated with a spiral fracture of the finger. Note the rotational displacement of the third fingernail.

the portion of the finger distal to the fracture site to rotate so that the fingernails are not in line with each other (Fig 15–31). Fractures that extended into the joint's articular surface can result in the long-term loss of ROM.

Finger fractures are managed similarly to metacarpal fractures.

Finger Avulsion Fracture

Mallet finger occurs when an avulsion or stretching of an extensor tendon results in the inability to fully extend the distal phalanx (see Box 15–2). This occurs when the DIP is forced into flexion, such as when the fingertip is struck with a ball. In addition to being unable to actively extend the finger, the distal phalanx, which rests at approximately 25 to 35 degrees of flexion, is painful. Active flexion is still present and the phalanx can be passively moved into extension.

An avulsion of the flexor digitorum profundus tendon off the palmar aspect of the DIP joint, **jersey finger,** results in the inability to flex the distal phalanx (see Box 15–2). This commonly occurs when an athlete grasps another athlete's jersey, forcing the finger into extension as the finger is attempting to flex and hold onto the opponent. The jersey finger injury is described as being one of three types.[20]

- **First degree:** The bony attachment is left intact and the ruptured tendon retracts to the PIP joint.
- **Second degree:** A portion of the bony attachment is avulsed and the tendon retracts to the palm.
- **Third degree:** A fragment of bone is avulsed with the tendon's insertion and retracts to the PIP joint.

On casual inspection and functional testing, the involved finger appears to be normal. The finger is painful, but little swelling or disfiguration is noted. The

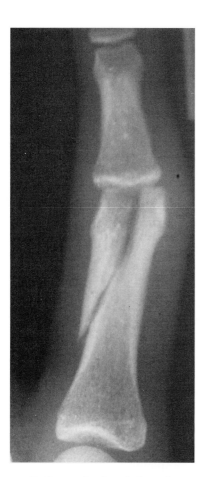

FIGURE 15–30. Radiograph of a phalanx fracture. Note that this is a spiral fracture involving the articular surface.

Table 15–12
EVALUATIVE FINDINGS: DeQuervain's Syndrome

Examination Segment	Clinical Findings	
History	***Onset:***	Insidious
	Pain characteristics:	Over the length of the extensor pollicis brevis and abductor pollicis longus, the radial styloid process and thenar eminence, possibly extending into the distal forearm; complaints of pain increased during radial and ulnar deviation
	Mechanism:	Repetitive stress often involving radial deviation
	Predisposing conditions:	Repetitive motion accompanied by poor biomechanics
Inspection	Swelling over the styloid process and in the involved tendons	
Palpation	Pain felt over the styloid process, thenar eminence, and the length of the extensor pollicis brevis and abductor pollicis longus muscles	
Functional Tests	***AROM:***	Wrist: pain with radial and ulnar deviation Thumb: pain with flexion and adduction and extension and abduction
	PROM:	Wrist: pain at the end range of ulnar deviation Thumb: pain with flexion and adduction
	RROM:	Wrist: pain with radial deviation Thumb: pain with extension and abduction
Ligamentous Tests	Not applicable	
Neurologic Tests	Not applicable	
Special Tests	Finkelstein's test	

AROM = active range of motion; PROM = passive range of motion; RROM = resisted range of motion.

fingers appear to flex and extend normally, with an increase in pain noted during flexion. The telltale sign occurs when the examiner stabilizes the PIP joint in extension and requests that the patient flex the DIP joint but the patient is unable to do so.

THUMB PATHOLOGY

The thumb is involved in most aspects of athletics and the position it assumes when gripping, catching, or in the "ready position" exposes it to potentially injurious forces in all planes. Unlike the other digits, the thumb is also susceptible to overuse conditions.

DeQuervain's Syndrome

DeQuervain's syndrome is a tenosynovitis of the extensor pollicis brevis and abductor pollicis longus tendons, which are encased by a fibrous sheath having a common synovial lining. Repetitive stress results in the compartment's becoming inflamed. Consequently, prolonged inflammation causes a thickening and narrowing of the tendon's sheath. A history of this condition reveals a mechanism of repetitive motions usually involving radial deviation.[21] Pain is located at the radial styloid process and dorsum of the thumb and radiates proximally into the forearm. Swelling may be located over the styloid process and thenar eminence. Radial and ulnar deviation of the wrist results in pain, as do

flexion, extension, and abduction of the thumb (Table 15–12). Although not conclusive, **Finkelstein's test** may be used to support or refute the presence of deQuervain's syndrome (Box 15–14).

Patients with deQuervain's syndrome are best treated with rest, ice, NSAIDs, and splinting to limit ulnar deviation. The use of iontophoresis may be helpful to decrease the inflammation in the tissues. Activity modification and long-term splinting may be needed to eliminate excessive stress on the tendons with repetitive ulnar deviation.

Thumb Sprains

The UCL of the thumb's MCP joint is injured 10 times more often than its radial counterpart is.[22] This structure may be acutely sprained by hyperabduction or hyperextension of the MCP joint or it may be traumatized secondary to a repetitive stress. In the case of acute trauma, an associated avulsion fracture may occur around the MCP joint. The term "gamekeeper's thumb" was coined to describe the stretching of this ligament suffered by individuals whose duty it was to snap the neck of small game that had just been captured during hunting. This injury is commonly seen in skiers, football players, and basketball players. UCL sprains limit opposition of the thumb and decrease grip strength.

The chief complaint is pain along the ulnar aspect of the MCP joint that hinders the ability to forcefully pinch or grasp smaller objects. Swelling, which can be

Box 15–14
FINKELSTEIN'S TEST FOR DEQUERVAIN'S SYNDROME

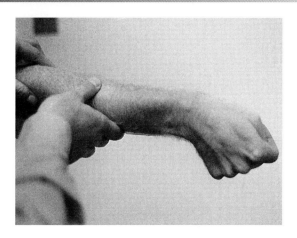

PATIENT POSITION	Seated or standing
POSITION OF EXAMINER	Standing in front of the patient
EVALUATIVE PROCEDURE	The patient tucks the thumb under the fingers by making a fist. The patient then ulnarly deviates the wrist.
POSITIVE TEST	Increased pain in the area of the radial styloid process and along the length of the extensor pollicis brevis and abductor pollicis longus tendons
IMPLICATIONS	deQuervain's syndrome (tenosynovitis of the extensor pollicis brevis and abductor pollicis longus tendons)
COMMENT	This test often produces false-positive results, so the results must be correlated with other findings of the evaluation.

extensive, is usually localized in the adductor compartment and thenar eminence. Ecchymosis may also be present. During palpation, tenderness is elicited over the UCL, with special attention paid to its proximal and distal attachments, noting for signs of an avulsion. Pain is produced and a strength deficit is noted during opposition of the thumb and index finger (Table 15–13). Valgus stress testing of the UCL demonstrates an increase in the amount of gapping present as compared with the uninjured hand. Stress testing should be carried out with the thumb extended as well as flexed to account for the geometry of the joint and to test the various bands of the UCL.[23]

The treatment of patients with sprains of the UCL of the first MCP joint is determined by the severity of the sprain. Instability of this joint will adversely affect ADLs as simple as gripping a soda can as well as more vigorous sports activities. Patients with incomplete tears with a firm endpoint and less than 30 degrees of opening compared with the opposite side during stress testing may be treated with a thumb spica splint for 4 to 6 weeks. Complete ruptures require early surgical repair to avoid long-term complications, but surgery can usually be attempted up to 3 weeks after the injury.[24]

Periods longer than 3 weeks after the injury may require a reconstruction of the ligament with a graft versus a primary repair of the tissue.

Metacarpophalangeal Joint Dislocation

Dislocation of the MCP joint is most common in the thumb and occurs when the volar plate is avulsed from the head of the first metacarpal.[25] The mechanism of injury is extension and abduction. A fracture of the proximal phalanx or first metacarpal joint may occur concurrently. The involved joint has obvious deformity and is unable to demonstrate AROM because of pain.

Thumb Fractures

Fractures of the first metacarpal are similar to the description given for metacarpal fractures of the hand. Fractures of the first metacarpal that extend into the articular surface are termed **Bennett's fractures** (Fig. 15–32). Because of the thumb's potential loss of function secondary to instability at the CMC joint, patients with this type of fracture often require internal or external fixation of the bony fracture.

Table 15–13
EVALUATIVE FINDINGS: UCL Sprains

Examination Segment	Clinical Findings	
History	*Onset:*	Acute or chronic
	Pain characteristics:	Along the ulnar aspect of the first MCP joint
	Mechanism:	Acute: hyperextension or hyperabduction (or both) of the first MCP joint
		Chronic: repetitive flexion or adduction (or both) of the joint
	Predisposing conditions:	Repetitive motion that applies a valgus force to the MCP joint
Inspection	Localized swelling in the adductor compartment and thenar eminence	
	Possible ecchymosis	
Palpation	Pain is felt along the ulnar border of the MCP joint	
	The examiner should note for the presence of bony fragments indicating an avulsion of the ligament.	
Functional Tests	*AROM:*	Pain during extension, abduction, and opposition of the thumb
	PROM:	Pain during thumb extension and abduction
	RROM:	Weakness experienced during flexion and adduction; pinch strength decreased
Ligamentous Tests	Test for ulnar collateral ligament instability	
	Valgus stress test for the MCP joint	
Neurologic Tests	Not applicable	
Special Tests	None	
Comments	UCL sprains should be referred to a physician for further evaluation to rule out an avulsion fracture	

AROM = active range of motion; MCP = metacarpophalangeal; PROM = passive range of motion; RROM = resisted range of motion; UCL = ulnar collateral ligament.

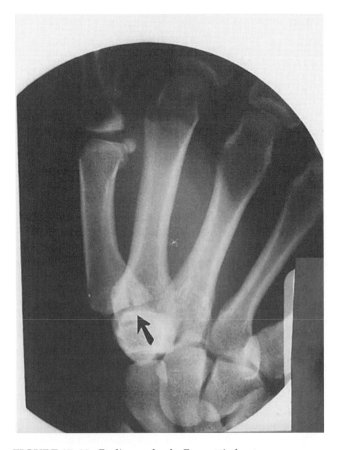

FIGURE 15–32. Radiograph of a Bennett's fracture.

◆ ON-FIELD EVALUATION AND MANAGEMENT OF WRIST, HAND AND FINGER INJURIES

Most often, athletes with a wrist, hand, or finger injury leave the field on their own, cradling and protecting the injured extremity. The examiner must carry out a complete inspection of the injured area, a task that is somewhat eased by the relatively superficial nature of the structures. With the exception of trauma to the carpal bones, deformity is usually obvious and may involve open or closed fractures or dislocation of the fingers.

Typically the injured hand and wrist are not covered by equipment. In certain sports such as football, ice hockey, and lacrosse, the athlete may wear a glove. In these cases, the glove is removed most easily, and with the least amount of pain, by the athlete.

WRIST FRACTURES AND DISLOCATIONS

Fractures of the radius or ulna as well as dislocations of the radiocarpal joint must be immobilized in the position in which they are found, using a vacuum-type splint (Fig. 15–33). Before splinting the area, the radial and ulnar arterial pulses must be evaluated. As with any fracture, the joint itself or the joint above and below the fracture site needs to be immobilized.

Suspected fractures or dislocations of the carpal bones can be carefully supported and the athlete moved off the

FIGURE 15–33. Wrist dislocation. Note that the radius and ulna are displaced posteriorly to the hand (relative to the anatomical position).

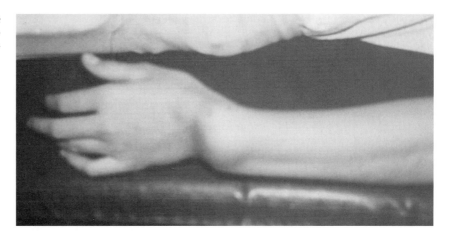

field for further evaluation. If a fracture is suspected, the wrist is immobilized as previously described.

INTERPHALANGEAL JOINT DISLOCATIONS

Dislocation of an IP joint results in obvious deformity. In some instances, the athlete instinctively reduces the dislocation by applying traction to the finger. However, the on-field reduction of these dislocations is discouraged because of the possibility of an underlying fracture or an avulsed piece of bone or ligament's becoming lodged within the joint space. The palmar aspect of the injured finger must be splinted in the position in which it was found. An ice pack is applied to the dorsal side, and the athlete is referred to a physician.

HAND AND FINGER FRACTURES

When fractures of the hand are suspected, the hand is splinted so that the wrist and fingers are also immobilized. However, the fingernails must remain uncovered so that their vascularity can be checked. Finger fractures are splinted in the position in which they are found using an aluminum splint that also immobilizes the MCP joint. Often a standard tongue depressor can be used to sufficiently splint the area. Table 15–14 describes the splinting position for other common finger injuries. Correct immediate management and proper

immobilization techniques reduce the chance that the injury will require surgical correction.

LACERATIONS

Because of the relatively superficial location of the tendons and nerves in the wrist, hand, and fingers, they are vulnerable to damage from even shallow lacerations. As with any cut, the possibility of infection exists, especially when the laceration involves the joints. Any laceration involving the fascia below the cutaneous level requires referral to a physician to rule out the possibility of trauma to the underlying tendons and nerves and determine the possible need for suturing.

 REFERENCES

1. Dawson, WJ: The spectrum of sports-related interphalangeal joint injuries. *Hand Clin*, 10:315, 1994.
2. Norkin, CC, and Levangie, PK: The wrist and hand complex. In Norkin, CC, and Levangie, PK (eds): *Joint Structure and Function: A Comprehensive Analysis* (ed 2). Philadelphia, FA Davis, 1992, p 267.
3. Daluiski, A, Rahbar, B, and Meals, RA: Russell's sign. Subtle hand changes in patients with bulimia nervosa. *Clin Orthop*, 343:107, 1997.
4. Frykman, GK, and Nelson, EF: Fractures and traumatic conditions of the wrist. In Hunter, J, et al (eds): *Rehabilitation of the Hand: Surgery and Therapy* (ed 3). St Louis, CV Mosby, 1990, p 267.
5. Trousdale, RT, et al: Radio-ulnar dissociation. A review of twenty cases. *J Bone Joint Surg Am*, 74:1486, 1992.
6. Palmer, AK, and Werner, FW: The triangular fibrocartilage complex of the wrist-anatomy and function. *J Hand Surg Am*, 6:153, 1981.
7. Phalen, GS: The carpal tunnel syndrome: Seventeen years' experience in diagnosis and treatment of 654 hands. *J Bone Joint Surg Am*, 48:211, 1966.
8. Phalen, GS: The carpal tunnel syndrome: Clinical evaluation of 598 hands. *Clin Orthop*, 83:29, 1972.
9. Inglis, AE, Straub, LR, and Williams, CS: Median nerve neuropathy at the wrist. *Clin Orthop*, 83:48, 1972.
10. Bechtol, C: Grip test: The use of a dynamometer with adjustable handle spacings. *J Bone Joint Surg Am*, 36:L820, 1954.
11. Zimmerman, GR: Carpal tunnel syndrome. *J Athletic Training*, 29:22, 1994.

Table 15–14
SPLINTING OF COMMON FINGER INJURIES

Deformity	Splinting Position
Jersey finger	DIP joint in flexion
Mallet finger	DIP joint in extension
Boutonnière deformity	PIP and DIP joints in extension

DIP = distal interphalangeal; PIP = proximal interphalangeal.

12. Colles, A: On the fracture of the carpal extremity of the radius. *Edinb Med Surg J*, 10:182, 1814.

13. Thoms, FB: Reduction of Smith's fractures. *J Bone Joint Surg Br*, 39:463, 1959.

14. Cave, EF: The carpus with reference to the fractured navicular bone. *Arch Surg*, 40:54, 1940.

15. Taleisnick, J, and Kelly, PJ: The extraosseous and intraosseous blood supply to the scaphoid bone. *J Bone Joint Surg Am*, 48:1126, 1966.

16. Dobyns, JH, and Linsheid, RL: Fractures and dislocations in the wrist. In Rockwood, CA, and Green, DP (eds): *Fractures in Adults* (ed 2). Philadelphia, JB Lippincott, 1984, p 411.

17. Campbell, RD, Lance, EM, and Yeoh, CB: Lunate and perilunate dislocations. *J Bone Joint Surg Br*, 46:55, 1964.

18. Rettig, RC, et al: Metacarpal fractures in the athlete. *Am J Sports Med*, 17:567, 1989.

19. Capo, JT, and Hastings H: Metacarpal and phalangeal fractures in athletes. *Clin Sports Med*, 17:491, 1998.

20. Leddy, JP, and Packer, JW: Avulsion of the profundus tendon insertion in athletes. *J Hand Surg Am*, 2:66, 1977.

21. Lipscomb, PR: Stenosing tenosynovitis at the radial styloid process. *Ann Surg*, 134:110, 1951.

22. Lane, LB: Acute grade III ulnar collateral ligament ruptures: A new surgical and rehabilitation protocol. *Am J Sports Med*, 19:234, 1991.

23. McCue, FC, Mayer, V, and Moran, DJ: Gamekeeper's thumb: Ulnar collateral ligament rupture. *J Musculoskel Med*, 5:53, 1988.

24. Langford, SA, Whitaker, JH, and Toby, EB: Thumb injuries in the athlete. *Clin Sports Med*, 17:553, 1998.

25. Rettig, AC: Hand injuries in football players: Soft-tissue trauma. *The Physician and Sportsmedicine*, 19:97, 1991.

C H A P T E R **16** ▷ The Eye

Resulting from a direct blow, impalement, or chemical invasion, trauma to the eye requires an accurate assessment so that proper management and further evaluation by an *ophthalmologist* can be initiated. Failure to recognize and properly manage eye trauma can result in permanent dysfunction, including blindness.

Racquet sports (in which the ball can reach speeds up to 140 mph), boxing, and golf are most often associated with catastrophic injury to the eye. However, traumatic injury to the eye can occur in all sports, with basketball being the most common.[1] An estimated 90 percent of all eye injuries can be prevented through the use of approved protective eye wear.

◆ CLINICAL ANATOMY

The eye, except for its anterior aspect, sits encased within the conical bony **orbit** (Fig. 16–1). In addition to protecting and stabilizing the eye, the orbit also serves as an attachment site for some of the extrinsic muscles acting on the eye. The **orbital margin** (periorbital region) comprises the **frontal bone,** forming the supraorbital margin; the **zygomatic bone** and a portion of the frontal bone, forming the lateral margin; and the zygomatic bone and **maxillary bone,** forming the infraorbital margin.

The anterior portion of the orbit's roof is formed by the frontal bone. A portion of the **sphenoid bone** forms its posterior aspect. Medially, the orbit is formed by the thin **lacrimal, ethmoid, maxillary,** and **sphenoid bones.** The floor is formed by the maxillary, zygomatic, and **palatine bones.** Laterally, the orbit is composed of the zygomatic bone and the sphenoid bone. Here the orbit is the thickest. The **superior orbital fissure,** an opening between the lesser and greater wings of the sphenoid bone, is located between the lateral wall and the roof. This fissure allows the cranial nerves, arteries, and veins to communicate with the eye. The orbit's posterior aspect is marked by the **optic canal,** the foramen through which the optic nerve passes to reach the brain.

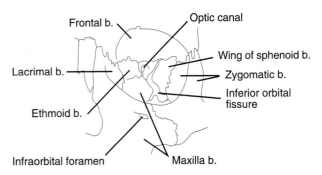

FIGURE 16–1. Bony anatomy of the orbit and orbital rim (periorbital region).

EYE STRUCTURES

The mass of the eye is a fibrous, fluid-filled structure collectively referred to as the **globe.** Its white layering, the **sclera,** encompasses the posterior five sixths of the globe and becomes continuous with the sheath of the optic nerve as the nerve continues posteriorly and merges with the brain's fibrous lining. The dark central aperture of the eye, the **pupil,** is surrounded by pigmented contractile tissue, the **iris** (Fig. 16–2). The **conjunctiva,** a thin mucous membrane, covers the sclera and lines the inside of the eyelids. Anteriorly, the conjunctiva is continuous with the transparent **cornea.** The cornea is the main structure involved in focusing light rays entering the eye.

Suspended by ligaments arising from the **ciliary body,** the **lens** is a clear elastic structure located behind the iris that serves to sharpen and focus visual rays on the globe's posterior surface, the **retina.** The area of the retina facing the center of the globe contains nervous tissues. The outer layer is composed of darkly

---

Ophthalmologist A medical doctor specializing in injury, diseases, and abnormalities of the eye.

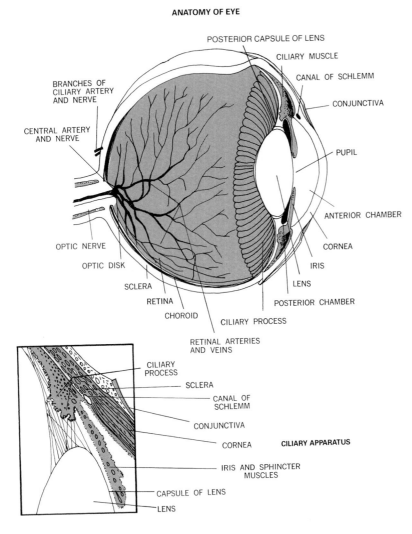

ANATOMY OF EYE

POSTERIOR CAPSULE OF LENS
CILIARY MUSCLE
CANAL OF SCHLEMM
CONJUNCTIVA
PUPIL
ANTERIOR CHAMBER
CORNEA
IRIS
LENS
POSTERIOR CHAMBER
CILIARY PROCESS
RETINAL ARTERIES AND VEINS
CHOROID
RETINA
SCLERA
OPTIC DISK
OPTIC NERVE
CENTRAL ARTERY AND NERVE
BRANCHES OF CILIARY ARTERY AND NERVE

CILIARY PROCESS
SCLERA
CANAL OF SCHLEMM
CONJUNCTIVA
CORNEA   CILIARY APPARATUS
IRIS AND SPHINCTER MUSCLES
CAPSULE OF LENS
LENS

FIGURE 16–2. Cross-sectional view of the anatomy of the eye with an enlargement of the ciliary apparatus.

pigmented vascular tissue, the **choroid.** Light rays strike the nervous tissues, stimulating the **rods** and **cones,** which are photoreceptors located on the globe's posterior surface. Each receptor passes its stimulus through a complex network of nerves until the impulses are collected and transmitted to the brain via the optic nerve. Rods and cones are absent at the **optic nerve,** thus causing a blind spot in the field of vision (Fig. 16–3).

Eyelids act as shutters to protect the eye from accidental direct contact by reflexively closing when an object comes close to the exposed globe and by preventing airborne dust and dirt from entering the eye. The con-

junctiva of the globe is continuous with the inner surfaces of the eyelids. The **blink reflex** aids in lubricating the eye's ocular surface.

MUSCULAR ANATOMY

Six muscles control the movement of the globe (Fig. 16–4). The inferior, medial, lateral, and superior **rectus muscles** rotate the globe toward the contracting muscle (e.g., the inferior rectus rotates the eye downward). The **inferior and superior oblique** muscles function to provide a torsion (circular) motion to the globe (Table 16–1).

FIGURE 16–3. Determining the blind spot in the field of vision. Close one eye and focus on the "X." Move the page toward or away from you until the round spot disappears, indicating the blind area in your field of vision.

Table 16–1
EXTRINSIC MUSCLES ACTING ON THE EYE

Muscle	Action	Origin	Insertion	Innervation	Root
Inferior rectus	Downward rotation of the globe	From a tendinous ring on the posterior aspect of the orbit	Middle of the inferior aspect of the anterior globe	Oculomotor	CN III
Superior rectus	Upward rotation of the globe	From a tendinous ring on the posterior aspect of the orbit	Middle of the superior aspect of the anterior globe	Oculomotor	CN III
Medial rectus	Medial rotation of the globe	From a tendinous ring on the posterior aspect of the orbit	Middle of the medial aspect of the anterior globe	Oculomotor	CN III
Lateral rectus	Lateral rotation of the globe	From a tendinous ring on the posterior aspect of the orbit	Middle of the lateral aspect of the anterior globe	Abducens	CN VI
Inferior oblique	Adduction of the globe Elevation of the globe Rotation of the globe when abducted	From the periosteum of the maxilla	Inferolateral quadrant of the globe	Oculomotor	CN III
Superior oblique	Abduction of the globe Depression of the globe Rotation of the globe when adducted	Greater wing of the sphenoid	Superolateral quadrant of the globe	Trochlear	CN IV

CN = cranial nerve.

569

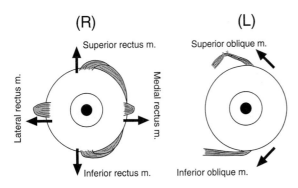

(R)   (L)

Superior rectus m.   Superior oblique m.

Lateral rectus m.   Medial rectus m.

Inferior rectus m.   Inferior oblique m.

FIGURE 16–4. Extrinsic muscles of the eye. The right eye is used to present the rectus muscles, which move the globe in the cardinal planes. The left eye describes the oblique muscles, which abduct and adduct the globe.

VISUAL ACUITY

Proper anatomy and correct geometry of the lens are required for perfect vision. The quality of vision, visual acuity, can be assessed using a **Snellen chart** (Fig. 16–5). This method determines the person's ability to clearly see letters based on a normalized scale. **Emmetropia,** 20/20 vision, is the ability to read the letters

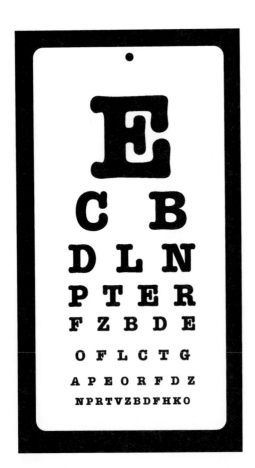

FIGURE 16–5. Snellen-type chart. This device is commonly used to determine an individual's visual acuity.

Table 16–2
SUPPLIES NEEDED FOR THE EVALUATION AND MANAGEMENT OF EYE INJURIES

Evaluation Supplies	Management Supplies
Snellen chart or similar	Eye shield
Occluder to cover the eye not being tested	Eye patch
Penlight	Tape
Cobalt blue light	Plunger for removing hard contact lenses
Small mirror	Sterile irrigation solution
Fluorescein strips	Sterile cotton swabs
Antibiotic eyedrops	Sterile guaze
Anesthetic eyedrops	Contact lens case
	Steri-Strips or butterfly bandages
	Telephone number of ophthalmologist
	Telephone number of hospital and poison control center

on the 20-ft line of an eye chart when standing 20 ft from the chart, indicating that the light rays are focused precisely on the retina. **Myopia,** or nearsightedness, occurs when the light rays are focused in front of the retina, making only objects very close to the eyes distinguishable. **Hypermetropia** (hyperopia), or farsightedness, results when the light rays are focused at a point behind the retina. Diminished visual acuity may require further assessment to enhance performance and ensure safe participation in sports through corrective methods such as eyeglasses or contact lenses.

◆ CLINICAL EVALUATION OF EYE INJURIES

Blunt trauma to the eye can result in injury to the globe and its related structures, laceration of the periorbital skin, or a fracture of the bony orbit. Infections, diseases, allergies, and brain trauma can also lead to dysfunction of the eye. Because of the eye's delicate nature, all maladies involving the eye must be managed with the utmost care and urgency. The supplies necessary for the evaluation and management of eye injuries are presented in Table 16–2.[2]

HISTORY

With the exception of dysfunction occurring secondary to infection, disease, or allergy, all eye injuries have an acute onset.

- **Location and description of the symptoms:** The patient may complain of *photophobia.* Complaints of

Photophobia   The eye's intolerance to light.

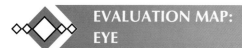

EVALUATION MAP: EYE

1. HISTORY

Location of the symptoms
Description of the symptoms
Injury mechanism
Prior visual assessment
Eyewear worn

2. INSPECTION

Periorbital Area
    Discoloration
    Gross deformity

Globe
    General appearance
    Eyelids
    Cornea
    Conjunctiva
    Sclera
    Iris
    Pupil shape and size

3. PALPATION

Orbital margin
Frontal bone
Nasal bone
Zygomatic bone
Soft tissue

4. FUNCTIONAL TESTS

Vision assessment
Pupil reaction to light
Eye Motility

5. NEUROLOGIC TESTS

Cranial nerve check (see chapter 18)
Numbness of lateral nose and cheek

6. SPECIAL TESTS

Corneal abrasion
    Fluorescein dye test

---

scratchiness or "something in the eye" may be caused by a foreign body, a displaced contact lens, or a **corneal abrasion.** Itching of the eye is usually associated with edema of the conjunctiva **(chemosis)** caused by an allergy. Disruption of the normal visual field may also be described. These findings are discussed in the "Functional Testing" section of this chapter.

- **Injury mechanism:** The size and elastic properties of the object striking the eye are key indicators of the subsequent injury (Table 16–3). Hard objects that are larger than the orbital rim transmit forces directly to the eye's bony margin. Elastic objects or objects smaller than the orbital margin may deliver forces directly to the eye. Elastic objects are of particular concern because the expansive force may be of a magnitude sufficient to rupture the globe.

Injury may also be caused by chemicals or other foreign substances entering the eye. In addition to dirt and sand, athletes commonly encounter substances

---

Table 16–3
MECHANISM OF INJURY AND THE RESULTING EYE PATHOLOGY*

Size Relative to the Orbit	Elastic Property	Resulting Pathology
Larger	Hard	Orbital fracture, periorbital contusion
Larger	Elastic	Blow-out fracture, ruptured globe, corneal abrasion, traumatic iritis, periorbital contusion
Smaller	Hard	Ruptured globe, corneal abrasion, corneal laceration, traumatic iritis
Smaller	Elastic	Ruptured globe, blow-out fracture, corneal abrasion, traumatic iritis

*All of these mechanisms of injury can result in subconjunctival hemorrhage and retinal pathology.

Table 16–4
FINDINGS SUFFICIENT FOR AN IMMEDIATE REFERRAL TO AN OPHTHALMOLOGIST

History	Inspection	Palpation	Functional Tests	Neurological Tests
Loss of all or part of the visual field	Foreign body protruding into the eye	Crepitus of the orbital rim	Restricted eye movement	Numbness over the lateral nose and cheek
Persistent blurred vision	Laceration involving the margin of the eyelid		Double vision occurring with eye movement	Pupillary reaction abnormality
Diplopia	Deep laceration of the lid			
Photophobia	Inability to open the eyelid because of swelling			
Throbbing or penetrating pain around or within the eye	Protrusion of the globe (or other obvious displacement)			
Description of mechanism for a ruptured globe	*Injected* conjunctiva with a small pupil			
Air escaping from the eyelid or pain when blowing the nose	Loss of corneal clarity			
	Hyphema			
	Pupillary distortion			
	Unilateral pupillary dilation or constriction			

such as lime (or other field marking agents), chlorine, and fertilizers and pesticides used for maintaining grass fields. If a foreign substance enters the eye, transport a sample of the substance to the hospital with the patient.

- **Prior visual assessment:** The patient's medical record is needed to ascertain prior visual acuity, the need for corrective lenses (glasses or contact lenses), and any relevant history of previous eye injuries.

INSPECTION

Because all but the most anterior portion of the eye is hidden from view, trauma to its external structures, the eyelid and the eyebrow, may mask underlying pathology. A relatively normal outward appearance of the eye does not correlate well with possible internal damage. The presence of the findings listed in Table 16–4 indicates the need for immediate referral for further assessment by an ophthalmologist.

Inspection of the Periorbital Area

- **Discoloration:** A simple **orbital hematoma** (or black eye) is common with blunt injuries and may have no consequence other than its abnormal appearance. However, external trauma to the eyelid, orbit, or conjunctiva may alter function and indicate trauma to the eye itself.[3]
- **Gross deformity:** Gross bony deformity of the orbit, although rare, indicates a significant condition re-

quiring immediate medical intervention. The loose skin surrounding the eye and eyelid is easily swollen after an injury, and the swelling is often less significant than it appears. Lacerations are common secondary to direct trauma and require management using the appropriate standard precautions.

Inspection of the Globe

- **General appearance:** The appearance of the globe is evaluated as it sits within the orbit relative to the uninvolved eye. Orbital fractures may cause the globe to be displaced medially, inferiorly, or posteriorly **(enophthalmos)** or to bulge anteriorly **(exophthalmos)** within the orbit.[4]
- **Eyelids:** The eyelids are inspected for signs of acute injury, such as swelling, ecchymosis, or lacerations, which may obscure serious underlying pathology of the globe (Fig. 16–6). A **stye,** an infection of a *ciliary gland* or *sebaceous gland,* is caused by bacteria. General eyelid edema, focal tenderness, and redness of the involved lid usually are observed.

Injected (injection) Congested with blood or other fluids forced into an area.

Ciliary gland A form of sweat gland on the eyelid.

Sebaceous gland Oil-secreting gland of the skin.

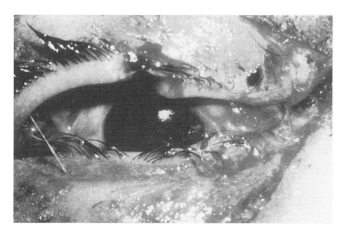

FIGURE 16–6. Laceration of the eyelid. This injury may also conceal underlying eye trauma.

- **Cornea:** Normally crystal clear, any discoloration of the cornea indicates trauma warranting the immediate termination of the evaluation and subsequent referral to an ophthalmologist. Increased intraocular pressure may result in corneal cloudiness. **Hyphema,** the collection of blood within the anterior chamber of the eye, is caused by the rupture of a blood vessel supplying the iris (Fig. 16–7).
- **Conjunctiva:** Normally, the conjunctiva appears transparent as it covers the white sclera anteriorly. To view the inferior portion of the conjunctiva, gently pull down on the eyelid as the patient looks upward. To view the upper conjunctiva, gently lift the upper eyelid while the patient looks downward. If a foreign body is suspected, the upper conjunctiva is viewed by gently inverting the upper eyelid using a cotton-tipped applicator. In some situations, the patient may be more comfortable doing this on his or her own (Fig. 16–8). Leakage of the superficial blood vessels, *subconjunctival hematoma,* is a common benign condition but is of concern because of its potential to conceal underlying pathology (Fig. 16–9).[5]

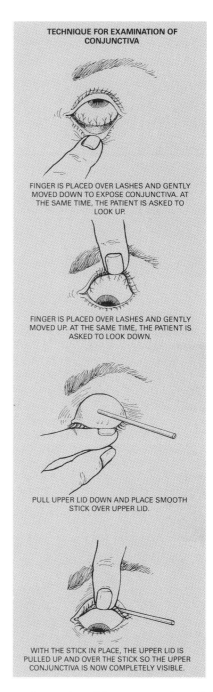

TECHNIQUE FOR EXAMINATION OF CONJUNCTIVA

FINGER IS PLACED OVER LASHES AND GENTLY MOVED DOWN TO EXPOSE CONJUNCTIVA. AT THE SAME TIME, THE PATIENT IS ASKED TO LOOK UP.

FINGER IS PLACED OVER LASHES AND GENTLY MOVED UP. AT THE SAME TIME, THE PATIENT IS ASKED TO LOOK DOWN.

PULL UPPER LID DOWN AND PLACE SMOOTH STICK OVER UPPER LID.

WITH THE STICK IN PLACE, THE UPPER LID IS PULLED UP AND OVER THE STICK SO THE UPPER CONJUNCTIVA IS NOW COMPLETELY VISIBLE.

FIGURE 16–8. Inspection of the upper surface of the eye. The upper eyelid is inverted around a cotton-tipped applicator to expose the upper portion of the sclera and conjunctiva.

- **Sclera:** The appearance of a black object on the sclera must be viewed with concern because it may actually be the inner tissue of the eye that is bulging outward through a wound.

Subconjunctival hematoma Leakage of the superficial blood vessels beneath the sclera

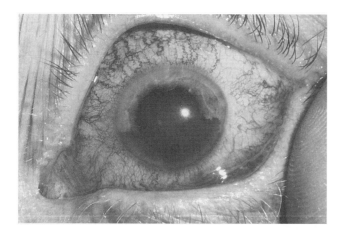

FIGURE 16–7. Hyphema, a collection of blood within the anterior chamber of the eye.

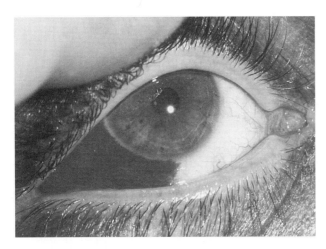

FIGURE 16–9. Subconjunctival hemorrhage. This condition by itself is usually benign but may conceal underlying pathology.

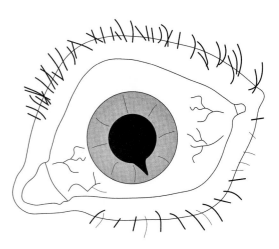

FIGURE 16–10. Teardrop pupil. This condition, or any other deviation in the normally round shape of the pupil, indicates serious underlying pathology such as a corneal laceration or ruptured globe.

- **Iris:** Marked conjunctival injection adjacent to the cornea indicates the presence of inflammation, **iritis.**
- **Pupil shape and size:** The pupils are normally equal in size and shape, but *anisocoria* may be congenital or associated with brain trauma. Any irregularity in the pupil's shape is an ominous sign of a serious injury. An elliptical or **"teardrop" pupil** is of serious concern because of the possibility of a **corneal laceration** or **ruptured globe** (Fig. 16–10).

PALPATION

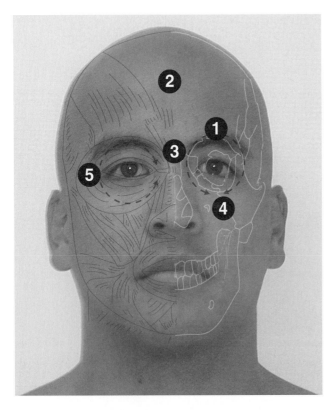

Assessment of eye injuries should not include palpation or probing of the globe itself. However, the superficial bony structures and the soft tissue surrounding the eye may be safely palpated for signs of an injury.

1. **Orbital margin:** Palpate the circumference of the orbital rim for signs of tenderness or crepitus indicating the presence of an orbital fracture. The bony prominence of the orbit may become obscured secondary to swelling.
2–4. **Related areas:** Include a general palpation of the frontal (2), nasal (3), and zygomatic (4) bones to rule out concurrent injuries caused by blunt trauma.
5. **Soft tissue:** Palpate the eyelid and skin surrounding the eye, if appropriate. Keep in mind that injury to these areas is usually apparent during inspection.

FUNCTIONAL TESTING

During the pre-participation physical examination, the athlete's visual acuity, required corrective devices (glasses or contact lenses), and history of previous eye injury must be documented and included as a part of the medical record. Any congenital pupillary changes, nystagmus (i.e., involuntary shaking of the eyes), or other deformity needs to noted so that the information is available for comparison with any subsequent examination findings.

Anisocoria Unequal pupil sizes; possibly a benign congenital condition or secondary to brain trauma.

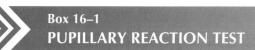

Box 16–1
PUPILLARY REACTION TEST

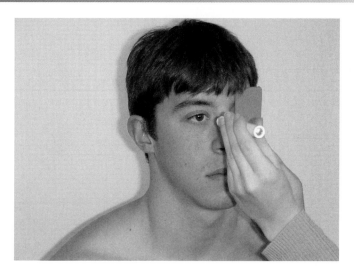

Checking for normal pupil reaction to light. If a penlight is not available, the eye tested can be covered and the pupil observed for constriction when the eye is exposed to light.

PATIENT POSITION	Sitting or standing
POSITION OF EXAMINER	Standing in front of the patient
EVALUATIVE PROCEDURE	A card, an occluder, or the patient's hand is held in front of the eye not being tested. A penlight is used to shine light into the pupil for 1 s and then removed. The examiner observes for the pupil constricting when the light is applied and dilating when the light is removed. This process is repeated for the opposite eye.
POSITIVE TEST	A pupil that is unresponsive to light or reacts sluggishly compared with the opposite eye
IMPLICATIONS	A mechanical or neurologic deficit of the iris

Vision Assessment

Vision can be assessed using the Snellen chart (see Fig. 16–5), a near-vision card, a newspaper, or a game program. Vision assessment is performed monocularly (one eye) and binocularly (both eyes). Individuals who require the use of glasses or contact lenses should be wearing these at the time of the vision assessment. A person younger than age 40 years who has 20/20 vision should be able to read standard newspaper print held 16 inches from the eye.[6] Individuals older than age 40 years may have 20/20 distance vision but may have *presbyopia* and require the use of reading glasses.

If the patient is unable to read the chart, fingers may be used. When testing, the fingers are held up at different distances and vision is evaluated. The lack of normal visual acuity or the onset of *diplopia* after an injury are signs that the patient requires a referral to an ophthalmologist for further evaluation.

Blurred vision that clears upon blinking the eye indicates the formation of mucus or other debris floating in the surface of the eye. This is not considered a significant finding.[2] Blinking that clears the vision momentarily can indicate a corneal abrasion. Loss of portions of the visual field, typically described as resembling a shade or curtain's being pulled over the eye, may indicate a detached retina. Diplopia may indicate an orbital fracture, brain trauma, damage to the optic or cranial nerves, or injury to the eye's extrinsic muscles.

Pupillary Reaction to Light

Pupillary dysfunction is also associated with significant head trauma and may include dilatation, diminished reactivity to light, or asymmetry (Box 16–1).

Diplopia Double vision.

Presbyopia Loss of near vision as the result of aging.

Box 16–2
TEST FOR EYE MOTILITY

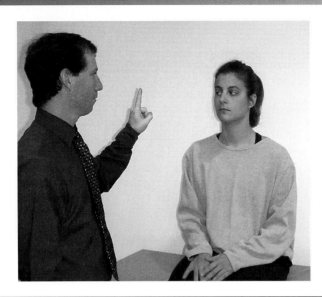

Field of gaze for eye motility

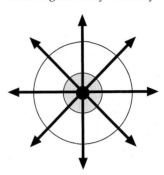

Checking the range of motion, motility, of the eye. The eyes should track smoothly and travel an equal distance.

PATIENT POSITION	Sitting or standing
POSITION OF EXAMINER	Standing in front of the patient, holding a finger approximately 2 ft from the patient's nose
EVALUATIVE PROCEDURE	The patient focuses on the examiner's finger. Patient is instructed to report any double vision experienced during test. The examiner moves the finger upward, downward, left, and right relative to the starting point. The patient follows this motion using only the eyes and is allowed to fix the gaze at the terminal end of each movement. The finger is then moved through the diagonal fields of gaze.
POSITIVE TEST	Asymmetrical tracking of the eyes or double vision produced at the end of the ROM.
IMPLICATIONS	Decreased motility of the eyes

ROM = range of motion.

Eye Motility

The eyes' ability to perform a complete sweep of the range of motion (ROM) in a smooth, symmetrical manner through the eye's field of gaze is a key examination finding (Box 16–2). Asymmetrical motion or movement that results in diplopia is considered significant.

NEUROLOGIC TESTING

The muscles of the eye are controlled sympathetically or parasympathetically by cranial nerves III, IV, and VI. A discussion of these nerves and their direct influence on the eyes is found in Chapter 18. Numbness in the cheek and lateral nose corresponds to the distribution of the infraorbital nerve and may indicate an orbital floor fracture.

 ## EYE PATHOLOGIES AND RELATED SPECIAL TESTS

Injury to the globe usually results in some degree of visual impairment, with or without outward signs of trauma. Periorbital injuries usually have no associated visual change. However, the potential for associated head trauma must be considered during the assessment of eye injuries.

ORBITAL FRACTURES

A blow to the periorbital area from an object that is larger than the orbit itself may result in a fracture of the frontal, zygomatic, or maxillary bones of the orbital rim. A deformable or irregularly shaped object, such as

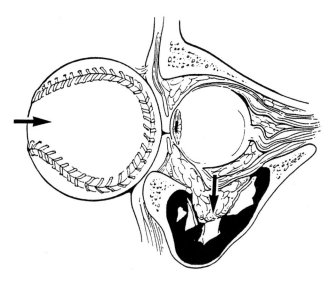

FIGURE 16–11. Mechanism for an orbital floor "blow-out" fracture. The object striking the eye causes the globe to expand downward, rupturing the relatively thin floor.

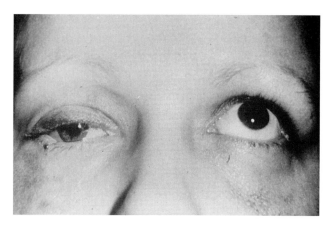

FIGURE 16–12. Restriction of eye motion following a blow-out fracture of the orbital floor. The person's right eye is unable to gaze upward, indicating an entrapment of the inferior rectus muscle.

a ball or an elbow, may also deliver force to the globe with a magnitude sufficient to cause the orbit to rupture at its weakest point, usually in the medial wall or the floor of the orbit (Fig. 16–11).[7] Fractures of the medial wall or floor are termed **blow-out fractures,** and fractures of the orbital roof are termed **blow-up fractures.**[8]

After an orbital fracture, the globe may be sunken, medially displaced, or retracted (enophthalmos) in relation to the location and magnitude of the fracture (i.e., a fracture of the orbital floor would cause the globe to sit low within the orbit). Numbness may also be present in the infraorbital area. However, none of these symptoms may be present.[9,10] Pieces of the maxillary portion of the orbital floor may entrap the inferior rectus muscle, mechanically limiting the ability to look upward (Fig. 16–12).

Initially, fractures of the medial wall of the orbit may be asymptomatic, remaining undiagnosed until the person attempts to blow his or her nose, at which time air escapes the nasal passage, enters the orbit, and exits from under the eyelids. A floor fracture or its subsequent swelling may cause infraorbital nerve entrapment, resulting in numbness in the lateral nose and cheek.

Any deformity of the orbit, caused by bony fractures, entrapment of a muscle, or edema can disrupt the eye's alignment and result in diplopia. Although not always associated with a blow-out fracture, fractures of the orbital rim may produce focal tenderness and crepitus during palpation (Table 16–5). The definitive diagnosis of orbital fractures may require radiographic examination, computed tomography (CT) scanning, or magnetic resonance imaging (MRI).

CORNEAL ABRASIONS

Scratching of the cornea may be caused by an external force directly striking the eye or by a foreign object such as sand or dirt being caught between the cornea and the eyelid. Contact lenses may also create a corneal abrasion. Subsequent blinking of the eyelids results in pain and the sensation of a foreign body on the eye, which may or may not still be present.

The eye sympathetically tears in an attempt to wash any invading particles from the eye. Subsequent exposure of the corneal nerves may result in a sharp, stabbing pain. If the abrasion involves the central visual axis, the vision may be blurred (Table 16–6). Under normal conditions, the abrasion is not visible to the unaided eye. Definitive diagnosis is made using fluorescein strips and a cobalt blue light. The fluorescein strips serve as a dye absorbed only by the cells exposed after a corneal laceration (Box 16–3). When a cobalt blue light is shined on the area, the abrasion becomes obvious.

An ophthalmologist will prescribe antibiotic and anesthetic eye drops. A patch may or may not be used to cover the eye.[11]

CORNEAL LACERATIONS

Direct trauma to the eye from a sharp object can result in partial- or full-thickness tears of the cornea.[12] Partial-thickness tears are similar in their signs and symptoms to corneal abrasions (see Table 16–6). However, with these lacerations, the actual trauma to the cornea may be visible. Full-thickness tears are readily apparent by the disruption in the normal translucent appearance of the cornea, a shallow anterior chamber, or the obvious opening of the laceration and subsequent spilling of its contents. An irregularly shaped (elliptical or teardrop) pupil is suggestive of a corneal laceration.

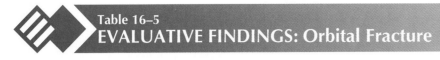

Table 16–5
EVALUATIVE FINDINGS: Orbital Fracture

Examination Segment	Clinical Findings	
History	***Onset:***	Acute
	Pain characteristics:	Oribital margin and possibly within the eye and orbit
		Asymptomatic or possible complaints of air escaping from beneath the eyelid
	Mechanism:	A direct blow to the periorbital area or the globe itself. A blow-out fracture occurs when a blow increases the amount of pressure within the orbit, causing the orbital floor or medial wall to fracture.
Inspection	Ecchymosis and swelling may be present in the periorbital area.	
	The eye may appear sunken inferiorly or posteriorly into the socket (enophthalmos), may bulge outward (exophthalmos), or may be medially displaced.	
	A laceration of the periorbital area or eyelid may be associated with trauma.	
Palpation	Possible tenderness in the periorbital area, but no tenderness may be elicited with a blow-out fracture.	
Functional Tests	***Vision:***	Diplopia, especially on end-gaze, is caused by an alteration in the shape of the orbit or possibly secondary to the bony impingement of the eye's intrinsic musculature or to edema; blurred vision may also be described.
	Motility:	Although not a prerequisite symptom, blow-out fractures may result in the affected eye's inability to look upward or outward.
Ligamentous Tests	Not applicable	
Neurologic Tests	Sensory testing of the cheek and lateral nose for infraorbital nerve involvement.	
Special Tests	Radiography, CT scan, or MRI is used to view the orbit.	
Comments	Individuals who are suspected of suffering from an orbital fracture should be referred to an ophthalmologist for further evaluation.	
	Patients suspected of suffering a blow-out fracture should be instructed to refrain from nose blowing.	

CT = computed tomography; MRI = magnetic resonance imaging.

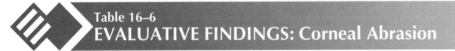

Table 16–6
EVALUATIVE FINDINGS: Corneal Abrasion

Examination Segment	Clinical Findings	
History	***Onset:***	Acute
	Pain characteristics:	Over the cornea and the surrounding conjunctiva, normally reported as "something in my eye;" pain possibly intense
	Mechanism:	Direct contact to the cornea or a foreign object (e.g., sand) between the cornea and the eyelid, causing an abrasion
Inspection	The eyes may water.	
	Conjunctival redness is present.	
	A small foreign object may be present.	
	The actual abrasion is not visible under normal conditions.	
Palpation	Not applicable	
Functional Tests	Possible sensitivity to light	
	Vision possibly blurred secondary to increased watering of the eye or to scratching of the central cornea	
Ligamentous Tests	Not applicable	
Neurologic Tests	Not applicable	
Special Tests	A corneal abrasion is definitively diagnosed through fluorescein strips and a cobalt blue light	
Comments	The visual symptoms of a corneal abrasion may momentarily clear when the surface is lubricated during blinking; however, the blurring of vision soon returns.	
	Patients suspected of having a corneal abrasion should be immediately referred to a physician, with the eye closed and patched.	

Box 16–3

FLUORESCENT DYE TEST FOR CORNEAL ABRASIONS

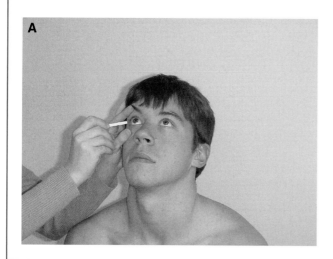

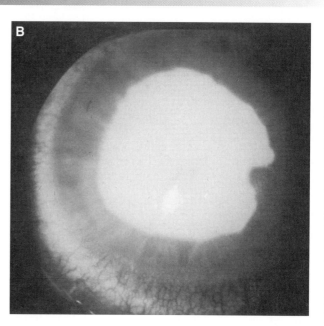

(A) A fluorescein strip is lightly touched to the conjunctiva. **(B)** A cobalt-blue light is shined into the eye to highlight the abraded area.

PATIENT POSITION	Seated or supine
POSITION OF EXAMINER	Standing in front of or beside the patient
EVALUATIVE PROCEDURE	Soak the fluorescein strip with sterile saline solution Lightly touch the wet fluorescein strip to the conjunctiva of the lower eyelid for a few seconds. Avoid placing the strip directly on the cornea. Ask the patient to blink the eye a few times to spread the solution. Darken the room and use a cobalt blue light to illuminate the eye.
POSITIVE TEST	When viewed with the cobalt blue light, corneal abrasions appear as a bright yellow-green pattern on the eye.
IMPLICATIONS	A corneal abrasion

IRITIS

Minor blunt trauma to the eye can activate an inflammatory reaction within the anterior chamber, resulting in the "red eye" appearance associated with iritis. Inflammation of the iris itself may occur without pain, but the sensation of pressure within the globe may be described along with marked sensitivity to light. On inspection, the involved pupil is constricted relative to the opposite side. In certain cases, however, the pupil appears dilated or normal.[13] The inflammatory cells within the anterior chamber may cause blurred vision. Assessment of pupillary reaction, determined with a penlight, reveals that the pupil reacts sluggishly when compared with the pupil of the uninjured eye (Table 16–7).

DETACHED RETINA

A jarring force to the head can result in an interruption in the communication of the retina and the choroid. Although this mechanism can be delivered to the head, the jarring motion associated with sneezing may also be sufficient. The actual detachment of the retina involves the interruption of the nerve pulses being relayed to the optic nerve, often occurring when the vitreous humor seeps between the retina and the choroid.

Table 16–7
EVALUATIVE FINDINGS: Traumatic Iritis

Examination Segment	Clinical Findings	
History	*Onset:*	Acute
	Pain characteristics:	Photophobia
	Mechanism:	A traumatic force to the eye that elicits an inflammatory response
Inspection	The conjunctiva adjacent to the cornea may be injected (profused with blood). The involved pupil may be constricted. On occasion, the pupil may be dilated or normal.	
Palpation	Not applicable	
Functional Tests	The pupil is sluggishly reactive to light. Photophobia is usually described.	
Ligamentous Tests	Not applicable	
Neurologic Tests	Pupillary reaction (CN III)	
Special Tests	Not applicable	
Comments	Blunt trauma can result in a tearing of the iris sphincter, leading to permanent pupillary deformity.	

CN = cranial nerve.

The patient may complain of flashes of light, halos, or blind spots within the normal field of vision. The patient may also describe a "curtain" or shape being pulled over the field of vision. Retinal detachment, only able to be diagnosed by an ophthalmologist, often requires surgical correction. Spontaneous retinal detachment may be indicative of Marfan syndrome (see Chapter 21).

RUPTURED GLOBE

The most catastrophic injury to the eye is a ruptured globe. Severe blunt trauma delivered to the globe itself (i.e., little or no force being dissipated by the orbital rim) can result in a rupture of the cornea or sclera, subsequently causing it to spill its contents. Commonly, these tears occur behind the insertion of the eye's extrinsic muscles (where the sclera is the thinnest) and therefore may not be visible. However, black specks on the sclera are indicative of the contents of the eye's spilling outward.

The primary complaints after a ruptured globe are pain and total or partial loss of vision. On inspection, the globe may appear disoriented in the orbit and the anterior chamber may seem unusually deep. The conjunctiva has marked edema (chemosis), and the pupil may be elliptical or teardrop shaped. Hyphema or a dark, coffee ground–like substance also may be viewed within the anterior chamber (Table 16–8). However, many ruptured globes are often outwardly asymptomatic.

Placement of an eye shield over the eye and immediate transport to the hospital are necessary for individuals suspected of suffering from a ruptured globe. Do not administer any type of eye drops or manipulate the eye. Because of the possibility of the need for immediate surgery, advise the person not to eat or drink.

CONJUNCTIVITIS

Conjunctivitis is the result of a viral or bacterial infection of the conjunctiva. The first symptoms of conjunctivitis are usually experienced upon waking in the morning. The eyelids may stick together and the eye burns and itches. The involved eye typically is red and swollen. The nature of the discharge usually dictates the etiology. A watery discharge accompanied by redness of the conjunctiva indicates a viral infection (pink eye), while a yellow or green discharge indicates a bacterial infection. The affected eye may also be sensitive to light (Table 16–9). Note that this condition may develop secondary to improper cleaning and care of contact lenses.

Patients with conjunctivitis, a highly contagious condition, must be instructed not to touch the affected eye to avoid spreading the contamination to the uninvolved eye. Likewise, athletes diagnosed with this condition must be barred from contact sports or from entering a swimming pool to prevent transmission of the disease to other athletes. Bacterial conjunctivitis is easily treated with antibacterial eyedrops. Therefore, individuals suspected of suffering from conjunctivitis are to be referred to a physician immediately.

FOREIGN BODIES

A foreign body in the eye is a troublesome but usually benign condition that clears after the object has been removed from the eye. On occasion, a foreign object can

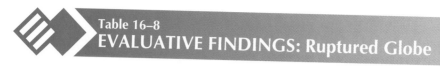

Table 16–8
EVALUATIVE FINDINGS: Ruptured Globe

Examination Segment	Clinical Findings	
History	*Onset:*	Acute
	Pain characteristics:	Throughout the eye; asymptomatic cases also reported
	Mechanism:	Severe blunt trauma to the globe
Inspection	The globe may be obviously deformed. The anterior chamber may appear deepened. Hyphema or a black, grainy substance may be visible within the anterior chamber. Elliptical or teardrop-shaped pupil may be observed. The contents of the globe may bulge outward through the sclera, appearing as a black "foreign object" on the eye.	
Palpation	Not applicable	
Functional Tests	Vision is lost or markedly decreased in the affected eye.	
Ligamentous Tests	Not applicable	
Neurologic Tests	Not applicable	
Special Tests	Not applicable	
Comments	Patients suspected of having a ruptured globe should immediately be transported to the hospital, with a shield covering the eye. Patches should not be used because direct pressure on the globe is to be avoided. No food or fluids should be permitted because immediate surgery may be required.	

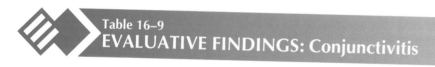

Table 16–9
EVALUATIVE FINDINGS: Conjunctivitis

Examination Segment	Clinical Findings	
History	*Onset:*	Acute; symptoms normally appearing on awakening
	Pain characteristics:	Itchy, burning sensation in the affected eye Photophobia also possible
	Mechanism:	Viral or bacterial infection; improper cleaning and care of contact lenses
Inspection	Reddening of involved eye Eyelid swelling possibly present Discharge commonly seen; if a discharge is present, the color should be noted: Clear or watery discharge; viral infection Yellow or green discharge; bacterial infection	
Palpation	Palpation is performed using latex gloves to prevent the infection from spreading to the examiner. The eyelids feel fluid filled and boggy.	
Functional Tests	Patient complaints of the eyelids sticking together upon awakening. Vision possibly hindered in the affected eye secondary to the inability to open the eye, swelling, and discharge.	
Ligamentous Tests	Not applicable	
Neurologic Tests	Not applicable	
Special Tests	None	
Comments	Viral conjunctivitis is highly contagious and will likely spread to the other eye. Individuals suffering from viral conjunctivitis should refrain from physical contact with other people or from entering a swimming pool. People suspected of suffering from conjunctivitis should be referred to a physician for further evaluation. The individual must refrain from wearing contact lenses.	

lead to corneal abrasions. Do not confuse foreign bodies with impalement of the eye by an object.

An attempt to locate the material causing the discomfort, as described in the section of this chapter on inspection, is necessary. After the particle has been located, it may be flushed out of the eye using a saline solution or water. A moistened cotton applicator or the corner of a gauze pad may also be used to blot the contaminant from the eye. Dry cotton should not be used on the eye because the fibers will stick to it, possibly inducing a corneal abrasion. Instruct the person to refrain from the instinct of rubbing the eye because this may worsen the problem. Discomfort may be reduced by having the person hold the upper eyelid outward, allowing the eye to tear, possibly washing the particle from the eye.

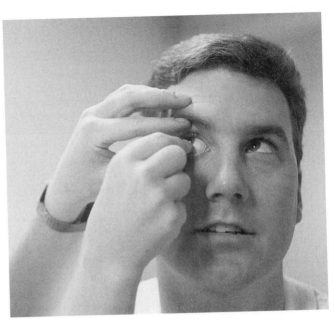

FIGURE 16–13. Removing a soft contact lens. Care must be taken not to insult the cornea or conjunctiva during this procedure.

 ## ON-FIELD EVALUATION AND MANAGEMENT OF EYE INJURIES

The correct initial management of eye injuries greatly increases the chances of the long-term viability of the eye. Likewise, improper management can worsen the severity of the injury and increase the likelihood of permanent disability.

CONTACT LENS REMOVAL

Trauma to the eye when swelling is imminent, such as with a periorbital contusion, requires that contact lenses be removed as soon as possible after the injury. Ideally, this is best performed by the athlete. However, in certain circumstances, the person may require assistance, because either the athlete is unable to do so or he or she cannot find the contact lens on the eye.

Hard contact lenses may be removed through the use of a plungerlike device or may be manually manipulated from the eye in the following manner:

1. The patient opens the eyes as wide as possible.
2. The examiner laterally pulls the outer margin of the eyelids.
3. While holding a hand under the eye to catch the lens, the patient blinks, forcing the lens out of the eye.

Never pluck soft contact lenses directly from the eye, especially when they are resting on the cornea. Doing so may result in serious trauma to the eye. The following procedure is recommended for the removal of soft contact lenses (Fig. 16–13):

1. The patient is asked to look upward.
2. A clean finger is placed on the inferior edge of the contact lens.
3. The lens is manipulated inferiorly and laterally, to where it can be pinched between the fingers and safely removed from the eye.

4. If the contact lens is torn, it is important to remove all pieces from the eye.

Do not attempt to remove the contact lens if a ruptured globe is suspected because of the risk of further damaging the cornea or other structures.

ORBITAL FRACTURES

Fractures to the orbital rim that are asymptomatic (other than pain) may require no extraordinary treatment other than ice packs loosely applied to the periorbital area, avoiding direct pressure on the globe.[14] Fractures that cause pain during eye movement need to be shielded with a plastic or metal guard, again avoiding direct pressure on the globe (Fig. 16–14). Because the eyes move in unison, the athlete is instructed to gaze straight ahead with the uninvolved eye, thus limiting voluntary eye movement.

PENETRATING EYE INJURIES

Eye shields, as described previously, are used to manage corneal lacerations and ruptured globes. Do not attempt to remove an object that is impaling the eye, and avoid applying direct pressure on the globe. If the object is protruding some distance outside of the eye, a foam, plastic, or paper cup may be used to cover and protect the eye. In this case, both eyes are covered to minimize movement. The patient must then be immediately transported to the hospital.

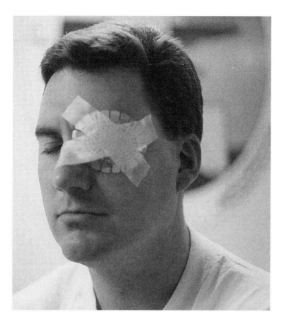

FIGURE 16–14. Protecting the eye with a metal shield. Because the eyes move in unison, it is recommended that the person close the uninvolved eye or stare straight ahead.

CHEMICAL BURNS

After a chemical burn, thoroughly irrigate the eye with large amounts of saline solution or water. Then patch the eye. The athlete, along with a sample of the invading substance, is immediately transported to a hospital.

 REFERENCES

1. Zagelbaum, B: Sports-related eye trauma: Managing common injuries. *The Physician and Sportsmedicine,* 21:25, 1993.
2. Whyte, DJ: Eye injuries. *Athletic Training: Journal of the National Athletic Trainers Association,* 22:207, 1987.
3. Sandusky, JC: Field evaluation of eye injuries. *Athletic Training: Journal of the National Athletic Trainers Association,* 16:254, 1981.
4. Halling, AH: The importance of clinical signs and symptoms in the evaluation of facial fractures. *Athletic Training: Journal of the National Athletic Trainers Association,* 17:102, 1982.
5. Jeffers, JB: Considerations of anatomy, physiology, and pathology of sports related ocular injuries. *Athletic Training: Journal of the National Athletic Trainers Association,* 20:195, 1985.
6. Erie, JC: Eye injuries. Prevention, evaluation, and treatment. *The Physician and Sportsmedicine,* 19:108, 1991.
7. Burm, JS, Chung, S, and Oh, SJ: Pure orbital blowout fracture: New concepts and importance of medial orbital blowout fracture. *Plast Reconstr Surg,* 103:1839, 1999.
8. Rothman, MI, et al: Superior blowout fracture of the orbit: The blowup fracture. *AJNR Am J Neuroradiol,* 19:1448, 1998.
9. Yab, K, Tajima, S, and Ohba, S: Displacements of eyeball in orbital blowout fractures. *Plast Reconstr Surg,* 100:1409, 1997.
10. Forrest, LA, Schuller, DE, and Strauss, RH: Management of orbital blow-out fractures. Case reports and discussion. *Am J Sports Med* 17:217, 1989.
11. Flynn, CA; D'Amico, F and Smith, G: Should we patch corneal abrasions? A meta-analysis. *J Fam Pract,* 47:264, 1998.
12. Belin, MW: Foreign bodies and penetrating injuries to the eye. In Catalano, RA (ed): *Ocular Emergencies,* Philadelphia, WB Saunders, 1992, p 203.
13. Bruckner, AJ: Diagnosis and management of injuries to the eye and orbit. In Torg, JS (ed): *Athletic Injuries to the Head, Neck, and Face* (ed 2). St Louis, Mosby-Year Book, 1991, p 659.
14. Seiff, SR, and Good, WV: Hypertropia and the posterior blowout fracture: Mechanism and management. *Ophthalmology,* 103:152, 1996.

17

The Face and Related Structures

Even when appropriate equipment is used, the face, nose, mouth, and ears are vulnerable to injury. However, rules requiring the use of facemasks and mouthguards have reduced the number and severity of injuries to the maxillofacial area. For maximum protection, these devices must be properly fitted. The use of mouthguards during practices and games should be encouraged, even in low-risk sports in which their use is not mandated.

Injuries to the facial structures are significant because of their relationship to neurologic function, the potential of permanent physical deformity and disability, and, in the case of throat injuries, the threat of compromising the airway. An accurate evaluation of injury to these areas is necessary to determine severity and initiate appropriate treatment and management immediately, lessening the probability of any long-term consequences.

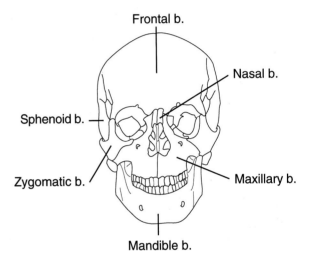

FIGURE 17–1. Bony anatomy of the face.

◆ CLINICAL ANATOMY

The face is formed by the **frontal, maxillary, nasal,** and **zygomatic bones** (Fig. 17–1). Comprising a large portion of the anterior face, the maxilla forms a portion of the inferior orbit of the eye, nasal cavity, and oral cavity. The superior row of teeth is fixed within the **alveolar process** along the maxilla's inferior border. The **zygoma** is fused to the maxilla anteriorly and the **temporal bones** posteriorly, forming the prominent **zygomatic arch** beneath the eyes. Providing the cheek with its surface structure, disruption of the zygomatic arch can drastically affect the face's physical appearance. The zygoma also serves an important role in ocular function by forming a portion of the lateral and inferior rim of the eye's orbit.

Anteriorly, the body of the **mandible** forms the chin. Diverging laterally from the point of the chin, the **ramus** of the mandible begins at the angle of the jaw and continues its course posteriorly and superiorly. The convex **mandibular condylar processes** are located at the end of the ramus, forming the inferior aspect of the **temporomandibular joint** (TMJ). Anterior to the

mandibular condylar process is the site of attachment of the temporalis muscle, the **coronoid process.** Injury to the mandible can potentially involve the alveolar process and thus affect the *occlusion* of the teeth.

TEMPOROMANDIBULAR JOINT ANATOMY

The TMJ joint is a synovial articulation located between the mandibular condylar process and the temporal bone. Pathology to the TMJ can result in *malocclusion* of the teeth, often cited as the cause of headaches, cervical muscle strain, and overall muscle weakness.[1,2] Correction of the malocclusion with

---

Occlusion   The process of closing or being closed.

Malocclusion   A deviation in the normal alignment of two opposable tissues (e.g., the mandible and maxilla).

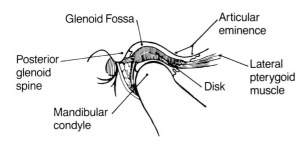

FIGURE 17–2. Anatomy of the temporomandibular joint. The joint structure allows the mandibular condyle to glide forward as the mouth is opened. Trauma to the disk results in a locking or catching as the mouth is opened and closed.

specially formed mouthpieces has been suggested to solve these problems.

Movement at the TMJ is necessary for communication and the *mastication* of food. The superior temporal articulation, from anterior to posterior, consists of the **articular tubercle, articular eminence, glenoid fossa,** and **posterior glenoid spine** (Fig. 17–2). The actual articulating area for the mandibular condylar process is the convex articular eminence. The anterosuperior portion of the mandibular condylar process and the articular eminence are covered with the thickest area of fibrocartilaginous tissue, enabling these surfaces to withstand the stresses associated with joint movement.

The entire TMJ joint is encased by a synovial joint capsule. An **articular disk** is located between the two bones. The disk is concave on both its superior and inferior surfaces, allowing for a smooth articulation between two convex bones. The disk has sturdy attachments to the mandible, attaching anteriorly and posteriorly to the capsule and surrounding tissues. Medially and laterally, there are no attachments to the joint capsule so that the disk has freedom of movement in the anteroposterior direction as the mouth opens and closes.[3]

THE EAR

The ear is composed of three sections: the external ear, middle ear, and inner ear (Fig. 17–3). The design of the ear permits it to focus acoustical energy and convert it into an electrical signal that can be interpreted by the brain. The ear also functions to maintain balance.

The External Ear

The shape of the external ear is maintained by an accumulation of cartilaginous tissue, the **auricle** (pinna). The shape of the external ear functions as a funnel, collecting and focusing sound waves into the **external auditory meatus** to be passed on to the middle ear. Although the auricle is sturdy enough to maintain the shape of the ear, the cartilage is capable of being deformed and quickly returning to its original shape, a

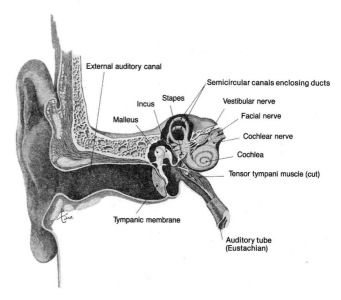

FIGURE 17–3. Anatomy of the ear. The external and middle ear are separated by the tympanic membrane. The middle and inner ear are divided by the oval window.

mechanism that efficiently disperses many of the forces to which the external ear is exposed.

The Middle Ear

The **tympanic membrane,** or eardrum, is the outer barrier of the middle ear. Functioning similar to a microphone that is picking up sound, sound waves strike the tympanic membrane, causing it to oscillate. Three small bones, the **auditory ossicles** consisting of the **malleus, incus,** and **stapes,** are aligned in a chain. These bones transmit the vibrations of the tympanic membrane to the **oval window** of the inner ear.

The middle ear is connected to the nasal passages by the **eustachian tube,** which regulates the amount of pressure within the middle ear.

The Inner Ear

Within the inner ear, the mechanical vibrations caused by sound waves are encoded into electrical impulses to be interpreted by the brain. The structures of the inner ear, the **cochlea** and the **semicircular canals,** sit within a bony, fluid-filled labyrinth formed within the temporal bone (Fig. 17–4). Acoustic signals are passed along the cochlea, a bony structure that moves up and down in response to these signals. This movement is detected by fine hair cells and subsequently translated into electrical impulses by the **vestibulocochlear nerve.**

The semicircular canals are filled with fluid. As the head moves, the fluid in the canals shifts. The feedback

Mastication The chewing of food.

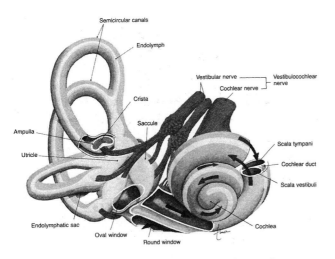

FIGURE 17–4. Inner ear. Here mechanical sound waves are converted into nervous impulses that are sent along to the brain for processing.

from this movement is provided to the brain, assisting in maintaining balance and an upright posture of the head and body.

THE NOSE

The paired, wafer-thin **nasal bones** arise off the facial bones to meet with extensions of the **frontal bones** and **maxillary bones,** forming the **nasal bridge.** The **nasal septum,** formed on its posterior half by the vomer bone and the perpendicular plate of the **ethmoid bone,** meets with the **nasal cartilage** anteriorly to separate the nasal passage into two halves. The floor of the nasal cavity is formed by the **hard palate** anteriorly and the **soft palate** posteriorly (Fig. 17–5).

The external nasal openings, the **nostrils,** allow air to flow into the nasal passages, through the inferior, middle, and superior **choanae,** and into the **pharynx** to be transmitted to the lungs via the **trachea.** The nasal passages are lined with **mucosal cells** that warm and humidify cool, dry air before inspiration into the lungs. These cells also produce mucus that acts in conjunction with the nasal hairs to trap foreign particles, preventing them from being passed along to the lungs.

THE THROAT

Because the **larynx** is the most superficial and prominent structure of the throat, it is the area most susceptible to traumatic injury. Covered superiorly by the prominent **thyroid cartilage** (Adam's apple) and inferiorly by the **cricoid cartilage,** the larynx is well protected from all but the most severe blows. Inferior to the cricoid cartilage, the **trachea**'s semicircular cartilage serves as its protective covering until it descends behind the sternum (Fig. 17–6).

The **hyoid bone,** located in the anterior neck between the mandible and the larynx, functions as the tongue's attachment site. This U-shaped bone is suspended by ligaments arising from the temporal bones. The hyoid bone, the only bone in the body that does not articulate with another bone, consists of a central body with two pairs of laterally and posteriorly projecting structures, the greater and lesser **cornua.**

THE MOUTH

Formed by connective tissue and a thin covering of skin, the lips contain a small layer of transparent cells over a network of vascular capillaries. The lips meet the

FIGURE 17–5. Cross section of the nasal passage.

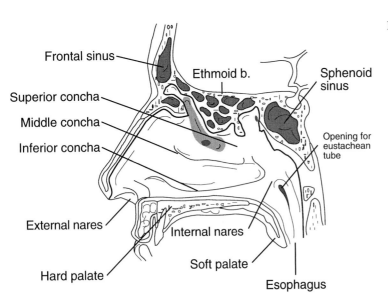

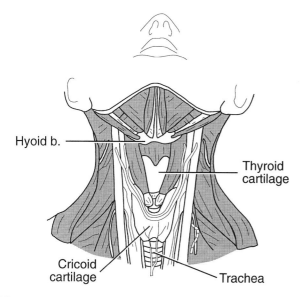

FIGURE 17–6. Anatomy of the upper trachea. The larynx lies behind the thyroid and cricoid cartilages.

Table 17–1
CLASSIFICATION AND FUNCTION OF THE TEETH PER ROW

Type	Number	Function
Incisors	4	Cutting
Cuspids (canines)	2	Tearing
Bicuspids (Premolars)	4	Crushing and grinding
Molars	6	Crushing and grinding

skin of the face at the **vermillum border.** The rest of the oral cavity is covered by a membrane that produces protective mucus throughout the digestive system (see Chap. 10). The mouth is divided into the **oral vestibule,** delineated as the area from the lips to the teeth, and the **oral cavity,** including everything past the teeth, leading to the trachea.

The tongue is a skeletal muscle covered by mucous membrane (Fig. 17–7). Its surface is covered with **papillae** and **taste buds.** The papillae are small, rough projections on the surface of the tongue that assist in the movement of food during chewing. The taste buds allow us to appreciate the flavor of whatever we are eating. The tongue is connected on its underside to the floor of the oral cavity by the **lingual frenulum.** This small piece of mucous membrane can be injured during trauma to the tongue or mouth.

THE TEETH

A total of 32 permanent teeth, divided equally into upper and lower rows, are normally present. Each row is formed by four different types of teeth, each serving a different function (see Fig. 17–7; Table 17–1). Individually, each tooth has three major anatomical areas: the **root,** the **neck,** and the **crown.** The roots are anchored to the alveolar process by **cementum** and small **periodontal ligaments.** The **gums** cover the alveolar process and root to the base of the tooth's neck.

Each tooth is formed by **dentin,** a hard, calcified substance covered by an even harder substance, **enamel.** The tooth's core is formed by the **pulp chamber,** housing a strong connective tissue **(pulp),** nerves, and blood vessels (Fig. 17–8). The nerves and blood vessels enter from the underlying bone through the apical foramen and course through the root canal up into the pulp cavity.

MUSCULAR ANATOMY

For the purposes of this chapter, the maxillofacial muscles are classified as being either the muscles of mastication or muscles of expression. Dysfunction of these muscles occurs secondary to lacerations, dislocations, fractures, or cranial nerve involvement. Additional facial muscles acting on the eye and eyelids are discussed in Chapter 16.

Muscles of Mastication

The primary muscle for flexing the jaw (closing the mouth) is the masseter, which spans the distance between the mandibular angle and the inferior portion of the zygomatic arch. The mouth is opened by the contraction of the **digastric, mylohyoid, medial pterygoid,** and **lateral pterygoid** muscles.

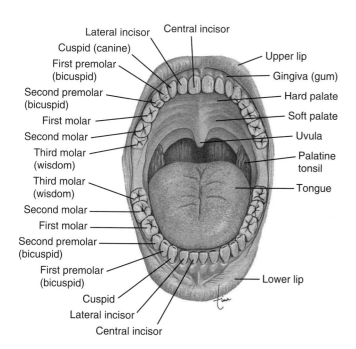

FIGURE 17–7. Oral cavity.

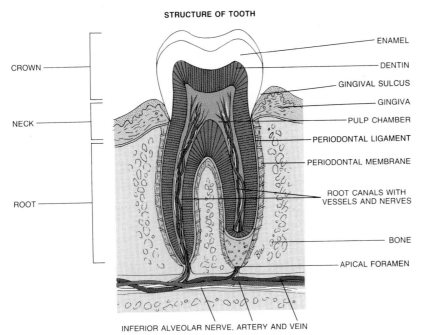

STRUCTURE OF TOOTH

CROWN

NECK

ROOT

ENAMEL
DENTIN
GINGIVAL SULCUS
GINGIVA
PULP CHAMBER
PERIODONTAL LIGAMENT
PERIODONTAL MEMBRANE
ROOT CANALS WITH VESSELS AND NERVES
BONE
APICAL FORAMEN

INFERIOR ALVEOLAR NERVE, ARTERY AND VEIN

FIGURE 17–8. Cross-sectional anatomy of a tooth.

Muscles of Expression

The muscles of expression—those that move the lips, cheeks, nose, eyebrows, and forehead—are presented in Table 17–2 and Fig. 17–9. The lack of symmetrical movement or hypertonicity of the facial muscles indicates that there is trauma or disease to one or more cranial nerves; this condition is known as *Bell's palsy.*

Bell's palsy Inhibition of the facial nerve secondary to trauma or disease, resulting in flaccidity of the facial muscles. In individuals suffering from Bell's palsy, the face on the involved side appears elongated.

FIGURE 17–9. The muscles of expression.

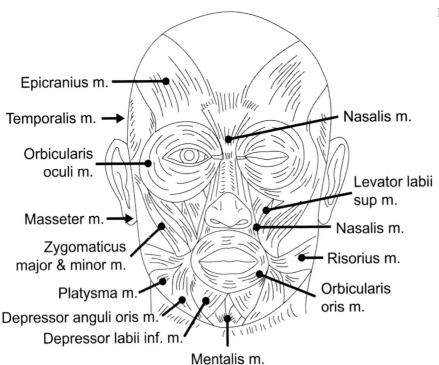

Epicranius m.
Temporalis m.
Orbicularis oculi m.
Masseter m.
Zygomaticus major & minor m.
Platysma m.
Depressor anguli oris m.
Depressor labii inf. m.
Mentalis m.
Nasalis m.
Levator labii sup m.
Nasalis m.
Risorius m.
Orbicularis oris m.

Table 17-2
MUSCLES OF EXPRESSION (PARTIAL LIST)

Muscle	Action	Origin	Insertion	Innervation	Root
Buccinator	Depresses the cheeks	Alveolar process of the maxilla and mandible.	Angle of the mouth	Facial	CN VII
Depressor anguli oris	Draws the angle of the mouth downward (frowning)	Oblique line of the mandible	Angle of the mouth	Facial	CN VII
Depressor labii inferioris	Lowers the mouth	Oblique line of the mandible	Lower lip	Facial	CN VII
Digastric	Opens mouth	Inferior border of the mandible	Superior aspect of the hyoid bone	Trigeminal	CN V
Geniohyoid	Opens mouth	Median ridge of the mandible	Body of the hyoid bone	Ansa cervicalis	CN I, CNII
Levator anguli oris	Raises each side of the mouth (a bilateral muscle)	Just superior to the canine teeth	Angle of the mouth	Facial	CN VII
Masseter	Aids in biting	**Superficial portion:** Zygomatic process of maxilla; anterior two-thirds of zygomatic arch **Profundus portion:** Posterior one-third of the zygomatic arch	**Superficial portion:** Inferior one-half of the lateral ramus of the mandible **Profundus portion:** Superior one-half of the ramus and coronoid process of the mandible	Trigeminal	CN V
Mentalis	Elevates the skin of the chin.	Incisive fossa of the mandible	Point of the mandible	Facial	CN VII
Mylohyoid	Opens mouth	Inferior border of the mandible	Superior aspect of the hyoid bone	Trigeminal	CN V
Orbicularis oris	"Puckers" lips	Originates off of the muscles surrounding the mouth	Skin surrounding the lips	Facial	CN VII
Procerus	Wrinkles the nose	Lower portion of the nasal bone Lateral nasal cartilage	Lower portion of the forehead between the eyebrow	Facial	CN VII
Temporalis	Aids in biting	Temporal fossa	Coronoid process and ramus of the mandible	Trigeminal	CN V
Zygomaticus major	Used for smiling	Zygomatic bone	Angle of the mouth	Facial	CN VII

CN = cranial nerve.

CLINICAL EVALUATION OF FACIAL INJURIES

The evaluation of a specific segment of the face need not encompass all aspects of otherwise unrelated structures. However, a secondary screen of these areas should be conducted to rule out concurrent injury.

HISTORY

Despite the presence of an obvious injury to a particular structure, trauma to adjacent areas must also be ruled out. Injuries to the larynx may impede the ability to speak.

History Involving the Ear

- **Location of the pain:** Direct blows to the external ear result in pain in the affected area. Complaints of pressure within the middle or inner ear indicate an infection or a tympanic membrane rupture. **Otitis externa,** the infection of the external auditory meatus, causes intense, chronic pain and itching.
- **Activity and injury mechanism:** Most ear injuries stem from a blunt trauma to the auricle, especially prevalent in sports in which headgear is not mandated. A **tympanic membrane rupture** can be caused by a slapping blow to the ear that produces pressure on the middle ear, thereby causing the membrane to rupture, an injury that is predisposed

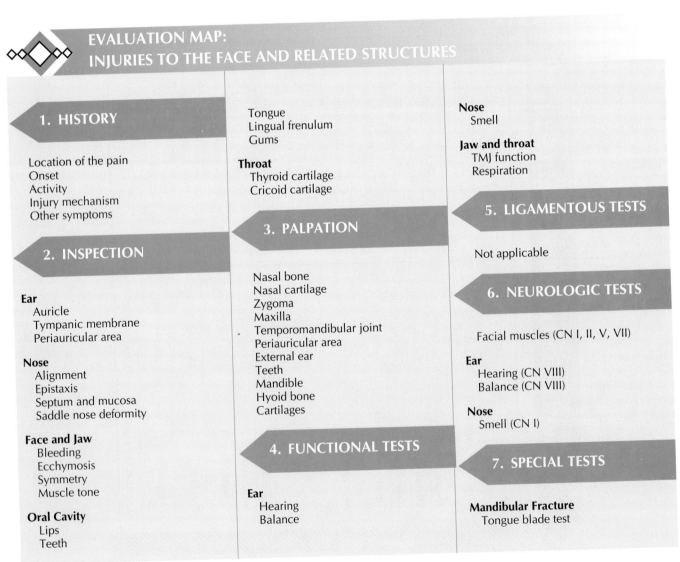

**EVALUATION MAP:
INJURIES TO THE FACE AND RELATED STRUCTURES**

1. HISTORY

Location of the pain
Onset
Activity
Injury mechanism
Other symptoms

2. INSPECTION

Ear
Auricle
Tympanic membrane
Periauricular area

Nose
Alignment
Epistaxis
Septum and mucosa
Saddle nose deformity

Face and Jaw
Bleeding
Ecchymosis
Symmetry
Muscle tone

Oral Cavity
Lips
Teeth

Tongue
Lingual frenulum
Gums

Throat
Thyroid cartilage
Cricoid cartilage

3. PALPATION

Nasal bone
Nasal cartilage
Zygoma
Maxilla
Temporomandibular joint
Periauricular area
External ear
Teeth
Mandible
Hyoid bone
Cartilages

4. FUNCTIONAL TESTS

Ear
Hearing
Balance

Nose
Smell

Jaw and throat
TMJ function
Respiration

5. LIGAMENTOUS TESTS

Not applicable

6. NEUROLOGIC TESTS

Facial muscles (CN I, II, V, VII)

Ear
Hearing (CN VIII)
Balance (CN VIII)

Nose
Smell (CN I)

7. SPECIAL TESTS

Mandibular Fracture
Tongue blade test

CN = cranial nerve; TMJ = temporomandibular joint.

by infection of the middle ear. A physical puncture of the tympanic membrane may occur from an object's entering the external auditory meatus. Infections to the middle ear are usually preceded by upper respiratory infections, resulting in inflamed mucous membranes that block the eustachian tubes. The tympanic membrane can also be injured secondary to external pressures during diving and airplane travel.

- **Other symptoms:** Because the inner ear plays a key role in the maintenance of equilibrium, *tinnitus* or dizziness may be described. With infection, pressure changes within the middle or inner ear cause the ear to feel congested. This condition may be aggravated by pressure changes associated with airplane travel.

History Involving the Nose

- **Location of the pain:** Pain may be located over the nose but may also radiate throughout the eyes, face, and forehead.
- **Onset:** The onset of injury is often, if not always, acute. The insidious onset of nasal symptoms is suggestive of diseases such as *sinusitis* or **upper respiratory infection.**
- **Activity and injury mechanism:** The mechanism of injury is a direct blow to the nasal bone or nasal cartilage. Spontaneous *epistaxis* may occur as the result of a hot, dry environment's drying out the highly vascularized nasal membrane.
- **Symptoms:** Pain and bleeding may be present. The patient requires evaluation for a possible concussion because the forces needed to fracture a nose may be sufficient to cause closed head trauma (see Chapter 18).
- **Medical history:** Questioning the patient about a history of past nasal trauma is important. A prior nasal fracture may result in deformity that can be mistaken for an acute injury.

History Involving the Throat

- **Location of the pain:** Acute throat trauma causes pain in the anterior portion of the neck. Pain arising from illness (e.g., sore throat) is described as being deep within the neck.
- **Onset:** Throat injuries typically have acute onsets.
- **Activity and injury mechanism:** The throat is usually injured when it is struck with an object such as a bat, ball, or an opponent's elbow.
- **Symptoms:** A blow that crushes the larynx may result in the inability to speak. Respiratory distress may occur secondary to an obstruction of the airway and may result in the patient's speaking in a hoarse, raspy voice. A crushing injury of the larynx may result in the patient's inability to speak.

History Involving Maxillofacial Injuries

- **Location of the pain:** Normally, the exact site of pain can be located. Dental injuries usually can be pinpointed to one or more teeth.
- **Onset:** Maxillofacial injuries are usually acute and the direct result of trauma. The exceptions are nonathletic dental problems (e.g., *dental caries*) and nerve conditions (e.g., **Bell's palsy,** *trigeminal neuralgia*).
- **Activity and injury mechanism:** The typical mechanism of injury is blunt trauma from an object or competitor. Balls, various forms of sticks and bats, and opponents all pose potential risks for inflicting maxillofacial injuries. Lacerating trauma to the lips or tongue can be self-inflicted as the patient accidentally bites these areas.
- **Other symptoms:** The facial bones are a large component of the eye orbit. The patient may complain of vision impairment and difficulty with eye movements. Initially, TMJ injuries may not be reported, but the patient may begin to notice pain or clicking in the TMJ while chewing. Malocclusion of the teeth also may be reported as difficulty chewing.

INSPECTION

Close inspection of the facial structures is vital for the accurate evaluation and management of injuries to this area. The primary inspection includes a check for obvious lacerations to the face and mouth because these injuries are usually found concurrently with other trauma. Because trauma to the face and mouth involves the respiratory system, the patency of the airway must also be immediately assessed. In cases of injury to the mouth, the oral cavity requires inspection for blockage by a mouthguard, piece of tooth, or other object that could become lodged in the airway.

Inspection of the Ear

- **The auricle:** Observe the outer ear for signs of a contusion or laceration. High-velocity impact of the auricle, as occurs when hit with a baseball, may cause a piece of the outer ear to be avulsed (Fig. 17–10).

Tinnitus   Ringing in the ears.

Sinusitis   Inflammation of the nasal sinus.

Epistaxis   A nosebleed.

Dental caries   A destructive disease of the teeth; cavities.

Trigeminal neuralgia   A painful condition involving cranial nerve V, with possible motor involvement to one side of the mouth and parasthesia in the cheek.

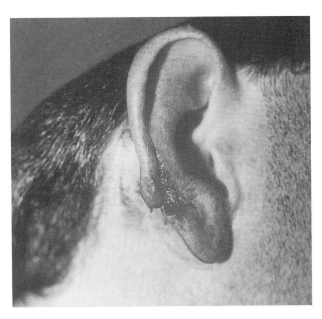

FIGURE 17–10. Laceration of the external ear. This injury requires suturing to prevent permanent deformity of the ear.

Formation of a hematoma within the auricle can result in the characteristic **pinna** or **auricular hematoma** (cauliflower ear) (Fig. 17–11). **Otitis externa** is evident as the external ear, including the external auditory meatus, is inflamed.

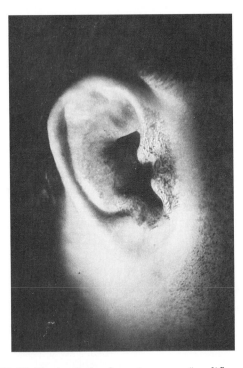

FIGURE 17–11. Auricular hematoma, or "cauliflower ear." This condition is shown in its acute stage. If the hematoma is allowed to develop, the underlying cartilage is destroyed, resulting in permanent deformity of the external ear. Hearing acuity is affected secondary to the decreased ability to funnel sound waves into the middle ear.

- **The tympanic membrane:** Inspect the eardrum using an otoscope (Box 17–1). The membrane normally appears shiny, translucent, and smooth without any perforations. Suspected disruption of the tympanic membrane or fluid within the auditory canal requires immediate referral for further medical evaluation. Infection of the middle ear causes the membrane to appear distended secondary to the collection of fluids, pus, and other debris. A collection of fluids may also be visible. These substances may also occlude the membrane.
- **Periauricular area:** Carefully inspect the area surrounding the ear for signs of a basilar skull fracture, characterized by ecchymosis around the mastoid process, known as **Battle's sign.** Locate the lymph nodes just inferior and posterior to the ear. They can become enlarged secondary to infection.

Inspection of the Nose

- **Alignment:** Inspect the nose for proper alignment and symmetry on each side of the sagittal plane. Asymmetry may be caused by a fracture or swelling. Any question regarding the presence of a deformity can be resolved by asking the patient to view his or her nose in a mirror to see if it looks "normal."
- **Epistaxis:** Observe for bleeding from the nose. Bleeding from the nasal passage is common after trauma to the nasal bones and is usually the result of mucosal laceration.[4,5] Light bleeding may indicate epistaxis from the anterior portion of the nose; moderate to heavy bleeding indicates posterior epistaxis.[6] Lacerations of the skin covering the nose are also common in patients with these injuries and may or may not have an associated fracture.
- **Septum and mucosa:** View the nasal septum and its mucosal lining using an otoscope (see Box 17–1) or penlight. On inspection, the septum appears symmetrical and straight; asymmetry or angulation of the nasal passage indicates a deviated septum.[7] Bony fragments may also be seen within the nasal passage.
- **Eyes and face:** Inspect the area beneath the eyes for the presence of ecchymosis. After a nasal or skull fracture, blood follows the contour of the bone to rest beneath the eyes (periorbital ecchymosis), a clinical sign termed **"raccoon eyes"** (Fig. 17–12).

Inspection of the Throat

- **Respiration:** Observe the patient's breathing pattern for signs of respiratory distress (see Chapters 12 and 18). Even relatively minor blows to the throat can disrupt breathing. Any difficulty in breathing must be considered a medical emergency.
- **Thyroid and cricoid cartilage:** Inspect these cartilages for deformity. Swelling may appear rapidly and obliterate the borders of the thyroid cartilage. Any deformity in this structure must be treated as a medical emergency because of the potential jeopardy to the airway.[8]

USE OF AN OTOSCOPE FOR INSPECTION OF THE EAR AND NOSE

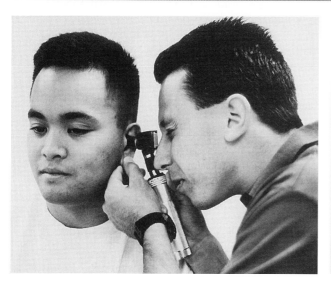
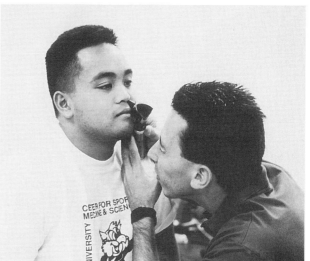

PATIENT POSITION	Seated or standing
POSITION OF EXAMINER	Position to easily access the patient's ear or nose
EVALUATIVE PROCEDURE	Use a speculum on the otoscope that will fit snugly into the opening. When inspecting the middle ear, open the auditory canal by gently pulling downward on the earlobe or upward on the apex of the external ear.

Inspection of the Face and Jaw

- **Bleeding:** Facial lacerations are often accompanied by profuse bleeding. Although controlling bleeding takes precedence, the possibility of underlying trauma must not be overlooked (see the section on on-field management of facial lacerations).

- **Ecchymosis:** The presence of periorbital ecchymosis may be the result of fracture to the nasal bones, maxilla, or zygoma. Additionally, it can occur without a fracture (e.g., "black eye"). Ecchymosis below the alveolar process and at the angle of the mandible is common after mandibular fracture.

- **Symmetry:** Inspection of the uninjured face usually reveals symmetry between the right and left halves. With facial pathology such as zygomatic fracture, TMJ injury, or mandibular fracture, this symmetry may be lost secondary to bony deformity or swelling. Inspection of the face also includes inspecting the patient's eye movements for equality. If the maxilla or zygoma is fractured, eye movement may be asymmetrical.

- **Muscle tone:** As the patient responds to your questions, the movements of his or her mouth, eyebrows, and forehead are inspected for symmetry. A unilateral paralysis of the facial muscles, **Bell's palsy,** is the result of traumatic or organic inhibition of the facial nerves.

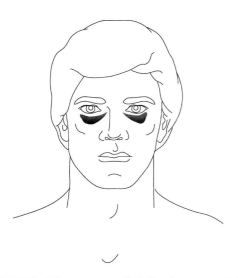

FIGURE 17–12. "Raccoon eyes." Following a nasal fracture, blood lost because of hemorrhage follows the contour of the face and pools beneath the eyes. This condition can also result from a skull fracture.

Inspection of the Oral Cavity

- **Lips:** Because of the high potential for infection and scarring, any laceration extending onto the lips requires a referral to a physician for further evaluation.

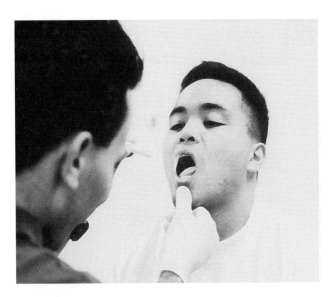

FIGURE 17–13. Inspection of the oral cavity to rule out tooth fractures and to locate the source of bleeding.

- **Teeth:** Although most types of tooth fractures are readily apparent during gross inspection, chipped teeth and fractures involving the root are more subtle. Both the inner and outer sides of the tooth's surfaces are inspected for chipped crowns. The use of a penlight and dental mirror assists in this process (Fig. 17–13).
- **Tongue:** The dorsal and ventral surfaces of the tongue are inspected for lacerations.
- **Lingual frenulum:** The integrity of the lingual frenulum is observed as the patient lifts the tongue (Fig. 17–14). This structure can become lacerated secondary to teeth fractures.
- **Gums:** The inner and outer border of the gums are inspected for lacerations, an abscess, or *gingivitis.*

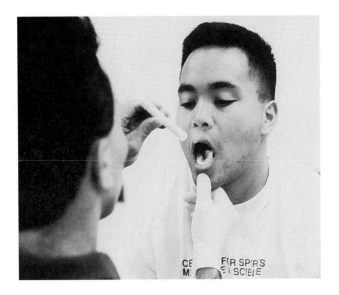

FIGURE 17–14. Inspection of the lingual frenulum. The patient is asked to lift the tongue to the roof of the mouth.

PALPATION

Because of the relatively subcutaneous location of the facial bones and mandible, these structures are easily palpated. Although the internal structures of the ears, nose, and throat cannot be palpated, the overlying and surrounding areas must be examined for tenderness and concurrent injury.

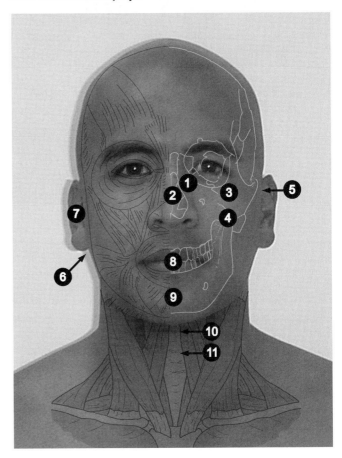

1. **Nasal bone:** Begin palpation of the nasal bone at the point that the zygomatic and maxillary bones merge beneath the medial portion of the orbit. Applying light yet firm pressure, continue to palpate medially to the base of the nasal bone and up to the bridge of the nose, noting painful areas or crepitus. From the upper boundaries of the nasal bone, proceed upward and laterally to palpate the frontal bone above the nose and eyes.
2. **Nasal cartilage:** From the bridge of the nose, continue palpating distal to the nasal cartilage at the tip of the nose. Normally, this structure should align with the center of the bridge.
3. **Zygoma:** Begin to palpate the face at the junction between the temporal and zygomatic bones, just anterior to the auditory canals and above the TMJ.

Gingivitis Inflammation of the gums.

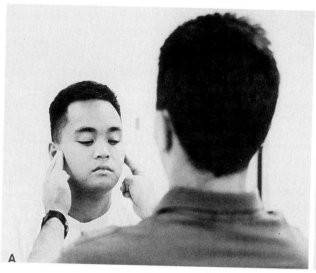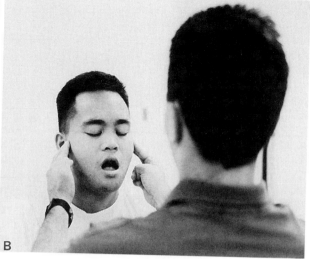

FIGURE 17–15. External palpation of the external temporomandibular joint. The temporomandibular joint is palpated while the mouth is opened and closed. Asymmetry of movement and clicking or locking of the joint are noted.

Palpate anteriorly and medially along the zygomatic arches as they pass beneath the eyes and merge with the maxillary bones bilaterally.

4. Maxilla: From the crest of the zygomatic arch, palpate upward along the maxillary bones. The fused joint where the maxillary and nasal bones join is marked by a sudden slope. Palpation continues to the crest of the nasal bones. Palpate the remainder of the maxillary bone by moving inferiorly from the nose and outward along the upper margin of the teeth.

5. TMJ: Open the jaw to move the coronoid process from under the zygomatic arch. Although this structure is often not directly palpable, the area can be palpated for underlying tenderness.

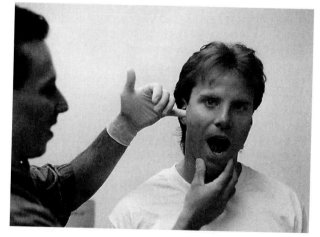

FIGURE 17–16. Palpation of the internal temporomandibular joint. Using rubber gloves, the examiner lightly places a finger in the outermost portion of the auditory canal to further palpate the mechanics of the temporomandibular joint as the mouth is opened and closed.

Placing the tips of the index and middle fingers over the TMJ, note the presence of any clicking or crepitus as the mouth is opened and closed (Fig. 17–15). These conditions are pathological, indicating a disruption of the joint's normal biomechanics. As the mouth is fully opened, a small depression is normally felt within the joint as the mandibular head and neck slide forward. Edema can fill this area.

Palpate the posterior aspect of the TMJ by placing the fifth finger in the opening of the external auditory meatus (Fig. 17–16). The bilateral movement of the TMJ normally is smooth and equal as the mouth is opened and closed. Any discrepancy in this motion may indicate TMJ dysfunction, a TMJ dislocation, or a mandibular fracture.

6. Periauricular area: To rule out the presence of a fracture, palpate the temporal bone surrounding the external ear and its mastoid process.

7. External ear: Palpate the auricle to determine tenderness and swelling. In cases of repeated trauma to the external ear, as commonly occurs in wrestlers, hard nodules may be felt within the auricle. Pain associated with a middle or inner ear infection is increased by tugging on the earlobe.

8. Teeth: Palpate the teeth after an oral injury with caution. Gentle pressure is sufficient to check the integrity of the tooth's attachment to the alveolar processes (Fig. 17–17). An alternative is to have the patient use the tongue to apply this pressure. Any suspicion of a loosened tooth warrants consultation with a dentist. The procedure for the management of a lost tooth is covered in the section on on-field management of these injuries.

9. Mandible: Begin the palpation of the chin at the mental protuberance (cleft of the chin). From here, progress posteriorly, palpating the lateral and pos-

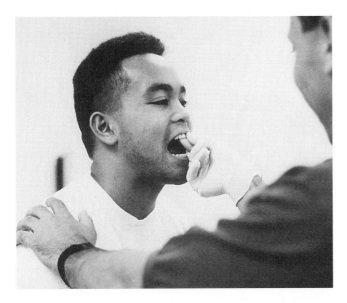

FIGURE 17–17. Palpation of the teeth. Because of the possibility of exposure to bloodborne pathogens, rubber gloves must be worn during this process.

terior portion of the mandible and the lower alveolar processes. The mandibular ramus and the lateral border of the angle of the mandible become obscured by the masseter muscle.

10. **Hyoid bone:** Palpate the hyoid bone, located approximately one finger's breadth superior to the thyroid cartilage. The integrity of the hyoid bone can be determined by gently grasping it between the thumb and index fingers. The bone glides downward as the patient swallows.

11. **Cartilages:** Begin the palpation of the cartilages at the sternal notch. Continue upward to find the series of depressions and hardened bands of the tracheal cartilage. Then proceed upward to find the cricoid cartilage and the thick body of the thyroid cartilage.

FUNCTIONAL TESTING

The functional tests for the ear, nose, and throat provide information about the pathology and impairment of hearing, balance, smell, and swallowing.

Tests for the Ear

- **Hearing:** Transitory hearing loss is to be expected immediately after a blow to the ear. Failure to regain normal hearing within 1 hour after injury is significant and warrants referral for further medical evaluation.
- **Balance:** The patient is questioned regarding balance and dizziness, each of which may occur secondary to either ear or brain trauma. Discussion of assessment of the sense of balance appears in Chapter 18.

Tests for the Nose

- **Smell:** The olfactory senses may be obscured by epistaxis but should return after the bleeding has subsided. The loss of olfactory function is more commonly attributed to brain trauma than to trauma directly to the nose itself.

Tests for Temporomandibular Involvement

Functional testing for TMJ pathology involves having the patient slowly open and close the mouth. Normally, the mouth can open wide enough to insert two knuckles (Box 17–2).[9]

To identify malocclusion, select a point, such as the junction between the two middle lower incisors, for use as a reference point (Fig. 17–18).[9] Normally, the jaw moves smoothly and evenly with no interruption. After injury to the TMJ, mandible, or maxilla, opening and closing the jaw may demonstrate a lateral deviation and the bite may be maloccluded.

Lateral excursion of the jaw may also be evaluated for distance and quality using the same reference point

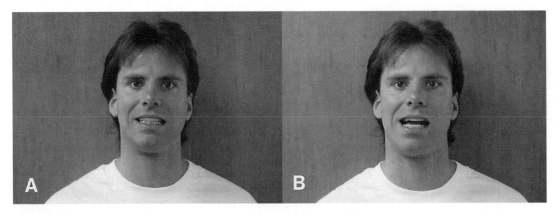

FIGURE 17–18. Observation for malocclusion of the teeth. **(A)** Normally, the mandible travels in a straight line. **(B)** Trauma to the temporomandibular joint or a fracture of the mandible causes the jaw to track laterally and results in a malalignment of the teeth.

Box 17–2
DETERMINATION OF TEMPOROMANDIBULAR JOINT RANGE OF MOTION

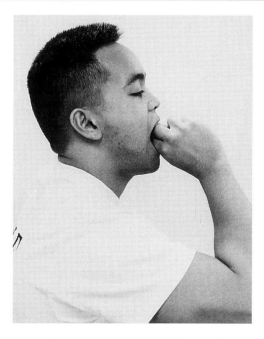

PATIENT POSITION	Seated or standing
POSITION OF EXAMINER	In front of the patient
EVALUATIVE PROCEDURE	The patient attempts to place as many flexed knuckles as possible between the upper and lower teeth.
POSITIVE TEST	The patient is unable to place a minimum of two knuckles within the mouth.
IMPLICATIONS	Decreased TMJ ROM

ROM = range of motion; TMJ = temporomandibular joint.

for the lower jaw. Then this can be compared with the point between the incisors of the upper jaw by asking the patient to move the jaw right and left. The distance that the lower reference point moves relative to the upper reference point is measured with a ruler and compared bilaterally. Normally, the movement is bilaterally equal and completed in a smooth and pain-free manner.

NEUROLOGIC TESTING

Loss of the associated special senses (hearing and smell) can indicate the presence of closed head trauma that has disrupted one or more cranial nerves. The evaluation of these conditions is described in Chapter 18.

◆ FACIAL PATHOLOGIES AND RELATED SPECIAL TESTS

Pathology to the ear, nose, and throat is relatively uncommon in athletes, largely because of the use of protective mouthguards and headgear. Also, rules have been implemented to decrease the possibility of injury by prohibiting blows to the face and head. Although limited in number, injuries to this area can involve major trauma with the potential for long-term complications of impaired hearing, smell, and speech. Laryngeal injury can be life threatening secondary to obstruction of the airway.

EAR PATHOLOGY

Most athletic-related ear injuries are the result of a single traumatic force or invading organisms and diseases. Although this trauma may be visible to the unaided eye, it may not be visible to untrained personnel. Thus, the decision to refer the patient to a physician is based on the complaints reported.

Auricular Hematoma

Repeated episodes of blunt trauma or shearing forces to the external ear can result in an auricular hematoma,[10]

	Table 17–3

EVALUATIVE FINDINGS: Auricular Hematoma

Examination Segment	Clinical Findings	
History	**Onset:**	Acute or chronic
	Pain characteristics:	The external ear
	Mechanism:	A single or repeated trauma to the external ear, resulting in a subcutaneous hematoma
Inspection	The external and possibly the middle ear appear violently red	
	Swelling secondary to a hematoma may be visible.	
Palpation	Palpation of an acute injury produces pain and confirms the presence of a hematoma.	
	Palpation of a chronic injury may reveal hardened nodules within the ear.	
Functional Tests	Hearing and balance should be checked.	
Ligamentous Tests	Not applicable	
Neurologic Tests	Impairment of cranial nerve VIII (acoustic nerve: hearing and balance)	
Special Tests	Hearing and balance	
Comment	Suspected auricular hematomas require an immediate referral to a physician.	

also termed "**cauliflower ear.**" Swelling within the skin of the outer ear develops within hours of the injury. Pooling of blood between the skin and the cartilage separates the two, depriving the cartilage of its source of nutrition. With time, the hematoma can scar, causing a deformed appearance to the external ear (see Fig. 17–11).[11]

The chief complaint is pain in the external and middle ear, accompanied by ecchymosis and swelling of the auricle. The external ear is inspected for open wounds and drainage from the middle ear. Palpation reveals increased tenderness and, initially, the "boggy" feel of swelling. Untreated cases with scarring appear smooth but feel hardened on palpation (Table 17–3). The inner ear is also examined using an otoscope (see information on the tympanic membrane).[12]

In cases caused by a blow to the head, brain trauma also must be ruled out. A concurrent basilar skull fracture may result in ecchymosis at the mastoid process (Battle's sign). Patients suspected of having a concurrent skull fracture must be immediately referred to a physician for a definitive diagnosis.

Often, the physician elects to drain the blood from within the hematoma, decreasing the amount of separation between the skin and the cartilage.[11] Chronic cauliflower ear may require surgical correction.[13] After this procedure is performed, or as a method of initial management of a patient with this condition, the ear may be casted with pieces of plaster casting material or gauze and *flexible collodion.*[14–16]

Tympanic Membrane Rupture

The mechanism of injury for a tympanic membrane rupture is a sudden change of air pressure on the tympanic membrane caused by blunt trauma or by a de-

creased ability to regulate inner ear pressure secondary to an infection. The use of hyperbaric oxygen chambers may increase the risk of tympanic membrane ruptures secondary to the high atmospheric pressures used in this procedure.[17] The membrane may also be ruptured through direct trauma, such as sticking a sharp object in the ear (Table 17–4).

An otoscope with a speculum that fits snugly within the ear canal, without causing pain, is used to inspect the tympanic membrane. The speculum needs to be placed only slightly into the ear canal to view the structures. Insertion into the external auditory meatus is eased by gently tugging down on the earlobe to better align the canal (some clinicians prefer to pull upward on the upper part of the ear).

Reddish-brown *cerumen* may be seen as the speculum enters the ear canal, possibly obscuring the view of the tympanic membrane. Any fluids in the canal are unusual and minimally indicate a rupture to the tympanic membrane. In a worst-case scenario, this is caused by a skull fracture. Disruption of the tympanic membrane warrants the referral for further examination by a physician.

The tympanic membrane's healing properties and process are different from those of other soft tissues. The defect tends to heal without first closing, resulting in a permanent fissure in the tympanic membrane.[18]

Flexible collodion   A mixture of ether, alcohol, cellulose, and camphor that dries to form a firm, protective layer.

Cerumen   A reddish-brown wax formed in the auditory meatus.

Table 17–4
EVALUATIVE FINDINGS: Tympanic Membrane Rupture

Examination Segment	Clinical Findings	
History	**Onset:**	Acute
	Pain characteristics:	Pain, often excruciating, in the middle ear, radiating inward and outward; tinnitus
	Mechanism:	A mechanical pressure (e.g., a slap to the ear or a blocked sneeze) that causes the tympanic membrane to burst or a mechanical intrusion through the membrane (e.g., cleaning the ears with a ballpoint pen)
	Predisposing conditions:	Upper respiratory infection, otitis media
Inspection	Blood or fluids may be seen leaking from the ear. Inspection with an otoscope reveals redness and the perforation may be visible.	
Palpation	Not applicable	
Functional Tests	There is a marked hearing loss in the involved ear. Valsalva maneuver may result in the audible escape of air from within the inner ear.	
Ligamentous Tests	Not applicable	
Neurologic Tests	Not applicable (in this case, hearing reduction is the result of a mechanical deficit)	
Special Tests	Hearing	
Comments	The resulting pain and inflammatory response may result in transient dizziness. The ear must be kept dry and the patient referred to a physician.	

Otitis Externa

Otitis externa is an infection of the external auditory meatus commonly termed "swimmer's ear" because of its prevalence in individuals who participate in water activities. The condition is usually caused by inadequate drying of the ear canal.[19,20] The dark, damp environment encourages the growth of bacteria or fungus, resulting in the inflammation of the external auditory meatus. The presence of psoriasis, eczema, excessively oily skin, and open wounds within the ear can predispose an individual to otitis externa. Overcleaning of the external auditory canal may inadvertently remove a protective chemical layer, also predisposing a person to otitis externa.[20] Additionally, a narrow inner ear can predispose an individual to otitis externa by preventing adequate drying and encouraging the growth of bacteria.[21]

The chief complaint is one of constant pain and pressure, possibly accompanied by itching in the ear. The patient may complain of a hearing deficit and dizziness. The area is red, and a clear discharge from the middle ear may be present. The lymph nodes around the ear may be enlarged. In severe cases, the mastoid process may be enlarged and tender to the touch. Tugging on the earlobe usually increases pain.

A physician may prescribe acid-based drops mixed with antibiotics or corticosteroids (or both). A wick may be placed in the ear to maintain dryness. For their own benefit, swimmers may be instructed to refrain from entering the water and other patients should be instructed to keep their ears dry.

Otitis Media

Upper respiratory infections and bacterial or viral invasion can cause an inflammation of the ear's mucous membranes, blocking the eustachian tubes and increasing the pressure within the inner ear. Upper respiratory infections, airplane travel, and seasonal allergies may predispose an individual to otitis media. In addition to having a history of upper respiratory problems, other complaints include a feeling of the ear's being blocked and pressure and pain within the inner ear. Inspection with an otoscope reveals fluid buildup and an opaque, reddened, and possibly bulging tympanic membrane. Otitis media may result in hearing loss in the affected ear. This hearing loss can be confirmed by striking a tuning fork and placing the stem on the center of the forehead (the **Weber test**);[20] in the presence of otitis media, the patient hears the vibration louder in the affected ear. Otitis media may also lead to tympanic membrane rupture.

Oral antibiotics are usually prescribed for patients who are suffering from otitis media. Decongestants and antihistamine medications may also provide symptomatic relief.

NASAL INJURIES

The nasal bones, the most commonly fractured bones of the face and skull, are fractured by direct blows to the nose.[22] Bleeding typically occurs immediately after the trauma but is usually easily controlled (see the section

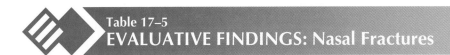

Table 17–5

EVALUATIVE FINDINGS: Nasal Fractures

Examination Segment	Clinical Findings	
History	***Onset:***	Acute
	Pain characteristics:	The bridge of the nose and nasal cartilage, possibly radiating into the frontal and zygomatic bones
	Mechanism:	A direct blow to the nose
Inspection	The nose may be visibly deformed. Bleeding normally accompanies nasal fractures. Ecchymosis may accumulate beneath one or both eyes ("raccoon eyes"). The internal nose requires inspection with an otoscope or penlight for the presence of a deviated septum.	
Palpation	Palpation of the traumatized area elicits pain. Crepitus may be felt over the fracture site.	
Functional Tests	The sense of smell and breathing through the nose may be obstructed by bleeding or a deviated septum (or both).	
Ligamentous Tests	Not applicable	
Neurologic Tests	Not applicable	
Special Tests	None	
Comment	Patients who have suffered a nasal fracture should also be screened for injury to the eyes and head.	

on on-field evaluation and management of nasal injuries). Athletes competing in contact or collision sports often have a history of nasal fractures. However, deformity of the nose should not be assumed to be preexisting.

Other than bleeding, the chief complaint is pain on and around the nose. On inspection, the nose may be visibly deformed, but the lack of a deformity does not conclusively rule out a nasal fracture. Swelling in and around the nose may obscure minor deformities, thus making palpation difficult. With time, ecchymosis develops and settles under the inferior aspect of the eyes ("raccoon eyes"). Palpation reveals tenderness at the fracture site and the surrounding areas. Crepitus may be identifiable at the fracture site as well (Table 17–5). Although radiographs are often used to identify the presence of a nasal fracture, their use has low reliability as a diagnostic tool.[23]

Repeated nasal trauma can result in necrosis of the nasal cartilage. As the cartilage dies, the bridge of the nose begins to collapse, resulting in a **saddle-nose deformity** when the nose is viewed in profile (Fig. 17–19).

The internal nose must be inspected for the presence of a **deviated septum** through the use of an otoscope or penlight. The patient should attempt to breathe through one nostril while holding the opposite one closed. The nostril should close during inhalation, and breathing should be unobstructed. The exhalation should be easy and unencumbered. If a nasal fracture or deviated septum is suspected, the patient requires a referral to a physician.

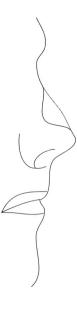

FIGURE 17–19. Saddle-nose deformity. Repeated trauma or other condition causing necrosis of the nasal cartilage can result in deformity of the nose.

THROAT INJURY

Trauma to this area often results in respiratory distress and the inability to speak, leading to agitation of the patient. The insulting blow to the anterior throat, if it includes the *carotid sinus*,[24] can result in the loss of

---

Carotid sinus An area near the common carotid artery that, when stimulated, results in vasodilation and a lowering of the heart rate. When this occurs suddenly, unconsciousness may occur.

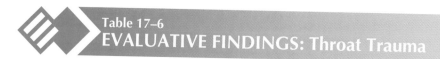

Table 17–6
EVALUATIVE FINDINGS: Throat Trauma

Examination Segment	Clinical Findings	
History	*Onset:*	Acute
	Pain characteristics:	Anterior neck, possibly radiating into the chest secondary to an obstructed airway
	Mechanism:	A crushing force to the anterior neck
Inspection	Bruising or other signs of trauma are present over the anterior throat. Swelling or deformity may be present. The mouth and throat may show bloody sputum. The patient may be coughing in an attempt to clear the airway. The patient's voice may be noticeably altered.	
Palpation	Palpation produces tenderness. Crepitus is present. Displacement of the cartilage or fracture of the hyoid bone may be felt.	
Functional Tests	The patient has difficulty breathing. There is an inability to speak or difficulty speaking **(aphasia)**.	
Ligamentous Tests	Not applicable	
Neurologic Tests	Not applicable	
Special Tests	Not applicable	
Comments	Immediate referral to a physician is indicated. Ice packs may be applied to control the swelling, but care must be taken not to compress the traumatized tissues. The vital signs require continuous monitoring.	

consciousness. Pain is increased during swallowing or while taking deep, gasping breaths of air. Bruising over and around the larynx is common, and the usual palpable definition of the larynx is lost because of deformity or swelling. There may be a noticeable change in the patient's voice.[25] The inside of the mouth is examined with the use of a penlight to detect the presence of bloody sputum, indicating an injury to the inside of the throat. Palpation may reveal a displaced cartilage and extreme tenderness or crepitus (Table 17–6). No attempt is made to correct any deviations because of the possibility of worsening the condition.[26] Immediate referral to a physician is indicated because airway compromise may develop as swelling continues.

FACIAL FRACTURES

Protective facial equipment, such as a football helmet's facemask or a catcher's mask, is useful in deflecting many otherwise injurious forces. However, most equipment leaves at least a portion of the face exposed to potential injury.

Mandibular Fractures

Mandibular fractures, the second most common type of facial fracture, ranking behind nasal fractures, are the result of a high-velocity impact to the jaw.[27] The chief complaint of a mandibular fracture is pain in the jaw that is increased by opening and closing the mouth. Difficulty with or discrepancies in jaw movement may also be noted by the patient (Fig. 17–20). Crepitus may be felt during palpation of the fracture site. Mandibular fractures typically result in a malocclusion of the jaw and teeth, a fact that warrants referral to a physician (Table 17–7). The **tongue blade test** may be used to reinforce the suspicion of a mandibular fracture (Box 17–3).[28]

Zygoma Fractures

Blows to the cheek and inferior periorbital area may result in a fracture of the zygomatic arch. Pain is described at the site of injury, and attempted eye movements may increase the pain or be performed with difficulty. Subconjunctival hematoma and periorbital swelling may be noted. Increased pain is elicited with palpation along the zygomatic arch and the lateral rim of the eye socket. Occasionally, a step-off deformity is noted during palpation of the fracture site.[27]

Maxillary Fractures

Fractures of the maxillae tend to occur concurrently with nasal fractures. Pain is described through the

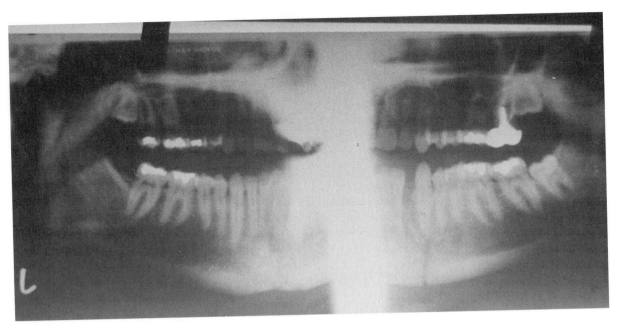

FIGURE 17–20. Radiograph of a mandibular fracture.

midportion of the face. Deformity found on inspection is rare, but ecchymosis and swelling along the alveolar processes are common. Crepitus may be elicited at the fracture site.

LeFort Fractures

The LeFort system is used to classify midface fractures. Because these fractures are normally the result of ex-tremely high-impact forces (e.g., automobile accidents), their incidence in athletes is unusual. Figure 17–21 pre-sents the LeFort classification system and identifies the bony segments involved. This type of fracture is so ex-tensive that when the upper teeth are pulled forward, the fractured segment and the associated portion of the face are also displaced forward, roughly resembling the anterior drawer test in the knee. Sinus fluid may also be observed running from the nose.

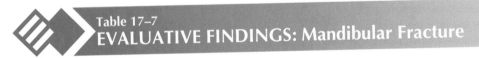

Table 17–7
EVALUATIVE FINDINGS: Mandibular Fracture

Examination Segment	Clinical Findings	
History	*Onset:* *Pain characteristics:* *Mechanism:*	Acute Ramus or mental protuberance of mandible Direct blow to the mandible on its anterior or lateral aspects
Inspection	Swelling or gross deformity may be seen over the fracture site. Malocclusion of the teeth may be noted.	
Palpation	Tenderness, crepitus, or bony deformity is present over the fracture site.	
Functional Tests	Pain is experienced when opening and closing the mouth, or this motion is prohibited secondary to pain. The mandible may track laterally.	
Ligamentous Tests	The structures of the TMJ may be affected. However, the integrity of these structures should not be checked in the presence of a known fracture.	
Neurologic Tests	Cranial nerves V or VII (or both) may be traumatized by the fracture (see Chapter 18).	
Special Tests	Tongue blade test	
Comments	Mandibular fractures may also be accompanied by a TMJ dislocation. Persons suspected of suffering a mandibular fracture or dislocation should be referred to a physician for further evaluation and treatment.	

TMJ = temporomandibular joint.

Box 17–3
TONGUE BLADE TEST

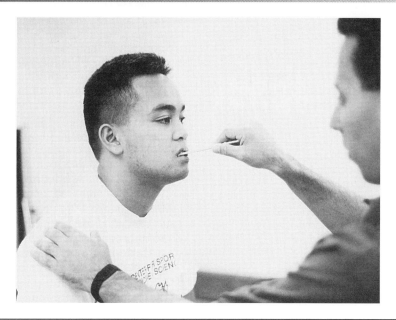

PATIENT POSITION	Seated
POSITION OF EXAMINER	Standing in front of the patient
EVALUATIVE PROCEDURE	A tongue blade (tongue depressor) is placed in the patient's mouth. As the patient attempts to hold the tongue blade in place, the examiner rotates (twists) the blade.
POSITIVE TEST	The patient is unable to maintain a firm bite or pain is elicited.
IMPLICATIONS	Possible mandibular fracture

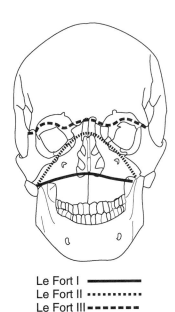

Le Fort I ——————
Le Fort II ···········
Le Fort III - - - - - -

FIGURE 17–21. Classification of LeFort fractures. Type I fractures involve only the maxillary bone; type II extend up into the nasal bone; type III cross the zygomatic bones and the orbit.

DENTAL CONDITIONS

Oral injury rates have been determined for both female and male intercollegiate athletes.[29,30] In female athletes, the injury rate ranges from 1.5 percent in softball players to 7.5 percent in basketball players; soccer, field hockey, and lacrosse players also have high rates. The highest oral injury rates for male athletes occur in basketball players, followed by ice hockey, lacrosse, football, soccer, baseball, and volleyball players. Patients with oral injuries must be carefully evaluated to ensure that their management is undertaken promptly and that physical deformity and disability are limited.

The pre-participation physical examination questionnaire should ascertain the presence of dental appliances such as crowns, caps, or porcelain implants. This dental work must be evaluated for loosening, fracture, or luxation along with the natural dental structures. The numeric system used by dentists in referencing the teeth is presented in Figure 17–22. With all dental injuries, the examiner must establish the presence of a suitable airway, rule out the presence of head injury and evaluate concurrent lacerations.

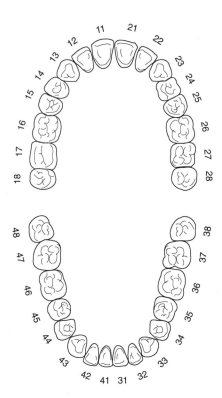

FIGURE 17–22. Numbering system for referencing the teeth. The upper right teeth are numbered by 10s, the upper left by 20s, the lower left by 30s, and the lower right by 40s.

Tooth Fractures

Tooth fractures, ranging from simple chips of the crown to full avulsions of the crown from its roots, are classified on a scale of I to IV (Fig. 17–23). Class I injuries, chip fractures, may be subtly noticed during eating, drinking, talking, or other activity in which the tongue is scraped across the teeth. These injuries may be self-evaluated by the patient's looking in a mirror. Class II, III, and IV fractures are more easily recognized secondary to pain, sensitivity to extreme temperatures of food or drink, or obvious deformity. The degree of sensitivity depends on the extent of the fracture. Fractures into the enamel are usually minor irritations. Fractures involving the dentin and the pulp cavity are painful and sensitive to hot and cold temperatures.

Tooth Luxations

A tooth luxation ranges from a tooth's being avulsed from the socket to its being driven into the bone (Fig. 17–24). A subtle tooth dislocation, one that is loosened in its socket, is not always visibly recognized. It may be discovered while the patient is chewing or applying pressure on it with the tongue. An **intruded tooth** is marked by its depression into the alveolar process relative to the contiguous teeth and to its match on the opposite side. An **extruded tooth** is partially withdrawn from the bone and may be tilted anteriorly or posteriorly or may be twisted. A **tooth avulsion** is marked by the intact tooth's being displaced from the alveolar process.

Another cause of a luxated tooth is the fracture of its root (Fig. 17–25). A fracture of the cervical third of the tooth may be repaired or permanently secured using dental hardware. Fractures to the middle third typically result in the loss of the tooth. The best prognosis occurs when the fracture occurs in the apical third (root) because the tooth is not greatly displaced in its socket.

The teeth can be evaluated for loosening through gentle palpation. If uncertainty exists as to whether a tooth has been partially dislodged, the patient may be given a mirror to conduct a self-assessment. A loose tooth should be left in place so that it can be properly managed by a dentist.

In the event of an avulsed tooth, the patient is keenly aware of the injury. Other types of tooth luxations result in pain, bleeding from the socket, and temperature hypersensitivity. After the condition is recognized, the patient must be properly managed to maximize the potential of saving the tooth. Management of the luxated tooth is found in the "On-Field Evaluation and Management of Injuries to the Face and Related Areas" section of this chapter.

Dental Caries

Also known as cavities and tooth decay, dental caries is a disease of the teeth that results in damage to the hard structures. The primary cause of tooth decay is *plaque,*

Plaque   Food, mucus, and bacteria that collect and harden on the exposed portions of the teeth; it can harden into tartar.

FIGURE 17–23. Classification scheme for tooth fractures.

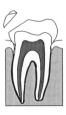 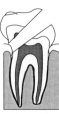 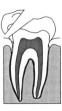 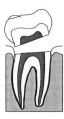

Class I   Class II   Class III   Class IV

FIGURE 17–24. Classification scheme for tooth luxations.

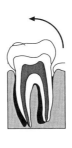 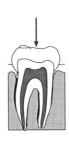 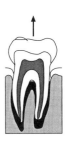 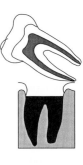

Partial displacement   Intrusion   Extrusion   Total avulsion

which adheres to the teeth. Bacteria within the plaque contain acids that begin to dissolve the tooth's enamel. High intakes of sugars and starches, consuming acid-rich food, and poor oral hygiene all contribute to the development of dental caries.

Most dental caries are initially painless and are only identified on radiographic examination. As the size of the decay enlarges and its depth into the tooth increases, the patient complains of the tooth's sensitivity to heat and cold. If the decay is allowed to progress, the defect will become visible to the unaided eye. In advanced cases, an abscess develops and the tooth's enamel and pulp are lost.

Gingivitis

Gingivitis is the inflammation or infection of the gums (gingiva) that is caused by the long-term accumulation of plaque that leads to bacteria's being released into the gums, causing an infection. The gums can also become inflamed by overbrushing or flossing the teeth or by the use of ill-fitting dental appliances. Poor oral hygiene, diabetes, pregnancy, and the use of birth control pills increase an individual's risk of acquiring gingivitis.

The initial complaint of gingivitis is a sore mouth or bleeding gums that is exacerbated by chewing or brushing the teeth. On inspection, the gums appear red and swollen with possibly a glossy appearance. Gingivitis may spread to involve the teeth's supporting structures, developing into **periodontitis.**

The treatment of gingivitis includes the removal of plaque and tartar from the teeth by a dentist or dental hygienist. Antibiotic or anti-inflammatory medications may be used to control the inflammation. The patient is then given appropriate oral hygiene regimen that may include tartar-reducing toothpastes or mouthwashes. Good oral hygiene is the best method of preventing the onset of gingivitis.

TEMPOROMANDIBULAR JOINT DYSFUNCTION

Injury to the TMJ may include sprains, cartilage tears, subluxations, or dislocations. Clinically, the determination of the specific pathology is less important than the need to identify that TMJ dysfunction exists.

Acutely, the TMJ is usually injured when a blow is received on the point of the chin or across the jaw. The initial complaint is jaw pain and possibly clicking at the joint. On inspection, the mouth may open and close in an asymmetrical fashion, causing the lower jaw to deviate in one direction. Palpation must be performed carefully to rule out a mandibular fracture. Palpation of the TMJ reveals localized tenderness and possibly crepitus or clicking at the joint (Table 17–8).

Dislocations often result in an observable displacement of the mandible. However, subtle subluxations that spontaneously reduce may be less evident (Fig. 17–26). The mechanism for this injury is a blow of suffi-

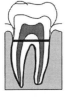 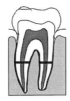 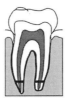

Cervical third   Middle third   Apical third

FIGURE 17–25. Classification scheme for root fractures.

Table 17–8
EVALUATIVE FINDINGS: TMJ Dysfunction

Examination Segment	Clinical Findings	
History	*Onset:*	Acute, insidious, or chronic
	Pain characteristics:	Area of the TMJ; possible clicking or locking of the joint
	Mechanism:	Trauma to the mandible or progressive joint degeneration
Inspection	Inspection of the joint may be unremarkable.	
	Swelling may be located over the joint.	
	Malocclusion of the jaw may be noted.	
Palpation	Tenderness exists over the joint surfaces.	
	Palpation of the external and internal structures may reveal clicking as the mouth is opened and closed.	
Functional Tests	Observation of the jaw for true inferior and superior movement as the mouth is opened or closed.	
	Any lateral deviation in the motion indicates joint pathology.	
Ligamentous Tests	Not applicable	
Neurologic Tests	Not applicable, but TMJ dysfunction has been implicated in causing headaches, decreased strength, and other symptoms.	
Special Tests	None	
Comments	Individuals suffering from persistent TMJ pain should be referred to a physician for further evaluation.	
	The patient is instructed not to eat hard foods (e.g., apples) that would cause pain during biting.	

TMJ = temporomandibular joint.

cient force to move the mandible laterally, such as being punched. The rotation of the mandible causes the joint opposite the direction of displacement to anteriorly dislocate. As previously described, the upper and lower teeth suffer a malalignment, and movement of the jaw may be significantly impaired.

Blows to the point of the mandible, driving the bone toward the skull, may result in a fracture along the mandibular ramus or, on rare occasion, the temporal bone. Similar to TMJ dislocations, mandibular fractures result in malocclusion of the teeth, crepitus and deformity over the fracture site, and the inability to normally open and close the mouth.

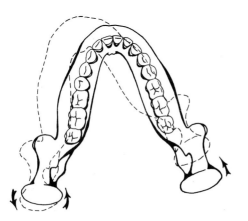

FIGURE 17–26. Malocclusion of the jaw following a mandibular dislocation. Correlate this illustration with Figure 17–18B.

◆ ON-FIELD EVALUATION AND MANAGEMENT OF INJURIES TO THE FACE AND RELATED AREAS

Owing to the proximity of the maxillofacial area to the airway, the presence of an unencumbered airway must be established. The athlete may concurrently sustain a laceration and injury to the maxillofacial structures. After establishing the presence of an airway, the responder must control bleeding before proceeding with a complete evaluation. As with all open wounds, the examiner must abide by the standard precautions for bloodborne pathogens.

LACERATIONS

Lacerations may mask underlying injuries. After the bleeding is controlled, the area around the laceration is palpated for tenderness, being careful to delineate between tenderness from the insulting blow that caused the injury and any actual fractures that may have occurred.

The presence of any foreign particles or objects within the laceration must be determined before any subsequent treatment. An imbedded object must be left in place. The surrounding area can be cleaned and dressed until the object can be removed and the wound can be further managed by a physician.

Next, the extent of the wound must be determined. As a general rule, any facial laceration requires a referral to a physician for possible suturing to limit the extent and visibility of any scars. The sooner the referral occurs, the better it is, but the physician should see the patient within 24 hours after the injury.[27] If the bleeding can be controlled and the wound closed and dressed with a sterile bandage, the athlete may return to competition. The bandage covering the wound must be sufficient to protect other competitors from contact with the athlete's blood.

In the case of lacerations of the throat, the athlete is assessed for difficulty with breathing and transported by trained personnel who can aid the athlete on route to the hospital. If the laceration avulses a piece of the ear, nose, or tongue, the avulsed tissue is cleaned with sterile water, wrapped in sterile gauze, put on ice, and transported with the athlete to the medical facility for possible reimplantation. Microsurgical techniques may be able to salvage these parts, giving the athlete a better cosmetic repair and normal function.

LARYNGEAL INJURIES

Laryngeal injuries present a difficult decision for the examiner because of their potential to become life threatening. Early signs of potentially catastrophic injury include progressive swelling (indicating bleeding), crepitation (indicating the presence of subcutaneous air), audible *stridor* (indicating a narrowing of the airway), and blood exiting the oral cavity.[31]

The decision must be made to move the athlete to the sideline before transport or to transport the athlete directly from the field. In cases in which the athlete has trouble breathing, it is prudent to stabilize the athlete and transport him or her to a hospital using emergency medical personnel capable of managing an obstructed airway. The athlete may first be moved to the sideline if no signs of breathing difficulty are noted. Ice may be applied to the anterior throat, but care must be taken not to compress the underlying structures. The pressure applied could be enough to displace the injured area, causing obstruction of the airway.

FACIAL FRACTURES

The forces required to fracture the facial bones (i.e., the zygoma, frontal, maxillary, and mandible bones) are usually of considerable magnitude. The athlete is not only "down" from the injury but may also be stunned or rendered unconscious by head injury from the incident. In this case, the head injury takes precedence and the examiner follows the evaluation and on-field management of the head injury (see Chapter 16).

LeFort fractures and other fractures around the nose and mouth can compromise the airway. In this case, maintaining an open airway is the highest treatment priority.[32] Athletes suffering stable facial fractures that do not jeopardize the airway can be care-

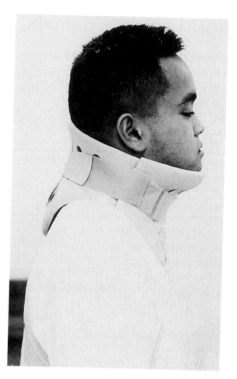

FIGURE 17–27. Use of a Philadelphia collar for immobilizing a suspected mandibular fracture. Applying too much pressure to the fracture site should be avoided.

fully moved to the sidelines. Athletes with suspected facial fractures can be removed to the sideline for further evaluation and treatment. If the athlete has an obvious fracture, movement of the athlete's head and neck is restricted. As long as it does not increase the athlete's discomfort, a Philadelphia collar can be used to stabilize the jaw and prevent unwanted motion while the athlete is transported to a medical facility (Fig. 17–27).

TEMPOROMANDIBULAR JOINT INJURIES

The TMJ may be injured along with the mandible from a blow to the jaw. If a fracture of the mandible is unlikely, the athlete can be carefully assisted to the sideline for a full assessment of the TMJ. Injuries that produce malocclusion warrant the removal of the athlete from participation immediately and referral to a physician or dentist. If the TMJ is dislocated the athlete can be immobilized with a Philadelphia collar as long as it does not create further pain. This athlete also requires a referral for immediate treatment.

Stridor A harsh, high-pitched sound resembling blowing wind that is experienced during respiration.

NASAL FRACTURE AND EPISTAXIS

Nasal fractures are usually accompanied by epistaxis, which must be controlled before further evaluation or management of the injury occurs. Although squeezing the nostrils and tilting the head forward is an adequate form of management for nasal bleeding, this method may be prohibited secondary to pain arising from the fracture. Applying a cold pack to the nose and surrounding area also may stop the bleeding. The nose may be packed with rolled gauze or a tampon that has been cut into quarters. (These should be precut and kept in the athletic trainer's medical kit.) Another technique to control bleeding involves placing a rolled cotton gauze pad between the anterior upper lip and gum. The pressure from the lip required to hold the gauze in place applies pressure on the arteries that supply the anterior nasal mucosa, potentially stopping bleeding.[6]

The nose, nasal cartilage, and adjacent maxillary, zygomatic, and frontal bones are palpated for tenderness and crepitus. If the nose is obviously deformed, the athlete is discouraged from viewing the injury in a mirror or feeling the deformity because doing so may increase his or her anxiety or cause the onset of shock. Suspected nasal fractures may be packed with a small bag of ice to assist in controlling pain and limiting the amount of bleeding until the athlete is seen by a physician.

DENTAL INJURIES

An athlete suffering tooth trauma usually reports to the sidelines for evaluation. Because continued participation can result in a complete tooth avulsion, athletes suffering from any form of tooth injury other than a class I fracture must be removed from competition and evaluated by a dentist (see Fig. 17–23).

Usually a fractured tooth is not a cause of immediate danger to the athlete unless the remaining portion is loose. If no loosening has occurred, the athlete can return to activity as long as a mouthpiece is used. However, follow up by a dentist must occur as soon as possible. The athlete should expect extreme discomfort, especially if the fracture penetrates the pulp cavity.

Every reasonable attempt must be made to find a tooth that has been luxated. With proper care, as recommended by the American Dental Association[33] and the American Association of *Endodontics*,[34] it is estimated that 90 percent of all avulsed teeth can be reimplanted for the life of the athlete.[35] The primary problem leading to failure of the tooth to survive involves the death of the periodontal ligament attached to the avulsed tooth. All treatment must focus on the survival of this ligament.[36–38] To improve the tooth's chances of survival, the emergency procedures found in Table 17–9 are recommended.[35] The team dentist should be consulted before the start of the season so that the protocol for these conditions can be established and followed.

Table 17–9
EMERGENCY MANAGEMENT OF DENTAL INJURIES

- Before reimplanting an avulsed tooth, rinse it off with a pH-balanced preserving solution or sterile saline solution. Allow the athlete to hold the tooth in its socket by biting on gauze. Make sure that the tooth is reimplanted in its proper orientation.
- If the tooth is not reimplanted immediately, store it in a secure biocompatible storage environment such as an emergency tooth preserving system or in fresh whole milk in a plastic container with a tightly fitting top.
- Do not attempt to clean, sterilize, or scrape the tooth in any way other than as noted above.
- Transport the athlete and the tooth to a dentist as quickly as possible.

◆ REFERENCES

1. Widmark, G, et al: Evaluation of TMJ surgery in cases not responding to conservative treatment. *Cranio*, 13:44, 1995.
2. Moss, RA, et al: Oral habits and TMJ dysfunction in facial pain and non-pain subjects. *J Oral Rehabil*, 22:79, 1995.
3. Bourbon, BM: Anatomy and biomechanics of the TMJ. In Krauss, SL (ed): *TMJ Disorders: Management of the Craniomandibular Complex.* New York, Churchill-Livingstone, 1988.
4. Jordan, L: Acute nasal and septal injuries. *The Eye, Ear, Nose, and Throat Monthly*, 53:51, 1974.
5. Olsen, K, Carpenter, R, and Kern, E: Nasal septal injury in children. *Arch Otolaryngol Head Neck Surg*, 106:317, 1980.
6. Weir, JD: Effective management of epistaxis in athletes. *Journal of Athletic Training*, 32:254, 1997.
7. Sitler, M: Nasal septal injuries. *Athletic Training: Journal of the National Athletic Trainers Association*, 21:10, 1986.
8. Bechman, SM: Laryngeal fracture in a high school football player. *Journal of Athletic Training*, 28:217, 1993.
9. Friedman, MH, and Weisberg, J: The temporomandibular joint. In Gould, JA, and Davies, GJ (eds): *Orthopaedic and Sports Physical Therapy.* St. Louis, CV Mosby, 1985, p 581.
10. Savage, R, Bevinino, J, and Mustafa, E: Treatment of acute otohematoma with compression sutures. *Ann Emerg Med*, 10:641, 1981.
11. O'Donnell, BP, and Eliezri, YD: The surgical treatment of traumatic hematoma of the auricle. *Dermatol Surg*, 25:803, 1999.
12. Fincher, AL: Use of the otoscope in the evaluation of common injuries and illnesses of the ear. *Journal of Athletic Training*, 29:52, 1994.
13. Vogelin, E, et al: Surgical correction of cauliflower ear. *Br J Plast Surg*, 51:359, 1998.
14. Keating, TM, and Mason, J: A simple splint for wrestler's ear. *Journal of Athletic Training*, 27:273, 1992.
15. Odom, CJ, and McCandless, R: Contour casting for cauliflower ear. *Athletic Training: Journal of the National Athletic Trainers Association*, 17:114, 1982.
16. Grosse, SJ, and Lynch, JM: Treating auricular hematoma. Success with a swimmer's nose clip. *The Physician and Sportsmedicine*, 19:98, 1991.
17. Plafki, C, et al: Complications and side effects of hyperbaric oxygen therapy. *Aviat Space Environ Med*, 71:194, 2000.

Endodontics The field of dentistry specializing in the management of injuries and diseases affecting the pulp of a tooth.

18. Gladstone, HB, Jackler, RK, and Varav, K: Tympanic membrane wound healing. An overview. *Otolarynol Clin North Am,* 28:913, 1995.
19. Schelkun, PH: Swimmer's ear. Getting patients back in the water. *The Physician and Sportsmedicine,* 19:85, 1991.
20. Davidson, TM, and Neuman, TR: Managing inflammatory ear conditions. *The Physician and Sports Medicine,* 22:56, 1994.
21. Goodman, RA, et al. Infectious disease in competitive sports. *JAMA,* 271:862, 1994.
22. Schendel, SA: Sports-related nasal injuries. *The Physician and Sportsmedicine,* 18:59, 1990.
23. Logan, M, O'Driscoll, K and Masterson, J: The utility of nasal bone radiographs in nasal trauma. *Clin Radiol,* 49:192, 1994.
24. Storey, MD, Schatz, CF, and Brown, KW: Anterior neck trauma. *The Physician and Sportsmedicine,* 17:85, 1989.
25. Bechman, SM: Laryngeal fracture in a high school football player. *Journal of Athletic Training,* 28:217, 1993.
26. Schuller, DE, and Schleuning, AJ: *DeWeese and Saunders' Otolaryngology-Head and Neck Surgery* (ed 8). CV Mosby, St. Louis, 1994, p 123.
27. Matthews, B: Maxillofacial trauma from athletic endeavors. *Athletic Training: Journal of the National Athletic Trainers Association,* 25:132, 1990.
28. Halling, AH: The importance of clinical signs and symptoms in the evaluation of facial fractures. *Athletic Training: Journal of the National Athletic Trainers Association,* 17:102, 1982.
29. Morrow, RM, and Bonci, T: A survey of oral injuries in female college and university athletes. *Athletic Training: Journal of the National Athletic Trainers Association,* 24:236, 1989.
30. Morrow, RM, et al: Report of a survey of oral injuries in male college and university athletes. *Athletic Training: Journal of the National Athletic Trainers Association,* 26:338, 1991.
31. Fabian, RL: Sports injury to the larynx and trachea. *The Physician and Sportsmedicine,* 17:111, 1989.
32. Lephart, SM and Fu, FH: Emergency treatment of athletic injuries. *Sports Dentistry,* 35:707, 1991.
33. Ad Hoc Committee on Treatment of the Avulsed Tooth. American Association of Endodontists: Recommended guidelines for the treatment of the avulsed tooth. *J Endodontics,* 9:571, 1983.
34. *Accepted Dental Therapeutics.* Chicago, American Dental Association, 1984, p 72.
35. Krasner, P: The athletic trainer's role in saving avulsed teeth. *Athletic Training: Journal of the National Athletic Trainers Association,* 24:139, 1989.
36. Andreasen, JO: Periodontal healing after reimplantation of traumatically avulsed human teeth. Assessment by mobility testing and radiography. *Acta Odontol Scand,* 33:325, 1975.
37. Andreasen, JO, and Kristersson, L: The effect of limited drying or removal of the periodontal ligament. Periodontal healing after reimplantation of mature permanent incisors in monkeys. *Acta Odontol Scand,* 39:1, 1981.
38. Andreasen, JO: Relationship between cell damage in the periodontal ligament after reimplantation and subsequent development of root resorption. A time-related study in monkeys. *Acta Odontol Scand,* 39:15, 1981.

18

Head and Neck Injuries

The greatest fear of every coach, parent, fan, and medical staff is that of an athlete suffering a catastrophic head or neck injury during sports participation. Fortunately, the overall rate of injury to these body areas is low. However, when it does occur, the outcome can be fatal.

Those sports in which blows to the head are commonplace—football, baseball, and ice hockey—have rules mandating the use of protective headgear. The use of helmets has greatly reduced the number and severity of head injuries in football, but various styles and brands have differing levels of effectiveness.[1–3] Ironically, the football helmet has been implicated in increasing the number of injuries to the cervical spine. A properly fitting mouthpiece can also prevent brain injury caused by a blow to the face or chin, and its use is recommended in all contact and collision sports.

Regular inspection of helmets is needed to ensure proper maintenance and continued protection. Athletes must be knowledgeable about the risks associated with participation in sports and be instructed in the proper techniques necessary to avoid serious head and neck injuries.

This chapter is dedicated to the immediate and follow-up evaluation and management of athletes with head and neck injuries. A well-organized procedure for the emergency management of head and neck trauma is crucial to this process and must be rehearsed regularly by the medical staff to ensure appropriate care. Chapter 11 describes the cervical spine's anatomy, evaluation of insidious cervical spine conditions, and injury to the brachial plexus.

◆ **CLINICAL ANATOMY**

With the exception of a small opening on the skull's base, through which the brain stem and spinal cord pass, the brain is almost fully encased in bone (Fig. 18–1). In adults, the cranial bones are rigidly fused by cranial sutures, making the skull a single structure. In infants and children, the sutures are more pliable because they are continually being remodeled during growth.

The skull's design allows for maximum protection of the brain. The density of the bone reduces the amount of physical shock transmitted inwardly. The rounded shape of the skull also has protective qualities. When an object strikes a rounded object, it tends to be deflected quickly. Consider, for example, two scenarios: dropping a brick on a tabletop and dropping a brick on a basketball. When the brick hits the tabletop, it stays there, transmitting its force into the table. When a brick is dropped onto a basketball, although some of the force is transmitted into the ball, the remaining force is removed as the brick deflects off the round surface. Lastly, the skin covering the skull increases the cranium's ability to protect the brain by absorbing and redirecting forces from the skull. The skin greatly increases the skull's strength, increasing its breaking force from 40 lb per square inch to 425 to 490 lb per square inch.[4]

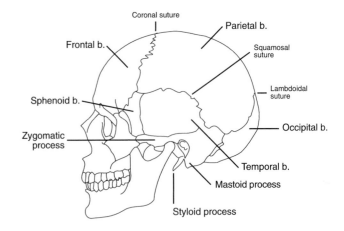

FIGURE 18–1. Lateral view of the bones of the skull.

Table 18–1
BRAIN FUNCTION BY AREA

Area	Function
Cerebrum	Motor function Sensory information (e.g., touch, pain pressure, temperature) Special senses (vision, hearing, smell, taste) Cognition Memory
Cerebellum	Balance and coordination. Smooth, synergistic muscle control.
Diencephalon	Routing of afferent information to the appropriate cerebral areas Body temperature regulation Maintenance of the necessary water balance Emotional control (anger and fear)
Brain stem	Heart rate regulation Respiratory rate regulation Control over the amount of peripheral blood flow

THE BRAIN

The brain is the most complex and least understood part of the human body. Its anatomy and function are presented in this chapter only as they relate to athletic injuries. Table 18–1 presents an encapsulated description of the major brain areas and their primary functions.

The Cerebrum

The largest section of the brain, the cerebrum is formed by two **hemispheres** separated by the **longitudinal fissure.** Each hemisphere is divided into **frontal, parietal, temporal,** and **occipital lobes,** which are separated by sulci and fissures and are named for the overlying cranial bones (Fig. 18–2).

The cerebrum is responsible for controlling the body's primary **motor functions,** both gross muscle contraction and coordination of the muscle contractions in a specific sequence. **Sensory information,** including temperature, touch, pain, pressure, and proprioception, is processed in this region of the brain, along with the **special senses:** visual, auditory, olfactory, and taste. **Cognition,** including spatial relationships, behavior, memory, and association, also occurs in the cerebrum.

With a few exceptions, the cerebrum communicates contralaterally with the rest of the body. The right hemisphere controls the motor actions and interprets much of the sensory input of the body's left side, and vice versa. So clinically, motor impairment of the body's left side usually reflects trauma to the brain's right hemisphere.

The Cerebellum

Designed to allow the quick processing of both incoming and outgoing information, the cerebellum provides the functions necessary to maintain **balance and coordination.** Visual, tactile, auditory, and proprioceptive information from the cerebrum is routed to the cerebellum for immediate processing. The outgoing information is relayed to the muscles via the cerebrum to properly orchestrate the necessary movements.

FIGURE 18–2. Regions of the brain, with insert showing the cerebral hemispheres.

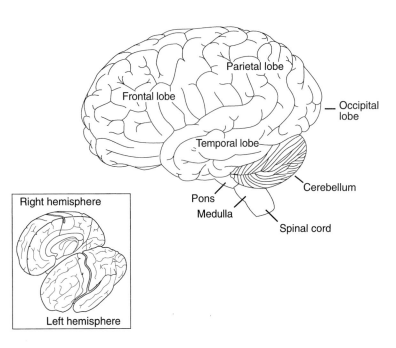

Fluid, synergistic motions, whether during performing a back flip in gymnastics or lifting a cup of coffee, are initiated and controlled by the cerebellum. Facilitative impulses are relayed from the cerebellum to the contracting muscles, and an inhibitory stimulus is sent to the antagonistic muscles. Individuals who have suffered trauma to the cerebellum are recognizable by their uncoordinated, segmental, robot-like movements. Cerebellar injuries are relatively rare in athletes. However, severe blows to the posterior aspect of the skull or acceleration and deceleration mechanisms that cause rotation of the brain stem can injure the cerebellum.

The Diencephalon

Formed by the **thalamus, hypothalamus,** and **epithalamus,** the **diencephalon** acts as a processing center for conscious and unconscious brain input. In its gatekeeping role, sensory information ascending the spinal cord is monitored by the thalamus, routing the specific types of information to the appropriate area of the brain. In addition to regulating some of the body's hormones, the hypothalamus is the center of the body's autonomic nervous system, regulating *sympathetic* and *parasympathetic nervous system* activity. Body temperature, water balance, gastrointestinal activity, hunger, and emotions are controlled by the hypothalamus.

The Brain Stem

Formed by the **medulla oblongata** (medulla) and the pons, the brain stem serves to relay information to and from the central nervous system (CNS) and controls the involuntary systems. Literally translating as "bridge," the **pons** serves to link the cerebellum to the brain stem and spinal cord, connecting the upper and lower portions of the CNS. Additionally, receptors in the pons regulate the respiratory rate.

The medulla serves as the interface between the spinal cord and the rest of the brain. Involuntary functions of heart rate, respiration, blood vessel diameter (vasodilation and vasoconstriction), coughing, and vomiting are regulated by the **medullary centers.**

THE MENINGES

The brain and spinal cord are buffered from the bony surfaces of the cranium and spinal column by three meninges: the **dura mater, arachnoid mater,** and **pia mater.** The progressive densities of the meninges support and protect the brain and spinal cord. Arterial and venous blood supplies are provided through these structures, as are the production and introduction of the cerebrospinal fluid (CSF).

The Dura Mater

Literally translating as "hard mother," the dura mater is the outermost meningeal covering, also serving as

the periosteum for the skull's inner layer. The **falx cerebri** is a fold in the dura mater in the longitudinal fissure between the two cerebral hemispheres. The void between the two cerebellar hemispheres is filled by another fold of the dura mater, the **falx cerebelli.**

Arteries in the dura mater, the **meningeal arteries,** primarily supply blood to the cranial bones. Blood supply to the dura mater is provided by fine branches from the meningeal arteries. At various points around the brain, the dura mater forms two layers. The space between these layers forms the **venous sinuses,** which serve as a drainage conduit to route used blood into the internal jugular veins in the neck.

The Arachnoid Mater

The name "arachnoid" is gained from this structure's resemblance to a cobweb ("arachne" is the Greek word for "spider"). Similar to a cobweb, the fibers forming the arachnoid are thin yet are relatively resilient to trauma. The arachnoid mater is separated from the dura mater by the narrow **subdural space.** Beneath the arachnoid is a wider separation, the **subarachnoid space,** containing the CSF.

The Pia Mater

The innermost meningeal membrane, the pia mater, envelops the brain, forming its outer "skin." This delicate membrane derives its name from the Latin word for "tender"; therefore, the pia mater is the "tender mother." The pia mater follows the brain's contour, protruding into its fissures and sulci.

CEREBROSPINAL FLUID

Originating from the **choroid plexuses** deep within the brain and secreted by cells surrounding the cerebrum's blood vessels, CSF slowly circulates around the brain and spinal cord within the subarachnoid space. From the lateral ventricles, CSF is forced into the third and fourth ventricles by a pressure gradient. After it is in the fourth ventricle, a small proportion of the CSF enters the central canal of the spinal cord. The remaining fluid flows down the spinal cord on its posterior surface and returns to the brain on the anterior portion of the subarachnoid space.

Because of the presence of the subarachnoid space and its watery content, the CNS floats within the body. This arrangement serves as another buffer against ex-

Sympathetic nervous system   The part of the central nervous system that supplies the involuntary muscles.

Parasympathetic nervous system   A series of specific effects controlled by the brain regulating smooth muscle contractions, slowing the heart rate, and constricting the pupil.

ternal forces being transmitted to the CNS. Although beneficial in dissipating the high-velocity impacts associated with collision sports, this protective configuration is most useful in buffering more repetitive forces, such as those seen when running.

BLOOD CIRCULATION IN THE BRAIN

When the body is at rest, the brain demands 20 percent of the body's oxygen uptake. For each degree (centigrade) the body's core temperature increases, the brain's need for oxygen increases by 7 percent. Blood supply to the brain is provided by the two **vertebral arteries** and the two **common carotid arteries.** Each common carotid artery diverges to form an **internal carotid artery** and an **external carotid artery.** The external carotid arteries continue upward to supply blood to the

head and neck, with the exception of the brain. The internal carotid arteries move toward the center of the cranium to assist in supplying the brain with blood.

The two internal carotid arteries and the two vertebral arteries converge to form a collateral circulation network, the **circle of Willis** (Fig. 18–3). If one of the cranial arteries is obstructed, the design of the circle of Willis permits at least a partial supply of blood to the affected area.

◆ EVALUATION OF HEAD AND NECK INJURIES

The ability to identify and properly manage patients with serious head and neck injuries may affect whether the athlete lives, dies, or becomes permanently disabled. Although some signs and symptoms of brain trauma

FIGURE 18–3. Blood supply to the brain. The circle of Willis provides collateral circulation to the brain's regions.

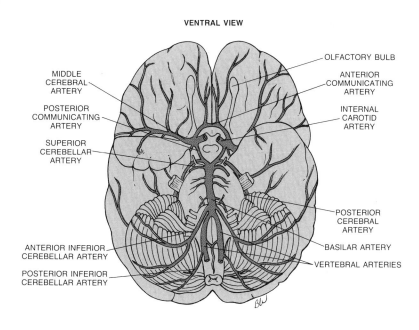

VASCULAR ANATOMY OF BRAIN

VENTRAL VIEW

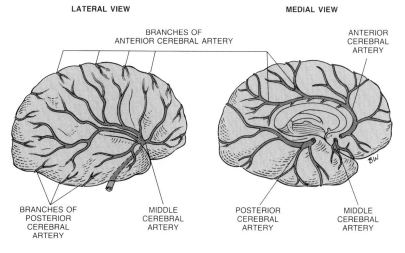

LATERAL VIEW   MEDIAL VIEW

are blatantly obvious, such as unconsciousness, some potentially catastrophic head injuries initially have few, if any, outward signs or symptoms. This section describes the signs and symptoms of brain and spine trauma. The following section describes the on-field management of athletes with these conditions. Many of these evaluative procedures are performed on the field.

EVALUATION SCENARIOS

Before discussing how to evaluate and manage athletes with head and neck injuries, the possible scenarios under which an evaluation may have to be performed must be considered. The best-case scenario is one in which the athlete is conscious and responsive to stimuli. The worst-case scenario is that of a prone, unconscious athlete who is devoid of an airway, breathing, or circulation (ABC). In either case, the decisions made by the medical staff are critical in the optimal management of athletes with catastrophic conditions.

A basic premise must be formed at this point and adhered to at all times: **All unconscious athletes must be managed as if a fracture or dislocation of the cervical spine exists until the presence of these injuries can be definitively ruled out.**

Ideally, athletes with head and neck injuries are evaluated on the field by at least two responders. One responder must ensure stabilization and immobilization of the athlete's head by grasping the sides of the head or helmet and applying **in-line stabilization** on the cervical spine until pathology has been ruled out. A second responder performs the necessary palpation, sensory, and motor tests (Fig. 18–4). One person acts as the leader and directs the actions of all others at the injury scene. In situations in which only one responder is present, other on-site personnel may be directed to assist in management of the athlete's condition. Prior discussion and practice are necessary to ensure orderly and precise action by the support staff.

EVALUATION OF THE ATHLETE'S POSITION

The initial assessment of an on-field head and neck injury may be further complicated by the position in which the athlete is found. A supine athlete is in the optimal position for subsequent evaluation and management. When athletes are in the sidelying or prone position, the evaluation is more difficult.

If, as determined in the next section, the athlete's vital signs are present, there is no need to move the athlete until a complete on-field evaluation is performed and the athlete's disposition is determined. However, when an athlete is prone or sidelying, the absence of vital signs takes precedence over the possibility of a spinal fracture. The athlete must be rolled into the supine position in the safest manner possible. These procedures are discussed in the "On-Field Management of Head and Neck Injuries" section of this chapter.

DETERMINATION OF CONSCIOUSNESS

When an athlete is "down" on the field or court, the first priority is to establish the athlete's level of consciousness. A moving and speaking athlete demonstrates that the ABCs are present and functioning. Even

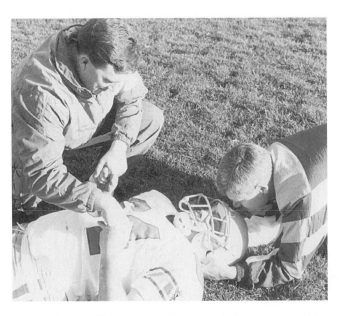

FIGURE 18–4. Head and neck trauma is best managed by two responders. One stabilizes the head while the second performs evaluative techniques.

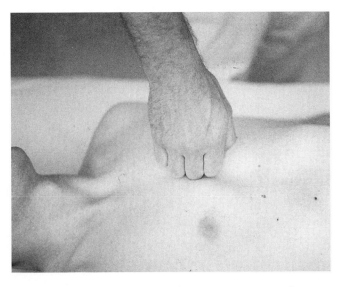

FIGURE 18–5. Attempting to elicit a pain response from an unconscious patient. This test is performed by squeezing the patient's fingernail, pinching the patient, or applying pressure with a knuckle to the sternum.

under these circumstances, however, a cervical fracture must be suspected, and the athlete's vital signs require regular monitoring. At the scene of a possible head or neck injury, the athlete's head is stabilized and immobilized by grasping the sides of the helmet or head and applying in-line stabilization on the cervical spine until pathology to the spine has been ruled out.

- **Level of consciousness:** While moving toward the scene of the injury, note whether the athlete is moving. At the scene, make an attempt to communicate with the athlete. If verbal communication fails, the athlete's responsiveness to painful stimuli is checked by applying pressure to the lunula of a fingernail or rubbing the sternum (Fig. 18–5).
- **Primary survey:** If the athlete is unconscious or unable to communicate, check the athlete's ABCs by looking, listening, and feeling for breathing (Fig. 18–6). If breathing is absent, use a modified jaw thrust to open the airway. In the event that no carotid or radial pulse is found, send someone to summon advanced medical assistance and initiate cardiopulmonary resuscitation. The "On-Field Management of Head and Neck Injuries" section of this chapter contains further discussion of this topic.
- **Secondary survey:** Although the suspicion of brain or cervical spine trauma takes precedence, do not overlook the possibility of other trauma to the body. Inspect the extremities and torso for bleeding or indications of fractures or dislocations.

The following components of an assessment of a head- or neck-injured athlete assume a sideline evaluation is being conducted. A descriptive on-field management procedure is detailed later in this chapter.

HISTORY

The history-taking process of an athlete with a head injury not only determines the injury mechanism but also assesses the athlete's level of brain function. Much of this portion of the evaluation is initially conducted when the athlete is on the field. Then this evaluation is repeated at regular intervals on the sidelines. In the event that the athlete becomes unconscious, proceed to the inspection phase of the evaluation while continuing to monitor the vital signs. Throughout the evaluation, the athlete must be questioned and observed for the presence of subtle signs and symptoms indicating a head injury (Table 18–2).

- **Location of symptoms:** The athlete is questioned regarding the location and type of pain or other symptoms experienced after the injury.

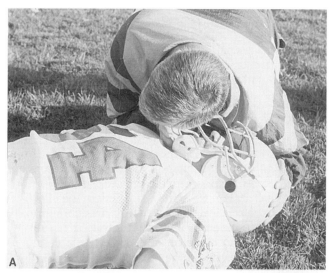

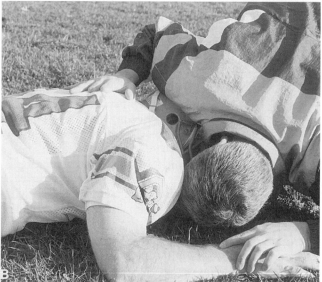

FIGURE 18–6. Establishing the presence of an open airway, breathing, and circulation. **(A)** Supine athlete. **(B)** Prone athlete.

Table 18–2
SIGNS AND SYMPTOMS OF A HEAD OR NECK INJURY TO OBSERVE FOR THROUGHOUT THE EVALUATION

Area	Signs and Symptoms
Brain	Amnesia (retrograde and anterograde) Confusion Disorientation Irritability Incoordination Dizziness Headache
Ocular	Blurred vision Photophobia Nystagmus
Ears	Tinnitus Dizziness
Stomach	Nausea Vomiting
Systemic	Unusually fatigued

○ **Cervical pain:** The most significant finding during this portion of the examination is cervical pain or muscle spasm. The significance of this finding is magnified when it is accompanied by pain, numbness, or burning, which may or may not radiate into the extremities.

○ **Head pain:** Diffuse headaches are a common complaint after brain trauma. Localized pain can indicate a contusion, skull fracture, or intracranial hemorrhage.

• **Mechanism of head injuries:** The type of injury inflicted to the head and cervical spine is somewhat dependent on the nature of the force delivered (Fig. 18–7). This information may be obtained by someone who witnessed the injury if the athlete is unconscious or groggy.

○ **Coup:** A coup injury results when a relatively stationary skull is hit by an object traveling at a high velocity (e.g., being struck in the head with a baseball). This type of mechanism results in trauma on the side of the head that was struck.

○ **Contrecoup:** A contrecoup injury occurs when the skull is moving at a relatively high velocity and is suddenly stopped, such as when falling and striking the head on the floor. The fluid within the skull fails to decrease the brain's momentum proportional to that of the skull, causing the brain to strike the skull on the side opposite the impact. This mechanism includes forces that are transmitted up the length of the spinal column, such as when falling and landing on the buttocks.

○ **Repeated subconcussive forces:** Athletes receiving repeated nontraumatic blows to the head (e.g., in boxing or while heading a soccer ball) have a higher degree of degenerative changes within the CNS.[5] A history of repeated concussions can result in cumulative neurologic and cognitive deficits by disrupting electroencephalographic (EEG) activity.[6]

○ **Rotational or shear forces:** Sudden twisting forces or acceleration and deceleration can disrupt neural activity and result in cerebral concussion symptoms.

• **Mechanism of cervical spine injuries:** Most of the forces directed toward the cervical spine are capable of being dissipated by the energy-absorbing properties of the cervical musculature and intervertebral disks.[7] The mechanisms of injury to the cervical spine involve flexion, extension, or lateral bending and may be accompanied by a rotational component.

Flexion of the cervical spine is the mechanism most likely to produce catastrophic injury.[7–11] As the crown of the head makes contact, the cervical spine and skull flexes. As soon as the neck is flexed to approximately 30 degrees, the cervical spine's lordotic curve is lost (Fig. 18–8). In this position, the effectiveness of the cervical spine's energy-dissipating mechanism is rendered ineffective, thus transmitting forces directly to the cervical vertebrae, creating an **axial load** through the vertical axis of the segmented columns (Fig. 18–9).

• **Loss of consciousness:** This portion of the history-taking process is closely related to the determination of the athlete's memory status. Record the responses given by the athlete immediately after the injury for future comparison. The athlete is questioned regarding a momentary loss of consciousness after the impact (e.g., "Do you remember being hit?"). The athlete may also describe "seeing stars" or "blacking out" at the time of the impact, both of which indicate transitory unconsciousness.

• **History of concussion:** A recent history of concussion increases the risk for subsequent concussions and **second impact syndrome.**[12] The history of concussions must be readily available from the athlete's medical file.

• **Complaints of weakness:** A general malaise is to be expected after a cerebral concussion. Reports of muscular weakness in one or more extremities is a more serious finding, possibly indicating trauma to the brain, spinal cord, or one or more spinal nerve roots.

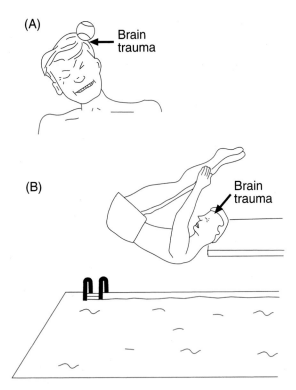

FIGURE 18–7. Mechanisms of an athletic head injury. **(A)** Coup mechanism caused by a moving object's striking the head, resulting in brain trauma on the side of the impact. **(B)** Contrecoup mechanism caused by a moving head striking a stationary object. Trauma occurs to the brain on the opposite side of the impact as it rebounds off the skull.

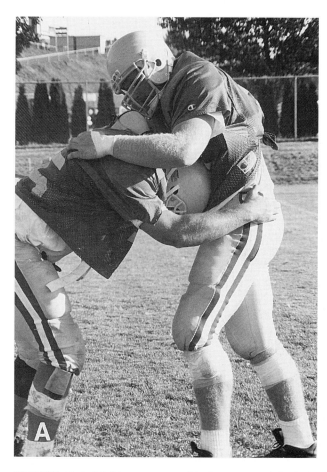
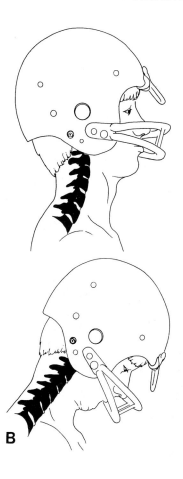

FIGURE 18–8. Making contact with the crown of the helmet results in axial loading, compressing the cervical vertebrae.

INSPECTION

If the athlete is wearing protective headgear at the onset of the inspection process, a decision must be made regarding whether and when to remove it. The helmet should not be removed if there is any lingering suspicion of a cervical spine fracture or dislocation. Much of the inspection and palpation process can be performed with the helmet still in place.

Inspection of the Bony Structures

- **Position of the head:** Observe the way in which the head is positioned. Normally the head should be upright in all planes. A laterally flexed and rotated skull that is accompanied by muscle spasm on the side opposite that of the tilt may indicate a dislocation of a cervical vertebra.
- **Cervical vertebrae:** Viewing the athlete from behind, observe the alignment of the spinous processes. A vertebra that is obviously malaligned (i.e., rotated or displaced anteriorly or posteriorly) can signify a vertebral dislocation.

- **Mastoid process:** Note any ecchymosis over the mastoid process, **Battle's sign,** which may indicate a basilar skull fracture.
- **Skull and scalp:** Inspect the athlete's skull and scalp for the presence of bleeding, swelling, or other deformities.

Inspection of the Eyes

- **General:** Note the general attitude of the athlete's eyes. A dazed, distant appearance may be attributed to mental confusion and disruption of cerebral function.
- **Nystagmus:** While observing both of the athlete's eyes simultaneously, look for the presence of involuntary cyclical movement, or nystagmus. This clinical sign, although it may normally occur, may indicate pressure on the eyes' motor nerves or disruption of the inner ear.
- **Pupil size:** Observe the equality of the pupils. A unilaterally dilated pupil is indicative of an intracranial hemorrhage's placing pressure on cranial nerve III.

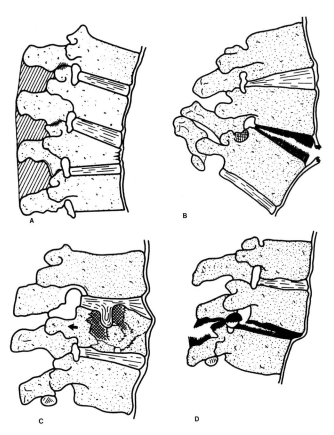

FIGURE 18–9. Mechanisms of cervical spine injuries and the resulting trauma. **(A)** Flexion mechanism resulting in compression of the vertebral body. **(B)** Extension mechanism resulting in tearing of the anterior longitudinal ligament and intervertebral disk. **(C)** Compression mechanism resulting in a posterior burst of the bone. **(D)** Flexion and rotation injury resulting in a dislocation of the cervical vertebrae.

Some athletes may normally display unequal pupil sizes, or anisocoria (Fig. 18–10). Although this condition is benign, its presence should be detected during the preparticipation physical examination and recorded in the athlete's medical file to avoid confusion during the evaluation of a head injury.

- **Pupillary reaction to light:** Refer to Box 16–1 and see the "Neurologic Testing" section of this chapter for the process and implications of negative pupillary reaction tests.

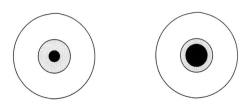

FIGURE 18–10. Anisocoria, or unequal pupil size. This condition may result from pressure on cranial nerve III or may be congenital.

Inspection of the Nose and Ears

Bleeding from the ears, even in the absence of CSF in the fluid, may indicate a skull fracture (Box 18–1). Bleeding from the nose could represent either a nasal fracture or a skull fracture. Ecchymosis under the eyes, "raccoon eyes," can indicate a skull fracture or nasal fracture.

PALPATION

Palpation should not be performed over areas of obvious deformity or suspected fracture, especially in the cervical spine and skull. Placing too much pressure on these structures may cause the bony fragment to displace, possibly resulting in catastrophic consequences. Refer to Chapter 11 for a detailed description of the palpation of the cervical spine.

Palpation of the Bony Structures

- **Spinous processes:** Position the patient sitting and leaning slightly forward. Standing behind the athlete, palpate the spinous processes of C7, C6, and C5 (Fig. 18–11). At approximately the C5 level, the spinous processes become less defined. Continue to palpate the area over the spinous processes of C4 and C3, noting for tenderness or crepitus.
- **Transverse processes:** Although the transverse processes of C1 are the only ones that are directly palpable (approximately two fingers' widths below the mastoid process), palpate the areas over the transverse processes of the remaining cervical vertebrae.
- **Skull:** Begin the palpation of the skull at the inion, the occipital bone's posterior process. Continue to palpate anteriorly toward the face, palpating the temporal bones and their mastoid processes, and the sphenoid, zygomatic, parietal, and frontal bones (see Fig. 18–1).

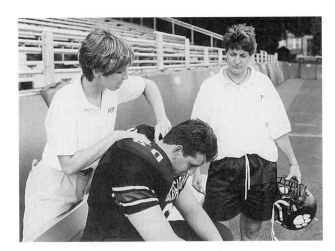

FIGURE 18–11. Sideline palpation of the cervical spine.

Box 18–1
HALO TEST

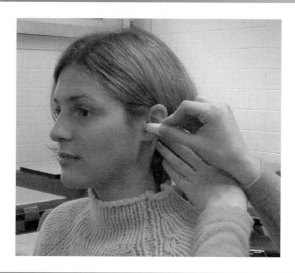
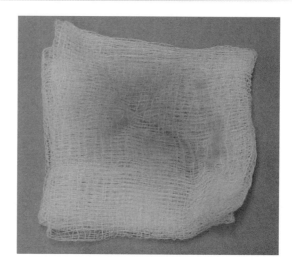

PATIENT POSITION	Lying or sitting
POSITION OF EXAMINER	Lateral to the patient's ear.
EVALUATIVE PROCEDURE	Fold a piece of sterile gauze into a triangle. Using the point of the gauze, collect a sample of the fluid leaking from the ear or nose and allow it to be absorbed by the gauze.
POSITIVE TEST	A pale yellow "halo" will form around the sample on the gauze.
IMPLICATIONS	Cerebrospinal fluid leakage.

Palpation of Soft Tissue

- **Musculature:** To identify muscular spasm, palpate the trapezius and sternocleidomastoid muscles. In addition to the muscle's reaction to a strain, spasm may result from insult to a cervical nerve root or may reflect the body's protective response to a cervical fracture or dislocation.
- **Throat:** Perform complete palpation of the anterior throat, if warranted, to rule out trauma to the larynx, trachea, or hyoid bone.

FUNCTIONAL TESTING

The goal of the functional testing of an athlete with a head or neck injury is to assess the status of the CNS. This portion of the examination begins with assessment of the athlete's airway, breathing, circulation, and level of consciousness. This section of the chapter assumes that the patient is conscious and capable of responding to the functional tasks presented. The cervical spine must be assessed first to rule out bone or joint dysfunction.

Memory

- One of the most obvious dysfunctions after brain trauma is the loss of memory. The inability to recall

events before the onset of the injury is termed **retrograde amnesia** (Box 18–2). When the athlete cannot remember events after the onset of injury, it is termed **anterograde amnesia** (Box 18–3) or posttraumatic amnesia (Fig. 18–12). Although significant retrograde amnesia is a cause of concern, fading or fogging memory identifies a progressive deterioration of the cerebral function. The patient should be questioned regarding the sequence of events after the injury:

- How did you get to the sidelines?
- Who has spoken to you since?
- Do you remember my asking you those questions before?

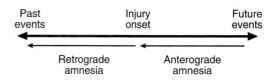

FIGURE 18–12. Types of amnesia. Loss of memory from onset backward in time is known as retrograde amnesia. Loss of memory after the onset of an injury is anterograde amnesia.

Box 18–2

DETERMINATION OF RETROGRADE AMNESIA

PATIENT POSITION	**On-field:** In the athlete's current position (see instructions regarding moving the athlete) **Sideline:** Standing sitting, or lying down
POSITION OF EXAMINER	In a position to hear the patient's response
EVALUATIVE PROCEDURE	The patient is asked a series of questions beginning with the time of the injury. Each successive question progresses backward in time, as described by the following set of questions: What happened? What play were you running? (or other applicable question regarding the patient's activity at the time of injury) Where are you? Who am I? Who are you playing? What quarter is it (or what time is it)? What did you have for a pregame meal (or what did you have to eat for lunch)? Who did you play last week?
POSITIVE TEST	The patient has difficulty remembering or cannot remember events occurring before the injury.
IMPLICATIONS	Retrograde amnesia, the severity of which is based on the relative amount of memory loss demonstrated by the inability to recall events Not remembering events from the day before is more significant than not remembering more recent events The same set of questions should be repeated to determine whether the memory is returning, deteriorating, or remaining the same. Further deterioration of the memory or acutely profound memory loss that does not return in a matter of minutes warrants the immediate termination of the evaluation and transportation to an emergency medical facility.
COMMENT	Record the patient's response and verify the answers with the athlete's teammates or coach.

Box 18–3

DETERMINATION OF ANTEROGRADE AMNESIA

PATIENT POSITION	Sitting or lying
POSITION OF EXAMINER	In a position to hear the patient's response
EVALUATIVE PROCEDURE	The athlete is given a list of four unrelated items with instructions to memorize them, for example: Hubcap Film Dog tags Ivy The list is immediately repeated by the patient to ensure that it has been memorized. The patient is asked to repeat the list to the examiner every 5 minutes.
POSITIVE TEST	The inability to completely recite the list
IMPLICATIONS	Anterograde amnesia, possibly the result of intracranial bleeding
COMMENT	This test is usually performed after the test for retrograde amnesia.

Table 18–3
NEUROPSYCHOLOGICAL ASSESSMENT TESTS USED FOR MILD HEAD-INJURED ATHLETES

Test and Publisher	Description
Trail Making Test A & B (Reitan Neuropsychological Laboratory, Tucson, AZ)	**Description:** The patient sequentially connects a series of numbers (Trail Making A) or series of alternating letters and numbers (Trail Making B) **Measurement:** The time required for successful completion **Assessment:** Visual conceptual, visuomotor tracking, general brain function
Wechsler Digit Span Test (WDST) (Psychological Corporation, San Antonio, TX)	**Description:** The patient is presented with a random list of single-digit numbers (0 to 9 with no repetition) and asked to repeat the list in the same order (Digits Forward) or reverse order (Digits Backwards). The first bout begins with three numbers and the next has four numbers, progressing up to 10. **Measurement:** The number of successful trials is recorded for each part. **Assessment:** Short-term memory, auditory attention, concentration
Stroop Color Word Test (Stoelting Co., Wood Dale, IL)	**Description:** Patients are presented with a list of 100 words (5 columns × 20 words each). The test itself consists of three trials, each 45 seconds in length. In the first trial, the patient is asked to read through the list as quickly as possible and read aloud the words "red," "green," and "blue," which are written in black ink. During the second trial, words are replaced with "XXXX" written in red, green, or blue ink, which the patient must identify the proper color. In the third trial, the words "red," "green," and "blue" are written in a color other than their own (e.g., "red" is written in blue ink and "blue" is written in green ink). The patient must identify the color the word is printed in, not the word itself. **Measurement:** Sum total of the number of correct responses in each subset **Assessment:** Cognitive processing speed, concentration ability to filter out distractions (inhibition)
Hopkins Verbal Learning Test (Johns Hopkins University, Baltimore, MD)	**Description:** The patient is read a list of 12 words grouped into three semantic categories of four words each three times. After each reading, the patient is asked to recall as many words as possible. After a 20-minute break, the patient is read a list of 24 words, 12 words from the original list, six words that are closely related, and six unrelated words. **Measurement:** The number of incorrect responses from the fourth trial subtracted from the total number of correct responses from the first three trials. **Assessment:** Language function, short-term memory
Symbol Digit Modalities Test (Western Psychological Services, Los Angeles, CA)	**Description:** Patients are given 30 seconds to memorize a list of nine symbols and their corresponding symbols. In one version of the test, the patient is asked to repeat the symbols corresponding to a four-digit number. An alternate form has the patient write the number that corresponds to a specific symbol. **Measurement:** The number of correct responses divided by the total number of completed responses **Assessment:** Psychomotor speed, concentration, visual speed, and visual perception
Controlled Oral Word Association Test (COWAT) (Psychological Assessment Resources, Inc. Odessa, FL)	**Description:** The patient is given three word naming trials based on two groups of letters, "C–F–L" and "P–R–W." In the first session, the patient is then asked to say as many words as possible that begins with that letter of the alphabet, starting with the first letter within the first code group and then progressing to the subsequent letter. The second code group is used in the second session. Proper names, numbers, and different variations of the same word (e.g., "count," "counting," "counted") are not allowed. This is repeated for three trials. **Measurement:** The raw score based on the total number of acceptable words produced in the three trials. The publisher of the COWAT provides formulas that allow the score to be adjusted based on the patient's age, gender, and level of education. **Assessment:** Verbal fluency

Cognitive Function

Trauma to the cerebrum can result in unusual communication between the patient and the examiner. This can manifest itself through inappropriate behavior, irrational thinking, and apparent mental disability or personality changes.

- **Behavior:** The individual's behavior, attitude, and demeanor may become altered after brain trauma. This may take the form of violent, irrational behavior; inappropriate behavior; and belligerence. After a head injury, the athlete may verbally or physically lash out at those attempting to assist.
- **Analytical skills:** The patient's analytical skills can be determined using **serial 7's.** The patient is asked to count backwards from 100 by 7's (e.g., 100, 93, 86, 79 . . .).
- **Information processing:** The athlete's ability to process the information and assimilate facts should

be noted. Confusion regarding relatively simple directions, such as "Sit on the bench," indicates profound cognitive dysfunction.

Neuropsychological Testing

Memory and cognitive testing provide a subjective assessment of the athlete's mental abilities. The use of objective neuropsychological tests and objective balance tests (see the information on the balance error scoring system in the next section) objectively quantify the amount of dysfunction demonstrated by the athlete.[13–19]

Table 18–3 presents a description of the six most commonly used neuropsychological tests in sports medicine.[15] Scores obtained from these tests during the preseason physical examination can reliably be used for baseline measures for post-head injury evaluation and return to play decisions.[14,17]

Box 18–4
ROMBERG TEST

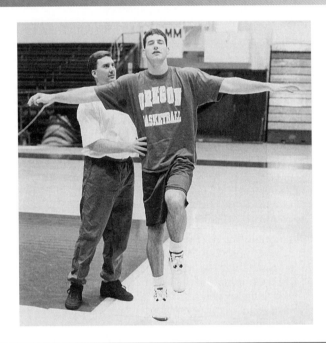

PATIENT POSITION	Standing with the feet shoulder width apart
POSITION OF EXAMINER	Standing lateral or posterior to the patient, ready to support the patient as needed
EVALUATIVE PROCEDURE	The patient shuts the eyes and abducts the arms to 90° with the elbows extended. The patient tilts the head backward and lifts one foot off the ground while attempting to maintain balance. If this portion of the examination is adequately completed, the patient is asked to touch the index finger to the nose (with the eyes remaining closed).
POSITIVE TEST	The patient displays gross unsteadiness.
IMPLICATIONS	Lack of balance and/or coordination indicating cerebellular dysfunction

Balance and Coordination

After a head injury, the athlete's balance and coordination may be hindered secondary to trauma involving the cerebellum or the inner ear. A profound loss of muscular coordination, ataxia, may be obvious as the athlete attempts to perform even simple tasks. The **Romberg test** (Box 18–4) and **tandem walking** (Box 18–5) are used to determine cerebellar function by determining the level of balance and coordination.

After a head injury, an electronic balance system can be used to objectively determine the amount of balance disruption. In the absence of these devices, a quantifiable clinical test should be used. The **balance error scoring system** (BESS), a newer clinical test that has been developed to evaluate impairment of balance and coordination, is more applicable and sensitive to the athletic population (Box 18–6).[20,21] In this procedure, balance is first tested on a firm surface and then again with the patient standing on foam.

Balance measurements should be obtained before the start of each season and used as a baseline for post–head injury evaluation. Baseline measurements should be conducted in a quiet, distraction-free environment. During baseline testing, the patient should be well rested and free from any lower extremity musculoskeletal injury. After injury, the BESS can be administered on the sidelines or in the clinic with the results then compared with the baseline measures. If baseline information is not available, the patient's BESS score can be compared with recovery curves for the normal population.[15, 20, 21]

Vital Signs

Techniques for determining the vital signs are described in Chapter 12. The following are qualitative parameters that are relevant after a head or neck injury.

Box 18–5
TANDEM WALKING

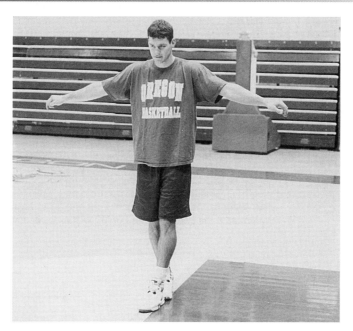

PATIENT POSITION	Standing with the feet straddling a straight line (e.g., sideline)
POSITION OF EXAMINER	Beside the patient ready to provide support
EVALUATIVE PROCEDURE	The patient walks heel-to-toe along the straight line for approximately 10 yd. The patient returns to the starting position by walking backward.
POSITIVE TEST	The patient is unable to maintain a steady balance
IMPLICATIONS	Cerebral or inner ear dysfunction that inhibits balance

Box 18–6
BALANCE ERROR SCORING SYSTEM (BESS)

Firm surface bout			**Soft surface bout**		

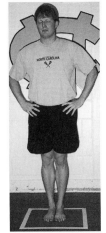 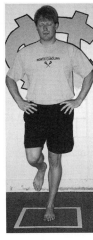 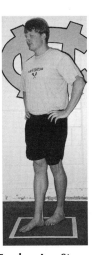 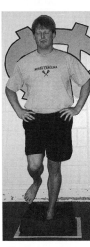 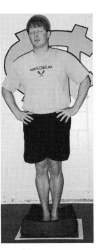 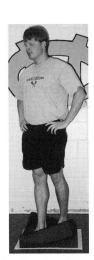

Double Leg Stance	**Single Leg Stance**	**Tandem Leg Stance**	**Double Leg Stance**	**Single Leg Stance**	**Tandem Leg Stance**

The balance error scoring system involves three different stances, each completed twice, once while standing on a firm surface and again while standing on a foam surface.

PATIENT POSITION	The patient is barefoot or wearing socks. The ankle must not be taped during the test. The patient assumes the following stances for each phase of the test: **Phase 1:** Double leg stance **Phase 2:** Single leg stance—standing on the nondominant leg. The non–weight-bearing hip is flexed to 20° to 30° and the knee is flexed to 40° to 50°. **Phase 3:** Tandem leg stance—The nondominant leg is placed behind the dominant leg and the patient stands in a heel–toe manner. The patient's hands are placed on the iliac crests. The eyes are closed during the test.
POSITION OF EXAMINER	The examiner stands in front of the athlete. A stopwatch is required to time the trials. A second clinician acts as a spotter.
EVALUATIVE PROCEDURE	The first battery of tests is performed with the patient standing on a firm surface. The patient assumes the double leg stance and attempts to hold the position for 20 seconds. The test is repeated using the single leg stance and then the tandem leg stance. The second battery of tests is performed with the patient standing on a piece of medium density foam (60 kg/m^3) that is 45 cm × 45 cm and 13 cm thick. The trial is incomplete if the patient cannot hold the testing position for a minimum of 5 seconds.

SCORING	One point is scored for each of the following errors:
	    Lifting hands off the iliac crest
	    Opening the eyes
	    Stepping, stumbling, or falling
	    Moving the hip into more than 30° of flexion or abduction
	    Lifting the foot or heel
	    Remaining out of the testing position for more than 5 seconds
	If more than one error occurs simultaneously, only one error is recorded.
	Patients who are unable to hold the testing position for 5 seconds are assigned the score of 10.

POSITIVE TEST	Scores that are 25 percent above the patient's baseline or the norm
IMPLICATIONS	Impaired cerebral function

• **Respiration:** In addition to the number of breaths per minute, the quality of the respirations are determined:

Type	Characteristics	Implications
Apneustic	Prolonged inspirations unrelieved by attempts to exhale	Trauma to the pons
Biot's	Periods of **apnea** followed by hyperapnea	Increased intracranial pressure
Cheyne-Stokes	Periods of apnea followed by breaths of increasing depth and frequency	Frontal lobe or brain stem trauma
Slow	Respiration consisting of fewer than 12 breaths per minute	CNS disruption
Thoracic	Respiration in which the diaphragm is inactive and breathing occurs only through expansion of the chest; normal abdominal movement is absent	Disruption of the phrenic nerve or its nerve roots

• **Pulse:** The pulse rate and quality must be monitored at regular intervals until the possibility of brain or spinal injury has been ruled out. Pulse abnormalities attributed to these conditions include:

Type	Characteristics	Implication
Accelerated	Pulse >150 beats per minute (bpm) (>170 bpm usually has fatal results).	Pressure on the base of the brain; shock
Bounding	Pulse that quickly reaches a higher intensity than normal, then quickly disappears	Ventricular systole and reduced peripheral pressure
Deficit	Pulse in which the number of beats counted at the radial pulse is less than that counted over the heart itself.	Cardiac arrhythmia
High tension	Pulse in which the force of the beat is increased; an increased amount of pressure is required to inhibit the radial pulse	Cerebral trauma
Low tension	Short, fast, faint pulse having a rapid decline	Heart failure; shock

• **Blood pressure:** Blood pressure readings should be taken concurrently or immediately after each pulse measurement. These measurements are recorded and repeated at regular intervals. Blood pressure is normally high after physical exertion. Blood pressure that does not decrease over time or continues to increase may be a sign of severe intracranial hemorrhage.

• **Pulse pressure:** To calculate the pulse pressure, the diastolic pressure is subtracted from the systolic pressure. The normal pulse pressure is approximately 40 mm Hg. A pulse pressure of greater than 50 mm Hg may indicate increased intracranial bleeding

NEUROLOGIC TESTING

Twelve pairs of cranial nerves (CNs), identified by Roman numerals (CN I to CN XII), arise from the brain and transmit both sensory and motor impulses (Table 18–4). Whereas the *ganglia* of the sensory component are located outside the CNS, the ganglia of the motor nerves are located within the CNS. Increased intracranial pressure results in impairment of the motor component of the cranial nerves involved but leaves their sensory component intact.

Cranial Nerve Function

An assessment of the cranial nerves must be conducted immediately after the injury and repeated in 15- to 20-minute intervals until the severity of the head injury has been determined. Accumulation of blood within the cranium places pressure on the cranial nerves, impairing their function. Information regarding the loss of many of these functions, such as vision, smell, and taste, is volunteered by the athlete. The following tests are ordered by the affected organ rather than by the cranial nerves themselves.

• **Eyes:** Vision (CN II) is assessed using a Snellen's chart (see Fig. 16–5) or by reading an object of reasonable size for normal vision, such as the amount of time remaining on the scoreboard. With the use of a penlight, the **pupil's reaction to light** (CN III) is determined by covering one of the athlete's eyes and briefly shining the light into the opposite pupil. Normally, the pupil should constrict when the light strikes it and dilate when the light is removed. Using a penlight, finger, or other object held approximately 2 ft from the athlete's nose, the equality of **eye movement** (CNs II, IV, and VI) is determined by moving the object up, down, left, right, and, finally, inward toward the athlete's nose.

  Diplopia experienced after the injury may indicate cerebral dysfunction; pressure on CN III, IV, or VI, causing spasm of the eye's extrinsic muscles; or a fracture of the eye's orbit. Diplopia that does not rapidly subside indicates the immediate need for advanced medical assistance.

Apnea   The temporary cessation of breathing.

Ganglion (nerve) (pl. **ganglia**)   A collection of nerve cell bodies housed in the central or peripheral nervous system.

Table 18–4
CRANIAL NERVE FUNCTION

Number	Name	Type	Function
I	Olfactory	Sensory	Smell
II	Optic	Sensory	Vision
III	Oculomotor	Motor	Effect on pupillary reaction and size Elevation of upper eyelid Eye adduction and downward rolling
IV	Trochlear	Motor	Upward eye rolling
V	Trigeminal	Mixed	Motor: muscles of mastication Sensation: nose, forehead, temple, scalp, lips, tongue and lower jaw
VI	Abducens	Motor	Lateral eye movement
VII	Facial	Mixed	Motor: muscles of expression Sensory: taste
VIII	Vestibulocochlear	Sensory	Equilibrium Hearing
IX	Glossopharyngeal	Mixed	Motor: pharyngeal muscles Sensory: taste
X	Vagus	Mixed	Motor: muscles of pharynx and larynx Sensory: gag reflex
XI	Accessory	Motor	Trapezius and sternocleidomastoid muscles
XII	Hypoglossal	Motor	Tongue movement

- **Face:** The athlete is asked to raise the eyebrows and forehead, smile, and frown (CN VII); clench the jaw (CN V); swallow (CNs IX and X); and stick out the tongue (CN XII).
- **Ears:** The functions of CN VIII include hearing, in which any disruption should be apparent. Tinnitus, which is determined in the history-taking portion of the examination, demonstrates possible malfunctions of CN VIII. Balance and equilibrium can be assessed through the Romberg test.
- **Shoulders and neck:** If the presence of a cervical injury has been ruled out, resisted range of motion testing of the cervical spine can be performed (see Box 11–1). Resisted shoulder shrugs are used to determine the integrity of CN XI.

Spinal Nerve Root Evaluation

A complete neurologic evaluation is required when brain or spinal trauma is suspected. A complete upper and lower quarter neurologic screen is necessary to test for normal sensory, motor, and reflex functions (see Chapter 1). The neurologic tests to be performed while the athlete is still down are less nerve root-specific and are explained in the "On-Field Management of Head and Neck Injuries" section of this chapter.

 ## HEAD AND NECK PATHOLOGIES AND RELATED SPECIAL TESTS

Organized football has a fatality rate of three deaths per 100,000 participants. The majority of these fatalities are attributed to head or cervical spine trauma.[22] However, head and neck trauma can—and does—occur in sports other than football. Therefore, emergency preparedness is not limited to the sport of football but, rather, should encompass all of an institution's or organization's athletic programs.

The ability to correctly identify and manage athletes with these conditions in a timely, safe, and efficient manner is a determining factor related to the successful management of a potentially catastrophic injury. Prudent decision making is necessary to determine the athlete's status and disposition. More so than any other type of injury described in this text, a consistent standardized plan of action must be implemented immediately in the management of these conditions.

HEAD TRAUMA

Protective headgear has greatly reduced the number and severity of brain injuries in sports mandating their use. The incidence of skull fractures and skin lacerations in areas directly protected by the helmet has been virtually eliminated. The symptoms of head injuries may increase with time, so even athletes who have been released in apparently good health after a head injury need to be given information about signs and symptoms of head injuries. These instructions should also be communicated to the athlete's parents, roommate, or spouse (see "Home Instructions").

Concussion

A cerebral concussion, a clinical syndrome of traumatic brain injury (also referred to as mild brain injury), is characterized by immediate but transient posttraumatic impairment of brain function.[23] Mental confusion, alteration of mental status, and amnesia are the hallmarks of concussion symptoms that may or may not also include the loss of consciousness.[24,25] Some brain cells are destroyed as a direct result of the concussive force, and other cells are placed at risk of further trauma secondary to changes in cerebral blood flow, increased intracranial pressure, and apnea.[26] After the trauma, a paradoxical period occurs that involves an increased demand for glucose to fuel cell metabolism along with a decrease in the blood flow needed to deliver these nutrients.[26] During this time, the risk for further brain trauma increases if the athlete is allowed to return to competition and suffers another head injury.[12]

Repeated head trauma may produce cumulative degenerative effects on brain function. Athletes with a history of multiple concussions can display the signs and symptoms of a current concussion in the absence of a recent history of head trauma.[27] Additionally, a concussion may produce lingering effects, be magnified by subsequent concussions, or mask underlying brain trauma.

No anatomic or physiologic findings exist on which to base a diagnosis of a concussion or determine its severity. The diagnosis of a concussion is based on the duration of the loss of consciousness (if any) and neuropsychological findings.[26] In the absence of a loss of consciousness, the immediate signs of a concussion are behavioral in nature (Table 18–5).[24] Approximately 85 to 90 percent of slight to mild concussions are not reported until after the practice or game.[15] Other symptoms associated with concussions include dizziness, tinnitus, nausea, memory loss, and motor impairment, with the symptoms occurring along a continuum ranging from no disruption to total disruption (Table 18–6). Severe cases may also be marked by convulsions, vomiting, and loss of bowel and bladder control (Table 18–7). Delayed symptoms may include personality changes, fatigue, sleep disturbances, lethargy, depression, and difficulty performing activities of daily living.[26] Magnetic resonance imaging (MRI) may be used to identify other forms of traumatic brain injury, and computed tomography (CT) scans may be used to image intracranial bleeding or swelling.[24,26]

Table 18–5
BEHAVIORAL SIGNS AND SYMPTOMS OF CONCUSSION

Sign	Behavior
Vacant stare	Confused or blank facial expression
Delayed verbal and motor responses	Slow to answer questions or follow instructions
Inability to focus attention	Easily distracted; unable to complete normal activities
Disorientation	Walking in the wrong direction; time, date, and place disorientation
Slurred or incoherent speech	Rambling, disjointed, incomprehensible statements
Gross incoordination	Stumbling; inability to walk a straight line
Heightened emotions	Appearing distraught, crying for no apparent reason, emotional responses that are out of proportion to the circumstances
Memory deficits	As evidenced by the retrograde and anterograde memory tests

The **Standardized Assessment of Concussion Instrument (SAC)** has been developed specifically for athletes (Box 18–7).[24,26,28] The SAC protocol is a useful adjunct to neuropsychological and balance testing, but does not replace formal neurologic testing or medical evaluation.

The magnitude of severely brain injured individuals can be quantified using the **Glasgow coma scale** (Table 18–8). The normal score on this battery is 15. Patients scoring 11 or higher on this instrument have an excellent prognosis for recovery. Scores of 7 or less represent serious brain dysfunction.

Concussion Rating Systems

Several different rating scales are used to quantify the severity of concussions. Table 18–9 presents four of the commonly used classification systems for athletic-related head trauma.[29–32] There is disparity among these systems, with different emphases on loss of consciousness and postconcussion symptoms. In one system, an athlete may be classified as having a grade III concussion, yet in another system this same person may only have a grade I concussion.[15] Likewise, the systems are considered to be overly conservative for the athletic population.[15]

These systems are presented as a framework of the different classification schemes that are used with an athletic population. Institutions should use these systems as the basis for their own standard operating procedures. To determine the extent of the injury, the findings of a cerebral concussion evaluation should be compared with the dysfunction guide in Table 18–6.

Table 18–6
DYSFUNCTION GUIDE FOR EVALUATING THE EXTENT OF CEREBRAL CONCUSSIONS

Function	Slight	Severe	Comments
Consciousness	No loss of consciousness	Unconscious for 10 seconds to 1 minute or altered consciousness for less than 2 minutes	Institutional standard operating procedures should identify the minimum duration of unconsciousness required to activate emergency medical services.
Memory	The patient is initially unable to remember the immediate events leading to the trauma	**Retrograde amnesia:** Inability to remember events before the mechanism of injury **Anterograde amnesia:** Inability to remember events after the injury	Transitory loss of memory of the injurious contact is to be expected and often associated with a brief loss of consciousness ("seeing stars" or "blacking out").
Cognitive function	Slight transient mental confusion ("What happened?")	Disorientation to person, place or time Demonstration of violent, aggressive, and otherwise inappropriate behavior or language Inability to process information "normally"	These traits may be expected immediately after the injury. Their continued presence is correlated with the severity of the injury.
Balance and coordination	Slight unsteadiness or unsteadiness that rapidly subsides	Profound disruption of balance and coordination; inability to walk without assistance and difficulty performing basic manual skills	These functions are based not only on the results of Romberg's test and the heel–toe walk but also on general observation.
Tinnitus	None or transitory	Prolonged tinnitus or tinnitus worsening over time	Ringing in the ears may be described immediately after the blow but should subside with time.
Pupil size	Equal; both pupils responsive to light	Dilated pupil that is unresponsive to light	Pupillary change indicates increased intracranial pressure on CN III. Unequal pupil size (anisocoria) may be normally present.
Nystagmus	Absent	Present	Nystagmus indicates increased intracranial pressure or inner ear dysfunction. This may be a normal finding.
Vision	Normal or initially blurred, which quickly subsides	Persistent blurred or double vision	The athlete's normal vision should be taken into account (i.e., if the athlete wears glasses).
Nausea	None or slight	Vomiting	Cumulative effect
Pulse	Within normal limits, possible decreasing with rest	Abnormally increasing or decreasing	Abnormal changes in pulse indicate intracranial hemorrhage.
Blood pressure	Within normal limits	Rapidly rising or falling	Rapid blood pressure changes suggest intracranial hematoma.
Respirations	Normal	Abnormal	See "Functional Testing" section of this chapter.

CN = cranial nerve.

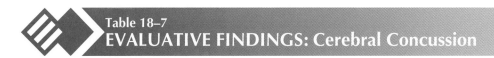

Table 18–7
EVALUATIVE FINDINGS: Cerebral Concussion

Examination Segment	Clinical Findings	
History	*Onset:*	Acute
	Chief complaints:	Headache, ringing in the ears, blurred vision, dizziness, unconsciousness (see Tables 18–2 and 18–4)
	Mechanism:	Blow to the skull or spinal column transmitting an injurious force to the brain
	Predisposing conditions:	A recent history of a cerebral concussion or a past history of repeated subconcussive forces to the head
Inspection	*Eyes:*	Generally may appear glazed or dazed
		Pupil sizes should be equal; a unilaterally dilated pupil may indicate pressure on CN III.
		Nystagmus may indicate pressure on the CNs or dysfunction within the inner ear.
	Nose and ears:	Fluid draining from the nose and ears is checked for the presence of CSF.
	General:	Severe concussions may result in convulsions.
		The entire skull requires inspection for secondary bleeding or contusions. The area over the mastoid process and the area beneath the eyes are checked for ecchymosis, indicating a skull fracture.
Palpation	If the athlete was not wearing a helmet at the time of injury, palpate the skull to determine areas of point tenderness, possibly indicating the presence of a skull fracture.	
Functional Tests	*Memory:*	Transient retrograde amnesia of the events leading up to the injury is possible. An increased scope of memory loss may indicate a severe concussion. The presence of anterograde amnesia warrants the immediate referral to a physician.
	Cognitive function:	The patient may display confused, violent, or aggressive behavior and may have diminished analytical function.
	Balance and coordination:	These functions are diminished immediately after the injury but should return rapidly.
	Eyes:	Blurred vision and unequal pupil size are present.
	Motor function:	Partial and transitory motor loss may occur secondary to trauma to the motor and premotor cortexes.
Ligamentous Tests	Not applicable	
Neurologic Tests	CN assessment, sensory testing, motor testing	
Special Tests	Monitor pulse, blood pressure, and respiration.	
	Retrograde amnesia test and anterograde amnesia test repeated at regular intervals.	
	Balance Error Scoring System	
	Romberg's test and heel–toe walk (balance and coordination)	
	Cerebral function tests (e.g., 100 minus 7)	
	Standardized Assessment of Concussion grade	
	Glasgow coma scale (used with profoundly head-injured patients)	
	Halo test	
Comments	The possibility of a cervical spine fracture must be assumed until such an injury can be ruled out.	
	When the severity of the injury is in doubt, refer the patient to a physician for further evaluation. Athletes who are unconscious for a measurable period of time must be cleared by a physician before returning to competition.	
	An athlete with a history of multiple head trauma or having symptoms after little or no physical trauma should always be referred for further assessment by a physician (see "Postconcussion Syndrome and Second Impact Syndrome" section).	

CN = cranial nerve; CSF = cerebrospinal fluid.

Box 18–7
STANDARDIZED ASSESSMENT OF CONCUSSION TOOL

Orientation (1 point each)

	Correct
Month	☐
Date	☐
Day of week	☐
Year	☐
Time (within 1 hr)	☐
Score	___ /5

Delayed Recall (1 point each)

	Correct
Word 1	☐
Word 2	☐
Word 3	☐
Word 4	☐
Word 5	☐
Score	___ /5

Immediate Memory (1 point for each correct response)

	Trial 1	Trial 2	Trial 3
Word 1	☐	☐	☐
Word 2	☐	☐	☐
Word 3	☐	☐	☐
Word 4	☐	☐	☐
Word 5	☐	☐	☐
Score			___ /15

Summary of total scores

Orientation	___ /5
Immediate memory	___ /15
Concentration	___ /5
Delayed recall	___ /5
TOTAL SCORE	___ /30

Concentration

Reverse digits (1 point each for each string length)

		Correct
3–8–2	5–1–8	☐
2–7–9–3	2–1–6–8	☐
5–1–8–6–9	9–4–1–7–5	☐
6–9–7–3–5–1	4–2–8–9–3–7	☐

Months of the year in reverse order (1 point for entire sequence correct)

	Correct
Dec–Nov–Oct–Sep–Aug–Jul	
Jun–May–Apr–Mar–Feb–Jan	☐
Score	___ /5

The following are performed between the Immediate Memory and Delayed Recall portions of the SAC, along with tests for memory, cerebral function, and strength.

Neurologic Screening

  Recollection of the injury

  Strength:

  Sensation:

  Coordination

Exertional Maneuvers (when appropriate)

  1 40-yard sprint

  5 sit-ups

  5 push-ups

  5 knee bends

Procedures (Administration time is approximately 5 minutes): Proper training is required for appropriate use.

Orientation	Patient is asked to identify the current place in time and receives 1 point for each correct response.
Immediate memory	The patient is asked to memorize a list of 5 random words. The list of words is repeated 3 times in succession, with 1 point being awarded for each correct response for a maximum total of 15 points. This list of words will be used for the delayed memory testing, but do not inform the patient as such.
Neurologic screening	The patient is evaluated for loss of consciousness, amnesia, etc.
Concentration	**Reverse digits:** The patient is given a sequence of numbers and asked to repeat them in reverse order (i.e., 2–8–3 would be recited as 3–8–2). If the patient correctly responds on the first attempt, progress to the next string length. If the patient incorrectly responds on the first attempt, use a second set of digits for the second attempt. If the patient incorrectly responds on the second attempt, move on to months of the year. **Months of year:** The patient is asked to recite the months of the year in reverse order.
Delayed recall	Approximately 5 minutes following the "Immediate Memory" test, the patient is asked to recall the list of words that were used for the immediate memory test. One point is awarded for each correct response.
Total	The scores for each of the four sections are totaled to yield an overall index of impairment.

Table 18–8
THE GLASGOW COMA SCALE

Response	Points	Action
Eye opening		
Spontaneously	4	Reticular system is intact; patient may not be aware
To verbal command	3	Opens eyes when told to do so
To pain	2	Opens eyes in response to pain
None	1	Does not open eyes to any stimuli
Verbal		
Oriented, converses	5	Relatively intact CNS; aware of self and surroundings
Disoriented, converses	4	Well articulated, organized, but disoriented
Inappropriate words	3	Random, exclamatory words
Incomprehensible	2	No recognizable words
No response	1	No audible sounds or intubated
Motor		
Obeys verbal commands	6	Readily moves limbs when told to
Localizes painful stimuli	5	Moves limb in an effort to avoid pain
Flexion withdrawal	4	Pulls away from pain with a flexion motion
Abnormal flexion	3	Exhibits decorticate rigidity
Extension	2	Exhibits decerebrate rigidity
No response	1	Demonstrates dypotonicity, flaccid: Suggests loss of medullary function or spinal cord injury

CNS = central nervous system.

Table 18–9
CONCUSSION RATING SYSTEMS

Rating System	Signs and Symptoms		
	Grade I	**Grade II**	**Grade III**
American Academy of Neurology[29]	No loss of consciousness Transient confusion Concussion symptoms resolve in **less than 15 minutes**	No loss of consciousness Transient confusion Concussion symptoms or mental status abnormalities on examination resolve in **more than 15 minutes**	Any loss of consciousness either brief (seconds) or prolonged (minutes).
American College of Sports Medicine Guidelines[30]	None or transient retrograde amnesia None to slight mental confusion No loss of coordination Transient dizziness Rapid recovery	Retrograde amnesia; memory may return slight to moderate mental confusion Moderate dizziness Transitory tinnitus Slow recovery	Sustained retrograde amnesia; anterograde is possible with intracranial hemorrhage Severe mental confusion Profound loss of coordination Obvious motor impairment Prolonged tinnitus Delayed recovery
Cantu Concussion Rating Guidelines[31]	No loss of consciousness Concussion symptoms resolving in less than 15 minutes Posttraumatic amnesia for less than 30 minutes	Loss of consciousness for less than 5 minutes Posttraumatic amnesia for more than 30 minutes but less than 24 hours	Loss of consciousness for more than 5 minutes Posttraumatic amnesia for more than 24 hours
Colorado Medical Society Concussion Rating Guidelines[32]	No loss of consciousness Transient confusion No amnesia	No loss of consciousness Transient confusion Amnesia	Loss of consciousness

Return-to-Play Criteria

Determining the time for the safe return to play after a head injury is a major concern of medical personnel. Some severe head injuries may not produce significant signs or symptoms for some time after the actual trauma. This fact alone suggests that it is better to err on the side of caution when making return-to-play decisions. The National Collegiate Athletic Association's *Sports Medicine Handbook* states that athletes who have been rendered unconscious for any period of time should not be returned to activity that day and should not return to activity while displaying postconcussion symptoms.[33]

An athlete who sustains a mild concussion may be allowed to return to participation after all the signs and symptoms have cleared. Athletes sustaining a moderate or severe concussion should not return to competition for several days, weeks, or months after the injury. Table 18–10 presents the recommended time to return to competition after cerebral concussions, assuming that all of the athlete's symptoms have cleared.[34]

External provocation tests can be used to determine if exercise will cause the symptoms to return.[29] The athlete performs exercises (e.g., a 40-yd sprints, 5 push-ups, 5 sit-ups) and is then evaluated for the presence or reoccurrence of concussion symptoms. The athlete should be withheld from competition if symptoms are present or if he or she is unable to complete the exercises.

Returning an athlete who has sustained a head injury to competition is ultimately a physician's decision. Prematurely returning an athlete to competition can increase the effects of postconcussion syndrome, increase the risk of subsequent concussions, and predispose the individual to second impact syndrome.[6] There is uni-versal agreement, however, that the athlete should not be returned to practice or competition while experiencing any concussion symptoms or be returned to competition on the same day in which consciousness was lost. After a grade I or grade II concussion, the athlete should be returned to activity under controlled conditions, progressively working toward unrestricted participation.[15]

Postconcussion Syndrome

Athletes suffering a cerebral concussion may describe a number of cognitive impairments for some time after the injury.[34] The extended duration of these symptoms is thought to be related to altered neurotransmitter function.[35] Postconcussion syndrome occurs more frequently in women than in men.

Postconcussion syndrome is characterized by decreased attention span, trouble concentrating, impaired memory, and irritability over both the short- and long-term (Table 18–11).[36] Exercise may cause headaches, dizziness, and premature fatigue.[35] Long-term consequences of postconcussion syndrome are balance disruptions and decreased cognitive performance.[37] These symptoms predispose the individual to second impact syndrome and may require that the patient be further evaluated by a neurosurgeon. The athlete should not be returned to competition until postconcussion syndromes have ceased. CT scans and neuropsychologic tests must show negative findings.

Second Impact Syndrome

A rare but possible consequence of returning an athlete to competition too soon after a concussion is an in-

Table 18–10
GUIDELINES FOR RETURNING TO PLAY AFTER A CEREBRAL CONCUSSION

Grade	1st Concussion	2nd Concussion	3rd Concussion
Grade 1 (mild)	May return to play if asymptomatic	Return to play in 2 wk if the athlete is asymptomatic during the previous week	Terminate season; may return to play the following season if asymptomatic
Grade 2 (moderate)	Return to play after being asymptomatic for 1 wk	Out a minimum of 1 mo; may return to play then if asymptomatic for 1 wk; consider terminating season	Terminate season; may return to play the following season if asymptomatic
Grade 3 (severe)	Out a minimum of 1 mo; may then return to play if asymptomatic for 1 wk	Terminate season; may return to play the following season if asymptomatic Consider terminating career	Terminate career in contact sports

Table 18–11
EARLY AND LATE SIGNS AND SYMPTOMS OF POSTCONCUSSION SYNDROME

Early	Late
Disorientation	Lack of concentration
Confusion	Poor memory
Headache	Irritability
Dizziness	Depression
Blurred vision	Anxiety
Nausea	Fatigue
Drowsiness	Headache
Sleep disturbance	Sleep disturbance

creased risk of second impact syndrome, the result of a second concussion's occurring while the individual is still symptomatic from an earlier concussion.[24] The second trauma, often a minor blow or contrecoup mechanism, increases cerebrovascular congestion, or a loss of cerbrovascular autoregulation, leading to brain edema and increased intracranial pressure.[24,38]

The second trauma is thought to disrupt the autoregulation of the brain's blood supply, resulting in vasodilation and the subsequent engorgement of the intracranial vasculature.[39] The increased blood flow and vascular expanse increase the intracranial pressure and quickly disrupt the brain stem's normal function. Outward signs of spinal and cranial nerve involvement occur within 2 minutes of the trauma.

Initially the athlete may display the signs and symptoms of a grade I concussion but quickly collapses in a semicomatose state. Pressure on the cranial nerves results in rapidly dilating pupils that are unresponsive to light and the loss of eye motion.[35] As the pressure continues to build, the athlete displays signs of respiratory distress secondary to disruption of phrenic nerve activity.

Intervention must be swift and concise. The physician, paramedic, or other qualified personnel should intubate the athlete and may induce hyperventilation to facilitate vasoconstriction secondary to decreased carbon dioxide in the bloodstream. Even in the best-case scenarios, second impact syndrome has a 50 percent mortality rate.[38] This severity emphasizes the importance of preventing this occurrence by prohibiting athletes from returning to athletic competition until all symptoms of a cerebral concussion have subsided and a physician has cleared the athlete's return to activity.

Intracranial Hematoma

Rupture of the blood vessels supplying the brain results in an intracranial hematoma, named relative to the meninges (Fig. 18–13). Intracranial hematoma may also develop after disruption of the sinus separating the two brain hemispheres. Subsequent hematoma formation within the enclosed space (the cranium) places pressure on the brain and may have catastrophic re-

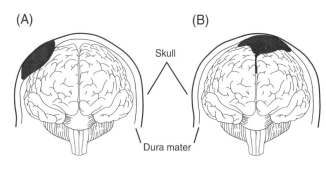

FIGURE 18–13. Intracranial hemorrhage. **(A)** Epidural hematoma, arterial bleeding between the skull and dura mater. **(B)** Subdural hematoma, venous bleeding between the dura mater and brain. The meningeal spaces have been enlarged for clarity.

sults (see Table 18–2). The length of time until the onset of symptoms varies, depending on the type of bleeding involved (arterial or venous) and the location relative to the dura mater (above or below it).

Epidural Hematoma

Arterial bleeding between the dura mater and the skull results in the rapid formation of an epidural hematoma, with the onset of symptoms occurring within hours after the initial injury. The mechanism of this injury is that of a concussion, a blow to the head that jars the brain. Because of the concussive mechanism, the athlete may be briefly unconscious and may show the signs and symptoms of mild concussion, although these are not prerequisite symptoms. These symptoms quickly subside, and the athlete progresses through a very *lucid* period (Table 18–12).

Table 18–12
PROGRESSON OF SYMPTOMS ASSOCIATED WITH AN EPIDURAL HEMATOMA

- Patient is unconscious or has other signs of a concussion (these are not prerequisite findings).
- The patient has a period of very lucid consciousness, perhaps eliminating the suspicion of a serious concussion.
- Patient appears to become disoriented, confused, and drowsy.
- Complaints of a headache that increase in intensity with time.
- Signs and signals of cranial nerve disruption.
- Onset of coma.
- If untreated, death or permanent brain damage occurs.

Lucid   Mentally clear.

As the size of the hematoma increases, the athlete's condition deteriorates at a rate proportional to the amount of intracranial bleeding. The individual becomes disoriented, displays abnormal behavior, and complains of or displays drowsiness. A headache of increasing intensity may be reported, indicating pressure on the periosteum of the skull or an insult to the dura mater. Continued expansion of the hematoma results in outward symptoms via the cranial nerves; a unilaterally dilated pupil is the most common sign.

Subdural Hematoma

Hematoma formation between the brain and dura mater usually involves venous bleeding. This type of injury accounts for the majority of deaths resulting from athletic-related head trauma.[40] Because venous bleeding occurs at a lower pressure than arterial bleeding and because the blood collects within the fissures and sulci, the symptoms occur hours, days, or even weeks after the initial trauma. Whereas acute subdural hematomas become symptomatic within 48 hours, chronic hematomas may not manifest symptoms until 30 days after the trauma.[41]

Subdural hematomas may be classified as simple or complex. No direct cerebral damage is associated with a simple subdural hematoma. Complex subdural hematomas are characterized by contusions of the brain's surface and associated cerebral swelling.

Initially after the injury, the individual is very lucid, even to the point of not displaying any of the signs or symptoms of a cerebral concussion. However, as blood accumulates within the brain, the patient begins to develop headaches, accompanied by a clouding of consciousness. Further hematoma formation results in the impairment of cognitive, behavioral, and motor ability, and signs of cranial nerve dysfunction may be observed. The potentially long duration between the trauma and the onset of symptoms illustrates the need for home instructions identifying the latent signs and symptoms of head injuries.

Skull Fractures

The prevalence of skull fractures is much higher in athletes who are not wearing headgear than in those who are. However, skull fractures can still occur in a head that is protected, especially in the bones around the helmet's periphery. Skull fractures are typically classified as **linear, comminuted,** or **depressed** (Fig. 18–14).

Linear fractures, referred to as hairline fractures in long bones, are caused by a blunt impact to the cranium. The subsequent swelling causes the loss of the skull's rounded contour in the traumatized area. Comminuted skull fractures result in the skull's fragmenting. A slight depression is felt during gentle palpation of the fractured area. If the blunt force is of enough intensity or fails to become deflected by the round shape of the skull, a depressed fracture can occur. The skull's indentation is obvious on gross inspection. Additional concern is focused around the possibility of the fractured pieces of bone's lacerating the meninges and brain.

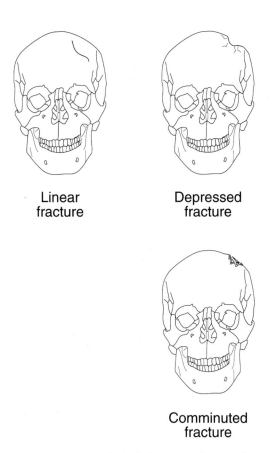

Linear fracture

Depressed fracture

Comminuted fracture

FIGURE 18–14. Types of skull fractures: linear, depressed, and comminuted.

Although depressed skull fractures are often obvious during inspection, linear and comminuted fractures are less evident. The traumatic impact often results in a laceration of the overlying skin. Although the bleeding must be controlled, no material or object should be inserted into the laceration or possible fracture site. Fractures of the ethmoid or temporal bones may result in the leakage of CSF from the nose or ears or in bleeding from the ears (see Box 18–1). With time, ecchymosis may accumulate beneath the eyes and over the mastoid process (Battle's sign) (Table 18–13). In addition to these symptoms, the patient may also describe the signs and symptoms of a concussion caused by the blow to the skull.

CERVICAL SPINAL CORD TRAUMA

The advent of protective football helmets made the use of the head an attractive weapon for blockers, tacklers, and ball carriers. The resulting axial load on the cervical spine caused a high rate of cervical fractures and dislocations, many producing catastrophic results. During the 1976 season, the National Collegiate Athletic Association (NCAA) and the National Federation of State High School Associations (NFHSA) adopted rules outlawing contact with opposing players using the top (crown) of the helmet, a rule change that drastically reduced the incidence of cervical injury in football play-

Table 18–13
EVALUATIVE FINDINGS: Skull Fracture

Examination Segment	Clinical Findings	
History	**Onset:**	Acute
	Pain characteristics:	Pain over the point of impact; a headache may be described secondary to the trauma
	Mechanism:	Blunt trauma to the head; either the skull's being struck by a moving object or the skull's striking a stationary object
Inspection	Bleeding may occur secondary to the blow. Ecchymosis under the eyes ("raccoon eyes") and over the mastoid process (Battle's sign) may be noted. The rounded contour of the skull over the impacted area may be lost.	
Palpation	Crepitus may be felt over the fracture site. Palpation should not be performed over areas of obvious fracture.	
Functional Tests	Not applicable	
Ligamentous Tests	Not applicable	
Neurologic Tests	Same as for evaluation of a cerebral concussion: Cranial nerve assessment, sensory testing, and motor testing	
Special Tests	Not applicable	
Comments	The presence of a cervical fracture or dislocation must be ruled out. No object should be inserted into the site of a skull laceration. A cerebral concussion may also be associated with this injury. Athletes suspected of suffering from a skull fracture should be immediately referred to a physician.	

ers.[7] Despite this ruling, reviews of game films estimate that spearing still occurs in 19 percent of football plays, most of which go unpenalized.[11]

Spinal cord function is inhibited by one of two mechanisms: (1) impingement or laceration secondary to bony displacement and (2) compression secondary to hemorrhage, edema, and ischemia of the cord.[42] Although the effects of pressure placed on the spinal cord, with no death of its cells, are often transitory and reversible, actual trauma to the spinal cord itself is rarely reversible and results in permanent disability.

Not all athletes suffering from bony cervical trauma remain on the field. In fact, an athlete who has suffered a cervical fracture or dislocation may walk off under his or her own power. With this in mind, any complaints of pain in the cervical spine, with or without symptoms radiating into the extremities, should always be thought of as a catastrophic injury until otherwise ruled out. Torg[43] has categorized risk groups, based on underlying trauma, as to their conditions predisposing the athlete to further cervical trauma (Table 18–14).

Jefferson's fracture   A fracture of a circular bone in two places; similar to breaking a doughnut in half.

Table 18–14
RISK FACTORS OF PREDISPOSING CONDITIONS RESULTING IN PERMANENT DISABILITY

Minimal Risk	Moderate Risk	Extreme Risk
Asymptomatic bone spurs	Acute lateral disk herniation	Acute large central disk herniation
Brachial plexus neurapraxia	Cervical radiculopathy–radial spur	Cervical cord anomaly
Certain healed facet fractures	Facet fractures	Occipitocervical dislocation
Healed disk herniation	Lateral mass fractures	Odontoid fracture
Healed lamina fracture	Nondisplaced healed ring of C1 fracture	Ruptured C1–C2 transverse ligament
Healed spinous process fracture	Nondisplaced odontoid fractures	Stenosis of the cervical canal
		Total ligamentous disruption of the lower cervical spine
		Unstable fracture or dislocation
		Unstable **Jefferson's fracture**

Trauma to the spinal cord above the C4 level has a high probability of death secondary to disruption of the function of the brain stem or the phrenic nerve. Trauma to the spinal cord anywhere along its length can result in the permanent loss of function of the nerves distal to the traumatized area.

The anatomy of the cervical spine is covered in Chapter 11. Before proceeding with this portion of the chapter, readers should take a moment to refresh their memory as to the important structures and anatomical relationships of this body area. Likewise, Chapter 11 also discusses injuries to the brachial plexus.

Cervical Fracture or Dislocation

The signs and symptoms of a cervical fracture and those of a dislocation are quite similar. Often these two conditions occur concurrently (Fig. 18–15). Cervical fractures alone do not cause spinal cord trauma. Rather, spinal cord trauma secondary to vertebral fractures results when a bony fragment lacerates the cord; swelling compresses the cord; ischemia affects the cord's cells; or the vertebra shifts, narrowing the spinal canal.

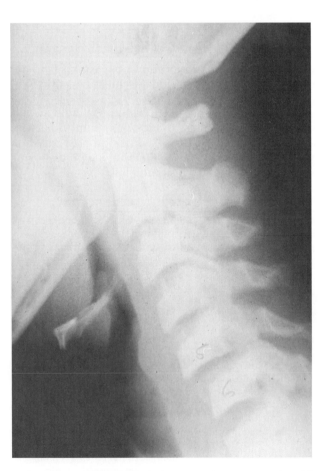

FIGURE 18–15. Fracture-dislocation of the C6 vertebra. Note the posterior displacement of the vertebral body relative to C5 and the fracture of the C6 spinous process.

Cervical dislocations represent a much more serious direct threat to the spinal cord. Most often affecting the lower cervical vertebrae (C4 to C6) when the neck is forced into flexion and rotation, the superior articular facet passes over the inferior facet. The resulting dislocation decreases the diameter of the spinal canal, often compressing the cord.

The signs and symptoms of a stretch or pinch of the brachial plexus can mimic many of those of a spinal cord injury. The primary differences are found in the relatively rapid fading of symptoms associated with brachial plexus trauma and the fact that the symptoms most often occur unilaterally.

Trauma to the cervical spine itself is identified by pain along its posterior and lateral structures and possible spasm of the surrounding muscles. If there is associated damage to the spinal cord or if displaced bone or swelling is compressing the cord, symptoms are manifested in the involved nerve distributions and in those nerves located distal to the site of the insult. Typically, these symptoms involve pain, burning, or numbness radiating into the extremities (Table 18–15). Fractures of the vertebral body may produce little or no symptoms unless the cervical spine and head are positioned in a manner that places a load on the involved body.[45]

Other than the actual physical trauma, the spinal cord tissue is further damaged by ischemia. Pharmacologically, the use of ganglioside (GM-1), methylprednisolone, and other medications has shown promise in limiting spinal cord trauma.[46,47] The strategy of medically increasing the patient's mean arterial blood pressure above 85 mm Hg has also been demonstrated to assist in reducing the long-term effects of spinal cord trauma.[48]

Transient Quadraplegia

Blows to the head that force the cervical spine into hyperextension, hyperflexion, or produce an axial load may result in transient quadriplegia, a body-wide state of decreased or absent sensory and motor function.[44,49–51] This results from neurapraxia of the cervical spinal cord and is predisposed by stenosis of the spinal foramen (especially at the C3-C4 level), congenital fusion of the cervical canal, abnormalities of the posterior arch, or cervical instability.[44] The risk of transient quadriplegia is increased when the ratio between the diameter of the spinal canal and the diameter of the vertebral body is 0.80 or less.[44,52] The narrowing of the spinal canal predisposes the spinal cord to compressive and contusive forces, a condition referred to as **spear tackler's spine.**[44]

Initially, the signs and symptoms of transient quadriplegia resemble those of a catastrophic cervical injury. Symptoms range from sensory dysfunction to burning pain, numbness, or paresthesia in the upper and lower extremities. Likewise, upper and lower extremity motor function is inhibited, ranging from muscular weakness to complete paralysis. However, these symp-

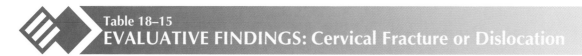

Table 18–15
EVALUATIVE FINDINGS: Cervical Fracture or Dislocation

Examination Segment	Clinical Findings	
History	*Onset:*	Acute
	Chief complaints:	Pain in the cervical spine
		Numbness, weakness, or paresthesia radiating into the extremities
		Cervical muscle spasm
		Chest pain
		Loss of bladder or bowel control
	Mechanism:	Fractures most commonly secondary to an axial load placed on the cervical vertebrae. Dislocations most commonly resulting from hyperflexion or hyperextension and rotation of the cervical spine.
	Predisposing conditions:	Increased risk of cervical fracture if the normal lordotic curve of the cervical spine is decreased.[44]
Inspection	Malalignment of the cervical spine may be observed.	
	The head may be abnormally tilted and rotated. Unilateral cervical dislocations result in the head's tilting toward the site of the dislocation. The muscles on the side opposite the dislocation (tilt) are in spasm. Those muscles on the side of the dislocation are flaccid.	
	Swelling may be present over the ligamentum nuchae.	
Palpation	Tenderness, crepitus, or swelling may be present over the cervical spine	
	Unilateral or bilateral muscle spasm may be present.	
Functional Tests	ROM testing should not be performed if numbness, weakness, or paresthesia radiating into the extremities or bowel and bladder signs are present.	
Ligamentous Tests	Not applicable	
Neurologic Tests	Upper quarter and lower quarter neurologic screens	
Special Tests	Not applicable in acute conditions in which a fracture or dislocation is suspected	
Comments	Athletes suspected of suffering a spinal cord injury should be immediately stabilized and transported	
	Trauma to the brain stem or phrenic nerve may result in cardiac arrest.	

ROM = range of motion.

toms clear within 15 minutes to 48 hours. Pain within the cervical spine is limited to burning paresthesia.[44]

The definitive diagnosis of transient quadriplegia is made through imaging and electrophysiologic testing. Radiographic examination is used to rule out fractures or congenital abnormalities of the cervical spine, and CT scans are used to gain a better definition of the cervical bony anatomy. The integrity of the spinal cord and its roots is determined through the use of MRI scans, *electromyelograms,* and nerve conduction velocity testing.

Return to Play Criteria

Athletes must not be returned to competition while neurologic symptoms including pain, motor weakness, paresthesia, or numbness are present. The cervical spine must demonstrate a pre-injury level of strength and range of motion. Clinical and radiographic examination should reveal no evidence of spinal stenosis, disc injury, or vertebral instability, and the cervical spine should have its normal lordotic curvature.

 ## ON-FIELD EVALUATION AND MANAGEMENT OF HEAD AND NECK INJURIES

The decisions made during a crisis situation are key to the proper management of head and neck trauma. It is the medical staff's responsibility to have a preplanned course of action that has been discussed and approved by the athletic training staff, physician, emergency medical service (EMS), and administration (Table 18–16).[53] Before the start of each season, these procedures must be reviewed by the involved parties, with each understanding not only his or her own roles but also those of the others. Furthermore, the techniques discussed in this text must be reviewed and rehearsed

Electromyelogram The recording of the electrical activity within a muscle.

Table 18–16
COMPONENTS OF AN EMERGENCY MEDICAL PLAN

Component	Considerations
Personnel	Athletic trainer Physician Emergency medical squad Emergency room personnel Institutional administrators
Communication	Members of the onsite medical team (athletic trainers and physicians) Emergency medical personnel Administrators and coaches
Equipment	Airway access (removal of facemask) Spinal stabilization Communication (walkie talkie, cellular phone, or location of nearest telephone) Compatibility of onsite equipment with the needs of the athletes Compatibility of onsite equipment with that of other medical personnel Location and accessibility of the emergency equipment

Facilities	Access for emergency vehicles and personnel
	Telephone location and accessibility
	Identification of the appropriate hospital because not all facilities are equipped
	   to handle advanced head trauma
	Determination of ground transportation or air lift
	Estimated time of arrival for the emergency medical squad and subsequent
	   transport time to the hospital

until each member is comfortable performing the techniques described. The procedures described in this section assume that more than one responder knowledgeable of the plan is present.

Because of the importance of not unnecessarily moving an athlete with a spinal injury and the potentially catastrophic ramifications of doing so, athletic trainers should conduct meetings with each team, instructing the athletes not to help injured players to their feet. In too many instances, these well-intentioned actions have resulted in an athlete's death or permanent paralysis.

This section assumes that the responder has a minimum of cardiopulmonary resuscitation (CPR) certification. The procedures discussed in this section are not intended to supersede formal CPR training.

EQUIPMENT CONSIDERATIONS

When, where, and how to remove a helmet after a spinal injury is a debatable issue.[54–58] The consensus opinion is the helmet should not be removed during the pre-hospital care of a patient with a spinal injury. The movement associated with removing the helmet places the spinal cord at too great of a risk for further injury, especially when the following are considered:

- The airway is still accessible by removing the face mask.[55]

- A cervical collar can be applied to the cervical spine while the helmet is still in place, although shoulder pads may make this difficult.

- The skull can be adequately secured to the spine board.

- Football helmets are radiographic translucent (Fig. 18–16); therefore, a definitive diagnosis can be made before removal.

- Removing the helmet without removing the shoulder pads results in the cervical spine's being placed in extension.[56]

In cases of improperly fitting helmets, the inability to remove the facemask, the inability to access the airway, or other extraordinary circumstances, the helmet and shoulder pads must be removed. These procedures are described in the following sections.

The strongest argument in support of removing the helmet and shoulder pads involves the necessity, or the potential necessity, of *defibrillating* the athlete.[56] Proper protocol for the use of a defibrillator requires that the athlete's chest be completely exposed and dry. The contact points for the defibrillator pads are over the apex of the heart and inferior to the right clavicle. If these pads were to come into contact with wet shoulder pads, the defibrillator's current could arc, an event that would not only decrease the defibrillator's effectiveness but could also defibrillate the operator. A standardized protocol for defibrillating athletes will be needed as the

Defibrillation (defibrillating) The process of restoring a normal heartbeat.

FIGURE 18–16. Radiograph of the cervical spine through a helmet. Note the metal snaps for the chin strap.

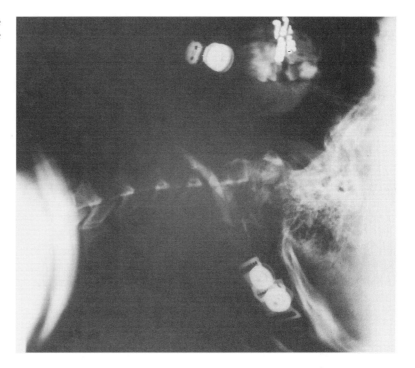

use of automated external defibrillators (AEDs) becomes more commonplace.

This section first discusses making the airway and chest accessible for CPR or the physical examination of these areas. Regardless of the athlete's condition, the helmet or shoulder pads must be removed at some point, whether on the field or in the hospital, and safely doing so is not an easy task. These techniques must be practiced and rehearsed before actually performing them on stricken athletes requiring assistance. Often it is necessary to assist hospital personnel with this procedure because they may be unfamiliar with the equipment.

Facemask Removal

An alternative to removing the athlete's helmet is to remove the facemask.[55] This device is commonly held in place by four plastic clips (Fig. 18–17). Unfastening the two lower clips allows the facemask to swing away from the athlete's face, making the mouth and nose accessible for assisted ventilation (Fig. 18–18). A scalpel, box opener, or other type of razor knife can be used to cut the clips, but this method carries with it the risk of cutting the athlete or the athletic trainer. Also, because the plastic hardens with age, older clips become harder to cut. Other methods of removing the facemask include unscrewing the bolts that attach the clips to the helmet or using a specifically designed cutting instrument.

Regardless of the method used to remove the facemask, this procedure requires two people. In-line stabilization of the head and neck must be maintained, and the cervical spine must be guarded against any movement that may occur during this process, especially avoiding hyperflexion of the cervical spine.

Chest Exposure

Auscultation of heart sounds and external cardiac compression during CPR require that the athlete's sternum be exposed. First the athlete's shirt is cut to expose the shoulder pads and, if the shirt is particularly tight fitting, it is cut along the anterior portion of the sleeves. Next, the clinician cuts or unfastens the rib straps on

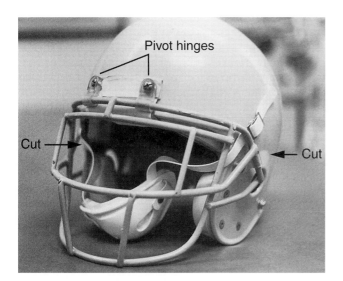

FIGURE 18–17. Clips attaching the facemask to the helmet. The lateral clips are cut, but the superior ones remain in place as pivot hinges for the facemask.

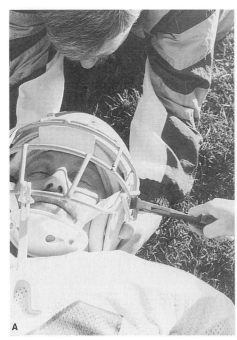

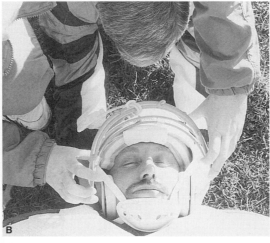

FIGURE 18–18. Cutting the clips attaching the facemask to the helmet and exposing the athlete's airway.

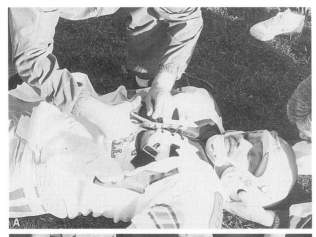

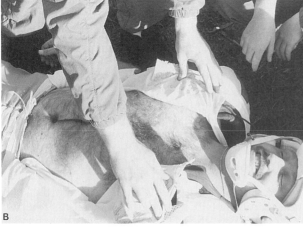

FIGURE 18–19. Exposing the athlete's sternum so that cardiopulmonary resuscitation can be performed. **(A)** The shirt and laces holding the shoulder pads together are cut. **(B)** The halves of the shoulder pads are spread.

the sternal portion of the pads and cuts the laces holding together the anterior portion of the pad. The halves are spread to expose the sternum (Fig. 18–19).

Helmet Removal

In cases necessitating the removal of the helmet, two people are necessary to perform the process in a manner that minimizes the amount of cervical spine motion (Fig. 18–20).[57] A semirigid collar can be fitted to the cervical spine before removing the helmet if the relationship of the helmet, shoulder pads, and surface provides sufficient room to do this with a minimum of movement; this may also require removing the shoulder pads (see the section on spine boarding the athlete).

While maintaining in-line stabilization, the other responder cuts the chin strap or straps. A flat instrument, such as the handle of a pair of scissors, is slid between the cheek pad and the helmet. A twist of this instrument causes the pad to unsnap and separate from the helmet. The pad is removed, and the procedure is repeated on the opposite side. The person who has been applying the in-line stabilization now slips a finger in each ear hole and spreads the helmet. As the helmet is slowly slid off the head, the second responder reaches behind the neck to support the cervical spine and provide a firm grip on the head.

Shoulder Pad Removal

The shoulder pads are removed only when the athlete's life is in jeopardy or such a state is imminent. This decision warrants that the immediate threat to the athlete's life outweigh the possibility of spinal cord injury that may result from moving the athlete. This decision should be made by a physician, if one is present. Other-

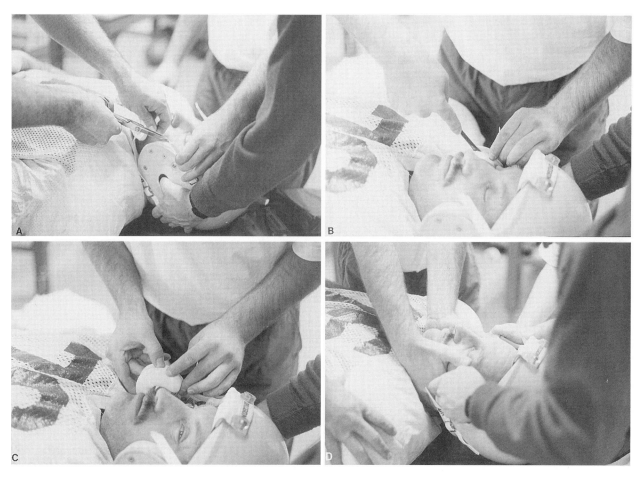

FIGURE 18–20. Removing a football helmet (the facemask has been fully removed for clarity). **(A)** In-line stabilization is maintained while the chin straps are cut. **(B)** Blunt object is used to unsnap the cheek guards. **(C)** Cheek guards are removed. **(D)** Secondary stabilization is applied to the cervical spine as the helmet is spread and slid off the athlete's head.

wise, the decision is made by the attending athletic trainer, emergency medical technician, or paramedic.

This procedure is most safely performed after the cervical spine has been stabilized by a hard or firm collar and the helmet removed. The responder begins this procedure by performing the steps described in the section on exposing the chest. After the anterior and axillary shoulder straps have been cut, the two halves of the shoulder pads may be widened. While one person continues to support the athlete's head, the shoulder pads are slid off the shoulders and over the head (Fig. 18–21).

INITIAL INSPECTION

The initial inspection encompasses contingencies that must be noted upon arrival at the accident scene. These factors provide clues to the severity of the injury and insight regarding the proper on-field management of the patient.

- **Encumbering circumstances:** Encumbering circumstances are factors that make the worst-case scenarios even more difficult to handle. Examples of these

include a diver who is still in the water, a football player who is lying on top of another player, or a hockey player whose head and neck are still against the boards.

- **Movement:** Any movement by the athlete must be noted. Unconscious athletes may be lying perfectly still or may have a seizure. Likewise, conscious athletes may lie still out of fear or grogginess.
- **Position:** Ideally, the athlete should be supine. Athletes who are sidelying or prone eventually must be rolled, but these initial assessments must be made before the decision to move the athlete is made.
- **Posture:** The alignment of the athlete's arms, legs, and cervical spine relative to the trunk is noted (Box 18–8). Splayed extremities must be aligned with the rest of the body if spine boarding or rolling the athlete is required. Male athletes who are suffering from a lesion of the spinal cord at the thoracic or cervical level may also demonstrate *priapism.*

Priapism   Spontaneous penile erection.

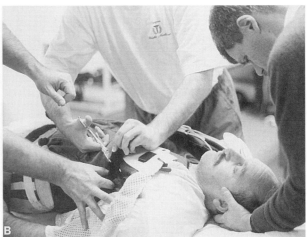

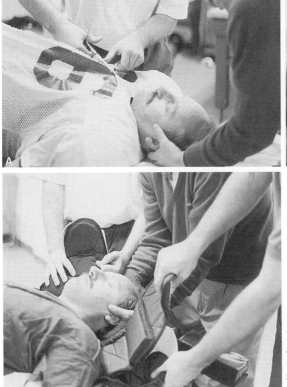

FIGURE 18–21. Removing the shoulder pads. **(A)** The athlete's shirt is cut along the middle of the sternum. **(B)** The axial straps are cut and the shoulder pad is spread. **(C)** The halves of the shoulder pads are slid from under the athlete. Note that in-line stabilization is maintained throughout this procedure.

INITIAL ACTION

After arriving at the scene, the responder's actions within the first 3 or 4 minutes strongly determine whether the athlete lives, dies, or becomes permanently disabled. Despite this urgency, the responder must not rush through these processes but must perform each with care and diligence.

- **Stabilize the cervical spine:** One responder must immediately assume control of the head by applying in-line stabilization. If the athlete is wearing a helmet, in-line stabilization is achieved by firmly grasping the sides of the helmet in the area of the ear holes and applying firm stabilization along the vertical axis of the cervical spine (Fig. 18–22). If the athlete is not wearing a helmet, stabilization is applied by grasping the skull beneath the occipital bone and mandible on each side, being careful not to alter the position of the spine and especially avoiding flexion.

  From this point until the situation resolves, either by the determination that no cervical spine injury exists or by the athlete's placement on a spine board, the person at the head maintains the in-line stabilization and directs the other individuals providing assistance. To protect the integrity of the spinal cord,

the motions of flexion and extension of the cervical spine must be avoided. Movement of the spinal column may result in a fragmented or displaced piece of bone's lacerating the spinal cord and causing death or permanent disability.

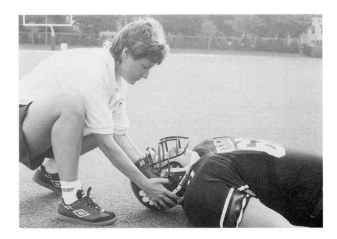

FIGURE 18–22. Applying in-line stabilization to the cervical spine.

Box 18–8
POSTURES ASSUMED AFTER SPINAL CORD INJURY

Decerebrate posture

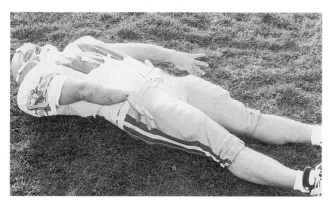

Posture
Extension of the extremities and retraction of the head

Pathology
Lesion of the brain stem; also possible secondary to heat stroke

Decorticate posture

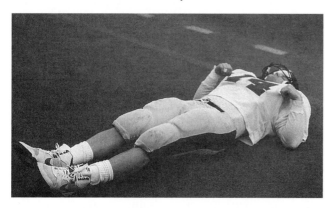

Posture
Flexion of the elbows and wrists, clenched fists, and extension of the lower extremity

Pathology
Lesion above the brain stem

Flexion Contracture

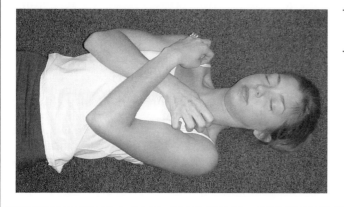

Posture
Arms flexed across the chest

Pathology
Spinal cord lesion at the C5–C6 level

- **Clear airway:** Remove the athlete's mouthpiece. Additionally, inspect the mouth for other objects that may become lodged in the athlete's airway.
- **Determine the level of consciousness:** In cases in which the athlete is not obviously responsive, the level of consciousness can be determined by calling the athlete's name and asking, "CAN YOU HEAR ME?" If this verbal stimulus fails to evoke a motor response, the athlete's response to a painful stimulus can be determined by applying pressure to the bed of a fingernail (see Fig. 18–5). Failure to evoke a response through either of these methods indicates that the athlete is unconscious. At this time, the athlete's ABCs should be reevaluated.
- **Inspect ears and nose:** Inspect the nose and ears for the presence of CSF, as described in the "Inspection" section of this chapter and in Chapter 17.
- **Secondary screen:** The torso and extremities are observed for any signs of additional trauma such as a fracture, joint dislocation, or bleeding. Of these pathologies, controlling bleeding takes the highest priority because of the need to preserve the athlete's blood pressure.

Management of the Unconscious Athlete

Figure 18–23 presents a flowchart describing the management of an unconscious athlete. Sustained unconsciousness (based on the institution's standard operating procedures) warrants the activation of the emergency medical system. If the athlete regains consciousness, follow the procedures described in the "Management of the Conscious Athlete" section. The athlete's cervical spine continues to be stabilized using in-line stabilization during these procedures.

- **Airway:** Permanent brain damage can occur within 4 minutes after oxygen deprivation. Establish that the athlete has an open airway by looking, listening, and feeling for breaths (see Fig. 18–6). Occlusion of the airway can occur secondary to intrinsic blockage (crushing or swelling of the larynx or trachea), extrinsic blockage (external hematoma), foreign body blockage (mouthpiece, gum), or central blockage (flaccid tongue) of the airway.[59] Foreign bodies must be manually dislodged from the athlete's airway; tongue forceps can be used for this purpose or to grasp the tongue and remove it from the airway. Complete obstruction of the airway owing to intrinsic and extrinsic blockage may require an emergency *tracheotomy*, a technique that must be performed only by trained personnel.
- **Breathing:** Breathing is determined by looking, listening, and feeling for signs of breathing. The absence of breathing or a respiratory rate of fewer than 10 or greater than 30 breaths per minute requires assisted ventilation:
- **Emergency roll:** Emergency rolls differ from standard spine boarding techniques and are used only in cases in which the athlete does not have a pulse or is not breathing. Bystanders must be recruited to quickly roll the athlete to the supine position, foregoing the immediate use of a spine board. Although this is done rapidly, in-line stabilization must be maintained with continued stabilization of the cervical spine. At this time, the chest must be exposed so that proper chest compressions may be performed on the sternum.

  - **Removal of the facemask:** The facemask is removed to access the athlete's mouth and nose.
  - **Jaw thrust:** A jaw thrust maneuver to open the airway is used rather than the head-tilt method.
  - **Ventilation:** The responder gives two quick breaths to ventilate the athlete. The use of a one-way mask or bag valve mask is recommended. If the athlete's gag reflex is absent, an oral–pharyngeal airway may be inserted by personnel who have been trained in this procedure.

- **Circulation:** Ideally, the carotid pulse is used to determine that the heart is beating. If the athlete's neck is inaccessible, either because of equipment or the athlete's position on the ground, the pulse can be identified over the radial, ulnar, or femoral or popliteal arteries. If the athlete is not breathing but has a heartbeat, then **rescue breathing** is initiated. If the athlete does not have a pulse, then **CPR** is begun.

Management of the Unconscious but Breathing Athlete

This section assumes that the athlete has an open airway and the cardiopulmonary system is functioning normally. Although these findings initially appear to be normal, they require continuous monitoring because the worst-case scenario involves the athlete's progressing to cardiac arrest. Lesions in the C1 region of the spinal cord alter brain stem function and result in almost immediate cardiac arrest. C2 to C4 lesions or subsequent hemorrhage and hematoma formation at these levels can interrupt the phrenic nerve, possibly resulting in a delayed onset of respiratory arrest.

- **Cervical spine evaluation:** Gently palpate the cervical spine for signs of gross bony deformity or swelling. The absence of these signs, however, does not rule out the possibility of cervical spine injury.
- **Blood pressure:** The athlete's blood pressure is monitored and recorded so that any change over time may

---

Tracheotomy A method of delivering air to the lungs by incising the skin and trachea and inserting a tube to form an airway; an emergency technique used only when the athlete's life is threatened by an immovable obstruction to the upper airway. Training is required to properly perform this technique.

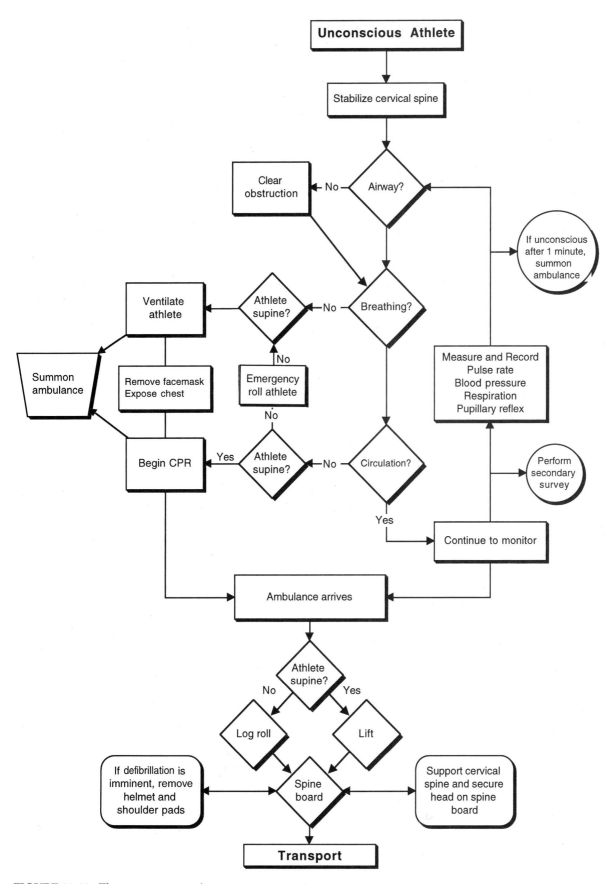

FIGURE 18–23. The management of an unconscious athlete.

be identified. If a blood pressure cuff is not immediately available, the athlete's blood pressure can be estimated based on where the pulses can be palpated:[60]

Palpable Pulse	Minimum Systolic Blood Pressure, mm Hg
Carotid artery	60
Femoral artery	70
Radial artery	90

- **Pupil responsiveness:** The athlete's eyelids are opened to observe for pupillary response. The act of opening the eyelids alone should cause the pupils to constrict. The absence of pupillary response indicates that the brain is not receiving oxygen or that substantial brain trauma has occurred.
- **Continuation of monitoring:** The athlete's respirations, blood pressure, pupillary reflex, and pulse are monitored and recorded every 5 minutes.[54] Decreased respiration, increased blood pressure, and decreased heart rate are signs of an expanding intracranial lesion.

Management of the Conscious Athlete

The on-field management described in this section assumes that the athlete has been determined to be conscious, in-line stabilization has been applied to the athlete's cervical spine, the athlete's mouthpiece has been removed, and the presence of an open airway has been established.

As long as the athlete displays stable vital signs, no attempts should be made to move the athlete until the possibility of a spinal fracture has been ruled out or the athlete is stabilized with a spine board and cervical collar. The athlete may express the desire to move or may attempt to do so. Either through verbal commands or gentle restraint, the athlete should not be allowed to move until the possibility of a fracture has been ruled out.

HISTORY

Question the athlete regarding any loss of consciousness, the mechanism of the injury, and any areas of pain or paresthesia in the cervical spine or radiating into the extremities. Any significant findings of pain or numbness radiating into the extremities or cervical pain warrant the immediate spine boarding of the athlete and transport to the hospital.

- **Loss of consciousness:** Determine if the athlete lost consciousness, even for a brief period of time. A transitory loss of consciousness may be described as "blacking out" or "seeing stars."
- **Mechanism of injury:** Identify how the injurious force was delivered. A direct blow to the head can result in either brain or cervical spine trauma. If this

mechanism forces the neck into flexion or extension, cervical spine trauma should be suspected. If the athlete cannot recall the onset of injury, bystanders or witnesses may be able to describe it.

- **Symptoms:** Question the athlete regarding the symptoms that indicate spinal pathology. Positive findings for any of the following support the assumption that a spinal cord or cervical vertebral injury is present:
  - Pain in the cervical spine
  - Numbness, tingling, or burning pain radiating through the upper or lower extremities
  - Sensation of weakness in the cervical spine, upper extremities, or lower extremities
  - Burning or aching in the chest secondary to cardiac inhibition

INSPECTION

This inspection process supplements the information gained during the observations made on the way to the scene and may be conducted concurrently with the previously described segments of the examination. If the athlete is supine, the inspection of the posterior cervical structures can be delayed until the athlete is moved to the sidelines or omitted if the athlete is being transported to the hospital.

- **Cervical vertebrae:** Observe the cervical vertebrae, if visible. They should display a normal alignment.
- **Cervical musculature:** Observe for the presence of muscle spasm indicating a cervical fracture, a dislocation, or a strain of the neck muscles.

PALPATION

Palpation is conducted to confirm any visual findings of malalignment and identify underlying pathology. Too much pressure during palpation must be avoided to prevent the possible displacement of a bony fragment. If the athlete is supine, palpation can be performed by reaching beneath the athlete. Certain pieces of equipment, such as cervical collars, can prohibit palpation while the athlete is in either the prone or supine position.

- **Cervical spine:** Palpate the area over the spinous and transverse processes for signs of vertebral malalignment, crepitus, or tenderness. Any of these signs signify the possibility of a cervical fracture or dislocation.
- **Cervical musculature:** Palpate the cervical musculature for signs of spasm in the upper portion of the trapezius, levator scapulae, or sternocleidomastoid muscles. Unilateral spasm is an indication of a cervical vertebral dislocation, especially when the skull is rotated and tilted toward the opposite side.

NEUROLOGIC TESTING

- **Sensory testing:** Although formal dermatome testing may be conducted while the athlete is on the field, the essential finding is that of normal and bilaterally equal sensation in the upper and lower extremities. Sensation may be compared by stroking along the following body areas:

Upper Extremity		Lower Extremity	
Area	Dermatome	Area	Dermatomes
Superior shoulder	C4	Lateral thigh	L1, L2, L3
Lateral humerus	C5	Lateral lower	
Lateral forearm	C6	leg and foot	L5, S1
Middle finger	C7	Medial lower	
Medial forearm	C8	leg and foot	L4
Medial humerus	T1		

- **Motor testing:** If no other signs and symptoms of cervical vertebral involvement exist, the athlete's ability to perform active motion of the upper and lower extremities and resisted movements of the upper extremity may be tested.
- **Active motion:** Active movements are first performed on the small joints because motion of the large joints (e.g., knees and hips) may result in a significant shift of the body. Begin by asking the athlete to wiggle the toes and fingers, progressing to movement of the ankles, wrists, knees, elbows, hips, and shoulders. Each of these motions should be performed smoothly and appear bilaterally equal.

◆ REMOVING THE ATHLETE FROM THE FIELD

Each on-field incident ends with the decision of how to remove the athlete from the field. The extremes of the possible scenarios range from the athlete's walking off the field without assistance to rolling and placing the athlete on a spine board. Cases that lie between these extremes require that the medical staff make a decision about the best method to safely remove the athlete.

Any suspected cervical spine trauma mandates that the athlete be placed on a spine board and transported to a hospital via an ambulance squad. The use of stretchers without a spine board is to be avoided in these cases. Additionally, if any doubt exists, the most conservative form of management should be chosen.

WALKING THE ATHLETE OFF THE FIELD

Removing athletes from the field under their own power is not as straightforward as standing the athlete up and having him or her walk off the field. After a head injury, the sudden change from a lying to a standing position may make the blood pressure drop suddenly, causing the athlete to faint or become unsteady.

The athlete's body should be allowed to gradually adjust to the change in positions, using a three-step process. First, the athlete is brought to a sitting position with the knees bent. The athletic trainer is positioned behind the athlete, providing support and being ready to assist the athlete if dizziness occurs. This position is maintained until the athlete feels comfortable with the position. The athlete then kneels forward on one knee and again waits, to ensure that dizziness does not occur. Finally, the athlete is brought to the standing position, with assistance being provided on either side. If the symptoms increase in any of these positions, the athlete should be transported in a supine or sitting position.

USING A SPINE BOARD

In-line stabilization is maintained throughout these procedures until the athlete's skull is securely affixed to the spine board. These procedures should be discussed and practiced with the emergency medical squad.

Cervical Spine Stabilization

The cervical spine is best stabilized using a semirigid collar, such as a **Philadelphia collar** (see Fig. 17–27). These devices are most easily applied when the athlete is not wearing shoulder pads or a helmet. Other types of collars, such as a vacuum splint cervical immobilizer, can be used for stabilization when the helmet and shoulder pads are still in place.[61]

After separating the two halves of the collar, the posterior shell is compressed and slid behind the cervical spine, taking care to prevent spinal movement. This section should fit snugly beneath the athlete's occipital and mastoid processes. The anterior shell is fitted so that it envelops the chin. Most models have an opening on the sternal pad that allows access to the trachea in case a tracheotomy must be performed.

The Athlete Who Is Supine

Spine boarding is best accomplished with a minimum of four people: the person who has been applying in-line stabilization (referred to as the leader) and a minimum of three people controlling the athlete's torso (Fig. 18–24). A fifth person may be recruited to manipulate the spine board. The leader maintains in-line stabilization throughout the roll and subsequent stabilization of the athlete on the spine board and is responsible for instructing and guiding the remaining personnel in the sequence to be performed.

The process of using a spine board for an athlete who is supine involves rolling the athlete to the side, sliding the board under the athlete, and then positioning the athlete on the board.

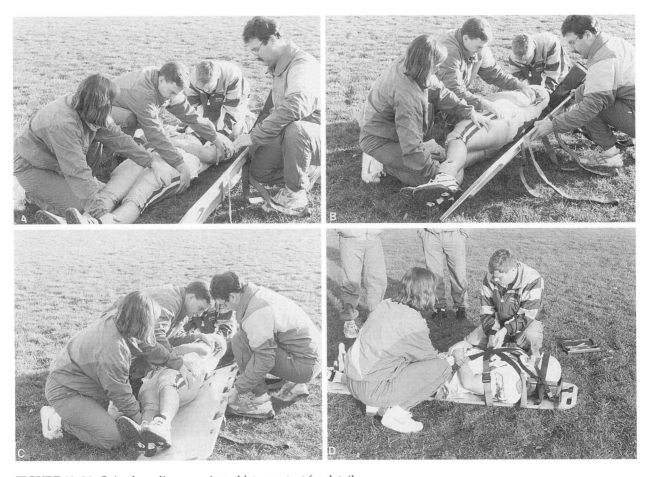

FIGURE 18–24. Spine boarding a supine athlete; see text for details.

1. **Align the athlete:** Before the athlete is placed on the board, the extremities must be aligned with the body. The arm on the side toward which the athlete is to be rolled is abducted to 180 degrees.
2. **Position the personnel:** When the minimum of three personnel is used at the torso, one is positioned at the shoulders, one at the hips, and one along the legs. The hands should be spaced along the athlete, gripping underneath the athlete. Tall, heavy, or large individuals may require more personnel to ensure safe movement.
3. **Roll to the side:** On the leader's instructions, the athlete is rolled 90 degrees. The following command is used: "On the count of three, we will roll the athlete toward you. Start and stop on my command. Ready? One, two, three, roll." The personnel used at the torso are responsible for maintaining axial alignment of the spinal column by staying with the leader's pace.
4. **Slide the spine board:** If a single person is given the responsibility of manipulating the spine board, it should be slid so that it is flat on the ground and resting against the athlete. The board is positioned longitudinally so that the head of the spine board is matched with the athlete's head. If the personnel used at the torso must position the spine board, the

individual at the hips should be given the responsibility of manipulating the board.
5. **Return the athlete:** After the leader is satisfied with the board's position relative to the athlete, he or she gives the command, "On the count of three, we will roll the athlete on the board. Start and stop on my command. Ready? One, two, three, roll." Again, it is the torso personnel who are responsible for meeting the pace of the leader. Minor adjustments may be needed after the athlete is positioned on the board.
6. **Secure the athlete:** After the athlete is properly positioned on the spine board, the torso is secured, using the strapping techniques applicable to the equipment being used. The cervical spine must be affixed, using the equipment supplied by the ambulance company or using commercially available equipment. If the helmet is left on, the head may be secured to the board by tape.

The Athlete Who Is Prone

Athletes in the prone position who are breathing but unconscious may be rolled onto the spine board in a safer and more orderly manner than that described in the section on the on-field management of an unconscious ath-

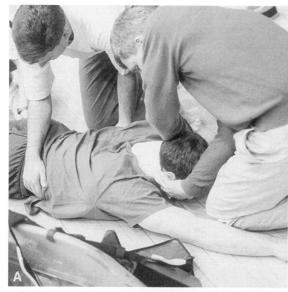

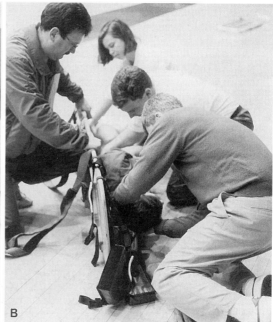

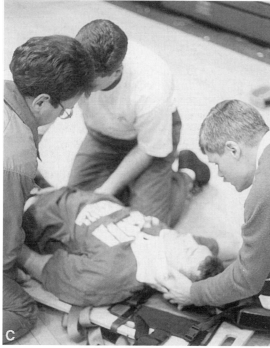

FIGURE 18–25. Spine boarding a prone athlete; see text for details. Note the cross-armed position of the leader applying in-line stabilization.

lete who is not breathing. The basic procedures are the same as those described for spine boarding an athlete in the supine position, but the athlete must be rolled 180 degrees rather than 90 degrees (Fig. 18–25). The person who is providing in-line stabilization to the cervical spine is again the operation's leader. A minimum of three additional people is necessary for this procedure to be safely performed. A fourth additional person is recommended to manipulate the spine board.

1. **Align the athlete:** Before the athlete is placed on the board, the extremities are aligned with the body. The arm on the side toward which the athlete is to be rolled is abducted to 180 degrees.

2. **Position the personnel:** When the minimum of three personnel is used at the torso, one is positioned at the shoulders, one at the hips, and one along the legs. The hands should be spaced along the athlete, gripping underneath the athlete. Tall, heavy, or large individuals may require more personnel in order to be moved safely.

3. **Roll to the side:** On the leader's instructions, the athlete is rolled 90 degrees. The command is given: "On the count of three, we will roll the athlete toward you. Start and stop on my command. Ready? One, two, three, roll." The personnel used at the torso are responsible for maintaining axial alignment of the spinal column by staying with the leader's pace.

4. **Slide the spine board:** If a single person is given the responsibility of manipulating the spine board, it should be slid so that it is resting against the athlete. The board is positioned longitudinally so that the head of the spine board is matched with the athlete's head. If the personnel used at the torso must position the spine board, the individual at the athlete's hips should be given the responsibility of manipulating the board.

5. **Placement:** After the leader is satisfied with the board's position relative to the athlete, he or she gives the command: "On the count of three, we will roll the athlete on the board. Start and stop on my command. Ready? One, two, three, roll." The torso personnel are responsible for meeting the pace of the leader. Minor adjustments may be needed after the athlete is positioned on the board.

6. **Secure the athlete:** The athlete is secured on the spine board as described in the previous section.

HOME INSTRUCTIONS

Because of the delayed onset of symptoms associated with intracranial hemorrhage, there is always the potential for a more serious condition to develop. The attending physician, in some cases, may elect to admit the athlete to the hospital for observation. In other cases, the athlete is allowed to return home.

It is good practice to inform the athlete's parents or roommates of the delayed progression of the signs and symptoms of head injuries and alert them to the appropriate course of action. A good method of doing this is through the use of a business card-sized instruction booklet. A list of emergency numbers (e.g., athletic trainer, physician, emergency room) is printed on the front cover. The card then opens to display a list of signs and symptoms to alert the individual to a deteriorating condition (Fig. 18–26).

Behavioral changes, forgetfulness, confusion, anger, aggression, and malaise are the most outward signs. Additionally, the athlete may describe nausea, vomiting, a headache with increasing severity, and a loss of appetite. Although these symptoms may be caused by other conditions, their presence after a head injury may be cause for concern. The onset of any of the other signs and symptoms of a cerebral injury may also indicate a severe head injury (see Tables 18–5 and 18–7).

Permission to take aspirin or other pain-relieving medication must be given by the physician. Many of these medications, as well as alcoholic drinks, inhibit the clotting mechanism, potentially increasing the rate of intracranial bleeding. Analgesic medications may also mask underlying symptoms, thus delaying their recognition. Prohibiting sleep after a concussion is largely founded in fiction rather than fact. Although it is necessary to keep the athlete conscious immediately after the injury, sleep should—and must—be permitted at night. The athlete's parents or roommate can be asked to check on the athlete at regular intervals. If enough doubt surrounds the athlete's condition to prohibit sleep, the physician will admit the athlete to the hospital for observation. The medical staff or emergency room personnel should be immediately contacted if any of the latent signs or symptoms of intracranial hemorrhage are manifested.

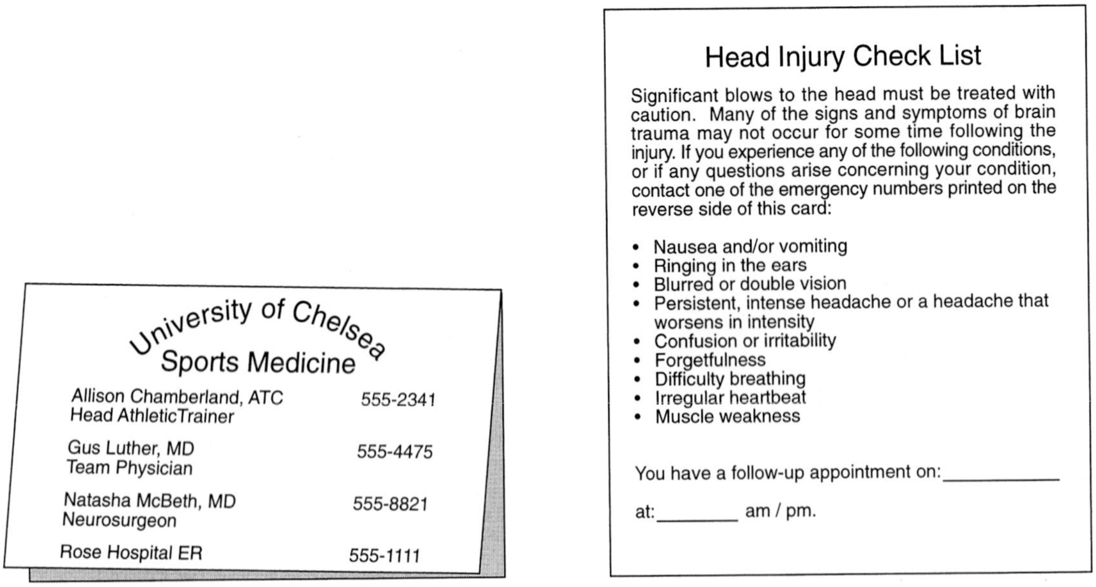

University of Chelsea Sports Medicine

Allison Chamberland, ATC Head AthleticTrainer	555-2341
Gus Luther, MD Team Physician	555-4475
Natasha McBeth, MD Neurosurgeon	555-8821
Rose Hospital ER	555-1111

Head Injury Check List

Significant blows to the head must be treated with caution. Many of the signs and symptoms of brain trauma may not occur for some time following the injury. If you experience any of the following conditions, or if any questions arise concerning your condition, contact one of the emergency numbers printed on the reverse side of this card:

- Nausea and/or vomiting
- Ringing in the ears
- Blurred or double vision
- Persistent, intense headache or a headache that worsens in intensity
- Confusion or irritability
- Forgetfulness
- Difficulty breathing
- Irregular heartbeat
- Muscle weakness

You have a follow-up appointment on:_____

at:_____ am / pm.

FIGURE 18–26. Business card method of communicating home instructions to a head-injured athlete.

◆ REFERENCES

1. Zemper, ED: Cerebral concussion rates in various brands of football helmets. *Athletic Training: Journal of the National Athletic Trainers Association*, 24:133, 1989.

2. Zemper, ED: Analysis of cerebral concussion frequency with the most commonly used models of football helmets. *J Athletic Training*, 29:44, 1994.

3. McWhorter, JM: Concussions and intracranial injuries in athletics. *Athletic Training: Journal of the National Athletic Trainers Association*, 25:129, 1990.

4. Nelson, WE: Athletic head injuries, *Athletic Training: Journal of the National Athletic Trainers Association*, 19:95, 1984.

5. Tysvaer, AT, and Lochen, EA: Soccer injuries to the brain. A neuropsychologic study of former soccer players. *Am J Sports Med*, 19:56, 1991.

6. Sports-related recurrent brain injuries: United States. *Morb Mortal Wkly Rep*, 14:224, 1997.

7. Torg, JS: Epidemiology, biomechanics, and prevention of cervical spine trauma resulting from athletics and recreational activities. *Operative Techniques in Sports Medicine*, 1:159, 1993.

8. Torg, JS: The epidemiologic, biomechanical, and cinematographic analysis of football induced cervical spine trauma. *Athletic Training: Journal of the National Athletic Trainers Association*, 25:147, 1990.

9. Otis, JS, Burstein, AH, and Torg, JS: Mechanisms and pathomechanics of athletic injuries to the cervical spine. In Torg, JS (ed): *Athletic Injuries to the Head, Neck, and Face* (ed 2). St Louis, Mosby-Year Book, 1991, p 438.

10. Torg, JS, et al: The epidemiologic, pathologic, biomechanical, and cinematographic analysis of football-induced cervical spine trauma. *Am J Sports Med*, 18:50, 1990.

11. Heck, JF: The incidence of spearing by high school football carriers and their tacklers. *J Athletic Training*, 27:120, 1992.

12. Guskiewicz, KM, et al: Epidemiology of concussions in collegiate and high school football players. *Am J Sports Med*, 28:643, 2000.

13. Oliaro, SM, Guskiewicz, KM, and Prentice, WE: Establishment of normative data on cognitive tests for comparison with athletes sustaining mild head injury. *J Athletic Training*, 33:36, 1998.

14. Onate, JA, et al: A comparison of sideline versus clinical cognitive test performance in collegiate athletes. *J Athletic Training*, 35:155, 2000.

15. Guskiewicz, KM: Concussion in sport: The grading system dilemma. *Athletic Therapy Today*, 6:18, 2001.

16. Bohnen, N, Twinjstra, A, and Jolles, J: Performance in the Stroop color word test in relationship to the persistence of symptoms following mild head injury. *Acta Neurol Scand*, 85:116, 1992.

17. Putukian, M, and Echemendia, RJ: Managing successive minor head injuries: Which tests guide return to play? *Physician and Sports Medicine*, 24:25, 1996.

18. Hinton-Bayre, AD, Geffen, G, and McFarland, K: Mild head injury and speed of information processing: A prospective study of professional rugby league players. *J Clin Exp Neuropsychol*, 19:275, 1997.

19. Iverson, G, Franzen, M and Lovell, M: Normative comparisons for the controlled oral word association test following acute traumatic brain injury. *J Clin Exp Neuropsychol*, 13:437, 1999.

20. Riemann, BL, and Guskiewicz, KM: Effects of mild head injury on postural stability as measured through clinical balance testing. *J Athletic Training*, 35:19, 2000.

21. Balance Error Scoring System (BESS) *User's Manual*. University of North Carolina, Chapel Hill, NC, Sports Medicine Research Laboratory.

22. Buckley, WE: Concussion injury in college football. An eight-year overview. *Athletic Training: Journal of the National Athletic Trainers Association*, 21:207, 1986.

23. Report of the Ad Hoc Committee to Study Head Injury Nomenclature: Proceedings of the Congress of Neurological Surgeons in 1964. *Clin Neurosurg*, 12:386, 1966.

24. Kelly, JP, and Rosenberg, JH: Diagnosis and management of concussion in sports. *Neurology*, 48:575, 1997.

25. Cameron, KL, Yunker, CA, and Austin, MC: A standardized protocol for the initial evaluation and documentation of mild brain injury. *J Athletic Training*, 34:34, 1999.

26. AOSSM Concussion Group: Concussions in sports. Rosemont, IL, American Orthopaedic Society for Sports Medicine, 1999 (*http://www.intelli.com/vhosts/aossm-isite/databases/Concussion.doc*).

27. Maroon, JC: Assessing closed head injuries. *The Physician and Sportsmedicine*, 20:37, 1992.

28. McCrea, M, et al: Standardized assessment of concussion in football players. *Neurology*, 48:586, 1997.

29. Practice parameter: The management of concussion in sports (summary statement). *Neurology*, 48:581, 1997.

30. Cantu, RC and Micheli, LJ (eds): American college of sports medicine guidelines for the team physician. Philadelphia, Lea & Febiger, 1991, p 93.

31. Cantu, RC: Guidelines to return to contact sports after cerebral concussion. *Phys Sports Med*, 14:76, 1986.

32. Colorado Medical Society: *Report of the Sports Medicine Committee: Guidelines for the Management of Concussion in Sports* (revised). Paper presented at the Colorado Medical Society, Denver, Co, 1991.

33. Potts, KA, and Dick, RW: NCAA guide line 2o: Concussion and second-impact syndrome. In Potts, KA, and Dick, RW (eds): *NCAA Sports Medicine Handbook*. Indianapolis, IN, National Collegiate Athletic Association, 2000, p 75–77.

34. Cantu, RC: Criteria for return to competition after a closed head injury. In Torg, JS (ed): *Athletic Injuries to the Head, Neck, and Face* (ed 2). St Louis, Mosby-Year Book, 1991, p 326.

35. Cantu, RC: Head and spine injuries in youth sports. The young athlete. *Clin Sports Med*, 14:517, 1995.

36. Erlanger, DM, et al: Neuropsychology of sports-related head injury. Dementia pugilistica to post concussion syndrome. *Clin Neuropsychol*, 13:193, 1999.

37. Geurts, AC; Knoop, JA and van Limbeek, J: Is postural control associated with mental functioning in the persistent postconcussion syndrome? *Arch Phys Med Rehabil*, 80:144, 1999.

38. Cantu, RC: Emergencies in sports. Second impact syndrome: Immediate management. *The Physician and Sportsmedicine*, 20:55, 1992.

39. Sanders, RI, and Harbaugh, RE: The second impact in catastrophic contact: Sports head trauma. *JAMA*, 252:538, 1984.

40. Muller, FO: Fatalities from head and cervical spine injuries occurring in tackle football: 50 years' experience. *Clin Sports Med*, 17:169, 1998.

41. White, RJ: Subarachnoid hemorrhage: The lethal intracranial explosion. *Emerg Med Clin North Am*, May:74, 1994.

42. Bailes, JE: Management of cervical spine sports injuries. *Athletic Training: Journal of the National Athletic Trainers Association*, 25:156, 1990.

43. Torg, JS: Criteria for return to collision activities after cervical spine injury. *Oper Techniques Sports Med*, 1:236, 1993.

44. Torg, JS, et al: Spear tackler's spine: An entity precluding participation in tackle football and collision activities that expose the cervical spine to axial energy inputs. *Am J Sports Med*, 21:640, 1993.

45. Khosla, R: An occult cervical spine fracture. *Physician and Sportsmedicine*, 24:69, 1997.

46. Geisler, FH: Clinical trials of pharmacotherapy for spinal cord injury. *Ann NY Acad Sci*, 845:374, 1998.

47. Seidl, EC: Promising pharmacological agents in the management of acute spinal cord injury. *Crit Care Nurs Q*, 22:44, 1999.

48. Vale, FL, et al: Combined medical and surgical treatment after acute spinal cord injury: Results of a prospective pilot study to assess the merits of aggressive medical resuscitation and blood pressure management. *J Neurosurg*, 87:239, 1997.

49. Scher, AT: Spinal cord concussion in rugby players. *Am J Sports Med*, 18:50, 1990.

50. Jordan, BD, et al: How to evaluate transient quadriparesis. *The Physician and Sportsmedicine*, 20:83, 1992.

51. Torg, JS: Cervical spine stenosis with cord neurapraxia and transient quadriplegia. *Athletic Training: Journal of the National Athletic Trainers Association*, 25:156, 1990.

52. Torg, JS, et al: The relationship of developmental narrowing of the cervical spinal canal to reversible and irreversible injury of

the cervical spinal cord in football players. *J Bone Joint Surg,* 78(A):1308, 1996.

53. Harris, AJ: Disaster plan-a part of the game plan? *Athletic Training: Journal of the National Athletic Trainers Association,* 23:59, 1988.
54. Nelson, WE, et al: Athletic head injuries. *Athletic Training: Journal of the National Athletic Trainers Association,* 19:95, 1984.
55. Putman, LA: Alternative methods for football helmet face mask removal. *J Athletic Training,* 2:170, 1992.
56. Feld, F: Management of the critically injured football players. *J Athletic Training,* 28:206, 1993.
57. Denegar, CR, and Saliba, E: On the field management of the potentially cervical spine injured football player. *Athletic Training: Journal of the National Athletic Trainers Association,* 24:108, 1989.
58. Potts, KA, and Dick, RW: NCAA guide line 4f: Guidelines for helmet fitting and removal in athletics. In Potts, KA and Dick, RW (eds): *NCAA Sports Medicine Handbook.* Indianapolis, IN, National Collegiate Athletic Association, 2000, p 75–77.
59. Pofeta, LM, and Paris, P: Emergencies in sports. Managing airway obstruction. *The Physician and Sportsmedicine,* 19:35, 1991.
60. Caroline, N: *Emergency Care in the Streets* (ed 3). Little, Brown, Boston, 25:147, 1990.
61. Ransone, J, Kersey, R, and Walsh, K: The efficacy of rapid form cervical vacuum immobilizer in the cervical spine immobilization of the equipped football player. *J Athletic Training,* 35:65, 2000.

19 > Environmental Injury

The onset of environmental injuries is not limited to temperature extremes or outdoor activities. The harmful gain or loss of heat from and to the external environment can occur during any physical activity. The body has the ability to adapt to exercise in most of the environmental extremes seen in athletics. Except for accidental exposure to very hot or very cold temperatures, environmentally related injuries are completely preventable.

◆ CLINICAL ANATOMY AND PHYSIOLOGY

Regulation of the body's core temperature primarily occurs in the hypothalamus and other brain centers. Normally, the skin temperature is higher than that of the surrounding environment. The body's core temperature is greater than that of the skin and extremities. As used in this text, the term "core temperature" is used to describe the actual temperature within the viscera.

Just as a furnace receives input from a thermostat, the hypothalamus receives input from thermoreceptors located in the skin, spinal cord, abdomen, and brain. In response to changes in the core temperature, the hypothalamus shunts blood toward or away from the skin, regulating the amount of cooling. Increasing blood flow to the skin decreases the core temperature. Conversely, decreasing blood flow to the skin increases the core temperature. Additionally, the core temperature is controlled by increasing mechanical and chemical heat production when the core temperature drops too low or increasing sweating when the core temperature rises too high (Fig. 19–1).

HEAT TRANSFER

Heat exchange to and from the body occurs through radiation, conduction and convection, and evaporation. Each of these mechanisms relies on a temperature gra-

dient between the body and the surrounding environment. The greater this difference, the greater the magnitude and rate of the exchange to and from the body.

Radiation

All objects emit heat in the form of infrared radiation. Normally, this exchange occurs in the form of the body's losing heat into the environment. However, when the body is placed in an exceedingly warm environment, such as on a hot, humid day; sitting in a sauna; or practicing in a wrestling room, the body gains heat through radiation.

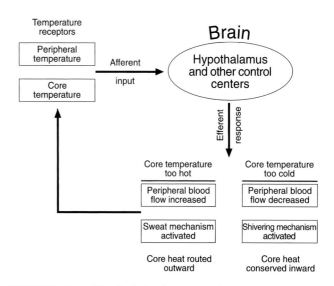

FIGURE 19–1. The body's thermoregulatory system. Thermoreceptors in the extremities, skin, and within the viscera monitor the body's temperature. High temperatures result in increased peripheral blood flow and activate the sweating mechanism to route the heat away from the core. Cold core temperatures activate a mechanism that conserves the core temperature.

Conduction and Convection

The body can gain or lose heat when it is in contact with an object that has a temperature warmer or cooler than itself Because the air contains molecules, the body can exchange heat directly with the atmosphere through **conduction.** The use of a hot pack or ice pack are examples of the body's gaining or losing heat through this mechanism. The efficiency of conduction in still, standing air is quite poor. Circulating the air across the body enhances the cooling process through the means of **convection.** The use of a room fan is an example of convective cooling.

Conduction and convection most commonly occur between the skin and the air. During swimming, water is the environmental medium through which most heat is lost. This explains why the temperature of competitive swimming pools is kept relatively low.

Evaporation

The evaporation of water from the skin carries heat with it, cooling the skin and subsequently lowering the core temperature. During physical exertion, the body depends primarily on evaporation for heat loss. In response to exercise, the body's perspiration rate increases, covering the body with fluids to be evaporated, thus removing heat.

Other Mechanisms

Heat is lost from the body through several other mechanisms, many of which are inconsequential or impractical during athletic competition. Respiration is the most common and applicable of these methods. As air passes into the lungs, it travels through warm, moist passages, humidifying it. During expiration, water and heat are lost. Elimination through urination, defecation, or vomiting also transfers heat from the body. However, these mechanisms also serve to dehydrate the body.

BLOOD FLOW AND HEAT EXCHANGE

To maintain its core temperature during exercise, the body must balance the amount of heat gained and heat lost. The body responds to a hot, humid environment by increasing the blood flow to the extremities and subcutaneous vessels. The vessels in the skin dilate, allowing more blood to carry heat away from the core to be released into the environment.

The proportion of heat lost via radiation, conduction, convection, and evaporation depends on the intensity of exercise, *relative humidity*, and *ambient* temperature.[1] Heat lost via conduction, convection, and radiation decreases as the ambient temperature increases. Increased humidity decreases the effectiveness of the sweating mechanism.

The total volume of the body's blood vessels is approximately four times greater than that of the heart's

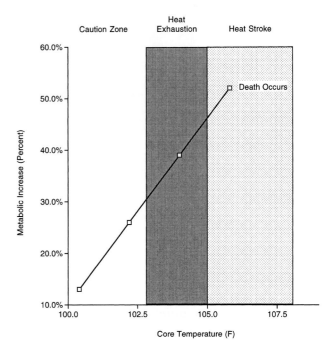

FIGURE 19–2. Linear relationship between core temperature and metabolism.

pumping capacity.[2] The body compensates for this disparity by routing more blood to the areas demanding oxygen and decreasing the supply to areas with a lesser demand. The brain receives the highest priority for oxygen.

During exercise, a worsening cycle occurs when the body's core temperature begins to increase above normal. Increased core temperature caused by exercise increases systemic metabolism. This, in turn, further increases the core temperature. For every 1 percent of body weight lost through sweating, there is a 0.27°C to 0.36°C (0.49°F to 0.65°F) increase in core temperature. The heart rate also increases 3 to 5 beats per minute.[1] As the core temperature rises above 40.0°C (104.0°F), a linear relationship between the core temperature and metabolic demands is developed (Fig. 19–2).[3] After the body's internal temperature reaches 42.0°C (107.6°F), the cardiovascular system can no longer meet the metabolic oxygen demand necessary to sustain life.

The brain is constantly monitoring the oxygen requirements of the exercising muscles, internal organs, and brain, making the adjustments necessary to maintain the viability of each while also keeping the core temperature within acceptable limits. Blood flow to the working muscles is increased, decreasing the supply of

Relative humidity   The ratio between the amount of water vapor in the air and the actual amount of water the air could potentially hold based on the current temperature.

Ambient   Pertaining to the local environment.

oxygen available to the other areas of the body. When this exertion occurs in a hot or humid environment, blood flow to the cutaneous vessels is increased to cool the core temperature. This rerouted blood draws more blood from the viscera and the brain, causing the core temperature to increase. Increased metabolism associated with the temperature rise and the exercising muscles further increases the core temperature.

SWEATING MECHANISM

Sweating reduces the body's internal temperature by carrying heat outward, where it can evaporate into the atmosphere. This process is inherently efficient because water conducts heat 25 times more rapidly than air.[4] Unfortunately, the sweating process is also self-depleting.

Sweat is not pure water. When sweat leaves the body, it also carries electrolytes, namely sodium (salt) and potassium, with it. The body's ability to efficiently sustain prolonged activity is directly related to the replacement of both water and electrolytes. When water is not replaced, the efficiency of the cooling mechanism is impaired. The plasma volume is reduced, decreasing blood pressure, causing the heart to work harder to deliver blood to the areas requiring it. When the electrolytes are not replaced, metabolic efficiency is hindered by depriving the body of essential substances required for normal physiologic function. The effects of increased core temperature and dehydration significantly alter cardiovascular function more so than dehydration or increased temperature occurring separate from the other.[5]

The total amount of sweat lost is based on the sweating rate, calculated as:[1]

$$\text{Sweat rate} = \frac{\left(\begin{array}{c} \text{pre-exercise body weight} \\ - \text{ Post-exercise body weight} \\ + \text{ fluid intake } - \text{ Urine volume} \end{array} \right)}{\text{Time in hours}}$$

Replenishing water before, during, and after exercise keeps the net fluid loss to a minimum, increases the efficiency of the sweating mechanism, and assists in preventing dehydration.

HEAT CONSERVATION

Just as excessive heat gain is harmful to the body, so is excessive loss of heat. The body conserves heat by reversing the process used to cool the body. Blood is routed away from the superficial vessels and the skin, maintaining the core temperature. When the temperature drops below 86°F, muscle tone increases and, eventually, shivering begins. The increased metabolism associated with these muscle contractions serves as a source of heat to rewarm the core. Chronic or prolonged exposure to a cold environment results in **chemical thermogenesis,** a process in which epinephrine is secreted into the bloodstream, increasing the metabolism of nonmuscular cells.[6]

INFLUENCE OF AMBIENT TEMPERATURE

The ambient temperature, humidity, wind velocity, and radiant heat all influence the risk of environmental injury.[7] The term "heat injury" is probably a misnomer because its onset is more directly related to the relative humidity (RH) than to the actual temperature of the air. Until the ambient air temperature exceeds 95°F or the relative humidity reaches 75 percent, sweating and evaporation account for most of the heat loss.[8] For every increase in air temperature of 5°F, the percentage at which relative humidity raises the risk of injury is decreased by 10 percent (i.e., at 70°F the humidity danger zone is 80 percent RH; at 90°F, the danger zone is 50 percent RH). After the relative humidity reaches 100 percent and the air temperature reaches that of the skin, the body can no longer lose heat into the environment.[9] The resulting core temperature can increase to fatally high levels.

Acclimatization

Physiologic systems can adapt to exercise in hot, humid environments through improved efficiency of the metabolic and cooling processes. "Acclimation" is used to describe physiologic changes that occur in a controlled environment. "Acclimatization" describes the physical adaptations that occur in a natural environment.[7] Acclimatization is achieved by gradually exposing the exercising athlete to the environmental condition over a period of several days to weeks, depending on the magnitude of the environmental change.

The process of making the body more efficient involves the modification of four individual components:[4]

1. Increased glycogen stores increases the amount of *adenosine triphosphate* (ATP) available to skeletal and cardiac muscle and provides an immediate source of energy.
2. The heart's efficiency is improved by increasing cardiac output and stroke volume, allowing the heart to deliver more blood to the working muscles at a lower pulse rate. The improved efficiency of cardiac and skeletal muscle contraction results in decreased metabolic heat production.
3. The body's sweat threshold temperature is lowered and the volume of sweat is increased, enhancing the rapid removal of heat from the body and preventing the core temperature from reaching the danger zone.
4. Improved renal function results in a decreased level of salt's being lost in the sweat, which, through osmotic properties, retains ECFs and plasma volume.

Adenosine triphosphate (ATP) An energy-yielding enzyme used during muscular contractions.

CLINICAL EVALUATION OF ENVIRONMENTAL INJURIES

The evaluative process of patients with environmental injuries requires knowledge of the symptoms and information about the environmental conditions and other factors that may predispose the individual to these injuries. Because of the relatively straightforward evaluation of patients with these conditions, the format of the evaluative process has been altered from those presented in previous chapters.

HISTORY

- **Environmental conditions:** The magnitude of environmental extremes decreases the duration of exposure required for the onset of symptoms. Heat exposure is compounded by humidity, and cold exposure is compounded by wind. These conditions, discussed in the "Environmental Pathologies and Related Special Tests" section, must be determined before competition or practice and influence whether or not the activity will be held or modified.
- **Weight loss:** Recent weight loss can increase the risk of environmental injury, especially when it is caused through water loss. The use of weight charts can identify individuals who are predisposed to heat injury secondary to water loss (see "Prevention of Heat Injuries").

- **Thirst:** The thirst response is triggered when the patient's body weight is decreased 1 to 2 percent by fluid loss.[7] Some systemic conditions may also alter the thirst response. Diets, especially those rich in salty and fried foods, may also increase the thirst response. Note that electrolyte depletion alone does not trigger the thirst response.
- **Recent history of illness:** Vomiting or diarrhea increases the amount of water and electrolytes lost from the body. Other illnesses increase the body's metabolic demands and decrease the body's resistance to stress by increasing the core temperature.
- **Nutrition:** Dieting or poor nutritional habits may increase the risk of environmental injury. Decreased intake of fluids and electrolytes decrease the plasma volume and may inhibit the metabolism necessary for athletic activity. High-protein diets may decrease the body's ability to cope with cold environments.
- **Other complaints:** Heat injury may cause the person to become confused and aggressive and have headaches. Individuals suffering from cold injuries express a desire to warm up or, in extreme cases, to sleep.
- **Conditioning level:** People who are poorly conditioned or are not acclimated are susceptible to heat injury. Proper conditioning assists in adapting to both hot and cold environments.
- **Body build:** Large muscle mass is a predisposition to heat injury secondary to increased metabolism.

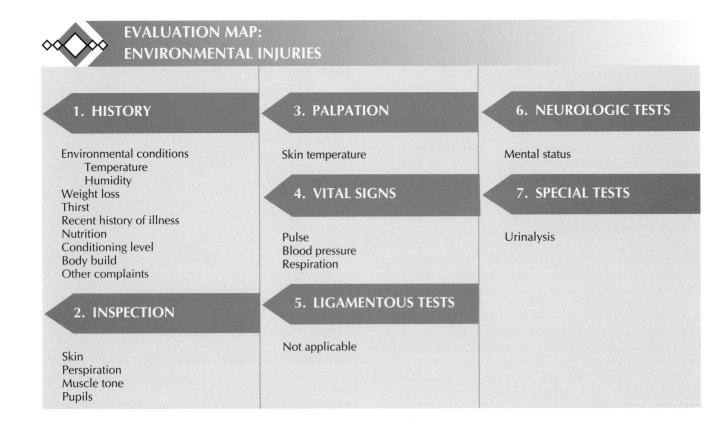

EVALUATION MAP: ENVIRONMENTAL INJURIES

1. HISTORY

Environmental conditions
    Temperature
    Humidity
Weight loss
Thirst
Recent history of illness
Nutrition
Conditioning level
Body build
Other complaints

2. INSPECTION

Skin
Perspiration
Muscle tone
Pupils

3. PALPATION

Skin temperature

4. VITAL SIGNS

Pulse
Blood pressure
Respiration

5. LIGAMENTOUS TESTS

Not applicable

6. NEUROLOGIC TESTS

Mental status

7. SPECIAL TESTS

Urinalysis

INSPECTION

- **Skin:** The color of the skin can provide evidence of the underlying condition. Minor heat-related injuries cause the skin to become pale. Heat stroke, a medical emergency, often results in dark or red skin. In the majority of athletic-related heat injuries, the athlete sweats profusely. Cold injury causes the skin to have a waxy appearance that is red in minor cases or pale in more severe cases.
- **Muscle tone:** As the core temperature increases, the muscle tone decreases to reduce the amount of metabolic heat produced and assist in routing the heat outward to the skin. The exception to this is heat cramps. The body responds to a cold environment by increasing muscle tone by shivering.
- **Pupils:** Exposure to extreme heat or cold causes pupillary dilation and decreased responsiveness to light, an indication of decreased brain function.

PALPATION

- **Skin temperature:** During heat exhaustion, the skin feels cool and clammy to the touch. During heat stroke, the skin feels hot. Cold exposure results in decreased skin temperature.

FUNCTIONAL TESTING

- **Pulse:** Heat injuries result in tachycardia in response to meet the body's demand for oxygen. Cooling of the core temperature causes the heart rate to become slow and weak.
- **Blood pressure:** During heat exhaustion and hypothermia, the blood pressure decreases and may result in syncope. Heat stroke causes an increase in the blood pressure.
- **Respiration:** Paralleling the findings of the heart rate, heat exposure increases the respiratory rate; cold exposure causes it to slow.
- **Mental state:** Prolonged increases or decreases of the intracranial temperature result in an altered cognitive function. Increased temperature results in dizziness, confusion, violent behavior, and unconsciousness. Cooling of the brain causes the individual to become drowsy, eventually drifting into unconsciousness.
- **Urinalysis:** Urine specific gravity (USG) of greater than 1.020 may indicate dehydration. Heat cramps are likely to occur when USG is greater than 1.016. A USG of less than 1.010 is considered adequate hydration.[1,7]

◆ ENVIRONMENTAL PATHOLOGIES AND RELATED SPECIAL TESTS

The delineation between heat and cold injuries is obvious. What is more difficult, however, is the delineation between the various types and severity of heat and cold injuries. The importance of preventing environmental injuries is emphasized throughout this chapter. Injuries from exposure to hot or cold environments are preventable, unlike the relatively unpreventable nature of most of the other injuries described in this text.

HEAT INJURIES

The effects of participating in a hot, humid environment, collectively referred to as **hyperthermia,** range from the relatively minor symptoms associated with heat cramps and heat exhaustion to the potentially fatal effects of heat stroke. These are not always progressive conditions. A person may collapse from heat stroke without displaying the signs and symptoms of the less serious conditions. A comparison of the signs and symptoms of heat cramps, heat syncope, heat exhaustion, and heat stroke is presented in Table 19–1.

The onset of heat-related injuries is directly related to the environment and based on the relationship between air temperature and humidity. The onset of heat injury is not limited to the summer or outdoor activities. Hot, humid gymnasiums, wrestling rooms, or even swimming pools can be the sites of heat injuries. Certain individuals may be predisposed to acquiring heat-related illnesses (Table 19–2). Despite the varying times and locations in which heat injuries can occur, they are all preventable through adequate rehydration and conditioning.

Heat Cramps

Heat cramps are easily recognized by the spasm or cramping of skeletal muscle, most often affecting the lower extremity muscles. The underlying cause of heat cramps is debatable, but the loss of electrolytes secondary to excessive sweating,[8] sodium depletion,[7] or a spinal neural mechanism[10] are most often implicated. Unconditioned individuals or otherwise conditioned athletes who are not acclimated to participating in a hot, humid environment are most susceptible to heat cramps. These conditions increase the athlete's sweating rate and volume, rapidly depleting the body of electrolytes.

Sodium lost through sweating or ingesting a hypotonic fluid results in a decrease in plasma sodium chloride (NaCl) concentrations, causing alterations in the sodium-potassium pump and in the action potential changes across the cell membrane.[7] Increased resting calcium levels cause more calcium to be released from muscle cells, producing random muscle contractions.[7]

Heat cramps can be differentiated from exercise-induced cramps by the location of the muscle spasm. Exercise induced cramps tend to involve the entire muscle or muscle group.[11] Heat cramps tend to affect individual muscle bundles.[7]

> **Table 19–1**
> # EVALUATIVE FINDINGS: Heat Illness

Evaluative Finding	Heat Cramps	Heat Syncope	Heat Exhaustion	Heat Stroke
Core temperature*	WNL**	WNL	103°F or above	102°F to 104°F or above
Skin color and temperature	WNL	WNL	Cool Pale	Hot Red
Sweating	Moderate to profuse	WNL	Profuse	Slight to profuse Sweat mechanism failing
Pulse	WNL	Rapid and weak	Rapid and weak	Tachycardia
Blood pressure	WNL	A sudden, imperceptible drop in blood pressure, which rapidly returns to normal	Low	High
Respiration	WNL	WNL	Hyperventilation	Rapid
Mental state	WNL	Dizziness Fainting	Dizziness Fatigue Slight confusion	Confusion Violent behavior Unconsciousness
Other findings	Cramping in one or more muscles		Headache Nausea Vomiting Thirst	Headache Nausea Vomiting Dilated pupils Decerebrate posture

WNL = within normal limits.
 *As determined by the rectal temperature.
 **Within normal limits for an exercising athlete.

Table 19–2
PREDISPOSING CONDITIONS TO HEAT ILLNESS

Predisposing Condition	Rationale
Large body mass	Large muscle mass increases the body's heat production. Large layers of adipose tissue decrease the heat exchange mechanism.
Age	The heat exchange mechanism of the young and old does not efficiently remove heat.
Conditioning level	Individuals who are poorly conditioned or conditioned athletes who are not acclimated to the environment produce increased levels of metabolic heat and are less efficient at dissipating the heat.
Poor hydration	Internal fluids are required for maximum efficiency of the heat transfer mechanism. Illnesses, especially those involving vomiting or diarrhea, dehydrate the body. Athletes should consume fluids before, during, and after exercise.
History of heat illness	A history of heat-related illness can indicate a chronically inadequate level of hydration or nutrition. An athlete with a recent history of heat-related illness may not have sufficient time to rehydrate.
Medications and other substances	Diuretic medications and alcohol promote fluid loss via urination. Creatine and anabolic steroids increase muscle mass and tend to increase the level of intramuscular fluids. Antihistamines, decongestants (pseudoephedrine), and amphetamines increase metabolism, cause vasoconstriction, or otherwise increase the risk of heat illness.

Heat Syncope

A fainting spell caused by hot, humid environments, heat syncope is sometimes included as a symptom of heat exhaustion.[10] Unlike fainting caused by heat exhaustion, the unconsciousness or dizziness associated with syncope occurs in the absence of an abnormally elevated core temperature unrelated to the depletion of fluids or electrolytes.[2,4] Vascular shunting routes the blood outward to the skin and extremities to lower the core temperature. A sudden shift in blood flow causes cardiac filling pressure and stroke volume to decline rapidly, decreasing cardiac output and blood pressure and depriving the brain of oxygen. Syncope can also have a metabolic, neurologic, or cardiovascular origin or can be the result of a drug reaction. These issues are discussed in Chapter 20.

Heat Exhaustion

Heat exhaustion is characterized by sudden, extreme fatigue as the body attempts to supply blood to the brain, exercising muscles, and skin. Unlike in heat stroke, the hypothalamus continues to function properly with heat exhaustion.

The physiologic effects of heat exhaustion can be traced to water or salt and electrolyte lost through sweating.[2,7] When these events are accompanied by profuse sweating and when fluids and electrolytes are not replaced, the body's volume of circulating fluid is depleted.

Heat exhaustion is classified according to its onset: water depletion or electrolyte depletion. Sweating, vomiting, diarrhea, and excessive urination without substantial rehydration cause a net water loss from the body, all predisposing conditions for heat stroke. Water depletion heat exhaustion has a rapid onset and, if untreated, can progress to heat stroke.[7]

Excessive loss of salt and electrolytes from the body causes a loss of ECF, reducing the plasma volume and subsequently reducing cardiac output and decreasing blood pressure. Severe cases of salt and electrolyte depletion results in peripheral vascular collapse, presenting the signs and symptoms of traumatic shock. Electrolyte depletion heat stroke tends to occur after several days of exercising in a hot environment.[7]

The presence or absence of thirst is a way of determining whether a heat illness is caused by water deprivation or salt deprivation. People who are water depleted describe thirst. Salt-depleted individuals have no such craving. Heat exhaustion caused by salt depletion is not resolved by the ingestion of plain water. Most athletic-related cases of heat exhaustion are caused by water depletion, but the two commonly occur in conjunction with each other.

Individuals suffering from heat exhaustion have a rectal temperature above 103°F and present with profuse sweating, causing the skin to feel cool and clammy. In response to cardiovascular demands, pulse and respiration are rapid, but the loss of fluids causes the pulse to feel weak and reduces the blood pressure.

The individual may complain of a headache and appear to be fatigued and confused.

Heat Stroke

A medical emergency, heat stroke represents the failure and subsequent shutdown of the body's thermoregulatory system. Heat stroke occurs when the body is unable to shed its excess heat into the environment, causing the core temperature to rise above 105°F. After this shutdown, the core temperature continues to increase, placing the cells of the internal organs and, most importantly, the brain, at risk. The body attempts to maintain arterial blood pressure at the expense of thermoregulation and blood flow to the skin, which is needed for cooling.[7] Subsequently, all of the body's systems begin to fail. If untreated, death can occur from heat stroke within 20 minutes.[9]

Heat stroke is classified as classic or exertional. **Classic heat stroke** most often affects infants and the elderly, occurring during a period when they are exposed to a hot environment and unable to rehydrate or cool themselves. These individuals are marked by the absence of sweat. This symptom is often, and incorrectly, correlated with **exertional heat stroke,** which most commonly affects athletes.[12]

Exertional heat stroke occurs within a matter of hours during exercise in a hot and humid environment. In this scenario, profuse sweating occurs and fluids are not replaced, depleting the body of water and electrolytes. Most athletes suffering from exertional heat stroke are sweating. Using the definition of classic heat stroke, athletes suffering from exertional heat stroke may be misevaluated because of the presence of sweating. However, exertional heat stroke may occur without significant dehydration.[7]

The athlete's probability of survival is directly related to the quick identification of heat stroke and the immediate initiation of treatment. The only practical difference between heat stroke and heat exhaustion that can be determined on the field is the athlete's mental state. Violent behavior followed by unconsciousness is a characteristic trait of heat stroke. The athlete's skin may feel hot compared with the expected finding of heat exhaustion, in which the skin tends to feel damp and cool. As brain function diminishes, the pupils become fixed and dilated and the athlete may assume a decerebrate posture (see Box 18–8). The attempt to maintain blood pressure may account for the incidence of liver and kidney failure associated with heat injuries.[2]

PREVENTION OF HEAT INJURIES

Table 19–3 presents a list of steps to reduce the incidence of athletic heat injuries and the rationale for doing so. Environmental heat conditions need to be determined before and during outdoor athletic competition. Traditionally, this has been done with the use of a sling psychrometer, a device that determines relative

Table 19–3
PREVENTION OF HEAT INJURY

Technique	Rationale
Acclimation	Improves the efficiency of muscle contraction, improves the efficiency of the cardiovascular system, lowers sweat threshold, and improves kidney function
Proper nutrition and hydration	Provides the body with the fluids and electrolytes to maintain homeostasis during exercise
Avoidance of environmental extremes	When practical, exercise in less hot or humid environments to maximize heat transfer from the body
Wearing appropriate clothing	Allows evaporation of perspiration to promote heat loss from the body when appropriate clothing is worn; therefore, full pads practices should not be conducted in extreme heat or humidity
Rest periods	Allows recovery and rehydration for athletes; includes activities such as cooling off in a cool area, consuming fluids, and allowing uniform changes during breaks

humidity through the temperatures derived from a dry thermometer and a wet one. The wet bulb temperature alone is often sufficient information to indicate the need to modify the activity. Practice should be suspended when the wet bulb temperature exceeds 82°F.[13] The temperature and humidity can also be obtained from local radio stations or dial-in weather services, but these reports may not accurately depict local weather conditions. High temperature and humidity require that the activity be modified accordingly (Table 19–4).

In regions where the temperature is normally hot and humid, practices should be regularly scheduled to avoid environmental extremes. However, in many regions, the summer months may be predominated by these conditions.[14] Altering the duration and intensity of the activity is also useful in preventing hyperthermia. Longer events performed at a slower pace have less risk of heat injury than do shorter, more intense activities held in the same environmental conditions.[15]

During two-a-day practices, the proportion of body weight lost because of dehydration can be calculated through the use of weight charts (Fig. 19–3). Athletes record their weight before and after each practice, with the percentage of body weight lost determining the risk of complications caused by the heat. Athletes who lose 3 percent of their weight from the start of one practice to the start of the next require continuous monitoring during practice. In addition, they are required to consume water frequently. Athletes displaying a 5 percent weight loss should be prohibited from practice. Those having a 7 percent drop in weight are in extreme danger and should be withheld from participation until the weight loss is reduced to 3 percent (see the following section on rehydration).

Table 19–4
GUIDELINES FOR MODIFICATION OF ATHLETIC COMPETITION IN HOT OR HUMID ENVIRONMENTS

Dry Bulb Temperature, °F	Wet Bulb Temperature, °F	Humidity, %	Consequences
80 to 90	68	<70	No extraordinary precautions are required for athletes not predisposed to heat injury. Athletes who are predisposed (e.g., unconditioned, unacclimated, or losing more than 3% of body weight from water loss) require close observation.
80 to 90 90 to 100	69 to 79	>70 <70	Regular rest breaks are necessary. Loose, breathable clothing should be worn, and wet uniforms require regular changing.
90 to 100 >100	>80	>70	Practice should be shortened and modified. The use of protective equipment covering the body should be curtailed.
	>82		Practice should be canceled

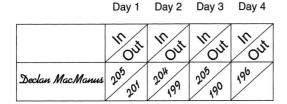

	Day 1	Day 2	Day 3	Day 4
Declan MacManus	In 205 / Out 201	In 204 / Out 199	In 205 / Out 190	In 196 / Out

FIGURE 19–3. Weight chart. Each athlete weighs "in" before practice and weighs "out" afterward. In the example, the athlete should have been restricted from practice on day 4 because of a 5 percent loss of body weight.

Sports gear made of substances that completely isolate the body from the external environment, such as neoprene or rubber, creates an environment with a temperature equal to or greater than the core temperature. Subsequent sweating raises the relative humidity within the suit to levels nearing 100 percent, actually predisposing the athlete to heat injury.

Athletes should report to practice physically fit and acclimated to the environment in which they will be competing. Athletes who have trained in a cool, dry environment are still predisposed to heat injury when moving to hot, humid areas.

Rehydration

Most heat-related injuries can be prevented by keeping athletes properly hydrated before, during, and after the activity (Table 19–5).[1] Proper hydration assists in heat dissipation by increasing blood flow to the skin and increasing the sweating rate, keeping the core temperature relatively low. Maintaining a proper fluid balance

maintains the central blood volume that sustains cardiac output and prevents plasma *hypertonicity*.[7]

The goal of pre-exercise hydration is to preload the body with fluid stores. During activity, the goal of hydration is to prevent the athlete from losing more than 2 percent of the body weight through water loss. Athletes are encouraged to drink beyond their thirst level at a rate of approximately 7 to 10 fluid oz every 10 to 20 minutes. After activity, athletes must be encouraged to consume fluids at a rate that is approximately 25 to 50 percent beyond that lost through sweating and urination. Ideally, water, carbohydrates, and electrolytes should be replenished within 2 hours after the activity.[1]

Simply ingesting fluids does not necessarily mean that the athlete will be rehydrated. Factors including the type, amount (volume), and *osmolality* of the fluid affect the body's ability to absorb—and therefore use—the fluid. After exiting the stomach, fluids are absorbed in the small intestine. The volume of the fluid must be large enough to trigger gastric emptying.[7] Often, the volume and osmolality of water consumption after exercise is not sufficient to rehydrate the body. Plain water, especially in small amounts, decreases osmolality, which limits the thirst response and increases urinary output. Including carbohydrates in the fluid increases the rate of intestinal absorption; the addition of a small amount of sodium may increase the thirst response.[7]

The use of carbohydrate drinks before exercise can assist in increasing glycogen stores. For maximum benefit, these drinks should contain a 6 percent concentration of carbohydrates. Carbohydrate concentrations above 8 percent can reduce gastric emptying and slow the absorption of fluids from the intestines.[1,16]

COLD INJURIES

Athletes who are competing outdoors in cold, damp environments are most predisposed to hypothermia. Indoor activities, except under the most unusual circumstances, do not normally predispose the athlete to cold injury. An exception to this is prolonged activity in a very cold swimming pool.

Hypothermia

Systemic cooling of the body, hypothermia, results from exposure to cold, damp air or immersion in cold water. The onset of hypothermia is not limited to subfreezing conditions. The body's core temperature begins to

Table 19–5 **REHYDRATION STRATEGIES**	
Strategy	**Comments**
Pre-exercise hydration	Two to three hours before competition: Consume 500 to 600 mL (17 to 20 fl oz) of water or sports drink Ten to twenty minutes before competition: Consume 200 to 300 mL (7 to 10 fl oz) of water or sports drink
Hydration maintenance	Every 10 to 20 minutes: Consume 200 to 300 mL (7 to 10 fl oz) of water or sports drink Prevent the athlete from losing more than 2% of body weight through water loss
Postexercise hydration	Within 2 hours: Replace water, carbohydrates, and electrolytes lost during activity

Hypertonic (hypertonicity) Having an increased osmotic pressure relative to the body's other fluids.

Osmolality A substance's concentration in a fluid affecting its tendency to cross a membrane (osmosis).

Table 19–6
EVALUATIVE FINDINGS: Hypothermia

Segment	Finding	
Onset	Gradual	
	A cold, damp windy environment predisposes athletes to hypothermia	
Pupils	Dilated in severe hypothermia	
Pulse	Slow and weak	
Blood pressure	Hypotension	
Respiration	Shallow and irregular	
Muscular function	*Slight:*	Shivering
	Mild:	Motor impairment
	Severe:	Extreme motor impairment followed by muscle rigidity
Mental status	*Slight:*	The athlete's mental focus begins to drift from the task at hand
	Mild:	Desire to warm up
	Severe:	Desire to sleep

decrease when the ambient temperature is less than the body temperature and influenced by other environmental conditions such as wind and water. Clothing that has become wet from rain, snow, perspiration, or other means conducts heat away from the core, increasing the risk of hypothermia.

After the core temperature drops below 95°F, shivering, the first sign of hypothermia, appears, providing a short-term source of heat by increasing the body's metabolism. Impairment of the body's regulatory systems occurs when the core temperature drops below 94°F, predisposing the individual to cardiac irregularities and impairing the heart's responsiveness to treatment.[17,18] A decreased cardiac stroke volume and an increased blood viscosity reduce the amount of blood reaching the brain, resulting in impaired mental function.

Cooling of the brain stem depresses the respiratory rate, resulting in body-wide anoxia. Systemic metabolism decreases, resulting in decreased metabolic heat production and further lowering of the core temperature. As the temperature continues to decrease, kidney function is impaired, disrupting the body's electrolyte balance.[17]

A core temperature between 90°F and 94°F is classified as **mild hypothermia.** Initially, the athlete complains of feeling cold, and the shivering response is initiated. Interest in the activity at hand wanes and is replaced by the desire to warm up. Signs of motor and mental impairment are indicated by decreased athletic performance. **Severe hypothermia,** a potentially fatal condition, results when the core temperature drops below 90°F. The athlete's desire to warm up is overrid-

den by the desire to sleep, causing the athlete to appear uncoordinated and have slurred speech. An examination of the vital signs reveals decreased heart rate, respiration, and blood pressure (Table 19–6).

Frostbite

Unlike hypothermia, frostbite occurs only when the body is exposed to subfreezing temperatures. In response to this environment, the body protects the integrity of the core temperature at the expense of blood flow to the extremities, with the toes and fingers being the most vulnerable sites. During competition, the nose and cheeks are often uncovered, increasing the possibility of frostbite's striking these areas. The freezing of the ECFs results in hypertonicity, dehydrating the cells by drawing the fluids out from the cell membrane via osmosis, an event that is more damaging than the actual extracellular ice formation.[19] However, ice forming within the cell results in the permanent disruption of the cell membrane.

The magnitude and rate of nerve transmission is reduced when the nerves are cooled. This interruption makes the athlete initially unaware of the potential damage to the skin. As the freezing progresses, the athlete experiences a cold, burning sensation that suddenly ceases and is replaced by a sensation of comfortable warmth, a warning sign of severe frostbite.

Frostbite occurs through progressing degrees of severity, based on the depth of tissues affected, with one stage preceding the next. Superficial frostbite affects only the outermost layer of skin and initially ap-

Table 19–7
CALCULATION OF THE WIND CHILL FACTOR

Wind Speed, MPH	Actual Thermometer Reading °F											
	50	40	30	20	10	0	−10	−20	−30	−40	−50	−60
	Wind Chill Factor °F											
Calm	50	40	30	20	10	0	−10	−20	−30	−40	−50	−60
5	48	37	27	16	6	25	−15	−26	−36	−47	−57	−68
10	40	28	16	4	−9	−24	−33	−46	−58	−70	−83	−95
15	36	22	9	−5	−18	−32	−45	−58	−72	−85	−99	−112
20	32	18	4	−10	−25	−39	−53	−67	−82	−96	−110	−124
25	30	16	0	−15	−29	−44	−59	−74	−88	−104	−118	−133
30	28	13	−2	−18	−33	−48	−63	−79	−94	−109	−125	−140
35	27	11	−4	−20	−35	−51	−67	−82	−98	−113	−129	−145
40	26	10	−6	−21	−37	−53	−69	−85	−100	−116	−132	−148
	Little danger				**Moderate danger**			**Extreme danger**				
					Skin freezes within 1 min			Skin freezes rapidly (< 1 min)				

pears with *hyperemia* and the development of edema within 3 hours. The superficial layer of skin *sloughs* within 1 week after the injury.

Deep frostbite initially presents with the same signs and symptoms of superficial frostbite. However, destruction of the skin's full thickness occurs. Blisters appear in 1 to 7 days. This tissue sloughs to expose a hard, black layer of tissue. Disruption of the blood supply to the affected body part and distal structures creates an environment that encourages the development of *gangrene*. The most severe cases of frostbite involve the total destruction of the tissues in the area, including bone.

PREVENTION OF COLD INJURIES

Common sense is the guide in preventing cold injuries. Environmental conditions are a combination of ambient air temperature and wind. **Wind chill** can quickly lower the air temperature equivalent to dangerously low levels capable of freezing the skin in a matter of minutes or even seconds (Table 19–7). In extremely cold temperatures, the athlete's skin should be covered as completely as possible and practical for the sport. Multiple layers of clothing provide better insulation from the external environment than a single layer (Table 19–8).

The athlete's diet may be a factor contributing to the onset or prevention of hypothermia.[20] High-protein diets must be avoided by individuals who face prolonged exposure to subfreezing environments. Compared with diets high in carbohydrates or fats, those that are high in protein increase an individual's metabolic water requirements, thus decreasing their tolerance to cold.

Hyperemia A red discoloration of the skin caused by an increased capillary blood flow.

Slough The peeling away of dead skin from living tissue.

Gangrene The death of bony or soft tissue resulting from a decrease in, or loss of, blood supply to a body area.

Table 19–8
NATIONAL COLLEGIATE ATHLETIC ASSOCIATION'S RECOMMENDED GUIDELINES FOR REDUCING COLD STRESS

Guideline	Comments
Layering clothing	Several thin layers of clothing are best to retain body heat; layers may be added or removed as needed
Covering the head	As much as 50% of the body's heat is lost through the head.
Protecting the hands	The use of mittens rather than gloves is recommended to protect the fingers from frostbite.
Staying dry	Water increases the rate of heat loss from the body. Rather than wearing clothes made of cotton, wearing those made of polypropylene, wool, or other material that wicks moisture away from the skin is recommended.
Staying hydrated	Fluids are needed to maintain the body's core temperature and are as important in preventing cold injuries as heat injuries.
Maintaining energy level	A negative energy balance increases the risk of hypothermia. Proper eating and consuming "energy snacks" and sports drinks helps maintain a positive energy balance.
Warming up thoroughly	A thorough warm-up is required before competition to elevate the core temperature.
Warming incoming air	The use of a scarf or mask across the mouth warms incoming air.
Avoiding alcohol, nicotine, and other drugs	These agents cause vasoconstriction or vasodilation of the superficial blood vessels, hindering regulation of the core temperature.
Never training alone	An injury that prevents the athlete from walking may be catastrophic in cold climates.

ON-FIELD EVALUATION AND MANAGEMENT OF ENVIRONMENTAL INJURIES

The premise for initial management of environmental injuries is to reverse the environmental extreme in which the athlete has been participating and return the core temperature to its normal range. Quick recognition, a rapid response, and transportation to a hospital are often necessary to keep the athlete alive.

HEAT INJURIES

The management of patients with all types of heat injuries requires rehydrating the athlete with cool water. Electrolytes, especially salt, often need to be replaced, but the use of salt tablets should be avoided because of their potentially counterproductive effects.[8] Dehydration, the root cause of many forms of heat injury, presents with a common set of symptoms (Table 19–9).[1]

Salt tablets delay gastric emptying and, if insufficient water is provided, fluids may be drawn from the extracellular space, causing further dehydration. Additionally, salt tablets are often poorly tolerated, irritating the stomach lining and possibly resulting in nausea and vomiting. The use of commercial electrolyte drinks before, during, and after competition may be an effective method of reducing heat injuries. However, drinking water should not be neglected.

Heat Cramps

Heat cramps are managed by controlling the symptoms and replacing fluids and electrolytes. While the athlete is on the field, the cramping muscle or muscles should be stretched until the spasm subsides (Fig. 19–4). After the athlete is returned to the sidelines, ice packs are applied to the involved area and the athlete's fluids and electrolytes are replenished. The athlete may return to competition after the symptoms have cleared and he or she has been rehydrated. These individuals should be frequently encouraged to consume fluids.

Table 19–9
SIGNS AND SYMPTOMS OF DEHYDRATION

Initial stages	Thirst
	Irritability
	General discomfort
Late stages	Headache
	Weakness
	Dizziness
	Cramps
	Chills
	Vomiting
	Nausea
	Decreased performance

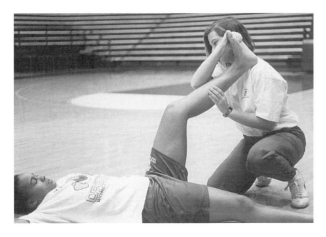

FIGURE 19–4. Treatment of heat cramp spasms by stretching the involved muscle group

Heat Exhaustion and Heat Stroke

The treatment goals for athletes suffering from heat exhaustion or heat stroke are to reduce the core temperature and replace fluids and electrolytes. In each case, **first aid cooling** must be initiated by moving the athlete from the hot environment to a shaded area or indoors; removing excess clothing; elevating the legs; and cooling the body through the use of ice packs, ice immersion, or fan-sprayed mist.

Patients with heat exhaustion can usually be adequately managed by applying ice packs to the superficial arteries located at the lateral neck, axilla, groin, and popliteal fossa (Fig. 19–5). A fan-sprayed mist has been used not only to treat but also to prevent heat injuries. These devices, often seen on football sidelines, spray a cool mist on the athlete to reduce the core temperature. However, their efficacy is questionable.[7] A cold shower

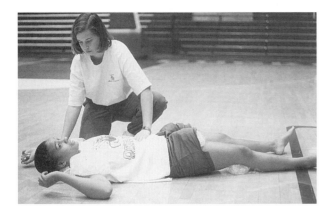

FIGURE 19–5. Emergency cooling of an athlete suffering from heat injury. Packing the areas in which arteries are relatively subcutaneous (i.e., the popliteal fossa, femoral triangle, axilla, and neck) serves to cool the core temperature.

is also an efficient method of reducing the core temperature, but the athlete should not be permitted to enter the shower unescorted.

Although ice packs may be used during the treatment of heat stroke, the ideal method of management of patients with this condition involves immersing the athlete in 8 to 10 inches of cold water with a temperature at or below 55°F.[13,21] A shallow animal watering trough or child's swimming pool filled with water and ice can be used for this purpose, but the use of deep whirlpools should be avoided because of the inherent risk of drowning. To prevent overcooling, the patient is removed from the cooling tub when the core temperature decreases to 102°F.[21]

If the athlete is conscious and cooperative, copious amounts of fluids are administered. In extreme cases of heat stroke, the physician orders *Ringer's lactate* to be administered intravenously. If the athlete's symptoms do not subside or if heat stroke is suspected, he or she must be immediately transported to the hospital because of the potentially fatal consequences.

COLD INJURIES

As with heat injuries, the management of patients with cold injuries involves removing the athlete from the insulting environment. In this case, the athlete must be placed in a warm, dry environment, allowing the body to return to its normal temperature.

Hypothermia

After the athlete has been placed in a warm environment, the wet clothing is removed and the body is dried. Then the athlete is dressed in dry clothing or wrapped in a blanket.

Techniques to rapidly rewarm the body, such as immersion in a hot bath, must be avoided. Rapid rewarming dilates the peripheral vessels, causing lactic acid to be routed to the core. This leads to rebound hypothermia, which can cause a further decrease in core temperature secondary to hypotension and ventricular fibrillation.[18] Athletes should not be allowed to sleep. Doing so decreases metabolism and delays rewarming of the core temperature. Warm drinks are not effective in raising the core temperature, and the use of alcoholic drinks must be avoided because of their depressant effects. The core may be quickly and safely rewarmed by having the athlete breathe in the mist of a humidifier or other source of hot, moist air.[22] Blankets, clothing, and so on can also be used to gently warm the individual.

Ringer's lactate A salt-based solution administered intravenously as a replacement for lost electrolytes.

Frostbite

Initially, frostbite can be limited by the athlete's keeping the affected body part moving, increasing the amount of metabolic heat production. When the athlete is still in the cold environment, frostbite of the fingers can be treated by the athlete's tucking the fingers in the axilla or crotch.[23] Once off the field, mild frostbite can be treated by immersing the body part in a warm (104°F to 110°F) bath. The affected area should never be rubbed and snow should not be applied.

Body parts with more significant frostbite should not be thawed if the risk of refreezing exists. After the frozen part thaws, the athlete must not be allowed to walk on or use the affected part. If the athlete is still in the cold environment, steps must be taken to prevent hypothermia. Athletes suspected of suffering from frostbite must be immediately referred to a hospital so that a definitive diagnosis may be made and proper treatment initiated.

 REFERENCES

1. Casa, DJ, et al: National Athletic Trainers' Association Position Statement: Fluid replacement for athletes. *Journal of Athletic Training*, 35:212, 2000.
2. Hubbard, RW, and Armstrong, LE: Hyperthermia: New thoughts on an old problem. *The Physician and Sportsmedicine*, 17:97, 1989.
3. Sheehy, SB: Environmental emergencies. In Sheehy, SB (ed): *Mosby's Manual of Emergency Care* (ed 3). St Louis, CV Mosby, 1990, p 300.
4. Davidson, M: Heat illness in athletics. *Athletic Training: Journal of the National Athletic Trainers Association*, 20:96, 1985.
5. Gonzalez-Alonso, J: Separate and combined influences of dehydration and hyperthermia on cardiovascular response to exercise. *Int J Sports Med*, 2(S):111, 1998.
6. Spence, AP, and Mason, EB: Metabolism, nutrition, and temperature regulation. In Spence, AP, and Mason, EB (eds): *Human Anatomy and Physiology* (ed 3). Menlo Park, CA, Benjamin/Cummings, 1987, p 754.
7. Casa, DJ: Exercise in the heat. II. Critical concepts in rehydration, exertional heat illness, and maximizing performance. *Journal of Athletic Training*, 34:253, 1999.
8. Birrer, RB: Heat stroke. Don't wait for the classic signs. *Emerg Med Clin North Am*, July:43, 1994.
9. Murphy, RJ: Heat illness in the athlete. *Athletic Training: Journal of the National Athletic Trainers Association*, 19:166, 1984.
10. Noakes, TD: Fluid and electrolyte disturbances in heat illness. *Int J Sports Med*, 2(S):146, 1998.
11. Schwellnus, MP: Skeletal muscle cramps during exercise. *Physician and Sportsmedicine*, 27:109, 1999.
12. Roberts, WO: Emergencies in sports. Managing heat stroke: On-site cooling. *The Physician and Sportsmedicine*, 20:17, 1992.
13. American College of Sports Medicine: Position stand on prevention of thermal injuries during distance running. *Med Sci Sports Exerc*, 16:ix, 1984.
14. Francis, K, Feinstein, R, and Brasher, J: Optimal practice times for the reduction of the risk of heat illness during fall football practice in the southeastern United States. *Athletic Training: Journal of the National Athletic Trainers Association*, 26:76, 1991.
15. Noakes, TD, et al: Metabolic rate, not percent dehydration, predicts rectal temperatures in marathon runners. *Med Sci Sports Exerc*, 23:443, 1991.
16. Potts, KA and Dick, RW: NCAA *Sports Medicine Handbook* (ed 13). Indianapolis, IN, National Collegiate Athletic Association, 2000.
17. Nelson, WE-Gieck, JH, and Kolb, P: Treatment and prevention of hypothermia and frostbite. *Athletic Training: Journal of the National Athletic Trainers Association*, 18:330, 1983.
18. Robinson, WA: Emergencies in sports. Competing with the cold. Part II: Hypothermia. *The Physician and Sportsmedicine*, 20:61, 1992.
19. Frey, C: Frostbitten feet. Steps to treatment and prevention. *The Physician and Sportsmedicine*, 20:67, 1992.
20. Askew, EW: Nutrition for a cold environment. *The Physician and Sportsmedicine*, 17:77, 1989.
21. Roberts, WO: Tub cooling for exertional heatstroke. *The Physician and Sportsmedicine*, 26:111, 1998.
22. Bowman, WD: Outdoor emergency care: *Comprehensive First Aid of Nonurban Settings*. Lakewood, CO, National Ski Patrol System, 1988, p 291.
23. Steele, P: Management of frostbite. *The Physician and Sportsmedicine*, 17:135, 1989.

20 Cardiopulmonary Conditions

Respiratory and cardiovascular injuries and illnesses are relatively rare in athletes. However, fatal episodes do occur, attracting a great deal of attention, especially when young, seemingly healthy individuals are stricken. Athletic trainers must be aware of the subtle early signs and symptoms, which may normally go unnoticed. However, recognizing them is essential to avert disaster. After an episode occurs, a swift but thorough evaluation and response must be made because the athlete's life is in imminent danger.

Although most athletic trainers and team physicians will never be faced with a life and death situation involving the cardiopulmonary system, many times they will be faced with managing the medical care of athletes with preexisting cardiac conditions.[1] Advances in the evaluation and medical management of cardiopulmonary conditions now allow individuals who would have once been withheld from exercise and competition to now compete. These advances include college students participating in intercollegiate athletics after heart transplantation.[2] The medical community has embraced exercise as a vital component of prevention and rehabilitation of these conditions.

All coaches, facilities coordinators, and other individuals who supervise athletic activities should maintain certification in cardiopulmonary resuscitation (CPR). In addition to standard CPR certification, athletic trainers should explore the feasibility of additional certification as an emergency medical technician (EMT), paramedic, or in the use of an Automated External Defibrillator (AED).

◆ CLINICAL ANATOMY

The heart and major vessels of the cardiovascular system lie within the mediastinum, between the lungs, from the first rib superiorly to the diaphragm inferiorly. The heart is lined by the fibrous and serous pericardium. The **fibrous pericardium** is the tough fibrous outer layer supporting the inner pericardial layer and the heart. The **serous pericardium** is further divided into a **parietal layer** lining the fibrous pericardium and

a **visceral layer** that sits tightly against the heart. The serous pericardium allows the heart to move freely within the chest and buffers forces to the heart.

The heart is a four-chambered muscular pump that delivers oxygenated blood to the tissues of the body. In the bloodstream, oxygen is exchanged for carbon dioxide, which is then returned to the lungs, where it is subsequently exhaled. The rate at which the heart beats is normally based on the metabolic needs of the body. The heart rate should increase to meet the metabolic demands of an exercising athlete.

The contraction of the cardiac musculature is controlled by an electrical system within the walls of the heart's chambers. This system allows for the synchronous contraction of the atria and ventricles, ensuring a smooth flow of blood through the cardiovascular system. Any disruption of the normal pattern of the heart's electrical stimulus can cause failure of the heart, potentially leading to death.

The **right atrium** of the heart receives deoxygenated blood from the head, neck, and upper extremities by way of the **superior vena cava.** The **inferior vena cava** delivers the deoxygenated blood from the trunk and lower extremities. As the right atrium contracts, the blood passes through the **tricuspid valve** and into the **right ventricle.** Contraction of the right ventricle causes the blood to pass through the **semilunar valves** into the **pulmonary arteries** and to the lungs, where it is oxygenated.

The newly oxygenated blood returns via the **pulmonary veins** into the **left atrium.** From the left atrium, the blood is passed through the **mitral valve** into the **left ventricle,** which contracts to distribute the blood to the body. As the left ventricle contracts, the blood is pushed out the **semilunar valves** and into the aorta. The left ventricle contains the greatest amount of cardiac muscle because it must provide the force needed to propel the blood throughout the body.

The valves of the heart all function as one-way valves (Fig. 20–1). The tricuspid and mitral valves are held tightly shut against the backflow of blood by the **chordinae tendinae** that are attached to **papillary muscles.**

667

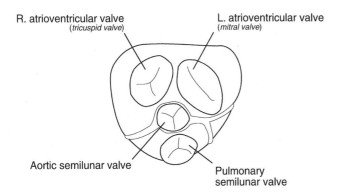

R. atrioventricular valve
(*tricuspid valve*)

L. atrioventricular valve
(*mitral valve*)

Aortic semilunar valve

Pulmonary
semilunar valve

FIGURE 20–1. Valves controlling blood entering and exiting the heart.

The muscles and cordinae tendinae mechanically prevent the valve from opening in the wrong direction. The semilunar valves contain no papillary muscles, relying on their mechanical shape to prevent reflux of blood. The backflow of blood causes the valves to form pockets that fill and shut tightly together.

Normally the heart makes "lubb" and "dupp" sounds as the valves open and close, respectively. Any reflux of blood through a faulty or leaking valve causes a decrease in the heart's ability to efficiently deliver the needed metabolites to the tissues of the body and alters the characteristic heart sounds (Table 20–1).

The structure and function of the lungs are described in Chapter 12.

 ## CLINICAL EVALUATION OF CARDIOPULMONARY INJURIES

Evaluation of athletes with cardiopulmonary injury and illness must be accomplished quickly and efficiently. Often the evaluation must be halted and man-

agement of the problem initiated before the examiner has a full understanding of the cause of the athlete's condition. After cardiopulmonary distress is recognized, the proper lifesaving techniques must be the first priority.

This chapter covers the evaluation of cardiac conditions and nontraumatic pulmonary injuries. The evaluation of traumatic pulmonary injuries such as pneumothorax and airway obstruction is covered in Chapter 12.

HISTORY

Athletes suffering catastrophic cardiovascular injuries usually have some unrecognized or unreported history of previous symptoms or have a family history of similar problems. Careful preparticipation screening may help to increase the awareness of symptoms, yet many other symptoms may go unrecognized. Table 20–2 describes the pertinent information to be obtained and recorded in the athlete's medical file and subsequently used to assist in identifying athletes who are potentially high-risk candidates for cardiopulmonary distress.[3]

Unfortunately, if the cardiopulmonary illness or injury is not recognized early, the results can be catastrophic. Sudden death can occur from a variety of cardiopulmonary conditions in athletes of all ages. Even when the signs and symptoms are quickly recognized, the athlete's life often cannot be saved without the use of advanced life support measures, which are often not standard equipment at the site of competition. Any report of symptoms, either related or unrelated to physical activity, warrants the referral of the athlete for a complete evaluation by a physician (Table 20–3).

Location of the Pain

Cardiac dysfunction results in intense pain, tightness, or squeezing in the center of the chest. Other signs of

Table 20–1 **HEART SOUNDS**		
Sound	**Status**	**Interpretation**
"Lubb"	Normal systole	Ventricular contraction; synchronous with the carotid pulse
"Dupp"	Normal diastole	Closure of the aortic and pulmonary valves
Soft, blowing "lubb"	Abnormal systole	Associated with anemia or other changes in blood constituents
Loud, booming "lubb"	Abnormal systole	Aneurysm
Sloshing "dupp"	Abnormal diastole	Incomplete closure of the valves; blood heard regurgitating backward
Friction sound	Abnormal	Inflammation of the heart's pericardial lining; pericarditis

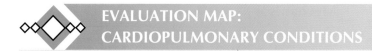

EVALUATION MAP:
CARDIOPULMONARY CONDITIONS

1. HISTORY

Location of the pain
Current symptoms
Prior symptoms
Onset
Mechanism

2. INSPECTION AND PALPATION

Unconscious Athlete
Airway
Breathing

Bradypnea
Tachypnea
Circulation

Conscious Athlete
Position of the athlete
Skin color
Airway
Breathing
Circulation
Sweating
Responsiveness
Nausea and vomiting

3. VITAL SIGNS

Pulse
Blood pressure
Respiration

4. SPECIAL TESTS

Peak flow meter

Table 20–2
CARDIOPULMONARY CHECKLIST FOR THE ATHLETE'S MEDICAL FILE

Family History	Personal History	General Information	Orthopedic Conditions
Episodes of syncope, dyspnea, or chest pain	Episodes of syncope or near syncope, dyspnea, or chest pain	Height	Elongated appendages
Premature atherosclerosis	Excessive, unexplained	Weight	Severe kyphoscoliosis
Seizures	shortness of breath or	Vital signs	Unsteady or irregular gait
Sudden death of a family	fatigue with exercise	Heart examination	Abnormal joint laxity
member who was younger	History of heart murmur	Lung examination	Club-shaped fingernails
than age 50 years	of hypertension	Dislocation of the	
Occurrence in family of	Premature atherosclerosis	optic lens	
hypertrophic cardiomyopathy,	Seizures		
dilated myopathy, long			
QT syndrome or Marfans			
syndrome			

Table 20–3
SIGNS AND SYMPTOMS OF CARDIOPULMONARY CONDITIONS

Cardiovascular	Both	Pulmonary
Panic	Chest pain	Congestion
Dizziness	Respiratory distress	Wheezing
Nausea		Fatigue
Vomiting		Anxiety
Sweating		Tingling in fingers and toes
Decreased blood pressure		Spasm in fingers and toes
Distended jugular vein		Periorbital numbness
Pallor		Pain in mid and upper posterior thorax
Clutching at chest		
Shoulder pain		
Epigastric pain		

ischemia to the cardiac tissues are manifested as referred pain into the left shoulder, arm, jaw, or epigastric area (see Fig. 12–15).

Pulmonary problems include difficulty with respiration, or pain, or both. The difficulty in breathing may cause the athlete to panic. Although pain may occur secondary to pulmonary obstruction, these problems are typically recognized by the shear labor required for the athlete to breathe. Excruciating, deep thoracic pain that develops in the middle and upper back is the most distinctive early sign of developing an aortic aneurysm, the typical cause of death associated with **Marfan syndrome** (see Chapter 21).[4,5]

Current Symptoms

Along with the intense chest pain and pressure associated with the ischemia of the cardiac musculature, the athlete may complain of dizziness, nausea, vomiting, and feeling faint. Although profuse sweating is a typical sign of cardiac arrest, this sign is often difficult to assess in an athlete who has been performing vigorous physical activity. Other symptoms of cardiac disorders that may be reported by the athlete include shortness of breath, lightheadedness, and fatigue. Disorders of the heart's electrical system may cause the sensation of the heart's skipping beats or racing abnormally fast. Syncope, a sudden transient loss of consciousness, is commonly related to a cardiac arrhythmia, often occurring with previously mentioned symptoms of cardiac distress.

Complaints related to pulmonary problems include chest congestion, fatigue, and minor difficulty in breathing before the onset of the traumatic respiratory problem. Otherwise, the athlete exhibits labored breathing, characterized by a quick wheezing breathing pattern, often accompanied by unusual sounds.

Prior Symptoms

Any previous episodes of symptoms associated with cardiopulmonary abnormalities recognized by the athlete should be noted and recorded in the athlete's medical record. Often athletes are reluctant to report a previous history of cardiopulmonary difficulties for fear of being disqualified from competition. Any individual with a history of cardiopulmonary symptoms should be examined by a physician before being allowed to participate because this history may be the only finding before sudden death.

Onset

Cardiopulmonary illness in athletes is usually congenital or acquired gradually over time, usually manifested as previously unrecognized conditions resulting in an acute climax of cardiopulmonary distress. Certain *arrhythmias* may be caused by a traumatic incident.

Mechanism

The mechanisms underlying the development of cardiopulmonary conditions are not fully understood, but a strong link exists between the onset of these problems and a family history of these conditions. The most common underlying condition leading to the onset of cardiac problems in middle-aged and older athletes is *atherosclerosis* of the cardiac arteries, leading to ischemia in the cardiac tissues. The mechanism for atherosclerosis is not fully understood but is associated with several risk factors, including family history, smoking, hypertension, decreased activity, obesity, high cholesterol levels, and even normal progressive changes caused by aging.

Pulmonary diseases once precluded a person from participating in sports, but with the advent of improved medications and treatment techniques, patients with pulmonary conditions such as cystic fibrosis and asthma are now participating in organized sports. Although the direct mechanism for pulmonary problems in athletes is the actual obstruction of the airway owing to mucus buildup or bronchospasm, underlying contributing causes are now being studied.

The incidence of **exercise-induced asthma** is seemingly on the rise. One explanation for this rise in frequency is increasingly poor air quality, especially in urban areas. The poor air quality triggers bronchospasm. Another school of thought relates increased cases of exercise-induced asthma to an increasing number of participants in athletic activities. As people become involved in exercise, the mechanism for triggering their asthma is induced. To determine causes of exercise-induced asthma, especially those leading to fatalities among athletes, the National Athletic Asthma Registry has been established at Temple University Hospital in Philadelphia.

INSPECTION AND PALPATION

The athlete suffering from cardiopulmonary problems undergoes inspection while being questioned about his or her complaints. In the case of an unconscious athlete, the examiner must always follow standard first-responder procedures, checking the airway, breathing, and circulation before any other assessment. In either case, the examiner must be prepared to perform lifesaving procedures if the athlete's condition warrants it. The examiner must use prudent decision making in a quick, precise fashion if the athlete is to have an optimal chance of survival.

Arrhythmia Loss of the normal heart rhythm; an irregular heart rate.

Atherosclerosis The buildup of fatty tissues on the inner arterial walls.

Because the athlete with a cardiopulmonary condition must be assessed quickly, the inspection and pertinent palpation that goes along with the inspection are covered together, just as they are carried out together during this type of evaluation.

Inspection and Palpation of the Unconscious Athlete

- **Airway:** The first area to be inspected in the unconscious athlete is the integrity of the airway. Before checking the airway, however, the cervical spine is stabilized in a neutral position if there is any possibility of head or neck injury (see Chapter 18). If the athlete is wearing a mouthpiece, it must be removed. The examiner then looks, listens, and feels for air being expired and observes for the rise and fall of the chest (see Fig. 18–6).
- **Breathing:** From the position used to inspect for a functional airway, the examiner assesses the breathing pattern and rate. A rate of fewer than 10 **(bradypnea)** or greater than 30 breaths per minute **(tachypnea)** requires assisted ventilation by properly trained personnel.[6] A labored, quick breathing pattern **(dyspnea)** is usually associated with some type of airway obstruction. Athletes with underlying pulmonary disease such as asthma or cystic fibrosis have labored breathing from obstruction by bronchospasm or excessive mucus formation. Athletes suffering from cardiac conditions may have difficulty breathing because of pain, but breathing is usually not as labored in these athletes as it is in those with pulmonary disorders.
- **Circulation:** The status of the circulation and thus the heart rate is assessed primarily by taking the pulse. While checking the airway and breathing, the examiner palpates for the carotid pulse. The method for palpating this pulse and the assessment of the findings are found in Chapter 10.

Inspection and Palpation of the Conscious Athlete

- **Position of the athlete:** The athlete with cardiac problems will most likely be clutching the chest, possibly bending over in pain. The athlete with a pulmonary problem may be bent over with hands on the knees so that the secondary muscles of respiration may be used to aid breathing. By putting the hands in a closed chain position, the sternocleidomastoid and pectoral muscles can aid in expanding the chest wall. In labored breathing, these muscles may be observed to be contracting forcefully. The athlete may recruit the secondary muscles of respiration by sitting with the elbows on the knees and the head hanging between the legs.
- **Skin color:** The color of the athlete's skin is normally flushed because of exercise. Cardiopulmonary distress results in pale or ashen skin. First appearing in the lips, the discoloration progresses to cyanosis as the skin's tissues are deprived of oxygen. An unexpected change in skin tone or color from that which is normally associated with exercise should be a "red flag" for the examiner.
- **Airway:** The fact that an athlete is conscious does not rule out an airway obstruction, but the athlete's ability to speak indicates a viable airway. It should be established that the athlete has not swallowed any part of the mouthpiece, food, or other material, by direct inspection and by simply asking the athlete if he or she has swallowed anything.
- **Breathing:** The breathing pattern is established for the conscious athlete suspected of having a cardiopulmonary problem. The method of establishing the rate and pattern of respiration is covered in Chapter 10.
- **Circulation:** Although it is obvious that the conscious athlete's heart is beating, circulation must be assessed for rate and quality at the carotid pulse, as outlined in Chapter 10. The pulse should be frequently monitored and should return to normal levels within 5 minutes after cessation of the activity. A pulse rate that remains elevated may indicate underlying cardiac pathology.
- **Sweating:** Anyone suffering from cardiac problems may perspire profusely. However, the athlete involved in vigorous physical activity normally exhibits perspiration as a result of the activity. In the absence of physical activity, complaints of chest pain and profuse sweating are classic symptoms of cardiac distress.
- **Responsiveness:** In general, the athlete suffering from a cardiac condition becomes lethargic and weak. Many conditions of the heart decrease left ventricular outflow, resulting in a decreased cardiac output and depriving the tissues of oxygen.[7] The athlete may also suffer from syncope, the causes of which are discussed later in this chapter.
- **Nausea and vomiting:** Acute myocardial infarction (MI) often brings about nausea and vomiting.[8]

During the assessment of a conscious athlete with symptoms of cardiopulmonary distress, deterioration in vital signs warrants immediate activation of an emergency medical system.

FUNCTIONAL TESTING

The special tests for cardiopulmonary distress are limited by the expertise of the caregiver. After it has been determined that the athlete is in acute distress, the athletic trainer becomes the provider of basic life support until assistance arrives.

The athlete's airway, breathing, and circulation must be established and appropriate actions taken if any or all of these functions are missing. Otherwise, the athlete's pulse, blood pressure, and respiration must be continuously monitored and recorded and appropriate actions must be taken in response to changes in these functions.

 ## CARDIOPULMONARY PATHOLOGIES AND RELATED SPECIAL TESTS

Unfortunately, many of the conditions predisposing athletes to cardiopulmonary distress go unnoticed or unreported until an acute attack occurs. Early identification and intervention provide the best opportunity for athletes suffering from cardiopulmonary conditions to safely participate in athletics as well as perform the activities of daily living.

SYNCOPE

Depending on its underlying cause, syncope can be an ominous sign of underlying cardiac abnormality, a symptom of heat illness, or simply a benign occurrence.[9,10] Initially, syncope may not be reported by the athlete. However, when it does occur, it should always be considered a sign warranting further assessment by a physician, particularly when it occurs during activity **(exertional syncope).** The five potential mechanisms of this event, shown in Table 20–4, are common in athletes during practice and competition. After the cause of the episode is determined, appropriate management and preventive measures against future episodes are indicated.

HYPERTROPHIC CARDIOMYOPATHY

Sudden death is a rare occurrence among athletes.[11] When an apparently healthy, active, and vibrant athlete is stricken, the results are especially devastating. The most common cause of sudden death in young athletes is hypertrophic cardiomyopathy, a condition that may not display any physical signs or symptoms.[12,13]

Hypertrophic cardiomyopathy is a condition that involves enlargement of the heart muscles without an increase in size of the heart's chambers. The ventricular septum is most often involved and becomes thickened (>15 mm) compared with that of the ventricular free wall. The left atrium and right ventricle may also be involved.[14] The enlarged muscles place an increased amount of force on an unchanged blood volume (the blood contained within the chambers), increasing the pressure on the interventricular septum and aorta. Acute failure may produce syncope, cardiac arrhythmia, or, in the most profound cases, a rupture of the septum or aorta, resulting in death.

Although the ability to evaluate and successfully treat the athlete who has suffered an acute episode is limited, the athletic trainer should be aware of the evaluative findings and predisposing factors leading to it.[15] The strongest indicator of an athlete's predisposition to sudden death is a family history of cardiovascular-related sudden death. The preparticipation examination's medical history questionnaire must be able to identify any history of cardiac-related sudden death. It should ask, "Has any family member suffered a heart attack or other heart condition?" Athletes must check off "Yes" or "No."

All "yes" answers require further investigation. A death that has occurred in a family member younger than age 50 years or during athletic activity indicates

---

Table 20–4
CAUSES OF SYNCOPE IN ATHLETES

	Vasovagal Reactions	Decreased Blood Volume	Metabolic Conditions	Cardiac Disorders	Drug Reactions
Cause	Venous dilation, increased vagal tone, and bradycardia after an anxiety-provoking event	Dehydration and electrolyte imbalance such as in heat illness Vomiting Diarrhea Prolonged fasting Hemorrhage	Hypoglycemia associated with diabetes	Arrhythmias associated with hypertrophic cardiomyopathy, atherosclerosis, or anomalous coronary arteries	Stimulant abuse; possibly masquerading as arrhythmia, dehydration, or vasovagal reactions
Signs and symptoms	Lightheadedness Dizziness Profuse sweating Nausea	Lightheadedness Dizziness Nausea Visual disturbances	Fatigue Headache Profuse sweating Trembling Slurred speech Poor coordination	Palpitations Irregular heartbeat	As associated with arrhythmia, dehydration, or vasovagal reactions

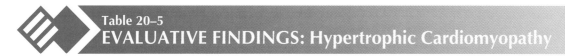

Table 20–5
EVALUATIVE FINDINGS: Hypertrophic Cardiomyopathy

Examination Segment	Clinical Findings	
History	*Onset:*	Congenital or acquired
	Pain characteristics:	Pain resembling that of a myocardial infarction
	Mechanism:	Hypertrophy of the heart's chambers, especially the left ventricle, increasing pressure on the interventricular septum and aorta
	Predisposing conditions:	Family history of cardiac sudden death. Significant heart murmur or arrhythmia; anomalous coronary circulation
Inspection	Fatigue, dizziness or exertional syncope	
Palpation	Arrhythmia during exercise	
Special Tests	Complete cardiovascular examination: electrocardiogram, ultrasound imaging, and so on	
Comments	Symptoms more likely to occur during exercise than at rest	

that the athlete should be examined and subsequently cleared for participation by a cardiologist.

A significant heart murmur or characteristics of Marfan syndrome (see Chapter 21) may also be present. In many cases of sudden death, evidence of previous arrhythmias has been documented in the athlete's history.[5,12,16] Associated congenital anomalous coronary circulation may also be discovered after the sudden death of a young athlete.[17]

Acutely, the athlete may experience excessive fatigue, exertional syncope, dizziness, dyspnea, or the sensation of chest pain and arrhythmias while exercising (Table 20–5). The symptoms of hypertrophic cardiomyopathy are more likely to occur during exercise than during rest.[16] Occasionally, these episodes occur after bouts of vigorous activity or during stoppage in play.[17]

Definitive diagnosis of this condition is complex because of the varying presence and inconsistent reporting of significant symptoms, extensive range of testing procedures, and their subsequent interpretation by cardiologists. The 16th Bethesda Conference on cardiovascular abnormalities established guidelines for competition eligibility that are often used when safe participation decisions must be made by a physician (Table 20–6).[18] Athletes displaying any of the previous symptoms should be referred to a physician for a complete medical work-up.

Table 20–6
RECOMMENDATIONS FOR ELIGIBILITY FOR EXERCISE IN ATHLETES WITH CARDIOVASCULAR DISEASE

Conditions contraindicating vigorous exercise	Acute myocarditis Congenital coronary artery anomalies Congestive heart failure Hypertrophic cardiomyopathy Left ventricle hypertrophy (idiopathic) Marfan syndrome Pulmonary hypertension Right ventricular cardiomyopathy Uncontrolled arrhythmias or valvular heart disease
Conditions requiring modified activity or continuous monitoring	Uncontrolled hypertension Uncontrolled atrial arrhythmias Aortic insufficiency Mitral stenosis Mitral regurgitation

MYOCARDIAL INFARCTION

Athletes suffering MI or heart attack during exercise have a better chance of survival than those collapsing from hypertrophic cardiomyopathy. The onset of MI is caused by blockage of the heart's coronary arteries, causing a depletion of oxygen to the cardiac muscle, eventually resulting in necrosis.

Athletic trainers must be aware of the *prodromal* symptoms in athletes who are at risk of a heart attack so that they can be referred and screened for coronary disease. Also, athletic trainers should be aware of the signs and symptoms of acute MI. Quick recognition of an acute attack and a rapid response provides the athlete with the best chance of survival. After a living heart attack victim enters a hospital, the chance of survival increases 50 percent.

Prodromal Pertaining to the interval between the initial disease rate and the onset of outward symptoms.

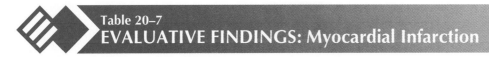

Table 20–7
EVALUATIVE FINDINGS: Myocardial Infarction

Examination Segment	Clinical Findings	
History	***Onset:***	Acute
	Pain characteristics:	Intense chest pain, possibly radiating to the jaw, left shoulder, and arm
	Mechanism:	Ischemia of the cardiac muscles
	Predisposing conditions:	Family history of cardiac disease, hypertension, high blood cholesterol level, being overweight or obese, smoking, known atherosclerosis
Inspection	The patient may sweat profusely, even in the absence of vigorous activity. Cyanosis is present. Nausea and vomiting may occur. Shallow, rapid respirations are present	
Palpation	Rapid, irregular pulse is found.	
Special Tests	Blood pressure testing reveals hypotension.	
Comments	Activate EMS. Continue to monitor the symptoms. If cardiac arrest occurs, initiate CPR. Treat the patient for shock.	

CRP = cardiopulmonary resuscitation; EMS = emergency medical service.

The athlete usually has had some previous symptoms, including chest pain, fatigue, and syncope. A strong family history of heart disease, hypertension, *hypercholesterolemia,* a history of smoking, excessive body weight, or a history of coronary artery disease are all considered risk factors for heart attack.

Individuals suffering MI complain of intense pain in the chest, often radiating to the jaw, left shoulder, and arm. A typical finding of MI is profuse sweating, but this may be an unreliable finding in an athlete involved in vigorous physical activity. The lips and fingernails may appear cyanotic. Nausea or vomiting may be experienced. The pulse may be abnormally high and irregular for some time after exercise has been discontinued, and respirations may be quick and shallow. Evaluation of the blood pressure reveals **hypotension** because the ailing heart is not able to produce sufficient output.

The symptoms presented in Table 20–7 indicate the need to immediately transport the athlete for further assessment and treatment. These symptoms may become progressively more severe and result in death quite rapidly.

ARRHYTHMIAS

Arrhythmias, or irregular heart rhythms, can be relatively common in the athletic population. Although many causes of arrhythmia are benign or can be controlled through the use of medications, other causes are potentially fatal. Any arrhythmia reported by an athlete or discovered during a physical examination requires further evaluation by a cardiologist to prescribe the appropriate management and determine the athlete's ability to safely participate in sports.

As described in Chapter 10, cardiac contusions or violent chest compression may also disrupt the athlete's normal heart rhythm.

BRADYCARDIA

Bradycardia, a heart rate lower than 60 beats per minute (bpm), is common in highly trained athletes and is often termed "athlete's heart." This condition was once considered pathological and recommendations were made for the individual to cease activity. However, it has been recognized that the decreased heart rate is associated with activities that enhance cardiovascular function.[19]

Occasionally athletes with a slow heart rate may experience syncope, especially when at rest. Normal sinus tachycardia takes over during exercise, decreasing or eliminating the manifestation of symptoms of bradycardia.[20,21] Any athlete with unexplainable bouts of syncope at rest and bradycardia should be examined by a physician to rule out significant cardiac implications.

TACHYCARDIA

Tachycardia, an increased heart rate, can be characterized as a normal response to a stressful circumstance. Other causes of tachycardia can result in sudden death.

Hypercholesterolemia A high blood cholesterol level caused by a high intake of saturated fats.

Clinically, athletes with tachycardia may become excessively fatigued, describe exertional syncope, and experience a sensation of the heart's "racing." Evaluation of the pulse can reveal sustained heart rates in excess of 200 bpm. The inefficient pumping action of the heart results in a decreased blood pressure.

An athlete suspected to be suffering from tachycardia and presenting with a normal *sinus rhythm* should be withheld from activity and referred for further evaluation by a physician. Sustained tachycardia indicates that the athlete should be transported to a medical facility by trained personnel because this condition can degenerate into ventricular fibrillation and result in sudden death.

MITRAL VALVE PROLAPSE

Approximately 5 percent of the population suffers from mitral valve prolapse (MVP).[22,23] Prolapse occurs after the valve has closed. The subsequent pressure from the backflow of blood causes the valve to collapse, resulting in the regurgitation of blood back into the ventricle. Many athletes with MVP are able to participate in vigorous activity. Athletes with documented arrhythmogenic syncope, family history of sudden death associated with MVP, experience tachycardia or ventricular arrhythmia with exercise, have documented moderate or marked mitral regurgitation, or have had a previous embolic event should be restricted to low-intensity athletic activities.[22–24]

HYPERTENSION

High blood pressure, the most common cardiovascular abnormality affecting athletes, is more prevalent in the African-American population than in other groups.[25] Additionally, hypertension is the most common cardiovascular condition in competitive athletes.[26] Increased peripheral vascular resistance to blood flow secondary to vasoconstriction increases the pressure required to force blood through the vessels.

Although systolic pressures greater than 140 mm Hg and diastolic pressures greater than 90 mm Hg are the clinical benchmarks for hypertension, the athlete's average blood pressure should be compared with the normative data reflecting the athlete's gender, age, height, and weight. Many variables influence blood pressure, including the possible anxiety associated with the procedure itself. Minimally, the blood pressure cuff must be 66 percent as wide as the upper arm from the top of the shoulder to the olecranon and encircle the arm completely.[26] The athlete should be seated and be at rest, and the arm should be supported at chest level. Elevated readings must be produced on several separate occasions for a diagnosis of hypertension to be made.

After the presence of hypertension has been established, its cause must be identified so that appropriate intervention can take place. Unregulated hypertension can result in MI, stroke, kidney failure, and distur-

bances in vision. Most athletes with controlled hypertension can safely participate in sports, assuming that no other associated organ damage has occurred and there is no evidence of concomitant cardiac disease. Athletes with unregulated hypertension should be limited to low-intensity activities and be closely monitored. Athletes with significant hypertension should have their blood pressure measured by their physician at least every 2 months to monitor the effects of exercise or medications on the disease.

ASTHMA

Asthma is caused by a narrowing of the bronchial tree, resulting in difficulty breathing. This narrowing results from an increase in mucosal secretions, bronchospasm, or both. Asthma can be divided into two groups, extrinsic or intrinsic asthma, as determined by the predisposing cause of the condition. **Extrinsic asthma** is caused by *allergens* such as hay fever, insect stings, pollen, animal *dander,* or foods. The cause of **intrinsic asthma** is less well defined, but the most common type in athletes is **exercise-induced asthma.**

Asthma is characterized by dry wheezing during respiration, an event that may be frightening to the athlete as well as to bystanders (Table 20–8). During an acute episode, the athlete experiences tightness in the chest during inspiration but usually has greater difficulty during expiration. If a partial obstruction occurs high in the airway, as with laryngeal injury, inspiration is commonly more difficult than expiration. It is not uncommon for an asthmatic athlete to experience repeated dry coughing during the asthma attack.

Athletes with extrinsic asthma have attacks precipitated by contact with one of the allergens. Intrinsic exercise-induced asthma is most commonly caused by exercise in a cold, dry climate, as the cool air triggers the bronchospasm. Athletes with exercise-induced asthma usually have fewer symptoms during activities with brief periods of intense work; with exercise in a relatively warm, humid environment; and with improvement in their aerobic condition.

Individuals with asthma often have knowledge of their condition before participating in organized sports. It is not unusual for high school athletes to use preparticipation medication or carry inhalers to control asthma attacks. This is important information for the athletic trainer to include in the athlete's medical

---

Sinus rhythm An irregular heartbeat characterized by an increased rate during inspiration and a decreased rate during expiration.

Allergen A substance that, when contacting the body's tissues, results in a state of sensitivity.

Dander Small scales from animal hair or feathers that cause allergic reactions in some individuals.

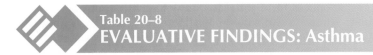

Table 20–8
EVALUATIVE FINDINGS: Asthma

Examination Segment	Clinical Findings	
History	***Onset:***	Congenital or acquired disease; acute attacks
	Pain characteristics:	In the chest, breathing is difficult, more so during expiration than inspiration.
	Mechanism:	Bronchospasm caused by allergens (extrinsic) or cold, dry air during exercise (intrinsic)
	Predisposing conditions:	Poor air quality or exposure to allergens
Inspection	Wheezing occurs with respiration. Repetitive dry coughing is present.	
Special Tests	Peak flow meter	
Comments	Many acute asthma attacks can be controlled quickly with the use of an inhaler.	

record, and it may necessitate carrying medication for the athlete in case of emergency.

Peak flow meters (PFMs) may be used to assist in diagnosing and monitoring asthma by determining the peak expiratory flow rate (PEFR) (Box 20–1). The PEFR represents the maximum velocity of air that can be forced from the lungs after taking a deep breath. This is directly affected by changes in the airways such as is found with increases or decreases in secretion buildup or bronchospasm.

The PEFR should remain steady or increase after an episode of exercise. After exercise, PEFR decreases of 15[27,28] and 10 percent[29] or greater from pre-exercise levels may indicate exercise-induced asthma. Unrecognized, this condition leads to increased fatigue and decreased performance.

In athletes with diagnosed asthma, routine measurements are compared with a baseline to monitor the condition. The baseline is a personal best measurement that represents the highest measurement the patient has attained over a 2- to 3-week period. After establish-

ing the personal best, the goal is to reach this baseline every day. Guidelines for management of asthma have been developed under the National Asthma Education Guidelines for the Diagnosis and Management of Asthma. These guidelines are color coded as green, yellow, and red, similar to a traffic light so they are easier to remember (Table 20–9).

HYPERVENTILATION

Conditions such as asthma, ***metabolic acidosis, pulmonary edema,*** and anxiety can increase the minute volume ventilation rate by increasing the athlete's

Metabolic acidosis Decreased blood pH caused by an increase in blood acids or a decrease in blood bases.

Pulmonary edema Swelling of the lung and its tissues.

Table 20–9
PEAK EXPIRATORY FLOW RATE GRADING

Color	Zone	Meaning
Green	80% to 100% of personal best	**All clear.** No asthma symptoms are present. Routine treatment plan can be followed. For patients who use medications on a daily basis, consistent measurements in the green zone may allow them to reduce their medications under their physician's guidance.
Yellow	50% to 80% of personal best	**Caution:** An acute attack may be present. Temporary increase in medications may be needed. Consistent readings in this zone may indicate that the condition is not being managed with the current dosage of medications and may need to be increased.
Red	Below 50% of personal best	**Medical alert.** Immediate use of bronchodilators is indicated. If levels do not return immediately to the yellow or green zone after use of the medication, the physician should be notified.

Box 20–1
PEAK FLOW METER (SPIROMETER)

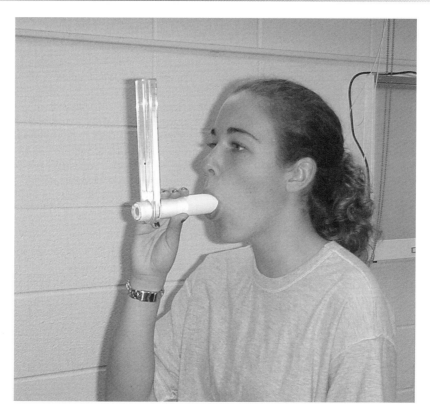

PATIENT POSITION	Standing
POSITION OF EXAMINER	Standing in front of the athlete
EVALUATIVE PROCEDURE	The patient takes as deep a breath as possible. The mouth is placed around the mouthpiece of the peak flow meter. The patient blows as hard and as fast as possible into the device.
POSITIVE TEST	**1.** Diagnostic: Decreases greater or equal to a 15% decrease in peak expiratory flow rate from pre-exercise to post-exercise. **2.** Monitoring: Daily percentage readings of 50 to 80% of personal best or less than 50% of personal best.
IMPLICATIONS	**1.** Exercise-induced asthma. **2.** Asthma attack requiring caution, possibly a temporary increase in bronchodilator dosage or immediate administration of bronchodilators and notification of the treating physician if levels do not return to at least 50% of personal best after medication administration
COMMENT	The patient must be careful not to block the mouthpiece opening with the tongue while performing the test.

respiratory rate. Subsequently, the body's oxygen and carbon dioxide levels are skewed by decreasing the level of carbon dioxide and increasing the level of oxygen. This imbalance results in dizziness, tracheal spasm, an increased heart rate, and, eventually, fainting. As soon as the oxygen and carbon dioxide levels are stabilized, the symptoms quickly subside.

◆ ON-FIELD EVALUATION AND MANAGEMENT OF CARDIOPULMONARY CONDITIONS

The most important aspects of the management of a patient with suspected cardiopulmonary injury or illness are the basic ABCs of first aid. The examiner must establish that the athlete has an airway, breathing is occurring, and circulation is present. Unfortunately for some of these athletes, such as those suffering from hypertrophic cardiomyopathy, illnesses not identified before participation may be fatal despite the most heroic lifesaving measures.

For other cardiac conditions in which breathing and a pulse have been established, the most important task of the athletic trainer is to initiate the emergency management system. Beyond this, the athletic trainer must take control of the situation and keep the athlete and bystanders as calm as possible. Vital signs should be continually monitored and documented until assistance arrives.

ASTHMA

Athletes with asthma can usually manage their own condition and may or may not require the athletic trainer's direct assistance. Proper management of these conditions includes having the athletes' medications on hand and marked as belonging to them and by quickly making them available to the athlete. These athletes are usually well versed and capable of dispensing their own medication but should be assisted as needed.

Under ideal circumstances, athletes suffering from asthma have been assessed and placed on a nonpharmacologic and pharmacologic treatment program as needed to control their disease.[29] Nonpharmacological treatment includes patient and family education and cardiovascular fitness evaluation. Pharmacologic treatments include the use of inhaled bronchodilators 15 minutes before exercise.

All athletes who have been previously identified as having asthma should carry an inhaler. In circumstances requiring the use of an inhaler, the athletic trainer should assist the athlete by ensuring that he or she is using the inhaler and is moved to the sidelines until the breathing becomes controlled.

If the athlete does not have an inhaler available, the situation must be managed as a pulmonary emergency. Because the primary problem is in exhaling rather than inhaling, the athlete should attempt to perform controlled diaphragmatic breathing, using the abdominal muscles to slowly, yet forcefully, push the air from the lungs. Placing the athlete in a sitting position with the arms resting on the knees assists in expiration.

Typically, the athlete suffering from an exercise-induced asthma attack experiences the symptoms approximately 10 minutes after beginning exercise. Managed with inhalers and cessation of exercise, the athlete's symptoms usually cease after 30 minutes. In some cases, the symptoms worsen before they clear.[30] More than half of athletes with exercise-induced asthma experience a refractory period after asthma attacks. During this 2-hour period, the athlete seems resistant to a recurrence of the symptoms while performing similar activities.[31]

HYPERVENTILATION

Athletes who are hyperventilating can be managed by controlling the rate at which carbon dioxide is lost from the body. The traditional method involves having the athlete breathe into a paper bag (not a plastic bag) held tightly around the mouth and nose (Fig. 20–2). An alternative method involves having the athlete breathe through only one nostril by holding the opposite nostril closed.

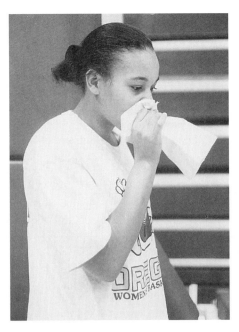

FIGURE 20–2. Controlling hyperventilation. Breathing into a paper bag recirculates carbon dioxide in the respiratory system and reestablishes the body's oxygen-carbon dioxide balance.

REFERENCES

1. Mangus, BC, and Finnecy, T: A pilot study of cardiac disorders in division I athletes. *Athletic Training: Journal of the National Athletic Trainers Association,* 25:237, 1990.
2. Finnecy, T, and Mangus, BC: Athletic participation after cardiac transplantation: A case study. *Athletic Training: Journal of the National Athletic Trainers Association,* 19:224, 1989.
3. Smith, AN, and Bell, GW: Hypertrophic cardiomyopathy and its inherent danger in athletics. *Athletic Training: Journal of the National Athletic Trainers Association,* 26:319, 1991.
4. Ballenger, M: Dissecting aneurysms. *Emergency Magazine,* 17:25, 1985.
5. Maron, BJ, Epstein, SE, and Roberts, WC: Causes of sudden death in competitive athletes. *J Am Coll Cardiol,* 7:204, 1986.
6. Feld, F: Management of the critically injured football player. *Journal of Athletic Training,* 28:206, 1993.
7. Cecil, LF: *Cecil's Essentials of Medicine.* Philadelphia, WB Saunders, 1986.
8. Erkkinen, JF: Nausea and vomiting. In Greene, HL, Glassock, RJ, and Kelley, MA (eds): *Introduction to Clinical Medicine.* Philadelphia, BC Decker, 1991, p 283.
9. Hargarten, K: Emergencies in sports: Syncope in athletes. Life-threatening or benign? *The Physician and Sportsmedicine,* 19:33, 1991.
10. Hargarten, KM: Syncope. Finding the cause in active people. *The Physician and Sportsmedicine,* 20:123, 1992.
11. Amsterdam, EA, Laslett, L, and Holly, R: Exercise and sudden death. *Cardiol Clin,* 5:337, 1987.
12. Maron, BJ, et al: Sudden death in young athletes. *Circulation,* 62:218, 1980.
13. Maron, BJ, Roberts, WC, and Epstein, SC: Sudden death in hypertrophic cardiomyopathy. *Circulation,* 65:1388, 1982.
14. Van Camp, SP: Exercise-related sudden death: risks and causes. *The Physician and Sportsmedicine,* 16:96, 1988.
15. Pipe, AL, Chan, K, and Rippe, JM: A case conference. Asymptomatic heart murmur in a professional football player. *The Physician and Sportsmedicine,* 16:53, 1988.
16. Burke, AP, et al: Sports-related and non-sports-related sudden cardiac death in young adults. *Am Heart J,* 121:568, 1991.
17. Thomas, RJ, and Cantwell, JD: Case Reports. Sudden death during basketball games. *The Physician and Sportsmedicine,* 18:75, 1990.
18. Munnings, F: The death of Hank Gathers: A legacy of confusion. *The Physician and Sportsmedicine,* 18:97, 1990.
19. Alpert, JS, et al: Athletic heart syndrome. *The Physician and Sportsmedicine,* 17:103, 1989.
20. Lichtman, J, et al: Electrocardiogram of the athlete. *Arch Intern Med,* 132:763, 1973.
21. Northcote, RJ, et al: Is severe bradycardia in veteran athletes an indication for a permanent pacemaker? *Br Med J,* 298:231, 1989.
22. 26th Bethesda Conference: Recommendations for determining eligibility for competition in athletes with cardiovascular abnormalities. *J Am Coll Cardiol,* 24:845, 1994.
23. Washington RL: Mitral valve prolapse in active youth. *Phys Sportsmed,* 21(1):136, 1993.
24. Moeller JL: Contraindications to athletic participation: cardiac, respiratory, and central nervous system conditions. *Phys Sportsmed,* 24(8):47, 1996.
25. Strong, WB, and Steed, D: Cardiovascular evaluation of the young athlete. *Pediatr Clin North Am,* 29:1325, 1982.
26. Kaplan, NM, Deveraux, RB, and Miller, HS: Task force 4: systemic hypertension. *J Am Coll Cardiol,* 24:885, 1994.
27. Kukafka, DS, et al: Exercise-induced bronchospasm in high school athletes via a free running test: incidence and epidemiology. *Chest,* 114:1613, 1998.
28. Feinstein, RA, et al: Screening adolescent athletes for exercise-induced asthma. *Clin J Sports Med,* 6:119, 1996.
29. Kyle, JM, et al: Exercise-induced asthma in the young athlete: guidelines for routine screening and initial management. *Med Sci Sports Exerc,* 24:856, 1992.
30. McFadden, ER: Exercise-induced asthma. Assessment of current etiologic concepts. *Chest,* 91:151, 1987.
31. Schoeffel, RE: et al: Multiple exercise and histamine challenges in asthmatic patients. *Thorax,* 35:164, 1989.

21

General Medical Conditions

Although orthopedic trauma is associated primarily with athletic participation, diseases can also impair an individual's ability to participate in strenuous physical activity. This chapter presents nonorthopedic conditions commonly seen by sports medicine specialists. Chapters 12 and 20 also discuss cardiovascular and respiratory diseases that can affect an athlete's performance or are a contraindication to athletic participation. In some instances, exercise can manifest symptoms of otherwise silent diseases.[1]

Many of the conditions presented in this chapter are considered reportable diseases to the state boards of health. These diseases represent a significant public health risk because of their prevalence, magnitude, or both. Physicians who treat a patient with a reportable disease are required to submit a written report or telephone report of the number of cases seen (Table 21–1).

Medications play an important role in the management of patients with most of the illnesses discussed in this chapter. Unfortunately, many common and otherwise therapeutic medications are banned by organizations such as the United States Olympic Committee (USOC) and the National Collegiate Athletic Associa-

tion (NCAA), which govern athletic competition. Physicians, athletic trainers, coaches, and athletes should be aware of those medications (and other substances) that are banned.

Additionally, over-the-counter medications should not be indiscriminately used. The use of aspirin in children with a viral illness is contraindicated because of the increased risk for developing *Reye's syndrome*. **Do not administer aspirin to patients of this age group without first consulting a physician and the child's parent.** Because of their side effects and interactions, keep records of athletes who are using prescription and nonprescription medication.

◆ RESPIRATORY INFECTIONS

Viral or bacterial infections can affect the upper or lower respiratory tracts. The various illnesses described in this section often are interrelated. A cause-and-effect relationship may lead to multiple conditions' occurring concurrently or sequentially. The organisms that cause respiratory infections are transmitted via the air (i.e., heavy breathing, coughing, sneezing), bodily contact, or contact with contaminated objects (i.e., wrestling mats, water bottles, towels).[2]

UPPER RESPIRATORY INFECTIONS

The term "upper respiratory infection" (URI) is used to describe a wide range of viral or bacterial infections of the nasal pathway, pharynx, or bronchi. Viral URIs, also referred to as the **common cold,** are caused by one

Table 21–1
DISEASES THAT MUST BE REPORTED TO STATE BOARD OF HEALTH*

Written Report Required	Number of Cases Seen Reported
AIDS	Influenza
Cancer	Mumps
Chlamydia	
Gonorrhea	
Hepatitis A, B, and C	
HIV	
Meningitis	
Pelvic inflammatory disease	
Syphilis	

*Only the diseases covered in the chapter are listed. Reportable diseases vary from state to state.

Reye's syndrome   A disorder of the liver, pancreas, heart, kidney, and lymph nodes; often seen in children younger than age 15 years; associated with acute viral infection and use of aspirin.

Table 21–2
SIGNS AND SYMPTOMS OF VIRAL UPPER RESPIRATORY INFECTIONS

Signs and symptoms	Nasal congestion Rhinitis Sore throat Coughing and/or sneezing Headache Fever (< 102°F) Muscle ache
Duration	10 to 14 days
Treatment	Managed most often through rest, analgesics, decongestants, antihistamine medications (to reduce nasal and ear congestion), and consuming increased fluids Antibiotics only prescribed if the cold results in a bacterial URI Antihistamines possibly administered to reduce nasal and ear congestion Possible reduction in risk for developing sinusitis with use of decongestants
Possible complications	Bronchitis, pneumonia, ear infections, sinusitis, bacterial infection, or LRIs.

LRI = lower respiratory infection; URI = upper respiratory infection.

Table 21–3
SIGNS AND SYMPTOMS OF INFLUENZA

Signs and symptoms	Fever and chills Muscle ache and joint pain Rhinitis Congestion Cough Sore throat Nausea Loss of appetite Sweating Fatigue Lethargy Headache Nausea, vomiting, or diarrhea
Duration	7 to 14 days
Treatment	Rest, analgesic medication Possible specific medication protocols for specific influenza strains Bacterial infections treated with antibiotic medication.
Possible complications	Bronchitis, pneumonia, bacterial infection

of more than 200 rhinovirus in adults and the corona virus in younger individuals. The rhinovirus is most prevalent during the autumn and spring. The corona virus is most common during the winter months.[3]

The signs and symptoms of colds, presented in Table 21–2, typically persist for 1 to 2 weeks. The physiological responses to submaximal and maximal exercise has little effect on pulmonary function in the presence of slight to moderate URIs.[4] However, severe URIs can significantly alter running gait, which can lead to orthopedic trauma.[5]

An individual's susceptibility to URIs is related to the level of physical activity. Sedentary individuals have an average risk of acquiring an URI. A moderate amount of strenuous physical activity decreases the risk. However, as the amount and intensity of physical activity increases, so does the risk of URI.[3,6] Repeated bouts of heavy exertion may adversely affect the body's immune system and increase the risk of acquiring a bacterial infection. However, the exact mechanism and effects are unclear.[3]

Influenza

Influenza is caused by a viral infection of the respiratory tract and is spread by water vapor and droplet transmission. Although influenza most commonly affects the upper respiratory tract, it may also involve the lower respiratory tract. Influenza viruses are classified as RNA myxovirus and fall into three groups. Type A is the most common, followed by types B and C.[7] This virus is constantly changing, producing annual epidemics. The yearly manifestation of the virus results in annual inoculations against the current strain.

The influenza virus attacks the respiratory tract's mucus lining, resulting in inflammation and necrosis of these tissues. As a result, the respiratory tract becomes vulnerable to bacterial infection. Influenza may have a sudden onset of symptoms (Table 21–3).

Sinusitis

Sinusitis, inflammation or infection of the nasal sinuses, disrupts the normal airflow in and out of the sinuses and blocks the normal fluid and mucus drainage from the sinus into the nose. The onset of sinusitis is traced to a bacterial infection that is often directly related to viral illness, allergy, or dental disease. Sudden changes in temperature or barometric pressure (e.g., in airplane travel) can increase the pressure and cause pain within the sinuses. Similarly, changes in body position such as bending over can increase pressure within the sinuses. Physical trauma that obstructs the nasal passages (e.g., a deviated septum) may also block fluid outflow from within the sinuses.

The signs and symptoms of sinusitis include headache and focal pain in the area of the nasal sinuses, representing the increase in pressure within the sinuses. In some instances, swelling or discoloration may be noted around the eyes ("allergic shiners"). Fever and chills also may be present along with possible production of a yellow or green nasal discharge. Postnasal drip can result in a sore throat and a persistent, dry nonproductive cough. Dryness of the nasal mucosa may result in epistaxis. Palpation over the sinus often elicits tenderness.

Oral or nasal decongestants are often prescribed to assist in sinus drainage and analgesic medication may be used for pain control. Sinusitis may become chronic. In this event, surgery may be required to clear the obstruction.

Laryngitis

One of the subsequent effects of an URI is inflammation of the larynx, called laryngitis. The enlargement of the vocal cords causes the voice to be weak, hoarse, or raspy. On occasion, the individual may be unable to speak. In rare instances, respiratory distress may develop. Laryngitis can also occur after direct trauma to the throat, allergies, gastroesophageal reflux, or a local tumor.

Laryngitis is treated by focusing on the underlying disease that brings about the symptoms. Resting the voice (which the patient often does voluntarily), taking throat lozenges, drinking cool drinks, and taking antacid medications (for cases caused by gastroesophageal reflux) are used to provide symptomatic relief.

Pharyngitis

Commonly referred to as a sore throat, pharyngitis involves the inflammation of the pharynx. Most forms of pharyngitis are caused by a virus. In rare cases, it is caused by bacteria. Pharyngitis is termed **strep throat** when it is caused by group A streptococcus. Sore throats may also be caused by **tonsillitis** when bacteria or viruses can invade the tonsils, large lymph nodes located at the back of the throat. The pharynx can become chronically inflamed secondary to smoking, alcoholism, or postnasal drip caused by URI.

In addition to a sore throat, pharyngitis is characterized by enlargement of the cervical and cranial lymph nodes, fever, and pain with swallowing. The diagnosis of strep throat and tonsillitis is made by physical examination of the oral cavity and culture of the throat cells. A definitive diagnosis of tonsillitis is made after a throat culture to identify the presence of the streptococcus (strep) bacteria. Tonsillitis may also be the result of viral invasion.

The treatment for pharyngitis is supportive. Gargling with salt water or commercial mouthwashes can assist in clearing the pharynx of the remnants of postnasal drip and provide soothing relief. Analgesics may be used to reduce pain and fever. A physician may prescribe antibiotic medication if the individual tests positive for streptococcus.

Allergic Rhinitis

Allergic rhinitis is a reaction to any one of many allergens found in the environment. Allergens can vary from naturally occurring irritants, such as pollen and dust, to human-made irritants such as chemicals. The most common irritant to athletes and people who are active outdoors is airborne pollen. The allergic reaction is commonly referred to as "hay fever," and several different types of pollen can trigger hay fever. Because the allergen, pollen, is transmitted through the atmosphere, hay fever is more likely to strike in hot, dry outdoor environments. When the weather is cool, damp, or rainy, the pollen is filtered out of the atmosphere, thus reducing the likelihood of transmission. Many weather forecasts give pollen counts to alert individuals with known problems with pollen to avoid outdoor activity when levels are increased.

During the cold months, different strains of mold replace pollen as the more common offending allergen. However, an individual who develops allergic rhinitis throughout the year is probably allergic to a broad spectrum of irritants. Athletes who exercise outdoors can be exposed to a wide spectrum of allergens, including pollen, that trigger allergic rhinitis.

Symptoms are produced when the allergen enters the body, triggering the release of histamine and antibodies. The range and magnitude of the symptoms vary according to the individual's sensitivity to the allergen. Excess mucus production causes rhinitis. The individual sneezes or coughs frequently as the body attempts to clear the air passages (Table 21–4). In severe cases, exercise while suffering from allergic rhinitis can trigger systemic muscle spasms and anaphylaxis that results in hives, swelling, and decreased blood pressure, a medical emergency.[6]

The treatment is symptomatic. Rhinitis is controlled through the use of antihistamines to decrease inflammation and decongestants to open the air passages. For

Table 21–4
SIGNS AND SYMPTOMS OF ALLERGIC RHINITIS

Signs and symptoms	Sneezing and coughing Clear or purulent discharge Nasal congestion Headache Sore throat Generalized itching Boggy eyes and nasal membranes
Duration	Symptoms persisting as long as the allergen is present
Treatment	Avoidance of prolonged exposure to any known allergens and use of nonsedating antihistamines, decongestants, corticosteriods
Possible complications	In severe cases, possible development of anaphylactic shock; drowsiness is possible with use of nonprescription antihistamines

hypersensitive individuals, behavioral modification is needed to limit the onset and severity of allergic rhinitis. Hay fever sufferers are encouraged to limit outdoor exposure when pollen counts are high. The use of air conditioning will decrease the humidity and lowers the pollen level. When possible, the individual's bedroom windows should be closed at night.

Mold- and dust-related allergic rhinitis requires regular cleaning of the person's living environment to decrease the accumulation of these allergens. Use of a dehumidifier to decrease the rate of mold growth may be helpful, especially in damp basements. Replacing natural down-filled pillows and comforters with non-organic microfiber filling and using vinyl casings around pillows is recommended. To kill dust mites, bed linens are to be washed regularly in hot water (> 130°F). Some individuals may have to limit their exposure to animals because the dander from cats and dogs can be a common allergen. In some cases, a series of desensitization injections may be required to increase the person's resistance to the specific allergen(s).

LOWER RESPIRATORY INFECTIONS

Although lower respiratory infections (LRI) are less common than URIs, their occurrence can be more problematic and result in an increased amount of time lost from physical activity. An inherent problem with LRIs is the actual air exchange within the lungs. Because the bronchi are involved, the overall efficiency of the lungs is reduced.

Bronchitis

Bronchitis is categorized as being either acute or chronic. **Acute bronchitis** is caused by a viral infection of the lower respiratory tract that inflames the bronchi. Once inflamed, the bronchi trap bacteria that cause a bacterial infection. Prolonged URIs can lead to bronchitis.

The long-term over production of bronchial mucus leads to **chronic bronchitis** (chronic obstructive pulmonary disease [COPD]). Long-term exposure to airborne pollutants, systemic infection, and cigarette smoke (including second-hand smoke) all can cause chronic bronchitis.

Because the bronchi are inflamed, passage of air into the lungs becomes partially obstructed. Individuals suffering from bronchitis complain of a shortness of breath that increases during activity and leads to premature fatigue. Deep breathing is often accompanied by wheezing or *crackles*. Coughing is triggered to expel mucus (sputum) from the lungs. Headaches are also often reported.

Prolonged pulmonary obstruction can result in swelling of the lower extremity. The face, palms, and mucous membranes of the mouth and nose may become red. If untreated, bronchitis may lead to pneumonia, emphysema, or other chronic diseases of the lungs.

Table 21–5
SIGNS AND SYMPTOMS OF PNEUMONIA

Signs and symptoms	Chest pain that is increased with coughing or deep breathing Rales Shortness of breath Cough producing mucus or green or yellow sputum Fever and chills Sweating Fatigue and malaise Nausea and vomiting Loss of appetite Headache
Duration	Approximately 2 weeks
Treatment	Bacteria-related pneumonia treated with antibiotics Severe cases possibly require respiratory therapy to assist with alveolar gas exchange.
Possible complications	Respiratory failure

Laboratory evaluation of bronchitis may include pulmonary function tests and determination of the level of arterial blood gasses. A chest radiograph may also be ordered.

Pneumonia

Pneumonia is a broad term used to describe an inflammation of the lungs. The causes and types of pneumonia are numerous and include bacteria, viruses, and chemical irritants. All forms of pneumonia have the commonality of being potentially life-threatening conditions. Pneumonia can occur as the result of a primary lung infection or secondary to other respiratory conditions that lower the lung's resistance to infection.[8]

The most common set of symptoms are presented in Table 21–5. Initially, the signs and symptoms of pneumonia can mimic those of URI.[8] Persistent coughing may lead to the irritation of the pleural membrane (pleurisy). Breathing may be difficult and the patient may display rales, wheezing, or shortness of breath. Diagnostic tests include a chest radiograph, mucus or sputum culture, arterial blood gas level, and a complete blood count.

Although rare, pneumonia has been traced as the source of sudden death during athletic competition. Normally, athletes can return to moderate workouts (50% of normal intensity) 7 days after the resolution of

---

Crackles   (rales) A crackling sound heard during inspiration and expiration caused by air passing over excessive secretions in the airway.

symptoms and continue to increase the intensity over the next 7 days if no complications are presented.[8]

MANAGEMENT OF ATHLETES WITH RESPIRATORY INFECTIONS

The decision on how to manage individuals suffering from respiratory infections is based on three factors: the chance of worsening the condition, the individual's physical ability to perform, and the risk of transmission to teammates.[2] The return to competition decision is relatively easy in minor or significant episodes of respiratory infections. The challenge lies in determining the status of athletes who are in the process of recovering from a respiratory infection.

As with most illnesses and injuries, physical activity may worsen the symptoms and delay recovery time.[2] Acute infections can alter cardiac output and decrease stroke volume, especially when the athlete exhibits a fever. Viral respiratory infections can inhibit pulmonary gas exchange.[2]

The effect of the medications' being used to treat the ailments must also be considered. Antihistamines can cause drowsiness and result in sedation and a dry mouth.[9] Although oral and topical decongestants are effective and seldom produce side effects, the use of topical decongestants can lead to dependency.[9]

After a mild URI, light to moderate training can be resumed a few days after the end of the symptoms. Infections that result in moderate fever, muscle aches, and enlarged lymph nodes may require a 2- to 4-week recovery period before the resumption of intensive exercise.[3]

VIRAL SYNDROMES

MONONUCLEOSIS

Mononucleosis is caused by the Epstein-Barr virus (EBV) or the cytomegalovirus (CMV), both forms of the herpes virus.[10] These viruses infect epithelial cells that, after a series of events, invade the secondary cells. There they remain latent, resulting in long-term infection and a proliferation of white blood cells (WBCs).[10] The epithelial cells of the nose and pharynx may also be involved, leading to pharyngitis. The EBV is most commonly transmitted by direct mouth-to-mouth contact, but it can also be transmitted by secondary routes such as sharing water bottles. In adults, CMV is most commonly transmitted by blood transfusion. Individuals between the ages of 15 and 35 years are most prone to acquiring mononucleosis.

There is an incubation period of up to 50 days between the initial infection and the onset of symptoms. The prodromal symptoms include malaise, fatigue, headache, weight loss, and *myalgia.* During the active period of infection, a triad of symptoms—fever, pharyngitis, and swollen lymph nodes, including en-

Table 21–6
SIGNS AND SYMPTOMS OF MONONUCLEOSIS

Prodromal symptoms	Malaise Fatigue Headache Muscle aches Weight loss Myalgia
Active symptoms	Fever Sore throat Lymph node enlargement Spleen enlargement Rash or hives Jaundice Chest pain Increased or irregular heart rate
Duration	Fever reducing within 10 to 14 days; lymph node swelling normally resolves within a month
Treatment	The treatment approach is supportive, emphasizing bed rest; analgesic medication for fever and pain; no specific medications used to treat patients with mononucleosis
Possible complications	Predispostion to splenic rupture (rare)

largement of the spleen—is present. (Table 21–6).[11] The signs and symptoms become more pronounced with age.[10] Diagnosis is made using a monospot test. However the results of this test may be negative when CMV is the causative organism. Liver enzyme analysis, WBC, and platelet counts may also be used diagnostically.[11]

Splenomegaly, or enlargment of the spleen, is a particular concern for athletes with mononucleosis. As the spleen enlarges, it hardens, predisposing it to rupture. Although rare, splenic rupture is the most common cause of death associated with mononucleosis, especially within the first three weeks of infection.[2,11,12]

No specific medication is used to treat patients with mononucleosis. Treatment consists of rest, increased fluid intake, acetaminophen or aspirin for pain and fever, and throat lozenges or other symptomatic treatment for sore throat.[10] Although athletes typically experience a faster recovery rate than nonathletes, the total recovery time is approximately 1 month.[10]

During the first three weeks of active infection, patients should be excluded from contact or streneuous noncontact activities. In noncontact sports, the patient is excluded as long as the spleen is large and palpable. In contact sports, the patient is withheld from competi-

Myalgia Muscle pain or tenderness.

tion for an additional week past the point where the spleen is no longer palpable. Ultrasonic imaging can be used to assist in the return to competition decision.[10,12] A flak jacket can be used for protection when the athlete returns to activity.[11]

MEASLES

Measles are a family of viral infections that present with systemic and skin-related symptoms. The two most common forms of measles, rubeola and rubella (German measles), are discussed in this section. Measles commonly affects individuals during infancy and early childhood. Immunizations against measles are typically given at 15 months of age with a follow-up vaccine administered between the ages of 4 to 6 years. After inoculated or infected, lifetime immunity is usually acquired.

Rubeola

Rubeola, caused by the paramyxovirus, is a highly contagious form of measles. The virus is spread by airborne droplets or direct or indirect mouth-to-mouth transmission. After it is in the body, the signs and symptoms develop within 1 to 2 weeks (Table 21–7). The initial symptoms resemble that of an LRI. Then the characteristic rash appears within 5 days, usually beginning at the head and progressing inferiorly. The rash first appears as areas of discolored splotches on the skin and other areas of raised red bumps. With time, these two dermatologic signs merge. White spots within the mouth, **Koplik's spots,** appear early in the disease process.

Although the diagnosis of rubeola is often made based on the signs and symptoms presented, blood work may be used to definitively diagnose the disease.

Rubella

Commonly known as the German measles, rubella is a milder form of measles and is less infectious than rubeola. The initial signs and symptoms persist for up to 5 days before the onset of the rash (Table 21–8). The signs and symptoms become more pronounced and severe with age.

Rubella is a concern for expectant women who contract the disease early during the first trimester of pregnancy. The chance of birth defects, mental retardation, and miscarriages can occur if the disease is acquired during this period.

MUMPS

A viral infection of the parotid glands, mumps is caused by the paramyxovirus (the virus that causes rubeola). The most common age for acquiring mumps is between the ages of 2 and 12 years. However, individuals of all ages can contract this disease. Immunizations against mumps are given concurrently with measles vaccines at 15 months of age. A follow-up vaccine is administered between the ages of 4 to 6 years.

The primary manifestation of the mumps is the enlargement of the parotid glands, causing swelling of the mandible and cheeks. The individual may complain of facial pain, headache, and a sore throat. A fever is also noted. Men may experience testicular pain, a lump on the testicles, and scrotal swelling. The central nervous

Table 21–7
SIGNS AND SYMPTOMS OF RUBEOLA

Signs and symptoms	Rhinitis Deep, moist cough Fever Sore throat Photophobia Generalized muscle ache Rash Koplik's spots within the mouth
Duration	Lasts approximately 9 days after the initial symptoms appears (rubeola is also referred to as the 9 day measles.)
Treatment	The treatment approach is supportive, consisting of bed rest; a humidifier is possibly helpful in relieving respiratory symptoms
Possible complications	Complications are rare; respiratory difficulties possibly causing lower respiratory infections or otitis media; untreated rubeola may lead to encephalitis, a potentially fatal disease.

Table 21–8
SIGNS AND SYMPTOMS OF RUBELLA

Signs and symptoms	Headache Rhinitis Malaise Fever less than 102°F Clouding of the cornea or conjunctivitis Skin rash (occurs in half of the cases)
Duration	The initial symptoms last up to 5 days; the rash, if present, persists for approximately 3 days
Treatment	Bed rest
Possible complications	Expectant mothers, if exposed to rubella especially in the first trimester, experience an increased risk of miscarriages and birth defects.

system (CNS), pancreas, prostrate, and breast may also become involved when mumps is contracted by older individuals.

Patients with mumps are treated with bed rest. Ice packs or moist heat may be used to alleviate facial pain. Mouthwashes and gargling with salt water can be used to decrease throat symptoms.

 SEXUALLY TRANSMITTED DISEASES

The primary age group for acquiring sexually transmitted diseases (STDs) is the late teens and early twenties, the age range of high school and college athletes.[13] Risk factors for acquiring STDs include multiple sexual partners, participating in unsafe sex, and the early onset of sexual activity.

In most states, cases of chlamydia, gonorrhea, and syphilis must be reported. This allows for follow-up evaluation and testing of sexual partners.

CHLAMYDIA

Chlamydia, microscopic parasites that live within cells, is the most common STD in the United States.[13] The primary organisms that trigger genital chlamydia include *Chlamydia trachomatis* and *Neisseria gonorrhoeae*.[14] Another type, *C. pneumoniae*, triggers respiratory infections such as pneumonia, bronchitis, and sinusitis. Although both genders can transmit this disease, men can transmit it more easily than women.[13]

Individuals who are infected with chlamydia may be asymptomatic for an extended period. Thus, infected individuals who participate in unprotected sexual intercourse may transmit the disease to their partner. Females infected with *C. trachomatis* typically remain asymptomatic for an extended period, often never showing outward signs.[13] The signs and symptoms of chlamydia are similar to those for gonorrhea (Table 21–9). Often the two diseases occur together. Definitive

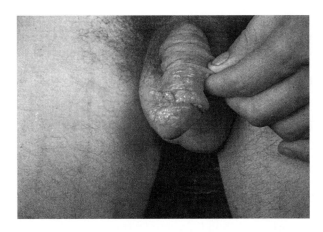

FIGURE 21–1. Genital warts of the penis.

diagnosis is made after a culture of the cervix in women or seminal fluid in men. Blood tests may also be performed to confirm the presence of chlamydia.

Oral antibiotic therapy is the standard treatment for patients with chlamydia infection. If left untreated, chlamydia can result in epididymitis and orchitis in men. In women, it can lead to pelvic inflammatory disease (PID), which is scarring of the fallopian tubes. Exposure to genital excretions can result in conjunctivitis.

GENITAL WARTS

Genital warts, caused by a strain of the human papillomavirus (HPV), are outgrowths of the skin of the sexual organs and anus (Fig. 21–1). In most cases, these growths are benign. However, some forms of genital warts are associated with the formation of malignant tumors such as cervical cancer.[13]

The primary sign of genital warts is one or more flat or fleshy, wartlike growths appearing on the genitals and vaginal walls and around the perianal area. The outward appearance of genital warts closely resembles that of another STD, **molluscum contagiosum** (Fig. 21–2). Other signs and symptoms include itching of the affected area, vaginal discharge, and abnormal vaginal bleeding. Although the diagnosis is often made based on visual inspection, blood test, serology, and biopsies may be used. A Papinacolaou (Pap) smear can also identify the presence of HPV in women.

Genital warts are transmitted by close physical contact with an infected person. The use of a condom greatly reduces the risk of transmission. Although genital warts may resolve without treatment, the HPV virus remains in the patient's system, increasing the likelihood of reoccurrence. In women, the presence of HPV and the herpes virus has been linked to the development of cervical cancer.[13] The physician may elect to remove the growth.

Table 21–9
SIGNS AND SYMPTOMS OF CHLAMYDIA

Common signs and symptoms	Burning during urination Frequent urination Pain or tenderness in the lower abdomen Fever Pain during intercourse
Female signs and symptoms	Vaginal discharge Menstrual irregularities
Male signs and symptoms	Discharge from the penis Testicular tenderness

FIGURE 21–2. Molluscum contagiosum of the inner thigh. This condition may resemble genital warts.

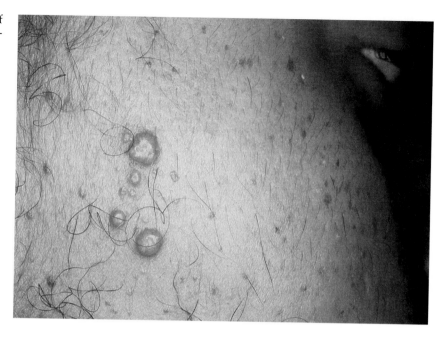

GONORRHEA

Gonorrhea, referred to as "the clap" in lay terms, is the second most common STD in the United States.[13] Caused by the bacteria *Neisseria gonorrhea*, the disease can infect the urogenital system, mouth, and rectum.

Patients infected with gonorrhea have about a 2- to 5-day incubation period. However, symptoms may take up to 2 weeks to appear. When the symptoms do occur, they often resemble those of chlamydia (Table 21–10). A Gram stain of the discharge from the female cervix or male urethra is used to diagnose infection. A positive stain is referred to as gram-negative diplococci. The results of the Gram stain are confirmed by a culture of the discharge. Long-term consequences of gonorrhea include epididymitis and pharangyitis. Women also are at risk for developing PID, infertility, and ectopic preg-

nancy. In cases that go untreated, the disease can infect the joints, heart, and brain.

Patients with gonorrhea are treated with oral or injected antibiotics. The individuals are usually also treated concurrently for chlamydia.

SYPHILIS

Caused by *Treponema pallidum*, syphilis is an STD that enters the body through lesions in the skin or mucous membrane. During its development, syphilis is marked by three distinct stages: primary, secondary; and tertiary (Table 21–11).

The primary stage, marked by the formation of a localized skin ulcer, occurs 3 to 5 weeks after the initial exposure (Fig. 21–3). The secondary stage is marked by the presence of *purulent* chancres on the trunk and mucous membranes. The systemic spread of the disease at this point may lead to hepatitis, arthritis, periosteitis, and other conditions. Between 3 to 13 weeks, secondary syphilis spontaneously resolves and the patient enters an asymptomatic latency period.[13] The patient may then experience a repeat of the secondary stage or progress onto the tertiary stage. Neurologic, cardiovascular, soft tissue, and skin symptoms emerge during the third stage of syphilis.

The definitive diagnosis of syphilis infection is made by the fluorescent treponemal antibody absorption (FTA-ABS) laboratory test. However, these tests do not produce positive findings until 4 to 6 weeks after infection.[13]

Table 21–10
SIGNS AND SYMPTOMS OF GONORRHEA

Common signs and symptoms	Painful urination Skin lesions
Female signs and symptoms	Vaginal discharge Urinary hesitancy Sore throat Mouth sores Painful intercourse
Male signs and symptoms	Increased urinary frequency Incontinence Inflammation of urethral opening Urethral discharge Testicular tenderness Proctitis

Purulent Containing pus.

Table 21–11
STAGES OF SYPHILIS

Stage	Onset (After exposure)	Symptoms
Primary	3 to 5 weeks	Chancres on the genitals, rectum, mouth, or fingers Swollen lymph nodes near the location of the sores
Secondary	6 to 13 weeks	Fever Fatigue Systemically swollen nontender lymph nodes Wide spread chancres Skin rash Ulceration of the mucous membranes Persistent headache Joint and muscle pain
Tertiary	9 to 25 weeks	Tumors (skin, bones, liver) Meningitis Deterioration of the cardiac aorta and/or valves CNS disorders

CNS = central nervous system.

Patients who test positive for syphilis also may be advised to be tested for HIV.

Antibiotic therapy is used to treat patients with syphilis. Each stage of the disease requires a different form of the antibiotic. If untreated, syphilis can lead to permanent disability or death.

HERPES SIMPLEX

Infection with the herpes simplex virus can cause type 1 (HSV1) and type 2 (HSV2) lesions. HSV1 affects the mouth, lips, and face. These lesions are commonly referred to as cold sores or fever blisters. The virus is transmitted by oral contact or by respiratory secretions. HSV2, most frequently associated with genital lesions, is spread via sexual contact. However, engaging in oral-genital sex can cause a cross-infection of HSV1 and HSV2 in which HSV2 affects the mouth or HSV1 affects the genitals.[15]

The herpes virus enters the body through breaks in the skin or mucous membranes. In some instances, pregnant women may pass the virus to the fetus in the womb or during childbirth. Once infected, the virus spreads via the CNS and then progresses to invade the mucous membranes. Herpes viruses that remain in the CNS may result in **herpes zoster** (Fig. 21–4).

After infection, the virus remains dormant and asymptomatic in the host tissues. Other diseases, physical or mental stress, sunlight, and certain foods or medications then trigger a symptomatic outbreak.

Most individuals become infected with HSV1 by the age of 20 years. HSV1 most commonly manifests itself through the characteristic cold sores or fever blisters (Fig. 21–5). Another consequence of HSV1 is **herpes gladiatorum,** a cutaneous infection of injured skin that is common in wrestlers.[16] In rare cases, HSV1 can also affect the eyes. Lesions on the genitals may occur secondary to cross-infection. Health care providers may develop a herpes infection of the fingers, **herpetic whitlow,** by exposure to oral secretions. HSV2 is characterized by burning lesions on the genitals. Both HSV1 and HSV2 may result in fever, sore throat, and swelling of the lymph nodes.

Although diagnosis may be made after visual inspection of the sores, blood analysis and samples of the lesions may be required to positively identify the disease. There is no cure for herpes simplex, and the treatment approach is symptomatic or cosmetic, using oral medication or topical ointments. Certain medications may

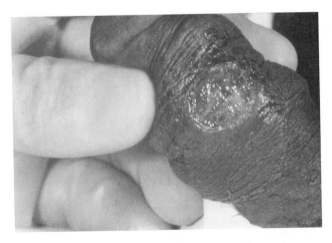

FIGURE 21–3. Primary syphilitic chancre of the penis.

FIGURE 21–4. Herpes zoster of the chest.

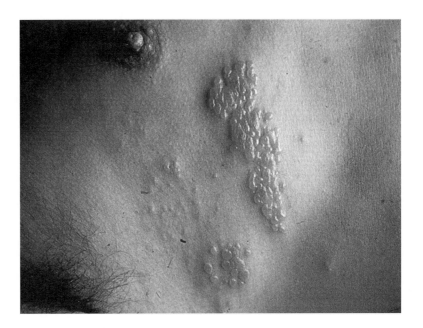

suppress the outbreak of lesions. Other medications may be used to prevent the outbreak of secondary lesions and prevent infection. However, petroleum-based ointments may delay healing.

Patients who are experiencing an active outbreak of herpes should refrain from physical contact with others. When lesions are present, the individual must be disqualified from sports that involve skin contact or contact with shared equipment. If the area is covered with clothing or the sport does not involve contact, participation is often permissible.[12] Likewise, care must be taken to avoid secondary transmission via other items, such as drinking glasses and towels.

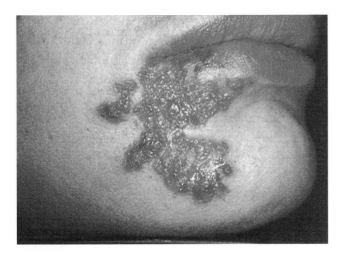

FIGURE 21–5. Herpes simplex 1 forming the characteristic "cold sore."

◆ BLOODBORNE PATHOGENS

Bloodborne pathogens cause a group of diseases that are primarily spread through contact with blood or contact with bodily fluids that contain blood. This section addresses hepatitis and the HIV. Most medical authorities agree that individuals who are affected with these diseases should be allowed to participate in all sports providing that their specific symptoms do not contraindicate intense physical activity.[17,18] Although precautions should always be taken to prevent accidental exposure to bloodborne pathogens (see Chapter 1), the risk of accidental transmission of these diseases during organized sporting activities is slight.

HEPATITIS

Inflammation of the liver, hepatitis, can be the result of viral or bacterial infection, drug or alcohol abuse, parasite infestation, or immune system disorders. Hepatitis occurs in one of five types: A, B, C, D, and E. Of these five types, hepatitis A, B, and C are most common, and hepatitis B and C are considered STDs. Hepatitis D typically occurs in patients who are infected with hepatitis B. Hepatitis E, similar to hepatitis A, is self-limiting and does not become chronic. Table 21–12 compares hepatitis A, B, and C. When undiagnosed or untreated, hepatitis can result in permanent liver damage and can lead to premature death. The common signs and symptoms of hepatitis include darkening of the urine and stool, fatigue, decreased appetite, generalized itching, jaundice, low-grade fever, and nausea and vomiting.

Hepatitis A and E are the most benign forms of hepatitis. These forms are most commonly seen as outbreaks associated with poor sanitary conditions or

Table 21–12
COMPARISON OF HEPATITIS A, B, AND C

Type	How Transmitted	Onset	Possible Complications
Hepatitis A	Fecal matter Exposure to body fluids	28 to 30 days	Little or none; usually self-limiting.
Hepatitis B	Sexual contact Blood exposure Needle reuse	60 to 90 days	Chronic hepatitis Cirrhosis Liver cancer
Hepatitis C	Blood tranfusion	10 to 77 days	Chronic liver disease

improper hand washing by those who are handling food. The clinical signs and symptoms of hepatitis A and E are generally mild and self-limiting. The treatment approach is supportive.

Hepatitis B

The hepatitis B virus (HBV) is the primary form of hepatitis contracted by athletes and other physically active individuals and the health care workers who care for them (HBV is also referred to as serum hepatitis). The primary modes of transmission of HBV are through unprotected sexual activity and accidental exposure to bodily fluids (including saliva, cerebrospinal fluid [CSF], and synovial fluids) or bodily wastes.[19] Intravenous (IV) drug users are at an increased risk of acquiring HBV. This disease can also be passed from infected pregnant mothers to their infants.

The incubation period between the initial exposure to the virus and the onset of symptoms is long, possibly up to 6 months. In addition to the common signs and symptoms of hepatitis, HBV also results in abdominal and joint pain, indigestion, tenderness of the liver, and abnormal tastes. Hepatitis B is a primary cause of chronic liver disease.[19] The hepatitis C and D viruses are commonly seen in the presence of HBV, further inflaming the liver and increasing the severity and duration of the symptoms. Because of the associated enlargement of the liver, individuals are predisposed to rupture of the liver after blunt abdominal trauma.[12]

Prevention Against Hepatitis

Hepatitis, primarily hepatitis B, C, and D, are considered bloodborne pathogens. Therefore, bloodborne transmission is a risk factor for health care practitioners. The use of the standard precautions for bloodborne pathogens serves to protect patients against blood-based hepatitis infection. Individuals who are regularly exposed to blood or bodily secretions or have the risk of accidental puncture by hypodermic needles should be vaccinated against the hepatitis A and the hepatitis B virus.[17] The general population is urged to practice safe sexual behavior. Additionally, care is necessary when handling needles to avoid inadvertent needlestick injuries. IV drug users are encouraged not to share needles to decrease the chance of accidental exposure to hepatitis. When performed improperly, receiving tattoos and body piercings are also potential sources of acquiring hepatitis.

To prevent transmission of the hepatitis A virus, food service workers and others handling food must thoroughly wash their hands after each trip to the restroom.

HUMAN IMMUNODEFICIENCY VIRUS

The human immunodeficiency virus (HIV) is a type I or II *retrovirus* that contains RNA. Type I HIV is prevalent in the United States. Type II HIV is most often found in Africa and Europe. The virus is thought to spread by entering a host cell where the RNA is changed to viral DNA. After it is inside the cell, the virus replicates and spreads to other cells. T-helper lymphocytes appear to be the primary target of HIV. Over time, the body's immune system is weakened, predisposing the individual to a wide range of infections.

HIV is transmitted by the same methods as hepatitis B. Unsafe sexual practices and sharing hypodermic needles are the primary modes of transmission in the United States. Pregnant women can also transmit HIV to the fetus *in utero*.

A latent period of approximately 1 month occurs between infection with HIV and the onset of symptoms. Because of their similarity to that of influenza and mononucleosis, the initial symptoms of HIV may not be recognized as such (Table 21–13). It may take up to 3 months for the infected person to test positive for the HIV antibody, commonly using the HIV ELISA or Western blot tests.[20] High-risk individuals who remain HIV negative should repeat these tests every 3 months.

Retrovirus   The generic name for the family of *Retroviridae* spp., viruses that contain RNA and may be associated with certain types of cancer.

Table 21–13
SIGNS AND SYMPTOMS OF HIV INFECTION AND AIDS

HIV
  Fever
  Fatigue
  Sore throat
  Enlarged lymph nodes
  Headache
  Diarrhea
  Body rashes
  Joint pain
  Muscle ache

AIDS
In addition to the possible signs and symptoms associated with HIV infection, the following are also common:
  Chronic, often debilitating fatigue
  Excessive sweating
  Cough
  Shortness of breath
  Mouth lesions
  Tumors, including Kaposi sarcoma
  Genital sores
  Vision difficulties
  Weight loss
  Muscular atrophy (wasting syndrome)
  Decreased or impaired cognitive function
  Predisposition to other infectious disease

ACQUIRED IMMUNODEFICIENCY SYNDROME

Most, but not all, HIV-infected individuals progress to develop **AIDS.** The diagnosis of AIDS is made when the CD4+ T-cell count, the marker for HIV infection, drops below $200/mm^3$ and the patient displays one of 25 specific clinical indicator conditions.

The onset of AIDS-related symptoms reflects the progressive deterioration of the body's immune system (see Table 21–13). At this time, there is no known cure for AIDS. However, several different treatment approaches, including new antiretroviral drugs, have been used to place the syndrome into remission.

The decision to allow participation in athletics is based on the individual's symptoms. The presence of HIV itself does not significantly hinder physical performance. Physical activity, which does help to enhance cardiovascular function, does not hinder the immune system.[21,22] Physical activity and athletic participation also has positive psychological benefits, improving the patient's overall quality of life.[21-23]

 ENDOCRINE SYSTEM DISORDERS

The endocrine system is a series of ductless organs that secrete hormones into the bloodstream and lymphatic system. The primary organs of the endocrine system include the pituitary, thyroid, parathyroid, and adrenal glands as well as the hypothalamus. A portion of the pancreas, the islands of Langerhans, is also part of the endocrine system. The ovaries and testicles are also part of this system; they are discussed in Chapter 12.

DIABETES MELLITUS

Diabetes mellitus (diabetes) is a metabolic disorder that affects the body's production and use of insulin. Insulin is hormone responsible for regulating carbohydrate metabolism, protein synthesis, and fat storage.[24] Insulin functions to store energy in the form of glucose in the muscles and glycogen in the liver. When carbohydrates are digested, they are turned into glucose that is absorbed by the bloodstream via the small intestine. Normally, the pancreas releases insulin proportionally to the level of glucose in the blood. However, with diabetes, blood glucose levels are increased, and the body is unable to use or store glucose. When it is untreated or poorly controlled, this disease can affect the cardiovascular, nervous, renal, ocular, and musculoskeletal systems.

Decreased insulin levels results in an increased level of glucose in the blood, called **hyperglycemia.** Water is lost from the body as glucose is excreted in the urine, resulting in excessive thirst. Because of the effects of strenuous exercise, diabetic athletes have an increased challenge of balancing insulin levels and carbohydrate intake and maintaining fluid levels.[25] **Hypoglycemia,** discussed later, occurs when the blood glucose level drops below 70 mg/dL.[24]

Types of Diabetes Mellitus

There are two primary types of diabetes, type 1 (formally known as insulin-dependent diabetes) and type 2 (formally known as noninsulin-dependent diabetes). Another type of diabetes, gestational diabetes, is related to pregnancy and is beyond the scope of this text.

The signs and symptoms of types 1 and 2 diabetes are quite similar. The individual's thirst is increased and need to urinate is frequent. Nausea and vomiting occur and, despite an increased appetite, weight loss may occur. The patient often reports feeling fatigued. Women may experience amenorrhea. Diabetes may also be marked by male impotence, blurred vision, and genitourinary and skin infection.

A diagnosis of diabetes is made after a urinalysis is done that identifies the level of glucose and ketone bodies, which are elevated in patients with diabetes. Fasting blood glucose levels greater than 140 mg/dL and random blood glucose levels greater than 200 mg/dL confirm diabetes. Other tests include insulin tests and tests to determine the level of glycosylated hemoglobin.

During exercise, hyperglycemia and *ketoacidosis* can occur, leading to diabetic coma or diabetic shock

---

Ketoacidosis An increase in the blood acid level caused by the accumulation of ketone bodies.

Table 21–14
SIGNS AND SYMPTOMS OF DIABETIC KETOACIDOSIS AND HYPOGLYCEMIC SHOCK

	Diabetic Ketoacidosis (Diabetic Coma)	Hypoglycemic Shock (Insulin Shock)
Onset	Gradual	Rapid
Pulse	Rapid, weak	Bounding
Blood pressure	Decreased	Normal
Respiration	Labored or deep	Normal or shallow
Mental state	Restlessness, confusion, stupor	Irritability Hostility
Skin	Dry Warm Possibly reddened	Cold Clammy Possibly pale
Other signs and symptoms	Intense thirst Dry mouth Nausea and vomiting Abdominal pain Fruity breath Coma	Dizziness Headache Hunger Profuse sweating Fainting Convulsions
Cause	Increased blood glucose levels	Decreased blood glucose levels

(hypoglycemia) (Table 21–14). Ketoacidosis, occurring when ketones collect in the body and causing a decrease in the pH level, usually takes several days to develop. When ketoacidosis occurs in the presence of dehydration, confusion, irritability, and coma occur.

Type 1 Diabetes

Type 1 diabetes most commonly affects individuals younger than age 30 years and previously has been referred to as "juvenile-onset diabetes." This form of diabetes is an autoimmune disorder in which the beta cells of the islets of Langerhans (the cells that secrete insulin) in the pancreas are destroyed or not functioning.[24] The absence of insulin in the bloodstream results in ketoacidosis. Because the body is unable to produce insulin on its own, the only way to truly control type 1 diabetes is through insulin injections or by the use of an insulin pump.

Patients must monitor their insulin levels and make the appropriate adjustments by increasing or decreasing the amount of insulin injected into the body. Insulin levels are also controlled by modifying the patient's diet and exercise. The blood glucose level should be maintained in the normal range of 80 to 120 mg/dL.[24]

Type 2 Diabetes

A decreased production of insulin or a decreased ability to use insulin is classified as type 2 diabetes. This form, the most common form of diabetes, typically affecting adults older than age 40 years, has a slow onset of symptoms.[26] Excess body fat causes an insulin resistance syndrome that leads to diabetes.[26] Type 2 diabetes is controlled through proper diet, weight control, exercise, oral medications, or insulin. The risk of develop-

ing type 2 diabetes is reduced by 6 percent for each 500-kcal increment in activity.

Metabolic Effects During Exercise

Exercise is beneficial for individuals with diabetes because it helps to manage weight, lower blood glucose levels, and increase blood insulin levels.[25–27] However, intense exercise and unregulated diet and insulin levels can worsen the condition. The muscles' demands for oxygen and metabolic substrates, including muscle and liver glycogen, muscle triglycerides, and free fatty acids, increase during exercise.[25]

The risk of hypoglycemia is greatest during exercise. Exercise must be preceded by increased caloric consumption or decreased insulin intake.[25] To prevent hypoglycemia in athletes with type 1 diabetes, precompetition insulin levels should be reduced 30 to 50 percent before exercise. In addition, carbohydrate intake must be increased.[12,26,28] During exercise, athletes should consume carbohydrates at the rate of 15 g for every half hour of exercise.[25]

Delayed post-exercise hypoglycemia also may be a problem with individuals who have type 1 diabetes. Repeated bouts of high-intensity, low-duration activity such as weight lifting increase post-activity insulin sensitivity.[26] Delayed hypoglycemia typically occurs at night, frequently within 6 to 15 hours after exercise, but the delay may be up to 28 hours later.[29] The onset has been associated with the inadequate replenishment of glycogen stores after bouts of exercise.[29] The risk of post-exercise hypoglycemia can be reduced by avoiding the use of intermediately acting insulin during the late afternoon and early evening or by using long-acting insulin.[25] Newer insulin pumps can also reduce the chance of onset.[25]

Risks Associated with Exercise

Hypoglycemia is the most immediate and serious risk associated with exercise, more so in individuals suffering from type 1 diabetes than those with type 2.[26,29] The site of insulin injection before exercise influences the blood glucose level. Injection into the primary exercising muscles, such as the quadriceps in runners or the deltoid in throwers, increases the rate of absorption. Increased blood insulin levels significantly decrease blood glucose levels, thus setting the stage for hypoglycemia. Injections within 2 hours of exercise should be given in the abdomen.[29] This not withstanding, athletes should regularly check their blood glucose levels during exercise.

Retinal damage caused by diabetes and generalized *retinopathy* are contraindications to intense exercise. Increased intrathecal pressure (Valsalva maneuver) can increase the intraocular pressure, subsequently causing hemorrhage into the vitreous humor.[25] Neurologic deficits and weakened muscles can increase the risk of metatarsal fractures and other biomechanical-related injuries.[30]

Individuals who are predisposed to or have a history of diabetic ketoacidosis or hypoglycemic shock should not participate in high-risk activities such as rock climbing, skydiving, and other sports that require high levels of coordination, vision, and sensory feedback, unless special precautions are taken to prevent injury (e.g., additional life lines or buddy jumping).[25]

Management of Diabetes-related Emergencies

Athletes with diabetes should be identified before competition. Diabetic athletes should also be encouraged to wear identification such as a Medic Alert tag that indicates they have diabetes. Diabetic emergencies occur secondary to hypoglycemia or hyperglycemia (see Table 21–14).

With mild hypoglycemia, administer 10 to 15 g of a fast-acting carbohydrate source. One serving (half of a can) of non-diet soda, 4 oz of orange juice, four packets of table sugar, or five to seven Life Savers candies can be administered to a conscious victim.[24] Chocolate and other high-fat foods should be avoided because the fat content will hinder the absorption of sugar. If the victim is unconscious or unable to swallow, glucagon injections or an oral glucose gel that is absorbed transcutaneously without swallowing must be administered. The procedures for administering the injections must be clarified with the patient and the patient's physician before the need to use them.[24]

After treatment, the victim's blood sugar should be rechecked every 15 minutes. If the blood glucose level remains below 70 mg/dL, another 10 to 15 g of carbohydrates should be administered. This process is repeated until the blood glucose returns to the low normal range.[24]

Table 21–15
SIGNS AND SYMPTOMS OF THYROID DISORDERS

Hyperthyroidism	Hypothyroidism
Nervousness	Weight gain
Weight loss	Fatigue
Increased appetite	Intolerance to cold
Excessive thirst	Depression
Intolerance to heat	Thinning of hair
Fatigue	Brittle fingernails
Excessive sweating	Pale skin color
Increased heart rate or bounding pulse	Slowing or slurring of speech
Constipation or diarrhea	Enlargement of the face, hands, and feet
Menstrual irregularities	Menstrual irregularities
Muscle cramps	
Tremor of the extended fingers	
Tremor of the tongue	
Possible visible enlargement of the thyroid gland (goiter)	

HYPERTHYROIDISM

Hyperthyroidism is a syndrome caused by the overproduction of thyroid hormone. The signs and symptoms of hyperthyroidism are varied (Table 21–15). The presence of the thyroid hormone accelerates the basal metabolic rate, necessitating the need (and physical desire) for increased caloric intake. Depending on its severity, hyperthyroidism can be a contraindication to athletic participation. Individuals suffering from hyperthyroidism have a reduced tolerance to heat. Additionally, the associated weight loss and fatigue may hinder muscular strength and cardiovascular endurance.

Hyperthyroidism can be caused by thyroid tumors, inflammation of the thyroid gland, or Graves' disease. The intake of excessive amounts of iodine has been linked to hyperthyroidism. Hyperthyroidism is initially managed using antithyroid medications. If this treatment approach fails, the gland is either removed or radioiodine is administered to ablate the thyroid. Its hormones are replaced using oral medications.

HYPOTHYROIDISM

Decreased thyroid activity, called hypothyroidism, results in a decreased basal metabolic rate. As a result, physical and cognitive functions may be impaired (see Table 12–15). Primary hypothyroidism occurs secondary to diseases of the thyroid gland. Secondary hypothyroidism is caused by failure of the pituitary gland to stimulate the thyroid to release an adequate level of hormones.

Retinopathy A general term used to describe a disorder of the eye's retina.

A primary consequence of hypothyroidism is obesity. Increased weight, slowed metabolism, and decreased muscle function all impair athletic function. Hypothyroidism is treated by replacing or supplementing the appropriate hormones.

PANCREATITIS

The pancreas is a gland that is connected to the duodenum at one end and the spleen at its opposite end, forming the **pancreatic duct** (see Fig. 12–4). Because it produces both internal and external secretions, the pancreas has both endocrine and exocrine function. The external secretion, **pancreatic juice,** is used in the digestion of food. Its endocrine functions include the production of insulin and glucagon (see the section on diabetes).

Inflammation of the pancreas, or **pancreatitis,** can be acute or chronic. Acute onset may be related to traumatic injury; gallstones; alcohol use; improperly cooked meats; or medications such as corticosteroids, acetaminophen, or tetracycline. Chronic pancreatitis often occurs concurrently with diabetes. Patients with chronic pancreatitis are treated with low-fat diets, the avoidance of alcohol or caffeine consumption, and other diet modifications.

The primary complaint of acute and chronic pancreatitis is severe pain in the upper left quadrant that radiates to the back and possibly increases when lying supine. The pain also may increase after meals, especially those that are high in fat, or after consumption of alcohol or caffeine. The patient may also complain of nausea, vomiting, intestinal gas, indigestion, and pale-colored stool. Clammy skin, sweating, fever, and abdominal distention also may be noted. A definitive diagnosis of pancreatitis is made after blood and urine analysis for increased levels of pancreatic enzymes. A computed tomography (CT) scan or ultrasonic imaging may show an increased size of the pancreas.

The management of pancreatitis is based on its cause. In mild cases, the treatment approach is symptomatic. Advanced cases may require the removal of the pancreas.

 SYSTEMIC DISEASES

MARFAN SYNDROME

An inherited condition, Marfan syndrome is characterized by cardiovascular, musculoskeletal, and ocular abnormalities observable during physical inspection. Classic physical findings of individuals suffering Marfan syndrome include an arm span greater than the person's height and elongated metacarpal and metatarsal bones, causing the hands and feet to appear disproportionately large.[31] Overall, there may be laxity throughout the joints. Kyphoscoliosis may be noted in the thoracic spine. **Steinberg's thumb,** in which the person is able to oppose the thumb beyond the ulnar border of the hand, is also a significant musculoskeletal determinant of Marfan syndrome.[32,33]

Although Marfan syndrome is a disease of the body's connective tissue, failure of the cardiac system usually leads to death. In this syndrome, the connective tissue providing strength to the aorta is decreased, leading to weakness of this tissue and the development of an aneurysm. Even when the syndrome is recognized and the individual is removed from strenuous activity, the person can suffer rupture of an aortic aneurysm, leading to immediate death.[34,35]

Although patients with Marfan syndrome are usually asymptomatic during exercise, Marfan syndrome can be detected during the physical examination (Table 21–16). Typically, the first finding leading to the diagnosis is that of a dislocated lens in the eye.[36] This finding, in conjunction with the physical appearance findings, warrants a full cardiac examination.

Table 21–16
EVALUATIVE FINDINGS: Marfan Syndrome

Examination Segment	Clinical Findings	
History	*Onset:*	Congenital
	Pain characteristics:	Possibly no complaints of cardiac disorder and no history of problems.
	Mechanism:	Congenital, deteriorating disease state
	Predisposing conditions:	A family history of Marfan syndrome
Inspection	Tall individuals whose arm span is greater than their height typify those with this syndrome. Elongation of the metacarpals and metatarsals is present. Kyphoscoliosis is noted. Dislocated lenses of the eye may be found.	
Ligamentous Tests	Laxity is present in multiple joints	
Special Tests	Cardiac examination reveals multivalvular disease and an abnormal aorta.	
Comment	Definitive diagnosis of Marfan syndrome is made by a physician.	

Cardiac testing may produce various abnormalities, the most common being an abnormal aorta and multivalvular deformities, leading to prolapse of the valves and aortic valve regurgitation.[32,35] The decreased amount of connective tissue in the aortic wall makes it susceptible to rupture because of the high pressure exerted on the weakened wall as pumped from the left ventricle. Aortic root dilation also is a prominent abnormality that eventually leads to dissecting aortic aneurysm.[37] Signs of an aneurysm are the most common finding on echocardiography.

Although medical clearance is determined on a case-by-case basis, individuals who have Marfan syndrome are restricted from participating in vigorous physical activity. An absolute disqualifying condition is an enlarged aortic root, a predisposition to aortic rupture.[12]

IRON DEFICIENCY ANEMIA

Iron is vital within the human body for various physiological functions, including oxygen transport in the blood. Iron deficiency anemia is the most common form of anemia. In children and adolescents, iron deficiency anemia is most commonly related to inadequate intake of iron in the diet. In adults, the deficiency may be linked to blood loss.

Patients with iron deficiency anemia often complain of fatigue, shortness of breath, weakness, and depleted energy during normal activities. These individuals may appear pale and their fingernails may be brittle. Definitive diagnosis is obtained through blood analysis for hemoglobin and serum ferritin levels. Several groups of patients, including women prone to excessive bleeding during menstruation, vegetarians, those with gastrointestinal (GI) blood loss, and those who abuse alcohol or are taking aspirin or nonsteroidal antiinflammatory drugs (NSAIDs) may be at higher risk to develop iron deficiency anemia.

Treatment of patients with iron deficiency anemia is usually managed by oral iron supplements. The supplements are usually continued for 4 to 6 months after hematocrit levels are restored to normal ranges. In rare cases, oral supplementation does not work and IV or intramuscular supplementation of iron must be used.

SICKLE CELL ANEMIA AND SICKLE CELL TRAIT

Sickle cell anemia (SCA) and sickle cell trait (SCT) are two genetic conditions that can be found in any race, but they occur more prevalently in people of African descent worldwide. In the United States, 8 to 10 percent of the African-American population demonstrates SCT, but less than 1 percent have SCA.[38]

The difference between SCT and SCA is found in the hemoglobin structure. In SCT, there is one normal hemoglobin gene (A) and one abnormal hemoglobin gene (S), leading to an (AS)-type hemoglobin. With SCA,

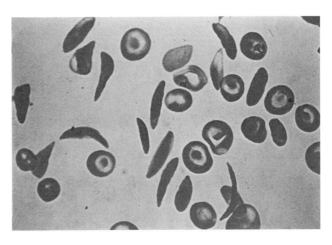

FIGURE 21–6. Sickle cell anemia. Note the elongated shape of the red blood cells, forming a sickled shape.

both hemoglobin genes are abnormal, type S, causing an (SS)-type hemoglobin.[38] SCT is acquired when one parent has the S gene. SCA is inherited when both parents have the S gene. SCT is not a disease in and of itself and must be distinguished from SCA, a potentially fatal disease.

Sickle Cell Anemia

Sickle cell anemia is an inherited, potentially fatal, disease that affects the function of the red blood cells (RBCs). Although this disease is present at birth, signs and symptoms do not appear until the age of approximately 4 months. Physical stress, such as infection, hypoxia, or dehydration, results in *acidosis,* causing the RBCs to collapse and form the characteristic sickle shape (Fig. 21–6). These cells soon die, causing the blood to thicken and clump, thereby decreasing the blood's oxygen capacity. The decreased delivery of blood and its oxygen soon affects the body's other systems (Table 21–17). Because of the high risk associated with SCA, affected individuals are often disqualified from athletic participation and restricted from most forms of physical exertion.

Care must be taken to prevent patients with SCA from being placed in situations that exacerbate the condition. Dehydration must be prevented by limiting physical activity; avoiding prolonged exposure to the sun, heat, and humidity; and encouraging proper hydration and nutrition. High altitude or low-oxygen environments (including during air travel) also increase the mass of the RBCs and the stress placed on the cardiovascular system.

Acidosis An increase in the blood's acid balance (lowering of pH) caused by the accumulation of acids or the loss of blood bases.

Table 21–17
SIGNS AND SYMPTOMS OF SICKLE CELL ANEMIA

Fatigue
Increased heart rate
Shortness of breath
Generalized weakness
Predisposition to infection
Fever
Nausea
Pain in the extremities and joints
Enlargement of the spleen
Abdominal and chest pain
Lower extremity ulceration
Jaundice
Excessive thirst
Priapism
Slowed physical maturation

Sickle Cell Trait

Unlike SCA, SCT is usually benign and does not require limitations on athletic participation. However, certain precautions must be followed.[38,39] In certain instances, particularly when athletes compete at altitudes above 5000 feet without prior acclimatization to the altitude, the risk of splenic *infarction* is increased.[38,40] In rare instances, SCT has been associated with, but not implicated in causing, exercise-related sudden death secondary to *rhabdomyolysis, hyposthenuria,* heat stroke, or cardiac arrhythmia.[38–42] Also, when competing at a high altitude, the risk of a splenic infarction increases, causing pain in the lower ribs, nausea, and weakness.[38]

The presence of SCT does not affect anaerobic exercise, but it can result in lower blood lactate concentrations that potentially may reduce recovery time.[42] Aerobic performance at high altitudes also tends to be reduced.[42] Other potential consequences of SCT during exercise include hypoxia, low blood pH, and the predisposition to dehydration.[12]

The *National Collegiate Athletic Association Sports Medicine Handbook* states that no restrictions should be placed on student-athletes who have SCT. However, precautions must be taken to avoid dehydration, and extra effort must be taken to acclimatize the athletes to heat, humidity, and altitude. Likewise, the individual should refrain from exercising during acute illness, especially those involving fever.[38]

LYME DISEASE

Lyme disease is a complex illness that affects multiple systems within the body. Caused by the *Borrelia burgdorferi* virus, it is transmitted to humans via the deer tick bite. If it is treated in its early stages, it can usually be well managed with limited progression of symptoms.

Not all tick bites transmit the disease. Imbedded ticks should be removed promptly because the tick may need to be attached for longer than 24 hours to transmit the infection. Individuals who are at risk to exposure should check for ticks on a routine basis. After removing the tick, the area should be observed carefully and medical attention should be sought if local symptoms appear.

An early manifestation of the disease is the development of an erythematous macule or papule at the site of the bite. Over a period of days, the infection spreads over the skin to create an erythematous migrans. Over time, the infection may spread via the blood. Secondary symptoms include fever, chills, headache, *arthralgias*, myalgias, and secondary skin site lesions. The disease can spread to the heart, creating carditis; the nervous system in the form of meningitis or cranial nerve palsy; and, very commonly, the joints in the form of unexplained pain and inflammation, often being confused with arthritis.[43] The knee is most commonly affected.

The diagnosis of Lyme disease is made primarily through clinical examination and serologic testing. Lyme disease progresses through three stages, but the symptoms may overlap between these stages (Table 21–18).[43]

In the early stages of the disease, blood tests may reveal that the patient has not become seropositive. After diagnosed, the treatment revolves around antibiotic therapy usually completed over a 2- to 3-week period. Although Lyme disease vaccine is currently available, it is not clearly determined who should absolutely have it. Individuals with a high risk of exposure to deer ticks should be vaccinated against Lyme disease.

CHRONIC FATIGUE SYNDROME

Chronic fatigue syndrome (CFS) is the name applied to a collection of symptoms that includes long-term fatigue as a part of the general diagnostic criteria. When this syndrome was identified in the 1980s, it was known as chronic EBV syndrome, a variant of mononucleosis.

Chronic fatigue syndrome may be the combined outcome of two separate entities, the presence of the EBV and clinical depression.[44] To be diagnosed with CFS, patients must have a history of disabling fatigue of unknown origin for at least 6 months.[44,45] The onset of fatigue often follows symptoms resembling those of the flu or mononucleosis. In addition to fatigue, the individual must display at least four of the eight possible symptoms to be diagnosed with CFS: sore throat,

---

Infarction (infarct) Necrosis of localized organ tissue caused by loss of the blood supply.

Rhabdomyolysis Acute, sometimes fatal disease marked by the destruction of skeletal muscle.

Hyposthenuria The inability to concentrate urine normally.

Table 21–18
STAGES OF LYME DISEASE

Stage	Onset After Exposure	Symptoms
1	3 to 30 days	A rash at the site of the bite (erythema migrans) Fever Headache Myalgias Arthralagias
2	Weeks to months	Increasing severity of illness with an increase in symptoms from stage 1 Malaise Neurologic symptoms (headache, cranial nerve palsies [especially Bell's palsy], lympocytic meningitis with or without radiculoneuropathy) Cardiovascular symptoms (carditis characterized by atrioventricular conduction abnormalitites)
3	Months to years	Synovial involvement Nervous system involvement (chronic neurologic Lyme disease, subtle encephalopathy, peripheral neuropathy, cognitive impairment most likely affecting short-term memory, paresthesias in a stocking or stocking/glove distribution) Systemic skin rashes Arthritis

lymph node swelling or tenderness, *arthralgias*, myalgias, sleep difficulties, cognitive difficulties, headaches, and an increase in symptoms within 24 hours of increased physical or mental activity. Because the symptoms can be vague and mimic other conditions, certain medical conditions such as hypothyroidism; sleep apnea; chronic active hepatitis; severe obesity; and psychiatric illnesses such as schizophrenia, dementia, bipolar affective disorder, eating disorders, and substance abuse must be ruled out.

Treatment of patients with CFS relies heavily on education about the syndrome and successful ways to manage it. The patient must develop coping skills to deal with the fatigue; enter a graduated exercise regimen, if possible; and use medications such as sleep aids, antidepressants, analgesics, and histamine blockers, as indicated to minimize the symptoms.

FIBROMYALGIA

Fibromyalgia is a pain syndrome characterized by at least 3 months of chronic pain, stiffness, and fatigue. This condition may be associated with CFS. The pain usually occurs at predictable anatomic sites (these painful sites are not to be confused with trigger points). Sleep disturbance, headache, psychological abnormality, reports of swelling, and varying degrees of functional disability may be present. Fibromyalgia is a noninflammatory condition. The presence of joint effusion, synovitis, warmth over the painful area, or deformity rules out fibromyalgia.[46]

To be diagnosed with fibromyalgia, the patient must meet two criteria.[46]. First, the patient must report widespread bilateral pain above and below the waist involving the axial skeleton and persisting for a minimum of 3 months. The second criterion is the patient must verbally declare pain during palpation in at least 11 of the 18 palpation sites (Table 21–19).

Table 21–19
COMMON SITES OF FIBROMYALGIA*

Occiput	At the insertion of the upper trapezius muscles
Cervical spine	Anterior aspect of the intertransverse spaces at C5 to C7
Trapezius	Superior to the vertebral border of the scapula
Supraspinatus	Origin near the scapular spine
Second rib	At the second costochondral junction
Lateral epicondyle	2 cm distal to the lateral epicondyles
Gluteus maximus	Upper, outer quadrant of the buttocks
Greater trochanter	2 cm posterior to the greater trochanter
Knee	At the medial fat pads of the knee

*All sites are bilateral.

Arthralgia Painful joints.

After a definitive diagnosis has been made, the first goal of treatment is to develop the patient's awareness of the syndrome's effects. The patient needs to understand that the syndrome is not progressively crippling or disabling. Symptomatic use of medications may be used. A holistic approach of meditation, relaxation exercises, biofeedback to decrease tension, and a graduated exercise program may all be used to decrease the affects of the syndrome.

 ## CANCER

Cancer refers to the uncontrolled growth and spreading of abnormal or atypical cells. A mass of growing cells is termed a tumor. Tumors are medically classified as being **benign** or **malignant.** Benign tumors consist of cells that resemble the original tissues. The mass of the tumor remains localized and tends to stay in an encapsulated structure with a relatively slow growth. Unless the tumor grows in an area that disrupts blood supply or in an enclosed area (e.g., within the skull), benign tumors are typically not fatal.[7] Benign tumors also are not considered cancerous.

Malignant tumors are a much more serious condition. Malignant tumors are formed by atypical cells that grow and spread. Malignant tumors are cancerous. Depending on the type and location of the neoplasm, the growth and spread can be rapid or slow. Because malignant tumors spread, they have a greater likelihood of having fatal outcomes.

The effects of malignant tumors occur secondary to obstructing anatomical structures, depriving healthy tissues of adequate blood supply, or both. Tumors that develop in the lungs, abdomen, or similar system can form physical obstructions that prevent normal physiological processes. For example, a tumor in the lungs may prevent the inflow of oxygen or an abdominal mass can disrupt intestinal or urogenital function. The tumor can also deprive the surrounding cells of oxygen, causing necrosis and infection, thereby triggering an inflammatory response. The affected cells also release collagenase, an inflammatory mediator that causes the breakdown of cells and further tissue destruction.[7]

There are more than 200 different forms of cancers classified by the types of tissues involved. **Carcinoma** primarily affects the epithelial cells that form the skin and lining body cavities. **Sarcomas** are associated with the mesenchymal cells that form connective tissues, blood, blood vessels, and the lymphatic system.

Cancer becomes fatal when its cells spread and invade other tissues or the tumor (neoplasm) directly disrupts the function of vital organs. Cancerous cells are characterized by the mutation of its DNA, resulting in uncontrolled growth or the progressive spread of the diseased tissues. Tumors develop when the body's normal regulatory functions no longer work and the tissue uncontrollably proliferates.

Cancerous or malignant tumors can spread in several manners. One way is by the direct **invasion** of the surrounding tissues. **Metastasis** occurs when cancerous cells are spread through the body by way of the bloodstream or lymphatic system. Cancer cells can also be transferred by certain body fluids or along membranes, resulting in seeding of the cells in other parts of the body.

SIGNS AND SYMPTOMS OF CANCER

The general signs and symptoms of cancer can be remembered using the mnemonic of "CAUTION":

C: Change in bowel or bladder habits
A: A sore that does not heal
U: Unusual bleeding or discharge
T: Thickening or lumps (in the breasts, testicles, and so on)
I: Indigestion or difficulty swallowing
O: Obvious change in warts or moles
N: Nagging cough or hoarseness

Specific forms of cancer may have unique signs, symptoms, and diagnostic tests. Some forms of cancer do not present with outward signs and symptoms until the disease has matured. This latent period causes a delay between the onset of the disease and the manifestation of symptoms.

The signs, symptoms, effects, disposition, and long-term consequences of cancer depend on its location in the body. As with many diseases, a family history of cancer is perhaps the strongest indicator of an individual's developing cancer. However, exposure to environmental concerns such as the sun, radiation (including those used in medicine and therapy), and chemicals can also cause cancer. The development of symptoms may take many years after exposure to the carcinogens.

LEUKEMIA

The uncontrolled proliferation of immature WBCs, leukemia originates in the bone marrow. The leukocytes produced in the presence of leukemia are nonfunctional. The proliferation of these cells decreases the bone marrow's ability to produce normal, functional cells. Leukemia affects people of all ages, but it is most commonly diagnosed in children and young adults.

Leukemias are categorized as being acute or chronic and are named according to the type of cell involved. A partial list of common leukemias is presented in Table 21–20. Acute leukemia involves a high proportion of immature, nonfunctional cells. Chronic leukemia involves a higher proportion of mature cells relative to acute leukemia and therefore has a better prognosis.[7]

The clinical signs and symptoms of leukemia reflect the diminished function of the red and WBCs. The individual is predisposed to infection (secondary to a decreased immune response), with possible low-grade

Table 21–20 **TYPES OF LEUKEMIA**	
Type	**Description**
Acute lymphocytic leukemia (ALL)	The incomplete development of white blood cells leads to malignant lymphocytes. Overtime, these cells replace healthy cells. ALL primarily affects children and has an exceptional survival rate with early detection.
Acute myeloid leukemia ([AML] **Acute nonlymphocytic leukemia)**	Granular leukocytes proliferate. As the disease progresses, the bone marrow ceases to function. AML affects adults and infants.
Chronic lymphocytic leukemia (CLL)	The WBC count slowly decreases, but the level of B lymphocytes proliferates. CLL primarily affects individuals older than age of 50 years.
Chronic myeloid Leukemia (CML)	Bone marrow proliferation involves all cell types Evidence of the Philadelphia chromosome, a genetic abnormality, is present in the majority of cases.
Hairy cell leukemia	Both red blood cell and WBC counts are reduced. A low platelet count increases the tendency to bleed.

WBC = white blood cell.

fever, lymph node swelling, and lethargy or fatigue. As the disease progresses, the spleen or liver becomes enlarged. The individual becomes anemic and has the tendency to bruise easily. Blood coagulation time also is prolonged. Women may experience irregular menstruation. A loss of appetite and subsequent weight loss may occur. Unexplained skin rashes, generalized itching, night sweats, and joint pain or pain within the bone may be reported.

The presence and type of leukemia is definitively diagnosed through laboratory blood analysis and bone marrow biopsy. During these diagnostic procedures, red blood cell and platelet levels are found to be low and the WBCs are immature or abnormal.[7]

Treatment consists of chemotherapy, blood marrow transplantation, or both. During the treatment period, the body's energy expenditure levels are decreased, possibly leading to post-treatment obesity.[47]

LYMPHOMAS

Two major classes of lymphoma occur, **non-Hodgkin's lymphoma** (NHL) and Hodgkin's lymphoma. A diverse range of malignant disorders, NHL primarily attacks the B lymphocytes of the lymph nodes and extranodal tissues. An aggressive disease, patients with NHL are more difficult to treat and have a lower long-term survival rate than Hodgkin's lymphoma

Hodgkin's Lymphoma

Hodgkin's lymphoma (Hodgkin's disease) is the growth of malignant tumors into the lymph nodes, bone marrow, spleen, and liver. In the early stages, Hodgkin's lymphoma starts within a single lymph node. As the disease progresses, the cancerous cells are spread by the bloodstream and appear in other lymphatic organs. Hodgkin's lymphoma is most prevalent in individuals between the ages of 15 and 35 years.

The severity of Hodgkin's lymphoma is based on the number and location of the lymph nodes that are affected using the Ann Arbor Staging System:

- **Stage I:** A single lymph node or region is affected.
- **Stage II:** Two or more lymph nodes or regions on the same side of the diaphragm are affected.
- **Stage III:** Lymph nodes on both sides of the diaphragm and the spleen are affected.
- **Stage IV:** The lymphoma spreads beyond the lymphatic system or extranodal organs (tissues other than the lymph nodes).

Clinically, the initial symptoms of Hodgkin's lymphoma are the painless swelling of lymph nodes, usually involving the groin, axilla, or cervical region. The patient may also complain of itching; neck pain; and excessive sweating, especially at night. As the body's immune system becomes weakened, the person may notice weight loss, fatigue, and fever. As the disease progresses, hair loss, splenic enlargement, and clubbing of the fingers or toes may be noted.

Hodgkin's lymphoma is marked by the presence of the Reed-Sternberg cell during laboratory analysis of blood. A definitive diagnosis of Hodgkin' lymphoma is made after a biopsy of the lymph nodes, bone marrow, or involved tissue.

Stage I and II Hodgkin's disease is treated with radiation therapy. Chemotherapy is administered for some forms of stage II Hodgkin's disease and for stages III and IV. The long-term prognosis for individuals with stage I or II lymphoma is excellent.

BRAIN TUMORS

Tumors that develop within the skull may be malignant (cancerous) or benign (noncancerous). Regardless of the etiology of the tumor, its growth within the confined space of the skull can be potentially fatal. As the size of the tumor increases, the intracranial pressure is increased, disrupting normal brain function. Tumors can also affect brain function secondary to inflammation or destruction of the brain cells. The actual number of cancerous tumors that originate in the brain is relatively low. More frequently, cancerous brain tumors occur as metastasis from other forms of cancer in other parts of the body.[48]

The signs and symptoms of brain tumors are similar to those of a subdural or epidural hematoma, which are described in Chapter 18. However, the duration between the onset of the disease and the manifestation of the symptoms is much longer. The initial signs of a brain tumor, usually behavioral, vary according to the location of the tumor. The individual may begin to display a gradual loss of balance and coordination, alterations in hearing or vision, changes in mood and personality, or subtle cognitive difficulties. As the tumor grows, headaches, gross motor dysfunction, and altered vital signs are possible. Seizures also may occur and are often the first indication of the tumor's presence.

MELANOMA

Melanoma, a form of skin cancer, involves the malignant growth of *melanin* cells of the skin or the eye (Fig. 21–7). Skin-based melanoma develops from a mole that was previously normal. Melanoma is an aggressive form of cancer that rapidly spreads to other areas.

Certain individuals are at an increased risk of developing melanoma. Those with a family history of melanoma, fair skin, freckles, moles, and a predisposition to sunburn are considered to be at a high risk of developing melanoma. A history of three or more episodes of severe blistering sunburns and a history spent outdoors between the ages of 10 and 24 years are additional risk factors for developing melanomas.

Individuals who are regularly exposed to direct sunlight are also at an increased risk of developing a melanoma and require regular screening for signs of a melanoma.[49] Although biopsies are required to diagnose a melanoma, moles should be inspected for the following signs of a melanoma:[50]

- **Asymmetry:** Irregularity in shape (increases suspicion of a melanoma because moles that are normal tend to be round and symmetrical)
- **Border:** Irregularly shaped borders
- **Color:** Nonuniform color; mottled
- **Diameter:** A diameter greater than 6 mm
- **Elevation:** The growth extending upward from the skin; elevation determined through palpation or side lighting the growth
- **Enlargement:** Increasing width over time

A mole that bleeds on a regular basis, is tender, or spontaneously appears in sunburn areas (e.g., face, neck, shoulder, back, arms) should promptly be evaluated by a physician.

At-risk athletes who regularly compete in the sun should take special precautions to decrease the risk of developing melanoma. When practical, practices

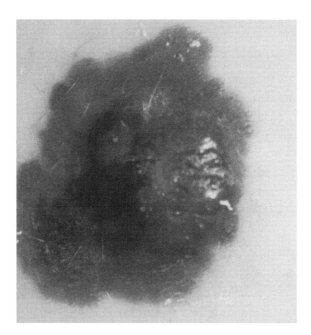

FIGURE 21–7. Nodular melanoma.

should be schedule to avoid peak sun exposures (a task that is more practical with individual sports such as track than team sports). When competing in the direct sunlight, encourage athletes to wear a sunblock with a sun protection factor (SPF) of 15 or higher or wear protective clothing. People considered at risk should perform self-examinations of their skin regularly and be examined by a physician on a regular basis.

ORAL CANCER

Oral cancer most commonly involves the lips, gums, tongue, or palate. Although strong causative relationships have not been substantiated, risk factors for developing oral cancer include the use of cigarettes and smokeless tobacco, denture use, excessive alcohol consumption, and poor oral hygiene.[51] A family history of oral cancer may be a strong predisposing factor in acquiring this disease.[52]

Initially, patients with oral cancer present with white or red lesions and nonhealing open wounds. Leukoplakia, precancerous cells, often form in the area of contact with smokeless tobacco (Fig. 21–8). The patient may complain of gingivitis-like symptoms, and the tongue may feel thick and swollen (angioedema). As the cancer progresses, the individual may experience difficulty swallowing and abnormal taste sensations.

Regular oral examinations for the signs of cancer should be conducted by a dentist or oral surgeon.[53] Self-examinations for the presence of leukoplakia or other prodromal signs of oral cancers should be performed monthly by at-risk individuals.[54]

Melanin The pigment produced by melanocytes that gives color to skin, hair, and eyes.

FIGURE 21–8. Leukoplakia of the tongue.

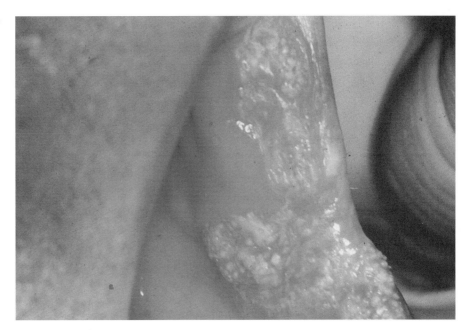

BREAST CANCER

Although breast cancer is most commonly associated with women, men may also develop the disease. Ductal carcinoma affects the lining of the breast ducts. Cancer that develops in the lobes is called lobular carcinoma. The risk of developing breast cancer increases with age.

Several factors may predispose an individual to the development of breast cancer, including the early onset of menses, lack of childbirth, late childbirth, obesity, and a delayed onset of menopause. A family history of breast cancer may be the strongest predictor of the risk for developing this disease.[55] The passing of mutated genes, *BCR1* and *BCR2*, may indicate that the predisposition to breast cancer is an inherited trait.[56]

Diet appears to play a role as both a predisposing factor and a preventive measure against breast cancer. High fat diets or diets in which the majority of the caloric intake is from fat may increase the risk of developing breast cancer.[57,58] Likewise, low-fat diets and diets high in fiber, garlic, and onion may decrease the risk.[57-59]

The initial symptom of breast cancer is often a lump discovered during a self-examination (Fig. 21–9). However, many masses found during self-examination are found to be benign, noncancerous fatty deposits. In the presence of cancer, as the size of the tumor increases, the size of the breasts may become asymmetrical, with the affected breast acquiring a firm feel.

Nipple retraction and areolar discoloration also may occur. The local lymph nodes and those in the axilla may become enlarged. The arm on the affected side may become swollen. A purulent, bloody, or clear discharge may occur from the nipple.

A mammogram is used to identify the presence of masses within the breast before it reaches a palpable size and evaluate the consistency of an existing palpable mass. Annual mammograms are recommended for all women older than age 40 years. The consistency of the mass (solid or fluid) can be determined noninvasively using ultrasound or thermal imaging techniques. A definitive diagnosis is made after biopsy of the mass.

Depending on the size and location of the tumor, patients with breast cancer may be treated through chemotherapy, radiation, hormones, or surgery (or a combination). Surgery may consist of removal of the lump (i.e., lumpectomy) and partial or total removal of the breast (i.e., mastectomy).

The American Cancer Society makes the following recommendation for the early detection of breast cancer:

- Women age 40 years and older should have an annual mammogram.
- A health professional should conduct a clinical breast examination every 3 years for patients age 20 through 39 years.
- Individuals older than age 20 years should perform monthly breast self-examinations.
- Changes in the breast such as the development of a lump, swelling, skin irritation, skin dimpling, nipple pain, nipple retraction, or unusual discharge should be evaluated by a physician.

FIGURE 21–9. Breast self examination.

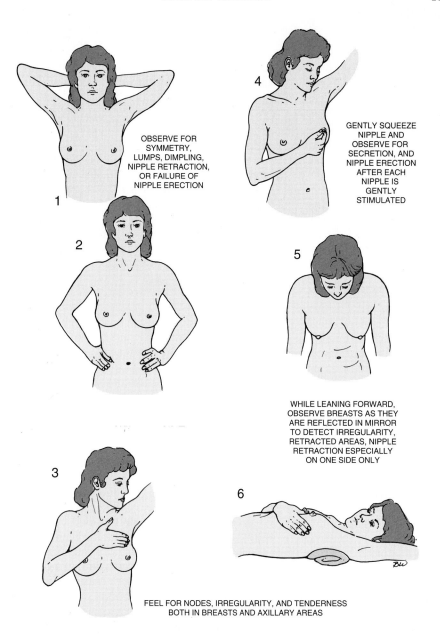

1 OBSERVE FOR SYMMETRY, LUMPS, DIMPLING, NIPPLE RETRACTION, OR FAILURE OF NIPPLE ERECTION

4 GENTLY SQUEEZE NIPPLE AND OBSERVE FOR SECRETION, AND NIPPLE ERECTION AFTER EACH NIPPLE IS GENTLY STIMULATED

5 WHILE LEANING FORWARD, OBSERVE BREASTS AS THEY ARE REFLECTED IN MIRROR TO DETECT IRREGULARITY, RETRACTED AREAS, NIPPLE RETRACTION ESPECIALLY ON ONE SIDE ONLY

3 FEEL FOR NODES, IRREGULARITY, AND TENDERNESS BOTH IN BREASTS AND AXILLARY AREAS

CERVICAL CANCER

Cancer of the uterine cervix usually evolves slowly, often taking years to fully develop. Initially, the superficial cells of the cervix become *dysplasic.* The abnormal cells then penetrate deeper into the lining of cervix, eventually invading the other pelvic and abdominal organs. The human papilloma virus (HPV), a sexually transmitted virus that is also associated with genital warts, is often implicated with cervical cancer.[60]

Cervical cancer presents no outward signs or symptoms during its early stages (often several years in duration). However, a **Pap smear** during this asymptomatic period can provide laboratory evidence of the presence of cervical cancer before cancerous lesions develop. In the event of positive Pap smears (note that Pap smears often produce false-positive results), the affected tissues can be surgically removed.

As the disease progresses, abnormal or unexpected vaginal bleeding and vaginal discharge may occur. The individual may complain of fatigue, pain in the legs or back, painful sexual intercourse, loss of appetite, and weight loss. In advanced stages, fistulas may develop, allowing urine or feces to escape through the vagina.

Dysplasic (dysplasia) Abnormal tissue development.

The survival rate for patients with cervical cancer is excellent when the disease is identified and the patient is treated in its early stage. As the disease spreads, the prognosis decreases. The American Cancer Society recommends annual Pap smears starting at age 18 years or when the individual becomes sexually active. The frequency of Pap smears can be performed less often after three consecutive negative tests.

OVARIAN CANCER

Ovarian cancer is an aggressive and rapidly spreading disease. The cancerous cells quickly spread from one ovary to the other. The physical location of the ovaries allows cancerous cells to seed the uterus, bladder, and intestines. Although the disease spreads rapidly, signs and symptoms typically do not occur until late in the disease.

Women who have a personal history of breast cancer or a family history of breast or ovarian cancer are at an increased risk of developing ovarian cancer. Other factors that increase the risk include infertility, repeated miscarriages, and high-fat diets.[61] Currently no screening test is available to detect ovarian cancer.

Several factors, including the absence of a screening test and the latent onset of symptoms, delay the diagnosis of ovarian cancer. The first symptoms include abdominal pain or abdominal "heaviness," oligomenorrhea, unexplained vaginal bleeding, loss of appetite, and weight loss. Excessive hair growth may be noted as the disease progresses. The American Cancer Society recommends annual pelvic exams for all women older than age 18 years or upon becoming sexually active.

TESTICULAR CANCER

Although younger or older age groups may be affected, testicular cancer is the most common form of cancer in men age 20 to 35 years. The signs and symptoms of testicular cancer include a lump on the testicle, testicular enlargement, and bloody ejaculate. Pain within the testicle itself is rare, but referred pain may be experienced in the abdomen (or an "empty" feeling in the abdomen) or back. As the disease progresses, *gynecomastia* may occur. Men with a history of an undescended testicle, mumps orchitis, or inguinal hernia are at an increased risk. Childhood vaccination against the mumps may reduce the risk factor of developing testicular cancer.[62] The rate of testicular cancer is reduced in men who have a moderate to high level of physical activity.[63]

Because the testicles are easily palpated, cancer of this region is often self-identified in its early stages. A monthly testicular self-examination is recommended for all postpubescent males. In part because of this early identification during self-examination, the long-term prognosis for testicular cancer is excellent. Further information regarding testicular cancer is presented in Chapter 12.

PROSTATE CANCER

Located inferior to the bladder and adjacent to the rectum, the prostate is a male sex gland that produces seminal fluids. The urethra passes through the prostate. Physiologically, the prostate must function with the bladder, urethra, and epididymis. Prostatic cancer can spread to these organs and then *metastasize* throughout the body, especially the lymphatic system, kidneys, and bones.

The prevalence of developing prostate cancer increases with age. Men younger than age 40 years are rarely affected; African-American males older than age 40 years are in the highest-risk group. Other factors that may contribute to the onset of prostate cancer include a family history of prostatic cancer, high-fat diets, and increased testosterone levels. Cardiovascular exercise may decrease the probability of developing prostate cancer.[64]

The early signs and symptoms of prostate cancer are experienced during urination and ejaculation, possibly mimicking a bladder infection or benign prostatic hypertrophy. Difficulty is experienced in starting and stopping the flow of urine, and the urge to urinate may become more urgent and frequent at night. Blood may also be visible in the urine. The individual may complain of pain during ejaculation. Pain may also be experienced during bowel movements and in the hips and low back.

The diagnosis of prostate cancer is made after tests for prostate-specific antigen (PSA). The diagnosis is confirmed by biopsy of prostate tissues. Although their efficacy has been called into question, an annual digital rectal examination is recommended for men older than age 40 years. Men older than age 50 years should also have an annual blood PSA test.

COLON CANCER

Cancer of the colon or rectum (**colorectal cancer**) is one of the most frequent types of cancer affecting men and women older than age 50 years. Noticeable signs of this disease may be absent until it is well developed. Some of the initial signs and symptoms of colorectal cancer resemble those of other GI disorders such as diarrhea, abdominal pain, intestinal gas, and weight loss. Microscopic or macroscopic blood may also be present in the stool leading to anemia. Constipation may develop secondary to obstruction of the bowel.

Gynecomastia Enlargement of the breasts in men and boys.

Metastasize (metastasis) Movement of cells, including cancer cells and bacteria, from one area of the body to another, thus spreading the disease.

The severity of colon cancer is based on the Duke's classification:[7]

- **Duke's A:** Involvement of the mucosa and submucosal tissues
- **Duke's B:** Involvement of the local tissues
- **Duke's C:** Regional lymph nodes are affected
- **Duke's D:** Metastases of the tumor

Early detection yields an excellent prognosis. An annual digital rectal examination is recommended for individuals older than age 40 years. Sigmoidoscopy should be performed every 3 to 5 years for individuals age 50 years and older. Colonoscopy may be recommended for patients with a significant family history of colon cancer.

EFFECT OF CANCER ON ATHLETIC PARTICIPATION

Most athletes who are suffering from cancer forego physical activity during treatment.[65] During this time, the body is adapting to the treatment. The lack of physical activity decreases muscular strength, muscular endurance, and cardiovascular function. Some patients prefer to resume light to moderate levels of physical activity as soon as possible to reduce the likelihood of contracting other health-related problems.[66]

A common side effect of the disease itself and the subsequent chemotherapy and radiation therapy is fatigue. The magnitude of this fatigue and the patient's ability to exercise is dependent on the type of cancer involved.[66] Cancer-related fatigue is more common after the earlier treatment bouts, possibly persisting for years after conclusion of the treatment.[67] Appropriate amounts of low-intensity activity may decrease the severity of cancer-related fatigue.[65]

Athletic participation after cancer treatment is often possible. Indeed, several high-profile professional athletes have returned to successful careers after cancer treatment. The reintegration back into sports should be progressive and based on the patient's current level of conditioning. The side effects experienced from chemotherapy and radiation may considerably weaken the patient, cause neuropathies, or weaken the heart. The rehabilitation process to return to normal activities of daily living may take months. As with anyone recovering from cancer, athletes should undergo frequent examinations to assess for any recurrence of the disease.

NEUROLOGIC DISORDERS

MIGRAINE HEADACHES

Migraine headaches are a recurrent form of profound headaches. The exact cause of migraine headaches is unknown, but this condition may be related to changes in the blood vessels of the brain and neck. These vessels constrict, reducing blood supply to the brain. The vasoconstriction is then followed by vasodilation, producing severe, often disabling headaches.

An aural period, marked by visual disturbances, such as blind spots in the field of vision, flashing lights, and hallucinations, may be experienced during the period of vasoconstriction.[68] Other prodromal symptoms may include paresthesia, aphasia, vertigo, or other neurologic or neuromuscular symptoms. Other signs and symptoms that indicate an upcoming attack include fatigue or excessive energy, GI symptoms, changes in eating habits, and mood changes.[68]

Migraine headaches are often brought on by triggering events. Such triggers include exercise, sexual intercourse, defecation, computer use, panic attacks, certain milk-based foods, meats, and alcohol.[68–70] In addition to the headache, migraine headaches may also be accompanied by pain in the eyes, dizziness, nausea, vomiting, fatigue, and irritability.

Although many individuals suffer from migraines throughout their lives, others may only experience an isolated time span during which the headaches occur.

Chronic migraine sufferers may be given prophylactic regimens to decrease the frequency and severity of onset. Relaxation techniques, avoiding known triggers, and taking medications such as cardiac beta-blockers, antidepressants, NSAIDs, and anticonvulsants may be used.

EPILEPSY

Epilepsy is a complex collection of syndromes with seizure as the primary manifestation of the disorder. A seizure is a sudden event involving the transient disturbance in the excitability in a group of the brain's neurons. The specific clinical manifestation of the seizure depends on the location of the event (e.g., a seizure in the motor cortex produces movement). Seizures can be caused by injuries and illness, including concussion, diabetes, kidney failure, drug dependency or withdrawal, or brain tumor.

The term "epilepsy" is used to describe a chronic seizure disorder that has no apparent cause. In certain instances, epilepsy can be acquired after a head injury.[71]

Epilepsy-related seizures can be related to emotional or physical stress or hormonal changes. Sensory stimuli such as flashing lights, sounds, or touch may also trigger a seizure. Often, seizures have no identifiable trigger. Seizures, described in Table 21–21, may be preceded by an aural period hours or minutes before the onset. The aural period is marked by a general feeling that a seizure is imminent, possibly consisting of olfactory, visual, auditory, or taste hallucinations.

Seizures are classified as being partial (localized) or generalized. Partial seizures arise from a discrete site in the brain. Generalized seizures originate from both cerebral hemispheres.[72]

Table 21–21
SIGNS AND SYMPTOMS OF EPILEPSY-RELATED SEIZURES

Type of Seizure	Absence Seizure (Petit Mal Seizure)	Tonic-Clonic Seizures (Grand Mal Seizure)	Partial Seizure (Focal Seizure)	Complex Partial Seizure
Signs and symptoms	The body remaining relatively motionless Unaware of physical surroundings Unresponsive to outside stimuli	Whole-body muscle contractions Loss of consciousness Apnea Incontinence Tongue or cheek biting	Localized muscle contraction (i.e., arm, leg) Sensory impairment Dilated pupils Sweating Possible nausea and vomiting	Automatic movement or behavior without conscious thought processes (automatism). Personality changes Sweating Nausea, vomiting Sensory impairment Inappropriate or unwarranted emotions (e.g. laughing, crying) Hallucinations False or imagined smells or tastes

The diagnosis of epilepsy is based on a history of recurrent seizures. Electroencephalograph (EEG) evaluation may reveal abnormalities in brain function. The other possible causes, such as tumors, brain trauma, or drug use, must also be ruled out. Some antiepileptic (anticonvulsant) medications are effective in reducing the frequency and magnitude of seizures.

The participation status of athletes with epilepsy is based on the magnitude and frequency of the seizures and the risk of the sport involved. Seizures are most likely to occur 15 minutes to 3 hours after activity.[72] Athletes who suffer from epilepsy should be disqualified from participating in high-risk activities such as solo airplane flying, hang gliding, parachute jumping, scuba diving, and mountain climbing. Sports such as gymnastics, boxing, motor sports, and football are also considered to be high risk for athletes with epilepsy.[72]

Management of Seizures

The primary goal of managing any seizure is to maintain an open airway and protect the individual from injury. Remove any equipment, furniture, or other objects that the victim may strike. In the event of vomiting, roll the person onto the side to allow drainage from the mouth. Techniques such as inserting an object in the mouth to prevent the victim from biting the tongue or restraining the victim should **not** be performed. A secondary survey should be done after the seizure to rule out the presence of lacerations, fractures, contusions, or other injuries.

BACTERIAL MENINGITIS

Bacterial meningitis, an inflammation of the meninges of the brain and spinal cord, may be caused by one of several bacteria. Currently, *Streptococcus pneumoniae* is the most common cause. Symptoms include fever, chills, general malaise, headache, vomiting, stiffness, and spasm. Deep tendon reflexes may be exaggerated. Additionally, examination reveals disproportional pain with movement of the head and spine. Definitive diagnosis rests on examination of the CSF for abnormalities.

Treatment of bacterial meningitis focuses on antibiotic therapy specific to the causative organism. The antibiotic usually is administered intravenously for at least 2 weeks. This is then followed by a course of oral antibiotics. Prophylactic treatment with antibiotics may be used in people who have had close contact with the infected individual.

DISORDERED EATING

Disordered eating is a global term used to describe the inadequate or inappropriate consumption of food. This behavior is characterized by dieting without regard to health, disorganized eating patterns, and overeating.[73] The three most common forms of disordered eating include anorexia nervosa, bulimia nervosa, and obesity. The onset of these conditions is influenced by biological, familial, and psychosocial factors.[74] Individuals with personality traits of high levels of anxiety, hostility, perfectionism, and social detachment and withdrawal are at an increased risk of displaying disordered eating patterns.[73,75]

Athletes competing in sports that place emphasis on physical appearance, such as gymnastics, ballet, swimming, and figure skating, are at increased risks of developing disordered eating.[76] Although disordered eating is often associated with competitive athletes, its prevalence in recreational athletes or women who regularly attend gyms may be higher.[75] Societal pressures of "thin is in," the quest for the perfect body, and conflicting dietary information may also play roles in disordered eating.[76,77]

Table 21–22
SIGNS AND SYMPTOMS OF ANOREXIA NERVOSA

Significant weight loss based on norms for height and weight
Abnormally low percentage of body fat
Decreased tolerance to cold
Muscular atrophy
Amenorrhea
Decreased blood pressure
Cardiac arrhythmia
Increased rate of dental caries
Constipation
Dry, brittle hair or hair loss

Disordered eating primarily affects women, but men can also be affected.[78] Disordered eating, along with amenorrhea and osteoporosis, are components of the **female athlete triad** (see Chapter 12).

ANOREXIA NERVOSA

Individuals who suffer from anorexia nervosa (anorexia) suffer from a psychologically induced self-starvation in an attempt to reduce body weight.[74] Anorexic behavior may also involve purging behaviors such as self-induced vomiting and the use of laxatives.[76] Anorexia may occur concurrently with *obsessive-compulsive disorder.*[79]

Anorexic patients have a morbid fear of being fat, a distorted body image, and an inability to maintain a body weight at least 85 percent of standardized values based on height and weight.[76] Amenorrhea occurs when the body fat level decreases below the threshold required to maintain the hormonal balance for menstruation (Table 21–22).

Treatment of anorexia involves physiological and psychological intervention. Depending on the severity of weight loss, the patient may be placed on controlled diets, fed intravenously, or fed nasogastrically to increase body weight. Psychological counseling addresses the underlying factors that led to the onset of anorexia. When left undiagnosed or untreated, anorexia nervosa can lead to death.

BULIMIA NERVOSA

Bulimia nervosa (bulimia) is characterized by episodes of binge eating followed by purging with the use of self-induced vomiting, laxatives, or diuretics. Actual purging may be substituted by periods of prolonged fasting and excessive exercise.[76] To meet the definition of clinical bulimia nervosa, the binging and purging must occur at least twice a week for a minimum of 3 months and occur independently from anorexia nervosa.[76] Similar to anorexia nervosa, individuals suffering from bulimia tend to be concerned with body shape and body weight. However, these individuals do not have a distorted body image and the person's body weight tends to stay within normal limits.[74,76] Those suffering from bulimia also tend to believe that they lack control over their eating.

Purging often occurs because of the guilt associated with overeating. The fact that the individual purges after eating is often unknown to friends, teammates, and family members. Individuals afflicted by bulimia may also be depressed and have family or psychosocial influences that lead to the disease. Boredom, loneliness, anger, and anxiety may precipitate the binging episodes.[74]

The signs and symptoms of bulimia include binge eating followed by purging (although the purging is done in secret). The repeated presence of gastric fluids in the mouth (as the result of vomiting) can lead to dental caries, gingivitis, or erosion of the teeth enamel. As the individual's body fat decreases, menstruation ceases. **Russell's sign,** abrasions, small lacerations, and callosities on the dorsal metacarpophalangeal and interphalangeal joints caused by the teeth abrading the fingers during self-induced vomiting, may also be present.[80]

OBESITY

Obesity, a body weight that is 20 to 30 percent above the average weight based on age, gender, and height, is one of the predominant health problems in our society. It is one of the most controllable causes of premature death.[81] The body cannot store protein or carbohydrates. When unused, protein and carbohydrates are converted to fat and stored as adipose tissue. As the amount of excess body weight increases, increased strains are placed on the cardiovascular and skeletal systems.

Although obesity is often related to the excessive consumption of calories or an inactive lifestyle, it may also be caused by certain diseases. Hypothyroidism, type 1 diabetes, endocrine dysfunction, and other metabolic disorders can decrease the body's metabolism, thereby decreasing caloric needs. In these cases, otherwise acceptable levels of caloric intake can lead to the production and storage of fat. Depression, excessive alcohol consumption, loneliness, food addiction, and improper eating habits may also lead to obesity.

Historically, the medical determination of obesity was made based on the percentage of body fat or total

---

Obsessive-compulsive disorder A behavioral condition characterized by unwarranted attention to detail, especially cleanliness. Individuals with this condition require a particular order to their lives.

body weight. Depending on the measure being used, obesity is used to describe a person who is 20 to 30 percent over the average weight based on gender, age, and height. Another measure is the body mass index (BMI).[82] The BMI, based on height and weight, is calculated by:

(Weight [lbs] × 705)/(height [in] × height [in])

Or

Weight (kg)/(height [m] × height [m])

A BMI of 27.0 is the most commonly used threshold to define obesity.[83] The National Center for Health Statistics proposes the following classification scheme for BMI, although other scales have been proposed:[82]

Overweight: ≥25.0
Pre-obese: 25.0 to 29.9
Class I obesity: 30.0 to 34.9
Class II obesity: 35.0 to 39.9
Class III obesity: ≥40.0

The accuracy of this scale for athletes has not been substantiated. For example, a person 6 feet tall (1.83 m) who weighs 200 lbs (90.7 kg) would have a BMI of 27.1 (90.7 kg/[1.83 m * 1.83 m]). This individual would fall into the pre-obese classification, even though he or she may have a low level of body fat. Therefore, the determination of obesity should be made on a case-by-case basis taking the individual's gender, height, weight, age, BMI, percent body fat, and level of activity into consideration.

The medical consequences of excessive, prolonged obesity are profound, being further complicated when the individual leads a sedentary lifestyle. Obese individuals are at an increased risk for developing type 2 diabetes, heart disease, and renal failure.[27] The treatment of obesity involves education and lifestyle modifications. The fundamentals of weight reduction, decreased caloric intake, and increased energy expenditure are supplemented with nutritional counseling. Psychological counseling may also be indicated when the weight gain is triggered by psychogenic disorders. Weight reduction medications and surgical remedies to obesity are only indicated in profound cases.

Obese children often grow up to be obese adults.[84] Early intervention with diet and exercise with children can elicit life-long behavioral changes and prevent adult obesity. Parental education may also be indicated, especially if the parents themselves are obese.

One pound of stored body fat equals approximately 3500 stored calories. Exercise programs should be structured to target weight loss at the rate of 1.5 lbs/wk. This represents increasing activity and decreasing caloric intake by 5250 cal/wk (750 cal/d).

The type of physical activity is an important consideration in the early stages of exercise. The adage, "Don't run to lose weight, lose weight so you can run" holds true. Walking is preferred to running because of the increased cardiovascular demands and increased orthopedic stresses associated with running. Obese individuals often forego exercise because of embarrassment and often are hindered because of a perceived lack of time to exercise.[83] Structured exercise programs that can be performed at home or in private may increase patient compliance.

 SKIN CONDITIONS

Disorders of the skin are a natural part of human existence. In many instances, dermatologic conditions cause *pruritus* and are cosmetic annoyances. In athletics, dermatologic problems can present a significant health risk, especially when the condition is communicable. A primary concern in the athletic health care environment is to identify which conditions are contagious and which are not.

For contagious cases, the source of the outbreak must be identified and the risk of transmission to other athletes must be minimized. Outbreaks among a group of athletes may be traced back to the **index patient**, the first person affected who then transmits the disease to others.

Several terms are used to describe the appearance of dermatologic conditions. Box 21–1 describes the most common of these terms. The location of specific conditions may be specified using anatomical suffixes (e.g., tinea pedis) (Table 21–23).

SKIN INFESTATIONS

The skin plays host to many different parasites (Box 21–2). In most instances, these infestations are harmless. However, on invading the skin, an inflammatory reaction is initiated.

Table 21–23
SUFFIX DESCRIPTORS FOR DERMATOLOGIC CONDITIONS

Body Area	Suffix
Head	_capitis
Eyebrows and eyelashes	_palpebrarum
Beard and facial hair	_barbae
Body	_corporis
Pubic area	_pubis
Feet	_pedis
Finger or toenails	_unguium

Pruritus Severe itching.

Box 21-1
COMMON DERMATOLOGICAL DESCRIPTORS

	Crusts	Macules	Papules and Plaques	Pustules	Scales
Appearance	Raised layers of dry, crusty skin layers	Flat	Raised Papules ≤ 1 cm in diameter Plaques > 1 cm in diameter Smooth, irregular, or scaly	Raised Possible head (pus) formation	Slightly raised Flaky
Color	Yellow-brown Black	Discolored relative to the surrounding skin	Brown to black	Red Yellow head (pus)	Tan
Cause	The collection of serum and inflammatory cells	Pigmentation disorder	Varied	Infection	The proliferation of the normal shedding of scales from under the skin

Box 21–2
SKIN INFESTATIONS

Scabies	Pediculosis (Lice Infestation)

Appearance

Burrows, linear path having a black dot (the scabie mite) at its terminal end Papules, vesicles, and pustules	Crusting Scaling Red eruptions on the skin The lice or their eggs possibly visible; the eggs resemble dandruff, but remain attached to the hair.

Common Sites

Hands Between the fingers Wrist and arm Axilla Genitals Inner thighs	Hair of the head (scalp, beard, eyebrows); infestations common behind the ears Body hair Pubic hair (crab lice)

Discharge

Pus in the late stages	Flaking of dry skin

Sensations

Severe itching	Severe itching

Cause

Infestation by an arachnid mite (Sarcoptes scabiei)	Infestation by lice

Communicable?

Yes Transmission via direct contact with an infected person; also by sharing clothing, bedding, and so on (rare)	Yes Disease transmission possible by direct contact, sharing of clothing, bedding, hairbrushes, and so on

Treatment

Use Permethrin 5% cream (or similar). Keep fingernails short to prevent infestation under the nails. Change bedding regularly. Keep clothes separated and wash at a high temperature.	Use over-the-counter shampoos and lotions or prescription medication (e.g., Kwell). Keep clothes separated and wash at a high temperature.

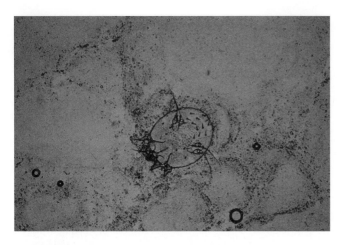

FIGURE 21–10. Scabies mite as viewed under a microscope.

Table 21–24
COMMON FORMS OF ACNE

Type	Description
Acne atrophica	Acne that causes scarring
Cystic acne	Acne that contains keratin and sebum
Keloid acne	Infection of the hair follicles of the posterior neck
Acne papulosa	Formation of papules, but with little or no inflammation
Steroid acne	Acne resulting form the use of anabolic steroids or other corticosteroid medications
Acne vulgaris	Common acne

Scabies

Scabies are mites that when viewed under a microscope resembles a spider (Fig. 21–10). The life cycles of a scabies mite consists of burrowing, feeding, and egg adhesion. Infestation occurs when impregnated females burrow beneath the skin and deposit their eggs in burrows. After a 3- to 5-day gestational period, larvae are formed and molt on the skin surface. Within 2 to 4 weeks, the larvae mature and mate, beginning a new cycle. The signs and symptoms associated with scabies represent an allergic reaction to the mite or its eggs (see Box 21–2). Diagnosis of scabies infestation is made by analyzing tissue scraped from the affected area.

Pediculosis (Lice Infection)

Lice are parasites that infest animals and humans. The lice's eggs, **nits,** adhere to body hair (e.g., scalp, beard, eyebrows, pubic hair) or clothing. Lice infestation is named according to the body area affected. For example, lice infestation of the head is termed pediculosis capitis (see Table 21–23). Pediculosis of the pubic hair is referred to as **crab lice.**

The lice (approximately 2 to 3 mm in length) may be visible. Nits appear as white spots, often resembling dandruff, but remain attached to the hair. Lice and nits may also be visible in clothing, especially in folds and seams. A secondary bacterial infection may occur after infestation.

INFLAMMATORY SKIN CONDITIONS

Inflammatory skin conditions are marked by redness of the skin as a result of contact with an irritant, allergy, or the buildup of skin oils. Box 21–3 presents common inflammatory skin rashes.

Acne Vulgaris

Acne vulgaris (pimples), the most common form of the acne family of skin conditions, involves the infection and inflammation of *sebaceous glands* and hair follicles. Other common forms of acne are presented in Table 21–24.

Although acne vulgaris most frequently affects adolescent boys, it can affect individuals of both genders and all ages. In adolescents, acne vulgaris is thought to reflect hormonal changes that affect the sebaceous glands in the skin. The menstrual cycle, use of birth control pills, and emotional stress can trigger an outbreak of acne vulgaris.

The severity of acne vulgaris is based on three grades:[85]

- **Grade 1:** Comedomal acne vulgaris, which is the presence of comedomes ("blackheads") caused by a buildup in the pores, limiting their ability to pass the body oils
- **Grade 2:** Papular acne vulgaris, which is the presence of red protrusions and pustules representing active inflammation and the collection of pus
- **Grade 3:** Cystic acne vulgaris, which is the formation of cysts, possibly leading to acne atrophica (Fig. 21–11).

In most cases, patients with acne vulgaris are treated by thoroughly washing the skin. If an individual has oily skin, specialized cleansers may be used. Antibiotic medication may be prescribed for chronic or recurrent cases of acne vulgaris. Acne that leaves permanent scars (e.g., acne atrophica) may require cosmetic surgical intervention such as dermabrasion.

Cellulitis

Cellulitis is the result of bacterial infection of the skin's connective tissue that is marked by edema, redness,

---

Sebaceous glands   Organs within the skin that secrete sebum, a fat-based oil.

Discharge	Pus	No discharge normally present. Secondary reactions (e.g., gangrene) possibly producing a discharge	Pus discharge from hair follicles possible	Clear seepage possible. Crusting frequent	No primary discharge	Usually no discharge, but pustules possibly forming in the affected area.
Sensations	May be painful	Pain Possible heat	Itching	Itching Burning	Itching	Dry skin related itching
Cause	Improper cleansing of the skin Heredity Consumption of certain foodstuffs Disruption in androgen-estrogen balance.	Bacterial infection Insect bite Postsurgery Postinjury	Staph or fungal infection Blockage of the hair follicle Exacerbation with shaving Hot tubs and whirlpool baths as possibly transmitting or causing folliculitis	The skin coming into contact with an irritant (e.g., poison ivy, soap, chemicals)	Histamine release Allergy or irritant Immune system deficiency Disease (e.g., lupus, mononucleosis, hepatitis)	The overproduction of skin cells. Factors such as too little or too much sunlight, stress, excessive alcohol consumption as triggers for outbreaks Plaques possibly occuring at the site of new trauma
Communicable?	No	No	Possibly	Not communicable, however, irritant can be transferred to other sites.	No	No
Treatment	Thorough cleansing of the skin Possible prescription of antibiotic or other acne medications	Antibiotics to treat the underlying infection Moist heat Elevation	Keeping area clean To avoid razor burn, changing the blade regularly	Medications such as Calamine lotion to dry the skin Possible antihistamine medications to control itching.	Treatment of underlying cause Possible antihistamines Cold soaks to reduce swelling and itching	Topical glucocorticoids that remove surface scales Ultraviolet light treatment

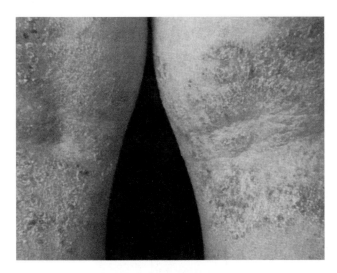

FIGURE 21–13. Eczema of the posterior legs.

may lead to skin ulcerations or gangrene. Atopic dermatitis, or **eczema,** causes the skin to become dry, scaly, and itchy (Fig. 21–13).

Urticaria (Hives)

Urticaria, commonly known as hives, is characterized by the formation of wheals. These red or skin-colored welts suddenly appear and disappear in response to an irritant or allergen. The causes of urticaria are numerous, including food allergies, pollen, animal dander, insect bites, medications, and stress.

Cholinergic urticaria can occur as the result of increased core temperature during exercise. Several 1- to 2-mm wheals appear within 30 minutes after starting the activity. The wheals and their associated itching resolve within 90 minutes after exercise.[4,86]

Urticaria is primarily more of a physical annoyance than a disability. The exception to this is when it affects the throat, which may compromise the airway.[4]

Psoriasis

Psoriasis is a chronic skin condition marked by raised red patches on the skin during periods of eruptions followed by periods of full or partial remission. An inherited, congenital condition that affects the body's immune or inflammatory mechanism, psoriasis results in the overproduction of epithelial cells, forming scales. During periods of remission, discoloration of the skin's pigment may be noted.

In most cases, the skin lesions associated with psoriasis are benign. The individual may complain of itching or pain if the scales crack. Cracked scales may become infected if the patient is not properly treated. Psoriasis

may be associated with psoriatic arthritis.[87] In severe cases, psoriasis can be life threatening.

Patients with mild to moderate forms of psoriasis are treated using topical ointments that slow the growth of the epithelial cells and decrease the redness and scaling associated with outbreaks. Other therapies include artificial long-wave ultraviolet therapy and sunlight exposure.

INFECTIOUS SKIN DISORDERS

Impetigo

Caused by a bacterial infection (staphylococcus or streptococcus), impetigo is a contagious skin disorder that is characterized by blisters and honey-colored crusting surrounded by red patches (Fig. 21–14). Impetigo outbreaks are usually localized and tend to occur around the mouth (often being confused with herpes simplex 1) or nostrils. Multiple lesions indicate a more powerful form of the infecting agent.[16] If untreated, the lesion may spread to other areas on the body.

Impetigo is caused by the staphylococcal or streptococcal bacteria. Breaks in the skin such as abrasions or insect bites allow the infecting agent to enter the subcutaneous tissues. Blisters form and then burst, forming the characteristic honey-colored crusts. Typically, the lesions are highly pruritic. Scratching can cause spread to the surrounding area or transmission to other body areas by the fingers.

Impetigo is treated by oral or topical antibiotic medication (or both). The use of antibiotic soap can be used as a prophylactic measure. Impetigo is highly contagious. Therefore, the individual's clothing, bedding, and towels should be handled with care and washed in very hot water. Athletes suffering from impetigo are disqualified from competition in sports that involve

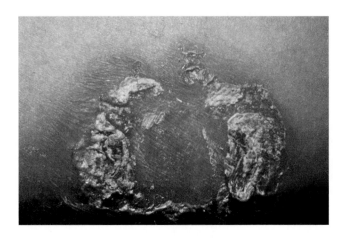

FIGURE 21–14. Impetigo, a contagious skin condition caused by bacteria.

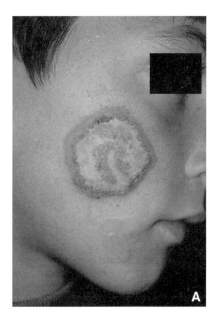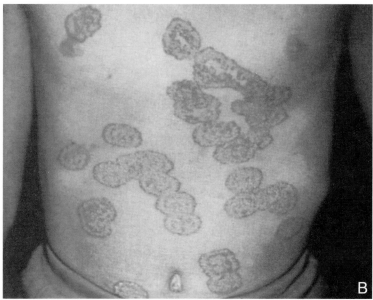

FIGURE 21–15. Ringworm of the face **(A)** and chest (tinea corporis) **(B).**

skin contact or contact with shared equipment (e.g., wrestling mats, gymnastics apparatus). If the area is covered with clothing or the sport does not involve contact, participation may be permitted after medical clearance by a physician.[12]

Tinea Infections

A fungal infection, tinea conditions can strike any portion of the body. The various forms of infection are named according to their body area. Most infections start as red, elevated, scaly patches. Vesicles or papules may also be present. The lesion spreads from the center outward, with the middle portion healing while the growth continues. This developmental pattern gives **tinea corporis** and **tinea capitis** its common name of "ringworm" (Fig. 21–15). Individuals may carry the fungus causing ringworm without developing the associated skin manifestations.[16]

Tinea pedis, "athlete's foot," and **tinea cruris,** "jock itch," are the most common tinea infections affecting athletes, primarily men and boys.[88] (Fig. 21–16). These conditions also may be caused by *Candida* fungi or filamentous fungi.[16] The body's immune system is often able to thwart tinea infection of the feet and groin. However, on occasion, the magnitude of the invasion may overwhelm the body's defense system, leading to an outbreak. Proper bathing, regularly changing socks and underwear, and keeping the areas dry help prevent the buildup of fungi.[89]

Topical corticosteroid agents can be used to provide symptomatic treatment for the lesions. When multiple sites of outbreak occur, systemic oral medication may be prescribed.[16] Individuals afflicted with tinea corporis or tinea capitis are disqualified from participating in contact sports such as wrestling as long as the skin lesions are deemed contagious. Topical or oral antifungal medication is administered for 4 to 6 weeks.[90] Before returning to competition, the lesions are covered with an occlusive dressing.[16]

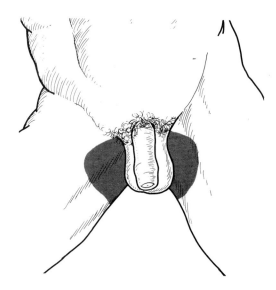

FIGURE 21–16. Tinea cruris (jock itch). This condition is characterized by a raised, red, and itching/burning patch.

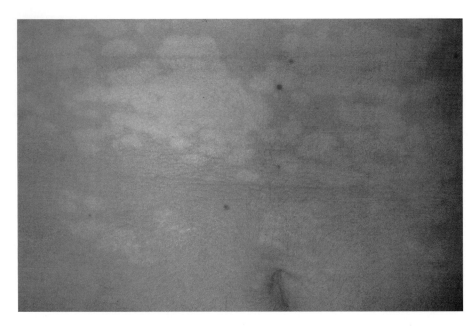

FIGURE 21–17. Tinea versicolor of the abdomen.

Tinea versicolor produces unique signs and symptoms relative to the other tinea infections. This condition is marked by brown papules and plaques that scale and flake when scratched (Fig. 21–17). Tinea versicolor most commonly afflicts adolescents and young adults. This condition can be treated by antifungal creams or shampoo containing selenium sulfide.

SKIN GROWTHS

Warts

Common warts, **verruca vulgaris,** are benign, hypertrophied areas of skin growth most commonly caused by the papillomavirus (Fig 21–18). Genital warts are discussed in the section on STDs in this chapter. Although warts may occur anywhere on the body, they are most commonly found on the hands, fingers, and feet. Warts present as raised, hard, fleshy lumps that typically differ in color (i.e., darker, lighter) from that of the surrounding tissue. Warts are not contagious.

Warts on the plantar aspect of the feet, **plantar warts** (verruca plantaris), have a different appearance than verruca vulgaris (see Figure 4–14). The thick callous on the feet cause plantar warts to appear to grow inward, creating a dark core within a depression on the bottom of the foot. Plantar warts can cause pain during weight-bearing activities and may disrupt gait.

Warts may spontaneously appear and disappear. Persistent warts can be successfully treated using over-the-counter wart medication containing salicylic or lac-

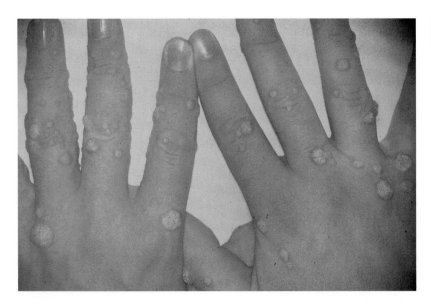

FIGURE 21–18. Verruca vulgaris (warts) of the hand.

FIGURE 21–19. Carbuncle of the posterior neck.

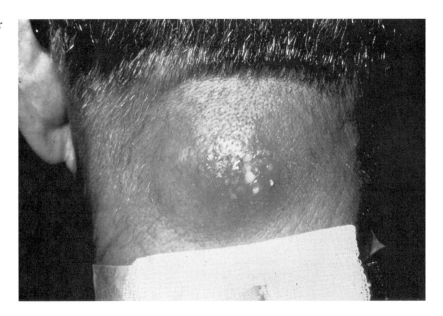

tic acid. Severe, widespread, or unrelenting warts may be removed by a physician or podiatrist using cryotherapy, electrocautery, or laser therapy.

Sebaceous Cysts

Sebaceous glands may fill with a fatty secretion (sebum), forming a sebaceous cyst. As the sebum collects within the gland, the size of the cyst increases and local circulation to the gland is hindered. Over time, the gland will *abscess* and possibly rupture, producing a foul-smelling discharge that resembles cottage cheese. Unless the affected gland is surgically excised, the cyst will likely reappear after drainage. The formation of a boil involving the sebaceous gland or hair follicle is termed a **carbuncle** (Fig. 21–19).

Sebaceous cysts most commonly form on the posterior neck and scalp, upper chest, back, and female genitals. The cyst itself is typically painless at first. As the size of the cyst increases, it may turn red and painful. Increased temperature may be noted during palpation.

◆ REFERENCES

1. Eichner, ER, and Scott, WA: Exercise as disease detector. *Phys Sports Med*, 26(3):41, 1998.
2. Primos, WA: Sports and exercise during acute illness: Recommending the right course for patients. *Phys Sports Med*, 24(1):44, 1996.
3. Nieman, DC: Risk of upper respiratory tract infection in athletes: An epidemiologic and immunologic perspective. *J Athletic Training*, 32:344, 1997.
4. Weidner, TG, et al: Effect of a rhinovirus-caused upper respiratory illness on pulmonary function test and exercise responses. *Med Sci Sports Exerc*, 29:604, 1997.
5. Weidner, TG, et al: Effects of viral upper respiratory illness on running gait. *J Athletic Training*, 32:309, 1997.
6. Blumenthal, MN, and Sherman, C: Managing allergies in active people. *Phys Sports Med*, 25(8):129, 1997.
7. Gould, BE: *Pathophysiology for the Health-Related Professions.* Philadelphia, W.B. Saunders Co., 1997.
8. Melham, TJ: Atypical pneumonia in active patients. Clues, causes, and return to play. *Phys Sports Med*, 25(10):43, 1997.
9. Swain, RA, and Kaplan, B: Upper respiratory infections: Treatment selection for active patients. *Phys Sports Med*, 26(2):85, 1998.
10. Eichner, ER: Infectious mononucleosis: Recognizing the condition, "reactivating" the patient. *Phys Sports Med*, 24(4):49, 1996.
11. Greenslade, RA: Presumed infectious mononucleosis in a college basketball player. *Phys Sports Med*, 28(6):79, 2000.
12. Moeller, JL: Contraindications to athletic participation: Spinal systemic, dermatologic, paired-organ, and other issues. *Phys Sports Med*, 24(9):47, 1996.
13. Clark, JR: Sexually transmitted diseases: Detection, differentiation, and treatment. *Physician and Sportsmedicine*, 25(1):76, 1997.
14. Bowden, FJ, et al: Estimating the prevalence of Trichomonas vaginalis, Chlamydia trachomatis, Neisseria gonorrhoeae, and human papillomavirus infection in indigenous women in northern Australia. *Sex Transm Infect*, 75:431, 1999.
15. Lafferty, WE, et al: Herpes simplex virus type 1 as a cause of genital herpes: Impact on surveillance and prevention. *J Infect Dis*, 181:1454, 2000.
16. Dienst, WL, et al: Pinning down skin infections: Diagnosis, treatment, and prevention in wrestlers. *Physician and Sportsmedicine*, 25(12):45 1997.
17. American Academy of Pediatrics: Committee on Sports Medicine and Fitness: Human immunodeficiency virus and other bloodborne viral pathologies in the athletic setting. *Pediatrics*, 104:1400, 1999.
18. Brown, SL, et al: HIV/AIDS policies and sports: the National Football League. *Med Sci Sports Exerc*, 26:403, 1994.
19. Buxton, BP, et al: Prevention of hepatitis B virus in athletic training. *J Athletic Training*, 29:107, 1994.
20. Mylonakis, E, et al: Report of a false-positive HIV test result and the potential use of additional tests in establishing HIV serostatus. *Arch Intern Med*, 160:2386, 2000.
21. Terry, L, Sprinz, E, and Riberio, JP: Moderate and high intensity exercise training in HIV-1 seropositive individuals: a randomized trial. *Int J Sports Med*, 20:142, 1999.
22. Shepard, RJ: Exercise, immune function and HIV infection. *J Sports Med Phys Fitness*, 38:101, 1998.

Abscess A localized collection of pus caused by a bacterial invasion.

23. Strigner, WW, et al: The effect of exercise training on aerobic fitness, immune indices, and quality of life in HIV+ patients. *Med Sci Sports Exerc*, 30:11, 1998.

24. Jimenez, CC: Diabetes and exercise: The role of the athletic trainer. *J Athletic Training*, 32:339, 1997.

25. Draznin, MB: Type 1 diabetes and sports participation. Strategies for training and competing safely. *Physician and Sportsmedicine*, 28(12):49, 2000.

26. Colberg, SR, and Swain, DP: Exercise and diabetes control. A winning combination. *Physician and Sportsmedicine*, 28(4):63, 2000.

27. Hough, DO: Diabetes mellitus in sports. *Med Clin North Am*, 78:423, 1994.

28. Fahey, PJ, Stallkamp, ET, and Kwatra, S: The athlete with type I diabetes: Managing insulin, diet and exercise. *Am Fam Physician*, 53:1611, 1996.

29. White, RD, and Sherman, C: Exercise in diabetes management. Maximizing benefits, controlling risks. *Physician and Sportsmedicine*, 27(4):63, 1999.

30. Wolf, SK: Diabetes mellitus and predisposition to athletic pedal fractures. *J Foot Ankle Surg*, 37:16, 1998.

31. Gocke, TV: Case report: Marfan's syndrome. *Athletic Training: Journal of the National Athletic Trainers Association*, 21:341, 1986.

32. Maron, BJ, Epstein, SE, and Roberts, WC: Causes of sudden death in competitive athletes. *J Am Coll Cardiol*, 7:204, 1986.

33. McKusick, V: *Heritable Disorders of Connective Tissue* (ed 4). CV Mosby, St Louis, 1972.

34. Anderson, RE, and Pratt-Thomas, HR: Marfan's syndrome. *Am Heart J*, 46:911, 1953.

35. Pan, CC, et al: Echocardiographic abnormalities in families of patients with Marfan's syndrome. *J Am Coll Cardiol*, 6:1016, 1985.

36. Allen, RA, et al: Ocular manifestation of Marfan syndrome. *Trans Am Acad Ophthalmol/Otolaryngol*, 71:18, 1967.

37. Ballenger, M: Dissecting aneurysms. *Emerg Mag*, 17:25, 1985.

38. Potts, KA, and Dick, RW: NCAA guide line 3c: The student-athlete with sickle cell trait. In Potts, KA, and Dick, RW (eds): *NCAA Sports Medicine Handbook*. Indianapolis, IN, National Collegiate Athletic Association, 2000, pp 59–60.

39. Shaskey, DJ, and Green, GA: Sports haematology. *Sports Med*, 29:27, 2000.

40. Thiriet, P, et al: Sickle cell trait performance in a prolonged rate at high altitude. *Med Sci Sports Exerc*, 26:914, 1994.

41. Kerle, KK, and Nishimura, KD: Exertional collapse and sudden death associated with sickle cell trait. *Mil Med*, 161:766, 1996.

42. Thiriet, P, et al: Hyperoxia during recovery from consecutive anaerobic exercises in the sickle cell trait. *Eur J App Physiol*, 71:235, 1995.

43. Wang, DH, and Goodman, JL: Joint pain and swelling: Could it be Lyme arthritis? *Phys Sports Med*, 25(2):26, 1997.

44. Cramer, CR: Fibromyalgia and chronic fatigue syndrome: An update for athletic trainers. *Journal of Athletic Training*, 33:359, 1998.

45. Shafran, SD: The chronic fatigue syndrome. *Am J Med*, 90:730, 1991.

46. Gremillion, RB: Fibromyalgia. *Phys Sports Med*, 26(4):55, 1998.

47. Reilly, JJ, et al: Reduced energy expenditure in preobese children treated for acute lymphoblastic leukemia. *Pediatr Res*, 44:557, 1998.

48. Isselbacher, KJ, et al: *Harrison's Principles of Internal Medicine* (ed 13). New York, McGraw-Hill, 1994, p 1221.

49. Dozier, S, et al: Beachfront screening for skin cancer in Texas Gulf coast surfers. *South Med J*, 90:55, 1997.

50. Fitzpatrick, TB, et al: *Color Atlas and Synopsis of Clinical Dermatology* (ed 3). New York, McGraw-Hill, 1997, p 970.

51. Bouquot, JE, and Meckstroth, RL: Oral cancer in a tobacco-chewing US population: No apparent increased incidence or mortality. *Oral Surg Oral Med Oral Pathol Oral Radiol Endod*, 86:697, 1998.

52. Ankathil, R, et al: Is oral cancer susceptibility inherited? Report of five oral cancer families. *Eur J Cancer B Oral Oncol*, 32(B):63, 1996.

53. Horowitz, AM, et al: Maryland adult's knowledge of oral cancer and having oral cancer examinations. *J Public Health Dent*, 58:281, 1998.

54. Mathew, B, et al: Evaluation of mouth self-examination in the control of oral cancer. *Br J Cancer*, 71:397, 1995.

55. Yang, Q, et al: Family history score as a predictor of breast cancer mortality: Prospective data from the cancer prevention study II, United States, 1982–1991. *Am J Epidemiol*, 147:652, 1998.

56. Hopper, JL, et al: Population-based estimate of the average age-specific cumulative risk of breast cancer for a defined set of protein-truncating mutations in BRCA1 and BRCA2 Australian breast cancer family study. *Cancer Epidemiol Biomarkers Prev*, 8:741, 1999.

57. Potischman, N, et al: Dietary relationships with early onset (under age 45) breast cancer in a case-controlled study in the United States: Influence of chemotherapy treatment. *Cancer Causes Control*, 8:713, 1997.

58. Simon, MS, et al: A randomized trial of a low-fat dietary intervention in women at high risk for breast cancer. *Nutr Cancer*, 27:136, 1997.

59. Challier, B, Peranau, JM, and Viel, JF: Garlic, onion and cereal fibre as protective factors for breast cancer: A French case-control study. *Eur J Epidemiol*, 14:737, 1998.

60. Schiffman, M, et al: HPV DNA testing in cervical cancer screening: results from women in a high-risk province of Costa Rica. *JAMA*, 283:87, 2000.

61. Kushi, LH, et al: Prospective study of diet and ovarian cancer. *Am J Epidemiol*, 149:21, 1999.

62. Forman, D, and Moller, H: Testicular cancer. *Cancer Surv*, 19–20:323, 1994.

63. Gallagher, RP, et al: Physical activity, medical history, and risk of testicular cancer. *Cancer Causes Control*, 6:398, 1995.

64. Olivera, SA, et al: The association between cardiorespiratory fitness and prostate cancer. *Med Sci Sports Exerc*, 28:97, 1996.

65. Schwartz, AL: Patterns of exercise and fatigue in physically active cancer survivors. *Oncol Nurs Forum*, 25:485, 1998.

66. Schwartz, AL: Patterns of exercise and fatigue in physically active cancer survivors. *Oncol Nurs Forum*, 25:485, 1998.

67. Courneya, KS, Mackey, JR, and Jones, LW: Coping with cancer. *Physician and Sports Medicine*, 28(5):49, 2000.

68. Diamond, S: Managing migraines in active people. *Physican and Sportsmedicine*, 24(12):41, 1996.

69. Bener, A, et al: Genetic and environmental factors associated with migraine in schoolchildren. *Headache*, 40:152, 2000.

70. Ossipova, VV, et al: Migraine associated with panic attacks. *Cephalagia*, 19:728, 1999.

71. McCrory, PR, and Berkovic, SF: Concussive convulsions Incidence in sport and treatment recommendations. *Sports Med*, 25:131, 1998.

72. Sirven, JI: Physical activity and epilepsy What are the rules? *Physician and Sportsmedicine*, 27(3):63, 1999.

73. Stephenson, JN: Medical consequences and complications of anorexia nervosa and bulimia nervosa in female athletes. *Athletic Training: Journal of the National Athletic Trainers Association*, 26:130, 1991.

74. Johnson, C, and Tobin, DL: The diagnosis and treatment of anorexia nervosa and bulimia nervosa among athletes. *Athletic Training: Journal of the National Athletic Trainers Association*, 26:119, 1991.

75. Augestad, LB, Saether, B, and Götestam, KG: The relationship between eating disorders and personality in physically active women. *Scand J Med Sci Sports*, 9:304, 1999.

76. Smith, AD: The female athlete triad: Causes, diagnosis, and treatment. *Physician and Sportsmedicine*, 24(7):67, 1996.

77. Clark, N: Food fight: Calling a truce with disordered eating. *Physician and Sportsmedicine*, 24(7):13, 1996.

78. Johnson, C, Powers, PS, and Dick, R: Athletes and eating disorders: The National Collegiate Athletic Association study. *Int J Eat Disord*, 26:179, 1999.

79. Gee, RL, and Telew, N: Obsessive-compulsive disorder and anorexia nervosa in a high school athlete: A case report. *J Athletic Training*, 34:375, 1999.

80. Daluiski, A, Rahbar, B, and Meals, RA: Russell's sign. Subtle hand changes with bulimia nervosa. *Clin Orthop*, HD(343):107, 1997.

81. Andersen, RE: What can physicians do about obesity? *Physician and Sportsmedicine*, 28(10):81, 2000.

82. Flegal, KM, et al: Overweight and obesity in the United States: Prevalence and trends, 1960–1994. *Int J Obes Relat Metab Disord*, 22:39, 1998.

83. Andersen, RE: Exercise, an active lifestyle, and obesity Making the prescription work. *Physician and Sportsmedicine*, 27(10):41, 1999.

84. Bar-Or, O: Juvenile obesity, physical activity, and lifestyle changes. Cornerstones for prevention and management. *Physician and Sportsmedicine*, 28(11), 2000.

85. Savin, RC, and Donofrio, LM: Aggressive acne treatment: As simple as one, two, three? *Physician and Sportsmedicine* 24(9):41, 1996.

86. Leshaw, SM: Itching in active patients: Causes and cures. *Physician and Sportsmedicine*, 26(1):47, 1998.

87. Camisa, C: Psoriasis: A clinical update on diagnosis and new therapies. *Cleve Clin J Med*, 67:105, 2000.

88. Burkhart, CG: Skin disorders of the foot in active patients. *Physician and Sportsmedicine* 27(2):88, 1999.

89. Ramsey, ML: Skin care for active people. *Physician and Sportsmedicine*, 25(3):91, 1997.

90. Hand, JW, and Wroble, RR: Prevention of tinea corporis in collegiate wrestlers. *J Athletic Training*, 34:350, 1999.

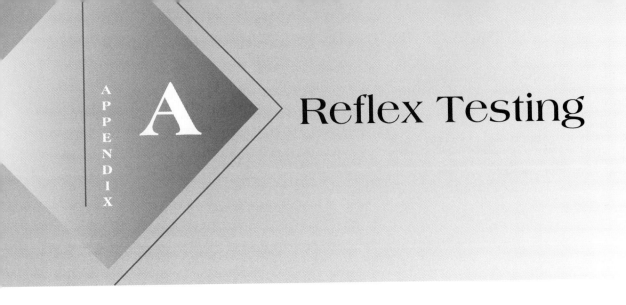

Deep tendon reflexes are elicited with a threshold response after a quick stretch of the muscle tendon that causes a reflexive muscular contraction. The procedure involves tapping the tendon with a reflex hammer with enough force to elicit the response. Practice is required to develop the right "touch" to elicit a reflex response. The amount of pressure required to elicit a response varies from reflex to reflex and from person to person. Obtaining a reflex response is facilitated by having the patient slightly tense an unrelated muscle during the reflex test (Fig. A–1). If the patient is anxious, instruct him or her to close the eyes so that he or she will not anticipate the test.

Reflexes must be checked bilaterally with each limb held at approximately the same position with equal

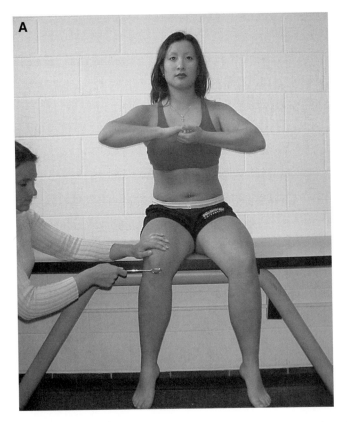
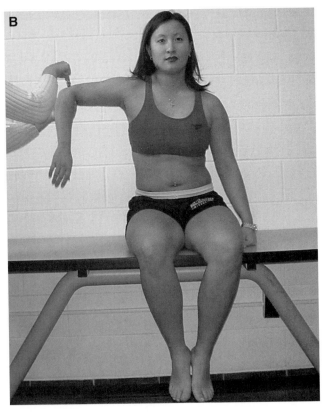

FIGURE A–1. (A) Muscle facilitation during lower extremity reflex testing. Have the patient attempt to pull the hands apart as shown. **(B)** Muscle facilitation during upper extremity reflex testing. The patient presses the medial aspect of the feet against each other.

amounts of muscular tension. The reflex can be graded on a four-point scale:

- **Grade 0**: No reflex elicited
- **Grade 1**: Reflex elicited with reinforcement (hypore-flexia)
- **Grade 2**: Normal reflex
- **Grade 3**: Hyperresponsive reflex

When assessing reflexes, evaluate all of the reflexes in the extremity being tested. Also test the same reflexes in the opposite extremity and compare the results. For example, in a patient who exhibits poor muscle tone, a reflex that must be elicited with reinforcement might be assessed as abnormal. However, further assessment would reveal that all of the the remaining reflexes are also grade 1. Therefore, this is the baseline assessment naturally found in this individual.

Box A–1
C5 NERVE ROOT REFLEX

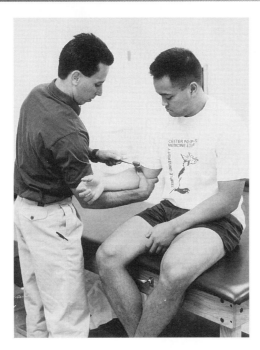

MUSCLE	Biceps brachii
PATIENT POSITION	Seated
POSITION OF EXAMINER	Standing to the side of the patient, cradling the forearm with the thumb placed over the tendon
EVALUATIVE PROCEDURE	The thumb is tapped with the reflex hammer.

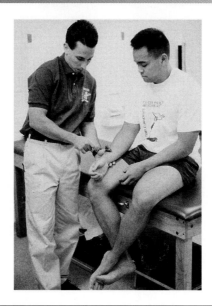

MUSCLE	Brachioradialis
PATIENT POSITION	Seated
POSITION OF EXAMINER	Cradling the patient's arm
EVALUATIVE PROCEDURE	The distal portion of the brachioradialis tendon is tapped with the reflex hammer. The proximal tendon may also be used.

Box A–3
C7 NERVE ROOT REFLEX

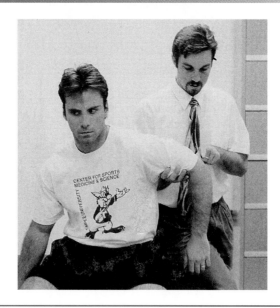

MUSCLE	Triceps brachii
PATIENT POSITION	Seated
POSITION OF EXAMINER	Supporting the athlete's shoulder abducted to 90° and the elbow flexed to 90°
EVALUATIVE PROCEDURE	The distal triceps brachii tendon is tapped with the reflex hammer.

L4 NERVE ROOT REFLEX

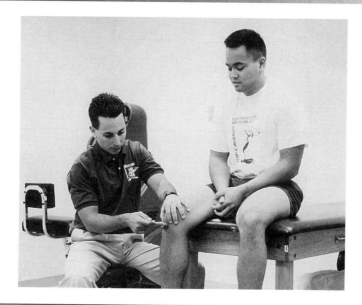

MUSCLE	Patellar tendon (quadriceps femoris)
PATIENT POSITION	Sitting with the knees flexed over the end of the table
POSITION OF EXAMINER	Standing or seated to the side of the athlete
EVALUATIVE PROCEDURE	The patellar tendon is tapped with the reflex hammer.

S1 NERVE ROOT REFLEX

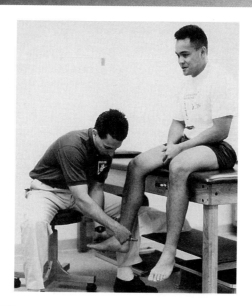

MUSCLE	Achilles tendon (triceps surae muscle group)
PATIENT POSITION	Sitting with the knees flexed over the edge of the table
POSITION OF EXAMINER	Seated in front of the athlete, supporting the foot in its neutral position
EVALUATIVE PROCEDURE	The Achilles tendon is tapped with a reflex hammer.

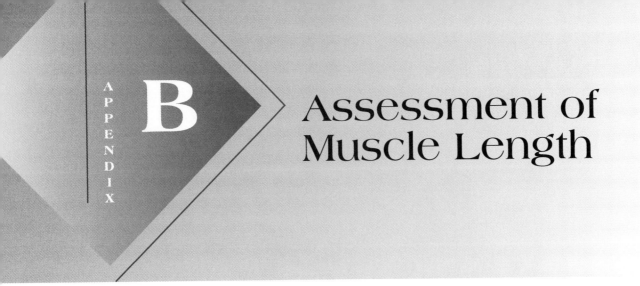

Assessment of Muscle Length

Muscle length assessment is used to objectively measure a muscle's normal length or flexibility (or both). If a muscle crossing a specific joint is shortened, abnormal stresses may be placed on the joint over which the muscle crosses or the necessary mobility required for normal function may be lacking. If a muscle crossing a specific joint is in an abnormally elongated position, the joint may also be affected by abnormal stresses or may lack the necessary stability required for normal function.

Muscles that cross more than one joint (two-joint muscles) have a greater tendency to become shortened during normal activities of daily living (ADLs) than do muscles crossing only one joint. The more common muscles that tend to adaptively shorten because of daily use are found in the lower extremities. Specific positions and measurements for these muscles are used to assist clinicians in objectively quantifying the degree of shortening that has taken place. Muscles that cross a single joint (one-joint muscles) are less likely to become shortened. Their length and flexibility is normally assessed during passive range of motion of the joint that the muscle crosses (normal joint range of motion measured with a goniometer represents the normal length of the one-joint muscle crossing that joint).

 ## ASSESSING FOR SHORTNESS OF THE LOWER EXTREMITY MUSCLES

When muscle shortening occurs, various postural deviations may result. These are highlighted in Table B-1. The specific procedures for assessing muscle length in selected lower extremity muscles are described in Boxes B–1 through B–4. The Ober test (see Box 6–22) and the Thomas test (see Box 8–5) are two additional tests for muscle length.

 ## ASSESSING FOR SHORTNESS OF THE UPPER EXTREMITY MUSCLES

When shortening occurs in upper extremity muscles, various postural deviations may result. These are highlighted in Table B–2. The specific procedures for assessing muscle length in selected upper extremity muscles are described in Boxes B–5 through B–7.

Table B–1
POSTURAL DEVIATIONS OF THE LOWER EXTREMITY AS THE RESULT OF MUSCLE SHORTNESS OR CONTRACTURE

Muscle	Posture (resting position except where noted)
Foot and Toes	
Abductor hallucis	Forefoot varus
	Extension of the first MTP joint
Adductor hallucis	Hallux valgus
Flexor hallucis brevis	Flexion of the first MTP joint
Flexor hallucis longus	Flexion of the IP joint of the first toe
Flexor digitorum longus	Flexion of the DIP joints of the lateral four toes
Extensor digitorum longus	Extension of the lateral four MTP joints
Extensor hallucis longus and brevis	Extension of the first MTP joint
	Depression of the head of the first MT
Ankle	
Tibialis anterior	Dorsiflexion of the talocrural joint; calcaneovarus
Tibialis posterior	Calcaneovarus, supination of the rearfoot
	Forefoot varus while bearing weight
Peroneus longus and brevis	Calcaneovalgus
Gastrocnemius and Soleus	Plantarflexion
Knee	
Gastrocnemius	Knee flexion
Biceps femoris	External tibial rotation (may become more apparent during RROM)
Semimembranosus and Semitendinosus	Internal tibial rotation (may become more apparent during RROM)
Popliteus	Internal tibial rotation
Hamstring group	Knee flexion
	Posterior pelvic tilt
	Loss of normal lumbar lordosis
	Pelvic tilt (unilateral contracture of the hamstrings)
Quadriceps group	Knee extension
Hip	
Iliopsoas	Hip flexion, hip adduction
	Increased lumbar lordosis
	Anterior pelvic tilt
Gluteus minimus	Internal femoral rotation, hip abduction
	When standing, pelvic tilt toward the side of the shortness (low side)
Gluteus medius	Hip abduction
	When standing, pelvic tilt toward the side of the shortness (low side)
Hip internal rotators	Internal rotation of the hip
Hip external rotators	External rotation of the hip
Adductor group	Adduction deformity
	When standing, pelvic tilt away from the side of the shortness (high side)
Sartorius	Flexion, abduction, and external rotation of the hip
	Flexion of the knee.

DIP = distal interphalangeal; IP = interphalangeal; MT = metatarsal; MTP = metatarsophalangeal; RROM = resisted range of motion.

MUSCLE LENGTH ASSESSMENT FOR THE GASTROCNEMIUS

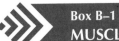

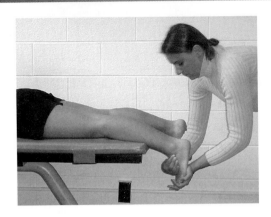

PATIENT POSITION	Prone with the foot off the edge of the table with the knee extended
POSITION OF EXAMINER	One hand palpating the subtalar joint The other hand grasping the foot
EVALUATIVE PROCEDURE	While maintaining the subtalar joint in the neutral position, the foot is taken into dorsiflexion.
POSITIVE TEST	Less than 10° of dorsiflexion for tightness may affect normal walking gait; less than 15° of dorsiflexion may affect normal running gait.
IMPLICATIONS	Tightness of the gastrocnemius can create overuse pathology at the foot, ankle, and knee.
POSSIBLE PATHOLOGIES	Plantar fasciitis, Sever's disease, Achilles tendinitis, calcaneal bursitis, patellofemoral pathology.

MUSCLE LENGTH ASSESSMENT FOR THE SOLEUS

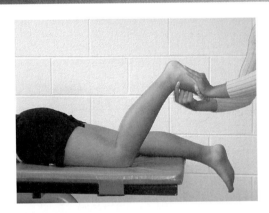

PATIENT POSITION	Prone with the foot off the edge of the table and the knee flexed at least 60°
POSITION OF EXAMINER	One hand palpating the subtalar joint The other hand grasping the foot
EVALUATIVE PROCEDURE	While maintaining the subtalar joint in the neutral position, the foot is taken into dorsiflexion.
POSITIVE TEST	Less than 10° of dorsiflexion for tightness may affect normal walking gait; less than 15° of dorsiflexion may affect normal running gait.
IMPLICATIONS	Tightness of the soleus can create overuse pathology at the foot, ankle, and knee.
POSSIBLE PATHOLOGIES	Plantar fasciitis, Sever's disease, Achilles tendinitis, calcaneal bursitis, patellofemoral pathology

Box B–3

MUSCLE LENGTH ASSESSMENT FOR THE HAMSTRING GROUP

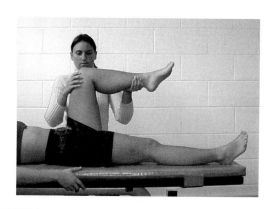
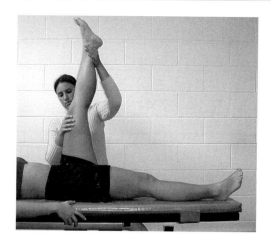

PATIENT POSITION	Supine
POSITION OF EXAMINER	Standing at the side of the patient; the leg being assessed is placed in 90° of hip flexion and 90° of knee flexion (90/90 position)
EVALUATIVE PROCEDURE	The upper leg is stabilized in 90° of hip flexion and the lower leg is extended at the knee.
POSITIVE TEST	Greater than 20° of full knee extension. In patients participating in athletic activities, degrees less than 20° of full knee extension may still be considered as a positive test.
IMPLICATIONS	Tightness of the hamstrings may affect the knee, thigh, hip, and spine.
POSSIBLE PATHOLOGIES	Muscle strains, patellofemoral dysfunction, ischial tuberostiy tendonitis, low back pain

Box B–4

MUSCLE LENGTH ASSESSMENT OF THE RECTUS FEMORIS

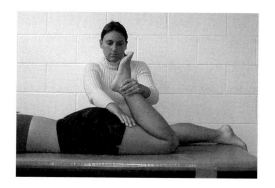

PATIENT POSITION	Prone
POSITION OF EXAMINER	At the side of the patient
EVALUATIVE PROCEDURE	The knee is flexed.
POSITIVE TEST	Less motion than available with ROM testing of the knee in the supine position or 10° or greater difference as compared with the nonaffected side.
IMPLICATIONS	Tightness of the quadriceps may affect the knee, thigh, hip, and spine.
POSSIBLE PATHOLOGIES	Muscle strains, patellofemoral dysfunction, hip pain, low back pain

ROM = range of motion

Table B–2
POSTURAL DEVIATIONS OF THE UPPER EXTREMITY AS THE RESULT OF MUSCLE SHORTNESS OR CONTRACTURE

Muscle	Posture (resting position except where noted)
Fingers and Thumb	
Adductor pollicis	Adduction contracture of the thumb
Flexor pollicis longus	Flexion of the interphalangeal joint of the thumb
Flexor pollicis brevis	Flexion of the first MCP joint
Abductor pollicis longus	Extension of first MT
	Slight radial deviation of wrist
Dorsal interossei	Abduction of the fingers relative to the third phalange
Palmar interossei	Adduction of the fingers relative to the third phalange
Lumbricales and Interossei	Flexion of the MCP joints
	Extension of the IP joints
Extensor digitorum	Hyperextension of the MCP joints (contracture).
	Hyperextension of the MCP joints during wrist flexion; extension of the wrist if the MCP joints are flexed (shortness).
Flexor digitorum superficialis	Flexion of the PIP joints (contracture)
	Flexion of the PIP joints if the wrist is extended; flexion of the wrist if the fingers are extended (shortness)
Flexor digitorum profundus	Flexion of the DIP joints (contracture)
	Finger flexion if the wrist is extended; wrist flexion if the fingers are extended (shortness)
Wrist and Hand	
Flexor carpi radialis	Radial deviation of the wrist
Flexor carpi ulnaris	Ulnar deviation of the wrist
Extensor carpi radialis longus and brevis	Wrist extension, radial deviation
Extensor carpi ulnaris	Wrist extension, ulnar deviation
Elbow and forearm	
Biceps brachii/Brachialis	Elbow flexion and forearm supination
Triceps brachii	Elbow extension
Shoulder	
Latissimus dorsi	Depression of the shoulder girdle; limitation in humeral elevation
	Kyphosis of the thoracic spine
Pectoralis major	Internal rotation and adduction of the humerus; scapular protraction (clavicular portion of pectoralis major)
	Forward shoulder posture and/or depression of the shoulder girdle (sternal portion)
Pectoralis minor	Forward shoulder posture
Teres major	Premature rotation of the scapula during glenohumeral abduction
Rhomboid major and minor	Retraction of the scapulae
Trapezius (upper fibers)	Unilateral bending of the cervical spine

DIP = distal interphalangeal; IP = interphalangeal; MCP = metacarpophalangeal; MT = metatarsal; PIP = proximal interphalangeal.

Box B–5
MUSCLE LENGTH ASSESSMENT OF THE SHOULDER ADDUCTORS

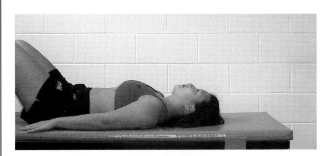

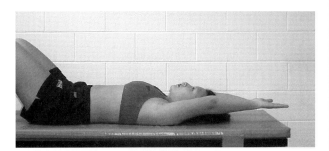

Starting Position	**Ending Position**

PATIENT POSITION	In the hook-lying position with the arms at the side
POSITION OF EXAMINER	At the side of the patient
EVALUATIVE PROCEDURE	The patient flexes the shoulders above the head and attempts to place the arms on the table.
POSITIVE TEST	The patient cannot flex the arms above the head or the lumbar spine lifts off the table.
IMPLICATIONS	Shortness of the latissimus dorsi and teres major muscles

Box B–6
MUSCLE LENGTH ASSESSMENT OF THE PECTORALIS MAJOR MUSCLES

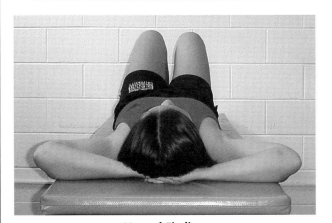

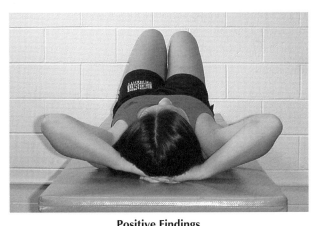

Normal Findings	**Positive Findings**

PATIENT POSITION	In the hook-lying position with the arms abducted, externally rotated, with the elbows flexed and the hands locked behind the head
POSITION OF EXAMINER	At the head of the patient
EVALUATIVE PROCEDURE	The patient attempts to position the elbows flat on the table.
POSITIVE TEST	The elbows do not rest on the table. To establish an objective baseline, measure (in centimeters) the distance from the posterior aspect of the acromion process to the tabletop.
IMPLICATIONS	Tight pectoralis major muscles may create rounded shoulders and subsequent forward head posture.

Box B–7

MUSCLE LENGTH ASSESSMENT OF THE PECTORALIS MINOR MUSCLES

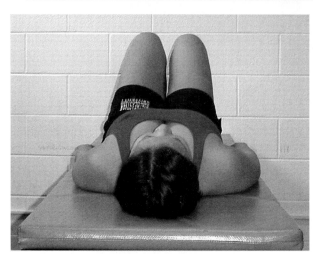

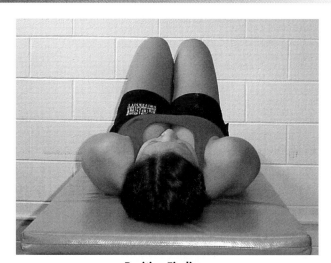

Normal Findings	Positive Findings

PATIENT POSITION	Supine with the arms at the side
POSITION OF EXAMINER	At the head of the patient
EVALUATIVE PROCEDURE	Observe the position of the shoulders in reference to the table.
POSITIVE TEST	The posterior shoulder does not rest on the table. To establish an objective baseline, measure (in centimeters) the distance from the posterior aspect of the acromion process to the tabletop.
IMPLICATIONS	Tight pectoralis minor muscles may create rounded shoulders and subsequent forward head posture.

Functional Testing of the Lower Extremity

Functional testing involves the application of controlled forces replicating the stresses that will be experienced during activity. The individual components of lower extremity function, including joint stability, range of motion, strength, and balance, are assessed during the evaluation of injury. The application of sport-specific functional tests assesses the patient's neuromuscular and proprioceptive status. Functional testing also challenges the athlete psychologically, requiring confidence that the limb can function under the stresses that will be placed on it during sports.

An athlete's functional status can be evaluated by using running, sprinting, and agility drills that emphasize quick starts, cutting, and stops. Actual sport skills such as backpedaling, cross-over steps, jumping, and so on may also be used. Additionally, specific tests have

been developed so that the injured leg's function can be assessed in the athletic training room, clinic, or physician's office. Although these tests may be sensitive in some patients, subjective complaints of difficulty with pivoting, cutting, and twisting may be the most sensitive determination of the ability to function. Patients who display gross joint laxity or muscle weakness should not perform these tests.

This appendix describes four common tests used for determining the functional ability of the lower extremity. These tests may be performed as a single set of one repetition on each limb or recorded as the average of three repetitions for each extremity. Positive tests indicate the presence of functional limitations that may suggest the inability to pivot, cut, and twist during activity.

Box C–1
SINGLE LEG HOP FOR DISTANCE

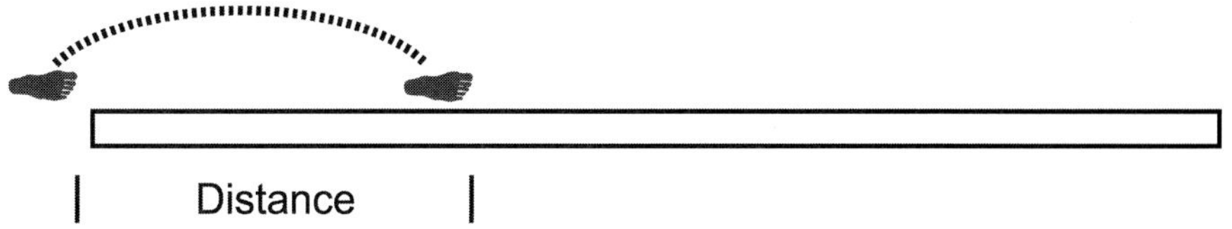

Distance

PATIENT POSITION	Standing on one leg
POSITION OF EXAMINER	At the side of the patient
EVALUATIVE PROCEDURE	The patient hops as far as possible, taking off and landing on the same leg. The first set is performed using the uninvolved leg. The second set is performed using the involved leg.
POSITIVE TEST	The distance hopped on the involved leg is less than 85% of the uninvolved leg.

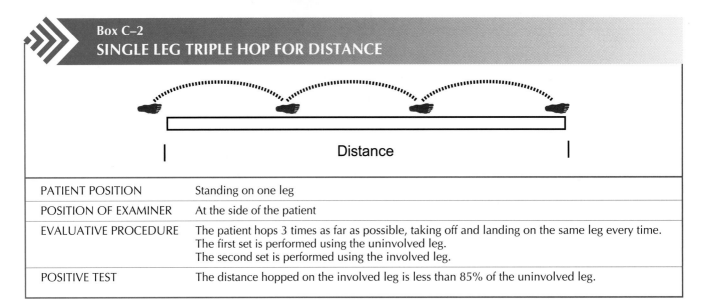

Box C–2
SINGLE LEG TRIPLE HOP FOR DISTANCE

Distance

PATIENT POSITION	Standing on one leg
POSITION OF EXAMINER	At the side of the patient
EVALUATIVE PROCEDURE	The patient hops 3 times as far as possible, taking off and landing on the same leg every time. The first set is performed using the uninvolved leg. The second set is performed using the involved leg.
POSITIVE TEST	The distance hopped on the involved leg is less than 85% of the uninvolved leg.

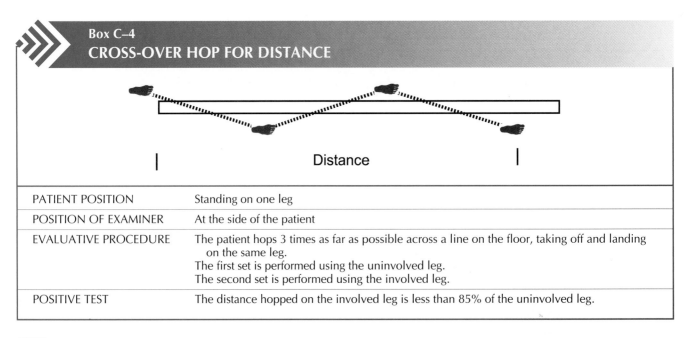

Box C–3
SINGLE LEG HOP FOR TIME

Time required to travel 18 feet

PATIENT POSITION	Standing on one leg
POSITION OF EXAMINER	At the side of the patient
EVALUATIVE PROCEDURE	The patient hops over a distance of 18 ft, taking off and landing on the same leg each time. The first set is performed using the uninvolved leg. The second set is performed using the involved leg.
POSITIVE TEST	The time it takes the patient to hop the distance on the uninvolved leg is less than 85% of the involved leg.

Box C–4
CROSS-OVER HOP FOR DISTANCE

Distance

PATIENT POSITION	Standing on one leg
POSITION OF EXAMINER	At the side of the patient
EVALUATIVE PROCEDURE	The patient hops 3 times as far as possible across a line on the floor, taking off and landing on the same leg. The first set is performed using the uninvolved leg. The second set is performed using the involved leg.
POSITIVE TEST	The distance hopped on the involved leg is less than 85% of the uninvolved leg.

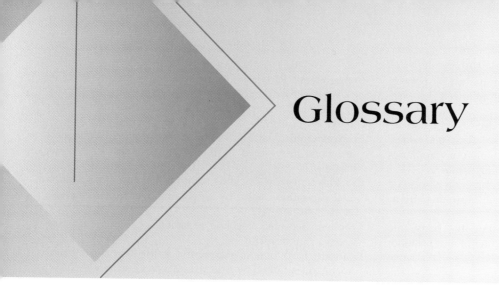

Glossary

Abduction: Lateral movement of a body part away from the midline of the body. In the feet, the movement is in reference to the midline of the foot.

Abscess: A localized collection of pus caused by a bacterial invasion.

Accessory motion: Motion that accompanies active movement and is necessary for normal motion but can not be voluntarily isolated.

Acidosis: An increase in the blood's acid balance (lowering of pH) caused by the accumulation of acids or the loss of blood bases.

Actin: A contractile muscle protein.

Activities of daily living (ADLs): The skills and motions required for the day-to-day activities of life.

Adduction: Medial movement of a body part toward the midline of the body. In the feet, the movement is in reference to the midline of the foot.

Adenosine triphosphate (ATP): An energy-yielding enzyme used during muscular contractions.

Adhesive capsulitis: Inflammation of a joint capsule that restricts its range of motion.

Allergen: A substance that, when contacting the body's tissues, results in a state of sensitivity.

Allograft: The tissues used to replace the ligament obtained from a cadaver.

Ambient: Pertaining to the local environment.

Amenorrheic (amenorrhea): The absence of menstruation.

Anatomical position: The position that the body assumes when standing upright with the feet and palms facing anteriorly.

Anisocoria: Unequal pupil sizes; possibly a benign congenital condition or secondary to brain trauma.

Ankylosis: Immobility of a joint.

Anorexia nervosa: A form of disordered eating characterized by the lack of appetite (or refusal to eat), depression, malaise, and distorted body image most commonly affecting young women between the ages of 12 and 21 years.

Anoxia: The absence of oxygen in the blood or tissues.

Antagonistic: In the opposite direction of movement (e.g., the antagonistic motion of extension is flexion).

Antalgic gait: A limp or unnatural walking pattern caused by pain, trauma, or dysfunction of the lower extremity.

Antalgic: Having a pain-relieving quality; analgesic.

Anteversion: A forward bending or angulation of a bone or organ.

Apnea: The temporary cessation of breathing.

Arrhythmia: Loss of the normal heart rhythm; an irregular heart rate.

Arthralgia: Painful joints.

Arthrokinematic: Action and reaction of articular surfaces as a joint travels through its range of motion.

Asymptomatic: Without symptoms.

Atherosclerosis: The buildup of fatty tissues on the inner arterial walls.

Atrophy: A wasting or decrease in the size of a muscle or tissue.

Autograft: The tissues used to replace the ligament harvested from the patient's body (e.g., bone–patellar tendon–bone, hamstring tendon).

Avascular necrosis: Death of cells secondary to lack of an adequate blood supply.

Axial load: A force applied through the long axis of a bone or series of bones.

Axonotmesis: Damage to the nerve tissue but without actually severing it.

Baseline measurements: The initial physical findings, either from the pre-season physical examination in the athlete or upon the initial evaluation during an injury or illness.

Bell's palsy: Inhibition of the facial nerve secondary to trauma or disease, resulting in flaccidity of the facial muscles. In individuals suffering from Bell's palsy, the face on the involved side appears elongated.

Biohazard: A substance that is toxic to humans, animals, or the environment.

Biomechanics: The effect of muscular forces, joint axes, and resistance on the quality and quantity of human movement.

Bleb: A large, loose blood vessel that has the potential to rupture.

Bolster: A support used to maintain the position of a body part.

Break test: An isometric contraction against manual resistance provided by the examiner; used to determine the athlete's ability to generate a static force within a muscle or muscle group.

Bulimia (bulimia nervosa): A condition marked by periods of insatiable appetite (binge eating) followed by self-induced vomiting (purging).

Bursa (pl. **bursae**): A fluid-filled sac that decreases friction between adjoining soft tissues or between soft tissue and bones.

Capillary perfusion pressure: Pressure within the capillaries that forces blood out into the surrounding tissues.

Capsular pattern: A pattern of decreased motion associated with injury of a joint's capsular tissue. Capsular patterns are specific to each joint.

Cardinal planes: Imaginary lines dividing the body into upper and lower (transverse planes), anterior and posterior (frontal plane), and left and right (sagittal plane) relative to the anatomical position.

Carotid sinus: An area near the common carotid artery that, when stimulated, results in vasodilation and a lowering of the heart rate. When this occurs suddenly, unconsciousness may occur.

Cartilaginous joint: A relatively immobile joint in which two bones are fused by cartilage.

Catastrophic: An injury that causes permanent disability or death.

Caudal (caudally): Moving inferiorly (toward the tail).

Center of gravity: Point inside or outside the body where all things are equally balanced or where gravitational pull is concentrated.

Cerebral palsy: A birth-related neurologic defect that results in motor dysfunction.

Cerumen: A reddish-brown wax formed in the auditory meatus.

Chlamydia: A family of microorganisms that produce infection in the genitals and are sexually transmitted.

Cholecystitis: Inflammation of the gallbladder.

Chondroblasts: A cell that forms cartilage.

Ciliary gland: A form of sweat gland on the eyelid.

Claudication: Pain arising in the lower leg as the result of inadequate venous drainage or poor arterial innervation.

Clawhand: Hand positioning characterized by hyperextension of the metacarpophalangeal joints and flexion of the middle and distal phalanges resulting from trauma to the median and ulnar nerves.

Closed-packed position: The point in a joint's range of motion at which its bones are maximally congruent; the most stable position of a joint.

Collision sports: Individual or team sports relying on the physical dominance of one athlete over another. By their nature, these sports mandate violent physical contact.

Compressive forces: A force applied along the length of a structure, causing the tissues to more closely approximate one another.

Concurrent: Occurring at the same time.

Congenital: A condition existing at or before birth.

Connective tissue: Tissue that supports and binds other tissue types.

Contractile tissue: Tissue that is capable of shortening and subsequently elongating; muscular tissue.

Contracture: A pathological shortening tissues causing a decrease in available range of motion.

Contraindication: Procedure that may prove harmful given the athlete's current condition.

Contralateral: Pertaining to the opposite side of the body or the opposite extremity.

Convergent: Two nerves combining together to form a single nerve.

Corticosteroid: A substance that permits many biochemical reactions to proceed at their optimal rates (e.g., tissue healing).

Crackles (rales): A crackling sound heard during inspiration and expiration caused by air passing over excessive secretions in the airway.

Crepitus: Repeated crackling sensations or sound emanating from a joint or tissue.

Cyanotic: Dark blue or purple tint to the skin and mucous membranes caused by a decreased oxygen supply.

Cystic fibrosis: A congenital condition of the exocrine glands that affects the pancreas, respiratory system, and other systems.

Dander: Small scales from animal hair or feathers causing an allergic reaction in some individuals.

Deconditioning: The loss of once existing cardiovascular or muscular endurance and strength.

Deep tendon reflex: An involuntary muscle contraction caused by a reflex arc in the spinal cord, initiated by the stretching of receptors within a tendon.

Defibrillation (defibrillating): The process of restoring a normal heartbeat.

Demyelination: Loss of a nerve's fatty lining.

Dental caries: A destructive disease of the teeth; cavities.

Dermatome: An area of skin innervated by a single nerve root.

Diaphysis: The shaft of a long bone.

Diffuse: Scattered; widespread.

Diplopia: Double vision.

Dislocation: The complete displacement of the articular surfaces of two joints.

Disposition: The immediate and long-term management of an injury or illness.

Distal: Away from the midline of the body, moving toward the periphery; the opposite of proximal.

Divergent: One nerve's splitting to form two individual nerves.

Dorsal (foot): The superior portion of the foot and toes.

Dorsal (upper extremity): The posterior aspect of the hand and forearm relative to the anatomical position.

Dorsiflexion: Flexion of the ankle; pulling the foot and toes toward the tibia.

Dysmenorrhea: Pain during menstruation.

Dysphagia: Difficulty or inability to swallow.

Dysplasic (dysplasia): Abnormal tissue development.

Dyspnea: Air hunger marked by labored or difficult breathing; may be a normal occurrence after exertion or an abnormal occurrence indicating cardiac or respiratory distress.

Dystrophy: The progressive deterioration of tissue.

Dysuria: Painful urination.

Eccentric muscle contraction: A contraction in which the elongation of the muscle is voluntarily controlled. Lowering a weight is an example of an eccentric contraction.

Ecchymosis: A blue or purple area of skin caused by the movement of blood into the skin.

Ectopic pregnancy: The formation of a fetus outside of the uterine cavity.

Efficacy: The ability of a protocol to produce the intended effects.

Electrolyte: Ionized salts, including sodium, potassium, and chloride, found in blood, tissue fluids, and cells.

Electromyelogram: The recording of the electrical activity within a muscle.

Elevation: Raising the arm in the scapular plane.

End-feel: The specific quality of movement felt by an examiner when moving a joint to the end of its range of motion.

Endodontics: The field of dentistry specializing in the management of patients with injuries and diseases affecting the pulp of a tooth.

End-point: The quality and quantity at the end of motion for any stress applied to a tissue.

Epineurium: Connective tissue containing blood vessels surrounding the trunk of a nerve, binding it together.

Epiphyseal line: The area of growth found between the diaphysis and epiphysis in immature long bones.

Epistaxis: A nosebleed.

Etiology: The cause of a disease; the study of the causes of disease.

Eversion: The movement of the plantar aspect of the calcaneus away from the midline of the body.

Exercise-induced asthma: Bronchospasm caused by exercise.

Extension: The act of straightening a joint and increasing its angle.

Extensor mechanism: The mechanism formed by the quadriceps and patellofemoral joint responsible for causing extension of the lower leg at the knee joint.

Extracapsular: Outside of the joint capsule.

Extravasate: Fluid escaping from vessels into the surrounding tissue.

Extrinsic: Arising from outside of the body.

Facet joints: An articulation of the facets between each contiguous part of vertebrae in the spinal column.

Facet: A small, smooth, articular surface on a bone.

Facetectomy: The surgical resection of a vertebral facet.

False joint: Abnormal movement along the length of a bone caused by a fracture or incomplete fusion.

Fascia: A fibrous membrane that supports and separates muscles and unites the skin with the underlying tissues.

Fine motor control: Specific control of the muscles allowing for completion of small, delicate tasks.

Flexible collodion: A mixture of ether, alcohol, cellulose, and camphor that dries to form a firm, protective layer.

Flexion: The act of bending a joint and decreasing its angle.

Force couple: Coordination between dynamic and isometric contractions of opposing muscle groups to perform a movement of a joint.

Forefoot varus: Inversion of the forefoot relative to the rearfoot.

Fossa: A depression on a bone.

Freedom of movement: The number of cardinal planes in which a joint allows motion.

Furunculosis (furuncle): A boil that is characterized by redness, leakage of pus, and necrosis of the involved tissue.

Gait: The sequential movements of the spine, pelvis, knee, ankle, foot, and upper extremity when walking or running.

Gait, antalgic: Abnormal or irregular walking or running pattern resulting from a biomechanical deviation or injury.

Gait, cosmetic: A walking or running pattern that has been corrected so that it has aesthetic quality for the patient.

Gait, functional: A walking or running pattern that has been corrected so that activities of daily living or sports can be performed; this does not imply a cosmetic gait.

Ganglion (nerve) (pl. ganglia): A collection of nerve cell bodies housed in the central or peripheral nervous system.

Gangrene: The death of bony or soft tissue resulting from a decrease in, or loss of, blood supply to a body area.

Gingivitis: Inflammation of the gums.

Gonad: An organ producing gender-based reproductive cells; the ovaries or testicles.

Goniometer: A device used to measure the motion, in degrees, that a joint is capable of producing around its axis.

Gout: A form of arthritis marked by inflammation and pain in the distal joints.

Graft: An organ or tissue used for transplantation. An allograft is a donor tissue transplanted from the same species. An autograft tissue is transplanted from within the same individual.

Gravity-dependent position: The extremity or body part is placed at a level that is lower than the heart, increasing intravascular pressure and hindering venous return.

Gross deformity: An abnormality that is visible to the unaided eye.

Ground reaction forces: Forces applied to the feet when there is contact with the floor or ground; equal, but in the opposite direction of the forces applied by the feet to the floor or ground.

Growth plates: The area of bone growth in skeletally immature individuals; the epiphyseal plate.

Gynecomastia: Enlargement of the male breasts.

Hemarthrosis: Blood within a joint cavity.

Hematoma: A collection of clotted blood within a confined space (*hemat* means *blood* and *oma* means *tumor*).

Hemodynamic: The process of blood's circulating through the body.

Hepatitis B virus (HBV): A virus resulting in inflammation of the liver. After a 2- to 6-week incubation period, symptoms develop, including gastrointestinal and respiratory disturbances, jaundice, enlarged liver, muscle pain, and weight loss.

Herniation: The protrusion of a tissue through the wall that normally contains it.

Heterotopic ossification: Misplaced and unwanted development of calcium.

Hook-lying: Lying supine with the hips and knees flexed and the feet flat on the table.

Human immunodeficiency virus (HIV): The virus that causes acquired immune deficiency syndrome (AIDS).

Hyaline cartilage: Cartilage found on the articular surface of bones, especially suited to withstand compressive and shearing forces.

Hypercholesterolemia: A high blood cholesterol level caused by a high intake of saturated fats.

Hyperemia: A red discoloration of the skin caused by an increased capillary blood flow.

Hyperhydrosis: Excessive or profuse sweating.

Hypermobile: Possessing excessive mobility.

Hyperreflexia: Increased action of the reflexes.

Hypertonic (hypertonicity): Having an increased osmotic pressure relative to the body's other fluids.

Hypertrophy: The increase in the cross-sectional size of a muscle, bone, or organ.

Hypoglycemia: The state of decreased levels of sugar in the blood, resulting in fatigue, restlessness, and irritability. Commonly associated with diabetes.

Hyporeflexia: A diminished or absent reflex response.

Hyposthenuria: The inability to concentrate urine normally.

Idiopathic: Of unknown origin.

Incontinence: A loss of bowel or bladder control.

Inert tissues: Noncontractile soft tissue, including joint capsule; ligaments supporting the joint capsule.

Infarction (infarct): Necrosis of localized organ tissue caused by loss of the blood supply.

Injected (injection): Congested with blood or other fluids forced into an area.

Insidious: Of gradual onset; with respect to symptoms of an injury or disease having no apparent cause.

Instability: Giving way or subluxation of a joint during functional activity that causes pain and inability to complete the activity.

Interosseous: Between two bones.

Intrathecal: Within the spinal canal.

Intrinsic: Arising from within the body.

Inversion: The movement of the plantar aspect of the calcaneus toward the midline of the body.

Ionizing radiation: Electromagnetic energy that causes the release of an atom's protons, electrons, or neutrons. Ionizing radiation is potentially hazardous to human tissue.

Iontophoresis: The use of a direct current to introduce medication into the body.

Ischemia: Local and temporary deficiency of blood supply caused by the obstruction of blood flow to a body area.

Isokinetic dynamometer: A device that quantitatively measures muscular function through a preset speed of movement.

Jefferson's fracture: A fracture of a circular bone in two places; similar to breaking a doughnut in half.

Joint reaction forces: Forces that are transmitted through a joint's articular surfaces.

Joint stability: The integrity of a joint when it is placed under a functional load.

Keloid: Hypertrophic scar formation secondary to excessive collagen.

Ketoacidosis: An increase in the blood acid level caused by the accumulation of ketone bodies.

Keystone: The crown of an arch that supports the structures on either side of it.

Kidney stones: A crystal mass formed in the kidney that is passed through the urinary tract.

Kienböck's disease: Osteochondritis or slow degeneration of the lunate bone.

Kinematic: The characteristics of movement related to time and space (e.g. range of motion, velocity, and acceleration); the effects of joint action.

Kinetic: The forces being analyzed; the causes of joint action.

Legg-Calvé-Perthes disease: Avascular necrosis occurring in children age 3 to 12 years, causing osteochondritis of the proximal femoral epiphysis and potentially decreasing the range of hip motion when they reach adulthood.

Long bones: A bone possessing a base, shaft, and head.

Lower motor neuron lesion: A lesion of the anterior horn of the spinal cord, nerve roots, or peripheral nerves resulting in decreased reflexes, flaccid paralysis, and atrophy.

Lucid: Pertaining to the state of mental clarity.

Lumina: The growth plate of a fingernail or toenail.

Lupus: A systemic disease affecting the internal organs, skin, and musculoskeletal system.

Lymph nodes: Nodules located in the cervical, axillary, and inguinal regions, producing white blood cells and filtering bacteria from the bloodstream. Lymph nodes become enlarged secondary to an infection.

Macrotrauma: A single force resulting in trauma to the body's tissues.

Malingering: Faking or exaggerating the symptoms of an injury or illness.

Malocclusion: A deviation in the normal alignment of two opposable tissues (e.g., the mandible and maxilla).

Marfan syndrome: A hereditary condition of the connective tissue, bones, muscles, and ligaments. Over time, this condition results in degeneration of brain function, cardiac failure, and other visceral problems.

Mastication: The chewing of food.

McKenzie exercises: A protocol of exercises involving spinal flexion and extension that is used during the treatment and rehabilitation of patients with back injuries; these are used to improve range of motion and strengthening the spine.

Median: Along the body's midline.

Melanin: The pigment produced by melanocytes that gives color to skin, hair, and eyes.

Menstruation (menstruating): The period of bleeding during the menstrual cycle.

Metabolic acidosis: Decreased blood pH caused by an increase in blood acids or a decrease in blood bases.

Metastasize (mestastasis): Movement of cells, including cancer cells and bacteria, from one area of the body to another, thus spreading the disease.

Microtrauma: Accumulation of subtraumatic forces at the cellular level that eventually causes injury to the tissue.

Moment of inertia: The amount of force needed to overcome a body's or body part's present state of rotatory motion.

Mononucleosis: A disease state caused by an abnormally high number of mononuclear leukocytes in the blood stream.

Morphologic: Changes in form and structure with regard to function.

Motor neurons: Neurons that send signals from the central nervous system to the muscular system.

Muscle guarding: Voluntarily or involuntarily assuming a posture to protect an injured body area, often through muscular spasm.

Musculotendinous unit: The group formed by a muscle and its tendons.

Myalgia: Muscle pain or tenderness.

Myelin sheath: A fatty-based lining of the axon of myelinated nerve fibers.

Myofascial tissues: A muscle and its associated fascia.

Myosin: A contractile muscle protein.

Nerve gliding: Movement of the nerve through surrounding tissues by placing the limb in various positions. The ability of the nerve to move freely during functional activity is assessed.

Neurapraxia: A stretch injury to a nerve resulting in transient symptoms of paresthesia and weakness.

Neurofibromatosis 1: Increased cell growth of neural tissues that is normally a benign condition; pain is possible secondary to pressure on the local nerves.

Neurotmesis: Complete loss of nerve function with little apparent damage to the nerve itself.

Neurovascular: Pertaining to a bundle formed by nerves, arteries, and veins.

Noncontractile tissues: Ligamentous and capsular tissue surrounding a joint.

Nonunion fracture: The incomplete healing of a bone that has not demonstrated signs of healing during the previous 3-month period.

Normative data: Normal ranges of data collected for comparison during the evaluation of an athlete. Athletes have norms different from the general population on many measures.

Nystagmus: An uncontrolled side-to-side movement of the eyes.

Objective data: Finite measures that are readily reproducible regardless of the individual who is collecting the information.

Obsessive-compulsive disorder: A behavioral condition characterized by unwarranted attention to detail, especially cleanliness. Individuals with this condition require a particular order to their lives.

Occlusion: The process of closing or being closed.

One-joint muscles: A muscle that only exerts force across one joint.

Open-packed position: The joint position at which its bones are maximally incongruent.

Ophthalmologist: A medical doctor specializing in patients with injuries, diseases, and abnormalities of the eye.

Orchitis: Inflammation of the testicle.

Orthoposition: Normal or properly aligned posture.

Osmolality: A substance's concentration in a fluid that affects its tendency to cross a membrane (osmosis).

Osteoblasts: Cells concerned with the formation of new bone.

Osteoporosis: Decreased bone density common in postmenopausal women.

Overpressure: A force that attempts to move a joint beyond its normal range of motion.

Overuse syndrome: Injury caused by accumulated microtraumatic stress placed on a structure or body area.

Painful arc: An area within a joint's range of motion that causes pain, representing compression, impingement, or abrasion of the underlying tissues.

Palliative: Serving to relieve or reduce symptoms without curing.

Pallor: Lack of color in the skin.

Parasympathetic nervous system: A series of specific effects controlled by the brain that regulate smooth muscle contractions, slow the heart rate, and constrict the pupils.

Paresthesia: The sensation of numbness or tingling, often described as a "pins and needles" sensation, caused by compression of or a lesion to a peripheral nerve.

Patency: The state of being freely open.

Pathology: A condition produced by an injury or disease.

Pathomechanics: Abnormal motion and forces produced by the body, most often occurring secondary to trauma.

Pelvic inflammatory disease: An infection of the vagina that spreads to the cervix, uterus, fallopian tubes, and broad ligaments.

Pericarditis: Inflammation of the lining surrounding the heart.

Periosteum: A fibrous membrane containing blood vessels covering the shafts of long bones.

Peripheral vascular disease (PVD): A syndrome involving an insufficiency of arteries or veins in maintaining proper circulation.

Peristalsis: A progressive smooth muscle contraction producing a wavelike motion that moves matter through the intestines.

Peroneal spastic flatfoot: A lowering of the medial foot caused by spasm of the peroneus longus muscle.

Phonophoresis: The use of therapeutic ultrasound to introduce medication into the body.

Photophobia: The eye's intolerance to light.

Plane synovial joint: A synovial joint formed by the gliding between two or more bones.

Plantar: The weight-bearing surface of the foot.

Plantarflexion: Extension of the ankle; pointing the foot and toes.

Plaque: Food, mucus, and bacteria that collect and harden on the exposed portions of the teeth; can harden into tartar.

Plumb line: A string and pendulum that hangs perpendicular to surface.

Postpartum: After childbirth.

Preiser's disease: Osteoporosis of the scaphoid, resulting from a fracture or repeated trauma.

Presbyopia: Loss of near vision as the result of aging.

Priapism: Spontaneous penile erection.

Prodromal: Pertaining to the interval between the initial disease rate and the onset of outward symptoms.

Prognosis: The course that a disease or injury is expected to take.

Pronation (forearm): Movement at the radioulnar joints allowing for the palm to be turned downward.

Proprioception: The athlete's ability to sense the position of one or more joints.

Protraction (scapular): Movement of the vertebral borders of the scapula away from the spinal column.

Proximal: Toward the midline of the body; the opposite of distal.

Pruritus: Severe itching

Pulmonary edema: Swelling of the lung and its tissues.

Purulent: Containing pus.

Radial deviation: Movement of the hand toward the radial (thumb) side.

Radicular pain: A sharp, shooting pain that tends to remain within a specific dermatome.

Radionuclide: An atom undergoing disintegration, emitting electromagnetic radiation.

Ramus: A division of a forked structure.

Ray: The series of bones formed by the metatarsal and phalanges.

Raynaud's phenomenon: A reaction to cold consisting of bouts of pallor and cyanosis, causing exaggerated vasomotor responses.

Referred pain: Pain at a site other than the actual location of trauma. Referred pain tends to be projected outward from the torso and distally along the extremities.

Reflex inhibition: A reflex arc prohibiting the contraction of a specific muscle or muscle group.

Relative humidity: The ratio between the amount of water vapor in the air and the actual amount of water the air could potentially hold based on the current temperature.

Resonant: Producing a vibrating sound or percussion.

Retinaculum: A ligamentous tissue serving as a restraining band to hold other tissues in place.

Retinopathy: A general term used to describe a disorder of the eye's retina.

Retraction (scapular): Movement of the scapular vertebral borders toward the spinal column.

Retrovirus: The generic name for the family of *Retroviridae*, viruses that contain RNA and may be associated with certain types of cancer.

Reye's syndrome: A disorder of the liver, pancreas, heart, kidney, and lymph nodes; often seen in children under the age of 15 years associated with acute viral infection and use of aspirin.

Rhabdomyolysis: An acute, sometimes fatal disease marked by the destruction of skeletal muscle.

Rigidity: A pathological loss of a joint's motion or a soft tissue's elasticity.

Ringer's lactate: A salt-based solution administered intravenously as a replacement for lost electrolytes.

Sarcomere: A portion of striated muscle fiber lying between two membranes.

Scapular dyskinesis: An improperly moving scapula.

Scapular tipping: The inferior angle of the scapula's moving away from the thorax while its superior border moves toward the thorax.

Sebaceous glands: Organs within the skin that secrete sebum, a fat-based oil.

Sensation: The ability to perceive sensory stimuli such as touch discrimination or temperature.

Sequestrated: Pertaining to a necrotic fragment of tissue that has become separated from the surrounding tissue.

Sesamoid bone: A bone that lies within a tendon.

Shear forces: Forces from opposing directions that are applied perpendicular to a structure's long axis.

Sign: An observable condition that indicates the existence of a disease or injury.

Sinusitis: Inflammation of the nasal sinus.

Sinus rhythm: An irregular heartbeat characterized by an increased rate during inspiration and a decreased rate during expiration.

Slip: A distinct band of tissue arising from the main portion of a structure.

Slipped capital femoris epiphysis: Displacement of the femoral head relative to the femoral shaft; common in children age 10 to 15 years and especially prevalent in boys.

Slough: The peeling away of dead skin from living tissue.

Soft tissues: Structures other than bone, including muscle, tendon, ligament, capsule, bursa, and skin.

Spina bifida occulta: Incomplete closure of the spinal vertebrae.

Spinal stenosis: A narrowing of the vertebral foramen through which the spinal cord or spinal nerve root pass.

Spondylolisthesis: The forward slippage of a vertebra on the one below it.

Sports medicine: The application of medical and scientific knowledge to the prevention (e.g., training methods and practices), care, and rehabilitation of injuries suffered by individuals participating in athletics.

Sprain: The stretching or tearing of ligamentous or capsular tissue.

Sputum: A substance formed by mucus, blood, or pus expelled by coughing or clearing the throat.

Stance phase: The weight-bearing phase of gait, beginning on initial contact with the surface and ending when contact is broken.

Standard (universal) precautions: Universally accepted guidelines concerning bloodborne pathogens in patient-clinician interactions.

Staphylococcal infection: An infection caused by the *Staphylococcus* bacteria.

Step length: The distance traveled between the initial contacts of the right and left foot.

Stride length: The distance traveled between two successive initial contacts of the same extremity

Stridor: A harsh, high-pitched sound resembling blowing wind that is experienced during respiration.

Subconjunctival hematoma: Leakage of the superficial blood vessels beneath the sclera.

Subluxation: The partial or incomplete dislocation of a joint, usually transient in nature; the joint surfaces relocate as the forces causing the displacement are relieved.

Sudden death: Unexpected and instantaneous death occurring within 1 hour of the onset of symptoms; most often used to describe death caused secondary to cardiac failure.

Sulcus: A groove or depression within a bone.

Supination (forearm): Movement at the radioulnar joints allowing for the palm to turn upward, as if holding a bowl of soup.

Swing phase: The non-weight bearing phase of gait that begins at the instant the foot leaves the surface and ends just before initial contact with the ground.

Sympathetic nervous system: The part of the central nervous system that supplies the involuntary muscles.

Symptom: A condition not visually apparent to the examiner, indicating the existence of a disease or injury. Symptoms are usually obtained during the history-taking process.

Syncope: Fainting caused by a transient loss of oxygen supply to the brain.

Syndesmosis joint: A relatively immobile joint in which two bones are bound together by ligaments.

Synostosis: The union of two bones through the formation of connective tissue.

Synovial hinge joint: A joint separated by a space filled with synovial fluid.

Synovial membrane: The membrane lining a fluid-filled joint.

Systematic: Orderly; based on a specific sequence of events.

Tendinosis: Lesions caused by decreased local blood flow (ischemia) secondary to peritendinitis.

Thrombophlebitis: Inflammation of a vein and the subsequent formation of blood clots.

Tinea pedis: A fungal infection of the foot and toes.

Tinnitus: Ringing in the ears.

Tracer element: A substance that is introduced into the tissues to follow or trace an otherwise unidentifiable substance or event.

Tracheotomy: A method of delivering air to the lungs by incising the skin and trachea and inserting a tube to form an airway; an emergency technique used only when the athlete's life is threatened by an immovable obstruction to the upper airway. Training is required to properly perform this technique.

Triage: The process of determining the priority of treatment.

Trigeminal neuralgia: A painful condition involving cranial nerve V, with possible motor involving one side of the mouth and paresthesia in the cheek.

Trigger point: A pathological condition characterized by a small, hypersensitive area located within muscles and fasciae.

Trophic: Pertaining to efferent nerves controlling the nourishment of the area they innervate.

Tuberosity: A nodulelike projection off a bone, serving as an attachment site for muscles and ligaments; referred to as a tubercle in the upper extremity.

Two-joint muscles: A muscle that exerts its force across two different joints and whose strength is dependent on the position of those joints.

Ulceration: An open sore or lesion of the skin or mucous membrane that is accompanied by inflamed and necrotic tissue.

Ulnar deviation: Movement of the hand toward the ulnar side of the forearm.

Uniplanar: Occurring in only one of the cardinal planes of motion.

Upper and lower quarter screen: Assessments of the neurologic status of the peripheral nervous system of the upper and lower extremities, respectively, through the evaluation of sensation, motor function, and deep tendon reflexes.

Upper motor neuron lesion: A lesion proximal to the anterior horn of the spinal cord that results in paralysis, loss of voluntary movement, spasticity, sensory loss, and pathological reflexes.

Valgus force: A lateral force applied toward the body's midline (medially).

Varicose veins: Enlargement of the superficial veins.

Varus force: A medial force applied from the body's midline outward (laterally).

Vasoconstriction: A decrease in a vessel's diameter.

Vasodilation: An increase in a vessel's diameter.

Vasomotor: Pertaining to nerves controlling the muscles within the walls of blood vessels.

Visceral: Pertaining to the internal organs contained within the thorax and abdomen.

Wallerian degeneration: Degeneration of a nerve's axon that has been severed from the body of the nerve.

Whorls: Swirl markings in the skin. Fingerprints are images formed by the whorls on the fingertips.

Winging (scapular): The inferior angle of the scapula's lifting away from the thorax.

Credits

CHAPTER 1

From Thomas, CL [ed]: Taber's cyclopedic medical dictionary, ed 17, Beth Anne Willert, MS, medical illustrator. FA Davis, Philadelphia, 1993, Fig. 1–5; From Rothstein, JM, Roy, SH, and Wolf, SL: The Rehabilitation Specialist's Handbook. FA Davis, Philadelphia, 1991, Fig. 1–9; Courtesy of the Biodex Medical Systems, Inc, Shirley, NY, Fig. 1–11; From Norkin, CC, and White, DJ: Measurement of Joint Motion: A Guide to Goniometry, ed 2. FA Davis, Philadelphia, 1995, Tables 1–3 and 1–4; From: Occupational Health and Safety Administration: Bloodborne pathogens. http://www.osha-slc.gov/SLTC/bloodbornepathogens/index.html, Table 1–10 (adapted); From Halpin, T and Dick, RW: NCAA Sports Medicine Handbook, 1999–2000 (ed 12). Indianapolis, National Collegiate Athletic Association, 1999, Box 1–2 (adapted).

CHAPTER 2

From Gross, MT: Chronic tendinitis: Pathomechanics of injury, factors affecting the healing response, and treatment. Journal of Orthopedic and Sports Physical Therapy 16:248, 1992, Table 2–2 (adapted).

CHAPTER 3

From Hoppenfeld, S: Physical examination of the elbow. In Hoppenfeld, S: Physical Examination of the Spine and Extremities. Appleton-Century-Crofts, New York, 1976, Adapted Fig. 3–7; From Novack, C and Mackinnon, S: Repetitive use and static postures: A source of nerve compression and pain. J Hand Ther, 10:151, 1997, Tables 3–11 and 3–13 (adapted). Table 3–6: Adapted from Greenfield, BH, et. al: The influence of cephalostatic ear rods on the positions of the head and neck during positional recordings. Am J Dentofacial Orthop. 95:312, 1989 and Molhave, A: A biostatic investigation of the human erect posture. Munkgard, Copenhagen, 1958.

CHAPTER 4

From Norkin, CC, and Levangie, PK: Joint Structure and Function: A Comprehensive Analysis, ed 2. FA Davis, Philadelphia, 1992, Fig. 4–1 (adapted), Figs. 4–9 and 4–18 and Table 4–1; From Rothstein, JM, Roy, SH, and Wolf, SL: The Rehabilitation Specialist's Handbook. FA Davis, Philadelphia, 1991, Fig. 4–3; From LifeART, Copyright 2000, Lippincott, Williams & Wilkins, Figs. 4–2, 4–5, 4–7, 4–24, and 4–30, Clinical Evaluation (Fig. 3), and Box 4–2 (Figs. 5, 6, 7, and 8; adapted); From Saltzman, CL, Nawoczenski, DA, and Talbot, KD: Measurement of the medial longitudinal arch. Arch Phys Med Rehabil, 76:45, 1995, Fig. 4–25 (adapted); From Dahle, LK, et al: Visual assessment of foot type and relationship of foot type to lower

extremity injury. J Orthop Sports Phys Ther 14:70, 1991, Table 4–6 (adapted); From Donatelli, RA: Biomechanics of the Foot and Ankle, FA Davis, Philadelphia, 1990, Box 4–3 (Figs. 5 and 6).

CHAPTER 5

From Rothstein, JM, Roy, SH, and Wolf, SL: The Rehabilitation Specialist's Handbook. FA Davis, Philadelphia, 1991, Fig. 5–3; From Norkin, CC, and Levangie, PK: Joint Structure and Function: A Comprehensive Analysis, ed 2. FA Davis, Philadelphia, 1992, Figs. 5–4 and 5–5. From LifeART, Copyright 2000, Lippincott Williams & Wilkins, Figs. 5–7(B), 5–20, and 5–27, Clinical Evaluation (Figs. 1, 2, 3, and 4), and Box 5–7 (Fig. 2); From Donatelli, R: Biomechanics of the Foot and Ankle. FA Davis, Philadelphia, 1990, Box 5–4 (Fig. 2B); From Coombs, JA: Peroneal nerve palsy complicating an ankle sprain. Athletic Training, 25:247, 1990, Table 5–5 (adapted); From Sollsteimer, GT and Shelton, WR: Acute atraumatic compartment syndrome in an athlete: A case report. Journal of Athletic Training. 32:248, 1997, Table 5–10.

CHAPTER 6

From LifeART, Copyright 2000, Lippincott Williams & Wilkins, Figs. 6–3, 6–4, 6–5, 6–10 and 6–22, Clinical Evaluation (Fig. 2), Box 6–4 (Fig. 2), Box 6–5 (Fig. 3), and Box 6–7 (Fig. 2); From Fu, F, et al: Biomechanics of knee ligaments. Basic concepts and clinical application. J Bone Joint Surg Am 75:1716, 1993, Fig. 6–7 (adapted); From Arms, SW, et al: The biomechanics of anterior cruciate ligament rehabilitation and reconstruction. Am J Sports Med 12:8, 1984, Fig. 6–8; From Greenfield, BH: Rehabilitation of the Injured Knee: A Problem-Solving Approach. FA Davis, Philadelphia, 1993, p 27, Fig. 6–9.

CHAPTER 7

Figure 7–5: From Ficat, P, and Hungerford, DS: Disorders of the Patello-Femoral Joint. Williams & Wilkins, Baltimore, 1977, Fig. 7–5; From Bloom, MH: Differentiating between meniscal and patellar pain. Physical and Sportsmedicine 17:95, 1989, Table 7–2.

CHAPTER 8

From Norkin, CC, and Levangie, PK: Joint Structure and Function: A Comprehensive Analysis, ed 2. FA Davis, Philadelphia, 1992, Figs. 8–4, 8–5, 8–6, and 8–8; From LifeART, Copyright 2000, Lippincott Williams & Wilkins, Fig. 8–12 and Clinical Evaluation (Fig. 4).

CHAPTER 9

Courtesy of Oxford Physical Therapy & Rehabilitation, Oxford, OH, with permission, Fig. 9–2; From Norkin, CC, and Levangie, PK: Joint

Structure and Function: A Comprehensive Analysis, ed 2. FA Davis, Philadelphia, 1992, Fig. 9–4 (adapted), Box 9–1 (Figs. 1 through 10), Box 9–2 (Figs.1 through 6), and Box 9–3 (Figs. 1 through 7), and Table 9–1.

CHAPTER 10

From LifeART, Copyright 2000, Lippincott Williams & Wilkins, Figs. 10–6, and 10–9; From Rothstein, JM, Roy, SH, and Wolf, SL: The Rehabilitation Specialist's Handbook. FA Davis, Philadelphia,1991, Fig. 10–10; From Hollingshead, WH, and Jenkins, DB: The organs and organ systems. In Hollingshead, WH, and Jenkins, DB: Functional anatomy of the limbs and back. WB Saunders, Philadelphia, 1991, Figs. 10–11 and 10–12 (adapted); From Norkin, CC, and Levangie, PK: Joint Structure and Function: A Comprehensive Analysis, ed 2. FA Davis, Philadelphia, 1992, Fig. 10–13; From Delitto, A; Erhard, RE and Bowling, RW: A treatment-based classification approach to low back syndrome: identifying and staging patients for conservative treatment. Phys Ther, 75:740, 1995 and Fritz, JM: Use of a classification approach to the treatment of 3 patients with low back syndrome. Phys Ther, 78:766, 1998, Table 10–9.

CHAPTER 11

From Norkin, CC, and Levangie, PK: Joint Structure and Function: A Comprehensive Analysis, ed 2. FA Davis, Philadelphia, 1992, Figs. 11–1, and 11–6; From Rothstein, JM, Roy, SH, and Wolf, SL: The Rehabilitation Specialist's Handbook. FA Davis, Philadelphia,1991, Fig. 11–4; From Figure 11–5: Adapted from Hollingshead, WH, and Jenkins, DB: The organs and organ systems. In Hollingshead, WH, and Jenkins, DB: Functional anatomy of the limbs and back. WB Saunders, Philadelphia, 1991, Fig. 11–5 (adapted); From Vereschagin, KS, et al: Burners. Don't overlook or underestimate them. The Physician and Sportsmedicine 19:96, 1991, Fig. 11–16 (B and C).

CHAPTER 12

From Otis, CL, et al: American College of Sports Medicine position stand. The female athlete triad. Med Sci Sports Exerc, 29:i, 1997, Table 12–9 (adapted).

CHAPTER 13

From Thomas, CL [ed]: Taber's Cyclopedic Medical Dictionary, ed 17. FA Davis, Philadelphia, 1993, p 1875, by Beth Anne Willert, MS, medical illustrator, Fig. 13–2; From Rothstein, JM, Roy, SH, and Wolf, SL, Rehabilitation Specialist's Handbook, FA Davis, Philadelphia, Fig. 13–3; From Norkin, CC, and Levangie, PK, The shoulder complex. In Norkin, CC and Levangie, PK. Joint Structure and Function: A Comprehensive Analysis. ed 2, FA Davis, Philadelphia, Figs. 13–7, 13–8, 13–9, and 13–10; From LifeART, Copyright 2000, Lippincott Williams & Wilkins, Fig. 13–11, Clinical Evaluation (Fig. 2), Box 13–18 (Figs. 1 through 4); From Rockwood, CA, and Young, DC: Disorders of the acromioclavicular joint. In Rockwood, CA, and Mastens, FA (eds): The Shoulder. Philadelphia, WB Saunders, 1990; and Bach, BR, VanFleet, TA, and Novak, PJ: Acromioclavicular injuries: Controversies in treatment. The Physician and Sports Medicine 20:87, 1992, Table 13–7; From Snyder, SJ, et al: SLAP lesions of the shoulder. Arthroscopy, 4:243, 1995, Table 13–13 (adapted); From Fleisig, S, Dillman, CJ, and Andrews, JR: Biomechanics of the shoulder during throwing. In Andrews, JR, and Wilk, KE (eds): The Athlete's Shoulder. Churchill Livingstone, New York, 1994 and Souza, TA: The shoulder in throwing sports. In Souza, TA (ed): Sports Injuries of the Shoulder. Churchill Livingstone, New York, 1994, Box 13–1.

CHAPTER 14

From Hoppenfeld, S: Physical examination of the elbow. In Hoppenfeld, S: Physical Examination of the Spine and Extremities.

Appleton-Century-Crofts, New York, 1976, Fig. 14–14; From Norkin, CC, and Levangie, PK: Joint Structure and Function: A Comprehensive Analysis, ed 2. FA Davis, Philadelphia, 1992, Fig. 14–15 (B); From Driscoll, SW, Bell, DF, Morrey, BF. Posterolateral instability of the elbow. J Bone Joint Surg. 1991, 73A:440–446, Box 14–5 (adapted).

CHAPTER 15

From Norkin, CC, and Levangie, PK, The shoulder complex. In Norkin, CC and Levangie, PK, Joint Structure and Function: A Comprehensive Analysis, ed 2, FA Davis, Philadelphia, 1992, Fig. 15–4; From Goldsmith, LA; Lazarus, GS and Tharp, MD: Adult and pediatric dermatology. A color guide to diagnosis and treatment. Philadelphia, FA Davis, 1997, Fig. 15–12. From Norkin, CC, and White, DJ: Measurement of Joint Motion: A Guide to Goniometry, ed 2. FA Davis, Philadelphia, 1995, Table 15–3 (adapted); From Stanley, BG and Tribuzi SM, Concepts in Hand Rehabilitation, FA Davis, Philadelphia, 1992, Box 15–2 (Figs. 2 and 3).

CHAPTER 16

From Thomas, CL [ed]: Taber's Cyclopedic Medical Dictionary, ed 17. FA Davis, Philadelphia, 1993, Fig. 16–2 and 16–8; From Matthews, B: Maxillofacial trauma from athletic endeavors. Athletic Training: Journal of the National Athletic Trainers Association 25:132, 1990, Fig. 16–11.

CHAPTER 17

From Norkin, CC, and Levangie, PK: Joint Structure and Function: A Comprehensive Analysis, ed 2. FA Davis, Philadelphia, 1992, Fig. 17–2; From Rothstein, JM, Roy, SH, and Wolf, SL, Rehabilitation Specialist's Handbook, FA Davis, Philadelphia, Figs. 17–3, 17–4, and 17–7; From Thomas, CL [ed]: Taber's Cyclopedic Medical Dictionary, ed 17, Beth Anne Willert, MS, medical illustrator. FA Davis, Philadelphia, 1993, Fig. 17–8; From Perry, JF, Rohe, DA, and Garcia, The Kinesiology Workbook, ed 2, FA Davis, Philadelphia, Fig. 17–26.

CHAPTER 18

From Thomas, CL [ed]: Taber's Cyclopedic Medical Dictionary, ed 17, Beth Anne Willert, MS, medical illustrator. FA Davis, Philadelphia, 1993, Fig. 18–3; From Torg, JS. The epidemiologic, biomechanical, and cinematographic analysis of football induced cervical spine trauma. Athletic Training: Journal of the National Athletic Trainers Association, 25:147, 1990, Fig. 18–8; From Mueller, FO, and Ryan, AJ, Prevention of Athletic Injuries: The Role of the Sports Medicine Team. FA Davis, Philadelphia, 1991, Fig. 18–9; From Kelly, JP and Rosenberg, JH : Diagnosis and management of concussion in sports. Neurology, 48:575, 1997, Table 18–5 (adapted); From Cantu, Criteria for return to competition after a closed head injury. In Torg, JS (ed): Athletic Injuries to the Head, Neck, and Face, ed 2. Mosby-Year Book, St Louis, 1991, Table 18–10 (adapted); From Torg, Criteria for return to collision activities after cervical spine injury. Operative Techniques in Sports Medicine 1:236, 1993, Table 18–14 (adapted); From McCrea, Michael, PhD, Box 18–7.

CHAPTER 19

From Casa, DJ, et al: National Athletic Trainers' Association Position Statement: Fluid replacement for athletes. Journal of Athletic Training, 35:212, 2000, Table 19–5 (adapted); From Sheehy, SB, Environmental emergencies. In Sheehy, SB: Mosby's Manual of Emergency Care, ed 3. CV Mosby, St Louis, 1990, Table 19–7 (adapted); From Potts, KA and Dick, RW: NCAA Guide Line 2m. Cold Stress. In NCAA Sports Medicine Handbook (ed 13). Indianapolis, IN, National Collegiate Athletic Association, 2000, Table 19–8 (adapted).

Index

Numbers followed by a "b" indicate boxes; numbers followed by an "f" indicate figures; numbers followed by a "t" indicate tables.